MEDICAL ONCOLOGY

A
COMPREHENSIVE
REVIEW

SECOND EDITION

MEDICAL ONCOLOGY

A

COMPREHENSIVE

REVIEW

RICHARD PAZDUR, MD EDITOR

From The University of Texas

M. D. Anderson Cancer Center

and the journal ONCOLOGY

Note to the reader

The information in this volume has been carefully reviewed for correctness of dosage and indications. Before prescribing any drug, however, the clinician should consult the manufacturer's current package labeling for accepted indications, absolute dosage recommendations, and other information pertinent to the safe and effective use of the product described. This is especially important when drugs are given in combination or as an adjunct to other forms of therapy. Furthermore, some of the medications described, as well as some of the indications mentioned, had not been approved by the US Food and Drug Administration at the time of publication. This possibility should be borne in mind before prescribing or recommending any drug or regimen.

For information on obtaining additional copies of this volume, contact the publishers, PRR, Inc., 17 Prospect Street, Huntington, NY 11743.

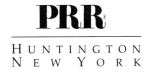

HUNTINGTON
NEW YORK

Publishers of ONCOLOGY
Oncology News International
Cancer Management
Primary Care & Cancer
The Journal of Myocardial Ischemia

Preface to the Second Edition

Medical Oncology: A Comprehensive Review, originally published in the fall of 1993, was a unique publishing experience. That volume is the only medical oncology textbook written exclusively by the medical oncology faculty of a single institution. This single-institution perspective demonstrates the breadth and strength of our faculty and provides an insight to how patients are treated at The University of Texas M. D. Anderson Cancer Center.

Although this text was written from the perspective of the discipline of medical oncology, we attempted to emphasize a multidisciplinary approach to cancer problems. The book's organization illustrates the disease site-specific teams of physicians who work on innovative cancer treatment. In 1996, M. D. Anderson Cancer Center will open disease-site clinics that demonstrate the institution's commitment to multidisciplinary care.

Another unique feature of this textbook is that most chapters have been jointly written by our faculty and fellows. This close collaboration between trainees and faculty reflects the commitment of our faculty to our medical oncology training program and to the academic development of our trainees. During their fellowships, trainees rotate through each of the clinical disease-site departments, providing them extensive experience in treating specific malignancies.

In designing the second edition of this book, some chapters from the first edition were completely or largely rewritten. In those cases, we bid farewell to former fellow-authors of the first edition chapters. Chapters updated for the second edition include the names of the former fellow-authors whose contributions remain reflected in the material. Our present trainees, who are the chapter's first authors, were responsible for updating and compiling the information in the current edition. As in many training programs, our former fellows are now practicing oncology in diverse locations ranging from our own backyard in Houston, to New York City, Mexico, Australia, Brazil, and Singapore. They work in universities, private practice settings, and in the pharmaceutical industry. We thank them for their contributions to this edition.

Because oncology is a rapidly changing field, this text was published within a year from the first organizational meeting for the second edition. Chapters were updated during production to ensure the timeliness of the information.

Many patients at M. D. Anderson are treated in clinical trials; however, this book was not designed as a forum for our clinical research. When therapies are discussed, the authors have presented nationally accepted approaches for a given disease. When controversial or innovative therapies are discussed, we provide the reader with the information needed to evaluate these treatments in the context of existing standards. To comply with length restrictions, we limited our perspective to that of the practicing medical oncologist. Therefore, details of radiation therapy and surgical procedures, as well as some medical oncology topics covered in detail in other subspecialty textbooks, are not provided here.

Some chapters were written by M. D. Anderson faculty who come from disciplines other than medical oncology but who work closely with us in caring for our patients. We wish to thank Sharon Weinstein for sharing her expertise in pain and symptom management, Kenneth Rolston for writing the infectious disease chapters, Ellen Manzullo for providing her insights on oncologic emergencies, Creighton Edwards for his unique views as a gynecologic oncologist, Rena Vassilopoulou-Sellin for her extensive experience with endocrine malignancies, and Victor Levin for his collaboration in writing the chapter on brain tumors. We are also grateful to Aman Buzdar and Hagop Kantarjian for their help in determining the scope of topics to be covered and author selection for some chapters.

This book could not have been realized without the assistance of the people of PRR, Inc., who collaboratively developed its concept, assisted in the editing, and provided the business development plan. Andrew Nash and Lois Friedman, with help from Roseanne Szczepanowski, provided editorial review of the manuscripts, and James F. McCarthy, Vice-President/Editorial, provided assistance in the book's organization. John A. Gentile, Jr., President of PRR, Inc., conceived a unique distribution system that allowed 20,000 US cancer specialists, 5,000 European oncologists, and 5,000 Japanese cancer physicians to receive copies of the first edition.

This book could not have been completed without the assistance of editors in the Department of Scientific Publications at M. D. Anderson Cancer Center. Diane S.

Rivera was the managing editor who organized the entire project, assisting with numerous chapter rewrites, coordinating manuscript preparation with the authors, the publisher, and support staff, and participating in numerous meetings with the authors.

During the year that this project was underway, the daily operations of educational programs in the Division of Medicine continued, even with the added pressures of developing, writing, and editing these chapters. We thank Pamela Connors, Maricela Malbrough, and Dean Anthony for providing the emotional and administrative "sanity" conducive to running the daily operations of one of the world's largest medical oncology training programs. Also during this period, the Division of Medicine acquired new leadership under Robert Bast, Jr., MD, and we thank him for his support of this endeavor. Finally, I would like to thank our medical oncology fellows for engaging in this educational venture with a sustained enthusiasm. To complete this project while actively engaged in research and patient care activities required sacrifice of personal time with friends and family.

This book was built on sharing. Our faculty contributors shared their vast clinical experience with our trainees, our former trainees shared the prior edition's manuscripts with current fellow-authors, and our editors shared their communication skills with our authors. This book is our way of bringing these collective experiences to you. Ultimately, we hope that you will share this information with your patients in delivering quality oncologic care.

Richard Pazdur, MD
Assistant Vice President for Academic Affairs
The University of Texas M. D. Anderson Cancer Center
Houston, Texas
November 1995

CONTENTS

SECTION 1

Leukemias & Lymphomas

Chapter 1
Acute Lymphocytic Leukemia   3
Jorge E. Cortes and Hagop Kantarjian

Chapter 2
Acute Myelogenous Leukemia   27
Habib M. Ghaddar and Elihu H. Estey

Chapter 3
Chronic Lymphocytic Leukemia   37
and Associated Disorders
Luis Fayad and Susan O'Brien

Chapter 4
Chronic Myelogenous Leukemia   57
Jorge E. Cortes, Moshe Talpaz, and Hagop Kantarjian

Chapter 5
The Indolent Lymphomas   73
Ali W. Bseiso and Peter McLaughlin

Chapter 6   Intermediate- and High-   99
Grade Non-Hodgkin's Lymphomas
Anton Melnyk and Alma Rodriguez

Chapter 7   Hodgkin's Disease   111
Gary P. Engstrom, David B. Sanford,
and Fredrick B. Hagemeister

Chapter 8
Multiple Myeloma and Other   127
Plasma-Cell Dyscrasias
Vali Papadimitrakopoulou and Donna M. Weber

Chapter 9
Allogeneic Marrow Transplantation   139
Paolo Anderlini and Donna Przepiorka

Chapter 10
Autologous Transplantation: 151
Basic Concepts and Controversies
Naoto T. Ueno and Richard E. Champlin

SECTION 2

Lung Cancer

Chapter 11   Small-Cell Lung Cancer   169
Marcos J. G. de Lima, Issa F. Khouri,
and Bonnie S. Glisson

Chapter 12
Non-Small-Cell Lung Cancer   181
Dimitrios Diamandidis, Martin Huber,
and Katherine Pisters

SECTION 3

Head & Neck Cancer

Chapter 13   Head and Neck Cancer   207
Edgardo J. Rodriguez-Monge, Dong M. Shin,
and Scott M. Lippman

SECTION 4

Gastrointestinal Carcinomas

Chapter 14
Carcinoma of the Esophagus   225
Philip Agop Philip and Jaffer Ajani

Chapter 15   Gastric Carcinoma   235
Philip Agop Philip and Jaffer A. Ajani

Chapter 16   Pancreatic, Hepatic,   247
and Biliary Carcinomas
Edgardo Rivera and James L. Abbruzzese

Chapter 17   Colorectal Cancer: 263
Diagnosis and Management
Enrique A. Diaz-Canton and Richard Pazdur

Chapter 18   Neuroendocrine Tumors   285
of the Gastrointestinal Tract
Nikolaos Touroutoglou, Anthony Arcenas, Jaffer A. Ajani

SECTION 5

Breast Cancer

Chapter 19   Early-Stage Breast Cancer   301
and Adjuvant Therapy
Juan Herrada, Pamela Hughes, and Aman Buzdar

Chapter 20
Metastatic Breast Cancer   311
Mary K. Crow, Edward Soo, and Frankie A. Holmes

Chapter 21   Special Issues in   329
Breast Cancer Management
Vance Wright-Browne and Richard L. Theriault

Contents continued on following page

CONTENTS *continued*

SECTION 6

Gynecologic Malignancies

Chapter 22 Ovarian Cancer 359
Eleni Diamandidou, John J. Kavanagh,
Creighton L. Edwards, and Andrzej P. Kudelka

Chapter 23
Gestational Trophoblastic Tumors 377
Ray D. Page, Andrzej P. Kudelka, Ralph S. Freedman,
and John J. Kavanagh

Chapter 24
Carcinoma of the Uterine Cervix 393
Arsenio Lopez, Andrzej P. Kudelka,
Creighton L. Edwards, and John J Kavanagh

Chapter 25
Tumors of the Uterine Corpus 407
Saraswati P. Reddy, Andrzej P. Kudelka, Cesar Gonzalez
de Leon, Creighton L. Edwards, and John J. Kavanagh

SECTION 7

Genitourinary Carcinomas

Chapter 26 Prostate Cancer 419
Philip Agop Philip and Randall Millikan

Chapter 27 Testicular Cancer 433
Chris B. Bringhurst and Robert Amato

Chapter 28 Bladder Cancer 449
Yung-Chang Lin and Shi-Ming Tu

Chapter 29 Renal-Cell Carcinoma 459
Gustavo A. Fonseca and Julie Ellerhorst

SECTION 8

Miscellaneous Tumors

Chapter 30 Brain Tumors 469
Edward W. Soo, Eugenio G. Galindo, and Victor A. Levin

Chapter 31 Endocrine Malignancies 483
Ana G. Ruiz Allison and Rena Vassilopoulou-Sellin

Chapter 32 Malignant Melanoma: 493
Biology, Diagnosis, and Management
Clay M. Anderson, Jacques Tabacof, and Sewa S. Legha

Chapter 33
Soft-Tissue and Bone Sarcomas 511
Danai Daliani and S.R. Patel

Chapter 34
Retrovirus-Associated Malignancies 531
Virginia Rhodes and Fredrick B. Hagemeister

Chapter 35
Unknown Primary Carcinomas: 559
Diagnosis and Management
Jean-Pierre M. Ayoub, Kevin P. Hubbard,
and Renato Lenzi

SECTION 9

Therapeutic Modalities & Supportive Care

Chapter 36 Biologic Therapy: 569
Interferons, Interleukin-2, and
Adoptive Cellular Immunotherapy
Jorge E. Cortes, John F. Seymour,
and Razelle Kurzrock

Chapter 37 Biologic Therapy: 587
Hematopoietic Growth Factors,
Retinoids, and Monoclonal Antibodies
Mohammad Qasim, Paula Marlton,
and Razelle Kurzrock

Chapter 38 Current Treatment of 599
Infection in the Neutropenic Patient
Kenneth V.I. Rolston

Chapter 39 Management of Fungal 607
and Viral Infections in Cancer Patients
Ricardo F. Garcia and Kenneth V.I. Rolston

Chapter 40
Management of Cancer Pain 615
Sharon M. Weinstein

Chapter 41 Management of 629
Nausea and Vomiting
Mary K. Crow, Habib M. Ghaddar, Richard Pazdur,
and Giuseppe Fraschini

Chapter 42 Oncologic Emergencies 643
Virginia Rhodes and Ellen Manzullo

Chapter 43 Epidemiology of Cancer 661
and Prevention Strategies
L. Arlene Nazario, Janet E. Macheledt,
and Victor G. Vogel

INDEX 673

SECTION I

LEUKEMIAS & LYMPHOMAS

CHAPTER 1   Acute Lymphocytic Leukemia

CHAPTER 2   Acute Myelogenous Leukemia

CHAPTER 3   Chronic Lymphocytic Leukemia
             and Associated Disorders

CHAPTER 4   Chronic Myelogenous Leukemia

CHAPTER 5   The Indolent Lymphomas

CHAPTER 6   Intermediate- and High-Grade
             Non-Hodgkin's Lymphomas

CHAPTER 7   Hodgkin's Disease

CHAPTER 8   Multiple Myeloma and Other
             Plasma-Cell Dyscrasias

CHAPTER 9   Allogeneic Marrow Transplantation

CHAPTER 10   Autologous Transplantation:
             Basic Concepts and Controversies

CHAPTER 1

Acute Lymphocytic Leukemia

Jorge E. Cortes, MD, *and* Hagop Kantarjian, MD

Department of Hematology, The University of Texas M. D. Anderson Cancer Center, Houston, Texas

Acute lymphocytic leukemia (ALL) is a malignant disorder resulting from the clonal proliferation of lymphoid precursors with arrested maturation.[1] The disease can originate in lymphoid cells of different lineages, thus giving rise to B- or T-cell leukemias or sometimes mixed-lineage leukemia.

The disease has historic relevance because it was one of the first malignancies reported to respond to chemotherapy[2] and was later among the first malignancies cured in a majority of children.[3] Since then, much progress has been made, not only in terms of treatment, but importantly, in deciphering the heterogeneity of ALLs.

As information accumulates about molecular aberrations, immunophenotyping, chromosomal abnormalities, and prognostic factors, more rational therapies have been designed. Because most cases are diagnosed in children,[4] our current knowledge has originated from studies in the pediatric population. As differences between childhood and adult ALL become apparent, more research is being conducted and progress is being made in ALL in adults.

EPIDEMIOLOGY

Every year, 3,000 to 5,000 new cases of ALL are diagnosed in the United States.[5,6] The median age at diagnosis is 12 years,[4] and nearly two thirds of cases are diagnosed in children, in whom it represents the most common malignancy, accounting for approximately one fourth of all childhood cancers.[7] In adults, ALL represents 20% of all leukemias[4] and 1% to 2% of all cancers.[8] ALL has a bimodal distribution with an initial peak incidence at age 3 to 5 years,[4,9] affecting 4.4 of 100,000 children. The incidence gradually decreases and remains low until about age 50, when the incidence increases steadily with age and reaches nearly 2 cases per 100,000 persons older than 65 years.[10]

Interestingly, the early age-specific peak is absent in some developing countries.[11,12] In all ages, the incidence is higher in males than in females[4,13] and higher in white than in African-American populations.[13] Although the overall incidence has remained stable over the past 10 to 15 years,[13,14] it may be increasing in some subgroups, such as white males[13] and children.[15]

ETIOLOGY

The etiology of ALL is not known, and although several studies have tried to identify risk factors for leukemic development, definite conclusions cannot be drawn.[16] However, some associations, such as genetic, parental, socioeconomic, and environmental factors, must be considered.

Genetic Factors: Reports have identified families with multiple members affected by leukemia.[17] When an identical twin is diagnosed with ALL, the other twin has a significantly higher risk of developing leukemia; as many as 20% of them will be diagnosed with the disease within 1 year,[18] but the risk is age dependent, decreasing from nearly 100% for the twins when the index case is diagnosed before the age of 1 year to a risk no different from that in other siblings when diagnosed after the age of 4 years. Siblings of patients with leukemia have a fourfold higher risk of developing leukemia than the general population.[19]

Several genetic syndromes have also been associated with leukemia, with the best characterized being Down's syndrome, which accounts for nearly 2% of all ALL cases in children.[20] Other syndromes, such as Bloom syndrome, ataxia telangiectasia, Wiskott-Aldrich syndrome, and Fanconi's anemia, are also associated with an increased risk of leukemia.[21,22]

Parental and Socioeconomic Factors: Maternal reproductive history is also important.[23] Children of mothers older than 35 years of age may have an increased risk of leukemia, only partially explained by the increased risk of having Down's syndrome.[24] A history of prior fetal loss, especially if there have been multiple miscarriages, has been identified as a risk factor for the offspring.[25] The association of increased weight at birth and childhood ALL has been reported consistently.[23,26] Parental occupational exposure to such agents as pesticides and benzene may increase the risk of leukemia in offspring, but most of these cases have been acute myelogenous leukemia (AML).[27] There may also be a higher risk for children with a better socioeconomic status, but this is not universally accepted.[28]

Environmental Factors: Exposure to radiation is associated with a definite risk of ALL. In utero exposure increases the risk of ALL over that of control populations.[29] Exposure to low-dose radiation, such as that used in diagnostic radiology, has not been proven to be leukemogenic, but exposure to high doses (like those used in radiotherapy) may be.[39,31] People exposed to radiation during the atomic disasters at Hiroshima and Nagasaki,[32,33] as well as people involved in other nuclear exposures[34–36] may have as much as a 10- to 20-fold higher risk of developing leukemia.

Exposure to different chemicals has also been associated with an increased risk of leukemia. The best characterized association involves benzene, although more than two thirds of these cases are AML.[37] The exposure to electromagnetic fields has been repeatedly linked to an increased risk of ALL,[38–41] but the evidence is inconclusive.

Several studies have suggested clustering of cases of childhood leukemia. This clustering usually represents a group of cases occurring within a population, whose incidence is higher than that expected for the general population.[42] This clustering of cases has been attributed to the proximity of environmental hazards, such as nuclear plants. However, evidence of this exposure is lacking in most cases. This and other epidemiologic data, such as the increased incidence of common ALL with higher socioeconomic status and isolation, have led to the hypothesis of an infectious etiology for common ALL in children.[43,44] According to this hypothesis, common ALL at childhood peak ages might arise after unusual patterns of exposure to common infectious agents. In more developed societies with better hygiene and fewer social contacts early in infancy, common infections are frequently delayed beyond the first year of life and until a higher level of social contacts is made.[43,44]

CLINICAL FEATURES

The signs and symptoms of ALL reflect the expansion of the leukemic clone in the bone marrow with impairment of normal hematopoiesis and the infiltration of nonhematopoietic tissues by the leukemic cells. The etiology of the suppression of normal hematopoiesis is not clear. Decreased numbers of normal progenitors, deficient production of normal hematopoietic growth factors, and production of inhibitory cytokines by the malignant clone have all been advocated as causes.[45,46]

The most common initial symptoms of ALL are attributable to anemia, neutropenia, and thrombocytopenia. They are manifested by fatigue, weakness, fever, weight loss, and bleeding. Frequently there is no detectable infectious cause of the fever,[47] which may be due to ALL itself.[48] The symptoms usually present abruptly but may be misdiagnosed as being related to an infectious process unless a detailed blood and bone marrow study is performed. Patients, especially children, may have severe pain resulting from an overgrowth of leukemic cells in the bone marrow; this most frequently affects the lower sternum and occasionally large joints[49] and sometimes is due to bone marrow necrosis.[50,51]

Almost 80% of patients with ALL have lymphadenopathy.[49] Lymph nodes are usually painless and movable. The spleen and the liver are also frequently enlarged, with up to 70% to 75% of patients presenting with hepatomegaly and/or splenomegaly.[49] Even when the liver is infiltrated, liver function is usually preserved. Lymph node, liver, and spleen enlargement is a representation of tumor burden and, therefore, when extensive, correlates with a poor prognosis.[52] Other organs, such as the kidney cortex (in one third of cases), may be involved but usually without functional impairment.[49] Less frequently, the lungs,[53] heart,[54] eyes,[55] and gastrointestinal tract are involved. Skin involvement is seldom seen and is almost always associated with the pre-B-cell phenotype.[56]

Central nervous system (CNS) involvement is seen in 5% of children and in less than 10% of adults with ALL. It is often seen among patients with mature B-cell ALL. However, many patients will eventually develop CNS disease if not adequately treated. Leukemia in the CNS presents with symptoms of increased intracranial pressure in 90% of cases, including headache, papilledema, nausea, vomiting, irritability, and lethargy. Signs of meningismus are common, and cranial nerves may also be affected, most frequently nerves III, IV, VI, and VII.

Testicular involvement is clinically evident in 1% of children with ALL at diagnosis, but it may be occult in as many as 25%.[57] The testicles represent a "sanctuary site," where disease can persist after systemic therapy. The testicles can be a frequent site of relapse, seen in up to 10% to 15% of children in some series,[58–61] but this is rare in adults. Disease in the testes presents as painless enlargement and firmness. Although involvement is usually unilateral, bilateral involvement is frequently diagnosed when a biopsy is performed.[62] The disease is characterized by interstitial involvement, but the seminiferous tubules are affected later.[62]

LABORATORY FEATURES AND DIAGNOSTIC WORKUP

The white blood cell (WBC) count is greater than 10×10^9/L in 50% to 60% of patients diagnosed with ALL and may be higher than 100×10^9/L in 10%. Another

30% to 40% have WBC counts lower than 10×10^9/L.[63] Despite high WBC counts, absolute neutrophil counts are frequently low.[63] The presence of blasts in the peripheral blood suggests the diagnosis of acute leukemia, but they are not always present and are not criteria for diagnosis. Despite very high WBC counts, symptoms of hyperleukocytosis are seldom seen.[64] Thrombocytopenia is the rule, with more than 90% of patients presenting with platelet counts less than 150×10^9/L and two thirds with less than 50×10^9/L.[63] Coagulopathies, including in situ ductal carcinomas, may be seen with ALL at presentation or during therapy.[65,66] Normocytic, normochromic anemia and reticulocytopenia are nearly universal.[63] Occasionally present at diagnosis is hypereosinophilic syndrome with tissue infiltration by eosinophils, which may lead to death from cardiorespiratory failure.[67]

Hyperuricemia and high levels of lactate dehydrogenase are common and reflect a large tumor burden, occasionally accompanied by urate nephropathy. Hypercalcemia is occasionally noted at diagnosis, whereas hypocalcemia, hyperkalemia, and hyperphosphatemia may be seen in association with tumor lysis syndrome. One third of patients have low levels of immunoglobulins (Igs), which may be a poor prognostic factor.[68,69]

The diagnosis of ALL requires the presence of at least 30% lymphoblasts[71,72] in bone marrow aspirates. The bone marrow is commonly hypercellular with few normal-appearing myeloid and erythroid precursors; rarely, it is hypoplastic or aplastic.[73] The diagnosis of ALL and its differentiation from AML made only on the basis of the morphologic appearance of the blasts are inaccurate, and additional discriminatory studies are needed. The most common way to determine the lymphoid origin of acute leukemia is by identifying its histochemical characteristics.

Histochemical Characteristics and Techniques

Stains: A combination of myeloperoxidase positivity of less than 3% of the blasts and a strong positive expression of terminal deoxynucleotidyltransferase (TdT) (less than 40% of the blasts) is indicative of a diagnosis of ALL. Positivity for TdT is noted in more than 95% of ALL cases.[74] TdT is a nonreplicative DNA polymerase that can elongate DNA chains on a template-independent basis.[74] TdT usually disappears upon lymphocyte maturation but is expressed on lymphoblasts. Patients with mature B-cell ALL are TdT-negative but express B-cell lineage (CD19 and CD20) and mature B-cell markers (surface Ig [sIg], kappa/lambda). TdT staining is not specific for ALL and is expressed in approximately 10% of patients with AML.[75]

A periodic acid-Schiff reaction may be positive in 40% to 70% of patients with ALL and represents liberation and oxidation of carbohydrates. Discrete granules can be seen in normal lymphocytes and megakaryocytes, and there is a diffuse positivity in granulocytes and monocytes. Block positivity for periodic acid-Schiff is seen in ALL, whereas diffuse cytoplasmic positivity for periodic acid-Schiff is noted in erythroleukemia.

Acid phosphatase is present in early T-cells, whereas B-cells have weak activity of this enzyme. Therefore, positivity to acid phosphatase, usually demonstrated as focal paranuclear concentrations, can differentiate T-cell ALL from non-T-cell ALL.[76]

Lymphoblasts are characteristically negative for myeloperoxidase, Sudan black B, and chloracetate esterase and may occasionally be faintly positive for nonspecific esterase.

Immunophenotype: The identification of differentiation antigens on leukemic cells by monoclonal antibodies has become an important element in the study of ALL. With this technique, the cell lineage can be determined (ie, B- or T-cell), as well as the state of differentiation within each lineage (Table 1), which may be relevant for therapeutic decisions. Knowledge of the immunophenotype can also aid in lineage determination in patients with acute leukemias that are morphologically undifferentiated and of mixed lineage or in patients with biphenotypic leukemias.

Molecular Techniques: These techniques can assist in identifying the clonality of the disease and the lineage of lymphoblasts.[77–81] They take advantage of the normal rearrangement that occurs among the variable, diverse, joining, and constant regions of the Ig and T-cell receptor (*TCR*) genes. In normal lymphocyte differentiation, these regions rearrange to produce different molecules (Ig and TCR) specific for the myriad antigens with which they will interact. Because each cell can produce an Ig (B-cells) or TCR (T-cells) that is reactive with only one specific antigen, lymphocytes from the peripheral blood of a normal individual show multiple rearrangements.[81] In patients with ALL, the clonal nature of the disorder results in lymphoblasts with the same rearrangement (ie, a clonal rearrangement).[81,82] However, the results of these molecular studies have to be interpreted with caution because nonspecificity has been identified,[83] with 10% to 20% of patients with T-cell ALL showing *Ig* gene rearrangement[84,85] and an equivalent proportion of patients with B-cell ALL bearing a *TCR-beta* gene rearrangement and even more frequently *TCR-gamma* and *TCR-delta* gene rearrangements.[86,87] A small percentage of patients with AML may have *Ig* or *TCR* gene rearrangements.[88]

TABLE 1

Expression of Differentiation Markers That Identify ALL Immunophenotype

B-cell lineage	HLA-DR	CD19	CD24	CD10	CD20	CD21	CD22	CD23	cIg	sIg
Early pre-B-cell	+	+	+	+	–	–	Cytoplasm	–	–	–
Pre-B-cell	+	+	+	+	+	+	+	–	+	–
Transitional B-cell	+	+	+	–	+	+	+	–	+	+[a]
Mature B-cell	+	+	+	–	+	+	+	+	–	+

T-cell lineage	CD7	CD2	CD5	CD1	CD4	CD8	CD3			
Early	+	+	+	–	–	–	–			
Intermediate	+	+	+	+	–	–	–			
Mature	+	+	+	–	+	+	+			

ALL = acute lymphocytic leukemia, cIg = cytoplasmic immunoglobulin, sIg = surface immunoglobulin   [a] Heavy chains but no light chains

These cross-lineage rearrangements are frequently nonproductive,[77,89] but some *Ig* gene rearrangements are also nonproductive in B-cell leukemias. Except in a few cases,[90] light-chain *Ig* gene rearrangement appears to be more B-cell specific than does heavy-chain *Ig* gene rearrangements.[91]

Electron Microscopy: Although not a routine element of the ALL workup, electron microscopy is a valuable adjunct in the classification of approximately 5% of leukemias that are otherwise undifferentiated. A small group of patients with ALL has cells that show myeloperoxidase positivity on electron microscopic scans. Such patients form an important subgroup because 85% of them have high-risk ALL.[92] Although 75% of these patients can achieve a complete response with ALL-type induction chemotherapy, the median duration is only 18 months.[92]

Diagnostic Workup

When the diagnosis of ALL is suspected, a complete workup should be initiated. It should include (1) a morphologic evaluation of peripheral blood and bone marrow aspirate and biopsy; (2) a histochemical evaluation of blast cells with stains for TdT, myeloperoxidase, esterase, and in some cases periodic acid-Schiff, acid phosphatase, and Sudan black B; (3) cytogenetic analysis; and (4) immunophenotypic analysis using B-lineage markers (CD19, CD20, cytoplasmic and surface Igs), T-lineage markers (CD1, CD2, CD3, CD7, CD5, CD4, and CD8), myeloid markers (CD13, CD33, CD14, CD15), common acute lymphocytic leukemia antigen (CALLA) (ie, CD10), the class II major histocompatibility complex

antigen (HLA-DR), and CD34. In some difficult cases, additional studies may be required for diagnostic purposes, including molecular studies to identify *Ig* or *TCR* gene rearrangements and electron microscopic scans.

CLASSIFICATION

ALL is a heterogeneous group of disorders comprising several subgroups that have distinct clinical and prognostic features. Several attempts to classify ALL have been made. The two most relevant ones are the morphologic and immunophenotypic classifications.

Morphologic Classification

The morphologic classification follows the guidelines defined by the French-American-British Cooperative Working Group.[71,72] It identifies three subgroups of ALL (Table 2): L_1, the most common variety in children (85% of cases), is only found in 30% of adults[93,94]; L_2, the predominant variety in adults (60% to 70% of cases), is found in less than 15% of children[93,94]; and L_3, which is found in less than 5% of cases. Cytoplasmic vacuoles are a prominent feature but are not pathognomonic of L_3 ALL.[95] The original French-American-British classification is not always reproducible, and a scoring system has been added to enhance concordance among observers.[72]

Immunophenotypic Classification

The immunophenotype is a more clinically relevant classification of ALL and is based on the expression of certain antigens on the surface of leukemic cells. Normal lymphocytes express specific antigens in an orderly

TABLE 2

French-American-British Classification of Acute Lymphocytic Leukemia

Type	Incidence (%) Adult	Children	Characteristics	Response rate (%)	3-year survival rate (%)
L$_1$	31	85	Small, homogeneous cells; round nucleus; scanty cytoplasm	85	40
L$_2$	60	14	Large, heterogeneous cells; irregular nucleus, cleft, nucleolus; more cytoplasm	75	35
L$_3$	9	1	Large, homogeneous; regular nucleus; vacuolated, basophilic cytoplasm; Burkitt's lymphoma; poor prognosis	65	10

Adapted, with permission, from Bennett JM, Catovsky D, Daniel M-T.[71,72]

fashion through their different stages of differentiation.[96] According to Greaves,[91] lymphoblasts represent an interruption at different steps of differentiation of normal lymphocytes. Therefore, expression of antigens on the cell surface indicates the specific step in differentiation where transformation occurred. Several classifications have been proposed for normal[97,98] and leukemic[99,100] lymphocytes. Table 3 presents the current immunophenotypic classification of ALL and the frequency of each subtype.

Although this classification is useful clinically, some cautionary notes must be added. The phenotype of the lymphoblasts may not correlate with any normal phenotype, including some cases with simultaneous expression of antigens normally present at different ends of the differentiation spectrum (ie, asynchronous antigen expression),[101] even though some of these lymphoblasts may actually have a rare normal counterpart.[102] Approximately 5% to 10% of children with ALL[103–105] and 30% of adults with ALL[106–108] express myeloid markers. It is not clear whether these cases represent transformation of a pluripotent cell or an as-yet-unidentified progenitor that coexpresses markers and features from several lineages.[109,110] It is clear that no marker is absolutely lineage-specific; in fact, CD19, CD2, and CD4 can be found in at least 50% of patients who have AML with t(8;21), acute promyelocytic leukemia, and AML with monocytic features, respectively.[111–113] Therefore, it has been suggested that two or more markers corresponding to a different lineage must be present to diagnose a mixed-lineage leukemia.[105]

Another cautionary factor is the presence of nonlineage-dependent markers. The most common marker is CD10 (ie, CALLA), which is a membrane-bound neutral endopeptidase[114,115] that can be expressed in both B- and T-cell leukemias.[116] CD34 is a marker of a very early pluripotential cell, including the stem cell,[117] and is most frequently expressed in non-T-cell, non-B-cell cases of ALL.[118] Coexpression of CD38 on CD34-positive cells is a marker for lineage commitment,[119] is present on 20% of normal bone marrow cells as well as activated plasma cells and T-cells, and is a common marker in both T-cell and B-cell leukemias.[120] CD71, another marker of activation, is more common in patients with T-cell than B-cell leukemias.[120]

The immunologic classification of ALL also correlates with clinical characteristics, with certain features associated with specific subtypes of B- and T-cells.

Early Pre-B-Cell ALL: Nearly 70% of children and adults with ALL have the early pre-B-cell type.[121] The immunophenotype is characterized by a lack of expression of cytoplasmic or surface immunoglobulins.[122] Patients are frequently young (1 to 9 years old) and have low WBC counts.[114,115] Nearly 50% of patients younger than 1 year old, 10% of older children, and 10% to 40% of adults do not express CD10.[123–125] Lack of expression of CD10 is associated with pseudodiploidy, high WBC counts, and poor prognosis. CD10-negative early pre-B-cell ALL probably represents a more immature counterpart of CD10-positive early pre-B-cell ALL.[126] More than three fourths of children with pre-B-cell ALL express CD34, a feature frequently accompanied by hyperdiploidy, a low incidence of CNS involvement at presentation, and good prognosis.[127,128]

Pre-B-Cell ALL: Approximately 20% of cases of ALL are pre B-cell ALL, which is identified by the expression

TABLE 3

Immunophenotypic Classification of Acute Lymphocytic Leukemia

Type	Markers	Incidence (%) Children	Adults	Observations
Early Pre-B	Cytoplasmic Ig–	65–70	50–60	Express at least one B-cell marker, CALLA + or –
Pre-B-cell	Cytoplasmic Ig+	15–20	15–25	Express at least one B-cell marker, CALLA + or –, worse prognosis than that for early pre-B-cell
B-cell	Surface Ig+	< 5	< 5	Extramedullary lymphomatous masses, CNS involvement, hyperuricemia, acute respiratory failure, Burkitt's leukemia
T-cell	CD2 CD3 CD5 CD7 CD4 CD8	10–15	20–25	High WBC count, CNS involvement, thymic mass

ALL = acute lymphocytic leukemia, CALLA = common acute lymphocytic leukemia antigen, CNS = central nervous system, WBC = white blood cell

of cytoplasmic Ig heavy chains[122,129]; almost all these patients also express CD10.[121] This subgroup includes more African-American patients than does the early pre-B-cell subgroup. These patients also have higher levels of lactate dehydrogenase and hemoglobin and higher WBC counts. Cytogenetic analysis often reveals pseudodiploidy, frequently associated with the t(1;19) abnormality and cells that are less likely to be hyperdiploid.[130-132] Poor prognostic characteristics and poor outcome are correlated with the t(1;19) abnormality.[133] Other studies suggest that among patients with the t(1;19) abnormality, a pre-B-cell immunophenotype correlates with a worse prognosis than an early pre-B-cell immunophenotype.[134]

Transitional Pre-B-Cell ALL: This newly characterized subtype accounts for approximately 1% of all cases of ALL. The hallmark is the expression of μ heavy chains on the surface with no light chains.[135] These patients have L_1 or L_2 morphology, low WBC counts, and hyperdiploidy; their outcome is better than that of patients with mature B-cell ALL.

Mature B-Cell ALL: Less than 5% of patients have mature B-cell ALL,[121] which represents a leukemic phase of Burkitt's lymphoma.[136] Mature B-cell ALL presents with bulky extramedullary disease, including abdominal lymphadenopathy and frequent CNS involvement.[137] Morphologically, mature B-cell ALL often represents the L_3 subtype of the French-American-British classification. Some cases of mature B-cell ALL do not show the L_3 morphology but instead exhibit lymphoma-like features and particular karyotypic abnormalities, such as 6q-, 14q+, t(11;14), or t(14;18).

T-Cell ALL: Nearly 15% to 20% of children[123] and adults[138] have T-cell ALL, but its incidence may decrease with age.[139,140] T-cell ALL is associated with males, high WBC counts, CNS involvement, and mediastinal masses[123,141]; mediastinal masses are associated with mature thymocyte phenotypes.[142] Patients with T-cell ALL with no expression of CD10 have a poor prognosis.[116]

PROGNOSIS

Several prognostic factors have been identified for children[143-145] and adults[146-148] with ALL, and risk categories have been defined to guide therapy. Some of the better-defined prognostic factors include age, WBC count, and cytogenetic characteristics and abnormalities.

Age: Infants younger than age 1 and children older than age 10 have a worse prognosis than patients 1 to 9 years old.[143,145,149] Adults have a worse prognosis than children, with the worst outcome associated with patients older than age 60.[146,147,150] The poor outcome in infants may be related to the frequent occurrence of other poor prognostic features in this group, including higher WBC counts; higher incidences of hepatomegaly, splenomegaly, and CNS involvement at diagnosis; CD10-negative disease[143]; and abnormalities in band 23 of the long arm of chromosome 11 in approximately 70% of patients.[151–153] Infants without 11q23 rearrangements may have an outcome comparable to that of children 1 year old or older.[152]

WBC Count: The WBC count at presentation is a highly significant prognostic variable. Patients with counts higher than 10×10^9/L have a worse prognosis.[145] The cutoff at which a good prognosis is defined in children varies in different centers,[154] but WBC counts higher than

50×10^9/L are clearly associated with a poor outcome,[126,154] and this value has been proposed by a National Cancer Institute (NCI)-sponsored workshop as the value with which to identify pediatric patients with a poor prognosis.[154] In adults, WBC counts are also an important prognostic factor for both the achievement[147] and duration[146,147,155] of a complete remission. The cutoff value for adults is not clear but is probably lower than that for children, ranging from 5 to 50×10^9/L.[155]

Cytogenetic Characteristics: Cytogenetic characteristics are probably the most important prognostic factor for ALL.[156] Cytogenetic abnormalities can be numeric or structural,[157,158] as shown in Table 4. In children, ploidy is the most important prognostic factor.[159–161] Patients with hyperdiploid ALL, in particular those with more than 50 chromosomes, have the best prognosis.[162–164] When analyzed by DNA index (ie, DNA content in leukemic cells vs that in normal cells), patients with an index higher than 1.16, which corresponds approximately to more than 50 chromosomes, have a better prognosis, with almost 90% of patients' having an event-free survival duration of 4 years.[159] The favorable outcome in patients with hyperdiploid common ALL may be due to an increased sensitivity to drugs, such as asparaginase (Elspar), mercaptopurine (Purinethol), cytarabine, and methotrexate.[165]

Hyperdiploidy is present in 25% to 30% of children with ALL[145] but in only 10% to 20% of adults. The index classification should be accompanied by regular cytogenetic analysis, because hyperdiploidy alone does not provide information on additional structural abnormalities and when they are present (as in 60% of hyperdiploid cases), the prognosis is not as good as when only the numeric abnormality is present.[166] Patients with a DNA index higher than 1.16 usually present with good prognostic features (ie, age 1 to 9 years, low WBC counts, early pre-B-cell phenotype).

Patients with high-risk features should be treated as good risks if hyperdiploid.[154] Hyperdiploid patients with nearly tetraploid cells (approximately 1% of all cases)[145,167,168] and patients with 47 to 50 chromosomes (ie, a DNA index between 1 and 1.16) (15% of all cases)[145] have an intermediate prognosis.[163] Patients with near tetraploidy are older and have a T-cell phenotype.[169] Patients with 47 to 50 chromosomes often have additional chromosomes 21, X, 8, and 10 and in 76% of cases also have additional structural abnormalities.[170] When trisomy 21 is the sole chromosomal abnormality, patients may have a particularly good prognosis, in part because of the association with other good prognostic features.[171]

Hypodiploid cases, most frequently from loss of chromosome 20,[172,173] represent 6% of all cases of ALL.[145]

TABLE 4
Cytogenetic Classification of ALL

	Cytogenetic abnormality	Incidence (%)	
		Children	Adults
Numeric abnormalities	Hyperdiploid	40–50	10–20
	47 to 50 chromosomes	15–20	5–10
	> 50 chromosomes	25–30	5–10
	Diploid	10–30	25–35
	Hypodiploid	7–10	5–10
Structural abnormalities	Pseudodiploid	40–50	50–60
	t(9;22)(q34;q11)	3–5	15–25
	t(8;14), t(8;2), and t(8;22)	3–5	5–10
	t(4;11)(q21;q23) (and others involving 11q23)	5	5
	t(1;19)(q23;p13.3)	5–7	< 5
	14q11 abnormalities	< 5	5–10
	7q35 abnormalities	< 5	< 5
	Others	5–15	5–15

ALL = acute lymphocytic leukemia

Although these patients commonly present with good prognostic features, they have an intermediate prognosis.[173] Patients with near-haploid ALL (less than 1% of all cases[145]) have a very poor prognosis.[174–176] Of all patients, 8% to 10% have a normal diploid karyotype,[145] but the frequency is as high as 30% in patients with T-cell ALL.[177] The prognosis of disease with a normal karyotype is intermediate.[163] Numeric chromosomal abnormalities (hyper- and hypodiploid) are less common in adults and have much less impact on outcome in adults than they do in children.[164] Adults with diploid ALL may have the best prognosis.[164]

A large percentage of patients have pseudodiploid ALL.[145,164] Overall, these patients have a poor prognosis. Some of the specific abnormalities observed in patients with pseudodiploid ALL are discussed.

Chromosomal Abnormalities: Translocation t(9;22)(q34;q11) or Philadelphia (Ph) chromosome is present in less than 5% of children with ALL[178–180] but is found in 15% to 30% of adults with ALL.[147,164,181] The incidence may be higher with more sensitive techniques; molecular studies for Ph-related abnormalities are positive in up to 30% of adults with ALL.[182,183] Ph-positive ALL is associated with older age, high WBC counts, and L_2 morphology[179,181]; in adults, it is also associated with a higher frequency of expression of CD10 and CD34.[181] Nearly one half of all patients with Ph-positive ALL may have additional chromosomal abnormalities, particularly monosomy 7.[184]

At the molecular level, the Ph chromosome in ALL may be different from the one seen in patients with chronic myelogenous leukemia (CML). In ALL, it involves band 34 of the long arm of chromosome 9, splicing the proto-oncogene c-*abl* to band 11 of the long arm of chromosome 22 in the *bcr* gene.[185] In 50% to 80% of cases of ALL, the breakpoint in 22q11 falls between exons b1 and b2 of the major breakpoint cluster region,[186] as opposed to between b2 and b3 or b3 and b4 in CML.[185] This translates into a different protein product of only 190 kDa (p190[BCR/ABL]) compared with that of CML (210 kDa, p210[BCR/ABL]).[185,186] Both proteins have increased tyrosine kinase activity.[187] Protein p190[BCR/ABL] can induce acute leukemia in transgenic mice[188] and may have a comparatively higher transforming potential than p210[BCR/ABL].[189] Of adults with Ph-positive ALL, 20% to 50% express p210 rather than p190[183]; some of these patients may have a blastic phase of a previously unrecognized CML.[190]

The outcome of patients with Ph-positive ALL is poor, with significantly low complete remission rates (75% in children and 50% to 70% in adults),[179,180] and long-term disease-free survival rates (less than 10%).[179,181,182]

Translocations t(8;14), t(8;2), and t(8;22) are present in most cases of mature B-cell ALL[191] and Burkitt's lymphoma.[192] The proto-oncogene c-*myc* present in band 24 of the long arm of chromosome 8 is juxtaposed to an Ig locus, most frequently the heavy chain (chromosome 14q32) but sometimes to the light chains kappa (2p12) or lambda (22q11).[193] This results in overexpression of MYC,[194] a transcription factor that interacts with other proteins (MAX and MAZ) and binds to DNA.[195] In transgenic mice, overexpression of c-*myc* driven by Ig enhancers induces lymphoid malignancies.[196] As previously mentioned, mature B-cell leukemia represents less than 5% of all cases of ALL,[121] is characterized by early CNS involvement and extramedullary disease, and carries a poor prognosis with conventional chemotherapy.[137] However, recent short-term dose-intensive regimens have significantly improved the outcome for patients with mature B-cell ALL.[197–202]

Translocation t(4;11) and other abnormalities in band 23 of the long arm of chromosome 11 (11q23) have become a focus of attention because an increasing number of patients being treated for ALL and other malignancies are developing the 11q23 abnormality that causes AML.[203–206] ALL with 11q23 abnormalities may present de novo and is seen in approximately 5% of children with ALL and less often in adults.[207] Patients with 11q23 abnormalities are frequently young and African-American, have high WBC counts,[207–208] are CD10 negative, and have early pre-B-cell disease,[209] and myeloid features. It is the most common chromosomal abnormality in infants with ALL,[210] affecting more than 70% of cases

at the molecular level.[211] Translocation t(4;11) carries a poor prognosis, but infants who do not have this chromosomal abnormality may have an outcome comparable to that of intermediate-risk childhood ALL; infants with 11q23 rearrangements have a 3-year event-free survival rate of 13%, compared with 67% for infants without this rearrangement.[212] The 11q23 abnormality codes for a gene called MLL or ALL-1.[213–214] It has an unknown function, but the fact that it is frequently involved in mixed-lineage and myeloid leukemias suggests that it plays a role in lineage differentiation.

Translocation t(1;19) is the most common (5% of cases) translocation in children with ALL[215–217] but is uncommon in adults. This translocation is frequently associated with a pre-B-cell immunophenotype.[132,218] Patients with this abnormality exhibit other poor prognostic factors (high WBC count and high lactate dehydrogenase level) and have a poor prognosis.[132] At the molecular level, translocation t(1;19) results in the fusion of E2A, an immunoglobulin enhancer-binding protein coded for in chromosome 19p13, with PBX, a homeobox protein that binds to DNA and is probably a transcription activation factor, coded for in chromosome 1q23.[219,220] This results in the constitutional expression in pre-B-cells of a gene (PBX) that is normally not expressed in these cells.

Regions 14q11 and 7q35 contain the loci for the alpha/delta and beta *TCR* gene, respectively. They are rearranged in patients with T-cell ALL.[221–226] The most common of these abnormalities is t(11;14)(p13;q11) (present in 7% of patients with T-cell ALL),[177,229] which fuses the *TCR* alpha/delta to a gene called rhombotin 2 (*Ttg2*).[227,228] A less common translocation, t(11;14)(p15;q11), present in only 1% of patients with T-cell ALL,[229] affects rhombotin 1 (*Ttg1*).[230] The rhombotin (*Ttg*) family of genes is involved in transcription regulation by means of a LIM-domain-mediated protein interaction, which in turn could prevent transcription activation by LIM-domain protein partners.[231] Other partner genes for *TCR* alpha/delta include *HOX11* in t(10;14), a homeobox gene[232,233] that binds DNA and activates gene expression; *TAL1/SCL* in t(1;14), a basic helix-loop-helix protein that binds DNA and can control transcription either directly or by dimerization with other DNA-binding proteins[234–236]; and c-*myc* in a t(8;14).[237–238] Translocations affecting *TCR* beta are less common.[237,238,240] Partner genes involved in these translocations include *TAL2*, similar to *TAL1/SCL*, in t(7;9)(q34;q32)[241]; *LYL1* in t(7;19), analogous to *TAL2*[234–236]; Ttg2 in t(7;11); and *TAN1* in t(7;9).[242]

Another abnormality found in the short arm of chromosome 9 occurs in 7% to 12% of children[243,244] and adults with ALL. This abnormality identifies a group of patients with high WBC counts, older age, T-cell immunophenotype, a high rate of extramedullary relapse,[245] and poor outcome. It affects 9p21-22, which contains the alpha and beta interferon (IFN-α and -β) genes.[246] Abnormalities in 6q occur in 6% of cases,[164] and their clinical and prognostic significance is uncertain.[247] The short arm of chromosome 12 is affected in 10% of cases of ALL in children,[248] usually of B-cell lineage, but there is great heterogeneity of the specific change. Patients with this abnormality may have a high incidence of CNS relapse.[249] Mutations of N-*ras* have been detected in 6% of children with ALL, clustered in codons 12 and 13, and may be a poor prognostic feature.[250]

Immunophenotype: Patients with T-cell ALL have a historically poor outcome, with a 5-year event-free survival rate of 50% in children[251] and 10% to 20% in adults. Recent studies have shown a similar or better outcome compared with that of other immunophenotypes,[146,147] probably from the inclusion of cyclophosphamide (Cytoxan, Neosar) and cytarabine in the treatment of this subgroup of patients.[252,253] Within the T-cell phenotype, patients with the pre-T-cell phenotype (CD7+, CD2–, CD1–, CD4–, CD8–) have a worse prognosis. CD10– T-cell ALL also carries a poor prognosis.[233]

Mature B-cell ALL is also associated with a poor prognosis. The introduction of hyperfractionated cyclophosphamide, high-dose methotrexate, and cytarabine has significantly improved the results, both in children[137,254] and in adults.[197] The best prognosis among B-cell-lineage ALL is associated with the early pre-B-cell phenotype, particularly when it is associated with CD10.[122,123]

The expression of myeloid markers has been difficult to evaluate as a prognostic factor, mostly because of different diagnostic criteria. Wide variations in the incidence of myeloid markers (from less than 20% to more than 40%) have been reported, most commonly in adults. Some investigators have reported an associated poor prognosis,[255] especially when adjusted for other poor prognostic factors,[108] but others have not.[256,257]

Other Prognostic Factors: CD34 expression has been correlated with a favorable outcome in children with the pre-B-cell phenotype[258] but has not in adults.[256] Expression of MDR (multidrug resistance)-associated protein P170 has also been reported to confer a poor prognosis for both children and adults.[259] Patients with MDR-positive ALL at diagnosis had lower complete response rates, higher relapse rates, and shorter survival than MDR-negative patients.[259] Males and African-Americans may have a worse prognosis.[260,261] Although not a feature that can be evaluated at diagnosis, a late response to therapy is a poor prognostic feature for all age groups.[146,147,262,263]

Prognostic Models: With all these risk factors, several prognostic models have been proposed. In children, an NCI-sponsored workshop has used age and WBC counts to define risk.[154] Patients aged 1 to 9 years with a WBC count lower than 50×10^9/L represent 68% of all children with B-cell-precursor ALL, and they have a 4-year event-free survival rate of approximately 80%. Patients older than age 10 or who have WBC counts higher than 50×10^9/L have a 4-year event-free survival rate of approximately 64%.[154] Moreover, there is a strong correlation between age and WBC counts. Almost 50% of infants have WBC counts of at least 50×10^9/L, whereas less than 20% of older children have WBC counts this high,[143] and 50% have counts lower than 10×10^9/L.[143,144] Twenty-five percent of all adults have WBC counts higher than 50×10^9/L.

Several prognostic models with similarities have been proposed for adults with ALL and are summarized in Table 5. High risk is associated with the majority of cases of adults with ALL. Hoelzer et al identified a time to complete response of longer than 4 weeks, age older than 35 years, WBC count higher than 30×10^9/L, and a null ALL phenotype as poor prognostic features.[146] Patients with none of these features (27% of cases) have a 5-year remission rate of 62%, compared with 28% for patients with at least 1 of these features.[146] Ph-positive ALL identifies a definitely poor prognostic group, whereas the prognosis of mature B-cell ALL is changing; favorable outcomes (complete response rates of 80% to 90% and long-term disease-free survival rates of 40% to 60%) have been reported with the use of recent short-term, dose-intensive regimens. The cutoff for WBC count depends on whether the particular model incorporates older age as a poor prognostic factor, because an inverse correlation is noted between age and WBC count. In the model by Hoelzer et al, age older than 35 years (more than 50% of patients) is a poor prognostic factor; thus, the cutoff for WBC count is high (30×10^9/L). In a model from the University of Texas M. D. Anderson Cancer Center (Table 5), age is not a poor prognostic factor, and so the cutoff for WBC count is lower (5×10^9/L).[155]

TREATMENT

Modern therapy has changed the outcome for patients with ALL. In children, ALL is now a highly curable disease, with cure rates ranging from 60% to 85%. Therapy for ALL in adults has followed the lead of that for children. Approximately 75% of adults with ALL (range, 65% to 90%) achieve a complete remission, but

TABLE 5

Prognostic Models Used for Adults With Acute Lymphocytic Leukemia

Risk category	Hoelzer et al[146]	Kantarjian et al[155]	Gaynor et al[147]
Standard			
Percentage of all patients	27%	28%	40%
Long-term disease-free survival rate	62%	70%	61%
Intermediate			
Percentage of all patients			22%
Long-term disease-free survival rate			43%
High-risk			
Percentage of all patients	73%	72%	38%
Long-term disease-free survival rate	28%	27%	30%
High-risk features	WBC count > 30 × 10⁹/L	WBC count ≥ 5 × 10⁹/L	WBC count > 20 × 10⁹/L
	Age > 35 years		Age > 60 years
	Null-cell ALL	B-cell ALL	Null- or B-cell ALL
	Complete resonse after > 4 weeks	Complete response after ≥ 2 induction courses	Complete response after > 5 weeks
		Ph-positive	Ph-positive
		CNS involvement	

ALL = acute lymphocytic leukemia, CNS = central nervous system, WBC = white blood cell

despite significant progress in the past 30 years, only 20% to 40% are cured.[264–266] Therapy for ALL includes induction, consolidation, maintenance, and CNS prophylaxis. The different phases are discussed separately, because modifications in each phase have been attempted and have resulted in improved outcome.

Induction Therapy

The first combination successfully used for induction chemotherapy in adults with ALL included vincristine (Oncovin) and corticosteroids, most frequently prednisone.[267–268] With this combination, 40% to 60% of patients achieved a complete response, but the median remission duration was only 3 to 7 months. Anthracyclines were then incorporated into this combination, and the complete response rate improved to 85% (range, 70% to 85%) compared with 47% without anthracyclines (P = .003).[269] This triple combination has become standard for induction of remission in adults with ALL. Doxorubicin (Adriamycin, Rubex) and daunorubicin (Cerubidine) are the commonly used anthracyclines and have produced similar results.[269,270] Mitoxantrone (Novantrone) may also be effective.[271] Among the corticosteroids, prednisone and methylprednisolone are the most frequently used agents; dexamethasone penetrates the CNS-blood barrier better and exhibits better in vitro antileukemic activity.[272] This triple-drug induction combination chemotherapy is associated with a low induction

mortality rate of approximately 10% or less.

Other chemotherapeutic agents, including cyclophosphamide, asparaginase, cytarabine, and, less frequently, etoposide (VePesid), teniposide (Vumon), and amsacrine, have been incorporated into induction regimens in an attempt to improve the rate and duration of complete response. The benefit from these modifications is difficult to determine, but overall results seem equivalent to those with vincristine, anthracyclines, and corticosteroids.

In one study, half of the patients who received induction therapy with vincristine, asparaginase, daunorubicin, and corticosteroids were randomized to receive additional cyclophosphamide induction. The complete response rate was 84% for both arms, and the continuous complete response rates at 3 years were also similar (47% vs 43%).[273] In another study, the addition of cyclophosphamide may have improved the outcome for patients with T-cell ALL.[274] The addition of high-dose cytarabine to the induction regimen has not improved the results and has been associated with increased toxicity and induction mortality rate.[275] Cytarabine at lower doses, together with thioguanine and daunorubicin, has been added to vincristine and prednisone, resulting in a complete response rate of 91%, but the median remission duration was only 15 months.[276] Cytarabine during induction therapy may selectively improve the outcome in T-cell ALL.[277] Asparaginase has been added to induction therapy with no improvement in complete response rates,[277–280] but remission duration may be prolonged in children.[281] In one study, asparaginase replaced anthracyclines in the induction regimen, resulting in a similar outcome but with the potential benefit of decreased cardiotoxicity.[282]. Using methotrexate instead of anthracycline produced equivalent results.[283]

More intensive regimens with growth factor support may induce rapid reductions in tumor burden and a potentially better outcome.[284] Preliminary results with such an approach are encouraging.[198,285] The duration of neutropenia may be shortened by using growth factors,[285,286] but there is the potential risk of growth factors stimulating the growth of leukemic cells.[287]

Some subsets of patients require a different induction approach. The improved outcome with cytarabine and cyclophosphamide for patients with T-cell ALL has been mentioned.[146,147,274,277] In patients with mature B-cell ALL, the use of hyperfractionated cyclophosphamide alternating with high-dose methotrexate and cytarabine has resulted in cure rates of 50% to 60% in children and in small series of adults.[197-202]

Consolidation Therapy

The use of intensive consolidation has demonstrated its value in children with ALL. High-dose methotrexate,[288] sometimes in combination with mercaptopurine[289,290] or teniposide and cytarabine,[291] and asparaginase[281] have significantly contributed to increasing the cure rate to 70% to 80% in children with ALL. Delayed intensification has also improved the outcome in children with ALL,[292] but it is difficult to demonstrate this benefit in adults. Some studies have failed to demonstrate that consolidation improves results,[293] whereas others conclude that it does improve outcome.[266] This discordance may be due to the difficulty in assessing the specific value of individual components or phases of overall treatment.

Some of the most effective regimens reported in the literature have included some form of consolidation, but its intensity varied from asparaginase alone,[280] to combinations including cyclophosphamide, cytarabine, mercaptopurine, and methotrexate.[146,147,156] These studies have resulted in median remission durations of 20 to 24 months and 3-year survival rates of 35% to 45%. One study randomized 61 patients to receive 3 monthly consolidation courses with doxorubicin, cytarabine, and asparaginase vs no consolidation and documented a 3-year disease-free survival rate of 38% and 0%, respectively.[294]

Other studies raised questions as to the benefit of this approach. The European Organization for Research and Treatment of Cancer randomized patients to receive a 3-month consolidation schedule with methotrexate, cytar-

abine, and thioguanine vs maintenance therapy after the induction of complete remission. No difference in the disease-free survival rate between the two groups was found.[295] Similarly, the Cancer and Leukemia Group B randomized patients after induction to receive two courses of cytarabine and daunorubicin vs maintenance with mercaptopurine and methotrexate. The duration of complete remission and the overall survival rate were similar for both arms.[296] There are important limitations in these studies, including (1) the limited time and intensity of the consolidation drugs used in these patients and (2) the use of schedules that did not include some of the most effective agents for consolidation in children with ALL, such as high-dose methotrexate and mercaptopurine, high-dose asparaginase, and cyclophosphamide with cytarabine.

High-dose cytarabine may be beneficial in some patients. Rohatiner et al found a trend for improved remission duration using high-dose cytarabine consolidation in patients with high blast-cell counts or T-cell morphology.[277] A German multicenter study used high-dose cytarabine with mitoxantrone for intensification in high-risk patients and found a continuous complete response rate at 4 years of 43%, compared with 23% for patients not receiving this therapy.[297] However, older patients were frequently not offered the high-dose therapy, and the difference in results may be at least partially explained by the presence of higher-risk patients in the control arm.[297] The Eastern Cooperative Oncology Group used high-dose cytarabine consolidation without improvement in outcome. However, some patients received very short induction regimens, and no patients received maintenance with mercaptopurine and methotrexate.[298]

Therefore, consolidation may be beneficial when adequate drugs at adequate doses are used. Some subsets of patients may benefit from specific agents (ie, patients with T-cell ALL from cyclophosphamide and cytarabine and patients with Ph-positive ALL or patients in high-risk groups from high-dose cytarabine).

Maintenance Therapy

Studies in children with ALL have established the value of maintenance therapy. This usually consists of mercaptopurine and methotrexate and is continued for 2 years. There is evidence that when adequate levels of these drugs are not achieved, the outcome may be as poor as when no maintenance is attempted.[299-300] Maintenance therapy with mercaptopurine and methotrexate-based regimens has also been used in adults with ALL,[146,147,155,280,301] but the schedules have varied. Some schedules have used relatively intensive maintenance, with regimens including high-dose methotrexate, daunorubicin, mercaptopurine, and prednisone[155] or with vincristine, prednisone, doxorubicin, mercaptopurine, oral methotrexate, dactinomycin (Cosmegen), cyclophosphamide, and carmustine (BiCNU).[301] Others have used simpler regimens with oral mercaptopurine and methotrexate reinforced by monthly doses of vincristine and prednisone and occasionally the addition of doxorubicin, or carmustine and cyclophosphamide.[147,280]

A few studies have omitted maintenance therapy altogether. The Cancer and Leukemia Group B used four intensification courses with several agents, including cytarabine, mercaptopurine, methotrexate, and asparaginase, but used no drugs for maintenance.[272] The median remission duration for these patients was only 11.2 months.[271] The Eastern Cooperative Oncology Group used consolidation therapy with high-dose cytarabine and methotrexate, asparaginase, cyclophosphamide, doxorubicin, vincristine, and prednisone without maintenance therapy and showed a 4-year disease-free survival rate of only 13%, with a median remission duration of 9.6 months.[298] One study from Italy randomized patients to receive conventional maintenance therapy or a more intensive schedule with mercaptopurine and methotrexate, alternating with the same drugs for consolidation therapy. No difference in disease-free survival was observed.[302] Therefore, conventional maintenance therapy with mercaptopurine and methotrexate could be as effective as more intensive regimens.

Maintenance therapy with mercaptopurine and methotrexate is not needed in patients with mature B-cell ALL, who are usually treated with dose-intensive therapy for 3 to 8 months, which results in disease-free survival rates of 40% to 60%. Patients with Ph-positive ALL probably do not benefit from maintenance therapy with mercaptopurine and methotrexate. Alternative investigations studying the use of IFN-α, high-dose cytarabine, immunomodulation, dose-intensive chemotherapy with autologous stem-cell transplantation with or without purging, and gene-targeted therapy are warranted in patients for whom allogeneic bone marrow transplantation (BMT) is not feasible in first complete remission.

CNS Prophylaxis and Treatment

Disease involving the CNS is present at diagnosis in only 5% of children and adults.[303,304] Without adequate prophylaxis, disease in 50% to 75% of patients with ALL will eventually involve the CNS.[305,306] CNS prophylaxis has reduced the incidence of relapses in the CNS to less than 10%.[212]

Different approaches have been used as prophylaxis for CNS disease, including cranial irradiation and intrathecal (IT) chemotherapy with methotrexate and cytarabine,[307–309] and are now standard for children with ALL.[305,310] These approaches can result in neurologic sequelae, including intellectual dysfunction, seizures, and dementia,[311] as well as extraneural complications, particularly slow growth in children.[312] Complications may be more common in patients receiving cranial irradiation,[311,313] and prophylaxis without cranial irradiation may be as effective, at least in patients who are at intermediate risk.[314]

Adults with ALL frequently receive CNS prophylaxis with IT chemotherapy and cranial irradiation in a manner similar to that for children. This has resulted in a lower incidence of relapse in the CNS.[315,316] The incidence of complications associated with CNS prophylaxis is similar to that in children, but the abnormalities observed are frequently asymptomatic and are detected only on electroencephalograms or computed tomography scans.[317] In a randomized study allocating patients to receive cranial irradiation and IT methotrexate or no CNS prophylaxis, the 3-year CNS relapse rate significantly decreased from 45% to 20% with prophylaxis. However, this did not translate into an improved survival rate.[315] In our studies, early intervention with IT chemotherapy and high-dose systemic chemotherapy without cranial irradiation is highly effective prophylactically in adults with ALL, particularly for patients at high risk for CNS relapse.[304] More recent studies have emphasized IT therapy plus high-dose systemic chemotherapy over cranial irradiation as CNS prophylaxis in both children and adults with ALL.

Several reports have identified risk factors for the development of CNS leukemia in children, including high WBC counts, T-cell or B-cell disease, young age, lymphadenopathy, thrombocytopenia, hepatomegaly, and splenomegaly.[305,318] In adults, a multivariate analysis identified a mature B-cell phenotype, high serum levels of lactate dehydrogenase, and a high proliferative index (ie, cells in $S+G_2M$ compartments greater than or equal to 14%) as risk factors for CNS disease.[319] Among patients with none of these factors (40%), the incidence of CNS leukemia at 1 year was 5%, compared with more than 50% in patients with high levels of lactate dehydrogenase and a high proliferative index.[319] The intensity of CNS prophylaxis could be adjusted to the risk of CNS disease according to this model.[304]

Patients who present with leukemia in the CNS should receive more aggressive therapy. One proposed therapeutic scheme includes IT methotrexate alternating with IT cytarabine twice weekly until the cerebrospinal fluid clears, then weekly for 1 month and once monthly thereafter for 2 years.[296] Cranial irradiation may be indicated in these patients.[201,296] For patients with a WBC count lower than 5×10^9/L and 15 WBC/μL in the cerebrospinal fluid together with blasts, prophylaxis as used for patients whose cerebrospinal fluid is blast-negative may be equally effective.[314] Patients with cranial nerve root involvement may benefit from selective irradiation to the base of the skull.

Allogeneic BMT

Allogeneic BMT is an effective alternative therapy for patients with ALL. The timing of the transplantation is controversial. Some groups have performed allogeneic BMT in patients who are in first remission and have reported long-term disease-free survivals in 22% to 60% of patients.[320–322] This wide range derives from the variability in patient selection because factors such as age, phenotype of the disease, WBC count, gender mismatch, and the type of prophylaxis used to prevent graft-vs-host disease significantly influence the outcome.[323]

The International Bone Marrow Transplant Registry reported a 5-year actuarial rate of leukemia-free survival of 44% for patients who received BMT during their first remission.[324] Several other studies have reported long-term disease-free survival for 40% to 70% of patients.[325–327] Patients undergoing allogeneic BMT usually represent a highly select population of young patients with no organ dysfunction.

To clarify the value of allogeneic BMT in patients in first remission, Horowitz et al conducted a retrospective analysis of patients who received intensive consolidation and maintenance therapies with the Berlin-Frankfurt-Munster regimen vs patients undergoing allogeneic BMT in first remission.[328] After accounting for age and lead time bias to BMT, the 5-year leukemia-free survival rate was 38% in patients who received chemotherapy and 44% in patients who underwent allogeneic BMT.[328] The causes of failure differed with these approaches. With chemotherapy, the 5-year probability of relapse was 59% and the probability of treatment-related death 4%; for patients treated with BMT, the probabilities were 26% and 39%, respectively.[328] The investigators were not able to identify subgroups of patients who benefited from BMT.[320]

In a prospective study by Fière et al, patients who had an HLA-identical sibling and who achieved remission were assigned to undergo allogeneic BMT if they were younger than 40 years; if older than 50 years, patients received consolidation with chemotherapy, and all others were randomized to autologous BMT or consolidation

with chemotherapy alone.[329] The estimated 3-year disease-free survival rate was 43% for patients undergoing allogeneic BMT, 39% for patients undergoing autologous BMT, and 32% for patients receiving chemotherapy (statistical difference not significant). The older patients had a significantly shorter 3-year disease free survival rate of only 24%.[329]

In a recent update of this study, the 5-year disease-free survival rate was 45% for the allogeneic BMT group and 31% for the control group, which combined the autologous BMT and chemotherapy groups ($P = .1$, Table 6).[330] When patients at high risk (ie, Ph-positive ALL, null or undifferentiated ALL, age older than 35 years, WBC count higher than 30×10^9/L, or time to complete response longer than 4 weeks) were analyzed separately, the 5-year disease-free survival rate was 39% for patients who underwent allogeneic BMT and 14% for patients who received other therapies ($P = .01$). For patients at standard-risk (62.5% of the total patient population), the 5-year disease-free survival rates were 48% and 43% for patients who underwent allogeneic BMT and patients who did not, respectively (nonsignificant difference). This study also showed the bias inherent in selecting patients for BMT: 62.5% of patients included had standard-risk ALL, whereas in most studies (Table 5), patients with standard-risk ALL comprise less than 30% of patients.

Barrett et al reported a 2-year disease-free survival rate of 38% in patients with Ph-positive ALL who underwent allogeneic BMT during their first remission.[331] These patients had a cure rate of less than 10% when treated with chemotherapy alone. Therefore, patients at high risk are likely to benefit from allogeneic BMT performed during first remission. However, this population must be selected carefully because treatment-related mortality is still significant with BMT and because the sequence of chemotherapy during the first complete response and BMT at the first relapse or subsequently may yield the best cumulative cure rate.

For patients with disease refractory to conventional therapy or in relapse or second remission, allogeneic BMT is the treatment of choice. In patients refractory to chemotherapy, the actuarial 3-year disease-free survival rate with allogeneic BMT was 23% in 1 study,[332] which is more than can be expected with salvage chemotherapy. For patients in second remission, several studies have reported long-term disease-free survival rates ranging from 18% to 45% (average, 30%).[320–323]

Patients experiencing relapse after allogeneic BMT may still respond to salvage chemotherapy. The outcome depends on the time from BMT to relapse: patients who

TABLE 6

Results With Allogeneic and Autologous BMT in Patients With ALL

	Allogeneic BMT	Autologous BMT
Number of patients included	116	95
Number undergoing BMT	95 (79%)	63 (66%)
3-year survival rate (%)	56	49
3-year disease-free survival rate (%)	44	39

ALL = acute lymphocytic leukemia, BMT = bone marrow transplantation

Adapted, with permission, from Gratwohl A, Hermans J, Zwaan F: Bone marrow transplantation for ALL in Europe, in Gale RP, Hoelzer D (eds): Acute Lymphoblastic Leukemia, pp 271–278. New York, Alan R. Liss, 1990.

experience relapse less than 100 days after BMT have a complete response rate of 18%, compared with 71% if the relapse occurs more than 1 year after BMT.[333] Remissions are usually short.

Autologous BMT

Two large studies have failed to demonstrate an advantage in disease-free survival for patients undergoing autologous BMT compared with chemotherapy alone.[323,339] A study from M. D. Anderson Cancer Center planned an intensive consolidation regimen that included autologous BMT for patients in complete remission.[155] Of 79 patients achieving complete remission, 32 experienced relapse before the time of BMT. Among the other 47 patients, 21 could not undergo BMT because of age, medical contraindications, or socioeconomic reasons. When the 26 patients who underwent BMT were compared with the 21 patients who did not, no significant difference in 3-year complete response rates (60% vs 49%, respectively) or survival rates (58% vs 62%, respectively) was evident. In the series from the French Group on Therapy for ALL, chemotherapy and autologous BMT produced comparable disease-free survival rates at 3 years (39% vs 32%; *P* = .8). However, late relapses (ie, after 3 years) were seen mainly in patients in the chemotherapy arm.[329]

These studies suggest that autologous BMT is not more effective than consolidation chemotherapy but may produce a plateau in disease-free survival after 3 years. Some patients, particularly those who are noncompliant or who are not willing to receive long-term therapy, may benefit from this one-time procedure. Several studies with autologous BMT also exemplify the problems with patient selection. Only 20% to 50% of patients for whom autologous BMT is planned can actually receive the transplant.[155,330]

For patients with refractory ALL or patients who experience relapse, autologous BMT can result in a long-term disease-free survival rate of 20% to 30%.[334–337] The best results (a disease-free survival rate of 40% to 50%) are achieved in patients who remain in first complete remission for longer than 1 year.[334] These patients may therefore benefit from autologous BMT. However, better methods of bone marrow purging are needed to reduce relapse rates to make this therapy a better alternative. One promising approach is in vivo purging by means of mobilization of normal hematopoietic precursors, which can be collected and later reinfused, after intensive chemotherapy.[338]

SURVIVAL

Long-term prognosis is excellent in children. More than 90% achieve a complete response and 60% to 70% will eventually be cured. In adults, the results are worse. When analyzing the outcome in adults with ALL, it is important to consider studies that have a long follow-up and the study inclusion criteria. The initial studies from Memorial Sloan-Kettering Cancer Center using the L_2 to L_{10}-M programs projected a long-term disease-free survival rate of more than 50%.[339] Linker et al initially reported long-term complete response and survival rates of 50% to 60% in patients younger than 50 years.[340] Both studies[339,340] excluded patients with Ph-positive disease. The follow-up from Memorial Sloan-Kettering, with less stringent inclusion criteria, indicated a long-term complete response rate of approximately 25%,[145] and the follow-up study from Linker et al demonstrated a long-term disease-free survival rate of 35%.[279] These and several other studies report a cure rate for adult ALL of 20% to 35%. Although a major improvement from results 3 decades ago, these findings pose a challenge for improving outcome toward what is now achievable in children with ALL.

BIOLOGIC AND PROGNOSTIC INVESTIGATIONS

Minimal Residual Disease

The availability of immunologic and molecular techniques has increased our ability to detect residual disease at levels below the sensitivity of morphologic evaluation. These techniques include flow cytometric sorting and immunophenotyping, clonogenic assays, and detection of leukemia-specific DNA or RNA sequences by Southern blot or polymerase chain reaction.[341] With these techniques, the presence of residual clonal cells may predict survival. In one study of patients treated with autologous BMT, all 42 patients with more than 51 malignant cells per 10^6 total cells (as measured by multiparameter flow cytometry and cell-sorting with assays for leukemic progenitor cells) experienced relapse within 1 year, but only 41% of patients with lower levels of residual disease experienced relapse.[342]

One approach for detecting minimal residual disease is to identify the rearrangement of *Ig* or *TCR* genes. As mentioned previously, the clonal nature of ALL is manifested by a specific and unique rearrangement of these genes in all malignant cells, whereas normal cells have a germline configuration.[81,82] Amplification of such a leukemia-specific marker by polymerase chain reaction can identify one leukemic cell among 10^5 normal cells.[343] The principle of this technique is based on amplifying and identifying the specific rearrangement that occurs during the differentiation of B- and T-cells in the Ig heavy chain (the hypervariable sequence known as the complementary determinant region III) and the TCR, respectively.

During induction chemotherapy, there is a 3- to 4-log reduction in the number of leukemic cells, but even after a complete response is achieved, some residual disease can be documented.[344] In some patients, an increase in leukemic cells can be demonstrated by polymerase chain reaction months before it becomes clinically evident.[344] The major limitation of this technique is that, because the specific rearrangement is unique for each clone, specific probes must be generated for each patient.

An alternative approach is the blast-colony assay, described by Estrov et al.[345] With this assay, in vitro growth of lymphoblastic colonies during complete remission was observed in patients who later experienced relapse. The presence of disease as detected by this method is not always associated with relapse, and a threshold for prediction of adverse outcome has not been established.

Multidrug Resistance Detection

The multidrug resistance (*MDR*) gene encodes for a membrane glycoprotein, p170, that is thought to function as an efflux pump.[346] The expression of this gene confers resistance to some chemotherapeutic agents, including vinca alkaloids, taxoids, anthracyclines, and epipodophylotoxins.[347] Of patients with ALL, 10% to 50% express *MDR* at diagnosis, and 15% to 60% express *MDR* at relapse.[348] In adults, the incidence of *MDR* positivity increases markedly after relapse (10% at diagnosis, 50% after relapse).[349] The expression of *MDR* is associated with a lower complete response rate (56% for *MDR*-

positive patients vs 93% for *MDR*-negative patients; $P = .05$) and a higher relapse rate (100% vs 46%, respectively; $P = .05$). This results in a survival advantage for MDR-negative patients.[349]

Expression of *bcl-2*

Oncogene *bcl-2* is involved in the regulation of cell death. Overexpression of *bcl-2* results in an inhibition of programmed cell death of hematopoietic cells.[350] B-cell precursor ALL cells overexpress *bcl-2*, and this results in prolonged survival of leukemic cells.[351] An association between *bcl-2* overexpression and glucocorticoid resistance has been reported.[352] Overexpression of *bcl-2* was documented in all patients with ALL, children and adults, studied by Gala et al, except in patients with Burkitt's phenotype.[353] The overexpression, however, was not associated with a poor prognosis.[353]

REFERENCES

1. Sawyers CL, Denny CT, Witte ON: Leukemia and the disruption of normal hematopoiesis. Cell 64:337–350, 1991.
2. Farber S, Diamond LK, Mercer RD, et al: Temporary remissions in acute leukemia in children produced by folic acid antagonist 4-aminopteroylglutamic acid (aminopterin). N Engl J Med 238:787–793, 1948.
3. George SL, Aur RJA, Maurer AM, et al: A reappraisal of the results of stopping therapy in childhood leukemia. N Engl J Med 300:269–273, 1979.
4. Brincker H: Population-based age- and sex-specific incidence rates in the four main types of leukaemia. Scand J Haematol 29:241–249, 1982.
5. Poplack DG: Clinical manifestations of acute lymphoblastic leukemia, in Hoffman R, Benz EJ Jr, Shattil SJ, et al (eds): Hematology: Basic Principles and Practice, pp 776–784. New York, Churchill Livingstone, 1991.
6. Lukens JN: Acute lymphocytic leukemia, in Lee GR, Bithell TC, Foerster J, et al (eds): Wintrobe's Clinical Hematology, 9th ed, pp 1892–1919. Philadelphia, Lea & Febiger, 1993.
7. Robinson LL: Epidemiology of childhood leukemia. ASCO Educational Book, pp 120–123, 1994.
8. Boring CC, Squires TT, Ting T, et al: Cancer statistics, 1994. CA Cancer J Clin 44:7–26, 1994.
9. Sather HN: Age at diagnosis in childhood acute lymphoblastic leukemia. Med Pediatr Oncol 14:166–172, 1986.
10. Baranovsky A, Myers MH: Cancer incidence and survival in patients 65 years of age and older. CA Cancer J Clin 36:26–41, 1986.
11. Amsel S, Nabembezi JS: Two-year survey of hematologic malignancies in Uganda. J Natl Cancer Inst 52:1397–1401, 1974.
12. Edington GM, Hendrickse M: Incidence and frequency of lymphoreticular tumors in Ibadan and the Western State of Nigeria. J Natl Cancer Inst 50:1623–1631, 1973.
13. Sandler DP: Epidemiology and etiology of acute leukemia: An update. Leukemia 6(suppl 4):3–5, 1992.
14. Call TG, Noel P, Habermann TM, et al: Incidence of leukemia in Olmsted County, Minnesota, 1975 through 1989. Mayo Clin Proc 69:315-322, 1994.
15. Birch JM, Marsden HB, Swindell R: Incidence of malignant disease in childhood: A 24-year review of the Manchester children's tumour registry data. Br J Cancer 42:215–223, 1980.

16. Sandler DP, Collman GW: Cytogenetic and environmental factors in the etiology of the acute leukemias in adults. Am J Epidemiol 126:1017–1032, 1987.

17. Gunz FW, Gunz JP, Vincent PC, et al: Thirteen cases of leukemia in a family. J Natl Cancer Inst 60:1243–1250, 1978.

18. De Oliveira MSP, El Seed FERA, Foroni L, et al: Lymphoblastic leukaemia in Siamese twins: Evidence for identity. Lancet 2:969–970, 1986.

19. Schmitt TA, Degos L: Leucémies familiales. Bull Cancer (Paris) 65:83–88, 1978.

20. Robinson LL, Nesbit ME Jr, Sather HN, et al: Down syndrome and acute leukemia in children: A 10-year retrospective survey from the Children's Cancer Study Group. J Pediatr 105:235–234, 1984.

21. Neglia JP, Robinson LL: Epidemiology of the childhood acute leukemias. Pediatr Clin North Am 35:675–692, 1988.

22. Aurebach AD: Fanconi anemia and leukemia: Tracking the genes. Leukemia 6(suppl 1):1–4, 1992.

23. Kaye SA, Robinson LL, Smithson WA, et al: Maternal reproductive history and birth characteristics in childhood acute lymphoblastic leukemia. Cancer 68:1351–1355, 1991.

24. Stark CHR, Mantel N: Effects of maternal age and birth order on the risk of mongolism and leukemia. J Natl Cancer Inst 37:687–698, 1966.

25. van Steensel-Moll HA, Valkenburg HA, Vandenbroucke JP, et al: Are maternal fertility problems related to childhood leukaemia? Int J Epidemiol 14:555–559, 1985.

26. Dailing JR, Staryk P, Olshan AF, et al: Birth weight and incidence of chilhood cancer. J Natl Cancer Inst 72:1039–1041, 1984.

27. Buckley JD, Robinson LL, Swotinsky R, et al: Occupational exposures of parents of children with acute nonlymphocytic leukemia: A report from the Children's Cancer Study Group. Cancer Res 49:4030–4037, 1989.

28. McWhirter WR: The relationship of incidence of childhood lymphoblastic leukaemia to social class. Br J Cancer 46:640–645, 1982.

29. Stewart A, Kneale GW: Radiation dose effects in relation to obstetric x-rays and childhood cancers. Lancet 1:1185–1188, 1970.

30. Court-Brown WM, Doll R: Mortality from cancer and other causes after radiotherapy for ankylosing spondylitis. Br Med J 2:1327–1332, 1986.

31. Simpson CL, Hempelmann LH, Fuller LM: Neoplasia in children with x-rays in infancy for thymic enlargement. Radiology 64:840–845, 1955.

32. Ishimaru M, Ishimaru T, Belsky JL: Incidence of leukemia in atomic bomb survivors belonging to a fixed cohort in Hiroshima and Nagasaki, 1950–1971: Radiation dose, years after exposure, age at exposure, and type of leukemia. J Radiat Res (Tokyo) 19:262–282, 1978.

33. Brill AB, Tomonaga M, Heyssel RM: Leukemia in man following exposure to ionizing radiation: A summary of the findings in Hiroshima and Nagasaki and a comparison with other human experience. Ann Intern Med 56:590–609, 1962.

34. Caldwell GG, Kelley DB, Zack M, et al: Mortality and cancer frequency among military nuclear test (Smoky) participants, 1957 through 1959. JAMA 250:620–624, 1984.

35. Land CE, McKay FW, Machado SG: Childhood leukemia and fallout from the Nevada nuclear tests. Science 223:139–144, 1984.

36. Caldwell GG, Kelley DB, Heath CW Jr: Leukemia among participants in military maneuvers at a nuclear bomb test: A preliminary report. JAMA 244:1575–1578, 1980.

37. Rinsky RA, Smith AB, Hornung R, et al: Benzene and leukemia: An epidemiologic risk assessment. N Engl J Med 316:1044–1050, 1987.

38. Savitz DA, Wachtel H, Barnes FA, et al: Case-control study of childhood cancer and exposure to 60-Hz magnetic fields. Am J Epidemiol 128:21–38, l988.

39. London SJ, Thomas DC, Bowman JD, et al: Exposure to residential electric and magnetic fields and risk of childhood leukemia. Am J Epidemiol 134:923–937, 1991.

40. Feychting M, Ahlbom A: Magnetic field and cancer in children residing near Swedish high-voltage power lines. Am J Epidemiol 138:467–481, 1993.

41. Sheikh K: Exposure to electromagnetic fields and the risk of leukemia. Arch Environ Health 41:53–56, 1986.

42. Alexander FE: Viruses, clusters, and clustering of childhood leukemia: A new perspective? Eur J Cancer 29A:1424–1443, 1993.

43. Greaves MF: A natural history of pediatric acute leukemia. Blood 82:1043–1051, 1993.

44. Greaves MF, Alexander FE: An infectious etiology for common acute lymphoblastic leukemia in childhood? Leukemia 7:349–360, 1993.

45. Moore MAS, Williams N, Metcalf D: In vitro formation by normal and leukemic human hematopoietic cells: Interaction between colony-forming and colony-stimulating cells. J Natl Cancer Inst 50:591–602, 1973.

46. Homans AC, Cohen JL, Barker BE, et al: Aplastic presentation of acute lymphoblastic leukemia: Evidence for cellular inhibition of normal hematopoietic progenitors. Am J Pediatr Hematol Oncol 11:456–462, 1989.

47. Peing LH, Keng TH, Sinniah D: Fever in children with acute lymphoblastic leukemia. Cancer 47:583–587, 1981.

48. Freeman AI, Pantazopoulos N, DeCastro L, et al: Infections in children with acute leukemia. Med Pediatr Oncol 1:167–173, 1975.

49. Henderson ES: Acute leukemia: General considerations, in Williams WJ, Beutler E, Erslev AJ, et al (eds): Hematology, 4th ed, pp 236–251. New York, McGraw-Hill, 1990.

50. Bevilacqua G, Abadessa A, Consolini R, et al: Bone marrow necrosis foreshadowing acute lymphoid leukemia. Am J Pediatr Hematol Oncol 7:223–228, 1985.

51. Niebrugge DJ, Benjamin DR: Bone marrow necrosis preceding acute lymphoblastic leukemia in childhood. Cancer 52:2162–2164, 1983.

52. Bakhshi A, Minowada J, Arnold A, et al: Lymphoid blast crises of chronic myelogenous leukemia represent stages in the development of B-cell precursors. N Engl J Med 31:826–831, 1983.

53. Corbaton J, Muñoz A, Madero L, et al: Pulmonary leukemia in a child presenting with infiltrative and nodular lesions. Pediatr Radiol 14:431–432, 1984.

54. Mancuso L, Marchi S, Pietro G, et al: Cardiac tamponade as first manifestation of acute lymphoblastic leukemia in a patient with echographic evidence of mediastinal lymph nodal enlargement. Am Heart J 110:1303–1304, 1985.

55. Taylor D, Day S: The eye as sanctuary in acute lymphoblastic leukemia. Lancet 1:452–453, 1980.

56. Miller DR, Steinherz PG, Feurer D, et al: Unfavorable prognostic significance of hand mirror cells in childhood acute lymphoblastic leukemia. Am J Dis Child 137:346–350, 1983.

57. Kim T, Hargreaves H, Byrnes R, et al: Pretreatment testicular biopsy in childhood acute lymphocytic leukemia. Lancet 2:657–658, 1981.

58. Nesbit ME Jr, Robinson LL, Ortega JA, et al: Testicular relapse in childhood acute lymphoblastic leukemia: Association with pretreatment patient. Cancer 45:2009–2016, 1980.

59. Kuo T-T, Tshang T-P, Chu J-Y: Testicular relapse in childhood acute lymphocytic leukemia during bone marrow remission. Cancer 38:2604–2612, 1976.

60. Land JL, Berry DH, Herson J, et al: Long-term survival in childhood acute leukemia: 'Late' relapses. Med Pediatr Oncol 7:19–24, 1979.

61. Eden OB, Hardisty RM, Innes EM, et al: Testicular disease in acute lymphoblastic leukemia in childhood. Br Med J 1:334–338, 1978.

62. Bowman P, Aur RJA, Hustu HA, et al: Isolated testicular relapse in acute lymphocytic leukemia of childhood: Categories and influence on survival. J Clin Oncol 2:924–929, 1984.

63. Boggs DR, Wintrobe MM, Cartwright GE: The acute leukemias. Analysis of 322 cases and review of the literature. Medicine 41:163–225, 1962.

64. Bunin NJ, Pui C-H: Differing complications of hyperleukocytosis in children with acute lymphoblastic or acute nonlymphoblastic leukemia. J Clin Oncol 3:1590–1595, 1985.

65. Sarris AH, Kempin S, Berman E, et al: High incidence of disseminated intravascular coagulation during remission induction of adult patients with acute lymphoblastic leukemia. Blood 79:1305–1310, 1992.

66. Sarris A, Kantarjian HM, Cortes JE, et al: Successful treatment of the DIC of adult ALL with fresh-frozen plasma, cryoprecipitate, and platelets. Blood 82(suppl 1):253a, 1993.

67. Nelken RP, Stockman JA: The hypereosinophilic syndrome in association with acute lymphoblastic leukemia. J Pediatr 89:771–773, 1976.

68. Leikin S, Miller DR, Sather HN, et al: Immunologic evaluation in the prognosis of acute lymphoblastic leukemia: A report from the Children's Cancer Study Group. Blood 58:501–508, 1981.

69. Hann IM, Jones PHM, Evans DIK, et al: Low IgG or IgA: A further indicator of poor prognosis in childhood acute lymphoblastic leukemia. Br J Cancer 42:317–319, 1980.

70. Hirsch-Ginsberg C, Huh YO, Kagan J, et al: Advances in the diagnosis of acute leukemia. Hematol Oncol Clin North Am 7:1–46, 1993.

71. Bennett JM, Catovsky D, Daniel M-T, et al: Proposals for the classification of the acute leukemias. Br J Haematol 33:451–458, 1976.

72. Bennett JM, Catovsky D, Daniel M-T, et al: The morphological classification of acute lymphoblastic leukaemia: Concordance among observers and clinical correlations. Br J Haematol 47:553–561, 1981.

73. Breatnach F, Chessells JM, Greaves MF: The aplastic presentation of childhood leukaemia: A feature of common ALL. Br J Haematol 49:387–393, 1981.

74. Stass SA, Dean L, Peiper SC, et al: Determination of terminal deoxynucleotidyltransferase on bone marrow smears by immunoperoxidase. Am J Clin Pathol 77:174–176, 1982.

75. Janossy G, Hoffbrand AV, Greaves MF, et al: Terminal transferase enzyme assay and immunological membrane markers in the diagnosis of leukaemia. Br J Haematol 44:221–234, 1980.

76. Catovsky D, Greaves MF, Pain C, et al: Acid-phosphatase reaction in acute lymphoblastic leukaemia. Lancet 1:749–751, 1978.

77. Krolewsky JJ, Dalla-Favera R: Molecular genetic approaches in the diagnosis and classification of lymphoid malignancies. Hematol Pathol 3:45–61, 1989.

78. Adriaansen HJ, Soeting PWC, Wolvers-Tettero ILM, et al: Immunoglobulin and T-cell gene receptor gene rearrangements in acute nonlymphocytic leukemias: Analysis of 54 cases and a review of the literature. Leukemia 9:744–751, 1991.

79. Felix CA, Wright JJ, Poplack DG, et al: T-cell receptor alpha-, beta-, and gamma- genes in T-cell and pre-B cell acute lymphoblastic leukemia. J Clin Invest 80:540–556, 1987.

80. Hara J, Benedict SH, Champagne E, et al: Relationship between rearrangement and transcription of the T-cell receptor alpha, beta, and gamma genes in B-precursor acute lymphoblastic leukemia. Blood 73:500–508, 1989.

81. Lieber MR: The mechanism of V(D)J recombination: a balance of diversity, specificity, and stability. Cell 70:873–876, 1992.

82. Waldmann TA, Davis MM, Bongiovanni KF, et al: Rearrangements of genes for the antigen receptor on T cells as markers of lineage and clonality in human lymphoid neoplasms. N Engl J Med 313:776–783, 1985.

83. Furley AJW, Chan LC, Mizutani S, et al: Lineage specificity of rearrangement and expression of genes encoding the T-cell receptor-T3 complex and immunoglobulin heavy chain in leukemia. Leukemia 1:644–652, 1987.

84. Kitchingam GR, Rovigatti U, Maurer AM, et al: Rearrangement of immunoglobulin heavy chain genes in T cell acute lymphoblastic leukemia. Blood 65:725–729, 1985.

85. Ha K, Minden M, Hozumi N, et al: Immunoglobulin μ chain gene rearrangement in a patient with T cell acute lymphoblastic leukemia. J Clin Invest 73:1232–1236, 1984.

86. Yagi-Yumura K, Hara J, Terada N, et al: Analysis of molecular events in leukemic cells at an early stage of T-cell differentiation. Blood 14:2103–2111, 1989.

87. Pelicci P-G, Knowles D, Dalla-Favera R: Lymphoid tumors displaying rearrangements of both immunoglobulin and T-cell receptor genes. J Exp Med 162:1015–1024, 1985.

88. Seremetis SV, Pelicci P-G, Tabilio A, et al: High frequency of clonal immunoglobulin or T-cell receptor gene rearrangements in acute myelogenous leukemia expressing terminal deoxyribonucleotidyltransferase. J Exp Med 165:1703–1712, 1987.

89. Felix CA, Poplack DG, Reaman GH, et al: Characterization of immunoglobulin and T-cell receptor gene patterns in B-cell precursor acute lymphoblastic leukemia of childhood. J Clin Oncol 8:431–442, 1990.

90. Hanson CA, Thamilarsan M, Ross CW, et al: Kappa light gene rearrangement in T-cell acute lymphoblastic leukemia. Am J Clin Pathol 93:563–568, 1990.

91. Greaves MF: Differentiation-linked leukemogenesis in lymphocytes. Science 234:697–704, 1986.

92. Preti A, Kantarjian HM, Estey EH, et al: Characteristics and outcome of patients with acute lymphocytic leukemia and myeloperoxidase-positive blasts by electron microscopy. Hematol Pathol 8:155–167, 1994.

93. Burns P, Armitage JO, Frey AL, et al: Analysis of the presenting features of adult acute leukemia: The French-American-British classification. Cancer 47:2460–2469, 1981.

94. Miller DR, Leikin S, Albo V, et al: Prognostic importance of morphology (FAB classification) in childhood acute lymphoblastic leukemia (ALL). Br J Haematol 48:199–206, 1981.

95. Lilleyman JS, Hann IM, Stevens RF, et al: Blast cell vacuoles in childhood lymphoblastic leukaemia. Br J Haematol 70:183–186, 1988.

96. Pui C-H, Behm FG, Crist WM: Clinical and biologic relevance of immunologic marker studies in childhood acute lymphoblastic leukemia. Blood 82:343–362, 1993.

97. Loken MR, Shah VO, Dattilo KL, et al: Flow cytometric analysis of human bone marrow. II: Normal B-lymphocyte development. Blood 70:1316–1324, 1987.

98. Reinherz EL, Kung PC, Goldstein G, et al: Discrete stages of human intrathymic differentiation: Analysis of normal thymocytes and leukemic lymophoblasts of T-cell lineage. Immunology 77:1588–1562, 1980.

99. Nadler LM, Korsmeyer SJ, Anderson KC, et al: B cell origin of non-T-cell acute lymphoblastic leukemia: A model for discrete stages of neoplastic and normal pre-B-cell differentiation. J Clin Invest

74:332–340, 1984.

100. Foon KA, Tood RF III: Immunologic classification of leukemia and lymphoma. Blood 68:1–31, 1986.

101. Hurwitz CA, Loken MR, Graham ML, et al: Asynchronous antigen expression in B lineage acute lymphoblastic leukemia. Blood 72:299–307, 1988.

102. Hurwitz CA, Gore SD, Stone KD, et al: Flow cytometric detection of rare normal human marrow cells with immunophenotypes characteristic of acute lymphoblastic leukemia cells. Leukemia 6:233–239, 1992.

103. Wiersman SR, Ortega J, Sobol RE, et al: Clinical importance of myeloid-antigen expression in acute lymphoblastic leukemia of childhood. N Engl J Med 324:800–808, 1991.

104. Kurec AS, Belair P, Stefanu C, et al: Significance of aberrant immunophenotypes in childhood acute lymphoid leukemia. Cancer 67:3081–3086, 1991.

105. Pui C-H, Raimondi SC, Head DR, et al: Characterization of childhood acute leukemia with multiple myeloid and lymphoid markers at diagnosis and at relapse. Blood 78:1327–1337, 1991.

106. Davey FR, Mick R, Nelson DA, et al: Morphologic and cytochemical characterization of adult lymphoid leukemias which express myeloid antigen. Leukemia 2:420–426, 1988.

107. Childs CC, Hirsch-Ginsberg C, Walters RS, et al: Myeloid surface antigen-positive acute lymphoblastic leukemia (My+ ALL): Immunophenotypic, ultrastructural, cytogenetic, and molecular characteristics. Leukemia 3:777–783, 1989.

108. Guyotat D, Campos L, Shi Z-H, et al: Myeloid surface antigen expression in adult acute lymphoblastic leukemia. Leukemia 4:664–666, 1990.

109. Greaves MF, Chan LC, Furley AJW, et al: Lineage promiscuity in hemopoietic differentiation and leukemia. Blood 67:1–11, 1986.

110. Smith LJ, Curtis JE, Messner HA, et al: Lineage infidelity in acute leukemia. Blood 61:1138–1145, 1983.

111. Kita K, Nakase K, Miwa H, et al: Phenotypical characteristics of acute myelocytic leukemia associated with the t(8;21) (q22;q22) chromosomal abnormality: Frequent expression of immature B-cell antigen CD19 together with stem-cell antigen CD34. Blood 80:470–477, 1992.

112. Claxton DF, Reading CL, Nagarajan L, et al: Correlation of CD2 expression with PML gene breakpoints in patients with acute promyelocytic leukemia. Blood 80:582–586, 1992.

113. Pui C-H, Schell MJ, Vodian MA, et al: Serum CD4, CD8, and interleukin-2 receptor levels in childhood acute myeloid leukemia. Leukemia 5:249–254, 1991.

114. Letarte M, Vera S, Tran R, et al: Common acute lymphocytic leukemia antigen is identical to neutral endopeptidase. J Exp Med 168:1247–1252, 1988.

115. LeBien TW, McCormack RT: The common acute lymphoblastic leukemia antigen (CD10)—Emancipation from a functional enigma. Blood 73:625–635, 1989.

116. Pui C-H, Rivera GK, Hancock ML, et al: Clinical significance of CD10 expression in childhood acute lymphoblastic leukemia. Leukemia 7:35–40, 1993.

117. Civin CI, Strauss LC, Brovall C, et al: Antigenic analysis of hematopoiesis. III: A hematopoietic progenitor cell surface antigen defined by monoclonal antibody raised against KG-1a cells. J Immunol 133:157–165, 1984.

118. Batinic D, Tindle R, Boban D, et al: Expression of haematopoietic progenitor cell-associated antigen BI-3C5/CD34 in leukaemia. Leuk Res 13:83–85, 1989.

119. Terstappen LWMM, Huang S, Safford M, et al: Sequential generations of hematopoietic colonies derived from single nonlineage-committed CD34+CD38- progenitor cells. Blood 77:1218–1227, 1991.

120. Koehler M, Behm FG, Hancock ML, et al: Expression of activation antigens CD38 and CD71 is not clinically important in childhood acute lymphoblastic leukemia. Leukemia 7:41–45, 1993.

121. Bain BJ: Immunological, cytogenetic, and other markers, in Bain BJ (ed): Leukemia Diagnosis: A guide to FAB Classification, p 64. Philadelphia, JB Lippincott, 1990.

122. Crist WM, Grossi CE, Pullen DJ, et al: Immunologic markers in childhood acute lymphocytic leukemia. Semin Oncol 12:105–121, 1985.

123. Coleman J: Carbonic anhydrase: Zinc and the mechanism of catalysis. Ann NY Acad Sci 429:26–48, 1984.

124. Greaves MF, Janossy G, Peto J, et al: Immunologically defined subclasses of acute lymphoblastic leukaemia in children: Their relationship to presentation features and prognosis. Br J Haematol 48:179–197, 1981.

125. Sallan SE, Ritz J, Pesando J, et al: Cell surface antigens: Prognostic implications in childhood acute lymphoblastic leukemia. Blood 55:395–402, 1980.

126. First MIC Cooperative Study Group: Morphologic, immunologic, and cytogenetic (MIC) working classification of acute lymphoblastic leukemias: Report of the workshop held in Leuven, Belgium, April 22–23, 1985. Cancer Genet Cytogenet 23:189–197, 1986.

127. Borowitz MJ, Shuster JJ, Civin CI, et al: Prognostic significance of CD34 expression in childhood B-precursor acute lymphocytic leukemia: A Pediatric Oncology Group study. J Clin Oncol 8:1389–1398, 1990.

128. Pui C-H, Hancock ML, Head DR, et al: Clinical significance of CD34 expression in childhood acute lymphoblastic leukemia. Blood 82:889–894, 1993.

129. Vogler LB, Crist WM, Bockman DE, et al: Pre-B-cell leukemia: A new phenotype of childhood lymphoblastic leukemia. N Engl J Med 298:872–878, 1978.

130. Crist WM, Boyett J, Jackson J, et al: Prognostic importance of the pre-B-cell immunophenotype and other presenting features in B-lineage childhood acute lymphoblastic leukemia: A Pediatric Oncology Group Study. Blood 74:1252–1259, 1989.

131. Pui C-H, Williams DL, Kalwinsky DK, et al: Cytogenetic features and serum lactic dehydrogenase level predict a poor treatment outcome for children with pre-B-cell leukemia. Blood 67:1688–1692, 1986.

132. Raimondi SC, Behm FG, Roberson PK, et al: Cytogenetics of pre-B-cell acute lymphoblastic leukemia with emphasis on prognostic implications of the t(1;19). J Clin Oncol 8:1380–1388, 1990.

133. Crist WM, Carroll AJ, Shuster JJ, et al: Poor prognosis of children with pre-B acute lymphoblastic leukemia is associated with the t(1;19) (q23;p13): A Pediatric Oncology Group study. Blood 76:117–122, 1990.

134. Pui C-H, Raimondi SC, Hancock ML, et al: Immunologic, cytogenetic, and clinical characterization of childhood acute lymphoblastic leukemia with the t(1;19)(q23;p13) or its derivative. J Clin Oncol 12:2601–2606, 1994.

135. Koehler M, Schell MJ, Behm FG, et al: Expression of a novel surface antigen MKW in childhood acute leukemia has prognostic significance. Leukemia 5:41–48, 1991.

136. Magrath IT, Ziegler JL: Bone marrow involvement in Burkitt's lymphoma and its relationship to acute B-cell leukemia. Leukemia Res 4:33–59, 1979.

137. Sullivan MP, Pullen DJ, Crist WM, et al: Clinical and biological heterogeneity of childhood B cell lymphocytic leukemia: Implications for clinical trials. Leukemia 4:6–11, 1990.

138. Sobol RE, Royston I, LeBien TW, et al: Adult acute lymphoblastic leukemia phenotypes defined by monoclonal antibodies. Blood

65:730, 1985.

139. Taylor PRA, Reid NM, Bown N, et al: Acute lymphoblastic leukemia in patients aged 60 years and over: A population-based study of incidence and outcome. Blood 80:1813–1817, 1992.

140. Zhou M, Findley HW, Ma L, et al: Effect of tumor necrosis factor-alpha on the proliferation of leukemic cells from children with B-cell precursor-acute lymphoblastic leukemia (BCP-ALL): Studies of primary leukemic cells and BCP-ALL cell lines. Blood 77:2002–2007, 1991.

141. Pui C-H, Behm FG, Singh B, et al: Heterogeneity of presenting features and their relation to treatment outcome in 120 children with T-cell acute lymphoblastic leukemia. Blood 75:174–179, 1990.

142. Bernard A, Boumsell L, Reinherz E, et al: Cell surface characterization of malignant T cells from lymphoblastic lymphoma using monoclonal antibodies: Evidence for phenotypic differences between malignant T cells from patients with acute lymphoblastic leukemia and lymphoblastic lymphoma. Blood 57:1105–1110, 1981.

143. Crist WM, Pullen DJ, Boyett J, et al: Clinical and biologic features predict a poor prognosis in acute lymphoid leukemias in infants: A Pediatric Oncology Group study. Blood 67:135–140, 1986.

144. Hammond D, Sather HN, Nesbit ME Jr, et al: Analysis of prognostic factors in acute lymphoblastic leukemia. Med Pediatr Oncol 14:124–134, 1986.

145. Ribeiro RC, Pui C-H: Prognostic factors in childhood acute lymphoblastic leukemia. Hematol Pathol 7:121–142, 1993.

146. Hoelzer D, Thiel E, Löffler H, et al: Prognostic factors in a multicenter study for treatment of acute lymphoblastic leukemia in adults. Blood 71:123–131, 1988.

147. Gaynor J, Chapman D, Little C, et al: A cause-specific hazard rate analysis of prognostic factors among 199 adults with acute lymphoblastic leukemia. J Clin Oncol 6:1014–1030, 1988.

148. Baccarani M, Corbelli G, Amadori S, et al: Adolescent and adult acute lymphoblastic leukemia: Prognostic features and outcome of therapy: A study of 293 patients. Blood 60:677–684, 1982.

149. Sather HN: Age at diagnosis in childhood acute lymphoblastic leukemia. Med Pediatr Oncol 14:166–172, 1986.

150. Cortes J, Kantarjian HM: Leukemia in the elderly. Cancer Bull 1995 (in press).

151. Pui C-H, Raimondi SC, Murphy SB, et al: An analysis of leukemic cell chromosomal features in infants. Blood 69:1289–1293, 1987.

152. Chen C-S, Sorensen PHB, Domer PH, et al: Molecular rearrangements on chromosome 11q23 predominate in infant acute lymphoblastic leukemia and are associated with specific biologic variables and poor outcome. Blood 81:2386–2393, 1993.

153. Kaneko Y, Shikano T, Maseki N, et al: Clinical characteristics of infant acute leukemia with or without 11q23 translocations. Leukemia 2:672–676, 1988.

154. Smith M: Towards a more uniform approach to risk classification and treatment assignment for children with acute lymphoblastic leukemia (ALL). ASCO Educational Book, pp 124–130, 1994.

155. Kantarjian HM, Walters RS, Keating MJ, et al: Results of the vincristine, doxorubicin, and dexamethasone regimen in adults with standard- and high-risk acute lymphocytic leukemia. J Clin Oncol 8:994–1004, 1990.

156. Bloomfield CD, Secker-Walker LM, Goldman AI, et al: Six-year follow-up of the clinical significance of karyotype in acute lymphoblastic leukemia. Cancer Genet Cytogenet 40:171–185, 1989.

157. Raimondi SC: Current status of cytogenetic research in childhood acute lymphoblastic leukemia. Blood 81:2237–2251, 1993.

158. Pui C-H, Crist WM, Look TA: Biology and clinical significance of cytogenetic abnormalities in childhood acute lymphoblastic leukemia. Blood 76:1449–1463, 1990.

159. Trueworthy R, Shuster JJ, Look TA, et al: Ploidy of lymphoblasts is the strongest predictor of treatment outcome in B-progenitor cell acute lymphoblastic leukemia of childhood: A Pediatric Oncology Group study. J Clin Oncol 10:606–613, 1992.

160. Look TA, Roberson PK, Williams DL, et al: Prognostic importance of blast cell DNA content in childhood acute lymphoblastic leukemia. Blood 65:1079–1086, 1985.

161. Katz J, Shuster JJ, Schneider N, et al: The significance of ploidy in childhood T-cell acute lymphoblastic leukemia: A Pediatric Oncology Group study. Proc Am Soc Clin Oncol 12:316, 1993.

162. Walker-Secker LM, Lawler SD, Hardisty RM: Prognostic implications of chromosomal findings in acute lymphoblastic leukaemia at diagnosis. Br Med J 2:1529–1530, 1978.

163. Williams DL, Tsiatis A, Brodeur GM, et al: Prognostic importance of chromosome number in 136 untreated children with acute lymphoblastic leukemia. Blood 60:864–871, 1982.

164. Bloomfield CD, Goldman AI, Alimena G, et al: Chromosomal abnormalities identify high-risk and low-risk patients with acute lymphoblastic leukemia. Blood 67:415–420, 1986.

165. Kaspers GJL, Smets LA, Pieters R, et al: Favorable prognosis of hyperdiploid common acute lymphoblastic leukemia may be explained by sensitivity to antimetabolites and other drugs: Results of an in vitro study. Blood 85:751–756, 1995.

166. Pui C-H, Raimondi SC, Dodge RK, et al: Prognostic importance of chromosomal abnormalities in children with hyperdiploid (more than 50 chromosomes) acute lymphoblastic leukemia. Blood 73:1963–1967, 1989.

167. Abe R, Raza A, Preisler HD, et al: Chromosomes and causation of human cancer and leukemia: IV. Near tetraploidy in acute leukemia. Cancer Genet Cytogenet 14:45–59, 1985.

168. Heerema NA, Palmer CG, Baehner RL: Karyotypic and clinical findings in a consecutive series of children with acute leukemia. Cancer Genet Cytogenet 17:165–179, 1985.

169. Pui C-H, Carroll AJ, Head DR, et al: Near-triploid and near-tetraploid acute lymphoblastic leukemia of childhood. Blood 76:590–596, 1990.

170. Raimondi SC, Roberson PK, Pui C-H, et al: Hyperdiploid (47–50) acute lymphoblastic leukemia in children. Blood 79:3245–3252, 1992.

171. Raimondi SC, Pui C-H, Head DR, et al: Trisomy 21 as the sole acquired chromosomal abnormality in children with acute lymphoblastic leukemia. Leukemia 6:171–175, 1992.

172. Betts DR, Kingston JE, Dorey EL, et al: Monosomy 20: A nonrandom finding in childhood acute lymphoblastic leukemia. Genes Chromosom Cancer 2:182–185, 1990.

173. Pui C-H, Williams DL, Raimondi SC, et al: Hypodiploidy is associated with a poor prognosis in children with acute lymphoblastic leukemia. Blood 70:247–253, 1987.

174. Pui C-H, Carroll AJ, Raimondi SC, et al: Clinical presentation, karyotypic characterization, and treatment outcome of childhood acute lymphoblastic leukemia with a near-haploid or hypodiploid less than 45 line. Blood 75:1170–1177, 1990.

175. Gibbons B, MacCallum P, Watts E, et al: Near haploid acute lymphoblastic leukemia: Seven new cases and a review of the literature. Leukemia 5:738–743, 1991.

176. Callen DF, Raphael K, Michael PM, et al: Acute lymphoblastic leukemia with a hypodiploid karyotype with less than 40 chromosomes: The basis for division into two subgroups. Leukemia 3:749–753, 1989.

177. Raimondi SC, Behm FG, Roberson PK, et al: Cytogenetics of childhood T-cell leukemia. Blood 72:1560–1566, 1988.

178. Ribeiro RC, Abromowitch M, Raimondi SC, et al: Clinical and biologic hallmarks of the Philadelphia chromosome in childhood

acute lymphoblastic leukemia. Blood 70:948–953, 1987.

179. Crist WM, Carroll AJ, Shuster JJ, et al: Philadelphia chromosome-positive childhood acute lymphoblastic leukemia: Clinical and cytogenetic characteristics and treatment outcome: A Pediatric Oncology Group study. Blood 76:489–494, 1990.

180. Fletcher JA, Lynch EA, Kimball VM, et al: Translocation (9;22) is associated with extremely poor prognosis in intensively treated children with acute lymphoblastic leukemia. Blood 77:435–439, 1991.

181. Preti HA, O'Brien S, Giralt S, et al: Philadelphia chromosome-positive adult acute lymphocytic leukemia: Characteristics, treatment results, and prognosis in 41 patients. Am J Med 97:60–65, 1994.

182. Westbrook CA, Hooberman AL, Spino C, et al: Clinical significance of the BCR-ABL fusion gene in adult acute lymphoblastic leukemia: A Cancer and Leukemia Group B study (8762). Blood 80:2983–2990, 1992.

183. Maurer J, Janssen JWG, Thiel E, et al: Detection of chimeric BCR-ABL genes in acute lymphoblastic leukemia by the polymerase chain reaction. Lancet 337:1055–1058, 1991.

184. Russo C, Carroll AJ, Kohler S, et al: Philadelphia chromosome and monosomy 7 in childhood acute lymphoblastic leukemia: A Pediatric Oncology Group study. Blood 77:1050–1056, 1991.

185. Heisterkamp N, Jenkins R, Thibodeau S, et al: The bcr gene in Philadelphia chromosome-positive acute lymphoblastic leukemia. Blood 73:1307–1311, 1989.

186. Kurzrock R, Gutterman JU, Talpaz M: The molecular genetics of Philadelphia chromosome-positive leukemias. N Engl J Med 319:999–1005, 1988.

187. Lugo TG, Pendergast A-M, Muller AJ, et al: Tyrosine kinase activity and transformation potency of bcr-abl oncogene products. Science 247:1079–1081, 1990.

188. Heisterkamp N, Jenster G, ten Hoeve J, et al: Acute leukaemia in bcr/abl transgenic mice. Nature 344:251–253, 1990.

189. McLaughlin J, Chianese E, Witte ON: Alternative forms of the BCR-ABL oncogene have quantitatively different potencies for stimulation of immature lymphoid cells. Mol Cell Biol 9:1866–1874, 1989.

190. Kantarjian HM, Talpaz M, Dhingra K, et al: Significance of the P210 versus P190 molecular abnormalities in adults with Philadelphia chromosome-positive acute leukemia. Blood 78:2411–2418, 1991.

191. Berger R, Bernheim J, Broquet JC, et al: t(8;14) Translocation in a Burkitt's type of lymphoblastic leukaemia (L3). Br J Haematol 43:87–90, 1979.

192. Magrath I: The pathogenesis of Burkitt's lymphoma. Adv Cancer Res 55:133–270, 1990.

193. Croce CM, Nowell PC: Molecular basis of human B-cell neoplasia. Blood 65:1–7, 1985.

194. Rabbitts TH, Forster A, Hamlyn P, et al: Effect of somatic mutation within translocated c-myc genes in Burkitt's lymphoma. Nature 309:592–597, 1984.

195. Blackwood EM, Eisenman RN: Max: A helix-loop-helix zipper protein that forms a sequence-specific DNA-binding complex with MYC. Science 251:1211–1217, 1991.

196. Adams JM, Harris AW, Pinkert CA, et al: The c-myc oncogene driven by immunoglobulin enhancers induces lymphoid malignancy in transgenic mice. Nature 318:533–538, 1985.

197. Fenaux P, Lai JL, Miaux O, et al: Burkitt cell acute leukaemia (L$_3$ALL) in adults: A report of 18 cases. Br J Haematol 71:371–376, 1989.

198. Kantarjian HM, O'Brien S, Beran M, et al: Modified Burkitt regimen for adult acute lymphocytic leukemia—The hyper-CVAD program. Blood 82:329a, 1993.

199. Hoelzer D: Therapy of acute lymphoblastic leukemia in adults. Leukemia 6(suppl 2):132–135, 1992.

200. Bowman WP, Shuster JJ, Cook B, et al: Improved survival for children with B-cell acute lymphoblastic leukemia and stage IV small noncleaved cell lymphoma. Proc Am Soc Clin Oncol 11:277, 1992.

201. Brecher M, Murphy SB, Bowman WP, et al: Results of Pediatric Oncology Group 8616: A randomized trial of two forms of therapy for stage III diffuse small noncleaved cell lymphoma in children. Proc Am Soc Clin Oncol 11:340, 1992.

202. McMaster ML, Greer JP, Greco A, et al: Effective treatment of small-noncleaved-cell lymphoma with high-intensity, brief-duration chemotherapy. J Clin Oncol 9:941–946, 1991.

203. Pui C-H, Behm F, Raimondi SC, et al: Secondary acute myeloid leukemia in children treated for acute lymphoid leukemia. N Engl J Med 321:136–142, 1989.

204. Prieto F, Palau F, Badia L, et al: 11q23 Abnormalities in children with acute nonlymphocytic leukemia (M4-M5): Association with previous chemotherapy. Cancer Genet Cytogenet 45:1–11, 1990.

205. Pedersen-Bjergaard J, Philip P: Balanced translocations involving chromosome bands 11q23 and 21q22 are highly characteristic of myelodysplasia and leukemia following therapy with cytostatic agents targeting at DNA-topoisomerase II. Blood 78:1147–1148, 1991.

206. Cortes J, O'Brien S, Kantarjian HM, et al: Abnormalities in the long arm of chromosome 11 (11q) in patients with de novo and secondary acute myelogenous leukemia and myelodysplastic syndromes. Leukemia 8:2174–2178, 1994.

207. Kaneko Y, Maseki N, Takasaki N, et al: Clinical and hematologic characteristics in acute leukemia with 11q23 translocations. Blood 67:484–491, 1986.

208. Raimondi SC, Peiper SC, Kitchingman GR, et al: Childhood acute lymphoblastic leukemia with chromosomal breakpoints at 11q23. Blood 73:1627–1634, 1989.

209. Furley AJW, Chan LC, Mizutani S, et al: Lineage specificity of rearrangement and expression of genes encoding the T-cell receptor-T3 complex and immunoglobulin heavy chain in leukemia. Leukemia 1:644–652, 1987.

210. Pui CH, Raimondi SC, Murphy SB, et al: An analysis of leukemic cell chromosomal features in infants. Blood 69:1289–1293, 1987.

211. Chen C-S, Sorensen PHB, Domer PH, et al: Molecular rearrangements on chromosome 11q23 predominate in infant acute lymphoblastic leukemia and are associated with specific biologic variables and poor outcome. Blood 81:2386–2393, 1993.

212. Pui C-H, Behm FG, Downing JR, et al: 11q23/MLL rearrangement confers a poor prognosis in infants with acute lymphoblastic leukemia. J Clin Oncol 12:909–915, 1994.

213. Kobayashi H, Espinosa R III, Thirman MJ, et al: Heterogeneity of breakpoints of 11q23 rearrangements in hematologic malignancies identified with fluorescence in situ hybridization. Blood 82:547–551, 1993.

214. Nakamura YGT, Alder H, Prasad R, et al: The t(4;11) chromosome translocation of human acute leukemias fuses the ALL-1 gene, related to Drosophila trithorax, to the AF-4 gene. Cell 71:701–708, 1992.

215. Carroll AJ, Crist WM, Parmley RT, et al: Pre-B cell leukemia associated with chromosome translocation 1;19. Blood 63:721–724, 1984.

216. Michael PM, Levin MD, Garson OM: Translocation 1;19—A new cytogenetic abnormality in acute lymphocytic leukemia. Cancer Genet Cytogenet 12:339–341, 1984.

217. Shikano T, Kaneko Y, Takazawa M, et al: Balanced and unbalanced 1;19 translocation-associated acute lymphoblastic leukemias. Cancer 58:2239–2243, 1986.

218. Crist WM, Boyett J, Jackson J, et al: Prognostic importance

of the pre-B-cell immunophenotype and other presenting features in B-lineage childhood acute lymphoblastic leukemia: A Pediatric Oncology Group study. Blood 74:1252–1259, 1989.

219. Nourse J, Melletin JD, Galili N, et al: Chromosomal translocation t(1;19) results in synthesis of a homeobox fusion mRNA that codes for a potential chimeric transcription factor. Cell 60:535–545, 1990.

220. Kamps MP, Murre C, Sun X-H, et al: A new homeobox gene contributes the DNA binding domain of the t(1;19) translocation protein in pre-B ALL. Cell 60:547–555, 1990.

221. Erikson J, Williams DL, Finan J, et al: Locus of the alpha-chain of the T-cell receptor is split by chromosome translocation in T-cell leukemias. Science 229:784–786, 1985.

222. Boehm T, Baer R, Lavenir I, et al: The mechanism of chromosomal translocation t(11;14) involving the T-cell receptor C delta locus on human chromosome 14q11 and a transcribed region of chromosome 11p15. EMBO J 7:385–394, 1988.

223. Champagne E, Takihara Y, Sagman U, et al: The T-cell receptor delta chain locus is disrupted in the T-ALL associated t(11;14) (p13;q11) translocation. Blood 73:1672–1676, 1989.

224. Croce CM, Isobe M, Palumbo A, et al: Gene for alpha-chain of human T-cell receptor: Location on chromosome 14 region involved in T-cell neoplasms. Science 227:1044–1047, 1985.

225. Chapelle A: The 1985 human gene map and human gene mapping in 1985. Cytogenet Cell Genet 40:1–7, 1985.

226. Raimondi SC, Pui C-H, Behm FG, et al: 7q32q36 Translocations in childhood T cell leukemia: Cytogenetic evidence of involvement of the T-cell receptor beta-chain gene. Blood 69:131–134, 1987.

227. Ribeiro RC, Raimondi SC, Behm FG, et al: Clinical and biologic features of childhood T-cell leukemia with the t(11;14). Blood 78:466–470, 1991.

228. Boehm T, Foroni L, Kaneko Y, et al: The rhombotin family of cysteine-rich LIM-domain oncogenes: Distinct members are involved in T-cell translocations to human chromosomes 11q15 and 11p13. Proc Natl Acad Sci U S A 88:4367–4371, 1991.

229. Pokora-Royer B, Loos U, Ludwig WD: TTG-2, a new gene encoding a cysteine-rich protein with the LIM motif, is overexpressed in acute T-cell leukaemia with the t(11;14)(p13;q11). Oncogene 6:1887–1893, 1991.

230. McGuire EA, Hockett RD, Pollock KM, et al: The t(11;14)(p15;q11) in a T-cell acute lymphoblastic leukemia cell line activates multiple transcripts, including Ttg-1, a gene encoding a potential zinc finger protein. Mol Cell Biol 9:2124–2132, 1989.

231. Rabbitts TH: Translocations, master genes, and differences between the origins of acute and chronic leukemias Cell 67:641–644, 1991.

232. Hatano M, Roberts CWM, Minden M, et al: Deregulation of a homeobox gene, HOX11, by the t(10;14) in T cell leukemia. Science 253:79–81, 1991.

233. Kennedy MA, Gonzalez-Sarmiento R, Kees UR, et al: HOX11, a homeobox-containing T-cell oncogene on human chromosome 10q24. Genetics 88:8900–8904, 1991.

234. Mellentin JD, Smith SD, Cleary ML: IyI-1, a novel gene altered by chromosomal translocation in T-cell leukemia, codes for a protein with a helix-loop-helix DNA binding motif. Cell 58:77–83, 1989.

235. Begley CG, Aplan PD, Davey MP, et al: Chromosomal translocation in a human leukemic stem-cell line disrupts the T-cell antigen receptor delta-chain diversity region and results in a previously unreported fusion transcript. Proc Natl Acad Sci U S A 86:2031–2035, 1989.

236. Hsu H-L, Cheng J-T, Chen Q, et al: Enhancer-binding activity of the tal-1 oncoprotein in association with the E47/E12 helix-loop-

helix proteins. Mol Cell Biol 11:3037–3042, 1991.

237. Erikson J, Finger L, Sun L, et al: Deregulation of c-myc by translocation of the alpha-locus of the T-cell receptor in T-cell leukemias. Science 232:884–886, 1986.

238. Shima EA, Le Beau MM, McKeithan TW, et al: Gene encoding the alpha-chain of the T-cell receptor is moved immediately downstream of c-myc in a chromosomal 8;14 translocation in a cell line from a human T-cell leukemia. Proc Natl Acad Sci USA 83:3439–3443, 1986.

239. Brito-Babapulle V, Matutes E, Parreira L, et al: Abnormalities of chromosome 7q and Tac expression in T-cell Leukemias. Blood 67:516–521, 1986.

240. Kaneko Y, Maseki N, Homma C, et al: Chromosome translocations involving band 7q35 or 7p15 in childhood T-cell leukemia/lymphoma. Blood 72:534–538, 1988.

241. Xia Y, Brown L, Yang CY-C, et al: TAL2, a helix-loop-helix gene activated by the (7;9)(q34;q32) translocation in human T-cell leukemia. Proc Natl Acad Sci U S A 88:11416–11420, 1991.

242. Ellisen LW, Bird J, West DC, et al: TAN-1, the human homolog of the Drosophila notch gene, is broken by chromosomal translocations in T-lymphoblastic neoplasms. Cell 66:649–661, 1991.

243. Chilcote RR, Brown E, Rowley JD: Lymphoblastic leukemia with lymphomatous features associated with abnormalities of the short arm of chromosome 9. N Engl J Med 313:286–291, 1985.

244. Carroll AJ, Castleberry RP, Crist WM: Lack of association between abnormalities of the chromosome 9 short arm and either 'lymphomatous' features or T-cell phenotype in childhood acute lymphocytic leukemia. Blood 69:735–738, 1987.

245. Murphy SB, Raimondi SC, Rivera GK, et al: Nonrandom abnormalities of chromosome 9p in childhood acute lymphoblastic leukemia: Association with high-risk clinical features. Blood 74:409–415, 1989.

246. Diaz MO, Ziemin S, Le Beau MM, et al: Homozygous deletion of the alpha and beta interferon genes in human leukemia and derived cell lines. Proc Natl Acad Sci U S A 85:5259–5263, 1988.

247. Hayashi Y, Raimondi SC, Look AT, et al: Abnormalities of the long arm of chromosome 6 in childhood acute lymphoblastic leukemia. Blood 76:1626–1630, 1990.

248. Raimondi SC, Williams DL, Callihan T, et al: Nonrandom involvement of the 12p12 breakpoint in chromosome abnormalities of childhood acute lymphoblastic leukemia. Blood 68:69–75, 1986.

249. van der Plas DC, Dekker I, Hagemeijer A, et al: 12p chromosomal aberrations in precursor B cell childhood acute lymphoblastic leukemia predict an increased risk of relapse in the central nervous system and are associated with typical blast cell morphology. Leukemia 8:2041–2046, 1994.

250. Lübert M, Mirro J, Miller CW, et al: N-ras gene point mutations in childhood acute lymphocytic leukemia correlate with poor prognosis. Blood 75:1163–1169, 1990.

251. Distelhorst CW, Lam M, Lisgaris M, et al: Dexamethasone induces increased synthesis of the glucose-regulated protein GRP78 in S49 mouse lymphoma cells. Leukemia 6:162, 1992.

252. Lauer SJ, Pinkel D, Buchanan GR, et al: Cytosine arabinoside/cyclophosphamide pulses during continuation therapy for childhood acute lymphoblastic leukemia. Cancer 60:2366–2371, 1987.

253. Wiley JS, Woodruff RK, Jamieson GP, et al: Cytosine arabinoside in the treatment of T-cell acute lymphoblastic leukemia. Aust N Z J Med 17:379–386, 1987.

254. Patte C, Philip T, Rodary C, et al: High survival rate in advanced-stage B-cell lymphomas and leukemias without CNS involvement with a short intensive polychemotherapy: Results from the French Pediatric Oncology Society of a randomized trial of 216 children. J Clin Oncol 9:123–132, 1991.

255. Sobol RE, Mick R, Royston I, et al: Clinical importance of myeloid antigen expression in adult acute lymphoblastic leukemia. N Engl J Med 316:1111–1117, 1987.

256. Preti A, Huh Y, O'Brien S, et al: Prognostic significance of positive myeloid markers in adult acute lymphocytic leukemia. Blood 82(suppl 1): 57a, 1993.

257. Boldt DH, Kopecky K, Head DR, et al: Expression of myeloid antigens in adult acute lymphoblastic leukemia: the Southwest Oncology Group experience. Proc Am Soc Clin Oncol 11:263, 1992.

258. Pui C-H, Hancock ML, Head DR, et al: Clinical significance of CD34 expression in childhood acute lymphoblastic leukemia. Blood 82:889–894, 1993.

259. Goasquen JE, Dossot J-M, Fardel O, et al: Expression of the multidrug resistance-associated P-glycoprotein (P-170) in 59 cases of de novo acute lymphoblastic leukemia: Prognostic implications. Blood 81:2394–2398, 1993.

260. Sather HN: Statistical evaluation of prognostic factors in ALL and treatment results. Med Pediatr Oncol 14:158–165, 1986.

261. Kalwinsky DK, Rivera G, Dahl GV, et al: Variation by race in presenting clinical and biologic features of childhood acute lymphoblastic leukaemia: Implications for treatment outcome. Leuk Res 9:817–823, 1985.

262. Miller DR, Coccia PF, Bleyer WA, et al: Early response to induction therapy as a predictor of disease-free survival and late recurrence of childhood acute lymphoblastic leukemia: A report from the Children's Cancer Study Group. J Clin Oncol 7:1807–1815, 1989.

263. Gaynon PS, Bleyer WA, Steinherz PG, et al: Day 7 marrow response and outcome for children with acute lymphoblastic leukemia and unfavorable presenting features. Med Pediatr Oncol 18:273–279, 1990.

264. Preti A, Kantarjian HM: Management of adult acute lymphocytic leukemia: Present issues and key challenges. J Clin Oncol 12:1312–1322, 1994.

265. Kantarjian HM: Adult acute lymphocytic leukemia: Critical review of current knowledge. Am J Med 97:176–184, 1994.

266. Hoelzer DF: Therapy of the newly diagnosed adult with acute lymphoblastic leukemia. Hematol Oncol Clin North Am 7:139–160, 1993.

267. Amadori S, Montuoro A, Meloni G, et al: Combination chemotherapy for acute lymphocytic leukemia in adults: Results of a retrospective study in 82 patients. Am J Hematol 8:175–183, 1980.

268. Hess CE, Zirkle JW: Results of induction therapy with vincristine and prednisone alone in adult acute lymphoblastic leukemia: Report of 43 patients and review of the literature. Am J Hematol 13:63–71, 1982.

269. Gottlieb AJ, Weinberg V, Ellison RR, et al: Efficacy of daunorubicin in the therapy of adult acute lymphocytic leukemia: A prospective randomized trial by Cancer and Leukemia Group B. Blood 64:267–274, 1984.

270. Stryckmans P, Debusscfer L: Chemotherapy of adult acute lymphoblastic leukaemia. Bailliere's Clin Haematol 4:115–130, 1991.

271. Cuttner J, Mick R, Budman DR, et al: Phase III trial of brief intensive treatment of adult acute lymphocytic leukemia comparing daunorubicin and mitoxantrone: A CALGB study. Leukemia 5:425–431, 1991.

272. Balis FM, Lester CM, Chrousos GP, et al: Differences in cerebrospinal fluid penetration of corticosteroids: Possible relationship in the prevention of meningeal leukemia. J Clin Oncol 5:202–207, 1987.

273. Mandelli F, Annino L, Vegna ML, et al: GIMEMA ALL 0288: A multicenter study on adult acute lymphoblastic leukemia: Preliminary results. Leukemia 6(suppl 2):182–185, 1992.

274. Schiffer CA, Larson RA, Bloomfield CD, for the CALGB: Cancer and Leukemia Group B (CALGB) studies in acute lymphocytic leukemia (ALL). Haematologica 76(suppl 4):106, 1991.

275. Weiss M, Telford P, Kempin S, et al: Severe toxicity limits intensification of induction therapy for acute lymphoblastic leukemia. Leukemia 7:832–837, 1993.

276. Kasparu H, Sreter L, Holowiiecki J, et al: Intensified induction therapy for ALL in adults: A multicenter trial. Onkologie 14(suppl 2):80, 1991.

277. Rohatiner AZS, Bassan R, Battista R, et al: High dose cytosine arabinoside in the initial treatment of adults with acute lymphoblastic leukemia. Br J Cancer 62:454–458, 1990.

278. Schaver P, Arlin ZA, Mertelsman R, et al: Treatment of acute lymphoblastic leukemia in adults: Results of the L-10 and L-10M protocols. J Clin Oncol 1:462–470, 1983.

279. Linker CA, Levitt LJ, O'Donnell M, et al: Treatment of adult acute lymphoblastic leukemia with intensive cyclical chemotherapy: A follow-up report. Blood 78:2814–2822, 1991.

280. Radford JE, Burns CP, Jones MP, et al: Adult acute lymphoblastic leukemia: Results of the Iowa HOP-L protocol. J Clin Oncol 7:58–66, 1989.

281. Clavell LA, Gelber RD, Cohen HJ, et al: Four-agent induction and intensive asparaginase therapy for treatment of childhood acute lymphoblastic leukemia. N Engl J Med 315:657–663, 1986.

282. Wiernick PH, Dutcher JP, Gucalp R, et al: MOAD therapy for acute lymphocytic leukemia. Proc Am Soc Clin Oncol 9:205, 1990.

283. Dutcher JP, Wiernick PH, Gucalp R: MOAD therapy for adult acute lymphocytic leukemia (ALL). Haematologica 76(suppl 4):66, 1991.

284. Hoelzer D: Acute lymphoblastic leukemia progress in children, less in adults. N Engl J Med 329:1343–1344, 1993.

285. Kantarjian HM, Estey EH, O'Brien S, et al: Intensive chemotherapy with mitoxantrone and high-dose cytosine arabinoside followed by granulocyte-macrophage colony-stimulating factor in the treatment of patients with acute lymphocytic leukemia. Blood 79:876–881, 1992.

286. Kantarjian HM, Estey EH, O'Brien S, et al: Granulocyte colony-stimulating factor supportive treatment following intensive chemotherapy in acute lymphocytic leukemia in first remission. Cancer 72:2950–2955, 1993.

287. Tsuchiya H, Adachi N, Asou N, et al: Responses to granulocyte colony-stimulating factor (G-CSF) and granulocyte-macrophage CSF in Ph' positive acute lymphoblastic leukemia with myeloid surface markers. Blood 77:411–413, 1991.

288. Pui C-H, Simone JV, Hancock ML, et al: Impact of three methods of treatment intensification on acute lymphoblastic leukemia in children: Long-term results of St. Jude therapy study X. Leukemia 6:150–157, 1992.

289. Abromowitch M, Fairclough D: Contribution of mercaptopurine intensification to improved outcome in patients with lower-risk ALL. J Clin Oncol 8:1442, 1990.

290. Camitta B, Leventhal B, Lauer S, et al: Intermediate-dose intravenous methotrexate and mercaptopurine therapy for non-T, non-B acute lymphocytic leukemia of childhood: A Pediatric Oncology Group study. J Clin Oncol 10:1539–1544, 1989.

291. Rivera GK, Raimondi SC, Hancock ML, et al: Improved outcome in childhood acute lymphoblastic leukaemia with reinforced early treatment and rotational combination. Lancet 337:61–66, 1991.

292. Tubergen DG, Gilchrist GS, O'Brien RT, et al: Improved outcome with delayed intensification for children with acute lymphoblastic leukemia and intermediate presenting features: A Children's Cancer Group phase II trial. J Clin Oncol 11:527–537, 1993.

293. Champlin RE, Gale RP: Acute lymphoblastic leukemia: Recent advances in biology and therapy. Blood 8:2051–2066, 1989.

294. Fiere D, Extra JM, David B, et al: Treatment of 218 adult acute lymphoblastic leukemias. Semin Oncol 14(suppl 1):64–66, 1987.

295. Stryckmans P, de Witte TH, Fillet G: Treatment of adult acute lymphoblastic leukemia-ALL-2 and ALL-3 EORTC studies. Haematologica 76(suppl 4):109, 1991.

296. Ellison RR, Mick R, Cuttner J, et al: The effects of postinduction intensification treatment with cytarabine and daunorubicin in adult acute lymphocytic leukemia: A prospective randomized clinical trial by Cancer and Leukemia Group B. J Clin Oncol 9:2002–2015, 1991.

297. Hoelzer D, Thiel E, Ludwig WD, et al: The German multicentre trials for treatment of acute lymphoblastic leukemia in adults. Leukemia 6(suppl 2):175–177, 1992.

298. Cassileth PA, Andersen JW, Bennett JM, et al: Adult acute lymphocytic leukemia: The Eastern Cooperative Oncology Group experience Leukemia 6(suppl 2):178–181, 1992.

299. Koren G, Ferrazini G, Sulh H, et al: Systemic exposure to mercaptopurine as a prognostic factor in acute lymphocytic leukemia in children. N Engl J Med 323:17–21, 1990.

300. Evans WE, Crom WR, Abromowitch M, et al: Clinical pharmacodynamics of high-dose methotrexate in acute lymphocytic leukemia: Identification of a relation between concentration and effect. N Engl J Med 314:471–477, 1986.

301. Hussein KK, Dahlberg S, Head DR, et al: Treatment of acute lymphoblastic leukemia in adults with intensive induction, consolidation, and maintenance chemotherapy. Blood 73:57–63, 1989.

302. Mandelli F, Annino L, Giona FMA: ALL 0183: A multicentric study on adult acute lymphoblastic leukemia in Italy, in Gale RP, Hoelzer D (eds): Acute Lymphoblastic Leukemia, pp 205–220. New York, Alan R Liss, 1990.

303. Bleyer WA: Central nervous system leukemia. Pediatr Clin North Am 35:789–814, 1988.

304. Cortes J, O'Brien S, Robertson LE, et al: The value of high-dose systemic chemotherapy and intrathecal therapy for central nervous system prophylaxis in different risk groups of adult acute lymphoblastic leukemia. Proc Am Soc Clin Oncol 14:335, 1995.

305. Pinkel D, Woo S: Prevention and treatment of meningeal leukemia in children. Blood 84:355–366, 1994.

306. Law IP, Blom J: Adult acute leukemia: Frequency of central nervous system involvement in long-term survivors. Cancer 40:1304–1306, 1977.

307. Bleyer WA, Coccia PF, Sather HN, et al: Reduction in central nervous system leukemia with a pharmacokinetically derived intrathecal methotrexate dosage regimen. J Clin Oncol 1:317–325, 1983.

308. Bleyer WA: Central nervous system leukemia, in Henderson ES, Lister TA (eds): Leukemia, 5th ed, pp 733–768. Philadelphia, WB Saunders Co, 1990.

309. Balis FM, Poplack DG: Central nervous system pharmacology of antileukemic drugs. Am J Pediatr Oncol Hematol 11:74–86, 1989.

310. Bleyer WA, Poplack DG: Prophylaxis and treatment of leukemia in the central nervous system and other sanctuaries. Semin Oncol 12:131–148, 1985.

311. Bleyer WA: Neurologic sequelae of methotrexate and ionizing radiation: A new classification. Cancer Treat Rep 65(suppl 1):89–98, 1981.

312. Shalet SM, Gibson B, Swindell R, et al: Effect of spinal irradiation on growth. Arch Dis Child 62:461–464, 1987.

313. Price RA, Jamieson PA: The central nervous system in childhood leukemia. II: Subacute leukoencephalopathy. Cancer 35:306–318, 1975.

314. Gilchrist GS, Tubergen DG, Sather HN, et al: Low numbers of CSF blasts at diagnosis do not predict for the development of CNS leukemia in children with intermediate-risk acute lymphoblastic leu-

kemia: A Children's Cancer Group report. J Clin Oncol 12:2594–2600, 1994.

315. Omura GA, Moffitt S, Vogler WR, et al: Combination chemotherapy of adult acute lymphoblastic leukemia with randomized central nervous system prophylaxis. Blood 55:199–204, 1980.

316. Henderson ES, Scharlau C, Cooper MR, et al: Combination chemotherapy and radiotherapy for acute lymphocytic leukemia in adults: Results of CALGB protocol 7113. Leuk Res 3:395–407, 1979.

317. Tucker J, Prior PF, Green CR, et al: Minimal neuropsychological sequelae following prophylactic treatment of the central nervous system in adult leukaemia and lymphoma. Br J Cancer 60:775–780, 1989.

318. Pavlovsky S, Eppinger-Helft M, Muriel FS: Factors that influence the appearance of central nervous system leukemia. Blood 42:935–938, 1973.

319. Kantarjian HM, Walters RS, Smith TL, et al: Identification of risk groups for development of central nervous system leukemia in adults with acute lymphocytic leukemia. Blood 72:1784–1789, 1988.

320. Doney K, Fisher LD, Appelbaum FR, et al: Treatment of adult acute lymphoblastic leukemia with allogeneic bone marrow transplantation: Multivariate analysis of factors affecting acute graft-versus-host disease, relapse, and relapse-free survival. Bone Marrow Transplant 7:453–459, 1991.

321. Gratwohl A, Hermans J, Zwaan F: Bone marrow transplantation for ALL in Europe, in Gale RP, Hoelzer D (eds): Acute Lymphoblastic Leukemia, pp 271–278. New York, Alan R. Liss, 1990.

322. Blume KG, Schmidt GM, Chao NJ: Bone marrow transplantation from histocompatible sibling donors for patients with acute lymphoblastic leukemia. Haematol Blood Transfus 33:636–637, 1990.

323. Barrett AJ, Horowitz MM, Gale RP, et al: Marrow transplantation for acute lymphoblastic leukemia: Factors affecting relapse and survival. Blood 74:862–871, 1989.

324. Christiansen NP: Allogeneic bone marrow transplantation for the treatment of adult acute leukemias. Hematol Oncol Clin North Am 7:177–200, 1993.

325. Chao NJ, Forman SJ, Schmidt GM, et al: Allogeneic bone marrow transplantation for high-risk acute lymphoblastic leukemia during first complete remission. Blood 78:1923–1927, 1991.

326. Vernant JP, Marit G, Maraninchi D, et al: Allogeneic bone marrow transplantation in adults with acute lymphoblastic leukemia in first complete remission. J Clin Oncol 6:227–231, 1988.

327. Mirsic M, Nemet D, Labar B, et al: Chemotherapy versus allogeneic bone marrow transplantation in adults with acute lymphoblastic leukemia. Transplant Proc 25:1268–1270, 1993.

328. Horowitz MM, Messerer D, Hoelzer D, et al: Chemotherapy compared with bone marrow transplantation for adults with acute lymphoblastic leukemia in first remission. Ann Intern Med 115:13–18, 1991.

329. Fiere D, Lepage E, Sebban C, et al: Adult acute lymphoblastic leukemia: A multicenter randomized trial testing bone marrow transplantation as postremission therapy. J Clin Oncol 11:1990–2001, 1993.

330. Sebban C, Lepage E, Vernant JP, et al: Allogeneic bone marrow transplantation in adult acute lymphoblastic leukemia in first complete remission: A comparative study. J Clin Oncol 12:2580–2587, 1994.

331. Barrett AJ, Horowitz MM, Ash RC, et al: Bone marrow transplantation for Philadelphia chromosome-positive acute lymphoblastic leukemia. Blood 79:3067–3070, 1992.

332. Biggs JC, Horowitz MM, Gale RP, et al: Bone marrow transplants may cure patients with acute leukemia never achieving remission with chemotherapy. Blood 80:1090–1093. 1992.

333. Mortimer J, Blinder MA, Schulman S, et al: Relapse of acute

leukemia after marrow transplantation: Natural history and results of subsequent therapy. J Clin Oncol 7:50–57, 1989.

334. Sallan SE, Niemeyer CM, Billett AL, et al: Autologous bone marrow transplantation for acute lymphoblastic leukemia. J Clin Oncol 7:1594–1601, 1989.

335. Soiffer RJ, Roy DC, Gonin R, et al: Monoclonal antibody-purged autologous bone marrow transplantation in adults with acute lymphoblastic leukemia at high risk of relapse. Bone Marrow Transplant 12:243–251, 1993.

336. Gilmore MJML, Hamon HG, Prentice F, et al: Failure of purged autologous bone marrow transplantation in high risk acute lymphoblastic leukemia in first complete remission. Bone Marrow Transplant 8:19–26, 1991.

337. Simonsson B, Burnett AK, Prentice HG, et al: Autologous bone marrow transplantation with monoclonal antibody purged marrow for high risk acute lymphoblastic leukemia. Leukemia 3:631–636, 1989.

338. Carella AM, Pollicardo N, Pungolino E, et al: Mobilization of cytogenetically 'normal' blood progenitor cells by intensive conventional chemotherapy for chronic myeloid and acute lymphoblastic leukemia. Leuk Lymphoma 9:477–483, 1993.

339. Schauer P, Arlin ZA, Mertelsmann R: Treatment of acute lymphoblastic leukemia in adults—Results of the L-10 and L-10M protocols. J Clin Oncol 1:462–470, 1983.

340. Linker CA, Levitt LJ, O'Donnell M, et al: Improved results of treatment of adult acute lymphoblastic leukemia. Blood 69: 1242–1248, 1987.

341. Potter MN: The detection of minimal residual disease in acute lymphoblastic leukemia. Blood Rev 6:68–82, 1992.

342. Uckun FM, Kersey JH, Haake R, et al: Pretransplantation burden of leukemic progenitor cells as a predictor of relapse after bone marrow transplantation for acute lymphoblastic leukemia. N Engl J Med 329:1296–1301, 1993.

343. Yamada M, Hudson S, Tournay O, et al: Detection of minimal disease in hematopoietic malignancies of the B-cell lineage by using third-complementary-determining region (CDR-III)-specific probes. Proc Natl Acad Sci U S A 86:5123–5127, 1989.

344. Yamada M, Wasserman R, Lange B, et al: Minimal residual disease in childhood B-lineage lymphoblastic leukemia: Persistence of leukemic cells during the first 18 months of treatment. N Engl J Med 323:448–455, 1990.

345. Estrov Z, Grunberger T, Dube ID, et al: Detection of residual acute lymphoblastic leukemia cells in cultures of bone marrow obtained during remission. N Engl J Med 315:538–542, 1986.

346. Chen CJ, Chin JE, Ueda K, et al: Internal duplication and homology with bacterial transport proteins in the MDR1 (P-glycoprotein) gene from multidrug-resistant human cells. Cell 47:381–389, 1986.

347. Fojo AT, Ueda K, Slamon DJ, et al: Expression of a multidrug resistance gene in human tumors and tissues. Proc Natl Acad Sci U S A 84: 265–269, 1987.

348. List A: Multidrug resistance: Clinical relevance in acute leukemia. Oncology 7:23–27, 1993.

349. Goasguen JE, Dossot JM, Fardel O, et al: Expression of the multidrug resistance associated P-glycoprotein (P-170) in 59 cases of acute lymphocytic leukemia—Prognostic implications. Blood 81:2394–2398, 1993.

350. Korsemeyer SJ: Bcl-2 initiates a new category of oncogenes: regulators of cell death. Blood 80:879–886, 1992.

351. Campana D, Coustan-Smith E, Manabe A, et al: Prolonged survival of B-lineage acute lymphoblastic leukemia cells is accompanied by overexpression of bcl-2 protein. Blood 81:1025–1031, 1993.

352. Smets LA, Van den Berg J, Acton D, et al: Bcl-2 expression and mitochondrial activity in leukemic cells with different sensitivity to glucocorticoid-induced apoptosis. Blood 84:1613–1619, 1994.

353. Gala JL, Vermylen C, Cornu G, et al: High expression of bcl-2 is the rule in acute lymphoblastic leukemia, except in Burkitt subtype at presentation, and is not correlated with prognosis. Ann Hematol 69:17–24, 1994.

CHAPTER 2

Acute Myelogenous Leukemia

Habib M. Ghaddar, MD, *and* Elihu H. Estey, MD

Department of Hematology, Section of Leukemia, The University of Texas M. D. Anderson Cancer Center, Houston, Texas

Acute myelogenous leukemia (AML) is a disorder marked by infiltration of the bone marrow by abnormal hematopoietic progenitors. These cells are unable to differentiate in a normal fashion into myeloid, erythroid, and/or megakaryocytic cell lines and, unlike normal progenitors, are capable of infiltrating vital organs. They also block the differentiation of the residual normal progenitors resulting in thrombocytopenia, anemia, and/or granulocytopenia. Without treatment, a patient only rarely survives more than 6 to 12 months; death results from complications of marrow failure.

AML is a rare malignancy that affects approximately 4 persons per 100,000 in the United States and England annually.[1,2] Despite the continued development of new therapies and increased understanding of its biology, AML remains fatal in approximately 80% of treated patients. With the introduction of cytogenetic banding, better characterization of various subsets of AML is now possible, and higher cure rates can be observed in certain subsets.[3–9] The cure rate for AML can potentially increase if different cytogenetic subsets are targeted with specific therapies[6,7] and if detection of clinically relevant minimal residual disease becomes practical.

PRESENTATION

Although AML occasionally is diagnosed on routine blood counts from asymptomatic patients, most patients are symptomatic at presentation. Commonly, the symptoms are those referable to various cytopenias or coagulopathies and consist mainly of weakness, bleeding, and infections. The infections most commonly seen are minor upper respiratory tract infections or vague flulike symptoms, although pneumonias occur in about 5% of cases. Bleeding is usually in the form of petechiae, which correlate with the degree of thrombocytopenia, or ecchymoses, which generally are caused by disseminated intravascular coagulation (DIC), commonly seen in patients with acute promyelocytic leukemia (APL).[10] Rare symptoms include bone pain presumed to be secondary to marrow expansion, skin lesions secondary to leukemic infiltration (leukemia cutis), gum hypertrophy (especially common in the monocytic subtypes of AML), and

abdominal pain caused by hepatosplenomegaly or adenopathy. Neurologic symptoms resulting from central nervous system (CNS) disease or leukostasis are also rare symptoms of AML.

DIAGNOSIS AND CLASSIFICATION

French-American-British Working Group

The diagnosis of AML is based on the revised criteria of the French-American-British (FAB) Working Group.[11] This classification relies entirely on morphologic features and cytochemical staining characteristics that can be seen by light microscopy. On rare occasions, electron microscopy and immunophenotyping are required to establish the diagnosis. The cytochemical stains used are myeloperoxidase (MPO), terminal deoxynucleotidyltransferase (TDT), nonspecific esterase (NSE), and Sudan black B (SBB). The diagnosis of AML is made when at least 30% of nucleated cells in the bone marrow or peripheral blood are blasts and when greater than or equal to 3% of these blasts are MPO positive by light microscopy, irrespective of the findings when other stains are used.

Instances of myeloid and lymphoid markers, found on the same or separate cells (lineage infidelity, biphenotypic leukemia), exist in a significant proportion of cases of AML, as we have defined the disease. Although they are not the focus of this chapter, such cases call attention to the arbitrary compartmentalization of acute leukemia as either AML or acute lymphocytic leukemia (ALL). Although SBB has been considered an alternative to MPO, due to the high rate of concordance when both stains are used, SBB should not be substituted, because 1.6% of ALL cases—MPO being negative by definition—are SBB positive. These cases would be misdiagnosed as AML.[12] It remains to be seen whether such cases would benefit more from ALL-type than AML-type therapy.

The FAB Working Group describes disease class M1 as acute myeloblastic leukemia without maturation. The blasts show a minimal tendency toward granulocytic maturation, with less than 10% of the marrow nucleated cells being progranulocytes or more mature granulocytes. In the M2 class, acute myeloblastic leukemia with maturation, maturation is more evident; the blasts show a lower nucleus-to-cytoplasm ratio, and more than 10% of the cells are progranulocytes or more mature granulocytes. M3, acute promyelocytic leukemia, occurs most commonly in its hypergranular form but also occurs in a variant or microgranular form.[13,14] Most cases have fewer than 30% blasts, but the number of progranulocytes is frequently greater than 75%. In M1, M2, and M3 classes, less than 20% of the cells are monocytic. Auer rods commonly are seen in M2 and especially M3, where they sometimes accumulate to form characteristic faggot cells. In M4 (acute myelomonocytic leukemia), M4Eo (M4 with abnormal eosinophils), and M5 (acute monoblastic leukemia), at least 20% of the bone marrow cells are monocytic; in M5, they are usually monoblasts. MPO can be negative in M5, but NSE is usually positive. In M6 (acute erythroleukemia), the MPO stain is negative, and cell-surface glycophorin A is positive[15]; at least 50% of the marrow cells are dysplastic erythroid cells, and at least 30% of nonerythroid cells are blasts. M7 is acute megakaryocytic leukemia. It is characterized by bone-marrow fibrosis, which makes aspiration difficult and impedes the diagnosis. It is the most common acute leukemia seen in patients with Down syndrome.[16] Because MPO also is negative in M7, the diagnosis should be based on the demonstration of platelet peroxidase by electron microscopy or glycoprotein IB or IIB/IIIA on the blast surface.[17] Rare cases wherein MPO, SBB, NSE, and TDT are negative but the cells express myeloid antigenic markers on the cell surface (CD13 or CD33) are classified as M0.[18] The incidence of the different FAB Working Group subtypes is reported as M1, 18%; M2, 28%; M3, 8%; M4, 27%; M5, 10%; M6, 4%; and M7, 5%.[19]

Cytogenetics

Although the FAB Working Group classification system has been widely adopted because it is easy to use, its prognostic value and hence clinical relevance are limited. More useful is the classification by leukemia cell karyotype.[5,20] In fact, the association of certain FAB Working Group subtypes with prognosis most likely results from their association with specific cytogenetic abnormalities: M3 with t(15;17),[21] M4Eo with inv(16),[22,23] M2 with t(8;21),[24] and M6 and M7 with complex karyotypes and frequent involvement of chromosomes 5 and/or 7.[25] These observations, together with recent data showing that various cytogenetic subsets benefit from different therapies[6,7] and data demonstrating the direct relationship between cytogenetic abnormalities and leukemogenesis,[26,27] make the cytogenetic classification of AML more clinically relevant than the FAB Working Group classification.

Of adults with AML, 60% to 90% were found to have cytogenetic abnormalities when tissue samples were studied with Giemsa or quinacrine banding.[3,28] This rate is dependent on factors such as the length of time in culture, banding techniques, and referral patterns of reporting centers.[29] High-resolution banding techniques suggest that almost all patients have cytogenetic abnormalities.[4]

Abnormalities such as inv(16), t(8;21), and t(15;17) occur in 5% to 10% of patients. Such patients have the best prognosis when treated with conventional doses of cytarabine and anthracycline combinations (the "3+7" regimen refers to the number of days each drug is administered).[5,30] These patients are younger than the average patient with AML and tend to have a lower incidence of antecedent hematologic disorders or prior exposure to cytotoxic therapy or radiation therapy. With the 3+7 regimen, complete remission (CR) rates are more than 90% for inv(16) and t(8;21) and nearly 70% for t(15;17). The 3-year disease-free survival rate is about 40% for all groups. Recent data have shown that the chimeric gene product resulting from the inversion in chromosome 16 is directly related to leukemogenesis.[26]

It is important to note that patients with inv(16) have a high likelihood of CNS relapse (about 35%) when treated with conventional-dose cytarabine-based regimens,[23] but this complication is almost completely eradicated when high-dose cytarabine is used.[6] Patients with t(8;21) and inv(16) have a higher cure rate (more than 50%), when high-dose cytarabine is used.[6,7] The abnormality t(15;17) involves the promyelocytic leukemia (PML) transcription unit on chromosome 15 and the retinoic acid receptor-alpha (RARA) gene on chromosome 17, resulting in the chimeric gene product PML-RARA.[30] Patients with t(15;17) respond dramatically, at least initially, to all-trans-retinoic acid (ATRA).[31–35] They commonly present with coagulopathy consistent with DIC or primary fibrinolysis,[10] a complication that accounts for most of the deaths occurring during induction therapy, which is the only cause of failure to enter CR in patients with APL.

Trisomy of chromosome 8 or deletions or losses of chromosomes 5 or 7, alone or with additional abnormalities, are seen in approximately one third of patients. These patients are generally older and have a higher incidence of antecedent hematologic disorders and prior exposure to alkylating agents or radiation therapy.[3,36,37] They have the worst prognosis when treated with conventional-dose cytarabine and anthracycline combinations (40% to 50% CR rate; less than 5% 2-year continuous complete remission [CCR] rate).

Translocations of chromosome 11 at the q23 breakpoint, seen in 5% of patients, involve the mixed-lineage leukemia gene.[38] These abnormalities commonly are seen in patients previously treated with topoisomerase II-reactive drugs.[39] In adults, the leukemia tends to be monocytic (M4/M5), but, unlike childhood cases of AML,[40] CNS disease and hepatosplenomegaly are not common features.[41] Adults with t(11q23) AML have a 60% CR rate and a 2-year CCR rate of less than 10%.

Nearly one third of patients have no cytogenetic abnormalities detected by Giemsa or quinacrine banding; these patients have an intermediate prognosis; 50% to 80% will achieve CR and 20% will remain in CR for more than 3 years when treated with the 3+7 regimen. It is unclear whether AML with a normal karyotype is a distinct entity or simply represents an abnormality missed by the techniques widely used. As techniques continue to improve, the decreasing incidence of AML with a normal karyotype tends to suggest that at least some of these cases represented undetected abnormalities.

When more than one cytogenetic abnormality is seen in the same patient, a hierarchic system that helps to assign such patients to various cytogenetic categories is generally used. This is especially important when treatment decisions are to be based on cytogenetics. Two systems are commonly used. The first system, devised by the Cancer and Leukemia Group B (CALGB), ranks abnormalities in the following order by decreasing priority: t(8;21), t(15;17), t(9;22), abnormal 16q22, abnormal 8q24, abnormal 11q23, 5q- or -5 and 7q- or -7, 5q-, -5, 7q-, -7, 6q-, +8, pseudodiploid, hyperdiploid, and hypodiploid.[9] The second system, suggested at the Sixth International Workshop on Chromosomes in Leukemia, follows a different order: abnormal 16, t(15;17), t(8;21), abnormal 5 and/or 7, abnormal 11q, pseudodiploid, hypodiploid, and hyperdiploid.[8] Given the limited information on the prognosis of patients with various combinations of abnormalities, both classifications are considered appropriate.

Finally, it should be noted that the different cytogenetic subsets themselves are prognostically heterogeneous. Although this heterogeneity may result, in part, from random variation, it is likely that other charcteristics, some unknown and others described later in this chapter, influence prognosis within each cytogenetic subset.

Immunophenotyping

The use of highly specific monoclonal antibodies (MABs) to differentiation antigens has aided in defining lineage and diagnosing rare subtypes of acute leukemias. Groups of MABs that recognize the same antigens are designated cluster groups of differentiation (CD).[42] CD positivity is defined arbitrarily as at least 20% of cells being reactive to the designated MAB. The myeloid-associated MABs are most valuable in cases of poorly differentiated AML, in which the diagnosis is unclear using standard morphologic and cytochemical analysis. The MABs against CD13, CD14, CD15, CD33, CD34, and human leukocyte antigen-DR (HLA-DR) are used most often to characterize AML. CD13, CD33, and HLA-DR are positive in most cases of AML except APL, where HLA-DR is almost always negative. This can aid in recognizing the microgranular variant of APL. The FAB Working Group classification incorporated immunophenotyping to aid in the diagnosis of FAB-M0 (negative cytochemical stains, myeloid markers positive),[18] M6 (glycophorin A antibody positive),[15] and M7 (platelet glycoproteins such as CD41, CD42, and CD61 positive).[25] Despite considerable interest in and increasing recognition of acute leukemias expressing various combinations of markers, there is no consensus regarding the definition, terminology, diagnostic criteria, or biologic implications. This is partly because of the heterogeneity of cases, which can range from cases expressing one aberrant marker in otherwise typical ALL or AML to the more extreme cases of acute mixed-lineage leukemia.

PROGNOSTIC FACTORS

Prognostic factors in AML, as in all diseases with relatively low cure rates, change continuously, as do treatment strategies and understanding of the biology of the disease. Because several of the reported prognostic factors are interrelated, their independent importance is often unclear, and the same factors are often not similarly prognostic in different studies. This lack of reproducibility probably results from technical considerations (eg, failure to account for interactions in regression analyses) and from the differences in population seen in different centers, again suggesting the heterogeneity of the disease.

Prognostic factors in AML can be divided into factors associated with death during chemotherapy and factors associated with resistance to chemotherapy, manifested either by failure to enter CR despite surviving induction therapy or by a short CR duration. Patient characteristics predictive of early death include poor performance status, age older than 60 years, and abnormal organ function.[43] The factors often associated with resistance to chemotherapy include pretreatment karyotype, age, performance status, prior myelodysplastic syndrome, prior exposure to chemotherapy or radiation therapy for another malignancy, and an antecedent hematologic disorder, defined as an abnormality in blood counts for one or more months prior to the diagnosis of AML.[5,43] Perhaps the most important prognostic factor is the pretreatment karyotype, as detailed previously in the section on cytogenetic classification. Other factors such as white blood cell count, percent bone marrow blasts, various measures of organ function, Auer rods, immunophenotyping (eg, CD34, CD19 positivity), or multidrug resistance (MDR) expression have not been consistently found to be predictive of resistance to chemotherapy.

TREATMENT

Marked improvement in the outcome of patients with newly diagnosed AML has been seen in the past three decades. AML was an invariably fatal disease 30 years ago; now, 25% of patients might be cured with current therapies. Although this advance could be secondary to improvements in supportive care, blood-product availability, and better treatment of infections, it is more likely related to advances in chemotherapy and improved treatment strategies.

Therapy generally is divided into remission induction and postremission components. All studies so far have treated all patients with AML in the same way and generally have focused on finding the best induction regimen and the best approach for postremission therapy. Given the marked heterogeneity of patients with AML, future studies are more likely to focus on finding the best treatment for each cytogenetically defined patient subset.

Remission Induction

The most commonly employed chemotherapy regimen is a combination of cytarabine, at conventional doses of 100 to 200 mg/m^2/d given intravenously (IV) by continuous infusion for 7 days, plus 3 days of an anthracycline, generally daunorubicin (Cerubidine), at 45 to 60 mg/m^2/d IV bolus. This is called the 3+7 regimen, and it results in a CR rate of 65% to 70%.[44–46]

In two randomized trials, inclusion of thioguanine in this regimen did not result in an improved CR rate.[47,48] The substitution of doxorubicin (Adriamycin, Rubex) for daunorubicin at equally myelotoxic doses resulted in a significantly greater appearance of necrotizing colitis in patients receiving doxorubicin, particularly in patients older than 60 years of age.[44]

The use of idarubicin (Idamycin), 12 to 13 mg/m^2/d for 3 days, instead of daunorubicin, 45 to 50 mg/m^2/d for 3 days, in combination with conventional-dose cytarabine resulted in higher CR rates in three randomized trials.[49–51] In addition, two of these trials reported that significantly fewer patients required two courses before entering CR in the idarubicin arm.[49,50] It is unclear

whether idarubicin and daunorubicin were used at equally myelotoxic doses, because one of the trials reported a significantly longer duration of myelosuppression with idarubicin.[50] Although most investigators agree that idarubicin is potentially superior to daunorubicin, some believe that more experience is needed before substitution of this more costly anthracycline for daunorubicin becomes routine.

The addition of etoposide (VePesid), 75 mg/m^2/d for 7 days, to the 3+7 regimen ("7+3+7") in a randomized trial by the Australian Leukemia Study Group (ALSG) resulted in a similar CR rate. Patients who received 7+3+7 instead of 3+7 had a higher frequency of stomatitis.[52] However, this study suggested that the remission duration of patients receiving 7+3+7 was longer. Longer follow-up is needed to evaluate the role of etoposide in AML therapy, especially because more recent data from the ALSG suggest inferior results with 7+3+7 in a subsequent cohort of patients.[53]

Because cytarabine seems to be a cornerstone in AML therapy, higher doses of cytarabine (HDAC) given in various schedules have been studied intensively. Its role in induction has been examined in two large, randomized trials by the ALSG and the Southwest Oncology Group (SWOG).[54,55] In both trials, no benefit of the HDAC regimen over the 3+7 regimen was observed. However, a follow-up report from the ALSG in which all patients were given the same postremission therapy indicated that the remission duration and the projected percentage of patients disease free at 5 years were significantly better in the HDAC arm.[53] Therefore, dismissal of HDAC from induction therapy seems premature at this time. Representative studies used in remission induction are summarized in Table 1.

Postremission Therapy

Evidence that postremission therapy in AML is needed comes from two randomized trials in which patients entering CR were assigned to either observation alone or low-dose cytarabine plus thioguanine.[56,57] Despite the modest doses of active drugs used and the short duration of therapy, prolonged remission duration in the treatment arm was observed in both trials.

The debate over what represents the best approach for postremission therapy continues. Strategies include maintenance therapy using doses lower than those used during induction, consolidation by repeating the induction regimen, intensification with a dose-intensified schedule of the drugs used during induction, or ablative therapy with allogeneic or autologous bone marrow transplantation (BMT).

TABLE 1

Representative Randomized Trials Addressing the Question of "The Best Induction Regimen" in AML

Source	Regimen	N	CR rate	Comments
Omura et al[47] 1982	"3+7" vs DAT	396	52% 50%	
				Thioguanine adds no benefit to "3+7"
Preisler et al[48] 1987	"3+7" vs DAT	427	53% 57%	
Yates et al[44] 1982	"3 dauno+7" "3 doxo+7"	440	60% 48%	Daunorubicin is superior to doxorubicin More enterocolitis with doxorubicin
Berman et al[49] 1991	"3 ida+7" "3 dauno+7"	120	80% 58%	
Wiernik et al[50] 1992	"3 ida+7" "3 dauno+7"	208	70% 59%	Idarubicin is a superior anthracycline Less patients required two courses to achieve CR with idarubicin in 2 studies[49,50]
Vogler et al[51] 1992	"3 ida+7" "3 dauno+7"	218	71% 58%	Duration of myelosuppression is longer with idarubicin
Bishop et al[52] 1991	"7VP+3+7" "3+7"	264	59% 56%	Etoposide does not improve CR rate, but increases CR duration. It results in more stomatitis. It does not enhance survival.
Bishop et al[53] 1994	HDAC+3+7VP" "7VP+3+7"	301	71% 74%	HDAC is not better for induction CR duration longer with HDAC
Weick et al[55] 1992	HDAC+3 dauno "3+7"	639	54% (< 50 y) 45% (> 50 y) 59% (< 50 y) 54% (> 50 y)	HDAC worse in patients 50 to 64 years of age

"3+7" = daunorubicin 45–50 mg/m2/d days 1–3 IV bolus + cytarabine 100[33–35,40] or 200[38,41] mg/m2/d CI days 1–7, DAT = "3+7" + thioguanine 100 mg/m2 orally twice daily for 5–7 days, dauno = daunorubicin, doxo = doxorubicin 30 mg/m2/d days 1–3 IV bolus, HDAC = 2 g/m2 every 12 hours × 8 doses,[39] or 2 g/m2 every 12 hours × 12 doses,[41] ida = idarubicin 12[14,16] or 13[15] mg/m2/d days 1–3 IV bolus, N = total number of patients evaluable in both arms, VP = etoposide 75 mg/m2/d days 1–7.

Even more controversial is the necessary duration of therapy. There has been no demonstrated advantage to continuing postremission therapy for more than one year compared with shorter lengths of time.[48,58] Most investigators administer two to four courses of chemotherapy in CR. Representative studies addressing the best postremission therapies are presented in Table 2.

Consolidation and Intensification

In a randomized trial by the Eastern Cooperative Oncology Group (ECOG), 283 patients entered CR after receiving cytarabine/daunorubicin/thioguanine (DAT). They then received either two courses of DAT as consolidation followed by 24 months of maintenance or the same maintenance regimen alone. This trial showed that the CR duration was significantly longer in the consolidation arm.[59] These results, with the CALGB observation of

similar disease-free survival in patients receiving 8 vs 36 months of maintenance as the only postremission therapy,[48] suggest that the use of higher doses for shorter periods postremission is superior to lengthy maintenance.

With this as a background, intensification was tested mostly with higher doses of cytarabine, the key drug in AML therapy. In a CALGB trial, 596 patients in CR were randomized to receive four courses of cytarabine at 100 mg/m2/d for 5 days by continuous infusion, 400 mg/m2/d for 5 days by continuous infusion, or 3 g/m2 every 12 hours twice daily every other day for six doses. After a median follow-up of 52 months, the 4-year CCR rate was significantly higher in the HDAC arm only in patients younger than 60 years of age.[45]

Similarly, in an ECOG trial, patients in CR were randomized to receive either HDAC plus amsacrine or

TABLE 2

Representative Randomized Trials Addressing the Question of "The Best Postremission Therapy"

Source	Induction therapy	CR rate	Postremission therapy	Number in CR	Median CR duration (months)	Number of patients remaining in CR	Comments
Cassileth et al[56] 1988	DAT	64%	Cytarabine, thioguanine vs no treatment	51	8.0 4.0	22% at 1 yr < 5%	Some maintenance is better than none
Embury et al[57] 1977	DAT	?	Cytarabine, thioguanine vs no treatment	26	10.3 6.7	30% at 1 yr 0	
Preisler et al[48] 1987	"3+7", DAT, or "3+10"	56%	DATOP for 8 mo vs DATOP for 36 mo	151	9.9 16.3	39% at 2 yr 39% at 2 yr	8 mo maintenance is equivalent to 36 mo
Cassileth et al[59] 1984	DAT	65%	DAT × 2 + maintenance for 24 mo vs no DAT + same maintenance	283	9.2 vs 7.8	28% at 2 yr 14% at 2 yr	Consolidation improves DFS
Mayer et al[45] 1994	"3+7"	64%	Cytarabine 100 mg/m²/d d1–5 CI	596		24% at 4 yr	HDAC improves DFS in intensification
			Cytarabine 400 mg/m²/d days 1–5 CI		29%		Effect varied by karyotype {inv (16) and t(8;21) benefit more from HDAC
			HDAC 3 g/m² every 12 hours every other day × 6 doses			44%	Benefit was limited to patients < age 60
Cassileth et al 1992[60]	DAT		Cytarabine, thioguanine × 24 mo	143		15% at 2 yr	HDAC consolidation is superior
			HDAC 3 g/m² every 12 hours every other day × 12 doses			28%	AMSA adds toxicity (12% toxic deaths in patients < age 60)

AMSA = m-amsacrine, CI = continuous infusion, DAT = "3+7" + thioguanine 100 mg/m² orally twice daily for 5–7 days, DATOP = daunorubicin, cytarabine, thioguanine, vincristine, prednisone, DFS = disease-free survival, HDAC = 2 g/m² every 12 hours × 8 doses,[39] or 2 g/m² every 12 hours × 12 doses,[41] "3+7" = daunorubicin 45–50 mg/m²/d days 1–3 IV bolus + cytarabine 100[33–35,40] or 200[38,41] mg/m²/d CI days 1–7.

conventional doses of cytarabine plus thioguanine.[60] The 2-year CCR rate was significantly higher in the HDAC arm. However, the death rate caused by the toxic effects of HDAC plus amsacrine intensification was very high (12% in patients younger than 60 years), suggesting that the addition of amsacrine to HDAC during intensification confers more harm than benefit.

Bone Marrow Transplantation

High-dose ablative chemotherapy with BMT support can be considered another form of postremission intensification. In addition to its ability to eliminate residual leukemic cells through its dose-intensified schedule, this schedule offers the presumed immune-mediated antileu-

kemic effect whereby donor lymphoid cells recognize and eradicate leukemic cells (the graft-vs-leukemia effect). Its usefulness in AML therapy, however, has been hampered by the multiple prerequisites needed for patients to be eligible. They include younger age, good performance status, normal organ function, absence of other comorbid conditions, and availability of HLA-matched siblings for allogeneic BMT. Most studies also require patients to be in the first CR after induction chemotherapy. These criteria, when applied to all patients with AML seen at two large centers, were met in only 6.2% to 8.6% of patients.[61,62]

This extreme preselection for BMT results in a group of patients who represent the best responders to standard chemotherapy and, thus, makes comparison between BMT and standard chemotherapy for patients in first CR very difficult. Moreover, event-free survival time in most BMT reports typically is calculated from the time the preparative regimen is started rather than from the time of CR. Therefore, patients who relapse very early, who, by definition, have more resistant disease or patients who die or have infectious complications while being screened for BMT are not included in the transplantation registries.

Allowing for these considerations, several prospective trials were undertaken to attempt to compare allogeneic BMT with postremission chemotherapy in patients in first CR.[60,63–70] Although all trials reported a greatly diminished likelihood of relapse in the transplant cohort, most studies[60,63–67] indicate that the increased treatment-related mortality rate in patients who underwent BMT results in similar or statistically insignificant differences in event-free and overall survival rates in the two groups.

The role of autologous BMT in first CR has been explored primarily by European centers. Advantages of this modality over allogeneic BMT include its applicability to older patients and use of unmatched donors. Disadvantages include the lack of the presumed benefit from the graft-vs-leukemia effect and the possible contamination of the harvested marrow with residual leukemic cells. The latter problem has been dealt with by treating the stored marrow with chemotherapeutic agents or antileukemic monoclonal antibodies (ie, purging).[71–74] Trials directly comparing autologous with allogeneic BMT found either a lower relapse rate and a longer disease-free survival rate with allogeneic BMT when purging was not used[69,75,76] or a similar disease-free survival rate and relapse rate when purging was used.[77] Comparisons between autologous BMT and intensive chemotherapy, in two small studies, revealed similar disease-free survival and relapse rates.[69,75]

A recent report compared patients assigned to undergo allogeneic BMT (160 patients) with patients randomized to receive either unpurged autologous BMT or intensive chemotherapy (254 patients) in first CR.[70] In an intention-to-treat analysis, relapse rates with allogeneic BMT, autologous BMT, and chemotherapy were 57%, 41%, and 24%, respectively. Disease-free survival rates in the two transplant arms were similar and were longer than those seen with chemotherapy. The overall survival rate, however, was similar in all three groups, because relapses after chemotherapy were salvaged with transplantation.

Therapy for Relapsed or Refractory AML

Most patients with newly diagnosed AML who achieve a complete remission later experience a relapse of the disease and die. Approximately 5% of all patients who are in first relapse or who were refractory to initial induction therapy and 15% of such patients who achieve a second CR are expected to be alive at 5 years.[78] The likelihood of achieving a second CR is heavily dependent on the duration of the first CR.[78–80] The CR rate in patients refractory to initial therapy or with a first CR shorter than 6 to 12 months is approximately 20%, compared with a CR rate of 60% in patients with a longer first CR.

The treatment of choice for patients with relapsed AML who are younger than 50 years of age is allogeneic BMT.[78] Patients who are not eligible for allogeneic BMT should receive investigational therapy if their first CR is shorter than one year or an induction regimen similar to that used initially if their first CR is longer than one year. Relapses after allogeneic BMT in first or second CR can be treated with a second allogeneic BMT[81] or an infusion of donor buffy coat or granulocyte-colony stimulating factor, which presumably stimulates the graft-vs-leukemia effect.[82]

Therapy for APL

The distinguishing features of APL (FAB Working Group M3) are as follows: younger median age of patients at presentation,[83] frequent presentation with leukopenia or pancytopenia,[84] life-threatening bleeding diathesis seen at presentation or relapse attributed to DIC or primary fibrinolysis,[10] an almost invariable association with t(15;17) detected either by banded cytogenetics or polymerase chain reaction,[21,85] achievement of CR without the obligatory chemotherapy-induced marrow aplasia,[86,87] increased sensitivity to anthracycline antibiotics,[88–92] and response to the differentiation agent ATRA in its oral[31–35] or liposomally encapsulated[93] form.

Complete response rates of 68% to 80% and in one study,[92] a CR duration of 24 months were observed in patients with APL treated with single-agent daunorubicin[89,92] or idarubicin.[88,91] Regimens including cytarabine in addition to anthracyclines did not result in higher CR rates or longer CR duration.[90,94–96] With chemotherapy, high promyelocyte or blast counts may persist in the marrow on day 21. However, further improvement to complete remission can be expected[86,87] unless DIC persists or recurs. With the use of ATRA, CR rates over 90% in otherwise untreated patients were observed.[35] In addition, coagulopathy appears to resolve more rapidly with ATRA than with chemotherapy.[31–34] ATRA generally is given at 45 mg/m^2/d until CR is achieved (average, 40 days). Despite the high CR rates achieved with ATRA, remissions maintained with ATRA alone have been brief,[35] and the administration of anthracycline-based chemotherapy is necessary. In a randomized trial in France, ATRA and chemotherapy (daunorubicin plus cytarabine) added either in CR or when leukocytosis developed during induction resulted in lower relapse and longer disease-free survival rates than those seen when chemotherapy alone was used for induction and maintenance.[97,98]

Induction therapy with ATRA can be complicated by two potentially life-threatening side effects: hyperleukocytosis and retinoic acid syndrome. Hyperleukocytosis, initially reported by the French group,[99] can lead to pulmonary and CNS toxicity. This can be controlled effectively by the early initiation of chemotherapy.[97,98] The second life-threatening side effect, retinoic acid syndrome, is seen in up to 25% of patients.[100] This is a constellation of findings that develop between days 2 and 28 of treatment. The syndrome is characterized by fever, respiratory distress, pulmonary infiltrates, pleuropericardial effusion, edema, and hypotension. Concomitant leukocytosis is common but not uniformly seen. The discontinuation of ATRA and treatment with high-dose steroids are necessary when severe symptoms are seen,[100] whereas low-dose steroid treatment (dexamethasone, 10 mg twice daily for 3 days) without discontinuation of ATRA is usually adequate if started at the earliest indication[30] of such side effects.

REFERENCES

1. Leukemia Research Fund: Leukemia and Lymphoma: Data collection study 1984–1988. London, Leukemia Research Fund, 1990.

2. National Cancer Institute: 1987 Annual cancer statistics review. NIH publication no. 88-2789. Washington, DC, US Department of Health and Human Services, 1988.

3. The Fourth International Workshop on Chromosomes in Leukemia: A prospective study of acute nonlymphocytic leukemia. Cancer Genet Cytogenet 11:251–252, 1984.

4. Yunis JJ, Brunning RD, Howe RD, et al: High-resolution chromosome as an independent prognostic indicator in adult acute nonlymphocytic leukemia. N Engl J Med 311:812–818, 1984.

5. Keating MJ, Smith T, Kantarjian H, et al: Cytogenetic pattern in acute myelogenous leukemia: A major reproducible determinant of outcome. Leukemia 2:403–412, 1988.

6. Ghaddar H, Plunkett W, Kantarjian H, et al: Long-term results following treatment of newly diagnosed acute myelogenous leukemia with continuous-infusion high-dose cytosine arabinoside. Leukemia 8:1269–1274, 1994.

7. Bloomfield CD, Lawrence D, Arthur DC, et al: Curative impact of intensification with high-dose cytarabine in acute myeloid leukemia varies by cytogenetic group. Blood 84:111a, 1994.

8. Arthur DC, Berger R, Golomb HM, et al: The clinical significance of karyotype in acute myelogenous leukemia. Cancer Genet Cytogenet 40:203–216, 1989.

9. Schiffer CA, Lee EJ, Takafumi T, et al: Prognostic impact of cytogenetic abnormalities in patients with de novo acute nonlymphocytic leukemia. Blood 73:263–270, 1989.

10. Tallman MS, Kwaan HC: Reassessing the hemostatic disorder associated with acute promyelocytic leukemia. Blood 79:543–553, 1992.

11. Bennett JM, Catovsky D, Daniel MT, et al: Proposed revised criteria for the classification of acute myeloid leukemia. Ann Intern Med 103:620–625, 1985.

12. Stass SA, Pui CH, Melvin S, et al: Sudan black B positive acute lymphoblastic leukemia. Br J Haematol 57:413–421, 1984.

13. Bennett JM, Catovsky D, Daniel MT, et al: A variant form of hypergranular promyelocytic leukemia. Ann Intern Med 92:261–280, 1980.

14. Golomb HM, Rowley JD, Vardiman JW, et al: Microgranular acute promyelocytic leukemia: A distinct clinical, ultrastructural, and cytogenetic entity. Blood 55:253–259, 1980.

15. Greaves MF, Sieff C, Edwards PAW: Monoclonal antiglycophorin as a probe for erythroleukemias. Blood 61:645–651, 1983.

16. Kojima S, Mutsuyama T, Sato T, et al: Down's syndrome and acute leukemia in children: An analysis of phenotype by use of monoclonal antibodies and electron microscopic platelet peroxidase reaction. Blood 76:2348–2353, 1990.

17. Bennett JM, Catovsky D, Daniel MT, et al: Criteria for the diagnosis of acute leukemia of megakaryocytic lineage (M7). Ann Intern Med 103:460–462, 1985.

18. Bennett JM, Catovsky D, Daniel MT, et al: Proposal for the recognition of minimally differentiated acute myeloid leukemia (AML-M0). Br J Haematol 78:325–329, 1991.

19. Blood, in Jandl JH (ed): Textbook of Haematology. Boston, Little Brown & Co, 1987.

20. Estey EH, Keating MJ, Dixon DO, et al: Karyotype is prognostically more important than FAB system's distinction between myelodysplastic syndrome and acute myelogenous leukemia. Hematol Pathol 1:203–208, 1987.

21. Larson R, Kondo K, Vardiman JW, et al: Evidence of a 15;17 translocation in every patient with acute promyelocytic leukemia. Am J Med 76:827–841, 1984.

22. Larson RA, Williams SF, Le Beau MM, et al: Acute myelomonocytic leukemia with abnormal eosinophils and inv(16) or t(16;16) has a favorable prognosis. Blood 68:1242–1249, 1986.

23. Holmes R, Keating MJ, Cork A, et al: A unique pattern of central nervous system leukemia in acute myelomonocytic leukemia associated with inv(16)(p13q22). Blood 65:1071–1078, 1985.

24. Sandberg AA: The Chromosomes in Human Cancer and Leukemia, 2nd ed. New York, Elsevier, 1990.

25. Olopade OI, Thangavelu MT, Larson RA, et al: Clinical, morphologic, and cytogenetic characteristics of 26 patients with acute erythroblastic leukemia. Blood 11:2873–2882, 1992.

26. Marlton P, Claxton DF, Liu P, et al: Molecular characterization of 16p deletions associated with inversion 16 defines the critical fusion for leukemogenesis. Blood 85:772–779, 1995.

27. de The H, Chomienne C, Lanotte M, et al: The t(15;17) translocation of acute promyelocytic leukemia fuses the retinoic acid receptor gamma gene to a novel transcribed locus. Nature 347:558–561, 1990.

28. Rowley JD: Recurring chromosome abnormalities in leukemia and lymphoma. Semin Hematol 27:122–136, 1990.

29. Yunis JJ: Recurrent chromosomal defects are found in most patients with acute nonlymphocytic leukemia. Cancer Genet Cytogenet 11:125–137, 1984.

30. Tallman MS, Rowe JM: Acute promyelocytic leukemia: A paradigm for differentiation therapy with retinoic acid. Blood Rev 8:70–78, 1994.

31. Huang ME, Ye YC, Chen SR: Use of all-transretinoic acid in the treatment of acute promyelocytic leukemia. Blood 72:567–572, 1988.

32. Castaigne S, Chomienne C, Daniel MT, et al: All-transretinoic

acid as differentiation therapy for acute promyelocytic leukemia: I. Clinical results. Blood 76:1704–1709, 1990.

33. Warrell RP, Frankel SR, Miller WH, et al: Differentiation therapy of acute promyelocytic leukemia with tretinoin (all-trans-retinoic acid). N Engl J Med 374:1385–1393, 1991.

34. Chen X, Xue Y, Zang R, et al: A clinical and experimental study of all-trans-retinoic acid-treated acute promyelocytic leukemia patients. Blood 79:1413–1419, 1991.

35. Fenaux P, Le Deley MC, Castaigne S, et al: Effect of all-transretinoic acid in newly diagnosed acute promyelocytic leukemia: Results of a multicenter, randomized trial. Blood 82:3241–3249, 1993.

36. Rowley JD, Golomb HM, Vardiman JW: Nonrandom chromosome abnormalities in acute leukemia and dysmyelopoietic syndromes in patients with previously treated malignant diseases. Blood 58:759–767, 1981.

37. Le Beau MM, Albain KS, Larson RA, et al: Clinical and cytogenetic correlation in 63 patients with therapy-related myelodysplastic syndromes and acute nonlymphocytic leukemia: Further evidence for characteristic abnormalities of chromosomes 5 and 7. J Clin Oncol 4:325–345, 1986.

38. Thirman MJ, Gill HJ, Burnett RC, et al: Rearrangement of the MLL gene in acute lymphoblastic and acute myeloid leukemias with 11q23 chromosomal translocations. N Engl J Med 329:909–914, 1993.

39. Pui C-H, Ribeiro RC, Hancock ML, et al: Acute myeloid leukemia in children treated with epipodophyllotoxins for acute lymphoblastic leukemia. N Engl J Med 325:1682–1687, 1991.

40. Sandoval C, Head DR, Mirro J Jr, et al: Translocation t(9;11)(p21;q23) in pediatric de novo and secondary acute myeloblastic leukemia. Leukemia 6: 513–519, 1992.

41. Cortes J, O'Brien S, Kantarjian H, et al: Abnormalities in the long arm of chromosome 11(11q) in patients with de novo and secondary acute myelogenous leukemias and myelodysplastic syndromes. Leukemia 8:2174–2178, 1994.

42. Knapp W: Leukocyte Typing IV: White Cell Differentiation Antigens. Oxford, Oxford University Press, 1989.

43. Estey EH, Smith TL, Keating MJ, et al: Prediction of survival during induction therapy in patients with newly diagnosed acute myeloblastic leukemia. Leukemia 3:257–263, 1989.

44. Yates J, Glidewell O, Wiernik P, et al: Cytosine arabinoside with daunorubicin or Adriamycin for therapy of acute myelocytic leukemia: A CALGB study. Blood 60:454–462, 1982.

45. Mayer RJ, Davis RB, Schiffer CA, et al: Intensive post-remission chemotherapy in adults with acute myeloid leukemia. N Engl J Med 331:896–903, 1994.

46. Vogler WR, Winton EF, Gordon DS, et al: A randomized comparison of post-remission therapy in acute myelogenous leukemia: A Southeastern Cancer Study Group Trial. Blood 63:1039–1045, 1984.

47. Omura GA, Vogler WR, Lefante J, et al: Treatment of acute myelogenous leukemia: Influence of three induction regimens and maintenance with chemotherapy or BCG immunotherapy. Cancer 49:1530–1536, 1982.

48. Preisler H, Davis RB, Krishner J, et al: Comparison of three remission induction regimens and two postinduction strategies for the treatment of acute nonlymphocytic leukemia: A Cancer and Leukemia Group B study. Blood 69:1441–1449, 1987.

49. Berman E, Heller G, Santorsa J, et al: Results of a randomized trial comparing idarubicin and cytosine arabinoside with daunorubicin and cytosine arabinoside in adult patients with newly diagnosed acute myelogenous leukemia. Blood 77:1666–1674, 1991.

50. Weirnik PH, Banks PLC, Case DC, et al: Cytarabine plus idarubicin or daunorubicin as induction and consolidation therapy for previously untreated adult patients with acute myeloid leukemia. Blood 79:313–319, 1992.

51. Vogler WR, Velez-Garcia E, Weiner RS: A phase III trial comparing idarubicin and daunorubicin in combination with cytarabine in acute myelogenous leukemia: A Southeastern Cancer Study Group study. J Clin Oncol 10:1103–1111, 1992.

52. Bishop JF, Lowethal R, Joshua D, et al: Etoposide in leukemia. Cancer 67:285–291, 1991.

53. Bishop JF, Matthews JP, Young GA, et al: High-dose cytosine arabinoside (ara-C) in induction prolongs remission in acute myeloid leukemia (AML): Updated results of a randomized phase III trial. Blood 84:232a, 1994.

54. Bishop JF, Young GA, Szer J, et al: Randomized trial of high-dose cytosine arabinoside (ara-C) combination in induction of acute myeloid leukemia (AML). Proc Am Soc Clin Oncol 11:849, 1992.

55. Weick J, Kopecky K, Appelbaum F, et al: A randomized investigation of high-dose (HDAC) versus standard dose (SDAC) cytosine arabinoside with daunorubicin (DNR) in patients with acute myelgoenous leukemia. Proc Am Soc Clin Oncol 11:856, 1992.

56. Cassileth PA, Harrington DP, Hines JD, et al: Maintenance chemotherapy prolongs remission duration in adult acute nonlymphocytic leukemia. J Clin Oncol 6:583–587, 1988.

57. Embury SH, Elias L, Heller PH, et al: Remission maintenance therapy in acute myelogenous leukemia. West J Med 126:267–272, 1977.

58. Kantarjian HM, Keating MJ, Walters RS, et al: Early intensification and short-term maintenance chemotherapy does not prolong survival in acute myelogenous leukemia. Cancer 58:1603–1608, 1986.

59. Cassileth PA, Begg CB, Bennett JM, et al: A randomized study of the efficacy of consolidation therapy in adult acute nonlymphocytic leukemia. Blood 63:843–847, 1984.

60. Cassileth PA, Lynch E, Hines JD, et al: Varying intensity of post-remission therapy in acute myeloid leukemia. Blood 79:1924–1930, 1992.

61. Berman E, Little C, Gee T, et al: Reasons that patients with acute myelogenous leukemia do not undergo allogeneic bone marrow transplantation. N Engl J Med 326:156–160, 1992.

62. Gamberi B, Bandini G, Visani G: Acute myeloid leukemia from diagnosis to bone marrow transplantation: Experience from a single center. Bone Marrow Transplant 14:69–72, 1994.

63. Schiller GJ, Nimer SD, Territo C, et al: Bone marrow transplantation versus high-dose cytarabine-based consolidation chemotherapy for acute myelogenous leukemia in first remission. J Clin Oncol 10:41–46, 1992.

64. Champlin RF, Ho WG, Gale RP, et al: Treatment of acute myelogenous leukemia: A prospective controlled trial of bone marrow transplantation versus consolidation chemotherapy. Ann Intern Med 102:285–291, 1985.

65. Appelbaum FR, Fisher LD, Thomas ED: Chemotherapy vs marrow transplantation for adults with acute nonlymphocytic leukemia: A five-year follow-up. Blood 72:179–184, 1988.

66. Horousseau JL, Milpied N, Briere J, et al: Double intensive consolidation chemotherapy in adult acute myeloid leukemia. J Clin Oncol 9:1432–1437, 1991.

67. Conde E, Iriondo A, Rayon C, et al: Allogeneic bone marrow transplantation versus intensification chemotherapy for acute myeloid leukemia in first remission: A prospective, controlled trial. Br J Haematol 68:219–226, 1988.

68. Zander AR, Keating M, Dicke K, et al: A comparison of marrow transplantation with chemotherapy for adults with acute leukemia of poor prognosis in first complete remission. J Clin Oncol 6:1548–1557, 1988.

69. Reiffers J, Gaspard MH, Maraninchi D, et al: Comparison of

allogenic or autologous bone marrow transplantation and chemotherapy in patients with acute myeloid leukemia in first remission: A prospective controlled trial. Br J Haematol 72:57–63, 1989.

70. Zittoun RA, Mandelli F, Willemze R, et al: Autologous or allogeneic bone marrow transplantation compared with intensive chemotherapy in acute myelogenous leukemia. N Engl J Med 332:217–223, 1995.

71. Yeager AH, Kaizer H, Santos GW, et al: Autologous bone marrow transplantation in patients with acute nonlymphocytic leukemia, using ex vivo marrow treatment with 4-hydroperoxycyclophosphamide. N Engl J Med 315:141–147, 1986.

72. Ball ED, Mills LE, Cornwall GG III, et al: Autologous bone marrow transplantation for acute myeloid leukemia using monoclonal antibody-purged bone marrow. Blood 75:1199–1206, 1990.

73. Robertson MJ, Soeffer RJ, Freedman AS, et al: Human bone marrow depleted of CD33-positive cells mediates delayed but durable reconstitution of hematopoiesis: Clinical trial of MY9 monoclonal antibody-purged autografts for the treatment of acute myeloid leukemia. Blood 79:2229–2236, 1992.

74. Gorin NC, Labopin M, Meloni G, et al: Autologous bone marrow transplantation for acute myeloblastic leukemia in Europe: Further evidence of the role of marrow purging by mafosfamide. Leukemia 5:896–904, 1991.

75. Amadori S, Testi AM, Arico M, et al: Prospective, comparative study of bone marrow transplantation and post-remission chemotherapy for childhood acute myelogenous leukemia. J Clin Oncol 11:1046–1054, 1993.

76. Lowenberg B, Verdovck LJ, Dekker AW, et al: Autologous bone marrow transplantation in acute myeloid leukemia in first remission: Results of a Dutch prospective study. J Clin Oncol 8:287–294, 1990.

77. Cassileth PA, Andersen J, Lazarus HM, et al: Autologous bone marrow transplant in acute myeloid leukemia in first remission. J Clin Oncol 11:314–319, 1993.

78. Keating MJ, Kantarjian H, Smith TL, et al: Response to salvage therapy and survival after relapse in acute myelogenous leukemia. J Clin Oncol 7:1071–1080, 1989.

79. Hiddemann W, Martin WR, Saverland CM, et al: Definition of refractoriness against conventional chemotherapy in acute myeloid leukemia: A proposal based on the results of retreatment by thioguanine, cytosine arabinoside, and daunorubicin (TAD9) in 150 patients with relapse after standardized first line therapy. Leukemia 4:184–188, 1990.

80. Angelov L, Brandevein JM, Baker MA, et al: Results of therapy for acute myeloid leukemia in first relapse. Leuk Lymphoma 6:15–24, 1991.

81. Barrett AJ, Locatelli F, Treleaven JG, et al: Second transplants for leukaemia relapse after bone marrow transplantation: High early mortality but favorable effect of chronic GVHD on continued remission, a report by the EBMT Leukaemia Working Party. Br J Haematol 79:567–574, 1991.

82. Giralt S, Escudier S, Kantarjian H, et al: Preliminary results of treatment with filgrastim for relapse of leukemia and myelodysplasia after allogeneic bone marrow transplantation. N Engl J Med 329:757–761, 1993.

83. Mertelsman R, Thaler HT, To L: Morphological classification, response to therapy and survival in 263 adult patients with acute nonlymphocytic leukemia. Blood 56:773–781, 1980.

84. Collins AJ, Bloomfield CD, Peterson BA, et al: Acute promyelocytic leukemia: Management of the coagulopathy during daunorubicin-prednisone remission induction. Arch Intern Med 138:1677–1680, 1978.

85. Biondi A, Rambaldi A, Alcalay M, et al: RAR-alpha gene rearrangment as a genetic marker for diagnosis and monitoring in acute promyelocytic leukemia. Blood 77:1418–1422, 1991.

86. Kantarjian HM, Keating MJ, McCredie KB, et al: A characteristic pattern of leukemia cell differentiation without cytoreduction during remission induction in acute promyelocytic leukemia. J Clin Oncol 3:793–798, 1985.

87. Stone RM, Maguire M, Goldberg MA, et al: Complete remission in acute promyelocytic leukemia despite persistence of abnormal bone marrow promyelocytes during induction therapy: Experience in 34 patients. Blood 71:690–696, 1988.

88. Avvisati G, Mandelli F, Petti, et al: Idarubicin (4-demethoxy-daunorubicin) as single agent for remission induction of previously untreated acute promyelocytic leukemia: A pilot study of the Italian cooperative group GIMEMA. Eur J Haematol 44:257–260, 1990.

89. Bernard J, Weil M, Boiron M, et al: Acute promyelocytic leukemia: Results of treatment by daunorubicin. Blood 61:489–496, 1973.

90. Rodeghiero F, Avvisati G, Castaman G, et al: Early deaths and anti-hemorrhagic treatments in acute promyelocytic leukemia: A GIMEMA retrospective study in 268 consecutive patients. Blood 75:2112–2117, 1990.

91. Rotoli B, for the GIMEMA Cooperative Group, Italy: The GIMEMA protocol LAP 0389 for the treatment of acute promyelocytic leukemia: Preliminary results (abstract #842). Abstracts of the 24th Congress of the International Society of Haematology, 1992.

92. Sanz MA, Jarque I, Martin G, et al: Acute promyelocytic leukemia: Therapy results and prognostic factors. Cancer 61:7–13, 1988.

93. Estey E, Cabanillas F, Rosenblum M, et al: Phase I and pharmacology study of liposomal (L)-all-trans-retinoic acid (ATRA). Blood 84:380a, 1994.

94. Kantarjian HM, Keating MJ, Walters RS, et al: Acute promyelocytic leukemia: M. D. Anderson Hospital experience. Am J Med 80:789–797, 1986.

95. Cunningham I, Gee TS, Reich LM, et al: Acute promyelocytic leukemia: Treatment results during a decade at Memorial Hospital. Blood 73:1116–1122, 1989.

96. Goldberg MA, Ginsburg D, Mayer RJ, et al: Is heparin administration necessary during induction chemotherapy for patients with acute promyelocytic leukemia? Blood 69:187–191, 1987.

97. Fenaux P, Castaigne S, Dombret H, et al: All-trans-retinoic acid followed by intensive chemotherapy gives a high complete remission rate and may prolong remissions in newly diagnosed acute promyelocytic leukemia: A pilot study of 26 cases. Blood 80:2176–2181, 1992.

98. Fenaux P, Robert MC, Castaigne S, et al: A multicenter trial comparing all-transretinoic acid plus chemotherapy (ATRA+CT) and CT alone in newly diagnosed acute promyelocytic leukemia. Proc Am Soc Clin Oncol 12:300, 1992.

99. Castaigne S, Chomienne C, Fenaux P, et al: Hyperleukocytosis during all-transretinoic acid for acute promyelocytic leukemia. Blood 76:260a, 1990.

100. Frankel SR, Eardley A, Lauwers G, et al: The 'retinoic acid syndrome' in acute promyelocytic leukemia. Ann Intern Med 117:292–296, 1992.

Chronic Lymphocytic Leukemia and Associated Disorders

Luis Fayad, MD, *and* Susan O'Brien, MD

Division of Medicine, The University of Texas M. D. Anderson Cancer Center, Houston, Texas

Chronic lymphocytic leukemia (CLL) is the most common adult leukemia in the Western hemisphere, accounting for 30% of the leukemias in this population. The disease results from a clonal expansion of small B-lymphocytes. CLL always involves the bone marrow and peripheral blood. The disease also can be demonstrated in lymph nodes, liver, and spleen. Bone marrow failure may occur as a late event. Staging systems (Rai and Binet) have been developed that correlate with survival, but there is still significant heterogeneity within subgroups. Cytogenetic and molecular analysis may provide information on disease development and prognosis. New therapeutic modalities such as nucleoside analogs and bone marrow transplantation have improved response rates in CLL and create expectations about potential cure of this disease.

EPIDEMIOLOGY

The incidence varies around the world, being more common in the Western hemisphere; in the United States, CLL constitutes 20% of all leukemias, whereas in Asiatic countries like Japan it accounts for only 2.5%.[1] The incidence is also age dependent,[2] with an increase from 5.2 per 100,000 persons older than 50 years to 30.4 per 100,000 in people older than 80.[3] The male to female ratio is 2:1. An increase in the incidence of CLL in the last 50 years was suggested by a recent study in a Minnesota population,[4] but was considered due to improved diagnostic techniques.[5]

ETIOLOGY

B-cell CLL (B-CLL) is the only leukemia that has not been associated with radiation exposure, chemicals or drugs.[6–8] On the other hand, an increased risk in relatives of patients with CLL has been found[9–15] that is between twofold to sevenfold higher than in a control population.[11,16] An increase in other lymphoid malignancies has been found as well.[12] Although the leukemic cells of family members sometimes express the same immunoglobulin (Ig) heavy-chain variable region gene,[17] the cells of each patient have different Ig heavy-chain variable region genes.[13,17,18]

Mitogens or phorbol myristate-acetate (PHA) can induce proliferation of B-CLL cells in vitro; with the use of G-banding and Q-banding techniques, almost 50% of the leukemic cells of CLL patients have been found to have clonal chromosomal abnormalities.[19–22] The most common cytogenetic abnormalities involve chromosomes 12, 13, and 14. Abnormalities involving chromosomes 6 and 11 are found less often.

Chromosome 12 Anomalies

The most common anomaly associated with CLL is trisomy 12,[20,23–25] which was found in 67 (17%) of 391 evaluable CLL patients in a study by Juliusson et al.[24] This trisomy can be found as the only anomaly in B-CLL but is often found with other chromosomal abnormalities. The presence of a complex karyotype may indicate clonal evolution.[26,27] Trisomy 12 may be also detected by using fluorescent in situ hybridization (FISH).[28–31] Escudier et al found that FISH is more sensitive in detecting this chromosomal abnormality than conventional cytogenetics,[30] but others did not demonstrate better sensitivity by FISH.[28] The significance of trisomy 12 as regards prognosis in B-CLL is controversial; some authors report a poor prognosis and advanced disease in patients with the anomaly,[27,30] or the presence of lymphocytes with a prolymphocytic-like morphology.[29] Other authors have not found a worse prognosis with this abnormally.[26,29]

Chromosome 13 Anomalies

Structural anomalies of chromosome 13 were found in 51 (13%) of 391 patients in the study done by Juliusson et al,[24] some of them involving the site of the retinoblastoma 1 gene (*RB1* gene). This anomaly confers a better outcome than trisomy 12 abnormalities, but is worse than diploid cytogenetics.[24]

Chromosome 14 Anomalies

Structural anomalies of chromosome 14 were found in 41 (10.5%) of 391 patients by Juliusson and colleagues.[24] Ten of those patients had t(11;14)(q13;q32). This translocation involved rearrangement of a proto-oncogene called *BCL-1* for B-cell leukemia-1,[46,47] and called later *PRAD1*, a proto-oncogene involved in the pathogenesis of mantle-cell lymphoma. B-CLL cases with *BCL-1*

TABLE 1

Diagnosis Criteria for Chronic Lymphocytic Leukemia

NCI WORKING GROUP

Lymphocytes > 5 × 10³/μL
"Atypical" cells < 55%
Duration of lymphocytosis ≥ 2 months
Bone marrow lymphocytes ≥ 30%

IWCLL

Lymphocytes > 10 × 10³/μL and either
    B phenotype *or*
    bone marrow involvement
Lymphocytes < 10 × 10³/μL and both bone marrow
    involvement + B phenotype
    Bone marrow lymphocytes > 30%

IWCLL = International Workshop on Chronic Lymphocytic Leukemia,
NCI = National Cancer Institute

rearrangement may represent the leukemic phase of mantle-cell lymphoma. This translocation involves chromosome 14 at band q32 that includes the Ig heavy chain locus. Other less frequent chromosomal anomalies include t(14;18)(q32;q21), t(14;19)(q32;q13.1) with high expression of the BCL-2 protein in the first case and expression of the proto-oncogene *BCL-3*. Most studies agree on the poor prognosis of either a 14q+ anomaly[24,34] or a complex chromosomal abnormality.[24,34]

Surface Antigen Phenotype

Freedman et al[35] studied the immunophenotype of 100 B-CLL patients and found that all cases expressed Ia, CD19, and CD20 (pan B-cell antigens). CD5, an antigen present on mature T-cells, was found in 95% of cases. In 90% of cases, CLL cells expressed the Epstein-Barr Virus (EBV) and CD21 (C3d complement) receptors. Surface immunoglobulin expression (sIg) was weakly expressed in 90% of CLL cases. The most common isotype was IgM plus IgD, seen in half of the patients, followed by IgM alone. The light chains were either κ or λ type. Expression of sIg is important for assessing the clonality of a lymphoid population. In addition, clonality can be proved by the detection of a specific cytogenetic abnormality and rearrangement of Ig heavy and light chains.

Cell of Origin

B-CLL cells may derive from a small subclone of normal, activated B-cells that develop clonal expansion by a mechanism that is not well understood. Those cells express the antigens described above. CD5+ B-cells are found in the periphery of the germinal centers of lymph nodes in the adult.

Clinical Characteristics and Laboratory Findings

At diagnosis, most patients are older than 60 years old, with more than 90% over 50 years. The diagnosis of CLL is often made incidentally, when an elevated absolute lymphocyte count (ALC) is found at the time of a complete blood count. Other patients may present with autoimmune disorders such as autoimmune hemolytic anemia (AHA), or autoimmune thrombocytopenia (ATP). Presenting symptoms may include infections, fatigue, malaise, or, rarely, B-symptoms. Physical examination may reveal cervical, axillary, or inguinal lymphadenopathy. Splenomegaly and hepatomegaly are also common.

Laboratory findings invariably show lymphocytosis. The ALC can range from 5 × 10³ to 500 × 10³/μL. During

TABLE 2

Immunophenotype of B-CLL and Other B-cell Related Disorders

	CD19/ CD20	SIg	CD5	CD10	CD11c	FMC7	CD25	TRAP	CD23
B-CLL	+ + +	weak	+ + +	−	−	±	+ +	−	+ + +
B-PLL	+ + +	strong	±	±	−	+ + +	−	−	−
Mantle-cell lymphoma	+ + +	strong	+	−	−	+ +	−	−	−
Follicular lymphoma	+ + +	strong	−	+ +	−	+ +	−	−	±
Hairy-cell leukemia	+ + +	strong	−	−	+ +	+ + +	+ + +	+ + +	−
Splenic lymphoma of villous lymphocytes	+ + +	strong	−	−	−	+ + +	+	−	−

CLL = chronic lymphocytic leukemia, PLL = prolymphocytic leukemia, SIg = surface immunoglobulin, TRAP = tartrate-resistant acid phosphatase smear preparation, abnormal lymphocytes are frequently damaged resulting in "smudge" cells. The degree of infiltration of the bone marrow varies between 30% and 99%, with a diffuse or nodular pattern of infiltration. The number of erythroid, myeloid and megakaryocytic precursors may be normal or decreased. Patients can present with anemia due to bone marrow infiltration or AHA. Pure red-cell aplasia has been described in 1% to 6% of the patients.[36]

Other features include thrombocytopenia due to hypersplenism, bone marrow failure or on an autoimmune basis. Patients may develop panhypogammaglobulinemia that progresses in frequency and severity with advancing disease.[37] Monoclonal gammopathy is also seen and the frequency varies according to the method used for diagnosis. Other laboratory findings include an increase in beta$_2$-microglobulin, and rarely serum lactate dehydrogenase (LDH) and hypercalcemia.

DIAGNOSIS

Diagnostic criteria were proposed by the International Workshop on Chronic Lymphocytic Leukemia (IWCLL) in 1989 and are summarized in Table 1.[38] An ALC of $10 \times 10^3/\mu$L or higher sustained for at least 4 weeks and involvement of 30% or more of the bone marrow with lymphocytes or evidence of clonality by immunophenotype is required. The National Cancer Institute-sponsored CLL Working Group (NCIWG) only required an ALC of $5 \times 10^3/\mu$L when the IWCLL bone marrow and clonality criteria are met.[39]

Morphologically, the lymphocytes are small and mature in appearance. When the number of larger, prolymphocyte-like cells is greater than 10% but less than 55% this has been considered a variant between CLL and prolymphocytic leukemia (PLL) and classified by the French-American-British group[40] and the NCIWG[39] as CLL/PLL. If more than 55% of the lymphocytes are prolymphocytes, the diagnosis is PLL.

Differential Diagnosis

Clinical, morphologic, immunophenotypic and cytogenetic methods help to make the differential diagnosis between B-CLL and and other diseases such as T-cell CLL (T-CLL), leukemic phase of non-Hodgkin's lymphoma (mantle cell, follicular and others), other mature B-cell lymphoproliferative disorders such as PLL, hairy-cell leukemia (HCL) and its variants, splenic lymphoma with villous lymphocytes (SLVL) and Waldenström's macroglobulinemia (WM) that can be confused with CLL. Table 2 summarizes the immunophenotypes in the differential diagnosis of these disorders.

TABLE 3

Rai Staging System for Chronic Lymphocytic Leukemia

Stage	Modified stage	Description	Median survival (years)
0	Low risk	Lymphocytosis only	> 10
I	Intermediate risk	Lymphocytosis and lymphadenopathy	> 8
2	Intermediate risk	Lymphocytosis and splenomegaly with and without lymphadenopathy	6
3	High risk	Lymphocytosis and anemia (hemoglobin < 11g/dL), with or without lymph-adenopathy or hepato-splenomegaly	2
4	High risk	Lymphocytosis and thrombocytopenia (platelets < 100 ×10³/µL), with or without anemia, lympha-denopathy or hepato-splenomegaly	2

TABLE 4

Binet Staging System for Chronic Lymphocytic Leukemia

Stage	Description	Median survival (years)
A	Two or fewer lymphoid-bearing areas[a]	> 10
B	Three or more lymphoid-bearing areas	6
C	Presence of anemia (hemoglobin < 10 g/dL) or thrombocytopenia (platelets < 100 × 10³/µL)	2

[a] Lymphoid-bearing areas include palpable cervical, axillary, or inguinofemoral lymph nodes plus the spleen and liver.

STAGING AND PROGNOSIS

The Rai[41] and Binet[42] are the most commonly used staging systems for CLL (Tables 3 and 4). Both systems evaluate the tumor burden by lymphadenopathy, hepatomegaly, splenomegaly, and bone marrow failure by anemia and thrombocytopenia. The original Rai system included five stages from 0 to 4; this has been modified to 3 stages by defining Rai stage 0 as low-risk, joining stages 1 with 2 to form an intermediate-risk group, and

TABLE 5

National Cancer Institute Response Criteria for Chronic Lymphocytic Leukemia

- Complete response

  Absence of lymphadenopathy, hepatosplenomegaly, and constitutional symptoms; normalization of CBC (neutrophils > 1.5 × 10³/μL, platelets > 100 × 10³/μL, hemoglobin > 11g/dL, lymphocytes < 4 × 10³/μL); bone marrow biopsy shows normal cellularity; lymphocytes < 30%; nodules and infiltrates in the bone marrow are permitted. Duration of response > 2 months.

- Partial response

  At least 50% reduction in absolute blood lymphocyte count and in lymphadenopathy and/or 50% reduction in splenomegaly or hepatomegaly; neutrophils > 1.5 × 10³/μL or 50% improvement over baseline; platelets > 100 × 10³/μL or 50% improvement over baseline; hemoglobin > 11g/dL (not supported by transfusions) or 50% over baseline. Duration of response: > 2 months.

- Stable disease

  No complete or partial response, or no progression.

- Progressive disease

  At least one of the following: > 50% increase in size of at least two lymph nodes, or new palpable lymph nodes; ≥ 50% increase in hepatomegaly or splenomegaly or appearance if previously absent; transformation to a more aggressive histology (Richter or PLL); > 50% increase of absolute peripheral blood lymphocyte count.

Adapted, with permission, from Cheson BD, Bennett JM, Rai KR: Am J Hematol 29:152–163, 1988.

stages 3 with 4 to be a high-risk group, with a median survival of > 12.5, 7, and 1.5 years for each risk group respectively.[43] The Binet staging system comprises three categories: A, with two or fewer lymphoid-bearing areas (LBA); B, with three or more LBA; and C, with a hemoglobin (Hb) < 10 g/dL and/or thrombocytopenia (100 × 10³ platelets/μL); with a median survival of > 10, 6, and 2 years respectively. Although both systems have correlated with survival in several prospective studies,[44–47] they fail to identify which patients in a given stage will have disease progression.

Several authors have described alternate prognostic factors. Montserrat et al[48] showed that patients with a lymphocyte doubling time (LDT) of less than 12 months had a median survival, independent of the stage, of 5 years, and, if the LDT was more than 12 months, the survival was more than 12 years. Other authors have confirmed this finding.[49] Expression of the proliferating cell nuclear antigen (PCNA), an estimate of proliferative

potential, has been found to correlate with the LDT.[50] Rozman et al[51] and Geisler et al[52] demonstrated that diffuse pattern of bone marrow infiltration was an independent poor prognostic factor in CLL.

The term "smoldering CLL" has been proposed for a subgroup of patients who belong to Binet stage A, with a lymphocyte count < 30 × 10³/μL, an LDT > 12 months, Hb level > 13g/dL, and a nondiffuse pattern (interstitial, nodular, and mixed) of the bone marrow.[53] The risk of progression in 3 years for this group was 5%, compared with 32% in other patients for stage A.

Monoallelic *p53* gene deletion has been found to be a strong adverse prognostic factor for survival and response to purine analogs in CLL patients.[53a] Gaidano et al[53b] reported mutations of *p53* in six (15%) of 40 cases of CLL and in three (43%) of seven patients with Richter's transformation. El Rouby and colleagues[53c] found *p53* gene mutations in 15% of 53 patients with CLL. While 27 (93%) of 29 treated patients without *p53* mutations responded to therapy, only 1 (14%) of 7 treated patients with *p53* mutations achieved a partial remission.

Other parameters with prognostic relevance in CLL patients are age and sex,[44,54,55] lymphocyte count,[53,56] serum LDH,[44] serum albumin,[57] free serum CD23 level,[58] presence of prolymphocytes,[59] absolute number of prolymphocytes > 15 × 10³/μL,[59] presence of myelomonocytic antigens on the lymphocytes,[60] karyotype,[24,61] beta$_2$-microglobulin,[62] absolute number of white blood cells in S phase in the peripheral blood,[63] and serum level of interleukin-2 (IL-2) receptors and CD8 antigen.[64,65]

TREATMENT

The time at which treatment should be initiated in a potentially indolent disease is unclear. De Rossi et al[66] reported a retrospective study of 133 patients with a median age of 46 years old and Rai stage 0 disease. They had a 60% likelihood of surviving longer than 10 years. In contrast, older patients had a median survival of 6 to 7 years. Other investigators found a group of patients with survival similar to the general population.[44,53,67,68]

Therefore, the treatment of patients in Rai stage 0 to 1 or Binet A is usually limited to those who present with severe hyperlymphocytosis or who have systemic symptoms such as fever, weight loss, night sweats, bulky disease, recurrent infections, immune mediated complications, LDT < 12 months or with diffuse infiltration of the bone marrow. Most investigators treat patients with Rai stage 3 or 4 or Binet stage C disease.

The National Cancer Institute[39] and the IWCLL[38] have proposed uniform guidelines for response criteria, which are summarized in Tables 5 and 6.

Chlorambucil

A nitrogen mustard derivative, chlorambucil (Leukeran) is the drug most commonly used in CLL. Chlorambucil schedules include 0.1 mg/kg/d, 0.4 to 1 mg/kg every 4 weeks, and 0.4 to 0.6 mg/kg every 2 weeks, alone or with prednisone. The drug is given orally and has excellent gastrointestinal absorption.

Chlorambucil was first used by Galton[69] in 1961, at a dose of 0.03 to 0.3 mg/kg/d for 4 to 8 weeks. He reported that 77% of patients responded to some degree. Other investigators report response rates between 38 and 75%.[70] The variations in response are due to the use of different doses and schedules of administration, the use of corticosteroids in some studies, and different criteria for response.

Two small randomized studies compared daily chlorambucil vs chlorambucil plus prednisone,[71,72] with a statistically significant difference in responses favoring the combination group. The 2-year survival was also better in the combination group but did not achieve statistical significance. Sawitzky et al[71] from the Cancer and Leukemia Group B (CALGB) performed a three-arm study in patients with Rai stage 3 and 4 disease, randomizing between prednisone, prednisone plus daily chlorambucil, or intermittent chlorambucil plus prednisone. He obtained response rates of 11%, 37%, and 47%, respectively.

Jaksic et al treated 181 CLL patients,[73] comparing intermittent chlorambucil plus prednisone vs chlorambucil, 15 mg/d, until remission or dose-limiting toxicity. The response rate was 90% (70% complete response [CR]) for chlorambucil alone vs 50%(31% CR) in the combination group. The total dose of chlorambucil in the daily-dose group was six times higher than in the intermittent group, showing that dose intensity is very important in alkylating agents

The French Cooperative Group in CLL (FCGCLL) randomized 612 patients with Binet stage A CLL to daily-dose chlorambucil or observation alone. The results did not show statistically significant difference in the 5-year survival between groups. In fact, the treatment group had a trend toward shorter survival when the disease progressed and an increased incidence of epithelial cancers.[67]

Almost all patients will become resistant to treatment with chlorambucil. Sulfhydryl groups, glutathione levels, and glutathione-S-transferase activity may be implicated in alkylator resistance.[74–76]

Cyclophosphamide

Cyclophosphamide (Cytoxan, Neosar) is as effective as chlorambucil in the treatment of CLL. Patients who

TABLE 6

International Workshop on Chronic Lymphocytic Leukemia (IWCLL) Response Criteria

- Complete response

  Resolution of lymphadenopathy, hepatosplenomegaly and constitutional symptoms; normalization of CBC (neutrophils > 1.5 × 10³/μL, platelets > 100 × 10³/μL, lymphocytes < 4 × 10³/μL); normalization of bone marrow findings (the presence of focal or nodular infiltrates is compatible with complete response)

- Partial response

  Change from stage C to A or B, or from stage B to A

- Stable disease

  No change in the stage of the disease

- Progressive disease

  Change from stage A to B or C, or from stage B to C

Adapted, with permission, from International Workshop on Chronic Lymphocytic Leukemia. J Clin Pathol 42:567–584, 1989.

TABLE 7

Chemotherapy Regimens for Chronic Lymphocytic Leukemia

Chlorambucil/prednisone
  Chlorambucil, 0.3 mg/kg on days 1–5
  Prednisone 40 mg/m² on days 1–5

COP
  Cyclophosphasmide, 300 mg/m² PO on days 1–5
  Vincristine, 1.4 mg/m² on day 1
  Prednisone, 40 mg/m² on days 1–5

CHOP
  Cyclophosphamide 750 mg/m² IV on day 1
  Vincristine 1.4 mg/m² IV on day 1
  Doxorubicin 25 mg/m³ on day 1
  Prednisone 40 mg/m² PO on days 1–5

Fludarabine
  25 to 30 mg/m²/d IV on days 1–5

Cladribine
  0.1 mg/kg/d IV by continous infusion days 1 to 7

Pentostatin
  4 mg/m² once every week for the first 3 weeks, then every other week for the next 6 weeks, then monthly

do not respond to chlorambucil may respond to cyclophosphamide. The usual dose is 100 mg/d. Other regimens include 500 to 750 mg/m[2] given intravenously (IV) or orally every 3 to 4 weeks.

Combination Chemotherapy

Various combination chemotherapies have been used in patients with CLL. For example, COP (cyclophosphamide, vincristine [Oncovin], and prednisone) has produced a response rate ranging from 44% to 82%.[77–80] In randomized trials, COP was neither better[79,80] nor inferior[81] to chlorambucil plus prednisone. CHOP (COP plus doxorubicin [Adriamycin, Rubex]) obtained better results than COP alone in advanced stages of disease[82,83] and better response rates than chlorambucil plus prednisone.[84,85] No survival differences were observed between patients randomized to CHOP or chlorambucil plus prednisone.[86]

Other combination chemotherapy regimens that have been studied in patients with CLL include M-2 (vincristine, carmustine [BiCNU], cyclophosphamide, doxorubicin, melphalan [Alkeran], and prednisone), CMP (cyclophosphamide, methotrexate, and prednisone), CAP (cyclophosphamide, doxorubicin, and cisplatin [Platinol]), and POACH (cyclophosphamide, doxorubicin, cytarabine, vincristine, and prednisone).[70] Although these regimens induce higher CR rates, they are more toxic and are not clearly better than the chlorambucil plus prednisone combination.[70]

Nucleoside Analogs

The most important nucleoside analogs in the treatment of CLL are fludarabine (Fludara), cladribine (Leustatin), and pentostatin (Nipent).

Fludarabine is the most extensively studied purine analog in CLL, but the agent's exact mechanism of action is unclear. Fludarabine is a fluorinated purine analog, dephosphorylated in the plasma to form 2-fluoro-ara-A,[87,88] which enters the cell by a carrier-mediated transport mechanism and is phosphorylated to 2-fluoro-ara-ATP. This is the form of the drug necessary for its cytotoxic effect. The rate-limiting enzyme in the phosphorylation is deoxycytidine kinase.[88] The accumulation of 2-fluoro-ara-ATP in the cell inhibits DNA synthesis[89] by interference with ribonucleotide reductase and DNA polymerase.

In clinical studies, fludarabine was first used by Grever and colleagues, in 26 previously treated CLL patients, at a dosage of 20 mg/m[2]/d for 5 days. One patient achieved CR, three had excellent partial responses (PR), and 15 had additional evidence of improvement.[90] Keat-

ing et al[91] used fludarabine at 25 to 30 mg/m[2]/d for 5 days every 3 to 4 weeks in 68 previously treated CLL patients, obtaining 13% CR and 44% PR rates. Using the NCI criteria that allowed persistence of residual nodules in the bone marrow, the CR rate was 29%, and the PR rate was 28%. At 36 months, median survival was the same for patients who achieved CR or nodular CR (nCR, defined as PR with only residual nodular disease of the bone marrow), and at 16 months, median survival of these patients was superior to that of patients achieving PR. The median duration of response was 21 months for the CR patients and 13 months for the PR patients. Ninety two percent of the responders achieved at least a PR after the first three courses. Following this study, 33 previously untreated CLL patients received fludarabine at M. D. Anderson.[92] A CR rate of 33% and PR rate of 45% was obtained. Using the NCI criteria including nCR, the CR rate increased to 72%.

In 1993, Keating et al[93] published the follow-up of 78 previously treated and 35 untreated CLL patients who received fludarabine. Using NCI criteria, the untreated group had a response rate of 80%, with a 74% CR rate. The previously treated group was divided into refractory patients, with 28% CR and 10% PR and nonrefractory patients, with an overall response rate of 93% and a CR rate of 57%. The response to the therapy correlated with the number of previous treatments, stage of disease, and whether the patients were refractory to alkylating agents.[93]

In another study, prednisone was added to fludarabine in a dosage of 30 mg/m[2] for 5 days in 256 CLL patients.[94] There was no increase in the response rate compared with fludarabine alone. An increase in the rate of opportunistic infections was noted in the combination therapy group, with 13 patients developing either *Listeria monocytogenes* or *Pneumocystis carinii* pneumonia. One patient developed both infections. Four patients died of *P carinii* pneumonia. Three of the *Listeria* cases occurred in patients who were in remission and not receiving treatment. In the same study, O'Brien et al noted a persistent decrease in CD4+ lymphocyte levels. In 217 patients for whom CD4 levels were available before the treatment, the median level before the initiation of FAMP and Pdn was 1,015/μL. After 6 months of therapy, the median level was 148/μL in 95 patients analyzed.[94] The main toxicity with the use of fludarabine was myelosuppression and infection. Nausea, vomiting, diarrhea, and neurotoxicity were present in 5% of the cases.

Robertson et al conducted immunophenotypic and molecular studies to assess the completeness of responses in 159 patients treated with six courses of fludarabine. No residual disease was detected by two-color flow cytometry in 89% of the CR, 51% of the nCR and only 19% of the PR patients. For complete responders having no residual disease by flow cytometry, the 2-year progression free survival was 84%, vs 39% in patients having residual disease ($P < .001$).[95]

Different fludarabine schedules of administration have been used. Puccio et al gave fludarabine at a loading dose of 20 mg/m^2 followed by a 48-hour continuous intravenous infusion of 30 mg/m^2/d (a total dose of 80 mg/m^2, compared with 150 mg/m^2 used in the daily $\times$ 5 schedule), repeated at 4-week intervals. Forty-two patients were evaluated for response. No patient achieved CR; 22 patients achieved PR, and 12% had stable disease.[96] A weekly schedule of 30 mg/m^2/wk was used at M. D. Anderson in 47 previously treated patients, with an overall response rate of 24%.[97]

A European cooperative group conducted a three-arm randomized study in 247 previously untreated CLL patients, comparing fludarabine at 25 mg/m^2/d for 5 days every 4 weeks with CAP (cyclophosphamide, 750 mg/m^2; doxorubicin, 50 mg/m^2; IV prednisone, 40 mg/m^2 on days 1 to 4) and miniCHOP (vincristine, 1 mg/m^2 IV, and doxorubicin, 25 mg/m^2 IV on day 1; plus cyclophosphamide, 300 mg/m^2, and prednisone, 40 mg/m^2, given orally on days 1 to 5). In 174 Binet stage B patients, a higher response rate was noted with fludarabine than with CAP and miniCHOP, with 48% CR and 40% PR in the fludarabine group, compared with 14% CR and 64% PR in the CAP group, and 32% CR and 45% PR in the miniCHOP arm ($P = .002$). In 73 Binet stage C patients, there was no significant difference in the response rate between the arms. Bone marrow was not assessed as part of the response.[98]

Hiddeman et al reported their preliminary results of a randomized trial comparing fludarabine vs CAP in 208 patients, 103 pretreated and 105 untreated, with an overall response of 58% for fludarabine and 42% for CAP. The response to fludarabine was 70% in untreated and 45% in pretreated patients, compared with 58% and 26% in the CAP arm.[99]

Deletion of the p53 gene has been associated with poor response to nucleoside analogs and short survival by Döhner et al.[53a] In their study, 100 patients (90 with B-CLL, 3 with Waldeström macroglobulinemia [WM], and 7 with PLL) were studied by in situ hybridization. Monoallelic deletion of the p53 gene was found in 17% (11 B-CLL, 1 WM, and 5 PLL). None of the 12 patients with p53 gene deletion, compared with 20 (56%) of 36 without a deletion, responded to therapy with fludarabine or pentostatin.

Finally, fludarabine was used in 15 CLL patients who relapsed after an initial response to the drug. Four patients achieved a second response (27%).[94]

Cladribine: Another purine analog with activity in CLL is cladribine, which has been used in a dosage of 0.1 mg/kg/d by continuous IV infusion for 7 days. A group of investigators from Scripps clinics used cladribine and reported an overall response of 55% in 18 previously treated CLL patients; 4 patients achieved PR (22%), and 6 patients (33%) achieved clinical improvement.[100] In 1991, the same group reported the response to cladribine in 90 previously treated patients, 82 of whom were Binet stage C, eight stage B, and one stage A. The treatment was repeated at 4-week intervals, and the patients received a median of two cycles, with some of the patients receiving bolus schedule. Four patients (4%) obtained CR, and 36 (40%) PR by NCI criteria. The median duration of the response was 4 months (range, 2 to 30 months). The main dose-limiting factor was myelosuppression with persistent thrombocytopenia in 24% of the cladribine-treated patients. Infections were present in 18% of the patients.[101]

Other investigators used cladribine 0.12 mg/kg/d over 2 hours for 5 days in 18 previously treated CLL patients and obtained 7 CR (39%) and 5 PR (28%).[102] Only 10 patients had Binet stage C disease in this study, and the patients received a median of four treatments.

Twenty previously untreated patients, eleven with Rai stage 3 or 4 disease, were treated with cladribine by the Scripps group. A median of four courses was given (range, 1 to 9). Using NCI response criteria, 5 patients (2 in Rai stage 2, 2 in Rai stage 3, and 1 in Rai stage 4) obtained CR (25%) and 12 patients (60%) achieved PR, for an overall response rate of 85%.[103]

Juliusson and colleagues retreated six CLL patients who previously responded to cladribine (two CR and four PR). The median time to retreatment was 19 months (range, 8 to 28 months). Responses included one CR, two PR, one minimal response, one death, and the last patient had no response. The main problem was hematologic toxicity with persistent cytopenias.[104]

Cross-resistance to cladribine in patients previously unresponsive to fludarabine has been studied. Juliusson reported four consecutive patients who responded to cladribine after they failed therapy with fludarabine. One CR and three PR were achieved.[105] Other investigators obtained poorer results with cladribine in this setting.[106–108] At M. D. Anderson, 28 fludarabine-refractory CLL patients were treated with cladribine. Two patients (7%) responded (by NCI criteria), and one had antitumor activity, with decrease of the peripheral blood and bone marrow lymphocytosis, but persistent thrombocytopenia. Overall, 65% of the treatment courses were complicated by febrile episodes, and 10 patients died within 60 days of starting cladribine therapy.[107]

Juliusson and colleagues used oral preparations of cladribine at doses of 10 mg/m²/d for 5 days every month for up to 6 months in 17 previously untreated CLL patients. Using NCI response criteria, 7 CR (41%), 5 PR (29%) and 5 treatment failures (29%) were seen.[109]

The ratio of deoxycytidine kinase to cytoplasmic 5′-nucleotidase—the enzymes that phosphorylate cladribine and dephosphorylate cladribine 5′-monophophate, respectively—was found to be predictive for cladribine responsiveness.[110]

Pentostatin is another nucleoside analog with significant activity in hairy-cell leukemia that has also been used in CLL. In 25 previously treated CLL patients, Grever found that pentostatin, at doses of 4 mg/m²/wk for 3 weeks, produced a 4% CR and 16% PR.[111] Dillman and colleagues[112] treated 39 patients, 26 previously treated and 13 untreated, obtaining one CR (3%) and 9 PR (23%). Six of the partial responders were previously untreated patients. The most significant toxicity was infection, with frequent stomatitis and rash.

Other Treatment Modalities

In patients refractory to conventional therapies, other investigational treatments have been used, including biologic response modifiers, monoclonal antibodies, and bone marrow transplantation.

Biologic Response Modifiers: Alpha interferon (IFN-α), used at doses of 1.5 to 3 million units three times a week, had less than a 50% response rate in stage A and B CLL patients, and less than 10%[113,114] in stage C patients.[115] It is possible that IFN alfa-2a (Roferon-A) may prolong chemotherapy-induced responses.[116,117] This last issue remains controversial, since in another recent study using IFN-α as maintenance in 31 B-CLL patients previously treated with FAMP, there was no difference in the time to progression of the disease compared with that in historical controls.[117a]

Recombinant Interleukin-2 (rIL-2) was used to activate natural killer cells, whose activity is decreased in CLL. Minor responses were obtained in two small studies with 12 and 8 patients respectively.[118,119]

Monoclonal antibodies (MoAbs) against antigens expressed on the surface of the malignant lymphocytes have been used therapeutically in patients with CLL. Antibodies against CD5 were used with few minimal responses.[120,121] Discouraged by the disappointing clinical results with unconjugated MoAbs, investigators decided to use them as a vehicle to deliver drugs, toxins, or radioisotopes directly to the tumor cell. MoAb-toxin conjugates, also

known as immunotoxins, have been examined in preclinical studies and recently incorporated in clinical trials. The antibodies used are directed against CD5, CD19, CD22, and CD25. The most commonly used toxins are the two-chain protein toxins, ricin and diphtheria toxin, and the single-chain toxin, *Pseudomonas exotoxin A.*

In clinical trials, the monoclonal antibody against CD19 (B4) conjugated to whole ricin was used by Grossbard et al in 25 patients with B-cell malignancies, obtaining one durable CR and two PR in patients with NHL.[128] Based on those studies, this conjugate was used in six CLL patients with only 1 PR.[122,123] LeMaistre et al used a ligand (IL-2) conjugated to modified diphtheria toxin (DAB486) in a patient with refractory CLL, obtaining a PR.[124] Others used IL-2 conjugated with *Pseudomonas* endotoxin.[125] The highly lytic CAMPATH was used by Janson and colleagues in two patients with refractory CLL, obtaining one CR and one PR.[126]

The most significant problems with the use of MoAbs are the lack of the expression of the tumor antigens and the development of antimouse antibodies.

Other Cytokines: Granulocyte colony-stimulating factor (G-CSF, filgrastim [Neupogen]) and granulocyte-macrophage colony-stimulating factor (GM-CSF, sargramostim [Leukine]) were used in CLL to ameliorate the neutropenia induced by chemotherapy or by the disease. GM-CSF increased the number of neutrophils 1.7- to 29-fold in patients with CLL,[127,128] with low doses superior to high doses in some cases.[128]

Allogeneic Bone Marrow Transplant: Allogeneic bone marrow transplant (BMT) can be effective in inducing long-term disease-free survival.[129–133] The European Group and the International Bone Marrow registry reported their experience with 47 CLL patients receiving allogeneic BMT from HLA-identical sibling donors. The median age was 42 years (range, 21 to 58); 56% had Rai stage 3 or 4 disease. Total body irradiation (TBI) was given to 96% of the patients as part of the conditioning regimen, and 64% received methotrexate and cyclosporine (Sandimmune) for prevention or treatment of graft-vs-host disease (GVHD). Forty-five patients were evaluated. Engraftment occurred in 43 (95%) and CR was obtained in 33 of 39 assessable patients (70%). Five patients (15%) relapsed between 4 and 54 months after transplant. Acute GVHD > grade 2 was experienced by 38% of the patients. Chronic GVHD was present in 47%, with extensive disease in 17% of the patients. GVHD was the most common cause of death. The projected leukemia-free survival at 5 years was 40%, with the most important prognostic factor being the stage of the CLL at the time of the transplant.[131]

Rabinowe and colleagues[132] performed T-cell depleted allogeneic BMT from HLA-identical siblings in eight patients with CLL. The median age was 40 years (range, 31 to 54). Seven patients had Rai stage 2, and one had Rai stage 4 disease. All the patients were treated to reduce the bulk of the disease, six of them receiving fludarabine. At the time of transplant, one patient was in CR, five had minimal disease in the bone marrow and lymph nodes, one had only disease in the bone marrow, and one had residual adenopathy. The conditioning regimen was cyclophosphamide plus TBI. There was one toxic death due to *P carinii* pneumonia. At a median follow up of 11.7 months (range 6 to 18), seven patients were in CR and one had progressive disease.

At M. D. Anderson, Khouri et al[133] performed allogeneic BMT in 11 CLL patients, nine with identical-HLA siblings, one with a one-antigen mismatch in the HLA-A locus, and one syngeneic transplant. The median age was 42 years (range, 25 to 55). All patients were treated previously with fludarabine, five were primary refractory to fludarabine, and two had refractory relapse. Eight patients had Rai stage 4 and one had Rai stage 3 disease at the time of BMT. Seven patients achieved CR, and one had a nodular CR. One patient died of disseminated *Aspergillus* infection at day 58. With a median follow-up of 10 months (range, 2 to 36), 10 patients are alive, with 7 patients still in CR, 2 in nodular CR (one was a PR who received a second allogeneic BMT). No acute GVHD > grade 2 occurred in any patient.

The incidence of GVHD in the American series was significantly less than that seen by the European group. Previous treatment with fludarabine in the American group was a common denominator. In contrast, in the European multicenter study, no patients were treated with fludarabine prior to the BMT. An association between pretreatment with fludarabine and lack of development of severe acute GVHD has been suggested.

Autologous BMT: New techniques, including allogeneic peripheral blood stem-cell transplantation are under investigation. Rabinowe et al[132] treated 12 patients with multiple MoAb purged autologous BMT, using cyclophosphamide plus TBI as a conditioning regimen. The median age was 45 years (range, 27 to 54). At the time of the transplant, two patients were in CR, and the rest had minimal disease. One patient died on day 62 with diffuse alveolar hemorrhage. At a median follow-up of 5 months (range, 2 to 31), five patients were in CR, one had persistent disease, and five were too early to be evaluated.

Khouri et al at M. D. Anderson[133] treated 11 patients with autologous BMT. Their median age was 59 years (range, 37 to 66). All patients responded; five patients achieved CR, four achieved nCR, and one achieved PR. At a median follow-up of 10 months (range, 2 to 29), six patients were alive, three in CR, two were relapsed, and one in PR. One patient died at day 100 of cytomegalovirus pneumonia in CR; another died in CR due to a complication of a liver biopsy 2 months after the BMT. Three patients developed Richter's transformation and died at 10, 10, and 11 months, respectively.

Splenectomy has been considered another therapeutic option in patients with CLL. With improved surgical techniques, the operative mortality has been reduced.[135-141] The indications for splenectomy can be summarized as hypersplenism with cytopenias unresponsive to treatment, autoimmune thrombocytopenia, hemolytic anemia, and massive symptomatic splenomegaly.

The results have varied between institutions and depending on the year of the study. In the Mayo Clinic, 57 splenectomized CLL patients were reviewed retrospectively, and 50 were analyzed; responses were noted in 77% of patients with anemia, 70% of patients with thrombocytopenia, and 64% of patients with anemia and thrombocytopenia. At 1 year, the response was sustained in more than 80% of responders. The operative morbidity was 20%, the mortality was 4%, and the median survival after splenectomy was 41 months in the responding group vs 14 months in the nonresponders.[140]

At M. D. Anderson, the outcomes of 55 splenectomized CLL patients were examined retrospectively. Hemoglobin values were increased by more than 3 g/dL in 25%, and platelets were increased by $50 \times 10^3/\mu L$ or more in 72% of patients. The mortality rate was 9%.[141]

Delpero et al[136] studied 44 CLL patients with splenomegaly and hypersplenism. Twenty-six had anemia and 36 had thrombocytopenia. The hemoglobin and platelet counts increased to normal in 85% and 92% of the patients, respectively.

Splenic irradiation (SI) has been used as an alternative to splenectomy, to alleviate cytopenias and symptomatic splenomegaly in patients whose surgical risk is considered unacceptable. SI helps to decrease the number of circulating lymphocytes and relieves the pain, but only improves the cytopenias in 25% of the patients in one series[142] and may aggravate the thrombocytopenia in some patients.[143] In one series, Roncandin et al[144] showed improvement in blood counts in 78% of patients and decrease in the size of the spleen by 50% or more in 63% of the patients.

Radiation has been used to palliate bulky lymphadenopathies when there is no response to the chemotherapy.

Intravenous Gammaglobulin (IVIG): Hypogammaglobulinemia occurs in 10% to 60% of B-CLL patients[145–147] and the severity of this condition has been associated with the stage of the disease, a diffuse pattern of bone marrow infiltration, and an increased incidence of infections.[148–152] An IgG level of < 700 mg/dL was associated with reduction in the survival.[148] In a study done in nine patients, deficiencies in IgG3 and IgG4 were the most significant findings, with only moderate reduction in IgG1 and IgG2.[159] This selective deficiency of IgG subtypes may explain the pattern of infections seen in CLL patients.

The etiology of the hypogammaglobulinemia in CLL patients is poorly understood and probably caused by multiple factors. Functional abnormalities in T-cells[153] or dysfunction of the nonclonal CD5-B cells may be implicated.[154] Jaksik et al noted no improvement in the serum Ig in 81% of 282 patients treated with chlorambucil.[155] In contrast, fludarabine improved IgM levels in patients who achieved CR.[156]

In 1988, an International Cooperative Group for the study of Immunoglobulins in CLL, initiated a prospective, double-blind, randomized study comparing placebo vs IVIG (400 mg/kg) every 3 weeks for 1 year. The IVIG-treated group had fewer bacterial infections than the placebo group (23 vs 42, P < .001). The infections prevented were of mild to moderate severity without differences found in the frequency of major infections or in survival.[157]

Weeks et al showed a gain of 0.8 quality-adjusted days per patient per year of therapy at a cost of $6 million per quality-adjusted 1 year gained[158] and an annual cost of $15,740 (in US$). To reduce the cost, selection of patients with a previous history of infections and hypogammaglobulinemia and home administration may be useful.

AUTOIMMUNE DISORDERS

Chronic lymphocytic leukemia has been associated with autoimmune hemolytic anemia (AHA), autoimmune thrombocytopenic purpura (ITP), aplastic anemia, pure red-cell aplasia and other autoimmune manifestations. Coombs positive AHA is observed in 1% of CLL at the time of the diagnosis,[160] but increases in frequency with the progression of the disease,[161] achieving a cumulative incidence of 7% to 35% during the course of the disease.[162,163] The origin of the autoantibodies causing hemolysis is not clear. In most cases, the autoantibodies are produced by the normal B lymphocytes rather than by the clonal B-CLL cells, but the abnormal clone was the origin of the antibodies in two patients.[164]

The autoantibodies causing the hemolysis in CLL patients are "warm" anti-red blood cell (RBC) antibodies (IgG)[165] and usually polyclonal in origin. Since the antibodies often react against a panel of RBC (pan-aggluti-

nins), blood banks may face difficulty in finding compatible blood. In a retrospective study that included 53 patients who had AHA,[166] patients who received transfusions did not have severe reactions or increased hemolysis. Therefore, if the anemia is symptomatic, transfusion with the most compatible blood is indicated. Appropriate treatment is prednisone, at doses of 1 to 2 mg/kg/d and then tapered over a few weeks, if possible. Patients who do not respond to prednisone or who require high doses of steroids may benefit from splenectomy,[167] splenic irradiation,[168] danazol,[169] or intravenous Ig.[170]

Autoimmune thrombocytopenia is less common and more difficult to demonstrate. The treatment includes steroids, IVIG, and sometimes splenectomy. Other therapeutic options include vincristine, immunosuppression, splenic irradiation, plasmapheresis, and recently, the use of the staphylococcal protein A column.

Pure red-cell aplasia occurs in 1% to 6%.[36] The combination of cyclosporine and prednisone was superior to treatment with prednisone alone.[171]

SECONDARY MALIGNANCIES

Patients with CLL have an increased risk of secondary malignancies. The most common solid tumors in CLL patients are melanoma, soft-tissue sarcoma, colorectal carcinoma, and lung cancer. A recent study showed an incidence of 8.9% of second malignancies in 9,456 cases studied. This was 28% higher risk than expected in a comparable population. The observed/expected ratio for Hodgkin's disease was 7.69; for ocular melanoma, 3.79; for malignant melanoma, 2.79; for brain tumors, 1.98; and for lung cancer, 1.90.[172]

TRANSFORMATION

Richter's Syndrome

In 1928, Maurice Richter described the association between CLL and "reticulum cell sarcoma."[173] Since then, many cases of this association have been reported. In general, the development of a higher-grade lymphoma, usually diffuse large-cell (DLCL) or immunoblastic variant occurs in 1% to 10% of the patients. Robertson et al[174] reported 39 cases of Richter's syndrome (RS) among 1,374 CLL patients seen between 1972 and 1992 (a 3% incidence). The presenting features, in order of frequency in this study were: increase in serum LDH (82%), progressive lymphadenopathy (64%), systemic symptoms (59%), monoclonal gammapathy (44%) and extranodal involvement (40%).

Ten patients had no evidence of CLL at the time of transformation. Three of these 10 were also free of disease as assessed by dual-color flow cytometry or restriction analysis for Ig gene rearrangement. The median survival was 5 months, despite treatment. Three of the eight patients who survived more than 1 year had de novo presentation of CLL and RS. Responders to treatment survive longer than nonresponders. Other studies showed similar clinical, laboratory, and survival characteristics.[175–177]

The association of Hodgkin's disease and CLL has been reported by some investigators.[178–179] Brecher and Banks called this association a Hodgkin's disease variant of RS.[178] The clinical presentation is similar to RS, and the median survival is 12 months.

CLL/PLL and Prolymphocytic Transformation

Up to 15% of patients with CLL present with a mixture of small lymphocytes and larger cells with prominent nucleolus called prolymphocytes (PL).[180–181] When PL in the peripheral blood measures between 11% and 55%, this is called CLL/prolymphocytic leukemia (PLL). Patients with CLL/PLL present with splenomegaly disproportionate to the degree of lymphadenopathy.

In a review by Melo et al, an absolute number of PL > than $15 \times 10^3/\mu L$ had an outcome and survival as bad as pure prolymphocytic leukemia (> 55% PL). A scoring system used by these investigators included as adverse prognostic factors: size of the spleen greater than 8 cm, absolute number of PL $> 15 \times 10^3/\mu L$, formation of rosettes 30% or less, and strong surface immunoglobulin stain.[181] Patients with more than two adverse factors had a median survival of 2.5 years.[181] The immunophenotype in CLL transforming to PLL, is the same as that in B-CLL.

Other Transformations

Rare cases of CLL transforming to acute leukemia have been reported.[182–185] Studies of some of these cases suggested that the blasts arise from the same B-cell clone as the CLL cells.[183–185] Isolated cases of CLL transformation into small noncleaved-cell lymphoma, lymphoblastic lymphoma, and hairy-cell leukemia have been reported.[186–188]

PROLYMPHOCYTIC LEUKEMIA

Prolymphocytic leukemia is another lymphoproliferative disorder characterized by massive splenomegaly, a high number of circulating lymphocytes, minimal lymphadenopathy, and median survival less than 3 years. The circulating lymphocytes may be B- or T-cell type and more than 55% of the circulating white cells should have typical morphologic characteristics. Prolymphocytes are larger and less homogeneous than CLL cells, have a clear and abundant cytoplasm, clumped nuclear chromatin, and a prominent nucleolus.

The B-cells in PLL have abundant immunoglobulins on the surface, usually do not express CD5, and are strongly positive for FMC-7. These features enable the differential diagnosis with CLL. PLL is associated with cytogenetic abnormalities such as t(11;14), t(6;12), and abnormalities involving chromosome 14.

In 20% of patients with PLL, T-cell markers are expressed. Splenectomy and combination chemotherapy (eg, CHOP) has been used, with short responses. Recently, purine analogs such as pentostatin and fludarabine showed activity in this disease.

T-CELL CHRONIC LYMPHOCYTIC LEUKEMIA

Less than 5% of CLL cases involve T-lymphocytes (T-CLL). The cells arise from the postthymic cell population and usually express either CD4 or CD8 on their surface. However, the malignant cells often display aberrations in their phenotype compared with normal T-cells. Many patients with T-CLL present with a prolymphocytic variant of the disease. The physical examination typically reveals minimal lymphadenopathy and prominent splenomegaly. Respose to treatment is usually poor, and survival is shorter than in B-CLL patients with similar stage disease.

LARGE GRANULAR LYMPHOCYTE PROLIFERATION

Large granular lymphocytes (LGL) are a morphologically recognizable lymphoid subset of peripheral blood mononuclear cells. LGL can be divided into two lineages: CD3+ and CD3–. CD3+ are T-cells that express the CD3/T-cell receptor (TCR) complex and rearrange TCR genes. CD3– are natural killer cells and do not express CD3/TCR complex.

T-LGL leukemia (T-LGLL) is characterized by clonal proliferation of CD3+ LGL and has also been called Tγ lymphocytosis. The median patient age at presentation is 57 years (range, 4 to 88 years).[188a] Recurrent bacterial infections, occurring as a consequence of neutropenia, and rheumatoid arthritis are the major reasons why these patients seek medical attention. The clinical picture may resemble that of Felty's syndrome. Splenomegaly is present in half of the patients, and hepatomegaly is not uncommon; lymphadenopathy is very rare. Severe neutropenia (< 500/μL) and anemia (Hct < 36%) are found in almost half of the patients, but thrombocytopenia is less common. Association with pure red cell aplasia has been reported. Bone marrow infiltration is found in 88% of patients.[188a] The typical T-LGL are bigger than normal lymphocytes and have a pale cytoplasm with prominent azurophilic granules. The T-LGL express CD3+ and often CD16+, CD57+, and CD8+; CD56 is usually negative. Most of the patients express TCRαβ+, whereas few of them express TCRγδ+.

The indolent course of this condition in the majority of patients makes observation the most common approach. Treatment is indicated in patients with recurrent infections, severe neutropenia, rapidly progressive disease, or severe autoimmune manifestations. Splenectomy, chlorambucil, cyclophosphamide, combination chemotherapy, low-dose methotrexate, and steroids have been used without significant success. G-CSF has been used for the treatment of neutropenia. One successful BMT in a patient with aggressive disease was recently reported.[188b]

CD3– LGL proliferation usually manifests as a chronic indolent condition with mild cytopenias and a lower incidence of autoimmune phenomena than T-LGL leukemia. Demonstration of clonality in these patients is difficult; in a study of seven women with chronic CD3– LGL leukemia who were heterozygous for certain X-linked loci, X-linked gene analysis did not demonstrate clonality.[188c]

A minority of CD3– LGL leukemia patients have a different presentation and prognosis from those of most patients with T-LGLL. The disease is also called natural killer-LGL leukemia (NK-LGLL). The median patient age is 39 years (range, 7 to 70).[188a] In contrast with T-LGLL, this group of NK-LGLL patients can present with fulminant disease, high fever without evidence of infection, and B-symptoms. Anemia and thrombocytopenia may be severe, but neutropenia is usually mild. Massive hepatomegaly and splenomegaly are common in these patients. Patients with fulminant disease usually die within 2 months due to multiorgan failure and coagulopathy. Some patients have chronic symptoms for long periods of time before they develop more aggressive disease. The phenotype of the LGL is CD3–, CD56+, CD15+, CD57–, CD8–, CD4–. Treatment options including steroids and combination chemotherapy are usually ineffective. Other malignancies such as some acute lymphocytic leukemias, lymphoblastic lymphomas, and other non-Hodgkin's lymphomas can express some LGL surface antigens, such as CD56, CD57, or CD16.

HAIRY-CELL LEUKEMIA

Hairy-cell leukemia is an uncommon B-cell malignancy usually associated with pancytopenia and splenomegaly and first described by Borouncle et al in 1958.[190] About 600 cases of HCL are diagnosed every year,[189] and the disease represents 2% of all adult leukemias. For many years, the only effective treatment was splenecto-my. However, in the last 10 years systemic therapy with interferon, and later with nucleoside analogs, has improved the prognosis of this disease and raised the possibility of cure.

Etiology and Pathogenesis

The etiology of HCL is unknown. Radiation exposure or Epstein-Barr virus (EBV) infection have been suggested by some investigators but denied by others. Fifteen cases of familial HCL have been published.[191-195] No specific cytogenetic abnormality has been described.

Based on immunologic and molecular studies, the cell of origin is believed to be of B-lymphocytic lineage.[196-199] Surface phenotype demonstrates expression of pan B-cell surface antigens, CD19, CD20, CD22, and monoclonal surface immunoglobulin. The cells often express heavy-chain isotypes. HCL cells also express CD25, CD11c, B-Ly-7, HC2, and other markers that have been helpful in the differential diagnosis.

Clinical Features

HCL is four times more common in males. The median age at presentation is 50 years. The patients may seek medical attention because of abdominal discomfort due to splenomegaly, weight loss, recurrent infections, or symptoms related to anemia. Splenomegaly is present in 90% of patients at the time of diagnosis, sometimes becoming massive. Palpable lymphadenopathy is uncommon, but Mercieca et al, using CT scans, reported enlargement of the mesenteric and/or retroperitoneal lymph nodes in 17% of patients at diagnosis and 56% at relapse.[200] Patients with HCL are more susceptible to infections usually caused by gram-negative bacteria, but infection with atypical mycobacterias are not infrequent. Rarely, patients can present with autoimmune complications like vasculitis and arthritis.

Laboratory Features

At the time of diagnosis, 80% of HCL patients have some degree of anemia and/or thrombocytopenia, with platelet count $< 100 \times 10^3/\mu L$. Only 10% have a platelet count $< 10 \times 10^3/\mu L$. Leukopenia with WBC $< 3 \times 10^3/\mu L$ is present in 50% of the patients, commonly associated with neutropenia and monocytopenia. Only 10% of patients present with leukocytosis (WBC $> 10 \times 10^3/\mu L$).

The malignant cells are larger than normal lymphocytes, with a diameter between 10 and 15 μm. The cytoplasm is pale blue and often has fine projections. The nucleus is round or ovoid with eccentric location, lacy chromatin, and often with a visible nucleolus. The hairy cells express high levels of CD19, CD20, CD22, CD25,

CD11c, sIg, B-Ly 7 and they are usually CD5–. The cells stain positively for tartrate-resistant acid phosphatase (TRAP). By electron microscopy, pseudopods and microvilli can be seen at the cell surface, and lamellar bodies are noted in 50% of cell samples.

The bone marrow is typically difficult to aspirate, and the presentation of a patient with pancytopenia, splenomegaly, and a difficult bone marrow aspiration (dry tap) should raise the suspicion for HCL, and appropriate stains and tests should be done. The bone marrow is usually hypercellular, and an increase in reticulin fibers is shown with silver stains.

The spleen can weigh more than 1,000 g in 51% of HCL patients.[201] Microscopic examination reveals infiltration by the malignant cells in the red pulp cords and sinuses. The white pulp is usually atrophic. Postmortem examinations and specimens obtained during splenectomies have revealed lymph-node infiltration by hairy cells.[189,201]

Erythropoietin levels are decreased in these patients, and free serum IL-2 receptor levels, serum tumor-necrosis factor (TNF)-alpha, serum IL-1-beta, and free serum CD8 levels correlate with outcome.[202–208]

Differential Diagnosis

HCL can be confused with malignant lymphomas, HCL variant (HCLv), splenic lymphoma with villous lymphocytes (SLVL), CLL, other non-Hodgkin's lymphoma in leukemic phase, and myelodysplastic syndromes.

HCLv is a disorder characterized by prolymphocytic-like cells, with a median WBC count of $90 \times 10^3/\mu L$. Cells are usually CD25– with CD11c and B-Ly 7 expressed less often. Neutropenia and monocytopenia are not usually present. The bone marrow is easier to aspirate than in typical HCL.

SLVL is a very rare B-cell low grade lymphoma recently included within the marginal zone group,[209] presenting with significant splenomegaly and minimal or no lymphadenopathy. Anemia and thrombocytopenia are common, but neutropenia and monocytopenia are rare. The cells express CD11c in 47%, CD25 in 25%, and almost never B-Ly-7 or HC2.[210] A score system has been proposed by Matutes et al,[210] giving 1 point for any of the four markers above. Approximately 98% of HCL cases have 3 or 4 points, whereas HCLv and SLVL cases have only 1 or 2. The SLVL cells are usually TRAP negative.

Other low-grade malignant B-cell lymphomas such as follicular and mantle-cell lymphomas in leukemic phase can be differentiated by the morphology of the cells as well as by the expression of CD10+ in follicular lympho-

mas, of CD5+ in mantle-cell lymphomas, and the absence of typical HCL markers in both disorders. In CLL, the morphology and immunophenotype usually makes the distinction easy.

Treatment

The indications for treatment are an absolute neutrophil count (ANC) < 1,000/μL, platelet count < $100 \times 10^3/\mu L$, or Hb < 10 g/dL; leukemic phase of HCL; symptomatic splenomegaly; recurrent infections; or autoimmune complications.

The criteria for a complete response (CR) require normalization of the complete blood count (CBC), with ANC > 1,500/μL, platelet count > 100,000/μL and Hb > 12 g/dL; regression to normal of organomegaly and bone marrow; and peripheral blood (PB) free of hairy cells. Partial responses require reduction of the hairy cells in the bone marrow to < 50%, < 5% hairy cells in PB, > 50% reduction in the organomegaly, and normalization of the CBC. Minimal response requires the normalization of at least one of the peripheral blood cell elements and decrease of the PB circulating cells by at least 50%.

Observation With No Treatment: A small group of patients having an indolent course can be observed without any treatment.[211] In general, in patients with one or two cytopenias without any other symptoms and not requiring transfusion, observation is a reasonable approach. At M. D. Anderson, only 2% of the HCL patients belong to that category. Few cases of spontaneous remission of HCL have been reported.[212,213]

Splenectomy: Splenectomy was the first-line treatment until systemic chemotherapy was started in 1984. The interpretation of the studies is difficult because no prospective studies have been done. Golomb and Verdiman[214] performed a retrospective study in 65 HCL patients who underwent a splenectomy. In their study, they note the adverse effect of bone marrow infiltration by the leukemic cells on response to splenectomy. Ratain et al showed that patients with bone marrow cellularity of < 85% and platelet count > 60,000/μL before splenectomy required further antileukemic treatment at a median of 56.5 months, as compared with less than 1 year in the other subset.[215]

Splenectomy is no longer necessarily front-line treatment in patients with HCL, and instead is reserved for special cases such as splenic rupture, infarcts, massively enlarged spleens, severe hypersplenism, or failure to systemic chemotherapy.

IFN-α: The initial observations on natural IFN-α were published by Quesada et al in 1984.[216] In that report, three of seven patients obtained a CR and four achieved a partial response. Since then, multiple studies were conducted using natural and recombinant IFN-α at daily doses of 3 million U/d by intramuscular or subcutaneous injections for 6 months, followed by 3 million U/d three times a week for 12 and 24 months.[217-222]

The overall results in 10 different studies and a total of 417 HCL patients were evaluated by Jaiyesimi and colleagues. The CR rate is 8%, PR rate 74%, minor responses 7%, and no responses 8%.[221] The median time to response was 6 months for patients achieving PR and 14 months to achieve CR. Patients frequently relapse between 12 and 24 months after discontinuation of therapy. Reinduction with IFN-α is successful in most previous responders.[219] The most common side effects of IFN-α are flu-like symptoms, fatigue, depression, neurologic symptoms, cytopenias, and elevation of hepatic enzymes. The presence of neutralizing antibodies against recombinant IFN-α has been associated with refractoriness to treatment.[223]

Purine Analogs, such as pentostatin and cladribine, have been shown to be potent and effective drugs in the treatment of HCL.

Pentostatin is a purine analog synthesized by *Streptomyces antibioticus.* This drug was developed based on the observation that patients with adenosine deaminase deficiency had a combined immunodeficiency with severely depressed levels of both T and B lymphocytes. Pentostatin binds to adenosine deaminase (ADA). The recommended dose is 4 mg/m² IV bolus every other week until CR is obtained. Usually, patients require a median of 8 courses (range, 4 to 15). The CR rate varies between 59% and 89% in different studies, and the PR between 4% and 37%. Responses can last for many years, and patients who relapsed often responded to retreatment with pentostatin.[227-229]

Cladribine is an active drug for the treatment of HCL, achieving similar activity to pentostatin. Due to this and the advantage of one cycle of a 7-day infusion, this drug is sometimes the first choice for treatment of this disorder. Cladribine inhibits ADA and results in selective accumulation of deoxypurine nucleotides, 2-deoxy ATP. Lymphocytes may accumulate deoxypurine nucleotides more than other cells, because the rate of deoxyadenosine phosphorylation exceeds the rate of nucleotide phosphorylation. Intracellular accumulation of 2′-chloro-deoxy ATP inhibits ribonucleotide diphosphate reductase, which inhibits DNA synthesis. In addition, inhibition of DNA polymerase and DNA ligase prevent DNA repair, resulting in increased DNA strand breaks, which, in turn, may accelerate the process of apoptosis.

The first (and later, the largest) clinical trial was performed by Piro and colleagues, who treated 144 HCL patients with cladribine, 0.1 mg/kg/d by continuous IV infusion for 7 days. A total response rate of 97% was obtained, with 85% CR and 12% PR. The response was independent of previous treatment with IFN or splenectomy, and three patients refractory to pentostatin were responsive to cladribine. With a median follow-up of 14.2 months (range, 8.1 to 68.3 months), only four patients relapsed. Fever was common, occurring in 43% of patients, usually on the sixth day of treatment and thought to be due to release of cytokines from dying cells. Recovery of the blood counts occurred by day 61 (range, 11 to 268 days).[224]

At M. D. Anderson, Estey et al treated 46 HCL patients and noted 78% CR, 11% PR, and one minimal response. Febrile episodes were present in 46% of the patients. In this study, the median CD4+ lymphocyte count before treatment was 588 cells/μL], and posttreatment decreased to 126 cells/μL.[225]

Four HCL patients who relapsed after responding to cladribine were retreated again with the same drug, resulting in two CR and one PR.[226]

There is very limited clinical data on the use of fludarabine in HCL.[230,231] Kantarjian et al treated three patients (two with HCL and one with HCL variant), observing two PR.

Other Treatments: Some patients occasionally responded to chlorambucil, cyclophosphamide, and combination chemotherapy. A successful syngeneic bone marrow transplantation has been reported.[232]

REFERENCES

1. Nishiyama H: Relative frequency and mortality rate of various types of leukemia in Japan. Gann 60:71–81, 1969.

2. Spier CM, Kjeldberg CR, Head DR, et al: Chronic lymphocytic leukemia in young adults. Am J Clin Pathol 84:675–678, 1985.

3. Cancer Statistic Review, 1983-1987. NIH publication no. 90-2789, MD National Cancer Institute, Division of Cancer Prevention and Control Surveillance Program. Bethesda, 1987.

4. Call TG, Phyliky RL, Noel P, et al: Incidence of chronic lymphocytic leukemia in Olmstead county, Minnesota, 1935 through 1989, with emphasis on changes in initial stage at diagnosis. Mayo Clin Proc 69:323–328, 1994.

5. Keating MJ: Leukemia whiter goest thou? Mayo Clin Proc 69:397–398, 1994.

6. Cronkite EP: An historical account of clinical investigations on chronic lymphocytic leukemia in the Medical Research Center, Brookhaven National Laboratory. Blood Cells 12:285, 1987.

7. Zahm SH, Weisenburger DD, Babbitt PA, et al: Use of hair coloring products and the risk of lymphoma, multiple myeloma, and chronic lymphocytic leukemia. Am J Public Health 82:990, 1992.

8. Inskip PD, Kleinerman RA, Stovall M, et al: Leukemia, lymphoma, and multiple myeloma after pelvic irradiation for benign disease. Radiat Res 135:108, 1993.

9. Schweitzer M, Melief CJ, Ploem JE: Chronic lymphocytic leukaemia in five siblings. Scand J Haematol 11:97, 1973.

10. Gunz FW, Gunz JP, Veale AM, et al: Familial leukaemia: A study of 909 families. Scand J Haematol 15:117, 1975.

11. Gunz FW: The epidemiology and genetics of the chronic leukaemias. Clin Haematol 6:3–20, 1977.

12. Conley CL, Misiti J, Laster AJ: Genetic factors predisposing to chronic lymphocytic leukemia and to autoimmune disease. Medicine 59:323, 1980.

13. Shah AR, Maeda K, Deegan MJ, et al: A clinicopathologic study of familial chronic lymphocytic leukemia. Am J Clin Pathol 97:184, 1992.

14. Cuttner J: Increase incidence of hematological malignancies in first-degree relatives of patient with chronic lymphocytic leukemia. Cancer Invest 10:103, 1992.

15. Linet MS, Van Natta ML, Brookmeyer R, et al: Familial cancer history and chronic lymphocytic leukemia. A case control study. Am J Epidemiol 130:655, 1989.

16. Heath CW Jr: The epidemiology of leukemia, in Schottenfeld D (ed): Cancer Epidemiology and Prevention: Current Concepts, pp 318–337. Springfield, IL, Thomas, 1975.

17. Shen A, Humphries C, Tucker P, et al: Human heavy-chain variable region gene family nonrandomly rearranged in familial chronic lymphocytic leukemia. Proc Natl Acad Sci USA 84:8563, 1987.

18. Brok-Simoni F, Rechavi G, Katzir N, et al: Chronic lymphocytic leukemia in twin sister: Monozigous but not identical (letter). Lancet 1:329, 1987.

19. Han T, Ozer H, Sadamori N, et al: Prognostic importance of cytogenetic abnormalities in patients with chronic lymphocytic leukemia. N Engl J Med 310:288, 1984.

20. Juliusson G, Gahrton G, Oscier D, et al: Cytogenetics abnormalities and survival in B-cell chronic lymphocytic leukemia. Second IWCCL compilation of data on 662 patients. Leuk Lymphoma 5S:21, 1991.

21. Losada AP, Wessman M, Tiainen M, et al: Trisomy 12 in chronic lymphocytic leukemia: An interphase cytogenetic study. Blood 78:775, 1991.

22. Crossen PE: Cytogenetics and molecular changes in chronic B-cell leukemia. Cancer Genet Cytogenet 43:143, 1989.

23. Gahrton G, Robert KH, Friberg K, et al: Extra chromosome 12 in chronic lymphocytic leukemia (letter). Lancet 1:146, 1980.

24. Juliusson G, Oscier DG, Fitchett M, et al: Prognostic subgroups in B-cell chronic lymphocytic leukemia defined by specific chromosomal abnormalities. N Engl J Med 323:720, 1990.

25. Juliusson G, Gahrton G: Chromosomal aberrations in B-cell chronic lymphocytic leukemia. Pathogenetic and clinical implications. Cancer Genet Cytogenet 45:143, 1990.

26. Han T, Henderson ES, Emrich LJ, et al: Prognostic significance of kariotypic abnormalities in B cell chronic lymphocytic leukemia: An update. Semin Hematol 24:257, 1987.

27. Juliusson G, Robert KH, Ost A, et al: Prognostic information from cytogenetic analysis in B-cell chronic lymphocytic leukemia and leukemic immunocytoma. Blood 65:134, 1985.

28. Qumsiyeh MB, Tharapel SA: Interphase detection of Trisomy 12 in B-cell chronic lymphocytic leukemia by fluorescence hybridization in situ. Leukemia 6:602, 1992.

29. Que TH, Marco JG, Ellis J, et al: Trisomy 12 in Chronic lymphocytic leukemia detected by fluorescence in situ hybridization: Analysis by stage, immunophenotype and morphology. Blood 82:571, 1993.

30. Escudier SM, Pereira-Leahy JM, Drach JW, et al: Fluorescent in situ hybridization and cytogenetic studies of trisomy 12 in chronic lymphocytic leukemia. Blood 71:2702, 1993.

31. Cuneo A, Wlodarska I, Sayed-Aly M, et al: Non-radiactive in situ hybridization for the detection and monitoring of trisomy 12 in B-cell chronic lymphocytic leukemia. Br J Haematol 81:192, 1992.

32. Motokura T, Bloom T, Kim HG, et al: A novel cyclin encoded by a BCL-1 linked candidate oncogene. Nature 350:512, 1991.

33. Seto M, Yamamoto K, Iida S, et al: Gene rearrangement and overexpression of PRADI in lymphoid malignancy with t(11;14)(q13:q32) translocation. Oncogene 7:1401, 1992.

34. Pittmann S, Catovsky D: Prognostic significance of chromosomal abnormalities in chronic lymphocytic leukemia. Br J Haematol 58:649, 1984.

35. Freedman AS, Boyd AW, Bieber FR, et al: Normal cellulae counterparts of B-cell chronic lymphocytic leukemia. Blood 70:418, 1987.

36. Chikkappa G, Zarrabi MH, Tsan MF: Pure red cell aplasia in patients with chronic lymphocytic leukemia. Medicine 65:339, 1986.

37. Fairley GH, Scott RB: Hypogammaglobulinemia in chronic lymphocytic leukemia. Br Med J 2:290, 1961.

38. International Workshop on Chronic Lymphocytic Leukemia: Recommendations for diagnosis, stage and response criteria. Ann Intern Med 110:236, 1989.

39. Cheson BD, Bennett JM, Rai KR, et al: Guidelines for clinical protocols for chronic lymphocytic leukemia. Am J Hematol 29:152, 1988.

40. Bennett JM, Catovsky D, Daniel MT, et al: Proposal for the classification of chronic (mature) B and T lymphoid leukemias. J Clin Pathol 42:567, 1989.

41. Rai KR, Sawitzky A, Cronkite EP, et al: Clinical staging of chronic lymphocytic leukemia. Blood 46:219, 1975.

42. Binet J-L, Auquier A, Dighiero G, et al: A new prognostic classification of CLL derived from multivariate survival analysis. Cancer 48:198, 1981.

43. Rai KR, Han T: Prognostic factors and clinical staging in chronic lymphocytic leukemia. Hematol Oncol Clin North Am 4:447, 1990.

44. Lee JS, Dixon DO, Kantarjian HM, et al: Prognosis of chronic lymphocytic leukemia: A multivariate regression analysis of 325 untreated patients. Blood 69:929, 1987.

45. Catovsky D, Fooks J, Richards S: Prognostic factors in chronic lymphocytic leukemia: The importance of age, sex and response to treatment in survival. A report from MRC CLL 1 trial MRC working party in leukemia in adults. Br J Haematol 72:141, 1989.

46. IWCLL/Working Group: Chronic lymphocytic leukemia in younger adults: Preliminary results of a study based in 454 patients. Blood 78 (suppl 1):273a, 1991.

47. Montserrat E, Gomis F, Vallespi T, et al: Presenting features and prognosis of chronic lymphocytic leukemia in younger adults. Blood 78:1545, 1991.

48. Montserrat E, Sanchez-Bisoni J, Vinolas N, et al: Lymphocyte doubling time in chronic lymphocytic leukemia: Analysis of its prognostic significance. Br J Haematol 62:567, 1986.

49. Molica S, Alberti A: Prognostic value of the lymphocyte doubling time in chronic lymphocytic leukemia. Cancer 60:2712, 1987.

50. Giglio AD, O'Brien S, Ford R, et al: Prognostic value of proliferating cell nuclear antigen expression in chronic lymphocytic leukemia. Blood 79:2717, 1992.

51. Rozman C, Montserrat E, Rodriguez-Fernandez JM, et al: Bone marrow histologic pattern—the best single prognostic parameter in chronic lymphocytic leukemia: A multivariate survival analysis of 329 cases. Blood 64:642, 1984.

52. Geisler G, Ralfkicer E, Mørk Hansen M, et al: The bone marrow histological pattern has independant prognostic value in early stage chronic lymphocytic leukemia. Br J Haematol 62:47, 1986.

53. Montserrat E, Vinolas N, Reverter JC, et al: Natural history of chronic lymphocytic leukemia: On the progression and prognosis of

early clinical stages. Nouv Rev Fr Hematol 30:359, 1988.

53a. Döhner H, Fischer K, Bentz M, et al: p53 gene deletion predicts for poor survival and non-response to therapy with purine analogs in chronic B-cell leukemias. Blood 85:1580–1589, 1995.

53b. Gaidano G, Ballerini P, Gong JZ, et al: p53 mutations in human lymphoid malignancies: Association with Burkitt lymphoma and chronic lymphocytic leukemia. Proc Natl Acad Sci USA 88:5413, 1991.

53c. El Rouby S, Thomas A, Costin D, et al: p53 gene mutation in B-cell chronic lymphocytic leukemia is associated with drug resistance and is independent of MDR1/MDR3 gene expression. Blood 82:3452–3459, 1993.

54. Mandelli F, De Rossi G, Mancini P, et al: Prognosis in chronic lymphocytic leukemia: A retrospective multicentric study from the GIMEMA group. J Clin Oncol 5:398, 1987.

55. Jaksic B, Vitale B, Hauptmann E, et al: The roles of age and sex in the prognosis on chronic leukemias. A study of 373 cases. Br J Cancer 64:345, 1991.

56. Rozman C, Montserrat E, Feliu E, et al: Prognosis of chronic lymphocytic leukemia: A multivariate survival analysis of 150 cases. Blood 59:1001, 1982.

57. Levis A, Ficara F, Marmont F, et al: Prognostic significance of serum albumin in chronic lymphocytic leukemia. Haematologica 76:113, 1991.

58. Reinisch W, Willheim M, Hilgarth M, et al: soluble CD23 reliably reflects disease activity in B-cell chronic lymphocytic leukemia. J Clin Oncol 12:2146, 1994.

59. Melo JV, Catovsky D, Gregory WM, et al: The relationship between chronic lymphocytic leukemia and prolymphocytic leukemia: IV. Analysis of survival and prognostic features. Br J Haematol 65:23, 1987.

60. Molica S, Dattilo A, Alberti A: Myelomonocytic associated antigens in B-chronic lymphocytic leukemia: Analysis of clinical significance. Leuk Lymphoma 5:139, 1991.

61. Rai KR, Sawitsky A: A review of the prognostic role of cytogenetic, phenotypic, morphologic, and immune function characteristics in chronic lymphocytic leukemia. Blood Cells 12:327, 1988.

62. Han T, Bhargava A, Henderson ES, et al: Prognostic significance of beta-2-microglobulin (b-2m) in chronic lymphocytic leukemia (CLL) and non-Hodgkin's lymphoma (NHL) (abstract). Proc Am Soc Oncol 8:270, 1989.

63. 63.Orfao A, Ciudad J, Gonzalez M, et al: Prognostic value of S-phase white blood cell count in B-cell chronic lymphocytic leukemia. Leukemia 20:47, 1990

64. Pavlidis NA, Manoussakis MN, Germanidis GS, et al: Serum-soluble interleukin-2 receptors in B-cell lymphoproliferative malignancies. Med Pediat Oncol 20:26, 1992.

65. Musolino C, Di Cesare E, Alonci A, et al: Serum levels of CD8 antigens and soluble interleukin 2 receptors in patients with B cell chronic lymphocytic leukemia. Acta Haematologica 85:57, 1991.

66. De Rossi G, Mandelli F, Corelli A, et al: Chronic lymphocytic leukemia (CLL) in younger adults: A retrospective study of 133 cases. Haematol Oncol 7:127, 1989.

67. The French Cooperative Group in Chronic Lymphocytic Leukemia: Effects of Chlorambucil and therapeutic decision in initial forms of chronic lymphocytic leukemia (Stage A): Results of a randomized clinical trial on 612 patients. Blood 1990, 75:1414, 1990.

68. French Cooperative Group on Chronic Lymphocytic Leukemia: Natural history of Stage A chronic lymphocytic leukemia untreated patients Br J Haematol, 76:45, 1990.

69. Galton DAG, Wiltshaw E, Szur L, et al: The use of chlorambucil and steroids in the treatment of chronic lymphocytic leukemia. Br J Haematol 7:73, 1961.

70. Keating MJ: Treatment of chronic lymphocytic leukemia, in Freireich EJ, Kantarjian H (eds): Therapy of hematopoietic Neoplasia, pp 175–204. New York, Dekker, 1991.

71. Sawitsky A, Rai KR, Glidewell C, et al: Comparison of daily versus intermittent Chlorambucil and prednisone therapy in the treatment of patients with chronic lymphocytic leukemia. Blood 50:1049, 1977.

72. Han T, Ezdinli EZ, Shimaoka K, et al: Chlorambucil vs combined chlorambucil– cortiscosteroid therapy in chronic lymphocytic leukemia. Cancer 31:502, 1973.

73. Jaksic B, Brugiatelli M: High dose continuous chlorambucil vs intermittent chlorambucil plus prednisone for treatment of B-CLL IGCI CLL-01 trial. Nouv Rev Fr Hematol 30:437, 1988.

74. Schisselbauer JC, Silber R, Papadopoulus E, et al: Characterization of glutathione-S-transferase expression in lymphocytes from chronic lymphocytic leukemia patients. Cancer Res 50:3562, 1990.

75. Begleiter A, Goldenberg GJ, Anhalt CD, et al: Mechanism of resistant to chlorambucil in chronic lymphocytic leukemia. Leuk Res 15:109, 1991.

76. Nagourney RA, Evans SS, Messenger JC: Glutathione, Glutathione-S-transferase and membrane potentials in drug resistant CLL and normal lymphocytes. Proc Am Assoc Cancer Res 32:2995, 1991.

77. Liepman M, Votaw ML: The treatment of chronic lymphocytic leukemia with COP chemotherapy. Cancer 41:1664, 1978.

78. Oken MM, Kaplan ME: Combination chemotherapy with cyclophosphamide, vincristine and prednisone in the treatment of refractory chronic lymphocytic leukemia. Cancer Treat Rep 63:441, 1979.

79. French Cooperative Group in Chronic Lymphocytic Leukemia: A randomized clinical trial of chlorambucil versus COP in stage B chronic lymphocytic leukemia. Blood 75:1422, 1990.

80. Raphael B, Andersen JW, Silber R, et al: Comparison of chlorambucil and prednisone versus cyclophosphamide, vincristine and prednisone as initial treatment for chronic lymphocytic leukemia: Long-term follow up of an Eastern Cooperative Oncology Group Randomized Clinical Trial. J Clin Oncol 9:770, 1991.

81. Montserrat E, Alcala A, Parody R, et al: Treatment of chronic lymphocytic leukemia in advanced stages. A randomized study comparing chlorambucil plus prednisone versus cyclophosphamide, vincristine, and prednisone. Cancer 56:2369, 1985.

82. French Cooperative Group on Chronic Lymphocytic Leukemia: Effectiveness of "CHOP" regimen in advsnced untreated chronic lymphocytic leukemia. Lancet 14:1346-1349, 1986.

83. French Cooperative Group on Chronic Lymphocytic Leukemia: Long term results of the CHOP regimen in stage C chronic lymphocytic leukemia (see comments). Br J Haematol 73:334, 1989.

84. French Cooperative Group on Chronic Lymphocytic Leukemia: CHOP regimen versus intermitent chlorambucil-prednisone in stage B chronic lymphocytic leukemia. Nouv Rev Fr Hematol 30:449, 1988.

85. Hansen MM, Andersen E, Christensen BE, et al: CHOP versus prednisone + chlorambucil in chronic lymphocytic leukemia (CLL): Preliminary results of a randomized multicenter study. Nouv Rev Fr Hematol 30:433, 1988.

86. Chevret S, Travade P, Chastang C, et al: for the French Cooperative Group on Chronic Lymphocytic Leukemia: the CHOP polychemotherapy in stage B chronic lymphocytic leukemia (CLL): Interim results of a controlled clinical trial on 287 patients (abstract). Proc Ann Meet Am Soc Clin Oncol 11:267, 1992.

87. Malpeis L, Graver MR, Starbus AE, et al: Pharmacokinetics of 2-F-ara-A (9-b-D-arabinofuranosyl-2 fluoroadenine) in cancer patients during the phase I clinical investigation of fludarabine phosphate. Semin Oncol 17:18, 1990.

88. Plunkett W, Chubb S, Alexander L, et al: Comparison of the toxicity and metabolism of 9-b-D-arabinofuranosyl-2-fluoroadenine

and 9-b-D-arabino-furanosyl adenine in human lymphoblastoid cells. Cancer Res 40:2349, 1980.

89. Cheson BD: New modalities of therapy in chronic lymphocytic leukemia. Crit Rev Oncol Hematol 11:167, 1991.

90. Grever MR, Kopecky KJ, Coltman CA, et al: Fludarabine phosphate: A potentially useful agent in chronic lymphocytic leukemia. Nouv Rev Fr Haematol 30:457, 1988.

91. Keating MJ, Kantarjian H, Talpaz M, et al: Fludarabine: A new agent with mayor activity against chronic lymphocytic leukemia. Blood 74:19, 1989.

92. Keating MJ, Kantarjian H, O'Brien S, et al: Fludarabine: A new agent with marked cytoreductive activity in untreated Chronic lymphocytic leukemia. J Clin Oncol 9:44, 1991.

93. Keating MJ, O'Brien S, Kantarjian H, et al: Long term follow-up of patients with chronic lymphocytic leukemia treated with fludarabine as a single agent. Blood, 81:2878, 1993.

94. O'Brien S, Kantarjian H, Beran M, et al: Results of fludarabine and prednisone therapy in 264 patients with chronic lymphocytic leukemia with multivariate analysis derived prognostic model for response to treatment. Blood 82:1695, 1993.

95. Robertson LE, Huh YO, Butler JJ, et al: Response assesment in chronic lymphocytic leukemia after fludarabine plus prednisone: Clinical, pathologic, immunophenotypic, and molecular analysis. Blood 80:29, 1992.

96. Puccio CA, Mittelman A, Lichtman SM, et al: a loading dose continuous infusion schedule of fludarabine phosphate in chronic lymphocytic leukemia. J Clin Oncol 9:1562, 1991.

97. Kemena A, O'Brien S, Kantarjian H, et al: Phase II clinical trial of fludarabine in chronic lymphocytic leukemia on a weekly low dose schedule. Leuk Lymphoma 10:187, 1993.

98. French Cooperative Group in Chronic Lymphocytic Leukemia: Comparison of Fludarabine (FDB), CAP and ChOP in previously untreated stage B and C chronic lymphocytic leukemia (CLL). First interim results of a randomized clinical trial in 247 patients. Blood (abstract suppl 1):84:461a, 1994.

99. Hiddemann W, Johnson S, Smith A, et al: Fludarabine versus cyclophosphamide, adriamycin and prednisone (CAP) for the treatment of chronic lymphocytic leukemia. Results of a multinational prospective randomized trial. Blood (abstract supp 1)82:199a, 1993.

100. Piro L, Carrera CJ, Beutler E, et al: 2-chlorodeoxyadenosine: An effective new agent for the treatment of chronic lymphocytic leukemia. Blood 72 (3):1069, 1981.

101. Saven A, Carrera CJ, Carson DA, et al: 2-chlorodeoxyadenosine in treatment of refractory chronic lymphocytic leukemia. Leuk Lymphoma, 5(suppl):133, 1991.

102. Juliusson G, Liliemark: High complete remission rate from 2-chloro-2'deoxyadenosine in previouly treated patients with B-cell chronic lymphocytic leukemia: Response predicted by rapid decrease of blood lymphocyte count. J Clin Oncol 11:679, 1993.

103. Saven A, Lemon RH, Kosty M, et al: 2-chlorodeoxyadenosine activity in patients with untreated chronic lymphocytic leukemia. J Clin Oncol 13:570, 1995.

104. Juliusson G, Liliemark J: Retreatment of chronic lymphocytic leukemia with 2-chlorodeoxyadenosine (CDA) at relapse, following CDA-induced remission: No acquired resistance. Leuk Lymphoma 13:75, 1994.

105. Juliusson G, Elmhorn-Rosenborg A, Liliemark J: Response to 2-chlorodeoxyadenosine in patients with B-cell chronic lymphocytic leukemia resistant to fludarabine. N Engl J Med 327:1056, 1992.

106. Saven A, Lemon RM, Piro LD: 2-chlorodeoxyadenosine for patients with B-cell chronic lymphocytic leukemia (letter). N Engl J Med 328 (11):812, 1993.

107. O'Brien S, Kantarjian H, Estey E, et al: Lack of effect of 2-chlorodeoxyadenosine therapy in patients with chronic lymphocytic leukemia refractory to fludarabine. N Engl J Med 330:319, 1994.

108. Delannoy A, Hanique G, Ferrant A: 2-chlorodeoxyadenosine for patients with B-chronic lymphocytic leukemia resistant to fludarabine. N Engl J Med 328 (11):812, 1993.

109. Juliusson G, Johnson S, Chrishausen I, et al: Oral 2-chlorodeoxyadenosine (CDA) as primary treatment for symptomatic chronic lymphocytic leukemia. Blood (abstract suppl 1)82:141a, 1993.

110. Kawasaki H, Carrera CJ, Piro LD, et al: Relationship of deoxycytidine kinase and cytoplasmic 5'nucleotidase to the chemotherapeutic efficacy of 2-chlorodeoxyadenosine. Blood 81:597, 1993.

111. Grever MR, Leiley JM, Kraut EH. et al: Low dose deoxycoformycin in lymphoid malignancy. J Clin Oncol 3:1196, 1985.

112. Dillman RO, Mick R, McIntyre OR: Pentostatin in chronic lymphocytic leukemia: A phase II trial of Cancer and Leukemia Group B. J Clin Oncol 7:433, 1989.

113. Pangalis GA, Griva E: Recombinant alpha-2b-interferon in untreated stages A and B chronic lymphocytic leukemia: A preliminary report. Cancer 61:869, 1988.

114. Pozzato G, Franklin F, Moretti M, et al: Low dose natural alpha-interferon in B-cell derived chronic lymphocytic leukemia. Haematologica 77:413, 1992.

115. Foon KA, Bottino GC, Abrams PG, et al. Phase II trial of recombinant leukocyte alpha interferon in patients with advanced chronic lymphocytic leukemia. Am J Med 78:216, 1985.

116. Ferrara F, Rametta V, Meli G, et al: Recombinant interferon-alpha-2a as manteinance treatment for patients with advance stage chronic lymphocytic leukemia. Am J Haematol 41:45, 1992.

117. Zinzani PL, Levrero HG, Lauria F, et al: A-interferon as maintenance drug after initial fludarabine therapy for patients with chronic lymphocytic leukemia and low grade non-Hodgkin's lymphoma. Haematologica 79:55, 1994.

117a. O'Brien S, Kantarjian H, Beran M, et al: Interferon maintenance therapy for patients with chronic lymphocytic leukemia in remission after fludarabine therapy. Blood 86:1296–1300, 1995.

118. Kay NE, Oken MM, Mazza JJ, et al: Evidence of tumor reduction in refractory or relapsed B-CLL patients with infusional interleukin-2. Nouv Rev Fr Hematol 30:475, 1988.

119. Allison MA, Jones SE, Mc Guffey P: Phase II trial of outpatient interleukin-2 in malignant lymphoma, chronic lymphocytic leukemia and selected solid tumors. J Clin Oncol 7:75, 1989.

120. Foon KA, Schroff RW, Bunn PA, et al: Effects of monoclonal antibody therapy in patients with chronic lymphocytic leukemia. Blood 64:1085, 1984.

121. Hertler AA, Schlossman DM, Borowitz MJ, et al: A phase I study of T101-ricin A-chain immunotoxin in refractory chronic lymphocytic leukemia J Biol Resp Mod 7:97, 1988.

122. Grossbard ML, Freedman AS, Ritz J, et al: Serotherapy of B-cell neoplasms with anti-B4-blocked ricin: A phase I trial of daily bolus infusion. Blood 79:576, 1992.

123. Grossbard ML, Nadler LM: Immunotoxin therapy of malignancy, in DeVita VT Jr, Hellman S, Rosenberg SA (eds): Important Advances in Oncology pp 11–135. Philadelphia, JB Lippincott, 1992.

124. LeMaistre C, Rosemblum MG, Reuben JM, et al: Therapeutic effects of genetically engineered toxin (DAB486-IL-2) in patients with chronic lymphocytic leukemia. Lancet 337:1124, 1991.

125. Kreitman RJ, Chaudhary VK, Waldmann TA, et al: Activity of anti-TAC (FV)-pseudomonas exotoxin derivatives against cells from patients with chronic lymphocytic leukemia and adult T-cell leukemia. Proc Am Assoc Cancer Res 32:1633, 1991.

126. Janson D, Nissel-Horowitz ES, Sattler M, et al: Complete and partial response in treatment of advanced refractory B-cell chronic lymphocytic leukemia using CAMPATH-1H. Blood (abst, suppl 1)82:139a, 1993.

127. Hollander AAMJ, Kluin-Melemans HC, Haak HR, et al:

Correction of neutropenia associated with chronic lymphocytic leukemia following treatment with granulocyte-macrophage colony-stimulating factor. Ann Hematol 62:32, 1991.

128. Kurzrock R, Talpaz M, Gomez JA, et al: Differential dose-related haematological effects of GM-CSF in pancytopenia: Evidence supporting the adventage of low- over high-dose administration in selected patients. Br J Haematol 99:352, 1991.

129. Michallet M, Corront B, Hollard D, et al: Allogeneic bone marrow transplantation in chronic lymphocytic leukemia: 17 cases. Report from the EBMTG. Bone Marrow Transplant 7:275, 1991.

130. Bandini G, Michallet M, Rosti G, et al: Bone marrow transplantation for chronic lymphocytic leukemia. Bone Marrow Transplant 7:251, 1991.

131. Michallet M, Archimbaud E, Bandini G, et al: HLA-identical sibling bone marrow transplants for chronic lymphocytic leukemia (CLL)–. A collaborative study of the European Bone Marrow Transplantation Group (EBMTG) and Internationa Bone Marrow Transplantation Registry (IBMTR). Blood (suppl 1, abstract)82:345a, 1993.

132. Rabinowe SN, Soiffer RJ, Gribben JG, et al: Autologous and allogeneic bone marrow transplant for poor prognosis patients with cell chronic lymphocytic leukemia. Blood 82:1366, 1993.

133. Khouri IF, Keating MJ, Vriesendorp H, et al: Autologous and allogeneic bone marrow transplantation for chronic lymphocytic leukemia: Preliminary results. J Clin Oncol 12:748, 1994.

134. Stein R, Weidert D, Reynolds V, et al: Splenectomy for end stage chronic lymphocytic leukemia. Cancer 59:1815, 1987.

135. Ferrant A, Michauz J, Sokal G: Splenectomy in advanced chronic lymphocytic leukemia. Cancer 58:2130, 1986.

136. Delpero J, Houvenaeghel G, Gastaut J, et al: Splenectomy for hypersplenism in chronic lymphocytic leukemia and malignant non-Hodgkin's lymphoma. Br J Surg 77:443, 1990.

137. Thiruvengadam R, Piedmonte M, Barcos M, et al: Splenectomy in advanced chronic lymphocytic leukemia. Leukemia 4:758, 1990.

138. Mentzer S, Starnes H, Canellos G, et al: Spleen enlargement and hyperfunction as an indication for splenectomy in chronic lymphocytic leukemia. Ann Surg 205:13, 1987.

139. Pegourie B, Sotto J, Hollard D, et al: Splenectomy during chronic lymphocytic leukemia. Cancer 59:1626, 1987.

140. Neal Jr TF, Tefferi A, Witzig T, et al: Splenectomy in advanced chronic lymphocytic leukemia: A single institution experience with 50 patients. Am J Med 93:435, 1992.

141. Seymour JF, Cusak J, Lerner S, et al: The hematologic and survival benefits of splenectomy in chronic lymphocytic leukemia: A case control study. Blood (suppl 1 abstract)84:461a, 1994.

142. Byhardt R, Brace K, Wiernick P: Role of splenic irradiation in chronic lymphocytic leukemia. Cancer 35:1621, 1975.

143. Gusney M, Liew K, Quong G, et al: A study of splenic irradiation in chronic lymphocytic leukemia. Int J Radiat Oncol Bio Phys 16:225, 1989.

144. Rocandin M, Arcicasa M, Trovo MG, et al: Splenic irradiation in chronic lymphocytic leukemia. Cancer 60:2624, 1987.

145. Fairley GH, Scott RB: Hypogammaglobulinemia in chronic lymphocytic leukemia. Br Med J 4:920, 1961.

146. Chapel HM, Buch C: Mechanism of infection in chronic lymphocytic leukemia. Semin Hematol 24:291, 1987.

147. Chapel HM: Hypogammaglobulinemia and chronic lymphocytic leukemia, in Gale RP, Rai K (eds): Chronic Lymphocytic Leukemia: Recent Progress, Future Directions, p 383. New York, Alan R. Liss, 1987.

148. Rozman C, Montserrat E, Vinolas N: Serum immunoglobulins in B-CLL: Natural history and prognostic significance. Cancer 64:279, 1988.

149. Itäla M, Helenius H, Nikoskelainèn J, et al: Infections and serum IgG in patients with chronic lymphocytic leukemia. Br J Haematol 47:539, 1992.

150. Foa R, Catowsky D, Brozovic M, et al: Clinical staging and immunological findings in chronic lymphocytic leukemia Cancer 44:483, 1979.

151. Whelan CA, Willoughby R, Mc Cann SR: Relationship between immunoglobulin levels, lymphocytes subpopulations and Rai staging in patients with B-CLL. Acta Haematol 69:217, 1983.

152. Montserrat E, Marques-Pereira JP, Gallant T, et al: Bone marrow histology and immunological findings in B-chronic lymphocytic leukemia. Cancer 54:447, 1984.

153. Apostopoulus A, Symeondis A, Zoumbos N: Prognostic significance of immune function parameters in patients with chronic lymphocytic leukemia. Eur J Haematol 44:39, 1990.

154. Dighiero G: Hypogammaglobulinemia and disordered immunity in CLL, in Cheson B (ed): Chronic Lymphocytic Leukemia: Scientific Advances and Clinical Developments, pp147–166. Marcel Dekker, New York, 1993.

155. Jaksic B, Rundek T, Planinc-Peraica A, et al: Changes in serum immunoglobulin concentration in B-chronic lymphocytic leukemia (B-CLL). XXII Congress of International Society of Hematology (abstract), p 323. Milan, August 28–Sept 2, 1988.

156. Keating MJ: Fludarabine phosphate in the treatment of chronic lymphocytic leukemia. Semin Oncol 17:49, 1990.

157. Cooperative Group for the Study of Immunoglobulin in Chronic Lymphocytic Leukemia: Intravenous immunoglobulin for the prevention of infections in chronic lymphocytic leukemia. N Engl J Med 319: 902, 1988.

158. Weeks JC, Tierney MR, Weinstein MC: Cost effectiveness of prophylactic intravenous immunoglobulin in chronic lymphocytic leukemia. N Engl J Med 325:81, 1991.

159. Copson ER, Ellis BA, Westwood NB, et al: IgG subclass levels in patients with B cell chronic lymphocytic leukemia. Leuk Lymphoma 14:471, 1994.

160. Dighiero G, Travade P, Chevret S, et al: B cell chronic lymphocytic leukemia: Present status and future directions. Blood 78:1901, 1991.

161. De Rossi G, Granati L, Girelli G, et al: Incidence and prognostic significance of autoantibodies against erythrocytes and platelets in chronic lymphocytic leukemia (CLL). Nouv Rev Fr Hematol 30:403, 1988.

162. Pirofsky B: Immunohemolytic disease: The autoimmune hemolytic anemias. Clin Hematol 4:168, 1975.

163. Lischner M, Prokocimer M, Zolberg A, et al: Autoimmunity in chronic lymphocytic leukemia. Postgrad Med J 64:590, 1988.

164. Sthoeger ZM, Sthoeger D, Shtalrid M, et al: Mechanism of autoimmune hemolytic anemia in chronic lymphocytic leukemia. Am J Hematol 43:259, 1993.

165. Leddy JP, Kakemeir RF: structural aspects of human erythrocyte autoantibodies. J Exp Med 121:1, 1965.

166. Salama A, Berghöfer H, Mueller-Eckhardt C: Red Blood cell transfusion in warm-type autoimmune haemolytic anemia. Lancet 340:1515, 1992.

167. Chertkow G, Dacie JV: Results of splenectomy in autoimmune haemolytic anemia. Br J Haematol 2:237, 1956.

168. Marcus H, Forfar JC: Splenic irradiation in treating warm autoimmune haemolytic anemia. Br Med J 293:839, 1986.

169. Ahn YS, Harrington WJ, Mylvaganam R, et al: Danazol therapy for autoimmune hemolytic anemia. Ann Int Med 102:298, 1985.

170. Besa EC: Rapid transient reversal of anemia and long-term effect of maintenance itravenous immunoglobulin for autoimmune hemolytic anemia in patients with lymphoproliferative disorders. Am J Med 84:691, 1988.

171. Chikkappa G, Pasquale D, Zarrabi MH, et al: Cyclosporine and prednisone therapy for Pure red cell aplasia in patients with chronic lymphocytic leukemia. Am J Hematol 41:5, 1992.

172. Travis LB, Curtis RE, Hankey BF, et al: Second cancers in patients with Chronic lymphocytic leukemia. J Natl Cancer Inst 16:1422, 1992.

173. Richter MN: Generalized reticullar cell sarcoma of lymp nodes associated with lymphatic leukemia. Am J Pathol 6:285, 1928.

174. Robertson LE, Pugh W, O'Brien S, et al: Richter's syndrome: A report of 39 patients. J Clin Oncol 11:1985, 1993.

175. Armitage JO, Dick FR, Corder MP: Diffuse hystiocytic lymphoma complicating chronic lymphocytic leukemia. Cancer 41:422, 1978.

176. Foucar K, Rydell RE: Richter's syndrome in chronic lymphocytic leukemia. Cancer 46: 118, 1979.

177. Harousseau JL, Flandrin G, Tricot G, et al: Malignant lymphoma supervening in chronic lymphocytic leukemia and related disorders (Richter's syndrome)—a study of 25 cases. Cancer 48:1302, 1981.

178. Brecher M, Banks PM: Hodgkin's disease variant of Richter's syndrome. Am J Clin Pathol 93:333, 1990.

179. Fayad L, Robertson LE, Hagemaister F, et al: Hodgkin's disease variant of Richter's syndrome. Blood (suppl 1, abstract) 84:451a, 1994.

180. Melo JV, Catovsky D, Galton D: The relationship between chronic lymphocytic leukaemia and prolymphocytic leukaemia. I. Clinical and laboratory features of 300 patients and characterization of an intermediate group. Br J Haematol 63:377, 1986.

181. Melo JV, Catovsky D, Galton D: The relationship between chronic lymphocytic leukaemia and prolymphocytic leukaemia. II. Patterns of evolution of "prolymphocytoid" transformation. Br J Haematol 64:77, 1986.

182. Zarrabi M, Grunwald HW, Rosner F: Chronic lymphocytic leukemia terminating in acute leukemia. Arch Intern Med 137:1059, 1977.

183. Brouet JC, Preud'homme JL, Seligmann M, et al: Blast cell with monoclonal surface immunoglobulin in two cases of acute blast crisis supervening on chronic lymphocytic leukemia. Br Med J, 4:23, 1973.

184. McPhedran P, Heath CW: Acute leukemia occurring during chronic lymphocytic leukemia. Blood 35:7, 1970.

185. Frenkel EP, Ligler FS, Graham MS, et al: Acute lymphocytic leukemia transformation of chronic lymphocytic leukemia: Substantiation by flow cytometry. Am J Hematol 10:391, 1981.

186. Litz CE, Arthur DC, Gajl Peczalska KJ, et al: Transformation of chronic lymphocytic leukemia to small non-cleaved cell lymphoma: A cytogenetic, immunological, and molecular study. Leukemia 5:972, 1991.

187. Pistoia V, Roncella S, Di Celle PF, et al: Emergency of a B-cell lymphoblastic lymphoma in a patient with B-cell chronic lymphocytic leukemia: Evidence for a single-cell origin of the two tumors. Blood 78:797, 1991.

188. Duchayne E, Delsol G, Kuhlein E, et al: Hairy cell transformation of a B-cell chronic lymphocytic leukemia: A morphological, cytochemical, phenotypic and molecular study. Leukemia 5:150, 1991.

188a. Loughran TP Jr: Clonal diseases of large granular lymphocytes. Blood 82:1–14, 1993.

188b. Scebach J, Speich R, Gmur J: Allogeneic bone marrow transplantation for CD3+/TCRγδ+ large granular lymphocyte proliferation (correspondence). Blood 85:853–854, 1995.

188c. Nash R, McSweney P, Zambello R, et al: Clonal studies of CD3– lymphoproliferative disease of granular lymphocytes. Blood 81:2363, 1993.

189. Bouroncle BA: Leukemic reticuloendotheliosis (hairy cell leukemia). Blood 53:412, 1979.

190. Bouroncle BA, Wisema BK, Doan CA: Leukemic reticuloendotheliosis. Blood 13:609, 1958.

191. Wylin RF, Greene MH, Palutke M, et al: Hairy cell leukemia in three siblings: An apparent HLA-linked diseases. Cancer 49:538, 1982.

192. Mylligan DW, Stark AN, Bynoe AG: Hairy cell leukemia in two brothers. Clin Lab Hematol 9:321, 1987.

193. Begley CG, Tait B, Crapper RM, et al: Familial hairy cell leukemia. Leuk Res 11:1027, 1987.

194. Ward FT, Baker J, Krishnan J, et al: Hairy cell leukemia in two siblings—a human leukocyte antigen-linked disease? Cancer 65: 319, 1990.

195. Gramatovici M, Bennett JM, Hiscock JG, et al: Three cases of familial hairy cell leukemia. Am J Hematol 42:337, 1993.

196. Foroni L, Catowsky D, Luzzato L: Immunoglobulin gene rearrangement in hairy cell leukemia and other chronic b-cell lymphoproliferative disorders. Leukemia 4:389, 1987.

197. Korsmayer SJ, Greene WC, Cossman J, et al: Rearrangement and expression of immunoglobulin genes and expression of Tac antigen in hairy cell leukemia. Proc Natl Acad Sci USA 80:4522, 1983.

198. Myers FJ, Cardiff RD, Taylor CR, et al: Hairy cell leukemia has a B-cell phenotype. Haematol Oncol 2:145, 1984.

199. Cleary ML, Wood GS, Warnke R, et al: Immunoglobulin gene rearrangements in haity cell leukemia. Blood 64:99, 1984.

200. Mercieca J, Puga M, Matutes E, et al: Incidence and significance of abdominal lymphadenopathy in hairy cell leukemia. Leuk Lymphoma 14(suppl 1):79, 1994.

201. Bouroncle BA: Thirty-five years in the progress of hairy cell leukemia. Leuk Lymphoma 14(suppl 1):1, 1994.

202. Steis RG, Marcon L, Clark J, et al: Serum soluble IL-2 receptor as a tumor marker in patients with hairy cell leukemia. Blood 71:1304, 1988.

203. Richards JM, Mick R, Latta JM, et al: Serum soluble interleukin-2 receptor is associated with clinical and pathological disease status in hairy cell leukemia. Blood 76:1941, 1990.

204. Lauria F, Rondelli D, Raspadori D, et al: Serum soluble interleukin-2 receptor levels in hairy cell leukemia. Correlation with clinical and hematological parameters and with a-interferon therapy. Leuk Lymphoma 7:103, 1992.

205. Ambrosetti A, Nadali G, Vinante F, et al: Soluble interleukin-2 receptor in hairy cell leukemia. Lab Res 23:34, 1993.

206. Cimino G, Annino L, Giona F, et al: Serum interleukin-1 beta levels correlate with neoplastic bulk in hairy cell leukemia. Leukemia 5:602, 1991.

207. Lindermann A, Ludwig WD, Oster W, et al: High-level secretion of tumor necrosis factor-alpha contributes to hematopoietic failure in hairy cell leukemia. Blood 73: 880, 1989.

208. Ho AD, Grossman M, Trümper L, et al: Clinical implications of increased plasma levels of CD8 in patients with hairy cell leukemia. Blood 75:1119, 1990.

209. Harris NL, Jaffe ES, Stein H, et al: A revised European-American classification of lymphoid neoplasm: A proposal from the International Lymphoma Study Group. Blood 84:1361, 1994.

210. Matutes E, Morilla R, Owusu-Ankomah K, et al: The immunophenotype of hairy cell leukemia, proposal for a scoring system to distinguish HCL from B-cell disorders with hairy or villous lymphocytes. Leuk Lymphoma 14:(suppl 1):57, 1994.

211. Bouroncle BA: The history of hairy cell leukemia: Characteristics of long term survivors. Semin Oncol 11(suppl 2):479, 1987.

212. Keefer MJ, Weber MJ, Bottomley SS, et al: Peripheral blood remission of hairy cell leukemia after transfusion hepatitis. Am J

Hematol 25:277, 1987.

213. Hersh EM, Murphy S, Zander A, et al: Host defense deficiency in hairy cell leukemia and its correction by leukocyte transfusion. Blood 56:526, 1980.

214. Golomb HM, Vardiman JW: response to splenectomy in 65 patients with hairy cell leukemia: An evaluation of spleen weight and bone marrow involvement. Blood 61:349, 1983.

215. Ratain MJ, Vardiman JW, Barker CM, et al: Prognostic variables in hairy cell leukemia after splenectomy as initial therapy. Cancer 62:2420, 1988.

216. Quesada JR, Reuben J, Manning JT, et al: Alpha interferon for induction of remission in hairy-cell leukemia. N Engl J Med 310:15, 1984.

217. Quesada JR, Hersh EM, Manning J, et al: Treatment of hairy cell leukemia with recombinant alpha interferon. Blood 68:493, 1986.

218. Foon KH, Maluish AE, Abrams PG, et al: Recombinant leukocyte A interferon therapy for advanced hairy cell leukemia. Therapeutics and immunologic results. Am J Med 80:351, 1986.

219. Italian Cooperative Group of Hairy Cell Leukemia: Long term results of interferon treatment in hairy cell leukemia. Leuk Lymphoma 14:457, 1994.

220. Golomb HM, Fefer A, Golde DW, et al: Sequential evaluation of alpha-2b-interferon treatment in 128 patients with hairy cell leukemia. Semin Oncol 14(suppl 2):13, 1987.

221. Jaiyesimi IA, Kantarjian HM, Estey EH: Advances in therapy for hairy cell leukemia. Cancer 72:5, 1993.

222. Flandrin G, Castaigne S, Sigaux F, et al: Results of treating 53 hairy cell leukemia patients with alpha-interferon. Leukemia 1:326, 1987.

223. Steiss RG, Smith JW, Urba WG, et al: Resistant to recombinant interferon alfa-2a in hairy cell leukemia associated with neutralizing anti-interferon antibodies. N Engl J Med 318:1409, 1988.

224. Piro LD, Douglas JE, Saven A: The Scripps Clinic experience with 2-chlorodeoxyadenosine in the treatment of hairy cell leukemia. Leuk Lymphoma 13(suppl 1):121, 1994.

225. Estey EH, Kurzrock R, Kantarjian HM, et al: Treatment of hairy cell leukemia with 2-chlorodeoxyadenosine (2-CdA). Blood 79:882, 1992.

226. Lauria F, Benfenati D, Raspadori D, et al: Retreatment with 2-CdA of progressed HCL patients. Leuk Lymphoma 14(suppl 1):143, 1994.

227. Cassileth PA, Cheuvart B, Spiers ASD, et al: Pentostatin induces durable remissions in hairy cell leukemia. J Clin Oncol 9:243, 1991.

228. Catowsky D, Matutes E, Talavera JG, et al: Long term results with 2'-deoxycoformycin in hairy cell leukemia. Leuk Lymphoma 14(suppl 1):109, 1994.

229. Annino L, Ferrari A, Giona F, et al: Deoxycoformycin induces long-lasting remissions in hairy cell leukemia: Clinical and biological results of two different regimens. Leuk Lymphoma 14(suppl 11):115, 1994.

230. Kraut EH, Hoo GC: Fludarabine phosphate in refractory hairy cell leukemia. Am J Hematol 37:59, 1991.

231. Kantarjian HM, Schachner J, Keating MJ: Fludarabine therapy in hairy cell leukemia. Cancer 67:1291, 1991.

232. Cheever MA, Fefer A, Greenberg PD, et al: Identical twin bone marrow transplantation for hairy cell leukemia. Semin Oncol 11(suppl 2):511, 1984.

CHAPTER 4

Chronic Myelogenous Leukemia

Jorge E. Cortes, MD, Moshe Talpaz, MD, *and* Hagop Kantarjian, MD

Department of Hematology, The University of Texas M. D. Anderson Cancer Center, Houston, Texas

Chronic myelogenous leukemia (CML) is a clonal myeloproliferative disorder resulting from the neoplastic transformation of the primitive hemopoietic stem cell.[1-4] The disease is monoclonal in origin, affecting myeloid, monocytic, erythroid, megakaryocytic, B-cell, and sometimes T-cell lineages.[4,5] Bone marrow stromal cells are not involved.[6] CML has a very significant historical relevance because it was the first disease in which a specific chromosomal abnormality was linked to its pathogenesis, implicating activation of a specific oncogene in the chromosomal rearrangement.[7-10] At the therapeutic level, it is also historically important because it is one of the first neoplastic diseases for which the use of a biologic agent (ie, interferon) could suppress the neoplastic clone[11] and prolong survival.[12] Some of the most impressive results with bone marrow transplantation (BMT) also come from studies of patients with CML.[13]

EPIDEMIOLOGY

CML accounts for 7% to 15% of all leukemias in adults, with approximately 1 to 1.5 cases per 100,000 population.[14-16] There is a male predominance, with a male to female ratio of 1.4–2.2 to 1.[15-17] The incidence of CML has remained steady for the last 50 years.[16] The median age at presentation is 50 to 60 years,[15,17] but the disease can be seen in all age groups. In earlier reports, 54% to 63% of patients were 60 years old and older,[15,18] but the incidence has decreased in more recent reports to as low as 12%.[3] This may be a consequence of earlier detection in recent years or the exclusion of patients having CML-like pictures (ie, other myeloproliferative disorders, Philadelphia chromosome-negative CML, chronic myelomonocytic leukemia) who are usually significantly older.

ETIOLOGY

The etiology of CML is not clear. There is little evidence for genetic factors linked to CML. Offspring of parents with CML do not have a higher incidence of CML than the general population.[19] There is also no correlation in monozygotic twins, suggesting that CML is an acquired disorder.[19] However, there may be some correlation with human leukocyte antigens (HLAs) CW3 and CW4.[20]

Survivors of the atomic disasters at Nagasaki and Hiroshima had a significantly higher incidence of CML.[21] Therapeutic radiation has also been associated with increased risk of CML.[22] This was the case in patients with ankylosing spondylitis treated with spinal irradiation[23] and in women with uterine cervical cancer given radiation therapy.[24] Chemicals have not been associated with increased risk for CML.

CLINICAL CHARACTERISTICS

The disease usually has a biphasic and sometimes triphasic course. The initial phase is the chronic phase, which is frequently asymptomatic. The incidence of asymptomatic cases has increased over the last decade from 15% to about 40% of all cases[3] as a result of more widespread use of routine blood testing. Patients with symptoms usually have a gradual onset of fatigue, anorexia, weight loss, increased sweating, left upper quadrant discomfort, and early satiety as a result of splenic enlargement.[25] Rare patients with very high counts of white blood cells (WBCs) may have manifestations of hyperviscosity, including priapism, tinnitus, stupor, visual changes from retinal hemorrhages, and even cerebrovascular accidents.[26] There are a few case reports of CML presenting as diabetes insipidus.[27] On physical exam splenomegaly was documented in approximately 70% of the patients in older series, but its incidence has decreased to 30% in more recent series. Sometimes the spleen may be massive. The liver is also enlarged in 10% to 40% of cases.

The accelerated phase is an ill-defined transitional phase[28] that is frequently asymptomatic. The diagnosis is made from changes in peripheral blood or bone marrow. Some patients may have fever, night sweats, and progressive enlargement of the spleen. At least 20% of patients enter a blastic phase without evidence of having had accelerated phase.[3]

Patients in the blastic phase are more likely to have symptoms, including weight loss, fever, night sweats, and bone pains.[17] Symptoms of anemia, infectious complications, and bleeding are commonly seen. Subcutaneous nodules or hemorrhagic tender skin lesions and lymphadenopathy are more common in this phase, and signs of central nervous system (CNS) leukemia can also be seen.[17] In the blastic phase, tissue infiltration can occur, most frequently to the lymph nodes, skin, subcutaneous tissues, and bone.

LABORATORY FEATURES

Peripheral Blood

The most common feature of CML is an elevated WBC count, usually above 25×10^9/L, and frequently above 100×10^9/L.[29] Some patients have wide cyclic variations in their WBC count, with peak counts every few days or separated by up to 70 days.[30] The WBC differential usually shows granulocytes in all stages of maturation, from blasts to mature granulocytes that look morphologically normal. The number of basophils is usually increased from that normally expected, but only 10% to 15% of patients have 7% or more basophils in peripheral blood; a very high proportion (ie, 20% or more) of basophils in the peripheral blood usually signals acceleration of CML.[28] The number of eosinophils is also frequently higher than normal, but to a smaller degree. The absolute lymphocyte count is usually elevated, mostly representing an expansion of T–lymphocytes.[31] The platelet count is elevated in 30% to 50% of patients and is higher than $1,000 \times 10^9$/L in a few patients. Thrombocytopenia can also be seen and usually signals acceleration of the disease.[28] Most patients have mild anemia at diagnosis, but untreated patients may be severely anemic.

The neutrophil function is usually normal or only mildly impaired.[32] Patients in the chronic phase do not have an increased risk for infections. However, the activity of their natural killer cells is impaired because of the defective maturation of these cells.[33] Platelet function is frequently abnormal as measured in the laboratory and most frequently shows a decreased secondary aggregation with epinephrine, but this usually does not have clinical significance.

Bone Marrow

The bone marrow is hypercellular, with cellularity of 75% to 90%, and very little fat. The myeloid to erythroid ratio is 10:1 to 30:1 rather than the normal 2:1 to 5:1.[34] The myelocyte is the predominant cell in the bone marrow during the chronic phase, with promyelocytes and blasts accounting for less than 10% of all cells. Megakaryocytes are increased early in the disease and may show dysplastic features. Cells mimicking Gaucher cells can be seen in 10% of cases, as can "sea–blue" histiocytes.[35] Fibrosis

may be evident at diagnosis and increases with disease progression.[36] Surprisingly, reticulin fibrosis grades 3 to 4 are seen in up to 30% to 40% of cases and has been associated with a worse prognosis.[36]

Other Laboratory Findings

The activity of leukocyte alkaline phosphatase is reduced in nearly all patients at diagnosis.[37] The significance of this finding is unclear, but interestingly, the activity can be restored after transfusing leukocytes from patients with CML to neutropenic patients, which suggests extrinsic regulation.[38] Granulocyte colony-stimulating factor can induce synthesis of leukocyte alkaline phosphatase in vitro.[39] The activity of leukocyte alkaline phosphatase also increases with infections, stress, and upon achievement of remission or progression to the blastic phase.

Serum levels of vitamin B_{12} and transcobalamin are increased, sometimes up to 10 times the normal levels. Although this is in part due to the high WBC count, these levels may remain high even after hematologic remission. Serum levels of uric acid and lactic dehydrogenase are also frequently elevated.

CML PHASES

As mentioned, CML has a bi- or triphasic course. There is an initial chronic phase that eventually leads to a blastic phase, sometimes preceded by an intermediate or accelerated phase. The chronic phase, if untreated, has a median duration of 3.5 to 5 years before evolving to the more aggressive phases. The diagnosis is based on the characteristics mentioned above.

The blastic phase resembles an acute leukemia. Its diagnosis requires the presence of at least 30% of blasts in the bone marrow or peripheral blood.[40] In some patients the blastic phase is characterized by extramedullary deposits of leukemia called myeloblastomas.[41] These usually appear in the CNS, lymph nodes, or bones and occasionally occur in the absence of blood or bone marrow evidence of blastic transformation. Most of these cases, however, will have hematologic manifestations within a few months.[42] Patients in the blastic phase usually die within 3 to 6 months. Approximately 50% of patients have a myeloid blastic phase, 25% lymphoid, and 25% undifferentiated.[43] Although median survival is slightly better for patients with a lymphoid blastic phase than for those who have myeloid or undifferentiated cases (9 vs 3 months), the outcome is still very poor.[43]

Seventy-five to 80% of patients go through an accelerated phase before entering the blastic phase.[3] The definition for the accelerated phase is not uniform.[28]

TABLE 1

Clinical Characteristics of Patients With Different Phases of Chronic Myelogenous Leukemia

	Percentage of patients with characteristics								
	Chronic phase			Accelerated phase			Blast phase		
Characteristics	Before 1983 (N=336)	Since 1983 (N=494)	P	Before 1983 (N=51)	Since 1983 (N=139)	P	Before 1983 (N=48)	Since 1983 (N=61)	P
Age ≥ 60 yr	18	12	.03	16	11	NS	13	21	NS
Asymptomatic	15	37	< .01	4	20	.02	8	24	NS
Hepatomegaly	46	18	< .01	51	19	< .01	60	22	.01
Splenomegaly	76	54	< .01	84	70	NS	91	56	.01
Hemoglobin < 12 g/dL	58	48	.01	50	55	NS	79	50	.05
WBC count ≥ 100 ×10⁹/L	69	56	< .01	67	64	.84	45	46	NS
Platelet count > 700 ×10⁹/L	28	19	< .01	20	14	NS	8	17	NS
Peripheral blasts	65	56	.03	48	41	NS	83	50	.03
Peripheral basophils ≥ 7%	17	14	NS	17	27	NS	14	13	NS
Marrow blasts ≥ 5%	16	9	< .01	35	34	NS	95	91	NS
Marrow basophils ≥ 3%	40	35	NS	57	52	NS	33	19	NS

NS = not significant, WBC = white blood cell

Specific criteria associated with a survival shorter than 18 months by multivariate analysis have been proposed, including the presence of 15% or more blasts in peripheral blood, 30% or more blasts and promyelocytes in the blood, 20% or more basophils in the blood, or a platelet count less than 100×10^9/L (Table 1).[28] Cytogenetic clonal evolution has been considered a criterion for acceleration. Recent analysis suggests that its prognostic effect depends on the specific abnormality, its predominance in marrow metaphases, and the time of appearance.[44] Patients with chromosome 17 abnormalities, 25% or more abnormal metaphases, clonal evolution longer than 25 months after diagnosis, and no prior therapy with alpha interferon (IFN-α) have the worst outcome. The median survival for patients with none of these features is 51 months compared with 24, 14, and 7 months when 1, 2, or 3 or 4 features, respectively, are present.[42]

STAGING OF CML

Several clinical characteristics have been identified to have prognostic significance in CML. These include age, spleen size, liver size, platelet count, WBC count, percentages of blasts and basophils in blood or bone marrow, number of nucleated red blood cells, and cytogenetic clonal evolution. These factors have been incorporated in staging systems.[45–48] A synthesis staging system has incorporated factors from all these systems and resulted in a simple model for staging that can identify four CML stages with different outcomes (Table 2).[49] The stage at diagnosis has been identified as one of the most important predictors of survival after treatment with IFN-α therapy[50,51] but is somehow less predictive for patients treated with chemotherapy alone.[52] The response to therapy with IFN-α is a significant prognostic factor for long-term survival and will be discussed later in this review.

Other factors have been suggested to be predictive of response to therapy and survival. The site of the breakpoint in the *bcr* gene has been thought to have prognostic significance,[53,54] but large studies show a lack of correlation with response to therapy or survival.[55]

CYTOGENETIC AND MOLECULAR CHANGES

Ninety to 95% of all patients with CML have the Philadelphia (Ph) chromosome.[56] Initially identified as a short chromosome 22, it actually represents a balanced translocation between the long arms of chromosomes 9 and 22, t(9;22)(q34;q11).[56] The c-*abl* proto-oncogene located on chromosome 9q34 is homologous to the transforming element of the Abelson murine leukemia

TABLE 2

Synthesis Staging System for Chronic Myelogenous Leukemia

Criteria	Stage	Definition
For chronic phase		
Age ≥ 60 years	1	0 or 1 characteristics
Spleen ≥ 10 cm below costal margin	2	2 characteristics
Blasts ≥ 3% in blood or ≥ 5% in marrow	3	≥ 3 characteristics
For accelerated phase	4	≥ 1 characteristic (regardless of characteristics for chronic phase)
Cytogenetic clonal evolution		
Blasts ≥ 15% in blood		
Blasts + promyelocytes ≥ 30% in blood		
Basophils ≥ 20% in blood		
Platelets < 100 × 10⁹/L		

virus, v-*abl*. It codes for a nonreceptor protein–tyrosine kinase expressed in most mammalian cells, but its normal function is unknown. In the Ph chromosome, the breakpoint occurs within the first intron of c-*abl*, therefore translocating exons 2 through 11 to chromosome 22.[56] In chromosome 22, the breakpoint occurs within the *bcr* gene, a large 70-kb gene with 20 exons. The breakpoint usually involves a 5.8-kb area known as the breakpoint cluster region, either between exons b3 and b4 or b2 and b3.[56] Therefore, two different fusion genes can be formed, both of them joining exon 2 of *abl* with either exon 2 of *bcr* (b2a2) or exon 3 of *bcr* (b3a2). This hybrid gene is then transcribed into an 8.5-kb mRNA, in contrast to the normal c-*abl*, which is 6 to 7 kb.[57]

Upon translation, a new protein is synthesized that has a molecular mass of 210 kDa (p210$^{bcr/abl}$); the normal c-*abl* is 145 kDa. The normal tyrosine kinase activity of c-*abl* is dysregulated as a consequence of its binding to *bcr*, with markedly increased autophosphorylating activity.[58] The binding to *bcr* also activates an actin-binding function associated with c-*abl*.[59] The expression of p210$^{bcr/abl}$ is sufficient to induce leukemic transformation of transfected cells[60] and can induce leukemia in transgenic mice.[61] Although the mechanism by which this new protein can induce transformation is not well known, recent data have clarified this issue to some extent. The first exon of *bcr* is essential for the transforming ability of *bcr/abl* and binds to an ABL SH2 domain in a phospho-

tyrosine-independent manner.[62] Disruption of this binding eliminates the transforming activity of *bcr/abl*. Upon autophosphorylation, several tyrosine residues are phosphorylated. The most critical one seems to be Y177, which then links p210$^{bcr/abl}$ to a 26-kDa protein with SH2 and SH3 domains called GRB-2.[63] This protein links tyrosine kinases to *ras* signaling.[64] *Ras* activation is in fact required for transformation by several tyrosine kinases,[65] and suggests that it also plays a major role in *bcr/abl* directed transformation. The actin-binding function of *abl* seems to be important for the transforming ability.[66] Other proteins may also be bound and phosphorylated by *bcr/abl*. One such protein is CRKL, which is the most abundant phosphorylated protein in some CML cell lines,[67] but its specific role in leukemic transformation is not yet clear. It is likely, however, that more than one pathway is involved in leukemic transformation after *bcr/abl* autophosphorylation. When the *bcr/abl* SH2 domain (ie, the major tyrosine autophosphorilation site of the kinase domain) is mutated, transforming activity is lost, but it can be restored by the overexpression of c-*myc*.[68] It is not known whether signals generated through GRB-2 feed into both pathways (ie, *ras* and *myc*) or whether other pathways are involved. It has also been suggested that the activation of the tyrosine kinase activity may suppress apoptosis in hemopoietic cells.[69]

The reciprocal fusion gene (ie, *abl/bcr*) is transcribed in approximately two thirds of patients with CML, but the significance of this event is not clear.[70]

As mentioned earlier, additional chromosomal abnormalities are a marker of acceleration of the disease. The most common events are the appearance of an additional Ph chromosome, trisomy 8, and isochromosome 17q. The molecular events of acceleration, however, are not well defined.[71] Mutations of *p53* have been found frequently by some investigators,[72] but others found mutations a less common event, whereas deletions and rearrangements may occur during the blastic phase.[73] Overall, loss of function of *p53* is probably associated with disease progression in approximately 25% of CML patients.[74]

Besides the intrinsic abnormalities of CML cells determined by the *bcr/abl* and associated intracellular signal elements, external regulatory factors are also affected in CML. Cells from CML patients have a defect in cellular adhesion to stromal cells that affects the regulation of myeloid cell growth.[75] CML progenitor cells are deficient in the expression of the cytoadhesion molecule lymphocyte function antigen-3.[76] This deficiency is corrected by exposure to IFN-α.[76] IFN-α can also increase adhesion to stroma by a mechanism that can be blocked by antibodies to integrins α4, α5, and β1.[77] This is not related to a deficient expression of the integrins but to a functional defect of these molecules.[77] More evidence for the dysregulation of CML cells by external influences was provided by studies on interleukin-1. Levels of interleukin-1-β have been reported to be elevated in patients with CML, and inhibitors of interleukin-1 can suppress CML clonogenic growth.[78] Elevated levels of interleukin-1 have been correlated with an adverse prognosis.[79]

THERAPY

Conventional Therapy and Other Chemotherapy

For a long time, therapy for CML has consisted mostly of busulfan (Myleran) or hydroxyurea (Hydrea). Busulfan allows long periods of hematologic control and is not expensive, making it attractive for use when socioeconomic issues are important or in patients for whom follow-up is erratic. Busulfan therapy is associated with lung, marrow and heart fibrosis and can cause Addisonlike disease; in 10% of patients, prolonged myelosuppression may be observed. The dose of busulfan is usually 0.1 mg/kg/d until the WBC counts decrease by 50%, and then the dose is reduced by 50%. Therapy is discontinued when the WBC count drops below 20×10^9/L and is restarted when it increases above 50×10^9/L.

Hydroxyurea has a lower toxicity profile but shorter control of hematologic manifestations, requiring more frequent follow-up.[80] It is usually given at a dose of 40 mg/kg/d and is reduced by 50% when the WBC count drops below 20×10^9/L. The dose is then adjusted individually to keep the WBC count at 5 to 10×10^9/L. One study used higher doses of hydroxyurea (2 g/m²/d) until the absolute neutrophil count reached $<1 \times 10^9$/L.[81] Patients achieving a cytogenetic response were given additional cycles until maximal response. Fourteen of 25 cycles administered to 14 patients in the chronic phase resulted in $\geq 25\%$ Ph-chromosome-negative cells. In one patient a complete cytogenetic remission was achieved. In all cases however, the responses were transient.[81]

Both drugs can control the hematologic manifestations of the disease in more than 70% of all patients. A recent large randomized study prospectively compared these two agents in patients with chronic-phase CML.[82] Patients treated with hydroxyurea had a longer median duration of the chronic phase (47 months vs 37 months, $P = .04$) and a longer overall survival (58 months vs 45 months; $P = .008$) than those treated with busulfan.[82] The toxicity profile was also better for hydroxyurea. Hematologic improvements were not accompanied by a significant reduction in the percentage of cells bearing the Ph

chromosome. Therefore, while disease control can be achieved with these agents, the ability to regress the disease to the acute phase remains unchanged.

One recent study used continuous infusion of low-dose cytarabine in patients with chronic-phase CML.[83] Five patients received 15 to 30 mg/m²/d of cytarabine. The hematologic manifestations of the disease were controlled in all patients, and all achieved some cytogenetic response, including one complete response and one partial response.[83] This approach, however, is still experimental. Other chemotherapeutic agents such as mercaptopurine (Purinethol), melphalan (Alkeran), and thioguanine have been used less frequently, sometimes in combination with busulfan.[84] Thiotepa has been used to treat excessive thrombocytopenia associated with CML.[85]

Homoharringtonine is a promising agent in CML. Patients in early chronic phase who have been treated with homoharringtonine have a complete hematologic response (CHR) rate of 95%, with 24% entering major cytogenetic remission.[86] In patients in the late chronic phase, these rates are 68% and 17%, respectively, despite the fact that two thirds of the patients were refractory to IFN-α.[87]

Interferon

In the early 1980s IFN-α was introduced into the therapy for CML, following observations of in vitro inhibition of myeloid colony formation when normal or CML progenitors were cultured in its presence.[88] The first reports in humans used partially pure IFN-α to treat 51 patients in chronic phase.[88] A CHR was achieved in 71%. More important, however, was the fact that cytogenetic responses (ie, suppression of the Ph-positive clone) were observed in 39% of patients.[89] Recombinant human IFN-α soon became available and had similar results to those achieved with natural IFN-α. This was confirmed in several trials. In the last update from The University of Texas M. D. Anderson Cancer Center, 274 patients treated with IFN-α-based were reported.[50] Eighty percent of the patients achieved a CHR with cytogenetic responses rates of 40% to 60% and a major cytogenetic response rate of 38%. Twenty-six percent of the patients achieved a complete cytogenetic response (Table 3). Cytogenetic responses are considered complete if Ph-positive cells constitute 0% of all cells, partial if they represent between 1% and 34% of all cells, and minor if they represent 35% to 90% of all cells. Complete and partial cytogenetic responses constitute major cytogenetic responses.[91] Other studies have used different criteria, making comparisons of results among studies difficult. Standard response criteria, as proposed in Table 4, will

TABLE 3

Results of Treatment With IFN-α for Patients in Early Chronic-Phase CML [a]

Response	Category	Number (%)
Hematologic	Complete	219 (80)
	Partial	19 (7)
	Resistant	36 (13)
Cytogenetic	Any [b]	159 (58)
	Complete	72 (26)
	Partial	32 (12)
	Minor	55 (20)

CML = chronic myelogenous leukemia, IFN-α = alpha interferon
[a] M. D. Anderson experience with 274 patients
[b] All with complete hematologic response

help such comparative studies in the future, because CHR and cytogenetic responses have prognostic relevance. The median time to achieve a hematologic remission is 6 to 8 months.[51,91] For cytogenetic responses, the median time is 22 to 24 months for a complete response, 12 to 18 months for a partial response, and 8 to 14 months for a minor response.[3,51,91] Responses may be faster with recombinant than with natural IFN-α.[91] The cytogenetic responses achieved with IFN-α are durable in > 50% of patients achieving them, or in about 25% to 30% of all patients in the early chronic phase.[3] The durability is greater in patients who achieve complete or partial responses than in those with lesser degrees of major cytogenetic responses. Several other groups have confirmed these observations, but the results vary.[51,92–96] In analyzing these results, several factors must be considered, including the dose, the patients selected for treatment trials and their phase of disease, the type of therapy given, and the toxic effects patients experience.

Dose: There is a dose-response effect with IFN-α in CML. The dose used in most studies that documented significant response is $5 \times 10^6/U/m^2/d$.[51] With lower doses the results are inferior.[3] In one study, patients were randomized to receive $2 \times 10^6 U/m^2$ three times a week or $5 \times 10^6 U/m^2$ three times a week.[97] The CHR rate was lower with the lower dose (24% vs 47%; $P = .06$). Patients who did not respond to the lower dose still achieved a CHR with the higher dose. The same group observed a CHR rate of 87% when they used a daily schedule.[97] One recent report suggests that low doses are as effective as high doses.[93] These results may be influenced by patient selection and should be considered cautiously. At this

point, the recommended dose is therefore $5 \times 10^6 U/m^2/d$ or the maximally tolerated individual dose not to exceed $5 \times 10^6 U/m^2/d$.

Patient Selection: Several patient characteristics are associated with failure to achieve a major cytogenetic response and with worse survival after treatment with IFN-α. These include poor performance status, the presence of symptoms at diagnosis, splenomegaly, anemia, leukocytosis, a high percentage of blasts in the peripheral blood, peripheral nucleated red blood cells, and marrow basophilia.[50] The stage of disease, whether staged with Sokal's model[47] or the synthesis staging system,[49] is strongly predictive of response and survival.[50] Patients at low risk have a CHR rate of 80% to 90%, with 40% having major cytogenetic responses compared with 50% to 60% and 20% to 30%, respectively, for patients at intermediate risk and 20% to 60% and 5% to 10%, respectively, for patients at high risk[3] (Table 5). Age is a significant survival factor, with patients 60 years old and older having a worse prognosis.[47,49] However, a recent report from M. D. Anderson Cancer Center suggests that patients in this age group may have responses to IFN-α similar to those in younger patients, albeit with more toxic effects.[98]

TABLE 4

Criteria for Response to IFN-α in CML

Response	Category	Criteria
Hematologic remission	Complete	Normalization of WBC counts to $< 9 \times 10^9$/L with normal differential
	Partial	Decrease in WBC to $\leq 50\%$ of pretreatment level and to $< 20 \times 10^9$/L, or Normalization of WBC with persistent splenomegaly or immature peripheral cells
Cytogenetic response	Complete [a]	No evidence of Ph-positive cells
	Partial [a]	5% to 34% of metaphases Ph-positive
	Minor	35% to 95% of metaphases Ph-positive
	None	Persistence of Ph chromosome in all analyzable cells

CML = chronic myelogenous leukemia, IFN-α = alpha interferon, Ph = Philadelphia chromosome, WBC = white blood cell   [a] Major cytogenetic response includes complete and partial cytogenetic responses

TABLE 5

Response to Alpha Interferon (IFN-α) Therapy With Different Dose Schedules

Study	IFN-α dose	Schedule	Number of patients	CHR (%)	Cytogenetic responses		
					Any	Major	Complete
MDACC	5×10^6 U/m²	Daily	274	80	58	38	26
Schofield et al	2×10^6 U/m²	Daily	27	70	33	22	7
Alimena et al	5×10^6 U/m²	TIW	30	63	NS	NS	NS
	2×10^6 U/m²	TIW	30	24	NS	NS	NS
Freund et al	5×10^6 U	TIW	10	33	0	0	0
Anger et al	3×10^6 U	TIW	9	22	20	0	0

CHR = complete hematologic response, MDACC = M. D. Anderson Cancer Center, NS = not stated, TIW = three times a week

CML Phase: The phase of the disease at the time of treatment is a major determinant of response. Patients in the chronic phase have the best response to IFN-α.[3] Among those in the chronic phase, patients treated within 1 year from diagnosis (ie, early chronic phase) have a CHR rate of 60% to 80%, and 20% to 30% of them have major cytogenetic responses compared with a CHR rate of 50% to 60% in fewer than 10% of patients treated more than 1 year from diagnosis. Patients in the accelerated or blastic phase have CHR rates of less than 40% and only occasionally have a cytogenetic response (Table 7).[3]

Several groups have documented a survival advantage for patients treated with IFN-α compared with conventional chemotherapy.[50,51,94–96] Time to progression to blastic phase was also prolonged. In all three randomized studies,[51,94,96] IFN-α produced higher rates of major and complete cytogenetic remission compared with conventional chemotherapy, but one of these studies showed no survival advantage over that achieved with hydroxyurea.[96] The recent update from the Italian Cooperative Study Group on CML,[51] which compared treatment with IFN–α vs conventional chemotherapy, documented a longer median survival for patients treated with IFN-α (median 72+ vs 52 months; $P = .002$). The 6-year survival rate was 50% vs 29% for patients treated with IFN-α and chemotherapy, respectively ($P = .002$). The time to the acceleration or blastic phase was also significantly prolonged for the IFN-α group (72+ vs 45 months; $P < .001$).[51] Similar results were reported by Allan et al.[94] A recent study by Hehlmann et al[96] randomized patients to receive IFN-α or conventional chemotherapy. Patients treated with IFN-α had a median survival of 5.5 years (5-year survival rate of 59%) compared with 3.8 years (32%) for those treated with busulfan ($P = .008$) and 4.7 years (44%) for those treated with hydroxyurea (not statistically significant).

Several points may explain the findings: (1) some patients entered on the IFN-α arm may not have been in the chronic phase (blasts up to 35%, platelets less than 100×10^9/L) (2) the actual dose–schedule of IFN-α delivered was 2×10^6 U/m²/d after the initial 4 weeks and (3) the complete and major cytogenetic response rates were low (7% and 10%, respectively). The latter two observations are important because some studies show superior survival only with achievement of a major cytogenetic response, which is enhanced by higher dose schedules of IFN-α.

Achievement of a cytogenetic response is associated with a survival advantage in several studies. However, two studies failed to document such a correlation.[92,96] These studies had a low rate of major cytogenetic responses, possibly because of the patients selected or because the actual doses of IFN-α administered were lower.[92,96] Two other studies show that patients who achieve a cytogenetic response have a survival advantage, whereas those who fail to achieve such a response have a survival similar to that of patients treated with conventional chemotherapy.[50,51] In a trial from the Medical Research Council, even though patients who did not respond to IFN-α had a shorter survival than did responders, they still showed a survival advantage over those treated with chemotherapy.[94] Multivariate analysis has not been completed in this study.[94]

Combination Therapy Using IFN: IFN-α-based combinations have attempted to improve on the results of single agent trials. Initial studies with IFN-γ documented a CHR rate of 23%, and some patients who were refractory to one type of IFN-(α or γ) responded to the other.[99] These results prompted the use of a combination of IFN-α and IFN-γ.[100,101] The combination is well tolerated, but the results are not better than those achieved with IFN-α alone.[100,101]

TABLE 6

Response to Alpha Interferon and Survival by Prognostic Groups

Prognostic group [a]	Cytogenetic response	Number of patients	Survival		P value
			3 years	5 years	
Good	Yes	73	93	79	< .01
	No	68	86	62	
Intermediate	Yes	25	95	82	< .01
	No	31	76	35	
Poor	Yes	9	100	83	< .01
	No	31	68	39	

[a] According to the prognostic synthesis model

Cytarabine has selective in vitro activity against CML, and preliminary studies reported cytogenetic responses in patients treated with it alone.[83] The combination of cytarabine and IFN-α in patients in late chronic phase achieved a CHR rate of 55% and a cytogenetic response rate of 15%, which compares favorably with the 28% (P < .01) and 5% (not significant), respectively, achieved with IFN-α alone. Survival rates were also better with the combination. For patients in the accelerated phase, no improvement in the response rate was observed.[102] Among patients in the early chronic phase, Arthur and Ma reported a CHR rate of 93%, a cytogenetic response rate of 67%, and a complete cytogenetic response rate of 30%.[103] Guilhot et al randomized patients to receive IFN-α alone or with low-dose cytarbine and reported a trend for a higher complete cytogenetic response rate in patients treated with the combination schedule (23% vs 14%; P < .24).[104]

Other combinations are less effective. The use of busulfan with IFN-α can be complicated by prolonged myelosuppression. Hydroxyurea can be given safely with IFN-α and is popular in clinical practice because CHR is achieved faster; however, the cytogenetic response rates are similar. With the results reported by Hehlmann et al,[96] this combination may be investigated further in future trials. Intensive chemotherapy can produce complete and major cytogenetic responses in 30% to 50% of patients who have chronic-phase CML,[105] but these responses are transient and last only for 3 to 9 months. The use of IFN-α as a maintenance drug following the induction of intensive chemotherapy does not improve the survival rate or the durability of cytogenetic responses over those achieved with IFN-α alone.[106]

Toxicity of IFN: Most patients treated with IFN-α experience a transient flu-like syndrome with fever, chills, malaise, fatigue, and anorexia. These are transient, not dose–limiting, and manageable symptomatically. Simple measures such as starting with 25% to 50% of the dose of IFN-α for the first week, giving it at night, reducing the initial WBC count to between 10 and 20 × 10^9/L with other chemotherapy before the start of IFN-α, and premedicating with acetaminophen can help control these symptoms.[3]

With long-term administration of IFN-α, late side effects occur that may be dose–limiting in 10% to 25% of patients.[3] The most common are chronic fatigue (61% of patients) and weight loss (50%). Less frequent (ie, less than 20%) side effects include diarrhea, alopecia, stomatitis, and neurotoxicity, usually in the form of recent memory loss or depression.[91] Patients 60 years old and older experience more side effects with IFN-α, particularly neurotoxicity.[98,107] Fewer than 2% of patients develop bone marrow aplasia, particularly when they had received prior busulfan therapy.[108] Autoimmune phenomena occur in fewer than 5% of patients and include hemolytic anemia, thrombocytopenia, hypothyroidism, Raynaud's phenomenon, arthritis, lupus erythematosus, and cardiac problems such as arrhythmias and congestive heart failure.[109] Interestingly, 91% of patients with hypothyroidism and 75% of those with diseases involving connective tissue had some degree of cytogenetic response.[109]

When side effects develop, dose reduction may be indicated as follows: (1) for grade 3 or 4 toxicity, hold therapy until recovery and restart at 50% of the dose; (2) for persistent grade 2 toxicity, reduce the dose by 25%; and (3) for WBC counts lower than 2 × 10^9/L or platelet counts less than 60 × 10^9/L, reduce the dose by 25%.

Allogeneic BMT

Another treatment used in patients with CML is allogeneic BMT, which is curative. Results are more encour-

TABLE 7

Response to Alpha Interferon by Chronic Myelogenous Leukemia Phase

		Cytogenetic response (%)	
Phase	CHR (%)	Any	Major
Early chronic	60–80	40–50	20–30
Late chronic	50–60	10–20	< 10
Accelerated	30–40	< 10	0
Blastic	20–30	< 10	0

CHR = complete hematologic remission

aging for patients in chronic than accelerated or blastic phase. Several studies have reported long-term survival rates of 50% to 80% and disease-free survival rates of 30% to 70% in patients with chronic-phase CML.[110-117] The results, however, are not uniform in all studies and are dependent on the patient's age at the time of BMT, the stage of disease, regimens used to prepare patients for BMT, and manipulation of bone marrow to enhance the chances of a good response.

Age at Time of Transplant: Younger patients have a better outcome with allogeneic BMT, but the age cutoff is controversial. Patients younger than 20 years have the best outcome, with long-term disease-free survival of 60% to 70% in most studies and a very low incidence of transplant-related mortality (approximately 10%) and leukemia relapse (20%).[110,115] With increased age, the rate of complications increases, but the relapse rate remains similar. Data from the International Bone Marrow Transplant Registry suggest that after age 20, there is a significant drop in the disease-free survival rate.[110,115] Data from a Seattle study show that selected patients age 50 to 60 years may have 4-year disease-free survival rates of greater than 80%.[13] Most studies, however, show a decline in long-term survival after age 20 to 30 years.[114,117] Until the results from Seattle can be reproduced more widely, patients older than 20 to 30 years, depending on the experience at each institution, should be considered to have a higher risk of transplant-related complications.

Stage of Disease: The results with allogeneic BMT are also better for patients in the chronic phase than for those in the accelerated or blastic phase. Long-term survival rates are 50% to 60%, 15% to 40%, and less than 15% for those three groups, respectively.[110,115] Among patients in the chronic phase, early transplantation is important in achieving good results. Some groups advocate that transplantation within 1 year from diagnosis produces better

results than later transplant.[111,116] This may be influenced by prior therapy: patients previously treated with busulfan do worse because of higher transplant-related morbidity; when these patients are excluded, the difference is less significant.[111] Prior treatment with IFN-α, however, does not adversely affect overall survival, disease-free survival, time to neutrophil or platelet recovery, incidence of graft-vs-host disease (GVHD), or the 100-day BMT-related mortality.[114] Data from the International Bone Marrow Transplant Registry show only a significant trend for better outcome for patients who undergo BMT within 1 year from diagnosis compared with those who have BMTs 1 to 3 years or more than 3 years after diagnosis,[114] but this has not been confirmed in the European Bone Marrow Transplant Registry.[110] Recent data from Seattle suggest that patients who undergo BMT 1 to 2 years after diagnosis have a similar outcome to those who have BMT within the first year of diagnosis.[11] Even when the difference is found to be significantly in favor of transplantation during the first year, the disease-free survival rate improves by less than 10%[118] and may be less with time.[119] Interestingly, this difference is not due to more resistant disease but to a higher BMT-related mortality.

Preparative Regimens: The initial studies of allogeneic BMT in patients with CML used conditioning regimens containing cyclophosphamide and total body irradiation.[115,116] An escalation in the dose of total body irradiation resulted in a decrease in the relapse rate but increased the risk of death due to causes other than relapse.[112] Substituting busulfan for total body irradiation resulted in an outcome comparable with that of patients whose regimens included total body irradiation.[111] In a randomized trial comparing the two alternatives, the busulfan-containing regimen resulted in a nonsignificant trend to better overall and disease-free survivals.[113] The use of total body irradiation was associated with significantly more patients with GVHD, fever, and prolonged hospitalization.[113] A recent report suggests that patients with advanced disease treated with busulfan may have more early toxic effects and increased transplant-related mortality.[120] Other preparative regimens produce similar results.[121]

Bone Marrow Manipulation: Several groups have used T-cell depletion in an effort to decrease the incidence of GVHD in patients undergoing allogeneic BMT.[122,123] Although this approach can in fact reduce the incidence of GVHD, it also leads to an increased risk of relapse and graft failure.[117,122,123] More selective depletion of specific subtypes of T-cells may preserve the cells responsible for the graft-vs-leukemia effect.[124] Selective

T-cell purging is an encouraging investigational trend.

Several approaches have become available for patients whose disease relapses after allogeneic BMT. A second transplant has been used with some success, particularly among patients who received a second BMT 1 year after the first.[125] Recent investigations have focused on immune-mediated mechanisms to control relapse. For instance, the infusion of leukocytes from the original bone marrow donor after disease relapses in patients with CML[126–130] has resulted in the disappearance of the malignant clone[126–129] even when assessed with the polymerase chain reaction (PCR).[126] Another approach is to give IFN-α therapy to patients whose disease recurs after BMT.[130,132] In two studies using this alternative, 6 of 18 patients who had a hematologic relapse and 8 of 11 who had a cytogenetic–only relapse[132] responded to IFN. A recent study combined IFN-α and donor leukocyte infusions to treat eight patients with chronic-phase CML that recurs after BMT.[133] PCR showed no evidence of cells bearing the Ph chromosome in six of these patients.[133]

Because only a small fraction of patients have donors for an allogeneic BMT, interest has focused on BMT using matched unrelated donors.[134,135] The 2-year disease-free survival rate is 37% to 45%,[134,135] with better results among patients who receive transplants when the disease is in the early chronic phase (45% vs 36%).[134] The best results are obtained in children.[135] Acute GVHD grades II to IV was seen in 77% to 82%,[134,135] and extensive chronic GVHD was seen in more than 50%. One disadvantage to this approach is the long time to identify a donor; in one study the median time from the start of the search to the BMT was 8.4 months.[135] Thus, although a promising alternative for patients without family donors, allogeneic BMT with matched unrelated donors is still a high-risk procedure with significant mortality and morbidity that is related to GVHD, which is most prevalent in patients 30 years or older and those with a mismatch of one or more antigens.

Autologous BMT

Some patients with CML have early progenitors (ie, CD34+, DR- cells) that do not express the bcr/abl gene and are thus probably unaffected by CML.[136] The early progenitors allow normal hematopoiesis to exist in these patients' bone marrows, even though the marrow is dominated by the malignant CML clone. The normal early progenitors can be collected by leukapheresis during early recovery following intensive chemotherapy.[137,138]

Cells collected in this way are more frequently Ph– negative than cells harvested from the bone marrow.[138]

This has led to investigations on autologous BMT as a therapeutic alternative in these CML patients. Although 40% to 70% of these patients can achieve some degree of suppression of Ph-positive cells upon engraftment after the transplant, this is usually a short-lived phenomenon, and disease in most patients eventually recurs.[137,139–142] The use of stem cells may enable faster engraftment but does not prolong survival.[142]

Interestingly, some patients previously refractory to IFN-α may regain sensitivity after autologous BMT.[139] Patients who receive a BMT with unpurged bone marrow show no survival advantage over those who receive conventional chemotherapy only.[143] Studies using retrovirus-marked autologous bone marrow have shown that the disease recurs at least in part from infused leukemic cells.[144] This suggests the need for better bone marrow purging. Several approaches have been used for this purpose,[145] including the use of a long-term bone marrow culture that can select Ph-negative cells,[146] although usually significant numbers of Ph-positive cells are still detectable.[147] In vitro purging with mafosfamide,[148,149] interferon-γ,[150] antisense oligodeoxynucleotides to c-myb[151] or bcr/abl,[152–154] and other immunologic approaches[155] are also used, as is in vivo purging using intensive chemotherapy and early stem-cell collection. The ideal purging technique is not yet known, and active research in this area is currently being conducted. The use of IFN-α for maintenance therapy after autologous BMT has not resulted in sustained remissions.

MINIMAL RESIDUAL DISEASE

With the availability of more sensitive techniques, detection of minimal residual disease in CML, which has the advantage of having a specific marker (ie, Ph chromosome), has become possible.[120] However, the information regarding methods to detect minimal residual disease and its significance may be confusing, and the clinician has to be careful with interpretation of the results.

After treatment with IFN-α, the bcr/abl gene can be detected in nearly all patients with the PCR,[156,157] even although a few patients do become negative for this gene.[158] However, most patients will remain in complete remission even if bcr/abl is still present.[157] This may be explained by the extreme sensitivity of this technique, which may detect bcr/abl-positive cells that are either not clonogenic or not myeloid (eg, T-cells) long-lived cells. Some investigators have advocated the use of a semi-quantitative PCR procedure that would identify an increase in the expression of bcr/abl, which may predict relapse.[159,160] The use of fluorescent in situ hybridization may reveal the Ph chromosome in proliferating cells, which may be more useful for predicting relapse,[161,162] but this hypothesis needs further testing. Hypermetaphase fluorescent in situ hybridization is a technique that allows the analysis of 500 or more metaphases and thus offers an intermediate level of sensitivity between cytogenetics and the PCR. Interestingly, patients treated with IFN-α may continue to show bcr/abl-positive cells on PCR tests for some time[158] after they achieve a cytogenetic response.[158] Some patients have turned negative as late as 5 years after the initial response, but even after becoming negative on PCR tests, residual disease may be detected in some patients by clonogenic assay,[158] which suggests a state of tumor dormancy.

Unlike the situation with IFN-α, the PCR test has been more predictive of long-term outcome when used on samples from patients who have had a BMT, particularly when done 1 year after the BMT. Ph-positive cells may be detected soon after BMT, but they frequently disappear.[163] Persistent or increasing proportions of Ph-positive cells, however, may herald a relapse.[163] Single positive results on PCR within the first 6 months after BMT do not predict relapse,[164-166] but positive PCR samples after 6 months may be predictive.[167] When serial studies are performed, persistent positivity on PCR tests will be followed by a relapse in 75% of patients, whereas disease in only 20% with both positive and negative results and in none with all negative results will recur.[168] Patients who receive unmanipulated BMT may still eventually become bcr/abl negative despite positive results on PCR tests after 1 year from the transplant.[169,170]

PATIENTS IN THE ACCELERATED OR BLASTIC PHASE

Patients in the accelerated or blastic phase of CML respond poorly to therapy. Regimens including high-dose cytarabine and daunorubicin induce remissions in only 25% to 35% of patients, with a median survival of 8 to 18 months for those in the accelerated phase and 3 months for those in the blastic phase.[171] Regimens that do not contain cytarabine produce similarly poor results in these patients.[172] Results with allogeneic BMT are also worse than for patients in the chronic phase. The 4-year survival rate is 20% to 40%.[111,173] Some studies report more optimistic results,[174] but patient selection may be different. Patients who are in the accelerated phase only on the basis of clonal evolution and who undergo BMT less than 1 year after diagnosis of CML have a 4-year probability of survival of 74%.[173] As mentioned earlier, this is a group with a good outcome.[44] Autologous BMT has been used with the intention of reinstituting a second

chronic phase.[175] Although most patients achieve this status, their disease eventually recurs after a median disease-free survival of 8 months.[175]

Ph-NEGATIVE CML

In 5% to 10% of patients with otherwise typical clinical features of CML, the Ph chromosome is not found in cytogenetic studies.[176-179] One third of these patients have evidence of the bcr/abl translocation when analyzed at the molecular level.[177] These patients have similar clinical features, response to IFN therapy, and long-term prognosis similar to those of patients with Ph-positive disease.[178] Patients without molecular evidence of the translocation are older, have a higher incidence of thrombocytopenia, lower WBC counts, and fewer basophils than Ph-positive or Ph-negative, bcr-positive patients. Their median survival is significantly shorter than that of patients with Ph-positive or Ph-negative, bcr-positive CML (25 months vs 73 and 68 months, respectively).[178] However, disease in these patients does not evolve to a blastic phase as it does in Ph-positive or Ph-negative, bcr-positive patients. Instead, their natural history is characterized by increasing leukemia burden, with progressive leukocytosis, organomegaly, extramedullary infiltrates, and bone marrow failure without a significant increase in blasts.[179]

REFERENCES

1. Silver RT: Chronic myeloid leukemia. A perspective of the clinical and biologic issues of the chronic phase. Hematol Oncol Clin North Am 4:319–335, 1990.

2. Champlin RE, Golde DW: Chronic myelogenous leukemia: Recent advances. Blood 65:1039–1047, 1985.

3. Kantarjian HM, Deisseroth A, Kurzrock R, et al: Chronic myelogenous leukemia: A concise update. Blood 82:691–703, 1993.

4. Fialkow PJ, Jacobson RJ, Papayannopoulou T: Chronic myelocytic leukemia: Clonal origin in a stem cell common to the granulocyte, erythrocyte, platelet and monocyte/macrophage. Am J Med 63:125–130, 1977.

5. Pialkow PJ, Gartler SM, Yoshida A: Clonal origin of chronic myelocytic leukemia in man: Proc Natl Acad Sci USA 58:1468–1471, 1967.

6. Greenberg BR, Wilson FD, Woo L, Jenks HM: Cytogenetics of fibroblastic colonies in Ph[1]-positive chronic myelogenous leukemia. Blood 51:1039–1044, 1978.

7. Nowell PC, Hungerford DA: Chromosome studies on normal and leukemic human leukocytes. J Natl Cancer Inst 25:85–109, 1960.

8. Rowley JD: A new consistent chromosomal abnormality in chronic myelogenous leukemia identified by quinacrine fluorescence and Giemsa staining. Nature 243:290–293, 1973.

9. Klein A, van Kessel AG, Grosveld G, et al: A cellular oncogene is translocated to the Philadelphia chromosome in chronic myelocytic leukemia. Nature 300:765–767, 1982.

10. Bartram CR, de Klein A, Hagemeijer A, et al: Translocation of c–abl oncogene correlates with the presence of a Philadelphia chromosome in chronic myelocytic leukemia. Nature 306:277–280, 1983.

11.Talpaz M, Kantarjian HM, McCredie KB, et al: Clinical investigation of human alpha interferon in chronic myelogenous leukemia. Blood 69:1280–1288, 1987.

12. Kantarjian HM, Smith TL, O'Brien S, et al: Prolonged survival following achievement of cytogenetic response with alpha interferon therapy in chronic myelogenous leukemia. Ann Intern Med 1995 (in press).

13. Clift RA, Appelbaum FR, Thomas ED: Treatment of chronic myeloid leukemia by marrow transplantation. Blood 82:1954–1956, 1993.

14. Morrison VA: Chronic leukemias. CA Cancer J Clin 44:353–377, 1994.

15. Brincker H: Population-based age- and sex-specific incidence rates in the 4 main types of leukaemia. Scand J Haematol 29:241–249, 1982.

16. Call TG, Noel P, Habermann TM, et a: Incidence of leukemia in Olmsted County, Minnesota, 1975 through 1989. Mayo Clin Proc 69:315–322, 1994.

17. Hughes TP, Goldman JM: Chronic myeloid leukemia, in Hoffman R, Benz EJ Jr, Shattil SJ, et al (eds): Hematology. Basic Principles and Practice, pp 854–869. New York, NY, Churchill Livingstone, 1991.

18. Baranovsky A, Myers MH: Cancer incidence and survival in patients 65 years of age and older. CA Cancer of Clin 36:26–41, 1986.

19. Lawler SD: The cytogenetics of chronic granulocytic leukaemia. Clin Haematol 6:55–75, 1977.

20. Bortin MM, D'Amaro J, Bach FH, et al: HLA associations with leukemia. Blood 70:227–232, 1987.

21. Heyssel R, Brill AB, Woodbury LA, et al: Leukemia in Hiroshima atomic bomb survivors. Blood 15:313–331, 1960.

22. Moloney WC: Radiogenic leukemia revisited. Blood 70:905–908, 1987.

23. Brown WMC, Doll R: Mortality from cancer and other causes after radiotherapy for ankylosing spondylitis. Br Med J 2:1327–1332, 1965.

24. Boice JD, Day NE, Andersen A, et al: Second cancer following radiation treatment for cervical cancer. An international collaboration among cancer registries. J Natl Cancer Inst 74:955–975, 1985.

25. Spiers ASD: The clinical features of chronic granulocytic leukaemia. Clin Hematol 6:77–95, 1977.

26. Lichtman MA, Rowe JM: Hyperleukocytic leukemias: Rheological, clinical, and therapeutic considerations. Blood 60:279–283, 1982.

27. Juan D, Hsu S–D, Hunter J: Case report of vasopressin–responsive diabetes insipidus associated with chronic myelogenous leukemia. Cancer 56:1468–1469, 1985.

28. Kantarjian HM, Dixon D, Keating MJ, et al: Characteristics of accelerated disease in chronic myelogenous leukemia. Cancer 61:1441–1446, 1988.

29.Canellos GP: Chronic granulocytic leukemia. Med Clin North Am 60:1001–1018, 1976.

30. Inbal A, Akstein E, Barak I, et al: Cyclic leukocytosis and long survival in chronic myeloid leukemia. Acta Haematol 69:353–357, 1983.

31. Dowding C, Th'ng KH, Goldman JM, et al: Increased T–lymphocyte numbers in chronic granulocytic leukaemia before treatment. Exp Hematol 12:811–815, 1984.

32. Cramer E, Auclair C, Hakim J, et al: Metabolic activity of phagocytosing granulocytes in chronic granulocytic leukemia: Ultrastructural observation of a degranulation defect. Blood 50:93–106, 1977.

33. Fujimiya Y, Chang WC, Bakke A, et al: Natural killer (NK) cell immunodeficiency in patients with chronic myelogenous leukemia.

Cancer Immunol Immunother 24:213–220, 1987.

34. Knox WF, Bhavnani M, Davson J, et al: Histological classification of chronic granulocytic leukaemia. Clin Lab Haematol 6:171–175, 1984.

35. Dosik H, Rosner F, Sawitsky A: Acquired lipidosis: Gaucher–like cells and "blue cells" in chronic granulocytic leukemia. Semin Hematol 9:309–316, 1972.

36. Dekmezian R, Kantarjian HM, Keating MJ, et al: The relevance of reticulin stain–measured fibrosis at diagnosis in chronic myelogenous leukemia. Cancer 59:1739–1743, 1987.

37. Rosner F, Schreiber ZR, Parise F: Leukocyte alkaline phosphatase. Arch Intern Med 130:892–894, 1972.

38. Rustin GJS, Goldman JM, McCarthy D, et al: An extrinsic factor controls neutrophil alkaline phosphatase synthesis in chronic granulocytic leukaemia. Br J Haematol 45:381–387, 1980.

39. Yuo A, Kitagawa S, Okabe T, et al: Recombinant human granulocyte colony–stimulating factor repairs the abnormalities of neutrophils in patients with myelodysplastic syndromes and chronic myelogenous leukemia. Blood 70:404–411, 1987.

40. Kantarjian HM, Keating MJ, Talpaz M, et al: Chronic myelogenous leukemia in blast crisis. Analysis of 242 patients. Am J Med 83:445–454, 1987.

41. Jacknow G, Frizzera G, Gajl–Peczalska K, et al: Extramedullary presentation of the blast crisis of chronic myelogenous leukemia. Br J Haematol 61:225–236, 1985.

42.Terjanian T, Kantarjian H, Keating M, et al: Clinical and prognostic features of patients with Philadelphia chromosome-positive chronic myelogenous leukemia and extramedullary disease. Cancer 59:297–300, 1987.

43. Derderian PM, Kantarjian HM, Talpaz M, et al: Chronic myelogenous leukemia in the lymphoid blastic phase: Characteristics, treatment response, and prognosis. Am J Med 94:69–74, 1993.

44. Majlis A, Kantarjian H, Smith T, et al: What is the significance of cytogenetic clonal evolution in patients with Philadelphia chromosome–positive chronic myelogenous leukemia? Blood 84(Suppl 1):150a (abstract #586), 1994.

45. Tura S, Baccarani M, Corbelli G et al: Italian Cooperative Study Group on Chronic Myeloid Leukemia. Br J Haematol 47:105–119, 1981.

46. Cervantes F, Rozman C: A multivariate analysis of prognostic factors in chronic myeloid leukemia. Blood 60:1298–1304, 1982.

47. Sokal JE, Cox EB, Baccarani M, et al: Prognostic discrimination in "good risk" chronic granulocytic leukemia. Blood 63:789–799, 1984.

48. Kantarjian HM, Smith TL, McCredie KB, et al: Chronic myelogenous leukemia: A multivariate analysis of the associations of patient characteristics and therapy with survival. Blood 66:1326–1335, 1985.

49. Kantarjian HM, Keating MJ, Smith TL, et al: Proposal for a simple synthesis prognostic staging system in chronic myelogenous leukemia. Am J Med 88:1–8, 1990.

50. Kantarjian HM, Smith TL, O'Brien S, et al: Prolonged survival following achievement of a cytogenetic response with alpha interferon therapy in chronic myelogenous leukemia. Ann Intern Med 1995 (in press).

51. The Italian Cooperative Study Group on Chronic Myeloid Leukemia: Interferon-α2a compared with conventional chemotherapy for the treatment of chronic myeloid leukemia. N Engl J Med 330:820–825, 1994.

52. Cervantes F, Robertson JE, Rozman C, et al: Long-term survivors in chronic granulocytic leukaemia: A study by the International CGL Prognosis Study Group. Br J Haematol 87:293–300, 1994.

53. Futaki M, Inokuchi K, Matsuoka H, et al: Relationship of the

type of BCR-ABL hybrid mRNA to clinical course and transforming activity in Philadelphia-positive chronic myelogenous leukemia. Leukemia Res 16:1071–1075, 1992.

54. Mills KI, Benn P, Birnie GD: Does the breakpoint within the major cluster region (M–bcr) influence the duration of the chronic phase in chronic myeloid leukemia? An analytical comparison of current literature. Blood 78:1155–1161, 1991.

55. Verschraegen C, Kantarjian H, Hirsch-Ginsberg C, et al: Prognostic relevance of 3' versus 5' breakpoints within the breakpoint cluster region of chromosome 22 in Philadelphia-positive chronic myelogenous leukemia. Blood 82:331a (abstract #1308), 1993.

56. Kurzrock R, Gutterman JU, Talpaz M: The molecular genetics of Philadelphia chromosome-positive leukemias. N Engl J Med 319:990–998, 1988.

57. Gale RP, Canaani E: An 8-kilobase abl RNA transcript in chronic myelogenous leukemia. Proc Natl Acad Sci USA 81:5648–5652, 1984.

58. Muller AJ, Young JC, Pendergast A-M, et al: BCR first exon sequences specifically activate the BCR/ABL tyrosine kinase oncogene of Philadelphia chromosome-positive human leukemias. Mol Cell Biol 11:1785–1792, 1991.

59. McWhirter JR, Wang JYJ: Activation of tyrosine kinase and microfilament-binding functions of c-abl by bcr sequences in bcr/abl fusion proteins. Mol Cell Biol 11:1553–1565, 1991.

60. Daley GQ, Van Etten RA, Baltimore D: Induction of chronic myelogenous leukemia in mice by the P210bcr/abl gene of the Philadelphia chromosome. Science 247:824–830, 1990.

61. Heisterkamp N, Jenster G, ten Hoeve J, et al: Acute leukaemia in bcr/abl transgenic mice. Nature 344:251–253, 1990.

62. Pendergast AM, Muller AJ, Havlik MH, et al: BCR sequences essential for transformation by the BCR-ABL oncogene bind to the ABL SH2 regulatory domain in a non-phosphotyrosine-dependent manner. Cell 66:161–171, 1991.

63. Pendergast AM, Quilliam LA, Cripe LD, et al: BCR-ABL–induced oncogenesis is mediated by direct interaction with the SH2 domain of the GRB-2 adaptor protein. Cell 75:175–185, 1993.

64. Lowenstein EJ, Daly RJ, Batzer AG, et al: The SH2 and SH3 domain-containing protein GRB2 links receptor tyrosine kinases to ras signaling. Cell 70:431–442, 1992.

65. Smith MR, DeGudicibus SJ, Stacey DW: Requirement for c-ras proteins during viral oncogene transformation. Nature 320:540–543, 1986.

66. McWhirter JR, Wang JYJ: An actin-binding function contributes to transformation by the Bcr-Abl oncoprotein of Philadelphia chromosome-positive human leukemias. EMBO J 12:1533–1546, 1993.

67. ten Hoeve J, Arlinghaus RB, Guo JQ, et al: Tyrosine phosphorylation of CRKL in Philadelphia+ leukemia. Blood 84:1731–1736, 1994.

68. Afar DEH, Goga A, McLaughlin J, et al: Differential complementation of Bcr-Abl point mutants with c-Myc. Science 264:424–426, 1994.

69. Evans CA, Owen-Lynch PJ, Whetton AD, et al: Activation of the Abelson tyrosine kinase activity is associated with suppression of apoptosis in hemopoietic cells. Cancer Res 53:1735–1738, 1993.

70. Melo JV, Gordon DE, Cross NCP, et al: The ABL-BCR fusion gene is expressed in chronic myeloid leukemia. Blood 81:158–165, 1993.

71. Ahuja H, Bar-Eli M, Arlin Z, et al: The spectrum of molecular alterations in the evolution of chronic myelocytic leukemia. J Clin Invest 87:2042–2047, 1991.

72. Nakai H, Misawa S, Toguchida J, et al: Frequent p53 gene mutations in blast crisis of chronic myelogenous leukemia, especially in myeloid crisis harboring loss of a chromosome 17p. Cancer Res 52:6588–6593, 1992.

73. Neubauer A, He M, Schmidt CA, et al: Genetic alterations in the p53 gene in the blast crisis of chronic myelogenous leukemia: Analysis of polymerase chain reaction based techniques. Leukemia 7:593–600, 1993.

74. Feinstein E, Cimino G, Gale RP, et al: p53 in chronic myelogenous leukemia in acute phase. Proc Natl Acad Sci USA 88:6293–6297, 1991.

75. Gordon MY, Dowding CR, Riley GP, et al: Altered adhesive interactions with marrow stroma of hematopoietic progenitor cells in chronic myeloid leukemia. Nature 328:342–344, 1987.

76. Upadhyaya G, Guba SC, Sih SA, et al: Interferon-α restores the deficient expression of the cytoadhesion molecule lymphocyte function antigen-3 by chronic myelogenous leukemia progenitor cells. J Clin Invest 88:2131–2136, 1991.

77. Bhatia R, Wayner EA, McGlave PB, et al: Interferon-α restores normal adhesion of chronic myelogenous leukemia hematopoietic progenitors to bone marrow stroma by correcting impaired β1 integrin receptor function. J Clin Invest 94:384–391, 1994.

78. Estrov Z, Kurzrock R, Wetzler M, et al: Suppression of chronic myelogenous leukemia colony growth by IL-1 receptor antagonist and soluble IL-1 receptors: A novel application for inhibitors of IL-1 activity. Blood 78:1476–1484, 1991.

79. Wetzler M, Kurzrock R, Estrov Z, et al: Altered levels of interleukin-1-α and interleukin-1 receptor antagonist in chronic myelogenous leukemia: Clinical and prognostic correlates. Blood 84:3142–3147, 1994

80. Rushing D, Goldman A, Gibbs G, et al: Hydroxyurea versus busulfan in the treatment of chronic myelogenous leukemia. Am J Clin Oncol 5:307–313, 1982.

81. Kolitz JE, Kempin SJ, Schluger A, et al: A phase II pilot trial of high-dose hydroxyurea in chronic myelogenous leukemia. Semin Oncol 19(suppl 9):27–33, 1992.

82. Hehlmann R, Heimpel H, Hasford J, et al: Randomized comparison of busulfan and hydroxyurea in chronic myelogenous leukemia: Prolongation of survival by hydroxyurea. Blood 83:398–407, 1993.

83. Robertson MJ, Tantravahi R, Griffin JD, et al: Hematologic remission and cytogenetic improvement after treatment of stable-phase chronic myelogenous leukemia with continuous infusion of low-dose cytarabine. Am J Hematol 43:95–102, 1993.

84. Shepherd PCA, Fooks J, Gray R, et al: Thioguanine used in maintenance therapy of chronic myeloid leukemia causes non-cirrhotic portal hypertension. Br J Haematol 79:185–192, 1991.

85. Renner D, Quei Ber U, Martinez C, et al: Treatment of excessive thrombocytopenia in chronic myeloid leukemia by thrombocytopheresis and intravenous Thio-TEPA. Onkologie 10:324–326, 1987.

86. O'Brien S, Kantarjian H, Feldman E, et al: Homoharringtonine produces high hematologic and cytogenetic response rates in Philadelphia-chromosome positive chronic myelogenous leukemia. Blood 80(suppl 1):358a (abstract #1421), 1992.

87. O'Brien S, Kantarjian H, Beran M, et al: Homoharringtonine produces high response rates in Philadelphia chromosome positive chronic myelogenous leukemia. Blood 78(suppl 1):170a (abstract #672), 1991.

88. Verma DS, Spitzer G, Gutterman JU, et al: Human leukocyte interferon preparation blocks granulopoietic differentiation. Blood 54:1423–1427, 1979.

89. Talpaz M, Kantarjian HM, McCredie KB, et al: Clinical investigation of human alfa interferon in chronic myelogenous leukemia. Blood 69:1280–1288, 1987.

90. Talpaz M, Kantarjian HM, McCredie K, et al: Hematologic remission and cytogenetic improvement induced by recombinant

human interferon alpha$_A$ in chronic myelogenous leukemia. N Engl J Med 314:1065–1069, 1986.

91. Talpaz M, Kantarjian H, Kurzrock R, et al: Interferon-α produces sustained cytogenetic responses in chronic myelogenous leukemia. Ann Intern Med 114:532–538, 1991.

92. Ozer H, George S, Pettenati M, et al: Subcutaneous α-interferon in untreated chronic phase Philadelphia chromosome positive chronic myelogenous leukemia: No evidence for significant improvement in response duration or survival (CALGB 8583). Blood 80(Suppl 1):358a (abstract #1422), 1992.

93. Schofield JR, Robinson WA, Murphy JR, et al: Low doses of interferon-α are as effective as higher doses in inducing remissions and prolonging survival in chronic myeloid leukemia. Ann Intern Med 121:736–744, 1994.

94. Allan NC, Shepherd PCA, Richards SM: Interferon-α prolongs survival for patients with CML in chronic phase: Preliminary results of the UK MRC randomized multicenter trial. Blood 84(suppl 1):382a (abstract #1513), 1994.

95. Kloke O, Niederle N, Qiu JY, et al: Impact of interferon-α-induced cytogenetic improvement on survival in chronic myelogenous leukemia. Br J Haematol 83:399–403, 1993.

96. Hehlmann R, Heimpel H, Hasford J, et al: Randomized comparison of interferon-α with busulfan and hydroxyurea in chronic myelogenous leukemia. Blood 84:4064–4077, 1994.

97. Alimena G, Morra E, Lazzarino M, et al: Interferon-α2b as therapy for Ph[1]-positive chronic myelogenous leukemia: A study of 82 patients treated with intermittent or daily administration. Blood 72:642–647, 1988.

98. Cortes J, Kantarjian H, O'Brien S, et al: Results of interferon-α therapy in patients with chronic myelogenous leukemia 60 years of age and older. Proc Am Soc Clin Oncol 19:339, 1995.

99. Kurzrock R, Talpaz M, Kantarjian H, et al: Therapy of chronic myelogenous leukemia with recombinant interferon-α. Blood 70:943–947, 1987.

100. Talpaz M, Kurzrock R, Kantarjian H, et al: A phase II study alternating α-2a-interferon and γ-interfeon therapy in patients with chronic myelogenous leukemia. Cancer 68:2125–2130, 1991.

101. Wandl UB, Kloke O, Nagel-Hiemke M, et al: Combination therapy with interferon α-2b plus low-dose interferon gamma in pretreated patients with Ph-positive chronic myelogenous leukemia. Br J Haematol 81:516–519, 1992.

102. Kantarjian HM, Keating MJ, Estey EH, et al: Treatment of advanced stages of Philadelphia chromosome-positive chronic myelogenous leukemia with interferon-α and low-dose cytarabine. J Clin Oncol 10:772–778, 1992.

103. Arthur CK, Ma DDF: Combined interferon α-2a and cytosine arabinoside as first-line treatment for chronic myeloid leukemia. Acta Haematol 89(suppl 1):15–21, 1993.

104. Guilhot F, Abgrall J-F, Harousseau J-L, et al: A multicenter randomised study of alfa 2b interferon and hydroxyurea with or without cytosine-arabinoside in previously untreated patients with Ph+ chronic myelocytic leukemia: Preliminary cytogenetic results. Leuk Lymphoma 11(suppl 1):181–183, 1993.

105. Kantarjian HM, Vellekoop L, McCredie KB, et al: Intensive combination chemotherapy (ROAP 10) and splenectomy in the management of chronic myelogenous leukemia. J Clin Oncol 3:192–200, 1985.

106. Kantarjian HM, Talpaz M, Keating MJ, et al: Intensive chemotherapy induction followed by interferon-α maintenance in patients with Philadelphia chromosome-positive chronic myelogenous leukemia. Cancer 68:1201–1207, 1991.

107. Quesada JR, Talpaz M, Rios A, et al: Clinical toxicity of interferons in cancer patients: A review. J Clin Oncol 4:234–243, 1986.

108. Talpaz M, Kantarjian H, Kurzrock R, et al: Bone marrow hypoplasia and aplasia complicating interferon therapy for chronic myelogenous leukemia. Cancer 69:410–412, 1992.

109. Sacchi S, Kantarjian H, Cohen P, et al: Immune–mediated and unusual complications during α-interferon therapy in chronic myelogenous leukemia. Blood 84(suppl 1):150a (abstract #587), 1994.

110. Gratwohl A, Hermans J, Niederwieser D, et al: Bone marrow transplantation for chronic myeloid leukemia: Long-term results. Bone Marrow Transplant 12:509–516, 1993.

111. Biggs JC, Szer J, Crilley P, et al: Treatment of chronic myeloid leukemia with allogeneic bone marrow transplantation after preparation with BuCy2. Blood 80:1352–1357, 1992.

112. Clift RA, Buckner CD, Appelbaum FR, et al: Allogeneic marrow transplantation in patients with chronic myeloid leukemia in the chronic phase: A randomized trial of two irradiation regimens. Blood 77:1660–1665, 1991.

113. Clift RA, Buckner CD, Thomas ED, et al: Marrow transplantation for chronic myeloid leukemia: A randomized study comparing cyclophosphamide and total body irradiation with busulfan and cyclophosphamide. Blood 84:2036–2043, 1994.

114. Goldman JM, Gale RP, Horowitz MM, et al: Bone marrow transplantation for chronic myelogenous leukemia in chronic phase. Ann Intern Med 108:806–814, 1988.

115. Speck B, Bortin MM, Champlin R, et al: Allogeneic bone marrow transplantation for chronic myelogenous leukemia. Lancet 1:665–668, 1984.

116. Thomas ED, Clift RA, Fefer A, et al: Marrow transplantation for the treatment of chronic myelogenous leukemia. Ann Intern Med 104:155–163, 1986.

117. Wagner JE, Zahurak M, Piantadosi S, et al: Bone marrow transplantation of chronic myelogenous leukemia in chronic phase: Evaluation of risks and benefits. J Clin Oncol 10:779–789, 1992.

118. McGlave PB: Therapy of chronic myelogenous leukemia with related or unrelated donor bone marrow transplantation. Leukemia 6:115–117, 1992.

119. Goldman JM, Szydlo R, Horowitz MM, et al: Choice of pretransplant treatment and timing of transplants for chronic myelogenous leukemia in chronic phase. Blood 82:2235–2238, 1993.

120. Ringden O, Ruutu T, Remberger M, et al: A randomized trial comparing busulfan with total body irradiation as conditioning in allogeneic marrow transplant recipients with leukemia: A report from the Nordic Bone Marrow Transplant Group. Blood 83:2723–2730, 1994.

121. Snyder DS, Negrin RS, O'Donnell MR, et al: Fractionated total-body irradiation and high-dose etoposide as a preparatory regimen for bone marrow transplantation for 94 patients with chronic myelogenous leukemia in chronic phase. Blood 84:1672–1679, 1994.

122. Marmont AM, Horowitz MM, Gale RP, et al: T-cell depletion of HLA-identical transplants in leukemia. Blood 78:2120–2130, 1991.

123. Scattenberg A, De Witte T, Preijers F, et al: Allogeneic bone marrow transplantation for leukemia with marrow grafts depleted of lymphocytes by counterflow centrifugation. Blood 75:1356–1363, 1990.

124. Barrett A, Jiang YZ: Immune responses to chronic myeloid leukemia. Bone Marrow Transplant 9:305–311, 1992.

125. Cullis JO, Scwarer AP, Hughes TP, et al: Second transplants for patients with chronic myeloid leukemia in relapse after original transplant with T-depleted donor marrow: Feasibility of using busulphan alone for reconditioning. Br J Haematol 80:33–39, 1994.

126. Bär BMAM, Schattenberg A, Mensink EJBM, et al: Donor leukocyte infusions for chronic myeloid leukemia relapse after allogeneic bone marrow transplantation. J Clin Oncol 11:513–519, 1993.

127. Kolb HJ, Mittermüller J, Clemm Ch, et al: Donor leukocyte

transfusions for treatment of recurrent chronic myelogenous leukemia in marrow transplant patients. Blood 76:2462–2465, 1990.

128. Cullis JO, Jiang YZ, Scwarer AP, et al: Donor leukocyte infusions for chronic myeloid leukemia in relapse after allogeneic bone marrow transplantation. Blood 79:1379–1381, 1992.

129. Jiang Y-Z, Cullis JO, Kanfer EJ, et al: T cell and NK cell mediated graft-versus-leukaemia reactivity following donor buffy coat transfusions to treat relapse after marrow transplantation for chronic myeloid leukaemia. Bone Marrow Transplant 11:133–138, 1993.

130. Drobyski W, Keevr C, Roth M, et al: Donor leukocyte infusions as treatment for relapsed chronic myelogenous leukemia after allogeneic bone marrow transplantation. Blood 80(suppl 1):66a (abstract #253), 1992.

131. Higano CS, Raskind WH, Singer JW: Use of alpha interferon for the treatment of relapse of chronic myelogenous leukemia in chronic phase after allogeneic bone marrow transplantation. Blood 80:1437–1442, 1992.

132. Higano C, Raskind W, Singer J: Alpha interferon treatment of cytogenetic-only relapse of chronic myelogenous leukemia after marrow transplantation. Proc Am Soc Clin Oncol 12:307 (abstract #1011), 1993.

133. Porter DL, Roth MS, McGarigle C, et al: Induction of graft-versus-host disease as immunotherapy for relapsed chronic myeloid leukemia. N Engl J Med 330:100–106, 1994.

134. McGlave P, Bartsch G, Anasetti C, et al: Unrelated donor marrow transplantation therapy for chronic myelogenous leukemia: Initial experience of the National Marrow Donor Program. Blood 81:543–550, 1993.

135. Gamis AS, Haake R, McGlave P, et al: Unrelated-donor bone marrow transplantation for Philadelphia chromosome-positive chronic myelogenous leukemia in children. J Clin Oncol 11:834–838, 1993.

136. Leemhuis T, Leibowitz D, Cox G, et al: Identification of BCR/ABL-negative primitive hematopoietic progenitor cells within chronic myeloid leukemia marrow. Blood 81:801–807, 1993.

137. Carella AM, Pollicardo N, Pungolino E, et al: Mobilization of cytogenetically "normal" blood progenitor cells by intensive conventional chemotherapy for chronic myeloid and acute lymphoblastic leukemia. Leuk Lymphoma 9:477–483, 1993.

138. Kantarjian H, Talpaz M, Hester J, et al: Collection of peripheral blood diploid cells from chronic myelogenous leukemia patients early in the recovery phase from myelosuppression induced by intensive chemotherapy. Blood 84(suppl 1):382a (abstract #1514), 1994.

139. Kantarjian HM, Talpaz M, LeMaistre CF, et al: Intensive combination chemotherapy and autologous bone marrow transplantation leads to the reappearance of Philadelphia chromosome-negative cells in chronic myelogenous leukemia. Cancer 67:2959–2965, 1991.

140. Brito-Babapulle F, Bowcock SJ, Marcus RE, et al: Autografting for patients with chronic myeloid leukemia in chronic phase: Peripheral blood stem cells may have a finite capacity for maintaining haemopoiesis. Br J Haematol 73:76–81, 1989.

141. Talpaz M, Kantarjian H, Khouri I, et al: Diploid cells collected from chronic myelogenous leukemia patients during recovery from conventional dose–induced myelosuppression generate complete cytogenetic remissions after autologous transplantation. Blood 84(suppl 1):537a (abstract #2135), 1994.

142. Reiffers J, Trouette R, Marit G, et al: Autologous blood stem cell transplantation for chronic granulocytic leukaemia in transformation: A report of 47 cases. Br J Haematol 77:339–345, 1991.

143. Khouri IF, Kantarjian HM, Talpaz M, et al: High-dose chemotherapy and unpurged autologous stem cell transplantation for chronic myelogenous leukemia: The M. D. Anderson experience. Blood 84(suppl 1):537a (abstract #2133), 1994.

144. Deisseroth A, Zu Z, Claxton D, et al: Retroviral marking studies show that infused exogenous marrow cells give rise to hematopoietic recovery after autologous transplant and that relapse after autologous transplant in CML may arise from Ph+ cells present in marrow at the time of transplant. Blood 82(suppl 1):454a (abstract #1800), 1993.

145. Dunbar CE, Stewart FM: Separating the wheat from the chaff: Selection of benign hematopoietic cells in chronic myeloid leukemia. Blood 79:1107–1110, 1992.

146. Turhan AG, Humphries RK, Eaves CJ, et al: Detection of breakpoint cluster region–negative and nonclonal hematopoiesis in vitro and in vivo after transplantation of cells selected in cultures of chronic myeloid leukemia marrow. Blood 76:2404–2410, 1990.

147. Brandwein JM, Dube ID, Laraya P, et al: Maintenance of Philadelphia–chromosome-positive progenitors in long-term marrow cultures from patients with advanced chronic myeloid leukemia. Leukemia 6:556–561, 1992.

148. Carlo–Stella C, Mangoni L, Piovani G, et al: In vitro marrow purging in chronic myelogenous leukemia: Effect of mafosfamide and recombinant granulocyte-macrophage colony-stimulating factor. Bone Marrow Transplant 8:265–273, 1991.

149. Rizzoli V, Mangoni L, Piovani G, et al: Mafosfamide purged autografts for chronic myelogenous leukemia. Blood 80(suppl 1):66a (abstract #254), 1992.

150. McGlave P, Miller J, Miller W, et al: Autologous marrow transplant therapy for CML using marrow treated ex vivo with human recombinant interferon gamma. Blood 80(suppl 1):537a (abstract #2134), 1992.

151. Ratajczak MZ, Hijiya N, Catani L, et al: Acute- and chronic-phase chronic myelogenous leukemia colony-forming units are highly sensitive to the growth inhibitory effects of c-myb antisense oligodeoxynucleotides. Blood 79: 1956–1961, 1992.

152. Szczylik C, Skorski T, Nicolaides NC, et al: Selective inhibition of leukemia cell proliferation by BCR-ABL antisense oligodeoxynucleotides. Science 253:562–565, 1991.

153. Mahon FX, Belloc F, Barbot C, et al: Chronic myelogenous leukemia: In vitro study with antisense oligomers. Blood 80(suppl 1):211a (abstract #834), 1992.

154. Martiat P, Lewalle P, Taj AS, et al: Retrovirally transduced antisense sequences stably suppress P210BCR/ABL and inhibit the proliferation of BCR/ABL-containing cell lines. Blood 81:502–509, 1993.

155. Chen W, Peace DJ, Rovira DK, et al: T-cell immunity to the joining region of p210BCR/ABL protein. Proc Natl Acad Sci USA 89:1468–1472, 1992.

156. Bilhou-Nabera C, Viard F, Marit G, et al: Complete cytogenetic conversion in chronic myelocytic leukemia patients undergoing interferon alpha therapy: Follow–up with reverse polymerase chain reaction. Leukemia 6:595–598, 1992.

157. Lee M-S, Kantarjian H, Talpaz M, et al: Detection of minimal residual disease by polymerase chain reaction in Philadelphia chromosome-positive chronic myelogenous leukemia following interferon therapy. Blood 79:1920–1923, 1992.

158. Talpaz M, Estrov Z, Kantarjian H, et al: Persistence of dormant leukemic progenitors during interferon-induced remission in chronic myelogenous leukemia. J Clin Invest 94:1383–1389, 1994.

159. Lion T, Izraeli S, Henn T, et al: Monitoring of residual disease in chronic myelogenous leukemia by quantitative polymerase chain reaction. Leukemia 6:495–499, 1992.

160. Malinge M-C, Mahon FX, Delfau MH, et al: Quantitative determination of the hybrid Bcr-Abl RNA in patients with chronic myelogenous leukemia under interferon therapy. Br J Haematol 82:701–707, 1992.

161. Zhao L, Kantarjian HM, Van Oort J, et al: Detection of residual proliferating leukemic cells by fluorescence in situ hybridization in CML patients in complete remission after interferon treatment. Leukemia 7:168–171, 1993.

162. Amiel A, Yarkoni S, Fejgin M, et al: Clinical detection of BCR-ABL fusion by in situ hybridization in chronic myelogenous leukemia. Cancer Genet Cytogenet 65:32–34, 1993.

163. Bilhou-Nabera C, Bernard Ph, Marit G, et al: Serial cytogenetic studies in allografted patients with chronic myeloid leukemia. Bone Marrow Transplant 9:263–268, 1992.

164. Hughes TP, Morgan GJ, Martiat P, et al: Detection of residual leukemia after bone marrow transplant for chronic myeloid leukemia: Role of polymerase chain reaction in predicting relapse. Blood 77:874–878, 1991.

165. Hughes TP, Ambrosetti A, Barbu V, et al: Clinical value of PCR in diagnosis and follow-up in leukaemia and lymphoma: Report of the third workshop of the Molecular Biology/BMT Study Group. Leukaemia 5:448–451, 1991.

166. Lee M, Khouri I, Champlin R, et al: Detection of minimal residual disease by polymerase chain reaction of bcr/abl transcripts in chronic myelogenous leukemia following allogeneic bone marrow transplantation. Br J Haematol 82:708–714, 1992.

167. Arnold R, Janssen JWG, Heinze B, et al: Influence of graft-versus-host disease on the eradication of minimal resdual leukemia detected by polymerase chain reaction in chronic myeloid leukemia patients after bone marrow transplantation. Leukemia 7:747–751, 1993.

168. Roth MS, Antin JH, Ash R, et al: Prognostic significance of Philadelphia chromosome-positive cells detected by the polymerase chain reaction after allogeneic bone marrow transplant for chronic myelogenous leukemia. Blood 79:276–282, 1992.

169. Guerrasio A, Martinelli G, Saglio G, et al: Minimal residual disease status in transplanted chronic myelogenous leukemia patients: Low incidence of polymerase chain reaction positive cases among 48 long disease-free subjects who recived unmanipulated allogeneic bone marrow transplants. Leukemia 6:507–512, 1992.

170. Miyamura K, Tahara T, Tanimoto M, et al: Long persistent bcr-abl positive transcript detected by polymerase chain reaction after marrow transplant for chronic myelogenous leukemia without clinical relapse: A study of 64 patients. Blood 81:1089–1093, 1993.

171. Kantarjian HM, Talpaz M, Kontoyiannis D, et al: Treatment of chronic myelogenous leukemia in accelerated and blastic phases with daunorubicin, high-dose cytarabine, and granulocyte-macrophage colony-stimulating factor. J Clin Oncol 10:398–405, 1992.

172. Dutcher JP, Eudey L, Wiernik PH, et al: Phase II study of mitoxantrone and 5-azacytidine for accelerated and blast crisis of chronic myelogenous leukemia: A study of the Eastern Cooperative Oncology Group. Leukemia 6:770–775, 1992.

173. Clift RA, Buckner CD, Thomas ED, et al: Marrow transplantation for patients in accelerated phase of chronic myeloid leukemia. Blood 84:4368–4373, 1994.

174. McGlave PB, Arthur DC, Weisdorf D, et al: Allogeneic bone marrow transplantation as treatment for accelerating chronic myelogenous leukemia. Blood 63:219–222, 1984.

175. Reiffers J, Trouette R, Marit G, et al: Autologous blood stem cell transplantation for chronic granulocytic leukemia in transformation: A report of 47 cases. Br J Haematol 77:339–345, 1991.

176. Kantarjian H, Kurzrock R, Talpaz M: Philadelphia chromosome-negative chronic myelogenous leukemia and chronic myelomonocytic leukemia. Hematol Oncol Clin North Am 4:389–404, 1990.

177. Dobrovic A, Morley AA, Seshadri R, et al: Molecular diagnosis of Philadelphia negative CML using the polymerase chain reaction and DNA analysis: Clinical features and course of M-bcr-negative and M-bcr-positive CML. Leukemia 5:187–190, 1991.

178. Cortes J, Talpaz M, Beran M, et al: Philadelphia chromosome-negative chronic myelogenous leukemia with rearrangement of the breakpoint cluster region. Cancer (in press), 1995.

179. Kurzrock R, Kantarjian HM, Shtalrid M, et al: Philadelphia chromosome-negative chronic myelogenous leukemia without breakpoint cluster region rearrangement: A chronic myeloid leukemia with a distinct clinical course. Blood 75:445–452, 1990.

CHAPTER 5

The Indolent Lymphomas

Ali W. Bseiso, MD, and Peter McLaughlin, MD

Division of Medicine, The University of Texas M. D. Anderson Cancer Center, Houston, Texas

The indolent non-Hodgkin's lymphomas constitute a heterogeneous group of lymphoproliferative disorders usually associated with relatively prolonged survival. They are categorized based on pathologic and cytologic features and with few exceptions,[1] they are almost exclusively of B-cell origin. The indolent lymphomas include follicular small cleaved, follicular mixed small- and large-cell, small lymphocytic, immunosecretory (Waldenström's), marginal-zone, and some cases of mantle-cell lymphoma (MCL). Marginal lymphoma includes mucosa-associated lymphoid tissue (MALT) and splenic (monocytoid) B-cell lymphomas (Table 1).

In the Working Formulation (WF),[2] most indolent lymphomas are classified as low-grade lymphomas, which include diffuse small lymphocytic, follicular small cleaved lymphomas (FSCL), and follicular mixed lymphomas (FML). Some of the new clinicopathologic entities, such as mantle-cell and marginal-zone lymphomas, do not easily fit within the confines of the subtypes of the WF, and this can be a source of confusion. Another source of confusion comes from the variable histology sometimes found in the same patient. This can happen in the same pathologic specimen, whereby two histologic subtypes are seen—a phenomenon referred to as composite lymphoma. More commonly, two distinct histologies are seen in specimens from two different sites—a discordant lymphoma.

Synchronous discordant lymphomas can be seen in 20% to 30% of newly diagnosed patients when more than one lymph-node biopsy is obtained simultaneously.[3] Another fairly common occurrence is the synchronous discordant pattern between the bone marrow, usually showing small cleaved cells, and a lymph node with diffuse large cells. By far, however, the most commonly recognized form of discordant lymphoma is asynchronous and is clinically referred to as transformation. This typically refers to an intermediate or high-grade lymphoma arising in a patient with prior low-grade histology.

BASIC CONCEPTS

Lymphocytes arise in the bone marrow from a pluripotent hematopoietic stem cell. For simplicity, their subsequent differentiation can be divided into two distinct stages: early, antigen independent and late, antigen driven. While early phases of T-cell differentiation occur in a specialized organ—the thymus—early B-cells undergo differentiation in the bone marrow.

The earliest sign of B-lineage commitment is the rearrangement of the immunoglobulin (Ig) heavy-chain locus on chromosome 14q32. This starts by the approximation of one of more than 20 D segments with a J_H segment creating a DJ region. This initial rearrangement occurs on both chromosomes. Subsequently, the DJ segment on one of the alleles is approximated with one of potentially several hundred V segments. The resulting VDJ segment then joins Cµ, and the rearranged heavy-chain gene is now ready to generate the heavy-chain protein. The successful production of the µ chain in the cytoplasm is the hallmark of pre-B-cell. Only if the rearrangement on the first chromosome was unsuccessful, will the second allele rearrange beyond the DJ stage (allelic exclusion). A failed rearrangement on the first allele can have potential pathogenic significance, as is the case with the t(14,18) translocation.

Once the heavy-chain locus successfully rearranges on either one of the two alleles, kappa light-chain gene rearrangement follows on chromosome 2(p11). The light-chain gene loci lack the D segment so that one of the variable genes will be directly approximated to one of five J_{kappa} regions. If the kappa gene rearrangement is unsuccessful, the other allele will rearrange, and only if that is unsuccessful will the lambda genes rearrange on chromosome 22(q11). Once a functional light chain is produced, it will bind to the µ heavy chain, producing a complete Ig molecule that will be expressed on the cell surface. The expression of surface immunoglobulin (sIg) is the hallmark of a mature B-cell.

The process of heavy-chain gene rearrangement requires an enzyme that joins the approximated splices by randomly adding nucleotides independent of a DNA template (N regions). These random processes add to the diversity of the Ig specificity and are mediated by the enzyme terminal deoxyribonucleotide transferase (TdT).

As the pre-B-cells express sIgM, they gradually change from the large, rapidly dividing cells (the "small noncleaved" cells) to the small resting ones and concomitantly lose TdT and CD10 reactivity. Called naive or virgin mature B-cells, they leave the bone marrow and circulate briefly before homing to the perifollicular lymphoid tissue or the splenic marginal zone. A fraction of these cells will express CD5 antigen. In humans, up to 17% of circulating B-cells are CD5 positive.[4] While in murine models there is evidence to suggest that these cells may arise from a separate ontogeny,[5] such evidence is lacking in humans, and CD5 expression may simply represent activation of naive B-cells upon antigen exposure.

Most mature B-cells entering a germinal center will undergo apoptosis or programmed cell death. For B-cells to survive and mature into postfollicle stages, they need a dual signal: The first comes through antigen engagement with surface immunoglobulin (sIg) receptor, and the second is mediated by T-cell help that follows antigen presentation. One molecular consequence of T-cell help is the interaction between CD40 on the antigen-presenting follicular B-cells and CD40 ligand, expressed on activated helper T-cells. In vitro data suggest that dual signalling via surface Ig receptor and CD40 rescues B-cells from apoptosis. For example, CD40 stimulation was shown to protect cells from Ig cross-linking-induced apoptosis in murine WEHI 231 cells.[6] Similarly, murine B-cells stimulated by CD40 alone were very sensitive to Fas-induced apoptosis, whereas those simultaneously stimulated by CD40 and anti-IgM were not.[7] Surviving cells undergo isotype switching and the progeny memory B-cells will circulate in blood.

One model of lymphomagenesis suggests that clonal B-cells carrying the t(14;18) translocation are subject to the same regulatory mechanisms as normal cells upon entry into the follicles, at least in the early phases of the disease. However, upon antigen exposure, these cells may behave differently, failing to differentiate further or undergo apoptosis. The outcome is the follicular lymphoma, a disease *initiated* by a specific chromosomal translocation, possibly *promoted* by an antigen-driven process,[8] and demonstrating *progression* with additional genetic abnormalities.

FOLLICULAR LYMPHOMAS

The follicular lymphomas are the most common human B-cell neoplasms in the Western hemisphere but are less common in the non-Western world; they constitute approximately 45% of all non-Hodgkin's lymphomas[2] and 80% of all indolent lymphomas. Follicular lymphomas are characterized by a relatively indolent course, with a median patient survival of approximately 8 to 10 years. They occur exclusively in adults and equally among males and females.

Approximately 80% to 90% of all patients present with advanced-stage disease (III or IV), with generalized adenopathy and a high incidence of bone marrow involvement. A characteristic of follicular lymphomas (as well as of diffuse small lymphocytic lymphomas) is the phenomenon of spontaneous regression, which occurred in up to 30% of patients in one series.[9] Such regressions, however, are usually partial and typically short-lived (1 to 2 years).

Cytologic and Pathologic Features

The follicular lymphomas usually grow in a nodular pattern, probably secondary to the expression of surface adhesion molecules, allowing homotypic adhesion or adhesion with dendritic reticulum cells. Among the prime molecular candidates to be involved (among many others) are the integrins LFA-1 (CD11a/18) and its ligand ICAM-1 (CD54). The concomitant expression of LFA-1 and ICAM-1 on neoplastic cells is shown to correlate with nodular growth pattern, whereas the lack of one or both molecules is associated with a diffuse growth pattern. Similarly, the lack of ICAM-1 expression is associated with a leukemic phase.[10]

The neoplastic nodules are generally of uniform size and can result in the total effacement of the normal nodal architecture. These nodules constitute homogeneous clumps of neoplastic cells, unlike normal lymphoid follicles, which display functional polarization with germinal centers and lymphoid cuff. The neoplastic cells resemble normal counterparts present in the normal germinal center; hence, the name "follicular center-cell lymphoma" in the Lukes-Collins classification. Scattered within the follicles is a dense meshwork of dendritic reticulum cells that are invariably present in follicular lymphomas. In the normal lymphoid follicle, the cells evolve through different stages with distinct cytologic features: small cleaved, large cleaved, and large noncleaved cells. The last cell type is more proliferative and, thus, is identified as a centroblast, as opposed to the small cleaved centrocyte under the Kiel classification.

The cytologic subtyping of follicular lymphomas can be difficult,[11,12] but they generally form a continuum from small cleaved predominance to mixed to large-cell predominance. The subtypes are divided based on the proportion of large cells in the nodules. The follicular small cleaved lymphoma should generally have no more than five large noncleaved cells easily identified per high-power field (HPF), while the FML has at least five large noncleaved cells per HPF.[12,13] The cutoff number between FML and follicular large-cell (FLC) lymphoma is somewhat arbitrary and may vary among different pa-

TABLE I

Classification of Non-Hodgkin's Lymphomas [a]

Working formulation	REAL classification	
Low-grade lymphomas	**B-cell**	**T-cell**
Small lymphocytic	B-CLL/SLL Prolymphocytic Mantle-cell Extranodal marginal zone (MALT) Nodal marginal zone Splenic marginal zone Lymphoplasmacytoid lymphoma	T-cell CLL Large granular leukemia/lymph (T-cell/NK cell)
Follicular small cleaved	FCL, follicular (grade I) Mantle-cell	
Follicular mixed	FCL (grade II)	
Intermediate-grade lymphomas		
Follicular large	FCL (grade III)	
Diffuse small cleaved	Mantle cell FCL, diffuse small-cell Extranodal marginal zone (MALT) Nodal marginal zone	Peripheral T-cell Angiocentric adult T-cell
Diffuse mixed	Mantle-cell Marginal zone (nodal and extranodal) Diffuse large B-cell	Peripheral T-cell lymph Adult T-cell leukemia/lymphoma Angioimmunoblastic Angiocentric
Diffuse large-cell	Diffuse large B-cell Primary mediastinal large B-cell	Same as under diffuse mixed
High-grade lymphoma		
Immunoblastic	Primary mediastinal large B-cell	Peripheral T-cell Angioimmunoblastic Adult T-cell leukemia/lymphoma Anaplastic large cell (T-cell/null cell)
Lymphoblastic	Precursor B-cell lymphoblastic lymphoma/leukemia	Precursor T-cell Lymphoblastic lymphoma/leukemia
Small noncleaved	Burkitt's/high-grade B-cell, Burkitt's like	

[a] As categorized under the Working Formulation with the corresponding subtypes as proposed by the Revised European American Lymphoma (REAL) classification
CLL = chronic lymphocytic leukemia, FCL = follicle center lymphoma, MALT = mucosa-associated lymphoid tissue, NK = natural killer, SLL = small lymphocytic lymphoma

thologists. Follicular large-cell lymphoma, constituting less than 10% of all follicular lymphomas, is typically included under intermediate-grade lymphoma of the WF because of its more aggressive clinical course. It typically consists of follicular large noncleaved cells as opposed to the less common category of follicular large cleaved; the latter probably maintains its indolent behavior and can be considered a low-grade lymphoma.

Under the Kiel classification, all three categories are lumped under centroblastic/centrocytic without identify-

ing subgroups, recognizing the fact that each subtype should, by definition, have both cell types, albeit in different proportions. More recently, the International Lymphoma Study Group proposed a Revised European American Lymphoma (REAL) classification. In the proposed schema, follicular lymphomas were categorized under "follicle center lymphomas" with cytologic grades referring to the proportion of large cells in the follicle (Table 1). Thus, grades I, II, and III form a continuum from follicular small cleaved-cell to large-cell predominance, without specific recommendations being made about cutoff criteria between grades.

A Southwest Oncology Group (SWOG) study recently suggested that Ki-67 expression may represent an objective reproducible method of delineating the subtypes of follicular lymphomas. Ki-67 is a nuclear protein detected throughout all phases of the cell cycle but not the G_0 phase.[14] It is, thus, a reliable marker of proliferation. In the SWOG study, the follicular small cleaved-cell lymphomas had a 5% proliferative rate, compared with 29% for follicular mixed lymphomas.[15]

Biology, Cytogenetics, and Immunophenotypic Characteristics

Follicular lymphomas are by definition derived from follicular center cells.[16] Immunologically, the neoplastic cells carry the characteristics of mature B-cells and express CD19, CD20, CD22, and sIg (mostly IgM/IgD but possibly also IgG or IgA). Being of follicular center-cell origin, the cells characteristically express CD10 and almost never express CD5. All subtypes of follicular lymphomas demonstrate heavy- and light-chain gene rearrangements,[17,18] whereas the TCR genes are almost never rearranged. A potential T-B-cell interaction may play a role in lymphomagenesis.

In one study, purified follicular lymphoma cells underwent vigorous in vitro proliferation when cultured with a CD4+ T-cell clone that recognized an alloantigen expressed by the lymphoma cells. As seen in normal T-cell/B-cell interactions, the lymphoma cell proliferation was MHC class II dependent. In the absence of T-cells, the lymphoma cells did not respond to lymphokines.[19] This suggests that the T-cells commonly seen infiltrating follicular lymphomas may contribute to neoplastic B-cell proliferation. The paradoxical observation that T-cell infiltration is more commonly associated with spontaneous regression may indicate an early phase of the disease when the B-cells are still T-cell dependent and not autonomous.

With conventional cytogenetic techniques, 65% to 75% of patients will be successfully karyotyped. This contrasts with the higher success rate usually obtained in more aggressive lymphomas.[20,21] Most of the successfully karyotyped specimens will show several chromosomal abnormalities with complex karyotypes, while up to 16% will be normal. The nature of karyotypic abnormality is somewhat histology dependent. Follicular small cleaved-cell lymphomas tend to be associated with hyperdiploidy, with a modal number of 47 or 48, whereas small lymphocytic lymphoma tends to be more commonly pseudodiploid.[22]

A variety of primary and secondary chromosomal aberrations have been described, with t(14;18)(q32;q13) being by far the single most common. This translocation, involving the bcl-2 gene, is most commonly seen in the follicular small cleaved histology, but its frequency declines as the proportion of large cells increases. It is almost always associated with other structural or numerical chromosomal aberrations.[23] Regional variation in the incidence of bcl-2 translocation has been described. In Japan, follicular B-cell lymphomas have been associated with a lower incidence of bcl-2 rearrangement.[24]

Interestingly, tonsils and lymph nodes with follicular hyperplasia and, more recently, peripheral blood have been shown to have bcl-2-Ig translocation in approximately half the cases in some series.[25–28] This suggests that the t(14;18) translocation may be a common event in normal lymphocyte physiology and that cells carrying the translocation are not necessarily committed to evolving into lymphoma.

Several cytogenetic abnormalities are associated with specific histologic subtypes. For example, while follicular small cleaved lymphoma is associated with t(14;18), follicular mixed lymphomas also show association with trisomy 8 and follicular large-cell with trisomy 7 and breaks in 17q21-q25.[22] Trisomy 12, on the other hand, is frequently accompanied by t(14;18) in diffuse large-cell lymphomas (DLCL), while as a solitary primary chromosomal abnormality, it is characteristically seen in chronic lymphocytic leukemia (CLL)/small lymphocytic lymphoma (SLL) and not follicular lymphomas.[21,29]

The loss of genetic material is a rather common secondary abnormality in low-grade lymphoma. A number of nonrandom deletions of chromosomal material have been described, including 1q, 3p, 6q, 11q, 14q, and 16q, areas that are speculated to carry as yet unidentified tumor-suppressor genes.[23] No major role for p53 mutations has been described in the early phases of the development of low-grade lymphoma.[30,31] However, p53 abnormalities do appear to play a role in some cases of histologic transformation.

Using molecular analysis, about 85% of all follicular lymphomas are shown to have the t(14;18)(q32;q21) translocation juxtaposing the bcl-2 gene from 18q21.3 with the Ig heavy-chain locus on 14q32.2.[32] The reciprocal event also happens such that the D segment, instead of joining the J segment on 14q32, is transposed to chromosome 18. While approximately 70% of the breakpoints occur at the 3′ untranslated region of bcl-2 gene (the major breakpoint region, MBR), about 20% will occur in a region 20 kb 3′ to the gene (the minor cluster region, MCR).[33,34] Oligonucleotide primers that span both breakpoint regions are being utilized in polymerase chain reaction (PCR) techniques in an attempt to monitor minimal residual disease following therapy.

Of interest, the t(14;18) translocation, like others in lymphomas, uses the same enzyme machinery that normally catalyzes Ig gene rearrangement, including recombinase, which joins the oligonucleotide segments, and TdT, which inserts N-regions between the joining segments. Therefore, it may be that while the neoplastic cells in follicular lymphoma have a mature B-cell phenotype, the translocation occurs at the pre-B-cell stage, probably in the bone marrow.

Bcl-2 is a mammalian homolog of the *Caenorhabditis elegans ced-9* gene.[35] It is formed by 3 exons, the first of which is untranslated. Exons 2 and 3 are separated by an intron more than 200 kb long. In t(14;18), the *bcl-2* gene is juxtaposed with an enhancer element in the Ig heavy-chain locus on 14q32, with the resultant constitutive overexpression of hybrid mRNA of two different sizes. The accumulating Bcl-2 protein, however, has normal size and function, with a molecular mass of 26 kDa and 239 amino acids. The carboxyl terminal end of the molecule is hydrophobic and serves as an integral membrane anchor.[36,37] The protein will associate with several subcellular membranes including the nuclear membrane, the endoplasmic reticulum, and mitochondrial membranes.[33,36]

The Bcl-2 protein accumulation, however, is not specific for follicular lymphomas. Indeed, a wide variety of lymphomas of both B- and T-cell origin, as well as normal mantle zone lymphocytes, overexpress the protein, while follicular hyperplasia and normal germinal centers do not.[38,39] The overexpression of Bcl-2 plays a critical role in blocking apoptosis, or programmed cell death, independent of affecting proliferation.[36,40] Normally, cells dying by apoptosis demonstrate membrane blebbing, volume contraction, nuclear condensation, and activation of a Ca^{2+}-dependent endonuclease, cleaving the DNA into nucleosomal length segments. This is reflected by the characteristic ladder pattern on DNA electrophoresis.

In vitro data suggest that deregulated *bcl-2* alone is insufficient to confer tumorigenicity to Epstein-Barr virus (EBV)-induced lymphoblastoid B-cells.[41] However, introducing *bcl-2* into a selected number of cell lines has an apoptosis-sparing effect after growth-factor withdrawal. This included cell lines dependent on interleukin (IL)-3, granulocyte-macrophage colony-stimulating factor (GM-CSF, sargramostim [Leukine]), IL-4, and IL-6.[40,42] Instead of undergoing apoptotic changes, the growth-factor-deprived cells simply enter G_0 and do not die. Cells could still be rescued with growth factor up to 30 days after factor deprivation.

Similarly, transfection of *bcl-2* protects a human pre-B-cell leukemia cell line by inhibiting apoptosis induced by several chemotherapeutic agents, including cytarabine, cisplatin (Platinol), etoposide (VePesid), and dexamethasone.[43] Although these agents inhibit proliferation in the *bcl-2*-transfected cell line, unlike the wild cell line, the cells demonstrate growth arrest but do not undergo apoptosis.[44] On the other hand, antisense-mediated reduction in *bcl-2* expression results in accelerated apoptosis in the setting of growth factor withdrawal.[45]

The above data indicate that whatever the promoting signal for apoptosis is (growth-factor deprivation, exposure to cytotoxic agents), Bcl-2 is a critical inhibitor of a final common pathway mediating the process.[46] This may explain why patients with the t(14;18) translocation are generally not cured with chemotherapy.

Transgenic mice bearing the *bcl-2/Ig* minigene will display "polyclonal" follicular proliferation that expands the IgM/IgD-expressing B-cell population. Upon activation, the cells will readily enter the cell cycle and display protracted proliferation.[47,48] Splenic cells from these mice demonstrate a remarkable survival advantage over B-cells from other mice; similar to the transfected cell lines, these cells mostly reside in G_0 but still proliferate in response to anti-IgM or lipopolysaccharide stimulation. Over time, these transgenic mice will progress from "polyclonal follicular hyperplasia" into a diffuse large-cell immunoblastic lymphoma.[49] As predicted, the transformation will invariably be associated with secondary genetic abnormalities. In this model, c-*myc* approximation with the immunoglobulin heavy-chain locus was observed as a secondary event in 50% of the mice.

Normal B-cells maintain high expression of Bcl-2 all through the pre-B phase and up to IgM/IgD expressing B-cell homing into the mantle zone. Subsequently, cells destined to die (eg, due to lack of T-cell help or failure to encounter their specific antigen within the follicle) maintain small cleaved morphology (centrocytes), downregulate Bcl-2 and undergo apoptosis within the follicle center. Even normal cells destined to survive will still partially downregulate Bcl-2, (compared with mantle zone cell levels) as differentiation proceeds.

Cells carrying t(14;18) entering the follicles with constitutive overexpression of Bcl-2 may not necessarily lead to follicular lymphoma. In fact, such cells are now commonly detected in the peripheral blood of normal individuals by PCR techniques, with higher titers correlating with advancing age.[28] Such aberrant expression of Bcl-2 by B-cells may lead to their prolonged survival within the follicle compared with normal counterparts, as suggested above. Antigen exposure,[8] T-cell help,[19] or further genetic abnormalities may add steps that permit lymphomagenesis. Subsequently, surviving cells will accumulate but, unlike their normal counterparts, will fail to differentiate to postfollicle stages like the immunoblast, plasma cell, and the memory B-cell.[42] This explains the original Rappaport terminology of "poorly differentiated lymphocytic lymphomas."

The accumulating cells will maintain some responsiveness to surrounding stimuli and will be liable for secondary genetic abnormalities that will mount an accelerated pace to the neoplastic process. Such genetic abnormalities may include the loss of tumor suppressor genes (like p53) or the activation of proliferation oncogenes. As detailed elsewhere, the clinical counterparts of genetic progression include refractory relapses, accelerated growth, and finally, frank transformation.[50] In fact, it is now clear that the transformed cells arise directly from a subclone of the follicular lymphoma, sharing with them the same idiotypic specificity and immunoglobulin heavy- and light-chain genes.[51]

The exact molecular mechanism of blocking apoptosis by Bcl-2 is not well understood and is beyond the scope of this review. Several areas of investigation have added to our knowledge in this regard, including the potentially important role of Bcl-2 in intracellular calcium partitioning, the newly described Bcl-2-related proteins like Bcl-x and Mcl-1, and the evolving crucial role of Bcl-2/Bax heterodimers in inhibiting the apoptotic effect of Bax homodimers.[52] In fact, the ratio between the two proteins may be more important than the absolute level of either.

Clinical Features, Diagnostic Workup, and Staging

Initial patient evaluation for follicular lymphoma involves history taking and physical examination. Patients should be closely questioned for the presence or absence of B symptoms. These symptoms occur in no more than 15% of patients with indolent lymphomas and include fever (38°C or above), drenching night sweats, and significant weight loss of more than 10% of baseline weight within 6 months. Patients may develop symptoms related to lymph-node enlargement, especially with bulky masses in the neck or the retroperitoneum.

Splenomegaly is more common in CLL/SLL than in follicular lymphomas. It may be the only sign of disease, such as in patients with primary splenic lymphoma. Splenic enlargement may lead to left upper quadrant discomfort and early satiety. Mediastinal lymph-node involvement may occur, but the occurrence of direct pressure symptoms (eg, superior vena cava syndrome) is extremely unlikely. Patients may have symptoms of anemia and, less commonly, thrombocytopenia. Symptoms of gastrointestinal tract involvement are nonspecific and include abdominal pain or discomfort, change in bowel habits, and gastrointestinal bleeding. The physical examination should include all lymph-node sites, including epitrochlear and postauricular lymph nodes. The abdominal examination may show a mass, splenomegaly, and, less commonly, hepatomegaly.

Excisional lymph-node biopsy is crucial to establishing the diagnosis. Fine-needle aspiration (FNA) is inadequate since it does not preserve the nodal architecture. Bilateral bone marrow biopsies are needed in the staging workup due to the patchy nature of involvement. The bone marrow characteristically shows paratrabecular infiltration with small cleaved cells.

Laboratory data may show anemia or thrombocytopenia. The cytopenias may result from direct marrow involvement, hypersplenism, or may be autoimmune in nature. The latter is more commonly seen in CLL/SLL than in follicular lymphomas, while hypersplenism may be more commonly seen in primary splenic (marginal) lymphoma and hairy-cell leukemia. Patients with anemia, however, should have a direct Coomb's test.

Platelet-associated antibodies may be positive in immune thrombocytopenia. The peripheral blood smear may be helpful if immune cytopenias are suspected. This smear may also show circulating neoplastic cells, especially in CLL where mature-looking lymphocytes are by definition increased. The serum lactate dehydrogenase (LDH) and beta$_2$-microglobulin levels may be elevated and are of prognostic significance.

Imaging studies should include a chest x-ray and a chest computed tomography (CT) scan if the x-ray result is suspicious. Abdominal and pelvic CT scans are essential, with their high sensitivity in detecting mesenteric lymphadenopathy. Lymphangiography is falling out of favor but remains a sensitive test to detect pelvic and para-aortic lymph node involvement, especially when lymph nodes are normal sized but have architecture abnormalities. It also provides an easy and accurate means to follow response to therapy with a plain abdominal film. A gallium scan is usually not indicated unless transformation is suspected.

The Ann Arbor Staging system is shown in Table 2. It was originally designed for the contiguously spreading Hodgkin's disease, as opposed to non-Hodgkin's lymphoma (NHL), which often spreads discontiguously. Thus, this staging system has drawbacks when applied to

TABLE 2

*Ann Arbor Staging System
for Non-Hodgkin's Lymphomas*

Stage I

A single lymph-node region or extralymphatic site

Stage II

Two or more lymph-node regions on the same side of the diaphragm or localized extralymphatic site with one or more lymph-node regions on the same side of the diaphragm

Stage III

Lymph-node regions on both sides of the diaphragm and possible localized involvement of an extralymphatic site or the spleen

Stage IV

Disseminated involvement of one or more extralymphatic organs or tissues

A or B

Denotes absence (A) or presence (B) of: unexplained weight loss > 10% body weight, unexplained fever > 38°C, or night sweats (*note*: pruritis is not a B symptom)

NHL—namely, the fact that most patients with indolent NHL have advanced disease (stage III or IV) at presentation and that even those with limited disease will have neoplastic cells detected in marrow and peripheral blood by sensitive molecular techniques.

Prognostic Factors

The importance of defining reliable prognostic factors in low-grade lymphomas becomes especially obvious in light of the great impact that patient selection can have on interpreting and comparing data among different trials. While histology is a major predictor in distinguishing clinical course between the low-grade and intermediate-grade lymphomas, most investigators found no clear difference in long-term survival among the different subtypes of low-grade histology (FSCL, FML, and SLL).[53,54]

Some data, however, suggest that patients with follicular mixed lymphomas have a more prolonged initial remission than those with follicular small cleaved lymphoma with potential curability.[55] Such data were contradicted by a different trial, making it difficult to reach any firm conclusions.[56] These differences may be due to the inconsistency in the criteria used by different pathologists in classifying follicular lymphomas.

A higher degree of nodularity has been associated in some reports with improved outcome,[57] but again, the issue remains controversial.[53,57–59] Other pathologic variables that may be associated with a favorable prognosis include the presence of interfollicular fibrosis[53] and the extent of helper T-cell infiltration.[60,61] In fact, the latter criterion was also associated with a higher rate of spontaneous regression.[61]

Laboratory criteria correlating with a poor prognosis include elevation of serum LDH[62] and beta$_2$-microglobulin levels[63] as well as increased expression of the nuclear proliferation antigen Ki-67, and the increased percentage of cells in S phase as determined by flow cytometry.[64] Some studies suggest that the presence of normal metaphases or the absence of abnormal ones correlates with a prolonged survival,[65,66] although this could not be confirmed by subsequent studies.[67]

The presence of structural breaks in either the short or long arm of chromosome 17 was shown by several groups to be a predictor of poor outcome, and seems to be an independent prognostic factor by multivariate analysis.[66,68] Patients with follicular small cleaved lymphoma with t(14;18) as a solitary abnormality typically have an indolent course, whereas those carrying additional karyotypic aberrations almost always have a more adverse outcome.[69] The ability to detect t(14;18) translocation by itself, on the other hand, has no impact on survival in patients with follicular lymphoma.[70]

Recently, there has been a growing interest in the detection of clonal cells in the peripheral blood in limited-stage disease as a potential prognostic factor. Early studies focused on detecting clonal excess (CE) by surface Ig staining with fluorescent monoclonal antibody (MoAb) against human kappa or lambda chains.[71,72] Several studies reported a higher incidence of CE in patients with low-grade histology as opposed to histologies of more aggressive disease.[73–75]

In the study by Johnson et al,[73] 27 patients with early-stage low-grade lymphoma in remission following involved-field (IF) radiation therapy were examined for CE. After a short median follow-up of 34 months, two of five patients with CE had relapsed, as opposed to none of 22 without CE (*P* < .0001). More sensitive techniques have been developed to detect clonal cells in peripheral blood, including Southern blot analysis[76] and, more recently, PCR techniques. PCR is a far more sensitive technique than the other two and is currently being investigated extensively as a potential predictor of relapse after high-dose and conventional chemotherapy.

Clinically, several variables have been shown to correlate with survival in follicular lymphoma. These include tumor burden, host factors, and response to therapy. Tumor burden can be defined in a variety of ways, utilizing variables including stage of disease, size of nodal disease, bone marrow involvement, beta$_2$-microglobulin level, and number of extranodal sites. Limited-stage disease is clearly associated with favorable outcome,[54,77,78] while the presence of two or more sites of extranodal involvement correlates with poor prognosis.[79] Adverse host factors include advanced age, B symptoms,[80] low hemoglobin level, male gender, and poor performance status.[77–79,81]

Attempts to design predictive models have been made,[83,79] but unlike the case in intermediate-grade lymphoma, no single system has gained wide acceptance. Recently, Lopez-Guillermo et al[82] examined the prognostic value of the International Index in predicting outcome in low-grade lymphoma. The International Index was devised for aggressive lymphomas and consists of five variables: age, performance status, Ann Arbor stage, extranodal involvement, and LDH level.[83] Lopez-Guillermo categorized 125 patients with low-grade lymphoma into three groups of low, intermediate, and high risk. While the International Index had no predictive value for response to therapy, there was a significant correlation with survival. The overall 10-year survival was about 75% for the low-risk group, 0% for the high-risk group, and approximately 50% for the intermediate-risk group. One important limitation of this system is that only 11% of the patients fell into the high-risk group, and most of these patients will probably have poor performance status and be poor candidates for aggressive therapy.

As shown by several series, response to initial therapy remains a powerful predictor of survival,[54] with more than 80% of complete responders living at 7 years compared with a median survival of 2 years among those failing to achieve a complete response (CR) in one study.[84]

At the time of relapse, favorable predictors for survival include having achieved a CR with initial treatment, a durable response to initial therapy of more than 1 year, and an age less than 60 years.[85]

SMALL LYMPHOCYTIC LYMPHOMAS

This category of the WF includes the classic nodal SLL, which is immunophenotypically and morphologically identical to chronic lymphocytic leukemia. It also has similar clinical features but lacks the characteristic absolute lymphocytosis. In addition, it also includes more recently characterized entities not specifically identified in the WF. These are the low-grade B-cell lymphoma of mucosa-associated lymphoid tissue (MALT lymphoma), monocytoid B-cell lymphoma, and extranodal SLL. The first two entities share similar pathologic and immunophenotypic characteristics and are thus encompassed together under the term marginal B-cell lymphomas.[13]

Indolent Lymphomas Arising From Mucosa-Associated Lymphoid Tissue

This group of indolent lymphomas has distinct clinical and pathologic characteristics. It probably includes many of the "pseudolymphomas" described in the old literature.[86] It is characterized by its localized nature, prolonged history, and good response to local therapy. It has been described at several extranodal sites including the gastrointestinal tract, lungs,[87] salivary glands, thyroid, thymus, breast, orbit, and conjunctiva.[88,89] Its potential for transformation into a high-grade histology is suggested by the significant number of high-grade gastric lymphomas that demonstrate a low-grade component in the background.[90] Dissemination is said to be rare and to occur late in the course.

Although most MALT lymphomas may be best categorized under SLL of the WF,[91] a recent study found the majority of MALT lymphoma patients to have previously been classified as having diffuse or follicular small cleaved lymphoma (30% each), while only a minority of the patients (5%) were described as having SLL.[91] Sometimes, within the same specimen, different cell types are grouped together and not intermingled, comprising a multiphasic histology.[88] Plasmacytoid differentiation is seen in one third of the patients.

With the exception of the Peyer's patches of the small intestines, MALT does not normally exist in any of the tissues in which MALT lymphomas arise. However, in response to an immune stimulus, MALT can arise as an ectopic tissue. The stimulus can be infectious in origin, like *Helicobacter pylori* in the gastric mucosa, or autoimmune in nature, as in Sjögren's syndrome[92] or Hashimoto's thyroiditis.[93] Whatever the underlying mechanism, the common pathophysiologic features of MALT are antigen recognition, T-cell help, and B-cell proliferation. If the proliferating B-cells show clonality, a MALT lymphoma is said to arise.

Both MALT and MALT lymphomas share constant pathologic features. They always have reactive lymphoid follicles. When lymphoma develops, tumor cells reside mostly in the area surrounding the mantle zone of the follicles; hence, the name marginal zone lymphoma. The marginal zone expands with diffuse cellular infiltrate, and the cells are of small lymphocyte or centrocyte morphology, explaining their WF classification. On occasion, neoplastic cells will "colonize" and even disrupt the follicles,[94] resulting in a pseudofollicular pattern to the tumor as a whole.

A second pathologic characteristic shared by both MALT and MALT lymphomas is lymphoepithelial invasion, in which the cells of the marginal zone are shown to invade into the overlying epithelium. Immunophenotypically, the neoplastic cells do not express CD5, CD10, or CD23 but mostly express surface IgM. Neither bcl-1 nor bcl-2 are rearranged, even when a pseudofollicular pattern is seen.[95] In the stomach, the pathologic recognition of MALT lymphoma may not be easy since the process constitutes a continuum along a spectrum from acute gastritis to MALT to MALT lymphoma. In one study,[96] the presence of dense lymphoid infiltrates, prominent lymphoepithelial lesions, moderate cytologic atypia, or Dutcher bodies were found to be highly suggestive of MALT lymphoma. Patients with gastric lymphoma arising in MALT may present with a previous history of gastritis or peptic ulcer disease. Other MALT-associated lymphomas will cause symptoms related to the anatomic site of the disease.

Recently there has been a great deal of interest in gastric lymphomas because of their association with *Helicobacter pylori*. Early studies correlated *H pylori* with gastric adenocarcinoma and gastric large-cell lymphoma.[97,98] A geographic correlation was also noted between *H pylori* infection and the incidence of gastric non-Hodgkin's lymphoma by several investigators.[97,99,100] In one study,[97] a comparison was made between the incidence of *H pylori* infection in gastric vs nongastric large-cell lymphomas; the odds ratio for the association of gastric lymphoma with *H pylori* was 6.3 as opposed to 1.2 for nongastric lymphoma, suggesting that *H pylori* may play a role in gastric lymphomagenesis.

Recently, more emphasis was put on studying the association between *H pylori* and MALT lymphoma, which constitutes a minority of primary gastric lymphomas. Wotherspoon et al[101] described MALT in 125 of 450 patients with *H pylori*-associated gastritis. Eight of the 125 had more pronounced lymphoepithelial invasion suggestive of MALT lymphoma. In a separate cohort of 110 patients with known gastric MALT, 101 of 110 patients had evidence of *H pylori* infection. While this suggests an association without proving a causal relationship, the observation that therapy for *H pylori* with antibiotics results in a dramatic reduction in gastritis-associated MALT was highly instructive.[101]

More recently, the same European group provided more convincing evidence of the causal relationship between *H pylori* and MALT lymphoma. In this study, Wotherspoon et al noted the complete disappearance of MALT lymphoma in five of six patients treated for *H pylori* infection.[102] In a recent update of their data, two more patients responded with regression of tumor, and remission was maintained up to 22 months after antibiotic therapy.[103] Stole et al[104] had less impressive results treating 32 patients with MALT lymphoma. Nineteen of the 32 had regression, 6 had full eradication, and 4 had persistence of the lymphoma.

Such clinical evidence was recently supported by laboratory investigation. Hussell et al[105] recently showed that cells from low-grade MALT lymphoma were stimulated by heat-killed *H pylori* in a strain-specific T-cell-dependent fasion in vitro. In contrast, extragastric MALT or gastric DLCL showed no such response. While the T-cells in this model demonstrate *H pylori* specificity, neoplastic B-cells did not, and in two cases there was a tissue autoantigen reactivity. This suggests that the B-cells may be autoreactive bystanders stimulated by nearby activated *H pylori* specific T-cells.[105,106]

Other gastrointestinal MALT lymphomas include a "Mediterranean" type referred to as immunoproliferative small intestinal disease (IPSID), which may share with gastric MALT a similar lymphomagenesis mechanism, being associated with gastrointestinal bacterial infections,[107] and demonstrating clinical responses to antibiotic therapy with tetracycline in the early phases of the disease.

Monocytoid B-cell lymphoma is the lymph-node counterpart of MALT lymphomas. The tumor consists of clear cells with reniform or oval nuclei. Instead of the lymphoepithelial lesions typical of MALT, these lymphomas have lymph-node growth pattern, with the neoplastic cells accumulating in confluent sinuses.

Early-stage marginal-zone lymphomas have an excellent prognosis with radiation therapy to the involved field. Advanced-stage marginal-zone lymphoma (MZL), on the other hand, has a comparable outcome to the other low-grade lymphomas. Among 43 patients with advanced-stage marginal zone lymphoma treated with CHOP and reported recently by Fisher et al,[91] the 10-year overall and failure-free survival was not significantly different from that of other categories of the WF studied, including SLL, FSC, FML, FLC, and diffuse small-cell (DSC) categories. When 19 patients with advanced-stage MALT lymphoma were compared with 21 patients with advanced monocytoid lymphoma, there were significantly worse overall (21% vs 53%, $P = .007$) and failure-free (21% vs 46%, $P = .009$) survivals among the MALT lymphoma patients at 10 years. In fact, advanced-stage MALT lymphoma fared worse than other low-grade categories of the WF studied. Therefore, in sharp contrast with early-stage MALT, the limited literature that exists suggests that advanced stages of MALT lymphoma may be worse than many other advanced-stage low-grade lymphomas.

MANTLE-CELL LYMPHOMA

Mantle-cell lymphoma is a relatively newly recognized clinicopathologic entity first recognized in the 1970s under the previously described categories "centrocytic lymphoma" of the Kiel classification and "intermediate differentiated lymphoma" or IDL of the modified Rappaport classification. The neoplastic cells arise from the mantle zone of secondary follicles[108,109] and usually give rise to a diffuse pattern of lymph-node involvement. Less commonly, a vaguely nodular pattern may be present (the mantle-zone lymphoma). As previously described, the WF does not recognize MCL as a specific entity, but it has most commonly been classified as diffuse small cleaved-cell lymphoma.

In a recent study, about 60% of MCLs were previously categorized as diffuse small cleaved, 25% as FSC, and the rest as SLL.[91] Presently, this lymphoma can be distinguished from lymphomas of follicular center-cell origin both morphologically and immunophenotypically. Mantle cells appear similar to the small cleaved lymphocytes with their scant cytoplasm and irregular nuclear contours, explaining their categorization under centrocytic lymphomas in the Kiel classification. But unlike the follicle-center lymphomas, which always contain large cells (centroblasts), mantle-cell lymphomas are more homogeneous morphologically. They also lack the dense organized meshwork of dendritic reticulum cells that characterizes follicle center-cell lymphomas.[110]

Immunophenotypically, mantle-cell lymphomas are almost always CD5 positive, like CLL and normal follicular mantle-zone cells, reflecting a prefollicle maturation with possible activation and distinguishing them from true follicle center-cell lymphomas that are virtually always CD5 negative. Otherwise, the cells typically express mature B-cell phenotype with CD19, CD20, CD22, and sIg, usually IgM, with a notable unexplained preference for lambda light chain. The cells also express CD43 but not CD10 or CD23. Such specific immunophenotypic features help distinguish this lymphoma from small lymphocytic lymphoma (CD23 positive) and follicle center-cell lymphomas (CD10 positive and CD43 negative). The absence of large or transformed cells, together with the mantle-zone phenotypic features of the

neoplastic cells, suggests that this tumor is a distinct entity unrelated to the spectrum of follicle center-cell lymphomas.[111]

The characteristic cytogenetic lesion of mantle-cell lymphoma is the t(11;14)(q13;q32) translocation, seen in about 73% of cases.[112–114] As a consequence of the translocation, a newly identified gene, *PRAD-1*, on 11q13 is juxtaposed to the Ig heavy-chain joining region on 14q32. The major breakpoint region on chromosome 11 is located approximately 110 to 120 kb centromeric to *PRAD-1* and is designated *bcl-1*. Unlike *bcl-2*, *bcl-1* simply represents the breakpoint region and does not represent an oncogene. Molecular probes to *bcl-1* can detect approximately 50% of all mantle-cell lymphomas, whereas probes to minor breakpoints will be needed to detect the rest.[115] As expected, the translocation will result in overexpression of *PRAD-1*,[116] a member of the cyclin family of proteins—hence, the other name of the protein, cyclin D1.[117] In fact, nuclear cyclin D1 can be detected in virtually all mantle-cell lymphomas using polyclonal antibody on paraffin-embedded sections.[118,119]

The role of cyclin D1 in oncogenesis is far from clear. The protein normally forms complexes with p21[waf1] and cyclin-dependent kinases and plays a role in cell-cycle progression. PRAD-1 was originally described in benign parathyroid adenomas as the oncogene rearranged to the parathyroid hormone locus.[119a] In addition to mantle-cell lymphoma, the gene is overexpressed in a considerable number of patients with breast cancer[119b] and head and neck squamous-cell carcinomas.[119c] Transgenic mice overexpressing the gene under the control of an immunoglobulin enhancer showed somewhat fewer mature T and B lymphocytes, albeit with normal cell-cycle activity and spontaneous lymphomas observed.[119d]

Mantle-cell lymphoma constitutes up to 10% of all NHL.[91] Patients are usually males older than 55 years who present with advanced-stage disease and generalized lymphadenopathy, bone marrow involvement, and a leukemic phase in up to 38% of cases. The liver, spleen, and Waldeyer's ring are frequently involved. Gastrointestinal tract involvement is seen in up to 20% of cases, with infiltration of the submucosa giving rise to multiple lymphomatous polyposis. This is distinct from lymphoepithelial involvement commonly seen in MALT lymphomas. Unlike other CD5-positive lymphoproliferative disorders, no autoimmune phenomena have been described in these patients.

The clinical course is heterogeneous, with some patients having very aggressive disease while other cases behave more like indolent lymphomas. In a small series of 23 patients at the National Cancer Institute (NCI), all patients presented with stage III or IV disease,[111] and liver involvement was an especially poor prognostic indicator. The pattern of growth may be prognostically important: A nodular pattern with residual germinal centers (mantle-zone lymphoma) appears to be indolent, while effacement of germinal centers or the entire node suggests a more aggressive behavior.[120,121] Likewise, blastic cytologic features or high Ki-67 expression may be adverse features, but all these observations need to be validated in large groups of uniformly treated patients. The usual prognostic factors (elevated LDH or beta$_2$-microglobulin levels, advanced stage, advanced age, and poor performance status) seem to be applicable to mantle-cell lymphomas.[122] Although the survival curves show patterns similar to those of low-grade lymphomas in that there is no plateau, the median survival is significantly shorter, ranging from 31 to 61 months.[115] The 10-year disease-free and overall survivals were 6% and 8% in one series, three to four times worse than corresponding survivals in indolent lymphomas reviewed.[91]

THERAPY FOR INDOLENT LYMPHOMAS

The vast majority of patients with advanced-stage low-grade NHL will respond to initial chemotherapy, with CR observed in one half to two thirds of patients. However, virtually all patients will ultimately relapse and most will die of their disease. While obvious responses and clinical effects may be seen using various therapeutic modalities, the hallmarks of advanced-stage disease (namely, its continuous recurring nature and incurability) remain unchanged.[111]

Assessment of new therapies for low-grade lymphomas can be difficult. First, the disease is heterogeneous, and differences in patient selection criteria can make comparison of data from different clinical trials difficult. Second, the disease has a long natural history, requiring long-term follow-up of patients before any final interpretation of data can be made. Surrogate biological markers that could reflect early therapeutic success are needed. PCR for bcl-2 may be such a marker, although further research is needed on this issue. Third, the frequency and stringency of restaging can affect the comparability of relapse-free survival in different series. Finally, the sequential utilization of multiple therapies in an individual patient confounds the analysis of each particular treatment intervention.

Limited-Stage Follicular Lymphoma

At time of presentation, about 15% to 20% of patients have limited-stage disease, and about half of these patients may be curable. Several series have reported that

approximately half of stage I-II patients achieve long-term disease-free survival following treatment with IF radiation.[123,124] Table 3 summarizes survivorship data from selected trials in patients with early-stage disease treated with radiation therapy alone or in combination with chemotherapy. In a recent update of the Stanford data,[123] the long-term failure-free survival (FFS) after definitive radiotherapy is 40%.[125] A subset of patients who received total-lymphoid irradiation (TLI) appeared more likely to be relapse free than those treated with involved-field or extended-field radiation. However, when laparotomy-staged patients were excluded from analysis, such a difference was no longer seen, suggesting that a disproportionate number of patients receiving TLI underwent laparotomy.

Recent insights perhaps make a systemic approach to early-stage disease appealing, given that bcl-2 gene rearrangement can be detected in marrow and peripheral blood with high frequency in both limited and advanced-stage disease.[126] The M. D. Anderson Cancer Center reported 76 patients with stages I-II disease who were treated with different modalities. Fifty patients received IF radiation alone, while 19 received combined modality with IF radiation and chemotherapy and the rest received chemotherapy alone. The overall 5-year failure-free survival was 47%. Those receiving combined modality therapy had a 5-year failure-free survival of 64% as opposed to 37% for those treated with IF radiation therapy alone, although no overall survival difference was seen.[127] A second retrospective analysis of 51 patients with stages I-II low-grade lymphoma treated at St. Bartholomew's hospital over a 13-year period also showed improved disease-free survival among those receiving combined-modality therapy compared with radiation alone, but again, no difference in overall survival was noted.[128]

Based on the encouraging results with combined-modality therapy in the retrospective studies, investigators at M. D. Anderson prospectively treated patients with stage I-II disease with 10 cycles of COP-Bleo (cyclophosphamide [Cytoxan, Neosar], vincristine [Oncovin], prednisone, bleomycin [Blenoxane]) or CHOP-Bleo (COP-Bleo plus doxorubicin [Adriamycin, Rubex]) with radiation to involved sites "sandwiched" after the third cycle. The 5-year disease-free survival was 77%, an apparent improvement over results with radiotherapy alone.[129] A prospective randomized trial also examined the efficacy of adding single-agent chlorambucil (Leukeran) for 6 months after radiation therapy with no improvement in disease-free or overall survival after up to 18 years of follow-up.[130]

TABLE 3

Treatment of Low-Grade Lymphomas, Stages I and II

Study	Treatment	Number of patients	Overall survival (%) 5-yr	10-yr	Failure-free survival (%) 5-yr	10-yr
Paryani, 1983	Radiotherapy	124	84	68	62	54
Gospodarowicz, 1984	Radiotherapy	190	75	66	55	53
McLaughlin, 1986	Radiotherapy	76	74		37	
	Chemotherapy with or without radiotherapy		73		64	
Lawrence, 1988	Radiotherapy or chemotherapy	54	83	69	60	48
Richards, 1989	Radiotherapy	57			61	
	Radiotherapy plus chemotherapy				94	
McLaughlin, 1991	Radiotherapy plus chemotherapy	44	88		74	

Experience is limited in the treatment of limited-stage MALT lymphoma and depends on the primary site. In general, long-term survival is attained with IF radiation with or without combination chemotherapy. As discussed elsewhere, antibiotic combinations have shown efficacy in the eradication of gastric MALT lymphoma in a large number of patients.

In summary, patients with limited-stage disease appear potentially curable, with overall long-term disease-free survival of approximately 50%. The role of radiation therapy in these patients is well established, and IF radiation remains the standard treatment. Total lymphoid irradiation may offer longer disease-free survival, although this is controversial and the subject of current investigation. The combined-modality approach has been intensively investigated, as discussed above. While adjuvant therapy with single agents did not improve outcome when added to radiation therapy, the addition of adjuvant or neoadjuvant combination chemotherapy may have an impact on disease-free survival, but large prospective trials to address this question are lacking.

Advanced-Stage Follicular Lymphoma

In patients with stages III and IV follicular lymphoma, the overall response rate with different chemotherapy programs is as high as 80% to 90%. The CR rate, however, varies widely, between 23% and 83% in various studies.[131-134] This is mostly explained by differences in patient selection criteria, techniques and diligence used to assess response, and the definition of response.

Recently, an attempt was made to standardize definitions of response and progression in Hodgkin's disease,[135] and the recommendations are generally applicable in non-Hodgkin's lymphoma as well. Complete response is defined as no clinical, radiologic, or other evidence of disease. Partial response (PR) is a decrease by at least 50% of the sum of the products of the largest perpendicular diameters of all measurable lesions. Progression is considered an increase in size of one or more measurable lesion by 25% or more. A new definition—CRu (unconfirmed/uncertain)—was introduced, referring to patients who have normal health but demonstrate some radiologic abnormality at the site of previous disease that is not consistent with the effect of previous therapy. This subset of patients has doubtlessly been classified in the past as CR in some trials and PR in others. The designation of CRu will hopefully improve the reliability and comparability of the data among different studies.

The impact of techniques used to assess response is best exemplified by the routine use of abdominal CT scan, which markedly increases the sensitivity of detecting mesenteric and upper abdominal lymph nodes. Thus, studies using such modalities to assess response may define CR more stringently and may have lower CR rates.

Because low-grade lymphomas are sensitive to radiation, radiation has been incorporated in primary therapy for some advanced stages of the disease. This has been best studied in patients with stage III disease. In updated results of a treatment program with central lymphatic irradiation initially reported by Cox et al,[136] the Milwaukee group demonstrated FFS rates of 40% at 15 years in stage III patients.[137] At Stanford, the FFS rates at 5 and 10 years were 60% and 40%, respectively, in 66 patients with stage III disease treated with TLI with or without chemotherapy. In a small subset of 16 patients prospectively randomized to receive TLI with or without CVP (cyclophosphamide, vincristine, prednisone), chemotherapy showed no significant advantage in survival or freedom from relapse.[138] Stage III patients at M. D. Anderson treated with CHOP-Bleo plus radiation to involved sites had a 5-year disease-free survival of 52%.[62] All these data strongly support a primary role for radiation therapy in stage III disease.

The role of radiation in patients with stage IV disease is less well understood. In one trial, 118 patients with advanced stage (III and IV) disease were randomized to receive combined modality therapy (TLI plus CVP or IF plus CVP) vs chemotherapy alone (CVP).[139] The 7-year relapse-free survival for patients in the combined modality groups (71% and 66% for TLI and IF, respectively) was significantly better ($P \leq .01$) than in patients receiving chemotherapy alone (33%). The overall survival was similarly improved, indicating a benefit for radiation therapy in advanced nodular lymphomas. This trial included both stage III and IV patients, however, and patients were not stratified according to stage when survival was examined. Other groups' experience with advanced-stage disease have failed to show any advantage for radiation therapy compared with or added to chemotherapy.

In a small randomized study by Hoppe et al, fractionated whole-body irradiation (with or without CVP) resulted in similar CR and overall survivals to those achieved with CVP or oral alkylating agents alone.[131] Whether radiation therapy will add to the effectiveness of more aggressive and dose-intensive regimens in stage IV patients remains to be seen. The Vancouver group is examining the efficacy of such an aggressive regimen, BP-VACOP (bleomycin, cisplatin, etoposide, doxorubicin, cyclophosphamide, vincristine, prednisone) with TLI in patients with bulky stage II, or stage III and IV disease.[140] Therefore, unlike stage III disease, the role of radiation therapy in stage IV follicular lymphoma is less well defined, and chemotherapy remains the mainstay of therapy in these patients.

Single-agent therapy with chlorambucil or cyclophosphamide (with or without prednisone) has long been considered a primary standard therapy in advanced low-grade lymphomas. Combination chemotherapy may result in more rapid responses than single-agent chlorambucil or cyclophosphamide,[131] but there is no clear evidence that it improves overall survival over single agents. Since response rates have been shown to correlate with survival, there has been emphasis on the CR rates of various chemotherapy programs. CVP was among the earliest combinations described and has gained wide acceptance.[141] The role of adding doxorubicin to the chemotherapy regimen remains controversial. CR rates and survivals seen in CHOP-treated patients were superior to those of a historical group of COP-treated patients at M. D. Anderson Cancer Center.[142] However, a large randomized study conducted by SWOG, reported no difference in outcome between CHOP-Bleo and COP-Bleo in indolent lymphomas.[143] Retrospective analysis of survival among 415 patients treated with CHOP in three SWOG trials also showed no advantage over results with less aggressive programs.[144] Similarly, CHOP has been compared with chlorambucil/prednisone,[145] and while more responses and shorter induction times were noted in the CHOP group, no survival difference was observed between the two groups.

In addition to CHOP and its variants (see Table 4), new programs incorporating different drugs have been developed. For example, procarbazine (Matulane)-containing regimens may be associated with more durable remissions in follicular mixed[55] and follicular small cleaved lymphoma.[146] Mitoxantrone (Novantrone) as a single agent had a high response rate of 95% in previously untreated[147] and up to 67% in relapsed patients.[148] Because of the synergism previously described between cytarabine and cisplatin in lymphoma,[149] the combination of etoposide, methylprednisolone, high-dose cytarabine, and cisplatin (ESHAP) was tested and shown to be effective in patients with relapsed low-grade lymphoma, with a CR rate of 35% and a PR rate of 40%.[150]

In keeping with the Goldie-Coldman hypothesis, 138 newly diagnosed patients were treated at M. D. Anderson with a sequential three-combination chemotherapy program (CHOD-B [CHOP-Bleo with dexamethasone instead of prednisone]/ESHAP/NOPP (mitoxantrone, vincristine, procarbazine, prednisone) for a total of 12 cycles. The overall CR rate was 65% with a projected 4-year survival of 94% and an FFS of 67%.[151] Though promising, the median follow-up of 27 months is too short to allow firm conclusions about this intensive regimen, but the follow-up PCR data for *bcl-2* gene rearrangement is provocative and encouraging. Several other aggressive combination chemotherapy and radiotherapy programs have been reported or are under investigation. To date, no single regimen has emerged as a standard, with 5-year failure-free survival ranging between 25% to 35% with most regimens (see Table 4).

TABLE 4

Treatment of Low-Grade Lymphomas, Stages III and IV

Study	Regimen[a]	Number of patients	Complete response (%)	5-yr Overall survival (%)	5-yr Failure-free survival (%)
Anderson, 1977	CVP C-MOPP BACOP	91	70	69	18 (DSL), 17 (FSC), 61 (FM)[b]
Jones, 1983	COP-Bleo CHOP-Bleo	77 75	71 72	50 57	29 38
Ezdinli, 1985	CP BCVP COPP	48 53 27	64 64 78	62 58 70	22 26 57
Steward, 1988	CVP CVP + maintenance	84 78	57 54	60 46	18 27
Young, 1988	ProMACE-MOPP + total nodal irradiation	43	78	84 (4-yr)	58 (4-yr)
McLaughlin, 1993	CHOP-Bleo + interferon alfa	127	73	74	47
McLaughlin, 1994	CHOD-B/ESHAP/NOPP	138	65	94 (4-yr)	67 (4-yr)

a CVP = cyclophosphamide, vincristine, and prednisone; C-MOPP = cyclophosphamide, vincristine, procarbazine, and prednisone; BACOP = bleomycin, doxorubicin, cyclophosphamide, vincristine, and prednisone; COP-Bleo = cyclophosphamide, vincristine, prednisone, and bleomycin; CHOP-Bleo = cyclophosphamide, doxorubicin, vincristine, prednisone, and bleomycin; CP = cyclophosphamide and prednisone; BCVP = carmustine, cyclophosphamide, vincristine, procarbazine, and prednisone; COPP = cyclophosphamide, vincristine, procarbazine, and prednisone; ProMACE-MOPP = prednisone, methotrexate, doxorubicin, cyclophosphamide, etoposide, mechlorethamine, vincristine, and procarbazine; CHOD-B = CHOP-Bleo with dexamethasone instead of prednisone; ESHAP = etoposide, methylprednisolone, high-dose cytarabine, and cisplatin, NOPP = mitoxantrone, vincristine, procarbazine, prednisone

b DSL = diffuse small lymphocytic lymphoma, FSC = follicular small cleaved cell lymphoma, FM = follicular mixed lymphoma

Because low-grade lymphomas have a long indolent course and since no therapy has clearly impacted on the continuous recurring nature of the disease, several investigators looked into the effect of withholding therapy in relatively asymptomatic patients until their symptoms warrant treatment—the so called "watch and wait" policy. Several reports in the literature suggest that this approach had no significant adverse impact on survival,[9,152,153] and some investigators recommend this as a standard approach in asymptomatic patients.[152]

To examine this concept further, the NCI conducted a study randomizing patients to receive intensive therapy with ProMACE-MOPP (prednisone, methotrexate, doxorubicin, cyclophosphamide, etoposide, mechlorethamine [Mustargen], vincristine, procarbazine) at the time of diagnosis or to defer therapy until the disease had progressed to a degree that could not be managed by radiation therapy alone in the watch-and-wait group.[154] The CR rate among those randomized to immediate therapy was higher than among those initially randomized to no therapy and later requiring treatment (75% vs 43%). Those who could not be randomized because they required intensive therapy at the time of

diagnosis also had a significantly worse CR rate of 57%. The lower CR rate in the watch-and-wait patients suggests that by the time the patients are symptomatic with bulky disease, a sufficient number of secondary genetic abnormalities may have accumulated to entail resistance to treatment. But with a median follow-up of 4 years, there was no survival difference among any of the 3 treatment groups. So far, therefore, it cannot be firmly concluded that early intensive chemotherapy will improve outcome. However, one of the preliminary conclusions of this trial has been a quality of life argument that, ironically, favors early intensive therapy: Those treated early enjoyed more time in remission off therapy than those managed with the palliative approach. An update of this trial is awaited.

Patients with follicular mixed lymphoma deserve special attention since several investigators have documented long-term disease-free survival in such patients treated with various regimens including C-MOPP (cyclophosphamide, vincristine, procarbazine, prednisone),[122] ProMACE-MOPP,[155] and CHOP-Bleo,[156] with long-term disease-free survival of up to 75%. This may be an argument for using early intensive therapy in this subgroup of patients. Glick et al,[157] on the other hand, failed to confirm such results using COPP.

A new class of drugs demonstrating remarkable activity in indolent lymphoproliferative disorders are the purine analogs. In particular, fludarabine (Fludara) and cladribine, or 2-chlorodeoxyadenosine (2-CdA, Leustatin) have been extensively studied and found to have significant activity. In addition to being antiproliferative, these agents can induce apoptosis.[158] This may explain their distinct effectiveness in indolent lymphoproliferative disorders as opposed to the more aggressive lymphomas. In addition, their resistance to the effect of adenine deaminase contributes to their efficacy compared with other nucleoside analogs.

Several phase II trials of fludarabine in low-grade lymphomas have been published. In general, when fludarabine is administered at a dose of 18 to 25 mg/m^2/d for 5 days repeated every 3 to 4 weeks, response is noted in one half to two thirds of previously treated patients with low-grade lymphoma. Those with intermediate-grade lymphomas, on the other hand, tend to show poor responses.[159,160] Redman et al treated 38 patients with relapsed or refractory low-grade lymphoma. The overall response rate was 55%; of the 21 patients with follicular small cleaved-cell lymphoma treated in this trial, four had a CR and nine had a PR. Other pathologic subtypes had less remarkable responses.

Similarly, in an Eastern Cooperative Oncology (ECOG) trial, 27 previously treated patients with low-grade lymphoma received fludarabine, with an overall response rate of 52% and CR noted in 5 of 27 patients.[160] In 16 previously untreated patients, Pigaditou et al demonstrated better overall and complete response rates of 75% and 60%, respectively.[161] The major dose-limiting toxicity of fludarabine in these trials was myelosuppression, mainly neutropenia, occurring in one third to one half of patients, with better tolerance noted among those without previous exposure to chemotherapy.[161]

Early trials with high doses of fludarabine (up to 125 mg/m^2/d for 7 days) for acute myelogenous leukemia (AML) were associated with significant neurotoxicity, but at the lower doses currently used for low-grade lymphomas and chronic lymphocytic leukemia (CLL), neurotoxicity is rare. However, Johnson et al recently described an unusual neurologic syndrome in five patients receiving fludarabine at standard dose for low-grade lymphoma. This included severe headache, hemiparesis, sensory abnormalities, and, in one patient, documented multiple brain infarcts. Therefore, patients receiving the drug should be carefully evaluated for any neurologic complications and the drug discontinued if necessary.[162]

With such a degree of activity as a single agent, fludarabine has been combined with other active agents. In a phase I[163] and a subsequent phase II trial, McLaughlin et al treated patients with recurrent low-grade or follicular large-cell lymphoma with the combination of fludarabine, mitoxantrone, and dexamethasone; in the phase II trial, the CR rate was 43% and PR rate was 51%, with durable responses.[164] The combination of fludarabine and chlorambucil was studied in phase I trials[165] and is currently being studied in a randomized trial in untreated CLL, comparing chlorambucil alone, fludarabine alone, and the combination of the two drugs. Other fludarabine-containing regimens are currently being evaluated with various drugs including cyclophosphamide, cytarabine, interferon,[166] and paclitaxel (Taxol).

The combined immunosuppressive effects of steroids and fludarabine may be of concern since the combination resulted in a higher incidence of serious infections including listeriosis in one report of CLL patients.[167] Cytomegalovirus and *Pneumocystis carinii* pneumonia (PCP) have also been reported.[168] Therefore, in more recent trials that combine fludarabine with steroids, prophylactic trimethoprim-sulfamethoxazole has been added, as was successfully done when the ProMACE-CytaBOM regimen was initially associated with a high incidence of PCP.[169]

Cladribine (2-CdA) has been less extensively studied in low-grade lymphomas. The standard dose is 0.1 mg/kg/d by continuous infusion for 7 days. Kay et al[170] demonstrated a response rate of 43% in patients with relapsed disease. Hoffmann et al demonstrated similar results, but there was a high incidence of myelotoxicity and infections.[171] Hickish et al[172] reported a somewhat better overall response of 75% in eight previously treated patients. As with fludarabine, previously untreated patients generally demonstrate better response rates. Emanuele et al[173] reported an impressive overall response rate of 82% in previously untreated patients. Liliemark et al[174] treated 20 patients with newly diagnosed low-grade lymphoma at a dose of 5 mg/m^2 as a 2-hour infusion for 5 days with cycles repeated every 28 days; there was a 60% overall response rate with 20% CR. Grade III/IV neutropenia was noted in up to 50% of patients.

Two other trials of cladribine reported similar overall response rates (50% and 66%) and toxicity profiles.[175,176] Responses to the drug have generally been brief. Cladribine is also being investigated in several combination regimens that include alkylating agents[177] or mitoxantrone. Important limitations of therapy with purine analogs include cumulative neutropenia and thrombocytopenia and an inversion in the CD4:CD8 ratio,[178] factors that limit the total number of cycles that can be delivered.

In summary, the purine analogs represent a highly promising group of compounds for therapy of indolent lymphomas. Their role in CLL is better established, but the data clearly show well-defined efficacy, especially for fludarabine, in the salvage of previously treated patients with indolent lymphomas. The role of purine analogs in various salvage combinations, as well as in primary therapy, is currently being extensively investigated. Their associated immune suppression and cumulative myelotoxicity may require dose or schedule modifications and prophylactic antibiotic therapy for PCP.

Given the recurring incurable nature of low-grade lymphoma, maintenance therapy has been an attractive modality to investigate. Although the initial remission duration may be prolonged, there is no evidence to suggest that either protracted single agents or maintenance with combinations of chemotherapy will prolong overall survival.[179,180] A biological agent, IFN, may also have an impact on remission duration in these patients.

Interferon

Interest in interferon therapy emerges from its unique mechanism of action and relatively mild self-limiting toxicity. In addition, it demonstrates activity in chemotherapy-resistant patients. The drug has been administered either as part of induction therapy or as maintenance after chemotherapy. It has been administered in a variety of doses and schedules with no clear superiority of one schedule over others. Its mechanism of action is discussed elsewhere.

As a single induction agent, the activity of IFN is substantial, both at diagnosis and relapse, with an overall response rate of about 50%, but the CR rate is only about 10%.[181-183,151] IFN has also been used in conjunction with chemotherapy as part of induction treatment. The ECOG conducted a trial showing that while response rates were similar among those receiving COPA (CHOP) alone vs COPA plus IFN. Patients in the IFN-containing induction arm had a significantly longer remission duration, compared with COPA alone ($P < .001$).[185] At 5-years, in 81% of those receiving COPA, disease had progressed, as opposed to 60% in the group receiving COPA and IFN ($P < .001$). A study by the Groupe d'Etude des Lymphomes Folliculaires (GELF)[186] supported these findings and also noted a survival advantage at 3 years in the IFN arm (86% vs 69%, $P = .02$). On the other hand, a randomized Cancer and Leukemia Group B (CALGB)-ECOG study has shown no benefit to date of adding IFN to single-agent cyclophosphamide in improving response rate, remis-

sion duration, or overall survival.[133] The latter study, however, treated patients at the time of initial diagnosis, unlike the ECOG and GELF studies, in which therapy was started after an initial "watch and wait" period.

Clinical studies have also investigated IFN in maintenance therapy. McLaughlin et al treated patients with stage IV low-grade lymphoma with CHOP-Bleo followed by IFN maintenance. At 5 years, 48% of patients treated with CHOP-Bleo and maintained on IFN for 2 years remain failure free, as opposed to 28% of historical controls treated with CHOP-Bleo alone ($P = .01$). However, similar to most other studies, there was no plateau in the relapse-free survival curve and no improvement in overall survival.[187] A trial by the European Organization for Research and Treatment of Cancer (EORTC) randomized patients into IFN maintenance therapy vs no therapy following eight courses of CVP and radiation therapy. There was a progression-free survival advantage noted in the IFN maintenance arm.[188] A British trial using chlorambucil with or without IFN[189] showed a significantly longer remission duration in the IFN maintenance arm without survival advantage.

In summary, the vast majority of programs that have integrated IFN into therapy for low-grade lymphoma have been associated with a benefit in prolonging remission duration, but the effect on survival is less convincing. Further studies and longer follow-up of ongoing trials will be required to establish the exact role of IFN in combination with various induction regimens and in different schedules as maintenance.

Mantle-Cell Lymphoma

To date, there is no accepted satisfactory treatment for mantle-cell lymphoma. As detailed above, the overall and disease free survival in patients treated with CHOP is rather poor.[91] Several reports have shown a fair frequency of achieving complete remission with standard CHOP-like therapy, averaging 40% to 50%.[190,191] but relapses are the rule and long-term survival is uncommon.[192] A recent retrospective review of 26 patients with centrocytic lymphoma suggested that the inclusion of doxorubicin was beneficial.[191] However, a German report[192] of 63 patients with centrocytic lymphomas who were randomized to receive COP or CHOP showed no significant improvement in survival in the CHOP-treated group.

Some of the discrepancies among studies may relate to differences in the pathologists' criteria in identifying the morphology of this relatively newly defined entity. Given their generally worse outcome, patients with mantle-cell lymphoma are being treated at several institutions with more intensive therapy with or without bone marrow transplantation (BMT). The efficacy of this strategy remains to be seen.

High-Dose Chemotherapy With Autologous Bone Marrow Support

Given the incurability of low-grade lymphoma with conventional-dose therapy, high-dose therapy has been investigated. Prolonged disease-free survival is attainable in a small fraction of patients with advanced indolent lymphomas. To date, however, there is no proof that any category of patients is cured, since survival curves continue to decline, with approximately 5% of patients dying each year. In general, more than 50% of the patients will ultimately relapse after autologous BMT.[193]

Bone marrow transplantation has mostly been reserved for young patients who have failed previous systemic therapy. The optimal high-dose regimen has not been identified. The sensitivity of follicular lymphomas to radiation therapy explains why most regimens have incorporated TBI as part of the preparative regimen. At the Dana-Farber Cancer Institute and St. Bartholomew's Hospital, patients with low-grade lymphoma mostly in second or subsequent remissions received high-dose cyclophosphamide and fractionated TBI, with autologous bone marrow rescue. The marrow was purged with MoAb and rabbit complement.[194] Recurrence rates were lower than expected at a median follow-up of 3.5 years, with only one third of patients relapsing,[195,196] when compared with a similar group of patients treated conventionally, but there was no improvement in survival and only those in second remission (as opposed to ≥ 3 remissions) seemed to have improvement in freedom from progression. A European group reported 52% failure-free survival at 5 years in patients with chemosensitive disease in CR or good PR. The median follow-up of the study is still short at 19 months.[197]

High-dose chemotherapy with autologous BMT has also been investigated in patients with transformed disease. Investigators from the University of Nebraska reported extremely poor outcome in patients transplanted after transformation. Most of their patients, however, had bulky advanced disease resistant to chemotherapy.[198] On the other hand, investigators from the Dana-Farber Cancer Institute did not report important differences in survival between those transplanted before or after transformation.[199] Their transformed disease patients, however, were sensitive to standard chemotherapy given before transplantation. Patient selection criteria, may explain the different results in these two studies.

High-dose chemotherapy with unpurged peripheral blood stem-cell (PBSC) support has also resulted in durable remissions in patients with relapsed indolent lymphomas.[200,201] An argument in favor of PBSC is that they may be less contaminated by neoplastic cells than is bone marrow.

Given the generally poor outcome once transformation occurs and given the encouraging preliminary results with BMT in relapsing patients, investigators are examining autologous BMT early in the course of the disease, ie, in first remission. Such trials are in their early phases, and longer follow-up will be required to show whether early BMT will have an impact on disease-free or overall survival.[198,202]

At present, high-dose chemotherapy with autologous rescue remains investigational. Although early data from the Dana-Farber Cancer Institute (DFCI)[203] suggested that those who achieved CR with conventional chemotherapy prior to BMT had better disease-free survival than those in PR, a recent update no longer shows a significant difference between the two groups.[204]

A recent study from Germany examined the assumption that PBSC may be less frequently contaminated with neoplastic cells than is the bone marrow and, thus, may serve as a better source for stem-cell support in conjunction with high-dose chemotherapy. The peripheral blood autografts were PCR positive in 22 of 30 patients (as opposed to the expected 100% yield from an unpurged bone marrow following standard chemotherapy). Of those who received PCR-positive autografts, 6 of 22 converted to PCR negative 6 to 16 months post-transplantation. This suggests that neoplastic cells may not be viable after peripheral blood stem cell collection and reinfusion. The median follow-up was too short to reach any conclusions beyond that.[205]

Allogeneic BMT has not been commonly employed in follicular lymphomas, but encouraging data do exist. In a recent trial, 8 of 10 patients with refractory or recurrent disease achieved remission and remain relapse-free at a median follow-up time of 816 days.[206] Though preliminary, these data seem to be an improvement over results with autologous transplant, suggesting a role for the graft-vs-lymphoma (GVL) effect. However, this has to be weighed against the increased transplant-related morbidity and mortality from possible graft-vs-host disease (GVHD). In addition, despite promising data from early clinical trials, laboratory data demonstrate that follicular lymphoma cells are poor stimulants of allogeneic T-cells in mixed lymphocyte reactions.[207] This may be explained by the follicular lymphoma cells lack of expression of the B7 family of molecules that initiate a necessary costimulatory signal in T-cells via CD28. It remains to be seen, however, whether this will translate into lack of clinically evident GVL effect in transplanted patients.

PCR in Assessing Response and Monitoring for Relapse

Molecular techniques using PCR amplification of bcl-2 minor and major breakpoints detect clonal cells in the bone marrow in most patients at the time of diagnosis, after remission induction with conventional therapy, and at the time of relapse.[208] PCR has also been used to assess efficacy of ex vivo purging of bone marrow. In a DFCI trial, all 114 patients in the study had PCR-positive bone marrow after treatment with CHOP at the time of harvest. Following purging with MoAb, 50% of the bone marrow turned PCR negative and such patients had a markedly more favorable disease-free survival posttransplant.[209,210] The group from St. Bartholemew's Hospital could not replicate such a high percentage of negative conversion following purging,[211] and three of the four patients whose bone marrow did turn negative with ex vivo purging relapsed. Such discrepancies may be explained by the fact that the British investigators used only one antibody to purge the bone marrow, whereas the DFCI investigators used three. This difference notwithstanding, overall survival of patients at the two centers is the same.[196]

PCR has also been used to monitor response after high-dose chemotherapy and autologous bone marrow rescue[212] as well as following conventional-dose chemotherapy.[151] Preliminary results from the DFCI group were encouraging in that those who were persistently PCR negative or became negative several months after BMT had no relapses (none of 77 patients at 6 years), while those who were persistently PCR positive ultimately relapsed (71% of 35 patients at 6 years). Similarly, McLaughlin et al[151] reported 19 patients with advanced-stage disease treated with three intensive sequential chemotherapy regimens. These 19 patients were originally positive in peripheral blood for bcl-2 rearrangement by PCR and had serial monitoring; 13 turned PCR negative after therapy, a superior result to what was previously observed with CHOP or other less intensive therapy.[213–215] Such "molecular remissions" seem to correlate with a lower likelihood of relapse (1 of 13 molecular remissions relapsed vs 2 of 6 patients with persistently positive PCR).

The above data indicate that some high-dose chemotherapy programs and some intensive standard-dose therapy are capable of converting patients into PCR-negative status. In the BMT patients, outcome also appears to depend on the successful purging of the autograft. The indication that PCR negativity correlates with disease-free survival may represent a breakthrough, since it identifies for the first time a surrogate molecular marker for long-term disease-free survival in patients who would otherwise require very long follow-up to show a favorable survival outcome.

A positive PCR for bcl-2 breakpoints may not be a highly specific predictor for relapse, however. The group from St. Bartholomew's Hospital reported six patients in remission for more than 10 years who are persistently PCR positive.[215] Similar observations were made by investigators from M. D. Anderson.[216] In addition, some groups[27] have obtained positive PCR results in the peripheral blood of normal individuals. In fact, recent data suggest that when peripheral blood cells from normal individuals were sorted for B-cells, more than half of the individuals tested were found to harbor t(14;18) breakpoints, and sometimes, of several unrelated clones in the same individual as demonstrated by DNA sequencing.[217] Therefore, it is not surprising that patients can be clinically disease free for a long time with persistently amplifiable fragments.

Nevertheless, a negative PCR may indeed be a highly specific predictor of favorable prognosis; this seems most convincing in the context of BMT, but the preliminary data described above with intensive conventional chemotherapy is also promising. One recent study[218] challenged this concept and concluded that PCR has no positive or negative prognostic significance. However, this study included only eight patients treated with conventional CVP (with or without radiation), and the whole argument is based on a single patient in whom, despite clinically progressive disease, PCR was always negative; the patient's PCR status at the time of diagnosis was not mentioned.

The premise that peripheral blood may be less contaminated by neoplastic cells than the marrow will have an impact on which source is used for disease monitoring (and harvest). The DFCI data looking at marrow and peripheral blood at the time of harvest and relapse indicates that peripheral blood is indeed less sensitive for monitoring disease.[208] At diagnosis, however, the PCR yield for bcl-2 is high in both peripheral blood and marrow, and the results are highly concordant.[126] After therapy, reversion to PCR negativity of either peripheral blood or marrow is prognostically favorable, although most strikingly so with marrow monitoring.[208] It remains to be seen whether the simplicity and practicality of peripheral blood monitoring is outweighed by the increased sensitivity of BM monitoring. Conceivably, the development of reliable quantitative PCR assays (titers) will provide another useful perspective on this threshold of detection issue.[219]

Conclusions

A number of factors can influence treatment decision for patients with newly diagnosed indolent lymphomas, including age, stage, histologic diagnosis, and the patient's general health and performance status. Prognostic factors are not as universally agreed upon as is the case in intermediate-grade lymphoma. The watch-and-wait policy is still an acceptable option in asymptomatic individuals without threatening disease. Older patients or those with poor performance status or other medical problems may be palliated with oral chlorambucil or cyclophosphamide. Oral purine analogs may also become available for this purpose.[220]

Younger patients with advanced-stage disease may warrant consideration of early intensive chemotherapy. However, no single regimen is demonstrated to be superior to others. The importance of including doxorubicin is not as clear as in the more aggressive lymphomas, but there are data to support the use of early intensive therapy in some subsets of patients, eg, those with follicular mixed lymphomas. The role of fludarabine-containing regimens as front-line therapy is not yet well defined and is currently being investigated in clinical trials. Integration of alpha interferon (IFN-α) into front-line therapy appears to result in improved relapse-free survival. The younger patient in relapse may benefit from high-dose therapy with bone marrow or peripheral stem-cell support in the context of a clinical trial.

HISTOLOGIC PROGRESSION AND CLINICAL TRANSFORMATION

In general, histologic progression corresponds with an accelerated clinical course. It usually evolves from follicular to diffuse histology with increasing numbers of large cells.[221] This histologic progression is associated with loss of the characteristic dendritic reticular cells constantly seen in follicular lymphomas. While approximately 30% of patients demonstrate progression on rebiopsy,[221] an autopsy study suggests that about 70% of patients with an initial diagnosis of follicular lymphoma who died with the disease had only a diffuse pattern at the time of death, while 6% had preserved follicular pattern. Cytogenetic analysis often indicates the acquisition of additional chromosomal abnormalities upon transformation. In one series, these included +7, +3, del(13)q32, and +18.[69] In addition, several series demonstrated *p53* mutations in a sizable number of patients with follicular lymphoma who undergo histologic transformation (up to 30% in one series).

Whether this simply represents a secondary phenom-enon or has a mechanistic role in progression is not clear at this time. The latter assumption is reasonable since loss of p53 leads to enhanced cycline dependant kinase (cdk) activity with subsequent increase in retinoblastoma protein phosphorylation; this leads to the release of transcription factor E2F, resulting in increased expression of several genes that contribute to S-phase entry, including c-*myc*, *fos*, and *myb* among others.[222,223]

The incidence of clinical transformation is difficult to assess, but approaches 40% to 70% at 8 to 10 years of follow-up, and its incidence does not seem to be affected by previous therapy.[224,225] Patients have clearly transformed without having received treatment. Indeed, the data from Ig-*bcl-2* transgenic mice suggests that transformation is an inherent feature. The time to transformation is highly variable, ranging between 8 months and 25 years, and, at least in the Stanford series, there does not seem to be a plateau in the rate of transformation in both initially treated and untreated patients. This extremely wide range of time to transformation is another demonstration of the high degree of heterogeneity in this disease.

In general, patients with histologic transformation have a poor prognosis, with survivals of less than 1 year often reported.[226,227] Prognostic factors at the time of transformation include disease bulk and response to chemotherapy.[228] In the Stanford data, the CR rate in transformed patients approached 40% with a median survival of 95 months for those complete responders.[228] The role of high-dose chemotherapy and autologous BMT in relapsed patients remains uncertain and is discussed elsewhere.

In summary, transformed patients should be treated with intensive chemotherapy regimens. As is the case for intermediate-grade lymphoma, there is no evidence that any regimen is superior to CHOP, but for those who have already received CHOP or other regimens during the indolent phase of the disease, it is probably advisable to select alternative non-cross-resistant regimens. While the definitive role of BMT in transformed lymphoma remains unsettled, patients demonstrating adequate response to conventional therapy should be good candidates for enrollment in clinical trials that incorporate BMT.

FUTURE DIRECTIONS

To date, most advanced-stage indolent lymphomas remain incurable and new approaches to therapy are clearly needed. High-dose chemotherapy with autologous bone marrow or PBSC support is being increasingly used earlier in the disease course. Purging techniques and

PCR monitoring are under investigation. New active drugs are being incorporated in combinations.[229,230]

Novel approaches to therapy are also being explored. Monoclonal antibodies[231] have been extensively investigated. These include unconjugated antibodies, radioimmunoconjugates, and immunotoxins. The exact role and efficacy of these agents remain to be established. Individualized therapy by generating anti-idiotype monoclonal antibodies has resulted in good responses, and the concept is being developed into stimulating endogenous anti-idiotype MoAbs by utilizing vaccines.[232–234] New biological agents are also being examined including IL-2, IL-4, and recombinant fusion toxins[235] (eg, $DAB_{486}IL-2$).

Recently, intense research has focused on understanding the molecular mechanisms of apoptosis in B lymphocytes. The demonstration that murine and human "immature" B-cells may undergo apoptosis instead of proliferation[236] in response to cross-linking surface immunoglobulin receptors raises interesting questions about exploiting similar signal transduction pathways to induce apoptosis in human follicle center lymphomas. Bcl-2 antagonism and Bax upregulation through manipulating signalling remain elusive therapeutic goals that may prove synergistic with direct triggering of apoptosis by chemotherapy or radiation. The role of Fas-FasL interaction in inducing apoptosis in B-cells[7,237] is becoming better understood and raises questions about how the enforced expression of *bcl-2* in follicular lymphomas may influence apoptotic signals through fas in neoplastic cells.

We still face many challenges in finding curative therapy for the indolent lymphomas. Future effective therapies will most likely emerge from a close interaction between basic scientists and clinical investigators, bringing knowledge acquired through fundamental research from the bench to the bedside.

REFERENCES

1. Suchi T et al: Histopathology and immunohistochemistry of peripheral T cell lymphomas: A proposal for their classification. J Clin Pathol 40:995–1015, 1987.

2. National Cancer Institute sponsored study of classification of non-Hodgkin's lymphoma: Summary and description of a Working Formulation for clinical usage. The non-Hodgkin's lymphoma pathologic classification project. Cancer 49:2112, 1982.

3. Fisher RI et al: Natural history of malignant lymphoma with divergent histologies at staging evaluation. Cancer 47:2022–2025, 1981.

4. Casali P et al: Human lymphocytes making Rheumatoid factor and antibody to ss DNA belong to Leu 1+ B-cell subset. Science 236:77, 1987.

5. Morris DL, Rothstein TL, in Snow EC (ed): Handbook of B and T cells, pp 421–445. San Diego, Academic Press, 1994.

6. Tsubata T, Wu J, Hongo T: B-cell apoptosis induced by antigen receptor crosslinking is blocked by a T-cell signal through CD40. Nature 364:645–648, 1993.

7. Rothstein TL, Wang Z, Boote L, et al: Protection against Fas-dependent Th1-mediated apoptosis by antigen receptor engagement in B cells. Nature 374:163–165, 1995.

8. Zelenetz A: Clonal expression in follicular lymphoma occurs subsequent to antigenic selection. J Exp Med 176:1137, 1992.

9. Horning ST, Rosenberg S: The natural history of initially untreated low grade non-Hodgkin's lymphomas N Engl J Med 311:1471–1475, 1984.

10. Stauder R: Expression of leukocyte function associated antigen-1 and 7F7-antigen, an adhesion molecule related to intercellular adhesion molecule-1 (ICAM-1) in non-Hodgkin's lymphomas and leukemias: Possible influence on growth pattern and leukemic behavior. Clin Exp Immunol 77:234–238, 1989.

11. Metter GE et al: Morphologic subclassification of follicular lymphoma. Variability of diagnoses among hematopathologists, a collaborative study between the Repository Center and Pathology Panel for Lymphoma clinical studies. J Clin Oncol 3:25–38, 1985.

12. Nathwani BN et al: What should be the morphologic criteria for the subdivision of follicular lymphomas? Blood 18:837–845, 1986.

13. Harris N et al: A revised European American Classification of lymphoid neoplasms: A proposal from the International Lymphoma Study Group. Blood 84:1361–1392, 1994.

14. Gerdes J: Production of a mouse monoclonal antibody reactive with a human nuclear antigen associated with cell proliferation. Int J Cancer 31:13–20, 1983.

15. Grogan T, Spier R, Fisher R: Refined Working formualtion (WF) categorization of lymphoma using phenotype and genotype analysis. A SWOG Control Repository Study (abstract #425). Lab Invest 64:73A, 1991.

16. Jaffe ES et al: Nodular lymphoma: Evidence for origin from follicular B lymphocytes. N Engl J Med 290:813–819, 1974.

17. Aisenberg A, Wilker B, Jacobson J, et al: Immunoglobulin gene rearrangements in adult non-Hodgkin's Lymphoma. Am J Med 82:738, 1987.

18. Williams ME et al: Immunoglobulin and T cell receptor gene rearrangement in human lymphoma and leukemia. Blood 69:79–86, 1987.

19. Umetsa D, Esserman L, Donlor J, et al: Induction of proliferation of human follicular (B type) lymphoma cells by cognate interaction with CD4+ T cell clones. J Immunol 144:2550, 1990.

20. Speaks SL: Chromosomal abnormalities in indolent lymphoma. Cancer Genet Cytogenet 27:335–334, 1987.

21. Offit K et al: Cytogenetic analysis of 434 consecutively ascertained specimens of NHL: Correlation between recurrent aberrations, histology and exposure to cytotoxic treatment. Genes, Chromosomes and Cancer 3:189–201, 1991.

22. Levine EG, Arthur D, Frizzera G, et al: There are differences in cytogenetic abnormalities among histologic subtypes of the non-Hodgkin's lymphomas. Blood 66:1414, 1985.

23. Mrozek K, Bloomfield C: Cytogenetics of indolent lymphoma. Semin Oncol 20(suppl 5):47, 1993.

24. Osada H et al: Bcl-2 gene rearrangement analysis in Japanese B-cell lymphoma: Novel bcl-2 recombination with immunoglobulin kappa chain gene. Jpn J Cancer Res 80:711–715, 1989.

25. Korsmeyer S: Bcl-2 initiates a new category of oncogenes: Regulators of cell death. Blood 80:879, 1992.

26. Limpens J: Bcl-2/JH rearrangement in benign lymphoid tissues with follicular hyperplasia. Oncogene 6:2271–2276.

27. Limpens J et al: Lymphoma-associated translocation t(14;18) in blood cells of normal individuals. Blood 85:2528–2536, 1995.

28. Liu Y, Hernandez A, Shibata D, et al: Bcl-2 translocation frequency rises in frequency with age in humans. Proc Natl Acad Sci

USA 91:8910–8914, 1994.

29. Cabanillas F, Pathak S, Trujillo J, et al: Frequent non-random chromosome abnormalities in 27 patients with untreated large cell lymphoma and immunoblastic lymphoma. Cancer Res 48:5557, 1988.

30. Gaidano G, Ballerini P, Gong J, et al: p53 mutations in human lymphoid malignancies: Association with Burkitt's lymphoma and chronic lymphocytic leukemia. Proc Natl Acad Sci USA. 88:5413–5417, 1991.

31. Ichikawa A, Hotta T, Takagi N, et al: Mutations of p53 and their relation to disease progression in B-cell lymphoma. Blood 79:2701, 1992.

32. Yunis J, Oken M, Kaplan, et al: Distinctive chromosomal abnormalities in histologic subtypes of non-Hodgkin's lymphoma. N Engl J Med 307:1231–1236, 1982.

33. Tsujimoto Y, Finger L, Yunis J, et al: Cloning of the chromosome breakpoint of neoplastic B-cells with the t(14;18) translocation. Science 226:1097, 1984.

34. Ngan BY, Nourse J, Cleary ML: Detection of chromosomal translocation t(14;18) with the minor cluster region of bcl-2 by PCR and direct genetic screening of the enzymatically amplified DNA in follicular lymphoma. Blood 73:1759–1762, 1989.

35. Hengartner MO, Horvitz R: C elegans survival gene *ced-9* encodes a functional homology of the mammalian protooncogene Bcl-2. Cell 76:665–676, 1994.

36. Hockenbery D, Nunez G, Korsmeyer J, et al: Bcl-2 is an inner mitochondrial membrane protein that blocks programmed cell death. Nature 348:334, 1991.

37. Chen-Levy Z: The bcl-2 candidate proto-oncogene product is a 24-Kd integral in membrane protein is highly expressed in lymphoid cell lines and lymphomas carrying t(14;18) translocation. Mol Cell Biol 9:701–710, 1989.

38. Pezzella F et al: Expression of the bcl-2 oncogen protein is not specific for the 14;18 chromosme translocation. Am J Pathol 137:225–232, 1990.

39. Zutter M: Immunolocalization of the bcl-2 protein with hematopoietic neoplasms. Blood 78:1062, 1991.

40. Nunez G, Hockenbery D, Korsmeyer S, et al: Deregulated bcl-2 gene expression selectively prolongs survival of growth factor-deprived hematopoietic cells. J Immunol 144:3602–3610, 1990.

41. Nunez G et al: Growth-and tumor-promoting effects of deregulated bcl-2 in human B- lymphoblastic cells. Proc Natl Acad Sci USA 86:4589–4593, 1989.

42. Vaux D: BCL-2 gene posseses haematopoietic cell survival and cooperates with c-myc to immortalize pre-B cells. Nature 335:440–442, 1988.

43. Miyashita T, Reed J: Bcl-2 gene transfer increases relative resistance of S49.1 and WEHI 7.2 lymphoid cells to cell death and DNA fragmentation induced by glucocorticoids and multiple chemoherapuetic drugs. Cancer Res 52:5407–5411, 1992.

44. Miyashita T, Reed JC: Bcl-2 Oncoprotein blocks chemotherapy-induced apoptosis in a human leukemia cell line. Blood 81:151–157, 1993.

45. Reed J, Stein C, et al: Antisense-mediated inhibition of bcl-2 proto-oncogene expression and leukemic cell growth and survival. Comparison of phosphodiester and phosphoorthoate oligodeoxynucleotides. Cancer Res 50:6565, 1990.

46. Reed JC: Bcl-2 and the regulation of programmed cell death. J Cell Biol 124:1–6, 1994.

47. McDonnell T: Bcl-2 immunoglobulin transgenic mice demonstrate extended B cell survival and follicular lymphoproliferation. Cell 57:79–88, 1989.

48. McDonnell T et al: Deregulated bcl-2 immunoglobulin transgene expands a resting but responsive immunoglobulin M and D-expressing B-cell population. Mol Cell Biol 10:1901–1907, 1990.

49. McDonnell T, Korsmeyer S: Progression from lymphoid hyperplasia to malignant lymphoma in mice transgenic for t(14;18). Nature 349:254, 1991.

50. Richardson M et al: Intermediate- to high-grade histology of lymphomas carrying t(14;18) is associated with additional nonrandom chromosome changes. Blood 70:444–447, 1987.

51. Zelenetz A, Chen T, Levy K: Histologic transformation of follicular lymphoma to diffuse lymphoma represents tumor progression by a single malignant B cell. J Exp Med 173:197, 1991.

52. Oltari Z, Milliman C, Korsmeyer J: Bcl-2 heterodimers in vivo with a conserved homologue, BAX, that accelerates programmed cell death. Cell 74:609–619, 1993.

53. Bastion Y, Coiffier B, et al: Follicular lymphomas: Assessment of prognostic factors in 127 patients followed for 10 years. Ann Oncol 2:123S.

54. Gallagher C et al: Follicular lymphoma: Prognostic factors for response and survival. J Clin Oncol 4:1470–1480, 1986.

55. Longo D et al: Prolonged initial remission in patients with nodular mixed lymphoma. Ann Intern Med 100:651–656, 1984.

56. Glick J et al: Nodular mixed lymphoma: Results of a prolonged trial failing to confirm prolonged disease-free survival with COPP chemotherapy. Blood 58:5, 1981.

57. Ezdinli E et al: Effects of the degree of nodularity on the survival of patients with nodular lymphoma. J Clin Oncol 5:413–418, 1987.

58. Warnike R et al: The coexistence of nodular and diffuse patterns in nodular non-Hodgkin's lymphoma. Cancer 40:1229–1233, 1977.

59. Hu E et al: Follicular diffuse mixed small-cleaved and large-cell lymphoma: A clinicopathologic study. J Clin Oncol 3:1183–1187, 1985.

60. Medeiros LJ et al: Numbers of host 'helper' T cells and proliferating cells predict survival in diffuse small-cell lymphoma. J Clin Oncol 7:1009–1017, 1989.

61. Strickler J et al: Comparison of "host cell infiltrate" in patients with follicular lymphoma with or without spontaneous regression. Am J Clin Pathol 90:257–261, 1988.

62. McLaughlin P et al: Stage III follicular lymphoma. Durable remisions with a combined chemotherapy-radiotheapy regimen. J Clin Oncol 6:867, 1987.

63. Litam P et al: Prognostic value of serum B2 microglobulin in low-grade lymphoma. Ann Intern Med 114:855–810, 1991.

64. Macartney JC et al: DNA flow cytometry of follicular non-Hodgkin's lymphoma. J Clin Pathol 44:215, 1991.

65. Kristoffersson U et al: Prognostic implication of cytogenetic findings in 106 patients with NHL. Cancer Genet Cytogenet 25:55–64, 1987.

66. Levine EG et al: Cytogenetic abnormalities predict clinical outcome in NHL. Ann Intern Med 108:14–20, 1988.

67. Schouten HC et al: Chromosomal abnormalities in untreated patients with NHL: Association with histology. Clinical characteristics and treatment outcome. Blood 7:1841–1847.

68. Cabanillas F, Grant G, Hagemeister F, et al: Refractoriness to chemotherapy and poor survival related to abnormalities of chromosome 17 and 7 in lymphoma. Am J Med 87:167–172, 1989.

69. Yunis J et al: Multiple recurring genomic defects in follicular lymphoma: A possible model for cancer. N Engl J Med 316:79–84, 1987.

70. Pezzella F, Jones M, et al: Evaluation of bcl-2 protein expression and t(14;18) translocation as prognostic markers in follicular lmphoma. Br J Cancer 65:87, 1992.

71. Ault K: Detection of small number of monoclonal B lymphoma in the blood of patients with lymphoma. N Engl J Med 300:1401–1405, 1979.

72. Ligler F, Smith G, Frenkel E, et al: Detection of tumor cells in the peripheral blood of non-leukemic patients with B-cell lymphoma: Analysis of "clonal excess". Blood 55:792–801, 1980.

73. Johnson A, Cavallin-Stahl E: Incidence and prognostic significance of blood lymphocyte clonal excess in localized non-Hodgkin's lymphoma. Ann Oncol 2(10):739–743, 1991.

74. Sobol RE, Dillman RO, et al: Application and limitation of peripheral blood by analysis of antigen receptor gene rearrangements: Results of a prospective study. Cancer 56:2005–2010, 1985.

75. Lindemalen C et al: Blood clonal B-cell excess (CBE) at diagnosis in patients with non-Hodgkin's lymphoma (NHL): Relation to clinical stage, histopathology and response to treatment. Eur J Cancer Clin Oncol 23:749–753, 1987.

76. Horning SJ et al: Detection of non-Hodgkin's lymphoma in the peripheral blood by analysis of antigen receptor gene rearrangement. Results of a prospective study. Blood 75:1139–1145, 1990.

77. Leonard RCF: The identification of discrete prognostic groups in low grade NHL. Ann Oncol 2:655–662, 1991.

78. Soubeyran P, Richaud P, Hoerni B, et al: Low grade follicular lymphoma: Analysis of prognosis in a series of 281 patients. Eur J Cancer 27:1606–1613, 1991.

79. Romaguera J et al: Multivariant analysis of prognostic factors in stage IV follicualr low-grade lymphomas: A risk model. J Clin Oncol 9:762, 1991.

80. Vuckovic J, Stula N, Capkun V, et al: Prognostic value of B-symptoms in low grade non-Hodgkin's lymphoma. Leukemia and Lymphoma 13:357–358, 1994.

81. Rudders RA et al: Nodular non-Hodgkin's lymphoma: Factors influencing prognosis and indications for aggressive treatment. Cancer 43:1143–1651, 1979.

82. Lopez-Guillermo A, Montserrat E, Basch F, et al: Low-grade lymphoma: Clinical and prognostic studies in a series of 143 patients from a single institution. Leuk Lymph 15:159–165, 1994.

83. Shipp MA, Harrington DP, Andrson JR, et al: A predictive model for aggressive NHL: The international NHL prognostic factors project. N Engl J Med 329:987–994, 1993.

84. Diggs C, Wiernick P, Ostrow S: Nodular lymphoma: Prolongation of survival by CR. Cancer Clin Trials 4:107–114, 1981.

85. Weisdorf D, Andersen J, et al: Survival after relapse of low-grade non-Hodgkin's lymphoma: Implications for marrow transplantation. J Clin Oncol 10:942–947, 1992.

86. Addis B, Hyjek E, Isaacson P: Primary pulmonary lymphoma: A re-appraisal of its histogenesis and its relationship to pseudolymphoma and lymphoid interstitial pneumonia. Histopathology 13:1–17, 1988.

87. Li G et al: Primary lymphoma of the lung: Morphological immunohistochemical and clinical features. Histopathology 16:519–531, 1990.

88. Isaacson PG: B cell lymphomas of mucosa associated lymphoid-tumor (MALT) Bull Cancer 78:203–205, 1991.

89. Isaacson PG: Lymphomas of mucosa-associated lymphoid tumor. (MALT). Histopathology 16:617–619, 1990.

90. Chan J, Ng C, Isaacson P: Relationship between high grade lymphoma and low grade B-cell mucosa associated lymphoid tissue lymphoma (MALToma) of the stomach. Am J Pathol 136:1153, 1990.

91. Fisher RI et al: A clinical analysis of two indolent lymphoma entities. Mantle cell lymphoma and marginal zone lymphoma (including mucosa-associated lymphoid tissue and monocytoid subcategories). A South West Oncology Group Study. Blood 85:1075–1082, 1995.

92. Hyjek E, Smith W, Isaacson P, et al: Primary B-cell lymphoma of salivary glands and its relationship to myoepithelial sialadenitis. Human Pathol 19:766–776, 1988.

93. Hyjek E, Isaacson P: Primary B-cell lymphoma of the thyroid and its relationship to Hashimoto's thyroiditis. Hum Pathol 19:1315–1326, 1988.

94. Isaacson P et al: Follicular colonization in B-cell lymphoma of mucosa associated lymphoid tissue. Am J Surg Pathol 15:819–828, 1991.

95. Pan L et al: The bcl-2 gene in primary B cell lymphoma of mucosa associated lymphoid tissue (MALT). Am J Pathol 135:7–11, 1989.

96. Zukerberg LR: Lymphoid infiltrate of the stomach evaluation of histologic criteria for the diagnosis of low-grade lymphoma on endoscopic biopsy specimens. Am J Surg Pathol 14:1087–1099, 1990.

97. Parsonnet J, Hansen S, Friedman G: Helicobacter pylori infection and gastric lymphoma. N Engl J Med 330:1267–1271, 1994.

98. Parsonnet JMB, Friedman G, et al: Helicobacter pylori infection and the risk of gastric carcinoma. N Engl J Med 325:1127–1131.

99. Doglioni C, Wotherspoon A, Isaacson P, et al: High incidence of primary gastric lymphoma in northeastern Italy: Lancet 339:834, 1992.

100. Tally N, Zinsmeister A, et al: Gastric adenocarcinoma and Helicobacter pylori infection: J Natl Cancer Inst 83:1734.

101. Wotherspoon A et al: Helicobacter pylori-associated gastritis and primary B-cell gastric lymphoma. Lancet 338:1175–1176, 1991.

102. Wotherspoon A: Regression of primary low grade B-cell gastric lymphoma of mucosa associated lymphoid tissue type after eradication of Helicobacter pylori. Lancet 342:575, 1993.

103. Wotherspoon AC, Isaacson P, et al: Antibiotic treatment for low grade gastric MALT lymphoma. Lancet 343:1503, 1994.

104. Stolte M et al: Healing gastric MALT lymphoma by eradicating Helicobacter pylori. Lancet 342:518, 1993.

105. Hussell T: The response of cells from low grade B cell gastric lymphomas of mucosa-associated lymphoid tissue type to Helicobacter pylori. Lancet 342:571, 1993.

106. Hussell T, Isaacson P, Spencer J, et al: Immunoglobulin specificity of low grade B-cell gastrointestinal lymphoma of mucosa-associated lymphoid tissue (MALT) type. Am J Pathol 142:285–292.

107. Khojaski A et al: Immunoproliferative small intestinal disease. A "third world lesion". N Engl J Med 308:1401–1405, 1983.

108. Raffeld M, Jaffe E: Bcl-1, t(11;14) and mantle cell-derived lymphomas. Blood 78:259–263, 1991.

109. Banks PM, Chan J, Warnke RA, et al: Mantle cell lymphoma: A proposal for unification of morphologic, immunologic, and molecular data. Am J Surg Pathol 16(7):137–140, 1992.

110. Harris N et al: Immunohistologic characterization of two malignant lymphomas of germinal center type (centroblastic/centrocytic and centrocytic) with monoclonal antibodies. Am J Pathol 117:262–272, 1989.

111. Bookman M, Jaffe E, Longo D, et al: Lymphocytic lymphoma of intermediate differentiation: Morphology, immunophenotype, and prognostic factors. J Natl Cancer Inst 82:742–748.

112. Weisenburger D et al: Intermediate lymphocytic lymphoma. Immunophenotypic and cytogenetic findings. Blood 69:1617–1621, 1987.

113. Athan E et al: Bcl-1 rearrangement: Frequency and clinical significance among B-cell chronic lymphocytic leukemia with NHL. Am J Pathol 138:591–599, 1991.

114. Williams M et al: Characterization of chromosome translocation breakpoints and the bcl-1 and PRAD-1 loci in centrocytic lymphoma. Cancer Res 52(suppl):5541–5544s, 1992.

115. Shiudazani R et al: Intermediate lymphocytic lymphoma. Clinical and Pathologic features of a recently characterized subtype of NHL. J Clin Oncol 11:802–811, 1993.

116. Rosenberg C, Bale A, Harris N, et al: PRAD-1, a candidate BCL-1 oncogene: Mapping and expression in centrocytic lymphoma. Proc Natl Acad Sci USA 88:9638–9642, 1991.

117. Motokusa T, Arnold A: PRAD 1/Cyclin D1 protooncogene: genomic organization 5' DNA sequence and sequence of a tumor-specific rearrangement breakpoint. Genes Chromoso Cancer 7:89–95, 1993.

118. Yang W, Arnold A, Harris N, et al: Cyclin D1 (Bcl-1, PRAD-1) protein expressed in low grade B cell lymphoma and reactive hyperplasia. Am J Pathol 145:86–96, 1994.

119. Case records of Massachusetts General Hospital, Case 43-1994. N Engl J Med 331:1576–1582, 1994.

119a. Motokura T, Bloom T, Kim HG, et al: A novel cyclin encoded by a bcl-1-linked candidate oncogene. Nature 350:512, 1991.

119b. Gillett C, Fantl V, Peters G, et al: Amplification and overexpression of cyclin D1 in breast cancer detected by immunohistochemical staining. Cancer Res 54:1812, 1994.

119c. Bartkova J, Lukas J, Strauss M, et al: Abnormal patterns of D-type cyclin expression and G1 regulation in human head and neck cancer. Cancer Res 55:949, 1995.

119d. Bodrug SE, Warner BJ, Adams JM, et al: Cyclin D1 transgene impedes lymphocyte maturation and collaborates in lymphomagenesis with the myc gene. EMBO J 13:2124, 1994.

120. Weisenburger D et al: Mantle cell lymphoma: A follicular variant of intermediate lymphocytic lymphoma. Cancer 47:1429–1438, 1982.

121. Majlis A, Pugh W, Cabanillias F: Three histologic variants of mantle cell lymphoma exhibit striking heterogeniety in clinical behaviour and histologic features. Blood 83: 388a Abs#1536, 1993.

122. Zucca E, Coiffier B: European Lymphoma Task Force (ELTF): Report of the workshop on mantle cell lymphoma (MCL). Ann Oncol 5:507–511, 1994.

123. Paryani SB: Analysis of non-Hodgkin's lymphoma with nodule and favorable histologies, stages I & II. Cancer 52:2300–2307, 1983.

124. Gospodarowicz M, Brown T, Chua T: Prognostic factors in nodular lymphomas: a multivariate analysis based on the Princess Margarett hospital experience. Int J Radiation Oncology Biol Phys 10:489–497, 1984.

125. Horning ST: Low grade lymphoma. 1993: State of the Art. Ann Oncol 5(suppl 2):523–527, 1994.

126. Berinstein NL, Klok RJ, Reis MD, et al: Sensetive and reproducible detection of occult disease in patients with follicular lymphoma by PCR amplification of t(14;18) both pre- and post-treatment. Leukemia 7:113–119, 1993.

127. McLaughlin P: Stage I-II follicular lymphoma. Cancer 58:1596–1602, 1986.

128. Richards MA et al: Management of localized non-Hodgkin's lymphoma. The experience of St. Bartholomew Hospital 1972–1985. Hematol Oncol 7:1–18, 1989.

129. Seymour J et al: Combined modality therapy may cure most patients with clinical stage I and II low-grade lymphoma (abstract #110). Blood 82:578a, 1993.

130. Kelsey SM et al: A British National lymphoma investigation randomised trial of single agent chlorambucil plus radiothrapy *versus* radiotherapy alone in low grade, localised non-Hoodgkin's lymphoma. Med Onc 11:19–25, 1994.

131. Hoppe RT, Rosenberg S, et al: The treatment of advanced stage favorable histology Non-Hodgkin's lymphoma: A preliminary report of a randomized trial comparing single agent chemotherapy, combination chemotherapy, and whole body irradiation. J Clin Oncol 58(3):592–598, 1981.

132. Solal-Celigny P et al: Recombinant IFN-2b combined with a regimen containing doxorubicin in patients with advanced follicular lymphoma. N Engl J Med 329:1608–1614, 1993.

133. Peterson BA, Oken M, Ozer H, et al: Cyclophosphamide vs cyclophosphamide and interferon-alpha 2b in follicular low grade lymphoma: A preliminary report of an intergroup trial (CALGB 8691 and EST 7486). Proc Am Soc Clin Oncol 12:1240–1241, 1993.

134. Smalley RV et al: Interferon alpha combined with cytotoxic chemotherapy for patients with non-Hodgkins lymphoma. N Engl J Med 327:1336–1341, 1992.

135. Lister TA et al: Report of a committee convened to discuss the evaluation and staging of patients with Hodgkin's disease: Cotswolds meetings. J Clin Oncol 7:1630–1636, 1989.

136. Cox J, Komaki R, Kun L, et al: Stage III nodular lymphocytic tumors (non-Hodgkin's lymphoma): Results of central lymphatic irradiation. Cancer 47:2247–2252, 1981.

137. Jacobs JP et al: Central lymphatic irradiation for stage III nodule malignant lymphomas: Long term results. J Clin Ocol 11:233–238, 1993.

138. Paryani S et al: The role of radiation therapy in the management of stage III follicular lymphoma. J Clin Oncol 2:841.

139. Avile A et al: Long term results in patients with low-grade nodular NHL. ACTA Oncologica 30, 1991.

140. Klasa RJ, Voss N, Connors J, et al: BP-VACOP and extensive lymph node irradiation for advanced stage low grade lymphoma (abstract #1117). Proc Am Soc Clin Oncol 11:328, 1992.

141. Luce J, Frei E III, Palmer R, et al: Combined cyclophosphamide, vincristine, and prednisone therapy of malignant lymphoma. Cancer 28:306, 1971.

142. Cabanillas F, Smith T, Bodey G, et al: Nodular malignant lymphomas: Factors affecting complete response rate and survival. Cancer 44:1983–1989, 1979.

143. Jones ST et al: Improved complete remission rates and survival for patients with large cell lymphoma treated with chemoimmunotherapy. A Southwest Oncology Working Group Study. Cancer 51:1083–1090, 1983.

144. Dana BW et al: Long term follow up of patients with low-grade malignant lymphomas treated with doxorubicin based chemotherpay or chemoimmunotherapy. J Clin Oncol 11:144–151, 1993.

145. Kimby E, Bjorkholm M, et al: Chlorambucil/prednisone vs CHOP in symptomatic low-grade non Hodgkin's lymphoma: A randomized trial from the Lymphoma Group of Central Sweden. Ann Oncol 5:567–571, 1994.

146. Ezdinli E et al: The effects of intensive intermittent maintenance therapy in advanced low-grade NHL. Cancer 10:156–160, 1987.

147. Hansen S et al: High activity of mitoxantrone in previously untreated low-grade lymphomas. Cancer Chemother Pharmacol 22:77–79, 1988.

148. Gams R et al: Mitoxantrone in malignant lymphoma. Investigational New Drugs 3:219–222, 1985.

149. Velasquez WS et al: Effective salvage therapy for lymphoma with CDDP in combination with high-dose ara-C and dexamethasone (DHAP). Blood 71:117–122, 1988.

150. Velasquez WS, McLaughlin P, Tacker S, et al: ESHAP—An effective chemotherapy regimen in refractory and relapsed lymphoma: A 4-year follow-up study. J Clin Oncol 12(6):1869, 1994.

151. McLaughlin P, Swan F, Younes A, et al: Intensive conventional dose chemotherapy for stage IV low grade lymphoma: High remission rates and reversion to negative of peripheral blood Bcl-2 rearrangement. Ann Oncol 5S2:S73–77, 1994.

152. Portlock C, Rosenberg S: No initial therapy for stage III and IV non-Hodgkin's lymphoma of favorable histologic types. Ann Intern Med 90:10–13, 1979.

153. Idestrom K, Kimby E, Wadman B, et al: Treatment of CLL and well-differentiated lymphocytic lymphoma with continuous low or intermittent high-dose prednimustine vs chlorambucil/prednisone. Eur J Cancer Clin Oncol 18:1117, 1982.

154. Young R: The treatment of indolent lymhomas. Watchful

waiting & aggressive combined modality treatment. Semin Hematol 25(suppl 2):11–16, 1988.

155. Longo DL: What's the deal with follicular lymphoma? J Clin Onc 11:202, 1993.

156. Peterson BA, Bloufield CD, Gottlieb AT, et al: Combination chemotherapy prolongs survival in follicular mixed lymphoma. Proc Am Soc Clin Oncol 9:259a, 1990.

157. Glick J, Ezdinli E, Bennett J, et al: Nodular mixed lymphoma: Results of a randomized trial failing to confirm prolonged disease-free survival wih COPP chemotherapy. Blood 58:920–925, 1981.

158. Robertson LE, Chubb S, Mega RE, et al: Induction of apoptotic cell death in CLL by 2-chlorodeoxyadenosine and 9 beta-D-Arabinosyl-2-fluoroadenine: Blood 81:143, 1995.

159. Redman JR, Cabanillas F, Velasquez W, et al: Phase II trial of fludarabine phosphate in lymphoma: An effective new agent in low grade lymphoma. J Clin Oncol 10:790.

160. Hochster H, Oken M, Oconnell M, et al: Activity of fludarabine in previously treated non-Hodgkin's low grade lymphoma: Results of an Eastern Cooperative Oncology Group Study. J Clin Oncol 10:28–32; 1992.

161. Pigaditou A, Rohatiner AZ, Lister T, et al: Fludarabine in low grade lymphoma. Semin Oncol 20(suppl 5):24–27, 1993.

162. Johnson PWM, Rohatiner A, Lister T, et al: Neurologic illness following treatment with fludarabine. Br J Cancer 70:966–968, 1994.

163. McLaughlin P et al: Phase I study of the combination of fludarabine, mitoxantrone, and dexamethasone in low grade lymphomas. J Clin Oncol 12:575–579, 1994.

164. McLaughlin P, Hagemeister F, et al: Fludarabine, mitoxantrone and dexamethasone (FND), for recurrent low grade lymphoma (LGL): A phase II trial (abstract #1318). Proc ASCO 13:387, 1994.

165. Weiss M, Berman E, Gee T, et al: Results of a phase I study of fludarabine monophosphate and chlorambucil in patients with CLL (abstract #914). Proc Am Soc Clin Oncol 11:276, 1992.

166. Foss F, Ihde D, Ghosh B, et al: Phase II study of FAMP and interferon-alpha-2A in advanced mycosis fungoides/Sezary syndrome (MF/SS). Proc Am Soc Clin Oncol 11:315, 1992.

167. O'Brien S, Kantarjian H, Keating M, et al: Results of Fludarabine and prednisone therapy in 264 patients with chronic lymphocytic leukemia with multivariate analysis-derived prognostic model for response to treatment. Blood 82:1695–1700, 1993.

168. Schilling P, Vadhan-Raj S: Concurrent CMV and PCP after Fludarabine therapy for CLL (letter). N Engl J Med 323:833–834, 1990.

169. Browne MJ et al: Excess prevalance of Pneumocystis carinii pneumonia in patients treated for lymphoma with combination chemotherapy. Ann Intern Med 104:338–344, 1986.

170. Kay AC, Saven A, et al: 2-Chlorodeoxyadenosine treatment of low grade lymphoma J Clin Onc 10:371–377, 1992.

171. Hoffman M, Tallman M, et al: 2-Chlorodeoxyadenosine is an active salvage therapy in advanced indolent non-Hodgkin's lymphoma. J Clin Oncol 12:788, 1994.

172. Hickish T, Oza A, Lister T, et al: 2-chlorodeoxyadenosine: Evolution of a novel predominantly lymphocyte selective agent in lymphoid malignancies. Br J Cancer 67:139–143, 1992.

173. Emanuele S, Saven A, Piro L: 2-CdA activity in patients with untreated low grade lymphoma (abstract #1002). Proc ASCO 94:13:306, 1994.

174. Liliemark J, Hagberg H, et al: Cladribine (2-CdA) for early low grade non-Hodgkin's lymphoma (abstract #658). Blood 84:10, 1994.

175. Taylor K, Grigg A, Stone J, et al: Short infusional 2-chlorodeoxyadenosine (2-CdA)-Effective therapy in relapsed or poor risk de novo low grade non-Hodgkin's lymphoma (abstract #659). Blood 84:168a, 1994.

176. Canfield V, Vose J, Nichols C: Phase II trial of 2-chlorodeoxy-adenosine (2-CdA) in patients with untreated low grade non-Hodgkin's lymphoma (abstract #657). Blood 84:168a, 1994.

177. Tefferi A, Witzig T, Reid J, et al: Phase I study of combined 2-chlorodeoxyadenosine and chlorambucil in CLL and low grade lymphoma. J Clin Oncol 12:569–574, 1994.

178. Boldt DH, Yon Hoff DD, et al: Effect on human peripheral lymphocyte of in vivo administration of 9-beta-D-arabinofuranoyl-G-fluroadenine-5 monophosphate. Cancer Res 44:4561–4566, 1984.

179. Ezdinli E, Harrington D, O'Connell M, et al: The effect of intensive intermittent maintenance therapy in advanced low grade non-Hodgkin's lymphoma. Cancer 60:156–160, 1987.

180. Steward W, Crowther D, Harris M, et al: Maintenance chlorambucil after CVP in the management of advanced stage low grade histologic type non-Hodgkin's lymphoma: A randomized prospective study with an assessment of prognostic factors. Cancer 61:411–447, 1988.

181. Horning S, Cabanillias F, Rosenburg S, et al: Human interfer-on alpha in malignant lymphoma and Hodgkin's disease. Cancer 56:1305–1310, 1985.

182. Gutterman J, Alexanian R, Hersh E, et al: Leukocyte interfer-on-induced tumor regression in human metastatic breast cancer, multiple myeloma and malignant lymphoma. Ann Intern Med 93:399–406, 1980.

183. Foon K, Sherwin S, Abrams P: Treatment of advanced non-Hodgkin's lymphoma with recombinant leukocyte A interferon. N Engl J Med 311:1148, 1984.

185. Smalley R, Andersen J, et al: Interferon-alpha combined with cytotoxic chemotherapy for patients with non-Hodgkin's lymphoma. N Engl J Med 327:1336, 1992.

186. Solal-Celigney P: Recombinant interleukin alpha 2b combined with a regimen containing doxorubicin in patients with advanced follicular lymphoma. Groupe d'Etude des Lymphomes de l'Adulte. N Engl J Med 329:1108–1114, 1993.

187. McLaughlin P, Cabanillias F, Hagemeister F, et al: CHOP-Bleo plus interferon for stage IV low-grade lymphoma. Ann Oncol 4:205–211, 1993.

188. Hagenbeek A, Van Hoof A, Conde P, et al: Interferon-alfa-2a vs control as maintenance therapy for low-grade non-Hodgkin's lymphoma: Results from a prospective randomized clinical trial on behalf of the EORTC Lymphoma Cooperative group. Proc Am Soc Clin Oncol 14:386, 1995.

189. Price CG, Rohatiner A, Lister TA, et al: Interferon-alpha 2b in addition to chlorambucil in the treatment of follicular lymphoma: Preliminary results of a randomized trial. Eur J Cancer 27(suppl 4):S34–36, 1991.

190. Weisenburger D, Kim H, Rappaport H: Mantle zone lymphoma: A follicular variant of intermediate lymphocytic lymphoma. Cancer 49:1429–1438, 1982.

191. Zucca E, Fontna S, Cavalli F: Treatment and prognosis of centrocytic (mantle cell) lymphoma: A retrospective analysis of twenty-six patients treated in one institution. Leu Lymph 13:105–110, 1994.

192. Meusers P, Engelhard M, Bartels H, et al: Multicenter randomized therapeutic trial for advanced centrocytic lymphoma: Anthracycline does not improve the prognosis. Hematol Oncol 7:365–380, 1989.

193. Freedman A, Anderson K, Nadler L, et al: Autologous Bone Marrow Transplantation in B-cell non-Hodgkin's lymphoma: Very low treatment-related mortality in 100 patients in sensetive relapse. J Clin Oncol 8:784–790, 1990.

194. Nadler LM, Bast RC, Canellos GP, et al: Anti-B-1 monoclonal antibody and complement treatment in autologous bone marrow transplantation for relapsed B-cell non-Hodgkin's lymphoma. Lancet 2:427–431, 1984.

195. Rohatiner AZ, Freedman A, Nadler L, et al: Myeloablative therapy with autologous bone marrow transplant as consolidation therapy for follicular lymphoma. Ann Oncol 5(suppl 2):143–146, 1994.

196. Rohatiner AZ, Price CG, Lister TA, et al: Myeloablative therapy with autologous bone marrow transplantation as consolidation therapy for recurrent follicular lymphoma. J Clin Oncol 12:1177–1184, 1994.

197. Schouten HC, Colombat PH, et al: Autologous bone marrow transplantation for low grade non-Hodgkin's lymphoma: The European Bone Marrow Transplant Group experience. Ann Oncol 5(suppl 2):S147–149, 1994.

198. Schouten HC, Bierman PJ, Armitage JO: Autologous bone marrow transplantation in follicular non-Hodgkin's lymphoma before and after histologic transformation. Blood 74:2579–2584, 1989.

199. Gribben J, Freedman A, Nadler L, et al: All advanced stage non-Hodgkin's lymphoma with amplifiable breakpoint of bcl-2 have residual cells containing the bcl-2 rearrangement at evaluation and after treatment. Blood 78:3275–3280, 1991.

200. Kessinger A, Vose J, Armitage J, et al: High dose therapy and autologous peripheral stem cell transfusion for patients with bone marrow metastasis and relapsed lymphoma: An alternative to bone marrow purging. Exper Hematol 19:1013–1016, 1991.

201. Bierman P, Vose J, Armitage J, et al: High dose therapy followed by autologous hematological rescue for follicular low grade lymphoma (abstract #1074). Proc ASCO 11:317, 1992.

202. Freedman A, Nadler L, Ritz J, et al: Autologous bone marrow transplantation in advanced low-grade non-Hodgkin's lymphomas in first remission (abstract #1313). Blood 10:332a (suppl 1), 1993.

203. Freedman AS, Ritz J, Anderson K, et al: Autologous bone marrow transplantation in 69 patients with a history of low-grade B-cell lymphoma. Blood 77:2524–2529, 1991.

204. Freedman A, Gribben J, Nadler L, et al: Autologous bone marrow transplant in relapsed low grade lymphomas (abstract 797). Blood 84:203a, 1994.

205. Hass R, Moos M, et al: Sequential high-dose therapy with peripheral blood progenitor cell support in low grade non-Hodgkin's lymphoma. J Clin Oncol 12:1685–1692, 1994.

206. van Besien, Koen W, et al: Allogeneic bone marrow transplantation for refractory and recurrent low grade lymphoma: The case for aggressive management. J Clin Oncol 13:1096–1102, 1995.

207. Schultz JL, Gribben J, Nadler L, et al: Most Follicular lymphomas do not stimulate an allogeneic T cell proliferative response. Blood 84(suppl 1):521a, 1994.

208. Gribben J, Neuberg D, Nadler L, et al: Detection of residual lymphoma cells by PCR in peripheral lymphocytic cells by PCR in PB is significantly less predictive for relapse than detection in bone marrow. Blood 83:3800–3807, 1994.

209. Gribben JG, Freedman A, Nadler L, et al: Immunologic purging of marrow assessed by PCR before autologous bone marrow transplantation for B-cell lymphoma. N Engl J Med 325(22):1525–1533, 1991.

210. Gribben J, Freedman A, Nadler L, et al: All advanced stage non-Hodgkin's lymphoma with amplifiable breakpoint of bcl-2 have residual cells containing the bcl-2 rearrangement at evaluation and after treatment. Blood 78:3275–3280, 1991.

211. Johnson PWM, Price CGA, Lister TA, et al: Detection of cells bearing the t(14;18) translocation following myeloablative treatment and autologous bone marrow transplant for follicular lymphoma. J Clin Oncol 12:798–805 1994.

212. Gribben J, Nadler L: Monitoring minimal residual disease. Semin Oncol 20(suppl 5):143–155, 1993.

213. Lee M, Cabanillias F, et al: Minimal residual circulating cells carrying the t(14;18) are present in patients with follicular or diffuse large cell lymphoma in long-term remission (abstract #898). Blood 72:247a, 1988.

214. Lee MS, Chang KS, Stass S, et al: Detection of minimal residual cells carrying the t(14;18) by DNA sequence amplification. Science 237:175–178, 1987.

215. Price C, Rohatiner A, Lister T, et al: The significance of circulating cells carrying t(14;18) in long remission from follicular lymphoma. J Clin Oncol 9:1527, 1991.

216. Lee M, Cabanillias F, et al: Detection of minimal circulating cells carrying the t(14;18) by PCR technique. Blood 81:151–157, 1993.

217. Limpens J, Stad R, et al: Lymphoma associated translocation t(14;18), in blood B cells of normal individuals. Blood 85:2528, 1995.

218. Lambrecht AC, Hupker PE, et al: Clinical significance of t(14;18)-positive cells in the circulation of patients with stage III and IV follicular non-Hodgkin's lymphoma during first remission. J Clin Oncol 12:1541–1546, 1994.

219. Meijerink J et al: Quantitation of follicular non-Hodgkin's Lymphoma cells carrying t(14;18) by competitive polymerase chain reaction. Br J Haematol 84:250–256, 1993.

220. Kemana A, Keating M, Plunkett W, et al: Plasma and cellular bioavailability of oral fludarabine (abstract #199). Blood 78:52a, 1991.

221. Hubbard S, Chabner B, DeVita V, et al: Histologic progression in non-Hodgkin's lymphoma. N Engl J Med 325:1525, 1991.

222. Sander CA, Yano T, Clark H, et al: p53 mutation is associated with progression in follicular lymphomas. Blood 82:1994–2004, 1993.

223. LoCoco F, Gaidano G, Louie D, et al: p53 mutations are associated with histologic transformation of follicular lymphoma. Blood 82:2289–2295, 1993.

224. Horning S, Rosenberg S: The natural history of initally untreated low grade lymphomas. N Engl J Med 1984; 311:1471–1475.

225. Ersboll J, Schultz H, Nissen N, et al: Follicular low grade non-Hodgkin's lymphoma: Long term outcome with or without tumor progression. Eur J Haematol 42:155–163, 1989.

226. Armitage J, Dick F, Corder M: Diffuse histiocytic lymphoma after histologic conversion: A poor prognostic variant. Cancer Treat Rep 65:413–418, 1981.

227. Ostrow S, Diggs C, Wiernik P, et al: Nodular poorly differentiated lymphocytic lymphoma: Changes in histology and survival. Cancer Treat Rep 65:929–933, 1981.

228. Yuen AR, Horning S: Long term survival after histologic transformation of low grade lymphoma (abstract #1236). Proc ASCO 12:365, 1993.

229. Straneo M, Gianni L: New active drugs in the treatment of lymphomas. Curr Op Onc 6:480–488, 1994.

230. Cheson B: New chemotherapeutic agents for the treatment of non-Hodgkin's lymphomas. Semin Oncol 20(suppl 5):96–110, 1993.

231. Grossbard M, Nadler L: Monoclonal antibody therapy for indolent lymphomas. Semin Oncol 20(suppl 5):118–135, 1993.

232. Miller R, Maloney D, et al: Treatment of B-cell lymphoma with monoclonal anti-idiotype antibody. N Engl J Med 306:517–522, 1982.

233. Kwak L, Campbell M, Levy R, et al: Induction of immune response against the surface immunoglobulin idiotype expressed by their tumors. N Engl J Med 327:1209–1215, 1992.

234. Brown S, Miller R, Horning S, et al: Treatment of B-cell lymphomas and anti-idiotype antibodies alone and in combination with alpha interferon. Blood 73:651–661, 1989.

235. LeMaistre CF, Deisseroth A, Parkinson D, et al: Phase I trial of an interleukin 2 (IL-2) fusion toxin ($DAB_{486}IL-2$) in hematologic malignancies expressing the IL-2 receptors. Blood 79:2547–2554, 1992.

236. Gottschall AR, Quintans J. Apoptosis in B lymphocytes. The WEHI-231 perspective. Immunol Cell Biol 73:8–16, 1995.

237. El-Khatib M, Stanger B, Ju ST, et al: The molecular mechanism of Fas L-mediated cytotoxicity by $CD4^+$ Th1 clones. Cell Immunol 163:237–244, 1995.

Intermediate- and High-Grade Non-Hodgkin's Lymphomas

Anton Melnyk, MD, *and* Alma Rodriguez, MD

Division of Medicine, The University of Texas M. D. Anderson Cancer Center, Houston, Texas

The non-Hodgkin's lymphomas (NHLs) are a collection of lymphoid malignancies with a diverse pathology and natural history. This diversity is illustrated by the different histologic subtypes and classifications of NHL that have appeared over the years. With the rapid progress in our understanding of the biology of lymphomas, new systems of classification have better described this group of diseases. Although the number of classification systems has caused some confusion, in the mid-1970s, the National Cancer Institute (NCI) initiated the NHL pathologic classification project with the aim of standardizing classifications through a Working Formulation (Table 1). This formulation is based on the largest single cohort of patients reported to date and is the framework for this chapter.[1,2]

The Working Formulation is useful as a source of prognostic information and a tool for treatment planning. However, several of its limitations deserve mention. First, nearly 10% of the lymphomas encountered in practice elude precise classification, particularly lymphomas presenting primarily in extranodal tissues where there is no lymph-node architecture. In these cases, clinical experience and certain tests can help to predict the natural history of the disease.

Second, within the broad histologic categories of low-, intermediate-, and high-grade lymphomas, there can be a wide spectrum of biologic behavior, as illustrated by the survival curves from the NCI project (Figure 1). Third, histopathologic classification alone is inadequate in some cases, as sometimes there is less-than-ideal interobserver agreement.[3] Immunophenotyping, cytogenetics, and specific oncogene studies have been found to be important factors in diagnosing clinically unique subtypes of NHL. Lymphomas not accounted for by the Working Formulation are listed in Table 1, with their unique immunophenotype or cytogenetic abnormalities, next to the histologic subtype with which they are typically associated.

Indeed, the limitations of the Working Formulation have prompted further discussion, and another classification system has now been introduced (Table 2).[4] This chapter, however, will follow the categorization of the Working Formulation.

EPIDEMIOLOGY AND ETIOLOGY

At present, there is an emerging unexplainable epidemic of NHL.[5] In the United States, the incidence has increased from 6.9 per 100,000 population in 1947 to 1950 to 17.4 per 100,000 population in 1984 to 1988. Changes in exposure to described risk factors (Table 3)[5–14] do not explain this increase, much of which is largely caused by a rise in intermediate-grade lymphomas among the elderly. Another unexplained phenomenon is the slight but consistent predominance of NHL incidence in men (male:female ratio 1.5 to 1.25:1).

Intermediate- and high-grade tumors comprise nearly 55% of NHLs, with a proportionately higher number of high-grade tumors in children and young adults.[1] Ninety percent of childhood NHLs are Burkitt's NHL, T-cell acute lymphoblastic lymphoma (T-ALL), or diffuse large-cell lymphoma with a Ki-1 immunophenotype.

Despite the variation with age in the incidence of certain types of NHL, the biology, including underlying molecular defects, appears relatively uniform within a histologic subtype. There is no single defect that alone causes a lymphoma. The etiology and pathogenesis of intermediate- and high-grade lymphomas are considered parts of a multistep process in which the malignant phenotype develops gradually. Hereditary and environmental factors contribute to this process. Hereditary factors, childhood lymphomas, and high-grade tumors are closely associated. Some of these associations and others, are presented in Table 3 and referenced.

Three factors appear common to the etiology of lymphomas. The first is that certain patients may be predisposed to develop a type of lymphoma because of a generalized or perhaps specific immune defect. This "host" defect frequently includes autoimmune diseases. The second factor is the occurrence of a specific infection that is difficult to eradicate and that may alter normal lymphoid tissues. The third factor is that a single specific mutation or a number of specific mutations or chromosome translocations can alter suppressor genes or oncogenes, respectively, and result in a lymphoma. With any specific lymphoma, any or all of these factors may be at work.

TABLE I

A Working Formulation for Non-Hodgkin's Lymphomas (NHL)

Classifiable non-Hodgkin's lymphomas	Unaccounted-for non-Hodgkin's lymphomas
Low-grade	
Small lymphocytic (CLL)	Mucosa-associated lymphomas, CD5–, CD10–
Follicular, predemoninantly small-cleaved cell	
Follicular mixed, small-cleaved and large-cell	
Intermediate-grade	
Follicular, predominantly large-cell	
Diffuse small-cleaved cell	Mantle-cell lymphoma CD5+, CD23–, t11;14 PRAD1
Diffuse mixed small- and large-cell epithelioid component	Lennert's lymphoma T-cell+
Diffuse large-cell cleaved, non-cleaved	T-cell variants Transformed from low-grade NHL, t14;18+
High-grade	
Large-cell, immunoblastic plasmacytoid, clear-cell, polymorphous, epithelioid	Anaplastic large-cell lymphoma, T-cell (rare B), Ki-1(CD30)+, t2;5
Small non-cleaved cell Burkitt's Follicular areas	
Miscellaneous	
Composite Mycosis fungoides/Sézary syndrome Histiocytic Unclassifiable	Other T-cell NHL HTLV-I lymphoma T-cell CLL Angioimmunoblastic lymphadenopathy with dysproteinemia Angiocentric-type Polymorphic reticulosis Lymphomatoid granulamatosis

CLL = chronic lymphocytic leukemia, HTLV = human T-cell leukemia virus

FIGURE I

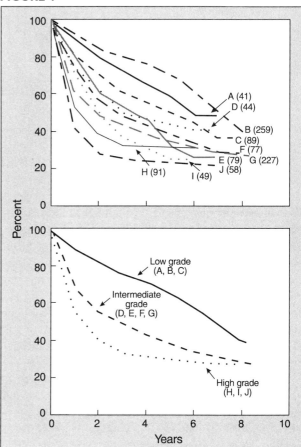

Actuarial survival curves for the 10 subtypes of the formulation shown individually (upper panel) and in the three prognostic categories (lower panel). Curves are discontinued when less than five patients are at risk. Adapted, with permission, from Cancer 1982.[1]

A number of specific diseases illustrate how immune factors contribute to lymphomagenesis. Duncan's syndrome, or X-linked lymphoproliferative syndrome, is a particularly interesting example.[15] Males with this syndrome are unable to mount an appropriate immunologic response to an Epstein-Barr virus (EBV) infection. They develop a fatal lymphoproliferative syndrome when first infected. The precise immune defect in these patients is not known.

Posttransplant lymphoproliferative syndrome is strikingly similar.[12] Immunosuppression following solid-organ transplantation can cause an EBV infection-related polyclonal lymphoproliferative disease that can develop into a typical NHL if immunosuppression is not stopped. The primary central nervous system (CNS) lymphomas associated with the human immunodeficiency virus (HIV) may develop in a similar fashion following EBV infection.[6] These examples show how an immune defect coupled with an infection can lead to a lymphoma.

Viruses such as EBV, human T-cell leukemia virus-1 (HTLV-1), and HIV are not the only infectious agents that can interact to cause lymphomas. *Helicobacter pylori* is a bacterium that has been found to cause gastric ulcers as well as gastric lymphomas.[9] The pathogenesis is still being determined, but it is possible to cure some gastric lymphomas with the triple antibiotic regimen used to eradicate *H pylori*. Thus, removing an infectious agent can possibly lead to curing a lymphoma. Similarly, in posttransplant lymphoproliferative disease, stopping the immunosuppression early in the process can prevent the development of a lymphoma. In both posttransplant lymphoproliferative disease and *H pylori* associated gastric lymphoma, beyond a certain point, reversing the offending agent does not lead to the resolution of the lymphoma. This suggests that another step occurs, conferring a nonreversible malignant phenotype.

In some cases, this last step may involve the mutation of a suppressor gene causing loss of tumor suppression, or a chromosome translocation, causing the abnormal expression of an oncogene. Both of these processes may in turn cause the loss of normal cellular responses. Tumor-suppressor genes have a number of functions, but many of them seem to suppress tumors by regulating the cell cycle and, in turn, proliferation. A good example of this is the transformation of typical low-grade follicular NHL into intermediate NHL through the development of a *p53* mutation.[16] Table 4 presents the known translocations and their oncogenes involved in lymphomagenesis.[17]

Perhaps the single best example of the modern paradigm of lymphomagenesis is the pathogenesis of African or endemic Burkitt's NHL.[7] Endemic Burkitt's NHL is found in areas of Africa with a high incidence of malaria. Malaria may cause a defect in the immune system of children residing in these areas, which results in their inability to resolve EBV infections successfully. Following EBV infection, which is serologically documented in more than 90% of cases of endemic Burkitt's lymphoma, the lymphoma finally develops when a chromosome translocation brings the c-*myc* oncogene on chromosome 8 into the proximity of an immunoglobulin gene on either chromosome 2, 14, or 22 and its regulatory sequences. The c-*myc* oncogene then becomes overexpressed through its abnormal transcription mediated by the immunoglobulin gene-regulatory sequences, causing cellular proliferation and Burkitt's lymphoma.

Nonendemic Burkitt's NHL has a different presentation from that of endemic Burkitt's NHL, it is less frequently associated with EBV, and it has a different translocation breakpoint between the c-*myc* and immu-

TABLE 2
Classification of Lymphoid Neoplasms

B-CELL NEOPLASMS

Precursor B-cell neoplasms

Precursor B-lymphoblastic leukemia/lymphoma

Peripheral B-cell neoplasms

B-cell chronic lymphocytic leukemia/prolymphocytic leukemia/small lymphocytic lymphoma

Lymphoplasmacytoid lymphoma/immunocytoma

Mantle-cell lymphoma

Follicle center lymphoma, follicular
• Provisional grades: 1 (small-cell), 2 (mixed), 3 (large-cell)
• Provisional subtype: diffuse, predominantly small-cell type

Marginal zone B-cell lymphoma
• Extranodal (MALT-type ± monocytoid B cells)
• Provisional subtype: Nodal (monocytoid B cells)

Provisional entity: Splenic marginal zone lymphoma (± villous lymphocytes)

Hairy-cell leukemia

Plasmacytoma/plasma-cell leukemia

Diffuse large B-cell lymphoma subtype: Primary mediastinal B-cell lymphoma

Burkitt's lymphoma

Provisional entity: High-grade B-cell lymphoma, Burkitt-like

T-CELL AND PUTATIVE NK-CELL NEOPLASMS

Precursor T-cell neoplasm

Precursor T-lymphoblastic lymphoma/leukemia

Peripheral T-cell and NK-cell neoplasms

T-cell chronic lymphocytic leukemia/prolymphocytic leukemia

Large granular lymphocyte leukemia
• T-cell type
• NK-cell type

Mycosis fungoides/Sézary syndrome

Peripheral T-cell lymphomas, unspecified

Angioimmunoblastic T-cell lymphoma

Angiocentric lymphoma

Intestinal T-cell lymphoma (± enteropathy associated)

Adult T-cell leukemia/lymphoma

Anaplastic large-cell lymphoma, CD30+, T and null-cell types

Provisional entity: Anaplastic large-cell lymphoma, Hodgkin's-like

HODGKIN'S DISEASE

Lymphocyte predominance

Nodular sclerosis

Mixed cellularity

Lymphocyte depletion

Provisional entity: Lymphocyte-rich classic Hodgkin's disease

MALT = mucosa-associated lymphoid tissue, NK = natural-killer

TABLE 3

Epidemiologic Risk Factors for Non-Hodgkin's Lymphoma (NHL)

Risk factors	Associated subtype of lymphoma
HEREDITARY	
Hereditary immuno-deficiency disorders	
Ataxia-telangiectasia	
Bruton-type agamma-globulinemia	
Severe combined immunodeficiency	
Wiskott-Aldrich syndrome	
Duncan's syndrome	
Chédiak-Higashi syndrome	
ACQUIRED	
Infections	
Human immunodeficiency virus (HIV) and Epstein-Barr virus (EBV)	Primary CNS lymphoma and aggressive poorly differentiated B-cell NHL[6]
EBV	African (endemic) Burkitt's NHL[7]
Human T-lymphocyte virus-I	Specific peripheral T-cell NHL[8]
Helicobacter pylori	Gastric mucosa-associated lymphoid tissue (MALT) lymphomas [9]
Autoimmune disorders	
Rheumatoid arthritis	Variable[10]
Sjögren's disease	Primary, salivary, and lacrimal gland NHL[11]
Hashimoto's thyroiditis	Primary thyroid gland NHL[11]
Celiac disease	Enteropathy-associated T-cell NHL
Drugs	
Immunosuppressants	Post-transplant lympho-proliferative disorder[12]
Chemotherapeutic agents	Secondary diffuse large-cell NHL
Phenytoin	Pseudolymphoma[13]
Blood transfusions	Variable[14]
Environmental toxins	
Herbicides Vinyl chloride Solvents Hair dyes	Variable[5]

CNS = central nervous system

noglobulin genes. All these factors suggest a different pathogenesis for nonendemic Burkitt's NHL.[18] The mechanism that causes one step to lead to the next still remains unknown. We are just beginning to scratch the surface of this complex problem, but as genes and their functions become better understood, it is likely that in the future, lymphomas will be diagnosed and treated based on their specific genetic abnormalities.

CLINICAL FEATURES AND DIAGNOSIS

Sites Of Presentation

The clinical manifestations of intermediate- and high-grade NHLs are diverse and depend on the site of disease involvement. These tumors have a rapid growth rate and present as masses that cause symptoms when they infiltrate tissues or obstruct organs. The more aggressive the lymphoma, the more frequently it is localized. Pain within an enlarged lymph node may also be noted if the tumor is rapidly growing.

Lymphomas appear most frequently in sites with the most lymphoid tissue. Thus, the lymphoid and reticuloendothelial system, which includes the lymph nodes, spleen, liver, and bone marrow, is most frequently involved, but any extranodal site may also be primarily involved. Certain lymphomas have classic anatomic presentations. However, these features are not invariably present, except perhaps in the cutaneous postthymic T-cell lymphomas, which include mycosis fungoides and Sézary syndrome. Endemic Burkitt's NHL frequently presents as a head and neck mass in a child. T-ALL frequently presents with a mediastinal mass in younger patients.[19]

Anaplastic large-cell lymphoma with positive Ki-1 staining (CD30+) in younger patients is another variant with frequent cutaneous presentation and a predilection for extranodal tissue.[20] A clinically distinct primary mediastinal B-cell diffuse large-cell lymphoma presents in young women.[21] The gastrointestinal tract is often involved in certain types of lymphoma. This is the case with many mucosa-associated lymphoid tissue (MALT) lymphomas, 15% of mantle-cell lymphomas, 10% of intermediate-grade lymphomas of Waldeyer's ring and sinuses, and rare lymphomas (enteropathy-associated T-cell NHL, immunoproliferative small-intestinal disease, and Mediterranean lymphoma).[22] Certain predisposing conditions will also have a classic extranodal tissue presentation. Patients with Hashimoto's thyroiditis are predisposed to primary thyroid lymphomas, patients with Sjogren's syndrome to primary salivary and lacrimal gland NHL, and patients with celiac disease to enteropathy-associated T-cell NHL.

TABLE 4

Translocations and Oncogenes Involved in Lymphomagenesis

Lymphoma type	Chromosome translocation	Affected gene
Burkitt's NHL	t(8;14) t(8;22) t(2;8)	c-MYC (8q24)
DLCL-NHL	t(3;14) t(3;4)	BCL-6 (3q27)
Mantle NHL	t(11;14)	BCL-1 (11q23)
Transformed NHL	t(14;18)	BCL-2 (18q21)
NHL-B and -T	Inv 14	TCR-Ca (14q11)
T-NHL	t(4;16)	IL-2 (4q26/ BCM (16p13.1)
Ki-1 anaplastic	t(2;5)	NPM (5q35/ ALK (2p23)

DLCL = diffuse large-cell lymphoma, NHL = non-Hodgkin's lymphoma

Involvement of "sanctuary" sites, which include the CNS and testicles, is more frequently associated with Burkitt's NHL and non-Burkitt's small-cell NHL, T-ALL, primary testicular diffuse large-cell lymphoma,[23] HIV-associated aggressive B-cell lymphoma, and HTLV-1 associated lymphoma.

Systemic Features

As with Hodgkin's disease, NHL also presents with systemic B symptoms, including fever, which may or may not have the Pel-Ebstein relapsing pattern; drenching night sweats; and more than 10% weight loss. Generalized pruritus may also be present.

Paraneoplastic syndromes may also develop with these types of lymphomas. Nonparathyroid hormone induced hypercalcemia occurs in approximately 10% of patients.[24] Hypercalcemia also is frequently associated with HTLV-1 T-cell lymphomas. Subacute motor neuropathy and polymyositis may also be linked with NHL.[25]

Diagnosis

A diagnosis of NHL as well as suspected relapses should be made based on the pathologic examination of a lymph node whenever possible. The accuracy of fine-needle aspiration (FNA) is variable. In one trial, lymphomas were diagnosed using FNA in 86% of cases and were accurately categorized into low, intermediate, or high grade in 68% of cases.[26] In some instances, it may be necessary to establish clonality to confirm malignancy. Clonality is established when one it can be proved that all cells in a lymphoma were derived from a single cell. In B-cell NHL, monotypic immunohistochemical staining for kappa or lambda light chain is often all that is needed to confirm clonality. In some cases, one may need to establish clonality by performing studies on either T-cell receptor rearrangement or J-H segment rearrangements of the B-cell immunoglobulin gene. Gene rearrangement studies are diagnostic and reliable in more than 96% of these cases.[27] Occasionally, a specific diagnosis can be made by cytogenetic analysis. Some of these specific chromosomal translocation fusion genes are amenable to polymerase chain reaction assays, which can then be used in studies of minimal residual disease (Table 4).[17]

STAGING AND TREATMENT

Staging allows clinicians to prognosticate and then treat appropriately. The staging of intermediate- and high-grade non-Hodgkin's lymphomas has become an area of intense research. For some time NHL was staged anatomically, like Hodgkin's disease. It has become clear, however, that unlike Hodgkin's disease, NHL does not spread anatomically to contiguous nodal regions and therefore cannot be reliably staged solely by anatomic methods.

The treatment of Hodgkin's disease and NHL has formed the modern paradigm of cancer chemotherapy. The basic concepts were first established for infectious diseases and then applied to oncology. Skipper and colleagues, followed by Goldie and Coldman, established the principles of tumor resistance and, in turn, combination chemotherapy and non-cross-resistant chemotherapeutic regimens.[28,29] The curability of advanced cancer ushered in the modern era of oncology.

Today, the principal treatment for NHL is combination chemotherapy and radiation therapy. Surgery is used chiefly as a diagnostic tool, with some unique exceptions. Combination chemotherapy with cyclophosphamide (Cytoxan, Neosar), doxorubicin (Adriamycin, Rubex), vincristine (Oncovin), and prednisone—the CHOP regimen—was developed at M. D. Anderson Cancer Center and introduced in the 1970s. Since then, a number of second- and third-generation regimens and combinations of non-cross-resistant regimens for intermediate- and high-grade NHLs have been developed. The benefit of these newer regimens is now in question, but some issues are not yet clearly resolved. Current trials of chemotherapy for NHL may hold the answers.

TABLE 5

Individual Prognostic Factors in Intermediate-Grade NHL

PROGNOSTIC FACTORS[30–33]

Host factors

Age
"B" symptoms
Performance status

Tumor burden

Ann Arbor stage
Number of extranodal sites
Bulky sites
Serum LDH level
Serum beta-2-microglobulin

Tumor biology

Pathogenicity
   B- vs T-cell
   S-phase percent
   Ki-67 expression
   CD-44 expression
   HLA-DR expression
   IL-10 serum concentration
   Soluble IL-2 receptor levels in serum
   Cytogenetics 7-, 17P-
   BCL-2 expression
   BCL-6 expression

Drug resistance
   Response after three cycles of chemotherapy
   MDR-1 gene expression

HLA = human leukocyte antigen, IL = interleukin, LDH = lactate dehydrogenase, NHL = non-Hodgkin's lymphoma

INTERMEDIATE GRADE NHL

Staging

A number of staging systems for intermediate-grade NHL have been developed based on retrospective evaluation of clinical, laboratory, radiologic, and pathologic data for patient cohorts. Table 5[30–33] lists the individual prognostic factors studied to date that have been related to outcome in intermediate-grade NHL.[30,34,35] These factors can be grouped into categories that reflect different aspects of the disease: host factors, tumor burden, and tumor biology as they relate to pathogenicity and drug resistance. Performance status, lactate dehydrogenase (LDH) level, and extent of tumor have been validated prospectively as reliable prognostic factors.[36]

Many of the other factors are still under investigation, and testing for some of the serologic parameters is not routinely performed. In the future, however, some of these factors may replace or complement existing ones, because even our best current prognostic models have less than desirable positive and negative predictive values.

At M. D. Anderson, disease is staged according to the "tumor score" system, which is compared in Table 6 with the other frequently used system, the International Index.[34,35] The main advantage of the M. D. Anderson tumor score is that it appears to separate more clearly tumors with a good prognosis from tumors with a poor prognosis (Table 7).

Localized and Good Prognosis Disease

It is possible to treat nonbulky, localized Ann Arbor stage I NHL with involved-field radiation therapy alone, which yields a 5-year disease-free survival (DFS) rate of 77% with salvage chemotherapy.[37] However, most physicians treat localized intermediate-grade NHL with chemotherapy plus involved-field radiation therapy. Pa-

TABLE 6

Comparison of Two Staging Systems for Intermediate- and High-Grade Non-Hodgkin's Lymphomas (NHL): International Index vs Tumor Score System

Factor	Prognostic models	
	International index	M. D. Anderson tumor score
Age > 60 years	Yes = 1 point	Not included
Ann Arbor stage: 3 or higher	Yes = 1 point	Yes = 1 point
2 or more extranodal sites	Yes = 1 point	Not included
2 or higher Zubrod performance status	Yes = 1 point	Not included
High LDH > 250 IU at MDA	Yes = 1 point	Yes = 1 point
Beta-2-microglobulin > 3.0 at MDA	Not included	Yes = 1 point
B symptoms	Not included	Yes = 1 point
Number of sites of bulky (> 7 cm diameter) NHL	Not included	Yes = 1 point
Total possible points	0 to 5 points	0 to 6 points

LDH = lactate dehydrogenase, MDA = M. D. Anderson Cancer Center

tients with good-risk stages I and II disease have achieved a 5-year DFS rate of 84% with 4 cycles of CHOP plus regional radiation therapy.[38,39] With the newer tumor staging systems, all these patients would have low scores and favorable disease, except the elderly and patients with bulky disease, who were shown in these studies to relapse more frequently. These latter patients with high-risk localized disease are now treated as patients with advanced disease at M. D. Anderson Cancer Center.

Localized extranodal NHL in the stomach, thyroid, sinuses, or Waldeyer's ring, unless the tumor is very small and localized, is best managed with combination chemotherapy and radiation therapy.[31,40] The issue of using prophylactic gastric resection to prevent perforation by chemotherapy in gastric lymphomas is still not resolved and will depend on the patient's condition.[41] Primary NHL of the CNS is a rare and not very favorable form of localized NHL, with a mean survival duration of approximately 19 months in patients without HIV.[42] Radiation therapy alone is standard treatment but has achieved disappointing results. The addition of high-dose intravenous methotrexate may improve the mean survival duration but increases the risk of leukoencephalopathy. Finally, testicular lymphoma frequently appears in the CNS or the contralateral testis; its management with prophylactic cranial and testicular irradiation has been debated.[23]

Advanced Disease

Developed in the late 1960s at M. D. Anderson Cancer Center and tested by the Southwest Oncology Group (SWOG) in the 1970s, CHOP was the first combination chemotherapeutic regimen to demonstrate cures in intermediate-grade NHL. During the 1980s, a number of trials showed improved survival with the newer, more complex second- and third-generation chemotherapeutic regimens. This prompted the SWOG phase III trial in patients with bulky disease Ann Arbor stage II or higher who were stratified for age, marrow development, histology, bulky disease sites, and LDH level. This trial compared CHOP with methotrexate, bleomycin (Blenoxane), doxorubicin, cyclophosphamide, vincristine, and dexamethasone (m-BACOD); prednisone, methotrexate, doxorubicin, cyclophosphamide, etoposide (VePesid), cytarabine, bleomycin, vincristine, and methotrexate (ProMACE-CytaBOM); and methotrexate, bleomycin, doxorubicin, cyclophosphamide, vincristine, and dexamethasone (MACOP-B).[43]

This trial showed that eight cycles of CHOP chemotherapy was capable of inducing a complete response (CR) rate of 44% and an estimated 3-year DFS rate of

TABLE 7

Comparison of M. D. Anderson Tumor Score vs International Index Score with Regard to Prognosis

M. D. Anderson tumor score	CR rate (%)	% Disease-free survival at 3 years
0 to 2	91	83
3 to 6	46	24

International index score	CR rate (%)	% Disease-free survival at 5 years
0 to 1	87	70
2	67	50
3	55	43
4 to 5	44	26

CR = complete response

41%. The other regimens did not produce statistically better results; instead, they had more fatal and life-threatening toxic effects. One debated conclusion of this trial is that increasing the dose intensity of chemotherapy does not improve results. Another is that CHOP remains the standard of care for advanced intermediate-grade NHL, even though the results are far from ideal. We can now fairly accurately predict which patients have only a 20% chance of surviving for 3 years, and the current problem is how to best treat those poor prognosis patients.

One group of patients who fares poorly are those more than 60 years old. There has been some question as to whether the biology of tumors in the elderly differs somehow from that of tumors in younger age groups. A recent study of prognostic factors in elderly patients who had undergone chemotherapy where dose intensity was maintained found that age did not alter survival.[44] Elderly patients, it appears, are underdosed to avoid increased toxicity, even when they present with good performance status and marrow function. Dose intensity may be important not only in the elderly but in all patients.[45,46] In a related issue, the use of growth factors in NHL may most reasonably be applied to the maintenance of standard dose intensity in the compromised patient, even though no survival benefit has yet been shown.[47] Dose intensity is also maintained by experience with a particular regimen. Removing these confounding variables may reduce the influence of age on treatment response and outcome.

In terms of chemotherapy, it would then seem that less is bad, but more is not necessarily better. Again, the issue of dose intensity is not so simple. There are a number of biologic variables that may confound the data and obscure cases in which more is better or in which nothing works. Some progress is being made in this regard. There is some evidence that second- or third-generation combination chemotherapeutic regimens improve CR and DFS rates in young patients with primary mediastinal B-cell diffuse large-cell lymphoma and Ki-1 anaplastic T-cell NHL.[48,49]

At M. D. Anderson, the alternating triple therapy (ATT) regimen, which consists of alternating non-cross-resistant regimens—ASHAP (doxorubicin, methylprednisolone, high-dose cytarabine, cisplatin), MBACOS (methotrexate, bleomycin, doxorubicin, cyclophosphamide, vincristine, solumedrol), MINE (mesna, ifosfamide, mitoxantrone, and etoposide)— has shown a significant benefit in the highest-risk patients, although further follow-up is needed.[50] Greater dose intensity is also being used to treat other subgroups of patients.[51] On the other hand, some lymphomas may be inherently resistant to current chemotherapy. T-cell variants of diffuse large-cell NHL have poorer response rates than B-cell types.[52,53] The diffuse mantle-cell NHL is another subtype with poor response.[54]

Patients who do not achieve a CR by the end of the first three cycles of the CHOP regimen also are at high risk.[55] One approach in these patients has been to switch therapy to a non-cross-resistant regimen and to include late dose intensification, which has shown some improvement over historic controls.[56] A recent investigation attempted to improve responses in these slowly responding patients by autologous bone marrow transplantation (ABMT), but no improvement in overall survival or DFS was shown at 3 years.[57] Further follow-up is needed, but at this stage, ABMT does not appear to be the answer.

In general approximately 45% of patients with the worst prognosis will obtain a CR, but many will then relapse; only about 25% will survive long term. A major area of focus has been consolidation treatments that can prevent relapse. Radiation therapy for sites of bulky disease seems to improve results in certain subsets of patients but not in others.[58] ABMT is currently being compared with sequential conventional-dose combination chemotherapy in these patients; initial reports of ABMT seemed favorable,[59] but a recent randomized trial of 464 patients did not show a benefit for ABMT overall.[60] Again, further follow-up is needed, and new approaches seem warranted.

Relapse and Primary Refractory Disease

In some patients, confirming the presence of persistent disease or early relapse can be difficult. Computed tomography scanning will readily identify residual masses in up to 40% of patients with bulky abdominal disease. Few of these patients, 5% in one review, actually had residual disease on laparotomy.[61] FNA biopsy may be inaccurate because of sampling errors, and gallium scans are operator-dependent.[62] These factors pose problems when interpreting results and managing some patients.

At present, there is no accepted standard of therapy for patients with primary refractory disease and relapsed disease. Current research has focused in two directions. The first approach has been high-dose chemotherapy with autologous stem-cell rescue to exploit the demonstrated dose-response curve of various chemotherapeutic agents. The second approach has been dose-intensive non-cross-resistant standard chemotherapeutic regimens to circumvent drug resistance. In the next few years, other avenues are likely to be explored.

ABMT is limited to patients younger than 60 years of age and has yielded 3-year DFS rates of 30% to 40% in patients who had a relapse after achieving a CR with conventional chemotherapy. Patients who had primary refractory disease and patients who achieved a partial response to conventional chemotherapy had 3-year DFS rates of 0% and 14%, respectively.[63]

Nearly 10% of patients who relapse will be able to achieve long-term DFS with current salvage combination chemotherapy regimens. A variety of reasonably successful salvage regimens have been developed, including MIME (mesna, ifosfamide, methotrexate, and etoposide),[64] DHAP (dexamethasone, high-dose cytarabine, and cisplatin),[65] and ESHAP (etoposide, methylprednisolone, high-dose cytarabine, and cisplatin),[66] which produce CR rates of 20% to 30%, and sequential MINE (mesna, ifosfamide, mitoxantrone, and etoposide)-ESHAP,[66] which produces a CR rate of 43%. These CR rates are seen primarily in patients with a better prognosis who previously achieved a CR with standard chemotherapy and relapsed with a low-volume of disease more than 6 months after stopping treatment. A recent phase III trial compared ABMT in a group of patients responding to salvage chemotherapy with another group who was continued on salvage chemotherapy. Although the results are preliminary, there appears to be no difference between the groups in the rate of DFS.[68]

Various new approaches include continuous-infusion chemotherapy,[69] the use of P-glycoprotein-blocking agents along with chemotherapy[70] and other biologic agents.[71] Allogeneic BMT has also been explored in a select subset of patients, with variable results.[72]

HIGH-GRADE TUMORS

Immunoblastic large-cell NHL is clinically indistinguishable from intermediate-grade NHL and is treated the same way. Lymphoblastic NHL, Burkitt's NHL, and non-Burkitt's NHL, on the other hand, behave more like ALL. These tumors double in size quicker than any other tumor, and they are rapidly fatal. The tumor lysis syndrome (see the chapter on Oncologic Emergencies) is commonly seen with the initiation of or even prior to therapy. Like ALL, these lymphomas have a predilection for the CNS. Prognostic factors are the same as those for ALL: age, LDH level, and CNS or bone-marrow involvement.

For adult lymphoblastic lymphoma, the treatment has been similar to that for adult ALL, which is based on vincristine, doxorubicin, and high-dose glucocorticoids.[19,73] CR rates have been as high as 95%, but DFS rates average 35% to 56%. These regimens are complex and protracted, with long maintenance phases, radiation therapy for the mediastinum, and CNS prophylaxis. See the chapter on ALL.

The treatment of adults with Burkitt's and non-Burkitt's NHLs is based on high-dose alkylating agents, usually cyclophosphamide, plus other cell cycle phase-specific agents.[74,75] In patients with a good prognosis, the overall CR rate is nearly 77% to 85%, and the 5-year DFS rate is about 60%. Favorable patients can also be treated with more standard chemotherapeutic regimens for lymphoma, such as ProMACE-CytaBOM, with good results.[76] Patients with a poor prognosis have a decidedly worse outcome, with a DFS rate of 20% to 30%. The role of bone marrow transplantation in these patients has not been established, but this therapy is often attempted in patients whose disease relapses.

Special Cases

Human Immunodeficiency Virus: Patients with HIV are at particularly high risk of developing intermediate- and high-grade NHL. Nearly 10% of patients with HIV will die as a result of a lymphoma. Poor prognostic factors for these patients have been a poor performance status, prior AIDS (acquired immunodeficiency syndrome)-defining illness, a low CD4 count, marrow involvement, and an elevated LDH level.[77,78] Treatment of these patients is difficult and quickly evolving. For intermediate-grade NHL, full-dose chemotherapy for less-debilitated patients can be tolerated and has achieved a CR rate of 77% and a 2-year survival rate of 34%. More advanced patients have been treated with low-dose M-BACOD. When this treatment was compared with regular-dose M-BACOD plus granulocyte-macrophage colony-stimulating factor (GM-CSF, sargramostim [Leukine]),[79] there was no difference between the two in CR or survival. Neither the role of CNS prophylaxis nor that of antiretroviral treatment has been established in this setting. The management of high-grade NHLs is based on individual factors because many patients cannot tolerate the intensive chemotherapy. Many high-grade lymphomas present as a primary CNS lymphoma in patients with HIV. In this situation, whole-brain radiation with a boost to the tumor is standard therapy and results in a CR rate of 50% and a mean survival duration of 2 to 4 months.[42] Survival is not altered in these cases, but quality of life is improved.

T-cell NHLs are a confusing group of diseases that are largely ignored by the working formulation but more clearly delineated by the new classification. Although some of these diseases have already been discussed (ALL, the Ki-1 [CD30+] anaplastic large-cell lymphoma, and the unspecified peripheral T-cell NHL), several others deserve mention.

Mycosis fungoides and Sézary syndrome are clinically distinct types of postthymic (mature) T-cell NHL characterized by cutaneous plaques of CD4+ T-cells progressing to nodal and visceral involvement in the former and by a generalized erythroderma with circulating abnormal lymphocytes progressing to visceral involvement in the latter. Both diseases are generally indolent (behaving like a low-grade NHL), with a mean survival duration of at least 10 years with cutaneous involvement and of only about 2 years when the viscera are involved.

Neither is curable with current therapy.[80] Both diseases are amenable to effective palliative therapy. There are numerous treatment options; the choice depends largely on the extent of the disease. In general, early disease confined to the skin is best treated with either topical mechlorethamine hydrochloride, oral psoralens and photopheresis, or whole-skin electron-beam radiation therapy. As the disease progresses, systemic therapy with single-agent chemotherapy, interferon, or retinoids may be attempted. Lastly, some form of combination chemotherapy is often used.[81] A conservative approach is supported by the results of the NCI randomized trial comparing combination chemotherapy plus electron-beam radiation with topical chemotherapy, which did not show a difference in survival despite differences in responses.[82]

HTLV-1-associated adult T-cell leukemia/lymphoma (ATLL) is another distinct type of T-cell lymphoma characterized by endemic regions of seropositivity for the virus in southwest Japan and the Caribbean, unique clinical features (including prominent systemic symptoms), frequent cutaneous involvement, hypercalcemia, and poor response to therapy. Several broad clinical stages of ATLL are recognized, from smoldering ATLL (in which a few circulating ATLL cells are present with transient skin lesions), through a chronic stage with lymphocytosis and mild nodal or visceral enlargement, to the acute form with marked lymphocytosis, hepatosplenomegaly, other organ involvement, systemic symptoms, and hypercalcemia. Another stage is characterized by the absence of lymphocytosis but the presence of prominent lymphadenopathy. This stage behaves aggressively, like the acute form.[83] Serum interleukin-2 receptor levels have been useful in separating patients with acute disease from patients with chronic disease and in predicting response to therapy.[84] The 2-year survival rate for the smoldering and chronic forms is 52% to 78% but only about 20% for the acute form.[83] Generally, no treatment is recommended for the smoldering and chronic forms, whereas combination chemotherapy has been attempted for the acute form, without appreciable improvement in survival.

CONCLUSION

Despite the great strides in our understanding of NHL, there remain many unanswered questions about its etiology in light of the current epidemic, its pathophysiology as it relates to advances in molecular biology, and its treatment in the case of patients with poor prognosis.

REFERENCES

1. National Cancer Institute-sponsored study of classifications of non-Hodgkin's lymphoma: Summary and description of a working formulation for clinical usage: The non-Hodgkin's Lymphoma Pathological Classification Project. Cancer 49:2112–2135, 1982.

2. Simon R, Durrlemann S, Hoppe RT, et al: The non-Hodgkin's Lymphoma Pathological Classification Project. Long-term follow-up of 1152 patients with non-Hodgkin's lymphomas. Ann Intern Med 109:939–945, 1988.

3. Sheibani K, Nathwani BN, Swartz WG, et al: Variability in interpretation of immunohistologic findings in lymphoproliferative disorders by hematopathologist: A comprehensive statistical analysis of interobserver performance. Cancer 62:657–664, 1988.

4. Harris NL, Jaffe ES, Stein H, et al: A revised European-American classification of lymphoid neoplasms: A proposal from the International Lymphoma Study Group. Blood 84:1361–1392, 1994.

5. Hartge P, Devesa SS: Quantitation of the impact of known risk factors on the trends in non-Hodgkin's lymphoma incidence. Cancer Res 52(suppl):5566–5569s, 1992.

6. Raphael BG, Knowles DM: Acquired immunodeficiency syndrome-associated non-Hodgkin's lymphoma. Semin Oncol 17:361–366, 1990.

7. Purtilo DT, Stevenson M: Lymphotropic viruses as etiologic

agents of lymphoma. Hematol Oncol Clin North Am 5:901–923, 1991.

8. Broder S, Bunn PA, Jaffe ES, et al: T-cell lymphoproliferative syndrome associated with human T-cell leukemia/lymphoma virus. Ann Intern Med 100:543–557, 1984.

9. Wotherspoon AC, Donglioni C, Diss TC, et al: Regression of primary low-grade B-cell gastric lymphoma of mucosal-associated lymphoid tissue type after eradication of Helicobacter pylori. Lancet 342:575–577, 1993.

10. Isomaki HA, Hakulinen T, Joutsenlahti U: Excess risk of lymphomas, leukemia, and myeloma in patients with rheumatoid arthritis. J Chronic Dis 31:691–696, 1978.

11. Fishleder A, Tubbs R, Hesse B, et al: Uniform detection of immunoglobulin-gene rearrangement in benign lymphoepithelial lesions. N Engl J Med 316:1118, 1987.

12. Chen JM, Barr ML, Chadburn A, et al: Management of lymphoproliferative disorders after cardiac transplantation. Ann Thorac Surg 56:527–538, 1993.

13. Hyman G, Sommers S: The development of Hodgkin's disease and other lymphomas during anticonvulsant therapy. Blood 28:416, 1966.

14. Cerhan JR, Wallace RB, Folsom AR, et al: Transfusion history and cancer risk in older women. Ann Intern Med 119:8–15, 1993.

15. Purtilo DT: Epstein-Barr virus infection in the X-linked recessive lymphoproliferative syndrome. Lancet I:798, 1978.

16. Sander CA, Yano T, Clark HM, et al: p53 Mutation is associated with progression in follicular lymphomas. Blood 82:1994–2004, 1993.

17. Rabbitts TH: Chromosomal translocations in human cancer. Nature 342:143–149, 1994.

18. Magrath I: The pathogenesis of Burkitt's lymphoma. Adv Cancer Res 55:133–270, 1990.

19. Coleman NC, Picozzi VJ, Cox RS, et al: Treatment of lymphoblastic lymphoma in adults. J Clin Oncol 4:1628–1637, 1986.

20. Kadin ME: Primary Ki-1-positive anaplastic large cell lymphoma: A distinct clinical entity. Ann Oncol 5(suppl 1):S25–30, 1994.

21. Jacobson JO, Aisenberg AC, Lamarre L, et al: Mediastinal large cell lymphoma: An uncommon subset of adult lymphoma curable with combined modality therapy. Cancer 62:1893, 1988.

22. D'amore F, Brincker H, Gronbaek K, et al: Non-Hodgkin's lymphoma of the gastrointestinal tract: A population-based analysis of incidence, geographic distribution, clinicopathologic presentation features, and prognosis. J Clin Oncol 12:1673–1684, 1994.

23. Doll DC, Weiss RB: Malignant lymphoma of the testis. Am J Med 81:515, 1986.

24. Seymour JF, Gagel RF, Hagemeister FB, et al: Calcitriol production in hypercalcemic and normocalcemic patients with non-Hodgkin's lymphoma. Ann Intern Med 121:633–640, 1994.

25. Stefansson K, Arnason BGW: Neurologic manifestations of systemic neoplasia, in Braunwald E, Isselbacher KJ, Petersdorf RG, et al (eds): Harrison's Principles of Internal Medicine, 11th ed, pp 1601–1604. New York, McGraw-Hill Book Company, 1987.

26. Das DK, Gupta SK, Datta BN, et al: FNA cytodiagnosis of non-Hodgkin's lymphoma and its subtyping under working formulation of 175 cases. Diagn Cytopathol 7:487–498, 1991.

27. Cossman J, Zehnbauer B, Garrett CT, et al: Gene rearrangements in the diagnosis of lymphoma/leukemia guidelines for use based on a multi-institutional study. Hematopathology 95:347–354, 1991.

28. Skipper HE, Schabel FH, Wilcox WS: Experimental evaluation of potential anti-cancer agents XII: On the criteria and kinetics associated with 'curability' of experimental leukemia. Cancer Chemother Rep 35:1–111, 1964.

29. Goldie JH, Coldman AJ: A mathematical model for relating the drug sensitivity of tumors to their spontaneous mutation rate. Cancer

Treat Rep 63:1727–1731, 1979.

30. Shipp MA: Prognostic factors in aggressive non-Hodgkin's lymphoma: Who has 'high risk' disease? Blood 83:1165–1173, 1994.

31. Doria R, Jekel JF, Cooper DL: Thyroid lymphoma. Cancer 73:200–206, 1994.

32. Stasi R, Zinzani PL, Galieni P, et al: Prognostic value of serum IL-10 and soluble IL-2 receptor levels in aggressive non-Hodgkin's lymphoma. Br J Haematol 88:770–777, 1994.

33. Yeun A, Sikic BI: Multidrug resistance in lymphoma. J Clin Oncol 12:2453–2459, 1994.

34. Shipp MA, Harrington DP, Anderson JR, et al: A predictive model for aggressive NHL: The International non-Hodgkin's Lymphoma Prognostic Factors Project. N Engl J Med 329:987, 1993.

35. Rodriguez J, Cabanillas F, McLaughlin P, et al: A proposal for a simple staging system for intermediate-grade lymphoma and immunoblastic lymphoma based on the 'tumor score'. Ann Oncol 3:711–717, 1992.

36. Coiffier B, Lepage E: Prognosis of aggressive lymphoma: A study of five prognostic models with patients included in the LNH-84 regimen. Blood 74:558–564, 1989.

37. Jeffery GM, Mead GM, Whitehouse JMA, et al: Involved field radiotherapy or chemotherapy in the management of stage I intermediate-grade non-Hodgkin's lymphoma. Br J Cancer 64:933– 937, 1991.

38. Tondini C, Zanini M, Lombardi F, et al: Combined modality treatment with primary CHOP chemotherapy followed by locoregional irradiation in stage I or II histologically aggressive non-Hodgkin's lymphomas. J Clin Oncol 11:720–725, 1993.

39. Connors JM, Klimo P, Fairey RN, et al: Brief chemotherapy and involved field radiation therapy for limited stage histologically aggressive lymphoma. Ann Intern Med 107:25–30, 1987.

40. Economopoulos T, Asprou N, Stathakis N, et al: Primary extranodal non-Hodgkin's lymphoma of the head and neck. Oncology 49:484–488, 1992.

41. Gobbi PG, Dionigi P, Barbieri F, et al: The role of surgery in the multimodal treatment of primary gastric non-Hodgkin's lymphoma: A report of 76 cases and review of the literature. Cancer 65:2528–2536, 1990.

42. Fine HA, Mayer RJ: Primary central nervous system lymphoma. Ann Intern Med 119:1093–1104, 1993.

43. Fisher RI, Gaynor ER, Dahlberg S, et al: Comparison of a standard regimen (CHOP) with three intensive chemotherapy regimens for advanced non-Hodgkin's lymphoma. N Engl J Med 328:1002–1006, 1993.

44. Grogan L, Corbally N, Dervan PA, et al: Comparable prognostic factors and survival in elderly patients with aggressive non-Hodgkin's lymphoma treated with standard-dose Adriamycin-based regimens. Ann Oncol 5(suppl 2):S47–51, 1994.

45. Meyer RM, Hryniuk WM, Goodyear MDE: The role of dose intensity in determining outcome in intermediate-grade non-Hodgkin's lymphoma. J Clin Oncol 9:339–347, 1991.

46. Lepage E, Gisselbrecht C, Haioun C: Relative received dose intensity (DIE) in poor risk lymphoma patients: Higher DIE correlates with longer survival: A study from GELA. Blood 80(suppl 1):158a, 1992.

47. Canellos GP: Critical review of the role of hemapoietic growth factors in dose intensification and outcome in the treatment of non-Hodgkin's lymphoma. Ann Oncol 5(suppl 2):S121– 122, 1994.

48. Toedeschini G, Ambrossetti A, Tecchio C, et al: Third-generation regimens are the therapy of choice in patients with mediastinal large B-cell lymphoma (MLBCL) with sclerosis. Blood 84(suppl 1):165a, 1994.

49. Toedeschini G, Tecchio C, Degani D, et al: Anaplastic large cell lymphoma CD30+ (ALCL); Clinical features and long-term response in 40 consecutive patients. Blood 84(suppl 1):165a, 1994.

50. Cabanillas F: Non-Hodgkin's lymphomas: A review of the M. D. Anderson experience. Semin Oncol 19:11–13, 1992.

51. Shipp MA, Schulman LN, Kaplan WD, et al: Intensified induction therapy for patients with 'high risk' aggressive NHL: High-dose CHOP. Blood 82(suppl 1):332a, 1993.

52. Armitage JO, Greer JP, Levine AM, et al: Peripheral T-cell lymphoma. Cancer 63:158–163, 1989.

53. Gasgoyne R, Tolcher A, Coupland R, et al: Prognostic significance of immunophenotype in diffuse large cell lymphomas. Lab Invest 70:109a, 1994.

54. Perry DA, Bast MA, Armitage JO, et al: Diffuse intermediate lymphocytic lymphoma: A clinicopathologic study and comparison with small lymphocytic lymphoma and diffuse small cleaved cell lymphoma. Cancer 66:1995–2000, 1990.

55. Armitage JO, Weisenburger DD, Hutchins M, et al: Chemotherapy for diffuse large-cell lymphoma: Rapidly responding patients have more durable remissions. J Clin Oncol 4:160–164, 1986.

56. Cabanillas F, Burgess MA, Bodey GP, et al: Sequential chemotherapy and late intensification for malignant lymphomas of aggressive histologic type. Am J Med 74:382–388, 1983.

57. Hagenbeek A, Verdonck L, Sonneveld P, et al: CHOP chemotherapy versus autologous bone marrow transplantation in slowly responding patients with intermediate- and high-grade malignant non-Hodgkin's lymphoma. Results from a prospective randomized phase III clinical trial in 294 patients. Blood 82(suppl 1):332a, 1994.

58. Shipp MA, Klatt MM, Yeap B, et al: Patterns of relapse in large-cell lymphoma patients with bulky disease: Implications for the use of adjuvant radiation therapy. J Clin Oncol 7:613, 1989.

59. Sweetham JW, Proctor SJ, Blaise D, et al for the Working Party of the European group for bone marrow transplantation: High-dose therapy and autologous bone marrow transplantation in first complete remission for adult patients with high-grade non-Hodgkin's lymphoma: The EBMT experience. Ann Oncol 5(suppl 2):S155–159, 1994.

60. Haioun C, Lepage E, Gisselbrecht C, et al for the groupe d'etude des lymphomes del'adulte: Comparison of autologous bone marrow transplantation with sequential chemotherapy for intermediate- grade and high-grade non-Hodgkin's lymphoma in first complete remission: A study of 464 patients. J Clin Oncol 12:2543–2551, 1994.

61. Surbone A, Longo DL, DeVita VT, et al: Residual abdominal masses in aggressive non-Hodgkin's lymphoma after combination chemotherapy: Significance and management. J Clin Oncol 6:1832–1837, 1988.

62. Kaplan WD, Jochelson MS, Herman TS, et al: Gallium-67 imaging: A predictor of residual tumor viability and clinical outcome in patients with diffuse large-cell lymphoma. J Clin Oncol 8:1966–1970, 1990.

63. Philip T, Armitage JO, Spitzer G, et al: High-dose therapy and autologous bone marrow transplantation after failure of conventional chemotherapy in adults with intermediate-grade or high-grade non-Hodgkin's lymphoma. N Engl J Med 316:1493–1498, 1987.

64. Cabanillas F, Hagemeister FB, Mclaughlin P, et al: Results of MIME salvage regimen for recurrent or refractory lymphoma. J Clin Oncol 5:407–412, 1987.

65. Velasquez WS, Cabanillas F, Salvador P, et al: Effective salvage therapy for lymphoma with cisplatin in combination with high-dose ara-C and dexamethasone (DHAP). Blood 71:117–122, 1988.

66. Velasquez WS, McLaughlin P, Tucker S, et al: ESHAP—an effective chemotherapy regimen in refractory and relapsing lymphoma: A 4-year follow-up study. J Clin Oncol 12:1169–1176, 1994.

67. Cabanillas F, Rodriquez MA: MINE-ESHAP salvage therapy

for recurrent and refractory lymphomas. Semin Hematol 31(suppl 2):30, 1994.

68. Philip T, Guglielmi C, Hagenbeek A, et al: The PARMA international randomized prospective study in relapsed non-Hodgkin's lymphoma: Second interim analysis of 172 patients. Blood 80(suppl 1):67a, 1992.

69. Wilson WH, Bryant G, Bates S, et al: EPOCH chemotherapy: Toxicity and efficacy in relapsed and refractory non-Hodgkin's lymphoma. J Clin Oncol 11:1573–1582, 1993.

70. Cobb P, Burris G, Weiss G, et al: Phase I trial of PSC 883 and doxorubicin, vincristine, cyclophosphamide, and prednisone (DCVP) in patients with refractory non-Hodgkin's lymphoma. Blood 84(suppl 1):167a, 1994.

71. Longo DL: Biological agents and approaches in the management of patients with lymphoma: A critical appraisal. Hematol Oncol Clin North Am 5(5):1067–1087, 1991.

72. Shepard JD, Barnett MJ, Connors JM, et al: Allogeneic bone marrow transplantation for poor prognosis non-Hodgkin's lymphoma. Bone Marrow Transplant 12:591–596, 1993.

73. Levine AM, Foreman SJ, Meyer PR, et al: Successful therapy of convoluted T-lymphoblastic lymphoma in the adult. Blood 61:92–98, 1983.

74. Lopez TM, Hagemeister FB, Mclaughlin P, et al: Small noncleaved cell lymphoma in adults: Superior results for stages I-III disease. J Clin Oncol 8:615–622, 1990.

75. Bernstein JI, Coleman CN, Strickler JG, et al: Combined modality therapy for adults with small noncleaved cell lymphoma (Burkitt's and non-Burkitt's types). J Clin Oncol 4:847–858, 1986.

76. Longo DL, Duffey PL, Jaffe ES, et al: Diffuse small non-cleaved-cell, non-Burkitt's lymphoma in adults: A high-grade lymphoma responsive to ProMACE-based combination chemotherapy. J Clin Oncol 12:2153–2159, 1994.

77. Hagemeister FB, Khetan R, Allen P, et al: Stage, serum LDH, and performance status predicts disease progression and survival in HIV-associated lymphomas. Ann Oncol 5(suppl 2):S41–46, 1994.

78. Levine AM, Louriero C, Sullivan-Halley J, et al: HIV-positive high- or intermediate-grade lymphoma: Prognostic factors related to survival. Blood 72;247a, 1990.

79. Levine AM: Acquired immunodeficiency syndrome-related lymphoma. Blood 80:8–20, 1992.

80. Sausville EA, Eddy JL, Makuch RW, et al: Histopathologic staging at initial diagnosis of mycosis fungoides and the Sézary syndrome: Definition of three distinct prognostic groups. Ann Intern Med 109:372–382, 1988.

81. Bunn PA, Hoffman SJ, Norris D, et al: Systemic therapy of cutaneous T-cell lymphomas (mycosis fungoides and the Sézary syndrome). Ann Intern Med 121:592–602, 1994.

82. Kaye FJ, Bunn PA, Steinberg SM, et al: A randomized trial comparing combination electron-beam radiation and systemic chemotherapy with topical therapy in the initial treatment of mycosis fungoides. N Engl J Med 321:1784–1790, 1989.

83. Shimoyama M, and members of the Lymphoma Study Group (1984–1988): Diagnostic criteria and classification of clinical subtypes of adult T-cell leukemia-lymphoma. Br J Haematol 79:428–437, 1991.

84. Shimoyama M, Ota K, Kikuchi M, et al: Major prognostic factors of adult patients with advanced T-cell lymphoma/leukemia. J Clin Oncol 6:1088, 1988.

CHAPTER 7

Hodgkin's Disease

Gary P. Engstrom, MD, David B. Sanford, MD, *and* Fredrick B. Hagemeister, MD
Section of Lymphoma, Department of Hematology, The University of Texas M. D. Anderson Cancer Center, Houston, Texas

Although there have been many advances in the treatment of Hodgkin's disease, diagnosis of the disease still rests on the identification of the Reed-Sternberg cell. This distinctive, though nonspecific cell was first described by Sternberg in 1898 and further elucidated by Reed in 1902. In most biopsies, the Reed-Sternberg cell accounts for only 1% of the cells present, with the remainder consisting of lymphocytes, granulocytes, histiocytes, plasma cells, and fibroblasts.[1]

The origin of the Reed-Sternberg cell remains a point of dissension. Theories on its origin have been based on structural and antigenic studies. Maksen et al have described similarities between the Reed-Sternberg cell and the macrophage system.[2] During the last decade, gene rearrangements and other biochemical markers have been studied; however, they have not helped clarify that cell's origin. The Leu-M1 and Ki-1 (CD30) antibodies identify T- and B-cell lymphomas as well as Reed-Sternberg cells. Both these markers, however, also identify a variety of benign cells.[3,4]

Recently, Carbone et al found that the CD40 antigen is strongly represented on the surface of Reed-Sternberg cells and can help in the distinction between nodular sclerosing Hodgkin's disease and other lymphoid malignancies.[5] Other nonspecific markers have been found in Hodgkin's disease, including interleukin-2 receptors, transferrin receptors, and HLA-DR. For these reasons, the diagnosis of Hodgkin's disease should be based on adequate tissue samples and on the opinion of expert hematopathologists.[6,7]

HISTOLOGIC CLASSIFICATION

In addition to recognition of the Reed-Sternberg cell, the background cells and their ratio to Reed-Sternberg cells are important in the classification of Hodgkin's disease.[1] The first such classification system, based on biologic characteristics, was developed by Lukes and Butler in 1963. That system was modified in 1966 at the Rye Conference. The Rye modification divides Hodgkin's disease into four histologic types, named according to their characteristic features: (1) lymphocyte-predominant, (2) nodular sclerosis, (3) mixed cellularity, and (4) lymphocyte-depleted.

Two variants of lymphocyte-predominant disease (nodular and diffuse) have been identified based on different phenotypes and behavioral characteristics. Nodular lymphocyte-predominant Hodgkin's disease is now widely regarded as a B-cell lymphoma and is the only subtype for which the cell of origin is known, although some investigators contest this conclusion.[6–8]

Nodular sclerosis Hodgkin's disease encompasses the lacunar cell variant of the Reed-Sternberg cell. Nodular sclerosis Hodgkin's disease may be difficult to distinguish from large-cell lymphoma, especially if there are many lacunar cells. MacLennan et al have divided nodular sclerosing Hodgkin's disease into grade 1 and grade 2 histology because they found differences in disease-free and overall survival rates between the two grades.[9] More recent investigations, however, have not demonstrated a correlation between a difference in grade and prognosis.[10–13]

The third type of Hodgkin's disease, mixed cellularity, has much more variation in cell type, has rare Reed-Sternberg cells, and may be confused with other lymphomas, especially peripheral T-cell lymphoma. Finally, the lymphocyte-depleted form of Hodgkin's disease is rare, partly because many of the cases described in the early literature were mistaken for large-cell lymphoma. A patient with this diagnosis should undergo a thorough pathologic review to ensure that the proper diagnosis has been made.[6,7]

EPIDEMIOLOGY

Hodgkin's disease is an uncommon disorder. Overall, 7,500 cases occur annually in the United States, accounting for 0.7% of all malignancies. The nodular sclerosing subtype has a female predominance, with the remaining subtypes occurring more commonly in men. Hodgkin's disease occurs more frequently in developed than in underdeveloped countries. The disease has a bimodal incidence pattern in both developed and underdeveloped countries, but for unknown reasons, the first peak occurs at an earlier age in patients in underdeveloped countries.

Investigators have performed multiple studies examining possible risk factors associated with Hodgkin's disease, including small family size, single family dwell-

TABLE I
Ann Arbor Staging Classification for Hodgkin's Disease

Stage I

Involvement of a single lymph-node region (I) or a single extralymphatic organ or site (I_E)

Stage II

Involvement of two or more lymph-node regions on the same side of the diaphragm (II) or localized involvement of an extralymphatic organ or site (II_E)

Stage III

Involvement of lymph-node regions on both sides of the diaphragm (III) or localized involvement of an extra-lymphatic organ or site (III_E), spleen (III_S), or both (III_{SE})

Stage IV

Diffuse or disseminated involvement of one or more extralymphatic organs, with or without associated lymph-node involvement; the organ(s) involved should be identified by a symbol: (P) pulmonary, (O) osseous, or (H) hepatic. In addition, (A) indicates an asymptomatic patient; (B) indicates the presence of fever, night sweats, or weight loss > 10% of body weight.

Adapted from Hellman S, Jaffe ES, DeVita VT: Hodgkin's disease, in DeVita VT Jr, Hellman S, Rosenberg SA (eds): Cancer: Principles and Practice of Oncology, p 1704. Philadelphia, JB Lippincott, 1989

ings, and high parental education. This series of factors may be explained by the delayed-infection hypothesis, which, although it may apply to young adults, may be less important in the pathogenesis of Hodgkin's disease in older patients. Epstein-Barr virus (EBV) has been implicated as a causative agent associated with the development of Hodgkin's disease because cases of this malignancy have occurred following bouts of infectious mononucleosis, and the EBV genome can be found in many of the cells present in involved lymph nodes. Immunodeficiency, induced by the human immunodeficiency virus type 1, has also been associated with the development of Hodgkin's disease, especially the mixed-cellularity subtype. The significance of this association, however, remains unclear.[6,14,15]

STAGING SYSTEM

Peters et al introduced the first clinically relevant system for staging this disease, based on results obtained with radiotherapy alone. Patients with stage I disease had a single site of involvement, those with stage II had two or more contiguous sites of involvement, and patients

with stage III disease had extensive nodal or visceral involvement. The concept of disseminated or stage IV Hodgkin's disease was introduced at the Rye Conference. The Ann Arbor System used today is based on these reports (Table 1).

At the Ann Arbor Staging Conference, the suffix letter "E" was introduced to designate patients with nodal involvement who had a limited degree of extension from diseased nodes into lung, bone, pericardium, and skin. Important modifications of the Ann Arbor System were developed at the Cotswalds Conference in 1989. At this time, it was recommended that patients who had bulky disease, including masses larger than 10 cm in their greatest dimension or mediastinal masses greater than one third the chest wall diameter, have a stage designated with the suffix "X," and that patients achieving greater than 90% partial response with stable adenopathy be designated as having achieved "CR_U" (complete response uncertain). Because there is no clear prognostic difference in subsets of patients with or without residual radiographic abnormalities, there is little clinical utility in creating an unduly complex staging system.[16]

Other recommendations made at the Cotswalds Conference included recognizing the importance of computed tomography in evaluating liver and spleen involvement and designating abdominal disease substages III_1 and III_2. Patients with stage III_1 disease have splenic involvement or lymphadenopathy involving the splenic hilar, celiac, or portal nodes. Disease involving the para-aortic, iliac, or mesenteric nodes is designated III_2. On the basis of our treatment experience, we at M. D. Anderson Cancer Center have designated patients with iliac or inguinal nodal involvement as having stage III_3 disease.[6,14]

PATIENT EVALUATION

The initial evaluation of patients with Hodgkin's disease has both prognostic and therapeutic significance. In addition to performing a hemogram, obtaining a chemical profile, measuring the beta-2-microglobulin level and erythrocyte sedimentation rate, and obtaining roentgenographic studies, other diagnostic procedures should be considered, depending upon the disease presentation and planned treatment (Table 2). Bilateral bone marrow biopsy should be routinely performed, although it is more likely to yield positive results in patients with B symptoms.

Lymphangiography remains a valuable diagnostic tool, especially in the evaluation of disease in the abdomen. Lymphangiography will detect early nodal disease that might be missed with computed tomographic imaging. In addition, nodal status can easily be serially evaluated on routine x-ray films to assess response both during and after therapy. The radiotherapist may also use these results to delineate treatment fields, although lymphangiography may be less essential for patients treated with chemotherapy alone.[7]

Staging by laparotomy remains a controversial subject. Various studies have examined clinical features predictive of abdominal involvement. Approximately 30% to 50% of patients with early-stage Hodgkin's disease will have microscopic abdominal involvement that is not detected by lymphangiography or computed tomography. For this reason, with few exceptions, all patients should be considered as having abdominal disease unless they have undergone a staging laparotomy that has shown otherwise.

Glatstein et al found that the presence of "B" symptoms (unexplained fever above 38°C, night sweats, and unexplained weight loss exceeding 10% of body weight) was predictive of abdominal disease.[17] At M. D. Anderson, male gender, age greater than 40 years, the presence of B symptoms, and mixed cellularity disease were correlated with higher-than-average risks of abdominal disease.[18] Investigators elsewhere have identified other features predictive of abdominal disease, including the number of nodal sites in the upper torso. However, there is currently no way to predict with total accuracy the presence of abdominal disease in a patient whose lymphangiogram is negative, except in patients with stage I disease above the cricoid cartilage, patients with lymphocyte-predominant stage I disease, and women with nodular sclerosis stage IA disease and a peripheral presentation.[7]

Other radiologic studies are of limited benefit in the management of Hodgkin's disease. Some authors have proposed that gallium scans may be used to detect complete response vs partial response to therapy. Hagemeister et al retrospectively reviewed 240 gallium scans from 165 patients with Hodgkin's disease. In untreated Hodgkin's disease, the sensitivity of this test was only 64%, with a specificity of 95%. In untreated patients or those in whom disease had recurred, gallium uptake was predictive for disease in specific sites. Unfortunately, 95% of predicted relapses were not detected by this study during routine follow-up.

The usefulness of the gallium scan, therefore, may be limited to confirming the diagnosis of Hodgkin's disease in new patients and in treated patients who have new or residual lesions.[19] Magnetic resonance imaging has not yet superseded computed tomographic scanning of the abdomen and chest in the evaluation of Hodgkin's dis-

TABLE 2

Recommended Procedures for Staging of Hodgkin's Disease Patients

History and examination

    Identification of B symptoms

Radiologic procedures

    Plain chest x-rays

    Computed tomograpy of thorax (unless chest film is normal)

    Computed tomograpy of abdomen and pelvis

    Bipedal lymphography

Hematologic procedures

    Full blood count with differential count

    Determination of erythrocyte sedimentation rate

    Bilateral bone marrow aspiration and biopsy

Biochemical procedures

    Liver function tests

    Serum albumin, lactate dehydrogenase, and calcium measurements

Procedures for use under special circumstances

    Laparotomy

    Ultrasound scanning

    Magnetic resonance imaging

    Gallium scanning

    Technetium bone scanning

    Liver-spleen scanning

Adapted, with permission, from Urba, Longo DL: N Engl J Med 326:679, 1992

ease. Bone scans should be considered only in patients with symptoms. Ultrasound of the spleen may play a role in the detection of occult splenic involvement.

TREATMENT OF EARLY DISEASE

Laparotomy Staged

Patients with laparotomy-staged supradiaphragmatic disease and no mass or a small mediastinal mass may be treated with radiotherapy alone. Initial investigations used low-dose involved-field radiation only. Patients responded well initially but had a high rate of disease relapse in a disseminated pattern, prompting investigation of higher doses of radiation, extended fields, and the use of prophylactic radiotherapy.[7]

Largely because of results from early clinical trials by investigators at Stanford, prophylactic abdominal irradiation for both pathologically and clinically early-staged supradiaphragmatic disease was initially standard therapy in the United States.[20-22] Later, questions arose concerning whether wider radiation fields were necessary. Patients receiving extended-field radiotherapy for pathologically early-staged disease were found to have excellent 10-year survival rates of 82% and 83% for stages I and II disease, respectively, with no reported adverse prognostic features.[23] However, it is unclear whether there was real benefit from the abdominal irradiation or whether the patients were simply of a more favorable group.

In studies comparing mantle vs extended-field radiotherapy, other investigators found that the addition of radiotherapy to the upper abdomen was not necessary in patients whose disease was staged by laparotomy.[24,25] Of note, patients in these studies were only offered single-modality radiotherapy if they lacked adverse features (eg, B symptoms, large mediastinal masses, or advanced age).

Lee et al added low-dose radiation to the lungs and liver to extended-field radiotherapy being done in patients with pathologically early-staged disease. They found that the 5-year disease-free survival rate was improved to 82%, compared with 58% in patients who received extended field radiation alone, with minimal or no added toxic effects.[26]

In studies done at M. D. Anderson and elsewhere for which favorable patients were not selected, the inclusion of abdominal irradiation did not decrease the low rate of abdominal relapse following single-modality radiotherapy for laparotomy-staged early disease in the upper torso.[27-29] At M. D. Anderson, a series of patients with pathologic early-stage Hodgkin's disease were treated with involved-field (including the mantle, if indicated), extended-field radiation, or involved-field radiation followed by six cycles of mechlorethamine (Mustargen), vincristine (Oncovin), procarbazine (Matulane), and prednisone (MOPP) chemotherapy.[27] Overall, the 5-year disease-free survival rate for those patients treated with involved-field radiation including the mantle was 72%, compared with 66% for patients treated with extended-field radiation.

Importantly, in studies of treatment options for pathologically staged early disease, including those mentioned above, several adverse prognostic features were identified that predicted for relapse if only radiotherapy was used. These included the presence of a mediastinal mass

greater than 7.5 cm or greater than one third the diameter of the chest, hilar lymphadenopathy, B symptoms, advanced age, extension of disease into pulmonary parenchyma, mixed cellularity histology, stage II disease, and increased number of nodal sites.[25-33] The major point to emerge from these trials was that the disease-free survival of patients with poor prognostic factors significantly improved with the use of combined modality chemotherapy and radiotherapy.

To compare chemotherapy alone with radiotherapy, Cimino et al treated patients who had pathologic stage I to IIA disease with extended-field radiotherapy or six cycles of MOPP.[34] The disease-free survival rates were 73% for patients treated with MOPP and 74% for those treated with radiotherapy. At 8-year follow-up, the radiotherapy arm had a significantly higher overall survival rate of 93%, compared with 56% for the chemotherapy arm. The respective rates of relapse-free survival were similar, at 70% and 71%. Lack of response to salvage treatment on the chemotherapy arm was thought to be the primary reason for the discordant survival rates. Adverse features for those treated with chemotherapy included bulky disease. The authors suggested that patients with early bulky disease be treated with combined-modality therapy.[34,35]

In contrast, investigators at the National Cancer Institute reported improved overall and disease-free survival rates with MOPP chemotherapy vs extended-field radiation.[36] The discrepancy is likely accounted for by the fact that the American trial included patients with stages IIB and III_1A disease, which have been shown to fare worse with single-modality radiotherapy, and excluded patients with peripheral stage IA disease.

As survival improved during the evolution of treatment methods, a new focus of therapy was the possibility that less intense or less toxic treatment could give equivalent results with decreased long- and short-term complications. A program was designed at M. D. Anderson to treat patients with poor-prognosis laparotomy-staged early disease with only two cycles of MOPP chemotherapy followed by radiotherapy.[37] The 4-year disease-free survival rate was 79% compared with 78% for patients who had favorable presentations and were treated with radiation alone. Toxic effects, including sterility and secondary malignancies, were reduced.

Horning et al treated patients with favorable pathologic stage IA, IIA, or IIIA disease with a combination of radiotherapy and a novel chemotherapy regimen of six cycles of vinblastine, bleomycin (Blenoxane), and methotrexate to avoid the toxic effects of MOPP chemotherapy.[38] The patients were randomized to either subtotal or total lymphoid irradiation or to involved-field radiation with vincristine, bleomycin, and methotrexate. The 5-year rates for freedom from disease progression were 70% for those treated with radiotherapy alone and 95% for those who received the combined-modality regimen. The outcome was comparable with reported results from studies of adjuvant MOPP treatments, and there was little adverse effect on fertility, although some reduction in pulmonary function was seen in patients who received irradiation plus bleomycin.

In summary, patients with laparotomy-staged early disease without large mediastinal masses can be treated with either involved or extended-field radiotherapy with equivalent results. The presence of B symptoms, bulky mediastinal disease, hilar involvement, extension into pulmonary parenchyma, or advanced age, especially in males, necessitates combined-modality radiotherapy and chemotherapy for optimal control of both local and abdominal recurrence, since there is a 10% to 15% risk of the latter even with the addition of splenic pedicle and para-aortic irradiation when radiotherapy is used alone. If adverse prognostic features are identified and the treatment approach instead focuses on combined modality therapy, staging by laparotomy becomes unnecessary.

Clinically Staged

The optimal therapy for patients with clinically staged I or II Hodgkin's disease remains controversial. Most centers recommend combined modality therapy. However, radiotherapy or chemotherapy alone may suffice in appropriate situations. One of the most challenging tasks in the treatment of clinically staged Hodgkin's disease is the identification of prognostic risk factors that will allow a therapeutic regimen to be tailored to any particular patient for maximum efficacy and minimal immediate and delayed toxic effects.

Sutcliffe et al investigated a large series of patients who had clinically staged I or II Hodgkin's disease. Based on the relapse rates following radiotherapy alone, the authors were able to define three groups. Group 1 consisted of patients who had disease above the cricoid cartilage. Group 2 comprised those patients who had stage IA disease below the cricoid cartilage or stage IIA lymphocyte-predominant or nodular sclerosis disease. Patients with early-stage disease and unfavorable histology or B symptoms were classified as group 3. Based upon disease relapse rates, the authors recommended that group 1 patients receive involved-field radiotherapy, that group 2 patients receive extended-field radiotherapy, and that group 3 patients receive combined-modality therapy (radiotherapy plus chemotherapy).[39]

Subsequently, Gospodarowicz et al expanded on this report with a larger number of patients treated at the same institution and identified subsets of patients who had favorable, intermediate, and unfavorable prognoses. Favorable prognosis included presentation of disease in the "high upper neck" that was nodular sclerosing stage IA disease in females, disease that had a lymphocyte-predominant histology, and disease that presented in the groin.[40] Patients with favorable features should achieve excellent disease-free survival rates with extended-field or even involved-field radiotherapy, because the likelihood of abdominal disease in these patients is low.[41]

Other investigators have studied the use of chemotherapy with or without radiotherapy. Pavlovsky et al treated patients who had clinically staged I and II Hodgkin's disease with cyclophosphamide (Cytoxan, Neosar), vincristine, procarbazine, and prednisone (CVPP) or CVPP plus radiotherapy. Patients with higher-risk features—age greater than 45 years, involvement of more than two nodal areas, a mediastinal mass larger than 10 cm in its greatest dimension, or peripheral lymphadenopathy greater than 5 cm—had freedom-from-progression rates of 34% with CVPP alone and 75% with combined-modality therapy. In the absence of these factors, patients had freedom-from-progression rates of 77% with CVPP and 70% with combined-modality therapy. The authors suggested that patients with adverse features receive combined-modality therapy.[42]

Although most investigators recommend combined-modality therapy in early clinically staged Hodgkin's disease, programs vary with respect to the amount of chemotherapy and radiotherapy delivered. Carde et al examined patients who had clinically staged I and II Hodgkin's disease with favorable or unfavorable characteristics. Those patients of advanced age, or with mediastinal involvement, unfavorable histologies, or bulky disease after laparotomy were included in the unfavorable group. The purpose of the study was to compare the efficacy of total lymphoid or subtotal lymphoid irradiation with that of combined-modality therapy consisting of six cycles of MOPP followed by mantle irradiation. Overall, the relapse-free survival rates were better for those treated with combined-modality therapy, although overall survival rates were identical because of salvage therapy.[24]

Zittoun et al studied patients who had clinically staged I and IIIA Hodgkin's disease treated with MOPP and radiotherapy. Those patients with favorable presentations received three courses of MOPP followed by involved-field or extended-field radiotherapy. Those patients with unfavorable characteristics received six courses of MOPP followed by radiotherapy. Most patients had a good outcome. However, patients with mixed-cellularity disease, men, and patients over 40 years old had a worse outcome. The investigators concluded that patients having unfavorable presentations should receive six courses of MOPP followed by extended-field radiotherapy.[43]

Nonetheless, in a study of 166 patients with clinically-staged I to IIA disease, Andrieu et al examined the efficacy of three cycles of MOPP followed by radiotherapy to varying fields, depending on the extent of disease. They reported a 5-year survival rate of 93% and a disease-free survival rate of 90% for patients who achieved a complete remission. Disease did not recur in the mediastinum among patients with mediastinal disease, and disease recurred in the abdomen among only a small percentage of patients, even without prophylaxis to this area. These authors thus concluded that a minimum of three courses of MOPP would be sufficient to prevent relapse in the mediastinum and abdomen.[44]

Another significant investigation was conducted by Ferme et al.[45] In that study, patients with clinically staged IB to III disease received three or six cycles of MOPP before radiotherapy. Complete responses were obtained in 96% of these patients after three cycles of MOPP and in 94% following six cycles.[45] This study was important because it illustrated the efficacy of three cycles of MOPP. The presence of a large mediastinal mass has also been confirmed in other studies as an adverse prognostic feature in patients treated with radiotherapy or chemotherapy alone or with combined-modality therapy.[46,47]

Infradiaphragmatic Presentation

Hodgkin's disease that presents initially in the abdomen is unusual. Some investigators have recommended chemotherapy based on the presence of B symptoms and bulky disease. However, patients with pathologic stage IA disease may receive "inverted Y" radiotherapy that includes the splenic pedicle. Patients with stage IIA disease should receive total lymphoid irradiation, and patients with stage IIB disease should receive combined-modality therapy.[48]

At M. D. Anderson, 60 patients with pathologic or clinical stage I to II Hodgkin's disease received radiotherapy with or without MOPP. The disease-free survival rate of the patients who received radiotherapy alone was 50%, compared with 92% for those who received combined-modality therapy. Radiotherapy alone may be adequate, however, in patients evaluated with lymphangiography who have pelvic, inguinal, or femoral involvement.[49]

TREATMENT OF STAGE III DISEASE

The optimal therapy for stage III Hodgkin's disease remains controversial. As with the other stages, treatment depends primarily on the extent of disease. Several studies have examined the role of certain factors that influence the outcome of treatment in stage IIIA Hodgkin's disease. Patients with stage III_1A disease have been observed to have improved overall and disease-free survival rates, compared with patients who have stage III_2A disease. Patients with stage III_1A and III_2A disease treated with radiotherapy alone had disease-free survival rates of 64% and 32%, respectively. The investigators noted that these patients showed a marked improvement in survival rates if they received combined-modality therapy, and concluded that patients with extensive disease should receive such therapy.[50]

Hoppe et al examined the significance of the number of splenic nodules in patients receiving radiotherapy alone.[51] Patients with fewer than five nodules had a 5-year disease-free survival rate of 90%, whereas patients with more than five nodules had a 5-year disease-free survival rate of only 30%.[51] Mazza et al also found that such patients with small lymphadenopathy had better disease-free survival rates than did those with larger nodes.[52] However, prognostic factors for these patients are different when the treatment is combined-modality therapy.

At M. D. Anderson, 102 patients with stage IIIA Hodgkin's disease received two cycles of MOPP followed by radiotherapy. A total of 73 patients received pelvic radiotherapy and 29 did not; the 10-year survival rates for these patient groups were 89% and 93%, respectively. Five-year survival and freedom-from-progression rates for the patients who did not receive pelvic radiotherapy were 93% and 85%, respectively. Twenty-three patients with stage III_2A disease were treated with two courses of MOPP and radiotherapy to involved sites. Five-year survival and freedom-from-progression rates were 85% and 79%, respectively. Twenty patients with stage III_3A disease treated with combined-modality therapy had 5-year-survival and freedom-from-progression rates of 82% and 85%, respectively. The results of this study indicated that the extent of abdominal involvement did not affect survival.[53]

Mauch et al identified a group of patients with stage III_1A disease (those with fewer than five splenic nodules) that can be adequately treated with total lymphoid irradiation alone. They recommended combined-modality therapy, however, for all other patients with stage IIIA Hodgkin's disease.[54]

Most investigators recommend chemotherapy with or without radiotherapy for stage IIIB Hodgkin's disease. Factors that might influence survival include advanced age, histologic tumor subtype, and tumor burden.[7] At M. D. Anderson, patients with stage IIIB Hodgkin's disease were treated with two courses of MOPP and radiotherapy. In this study, patients who had stage III_1B or III_2B disease had similar good outcomes, but patients with stage III_3B disease had inferior results. Therefore, patients with stage III_3B disease should be treated more intensively.[55,56]

In another study, Bonadonna et al randomized patients with stage IIB, III, or IV Hodgkin's disease to receive MOPP or doxorubicin, bleomycin, vinblastine, and dacarbazine (ABVD) followed by radiotherapy. Radiotherapy increased the complete response rate of patients treated with ABVD from 69% to 94%, and for those treated with MOPP, from 66% to 95%. Freedom-from-progression rates were 81% for the ABVD group and 63% for the MOPP group.[57] Other studies utilizing different chemotherapeutic regimens and radiotherapy sequences have yielded similar results. Therefore, stage IIIB disease should be treated with combined-modality therapy, although the extent of disease may play a role in the number of cycles of chemotherapy needed to achieve good results.[7]

TREATMENT OF STAGE IV DISEASE

Multiple prognostic factors for treatment outcome in stage IV Hodgkin's disease have been studied. Investigators at M. D. Anderson, the National Cancer Institute, and other centers have identified B symptoms, dose of vincristine administered, extent of extranodal lesions, mechlorethamine dose, bone marrow involvement, anemia, elevated erythrocyte sedimentation rate, and advanced age as factors that influence prognosis.[58–60]

Longo et al examined 158 patients with stage IV Hodgkin's disease, 84% of whom achieved a complete response and 45% of whom were alive without disease at 9-year follow-up. Factors influencing complete response were lack of B symptoms and vincristine dose intensity. Factors noted to affect duration of remission were B symptoms, pleural disease, advanced age, and increased number of extranodal sites.[58]

At M. D. Anderson, among 53 patients treated with MOPP, the complete response rate was influenced by the number of extranodal sites. Of patients with one extranodal site, 75% entered complete remission compared with 25% of those with two or more extranodal sites. Overall survival was also influenced by this factor. Patients who received more than 80% of the planned dose

of mechlorethamine also had higher disease-free and overall survival rates.[60]

Alternative treatments for advanced Hodgkin's disease have also been proposed (Table 3). The ABVD regimen was examined as first-line therapy for advanced Hodgkin's disease by Bonadonna et al.[61] They showed that ABVD was equivalent to MOPP in achieving a complete response rate but that disease-free survival rates appeared to be superior with ABVD.[61] The Cancer and Leukemia Group B (CALGB) also investigated MOPP vs ABVD and noted a complete response rate of 47% for the MOPP group and 83% for the ABVD group. The disease-free survival rate was also better with ABVD.[62] Bonadonna et al also examined the efficacy of MOPP-ABVD in stage IV Hodgkin's disease and found that the complete response rate was better for MOPP-ABVD than for MOPP alone.[61] However, only 44% of patients in the MOPP group received more than 80% of the planned dose, whereas 64% of patients in the MOPP-ABVD group received more than 80% of the planned dose, and, as previously stated, the amount of drug delivered may affect outcome. In a three-armed study, CALGB treated 38 patients with MOPP-ABVD, ABVD, or MOPP alone. Patients in the MOPP-ABVD and ABVD groups had better overall survival rates as well as better complete response rates than did those in the MOPP group.[62] Connors and Klimo modified the MOPP-ABVD regimen. They gave patients a regimen of MOPP plus a combination of doxorubicin, bleomycin, and vinblastine, with patients receiving all seven drugs each month, and showed that this regimen yielded similar results to MOPP-ABVD.[53]

The use of combined modality therapy in stage IV Hodgkin's disease remains controversial. Studies at the National Cancer Institute revealed that patients treated with adjuvant radiotherapy after MOPP therapy had no significant improvement in overall survival.[7] At Memorial Sloan-Kettering Cancer Center, Yahalom et al examined the effect of adjuvant radiotherapy in patients with advanced-stage Hodgkin's disease treated with combined chemotherapy. They found that the majority of relapses occurred in previously unirradiated sites and, therefore, concluded that radiotherapy in combination with chemotherapy could improve survival and decrease relapse in patients with advanced Hodgkin's disease.[64]

SALVAGE THERAPY

The optimal selection of salvage therapy for relapsed Hodgkin's disease depends primarily on the initial therapy. Patients in whom disease recurs after radiotherapy for early-stage Hodgkin's disease may receive any che-

TABLE 3

Combination Chemotherapy Regimens for the Treatment of Advanced Hodgkin's Disease

Regimen	Dose (mg/m²)	Route	Days
MOPP			
Mechlorethamine	6	IV	1, 8
Vincristine	1.4	IV	1, 8
Procarbazine	100	PO	1–14
Prednisone	40	PO	1–14
MVPP			
Mechlorethamine	6	IV	1, 8
Vinblastine	6	IV	1, 8
Procarbazine	100	PO	1–14
Prednisone	40	PO	1–14
LOPP			
Chlorambucil	6	PO	1–14
Vincristine	1.4	IV	1, 8
Procarbazine	100	PO	1–14
Prednisone	40	PO	1–14
CHLVPP			
Chlorambucil	6	PO	1–14
Vinblastine	6	IV	1, 8
Procarbazine	100	PO	1–14
Prednisone	40	PO	1–14
ABVD			
Doxorubicin	25	IV	1, 15
Bleomycin	10	IV	1, 15
Vinblastine	6	IV	1, 15
Dacarbazine	375	IV	1, 15
MOPP/ABVD			
Alternating months of MOPP and ABVD			
MOPP/ABV			
Mechlorethamine	6	IV	1
Vincristine	1.4	IV	1
Procarbazine	100	PO	1–7
Prednisone	40	PO	1–14
Doxorubicin	35	IV	8
Bleomycin	10	IV	8
Vinblastine	6	IV	8

Adapted, with permission, from Longo DL: Semin Oncol 17:717, 1990

motherapeutic regimen with an 80% to 90% chance of achieving complete remission.[7] Patients in whom disease recurs after achieving complete response with chemotherapy may be treated again with another regimen (Table 4).

Fisher et al studied a series of patients whose disease recurred after treatment with MOPP. Patients whose disease recurred 1 year or more after they had achieved complete remission had a greater than 90% chance of achieving a second complete remission. Those patients in whom MOPP treatment failed to induce a complete remission had a poor prognosis. Patients whose disease recurs less than 1 year after they achieve a complete remission may be retreated with a second regimen, but results may vary depending on prognostic features. Patients may also be considered for high-dose chemotherapy followed by autologous or allogeneic bone marrow transplantation.[65,66]

COMPLICATIONS OF TREATMENT

The treatment of Hodgkin's disease may predispose patients to secondary malignancies. The use of chemotherapeutic agents, especially alkylating agents, is associated with an increased incidence of hematologic malignancies, whereas radiotherapy has been associated with an increased incidence of solid tumors. Patients with Hodgkin's disease may also experience endocrine dysfunction, cardiopulmonary complications, and musculoskeletal abnormalities as a result of treatment (Table 5).

Secondary Malignancies

Almost any type of malignancy may occur after chemotherapy for Hodgkin's disease. The most common are acute nonlymphocytic leukemia, myelodysplastic syndrome, non-Hodgkin's lymphoma, and solid tumors. The overall risk of occurrence of acute nonlymphocytic leukemia is 0.5% to 2.0% per year. The cumulative risk is 10% to 15%.[67]

Risk factors associated with the development of acute nonlymphocytic leukemia include prolonged exposure to alkylating agents and advanced patient age. Diffuse non-Hodgkin's lymphoma is the next most common secondary malignancy, with a cumulative 10-year risk of 4% to 5%.[68] Although most secondary malignancies are thought to be related to therapy, the incidence of non-Hodgkin's lymphoma may also be increased in untreated patients.[69]

Unlike the hematologic malignancies, the occurrence of solid tumors in patients with Hodgkin's disease appears to be related to radiotherapy. The incidence of secondary solid tumors is highest approximately 7 years after treatment.[70] The cumulative incidence of solid

TABLE 4

Conventional Dose Salvage Combination Chemotherapy Regimens for Relapsed Resistant Hodgkin's Disease

Regimen	Number of patients	Complete remission rate (%)	Duration of remission (mo)
VABCD	18	8 (45)	30
Vinblastine, 6 mg/m² IV every 3 wk Doxorubicin, 40 mg/m² IV every 3 wk Dacarbazine, 800 mg/m² IV every 3 wk Lomustine, 80 mg/m² PO every 6 wk Bleomycin, 15 U IV once a week			
ABDIC	34	12 (35)	47
Doxorubicin, 45 mg/m² IV on day 1 Bleomycin, 5 U/m² IV on days 1 and 5 Dacarbazine, 200 mg/m² IV on days 1 through 5 Lomustine, 50 mg/m² PO on day 1 Prednisone, 40 mg/m² PO on days 1 through 5 Repeat every 28 days			
CBVD	20	9 (45)	10
Lomustine, 120 mg/m² PO on day 1 Bleomycin, 15 U IV on days 1 and 22 Vinblastine, 6 mg/m² IV on days 1 and 22 Dexamethasone, 3 mg/m² PO on days 1 through 21 Repeat every 6 wk			
PCVP	11	8 (72)	6 to 16 +
Vinblastine, 3 mg/m² IV every 2 wk Procarbazine, 70 mg/m² PO every other day Cyclophosphamide, 70 mg/m² PO every other day Prednisone, 8 mg/m² PO every other day Repeat for 1 yr			
CEP	58	23 (40)	15 +
Lomustine, 80 mg/m² PO on day 1 Etoposide, 100 mg/m² PO on days 1 through 5 Prednimustine, 60 mg/m² PO on days 1 through 5			
CEP/ABVD	21	14 (67)	24 +
CEP (as above)	15	4 (27)	4 to 18 +
EVA	19	6 (32)	Not stated
Etoposide, 200 mg/m² PO on days 1 through 5 Vincristine, 2 mg IV on day 1 Doxorubicin, 50 mg/m² IV on day 1			
LVB	63	30 (48)	24 +
Lomustine Vindesine Bleomycin			

Table 4 continues on the following page

TABLE 4 *continued*

Conventional Dose Salvage Combination Chemotherapy Regimens for Relapsed Resistant Hodgkin's Disease

Regimen	Number of patients	Complete remission rate (%)	Duration of remission (mo)
MIME	47	11 (23)	23% at 19
Methyl GAG, 500 mg/m^2 IV on days 1 through 14 Ifosfamide, 1 g/m^2 IV on days 1 through 5 Methotrexate, 30 mg/m^2 IV on day 3 Etoposide, 100 mg/m^2 IV on days 1 through 3 every 3 wk			
MTX-CHOP	11	4 (36)	4, 15, 24, 94 +
Methotrexate, 30 mg/m^2 IV every 6 h for 4 days, beginning on days 1 and 8, with rescue Cyclophosphamide, 750 mg/m^2 IV on day 15 Vincristine, 1 mg/m^2 IV on days 15 and 22 Prednisone, 100 mg/m^2 PO on days 22 through 26 Doxorubicin, 50 mg/m^2 IV on day 15 every 4 wk			
CEM	32	4 (13)	7 +, 10, 41 +, 51 +
Lomustine, 100 mg/m^2 PO on day 1 Etoposide, 100 mg/m^2 PO on days 1 through 3 and 21 through 23 Methotrexate, 30 mg/m^2 PO on days 1, 8, 21, and 28 every 6 wk			
CEVD	32	14 (44)	10 +

Lomustine, 80 mg/m^2 PO on day 1
Etoposide, 120 mg/m^2 PO on days 1 through 5
   and 22 through 26
Vindesine, 3 mg/m^2 IV on days 1 and 22
Dexamethasone, 3 mg/m^2 PO on days 1 through 8,
   followed by 1.5 mg/m^2 PO on days 9 through 26 every 6 wk			

MOPLACE	30	5 (21)	5
Cyclophosphamide, 750 mg/m^2 IV on day 1 Etoposide, 80 mg/m^2 IV on days 1 through 3 Prednisone, 60 mg/m^2 PO on days 1 through 14 Methotrexate, 120 mg/m^2 IV on days 15 and 22, with rescue Cytarabine, 300 mg/m^2 IV on days 15 and 22 Vincristine, 2 mg IV on days 15 and 22 every 4 wk			
CAVP	31	8 (26)	10
Lomustine, 90 mg/m^2 PO on day 1 Melphalan, 7.5 mg/m^2 PO on days 1 through 5 Etoposide, 100 mg/m^2 PO on days 6 through 10 Prednisone, 40 mg/m^2 PO on days 1 through 10 every 6 wk			
EVAP	27	9 (33)	6
Etoposide, 120 mg/m^2 IV on days 1, 8, and 15 Vinblastine, 4 mg/m^2 IV on days 1, 8, and 15 Cytarabine, 30 mg/m^2 IV on days 1, 8, and 15 Cisplatin, 40 mg/m^2 IV on days 1, 8, and 15, every 4 wk			

Adapted, with permission, from Longo RL: Semin Oncol 17:728–729, 1990

tumors is 9% at 10 years.[71] Solid tumors that show an increased incidence include carcinoma of the head and neck, melanoma, and female breast cancer.[72-77]

Endocrine Complications

Patients treated for Hodgkin's disease may experience endocrine abnormalities that are primarily limited to thyroid and gonadal dysfunction. Patients may develop thyroid hyperplasia, which may need to be distinguished from malignancy.[78] Clinical hypothyroidism occurs in 6% to 25% of patients treated with mantle or cervical radiotherapy. Chemotherapy has little or no role in the development of thyroid dysfunction. Thyroid malignancy may develop in patients treated for Hodgkin's disease, especially those who receive partial thyroid ablation with radiation, thereby causing excessive stimulation of residual thyroid tissue by thyroid-stimulating hormone.[79,80]

Because some patients with Hodgkin's disease attain prolonged disease-free survival, the issue of fertility has become important. Approximately 30% to 50% of men have suboptimal semen analyses before therapy.[71] Radiotherapy or its scatter may affect testicular function. Recovery of that function and the length of time to optimal recovery are related to radiation dose. Testicular shielding will reduce exposure.[76,81]

Alkylating agents are the most important agents affecting male fertility. These agents include cyclophosphamide, chlorambucil (Leukeran), mechlorethamine, and procarbazine.[82] MOPP therapy results in prolonged testicular dysfunction in 80% of patients. Only 10% of patients will show partial recovery within 1 to 7 years of treatment. Patients who receive less than four cycles of MOPP have a more rapid recovery.[83] Studies of ABVD have shown that 54% of men have impaired spermatogenesis but that all patients recover adequate function within 2 years.[84]

Women are also affected by chemotherapy. Menopausal symptoms may develop several years after chemotherapy. Ovarian dysfunction may be heralded by irregular or anovulatory cycles. However, even with preexisting ovarian damage, pregnancy can occur and, thus, should not be considered a sign of adequate ovarian function.[71,85]

As with the testis, the ovary appears to be more affected by alkylating agents. In general, the ovary tolerates radiotherapy better than the testis does. Patients nearer to menopause will experience primary amenorrhea at lower radiotherapy doses than will other patients.[71] Ovarian shielding and oophoropexy may be useful for preventing an excessive radiation dose to the ovary. Of all women treated for Hodgkin's disease, 80% will have some ovarian dysfunction and 20% to 30% will have permanent amenorrhea. Patients who receive combined modality therapy and radiotherapy have a higher incidence of dysfunction.[86] Ovarian failure has been correlated to the age of the patient during the period of treatment. Eighty to 100% of patients over 25 years old will experience ovarian failure compared with 25% to 30% of women under 25.[71]

Cardiovascular Complications

Both radiotherapy and chemotherapy may have deleterious effects on the heart. Pericarditis resulting from mantle irradiation is the most common cardiovascular side effect of radiotherapy; its incidence is related to the dose, rate, and anatomic volume treated. Use of anterior-posterior ports contributed significantly to cardiac toxicity in early trials. The highest incidence of pericarditis occurs 5 to 9 months after completion of radiotherapy.[87,88] Most patients with pericarditis are asymptomatic, but others may present with cardiomegaly, friction rub, effusion, tamponade, fever, electrocardiographic changes, and pleuritic pain.

Multiple modes of therapy for acute pericarditis exist, depending upon symptomatology. For symptomatic relief, nonsteroidal agents, digoxin, and diuretics have been used. For patients with hemodynamic compromise, pericardiocentesis and pericardiectomy may be utilized. Pericardial effusions develop in 25% to 30% of patients. This usually occurs within 2 years of therapy, but may arise later.[89] Chronic pericarditis occurs 53 to 124 months after therapy.[90] These patients usually present with dyspnea on exertion. This form of pericarditis is usually constrictive and is treated with pericardiectomy.

Myocardial damage may also be experienced after radiotherapy. Brosius et al conducted a postmortem study of 16 patients who received greater than 3,500 cGy to the heart. Fifteen of these patients had signs of myocardial damage.[91] Utilizing radionuclide ventriculography, Burns et al examined ventricular function after radiotherapy in 12 of 21 asymptomatic patients and 10 historical controls. Right-ventricular ejection fraction dysfunction was the most common finding. The authors concluded that the right ventricle may experience more damage because of its location.[92]

Other studies utilizing patients who underwent radiotherapy with various cardiac-shielding techniques showed objective evidence of myocardial damage in the absence of clinical symptoms, suggesting that newer techniques may decrease the severity of myocardial damage. Valvular abnormalities have also been seen in patients with

TABLE 5

Long-term Complications in Patients Cured of Hodgkin's Disease

Complication	Etiology/risk factors	Management and prevention
Immune dysfunction	Hodgkin's disease; treatment	Appropriate vaccinations
Herpes zoster/varicella	Hodgkin's disease; treatment	Systemic antiviral therapy; zoster immune globulin
Pneumococcal sepsis	Splenectomy; asplenia following radiotherapy	Pretreatment pneumococcal vaccine; selected antibiotic prophylaxis; avoid unnecessary splenectomy
Nonlymphocytic leukemia	Treatment; age above 40	Avoid combined modality treatment for Hodgkin's disease; supportive care, low-dose treatment; aggressive antileukemic treatment; bone marrow transplantation
Myelodysplastic syndromes	Treatment; age above 40	Same as above
Non-Hodgkin's lymphoma	Treatment	Aggressive chemotherapy
Solid tumors	Direct/indirect radiotherapy	Conventional management
Thymic hyperplasia	Hodgkin's disease; treatment	Resection
Hypothyroidism	Direct/indirect radiotherapy	Hormone replacement; ? thyroid suppression during treatment
Thyroid cancer	Direct/indirect radiotherapy; chronic TSH stimulation	Thyroid suppression
Male infertility	Hodgkin's disease; treatment	Attempt sperm storage; testicular shielding during radiotherapy; ? suppression of spermatogenesis during chemotherapy; alternative chemotherapy
Male impotence	Hodgkin's disease; treatment	Counseling; trial of testosterone
Female infertility	Treatment	Oophoropexy; ? ovarian suppression during treatment; cyclic estrogen replacement
Female impotence	Hodgkin's disease; treatment	Counseling; cyclic estrogen replacement
Pericarditis, acute	Mediastinal treatment; chemotherapy recall post-irradiation	Appropriate treatment technique; avoid doxorubicin post-irradiation anti-inflammatory medication; pericardiocentesis
Pericarditis, chronic	Mediastinal radiotherapy	Appropriate radiotherapy technique; pericardiectomy
Cardiomyopathy	Mediastinal radiotherapy; doxorubicin; chemotherapy recall post-irradiation	Appropriate radiotherapy technique; avoid doxorubicin post-irradiation; monitor for early toxicity; limit cumulative doxorubicin dosage; provide medical support
Pneumonitis, acute	Direct/indirect radiotherapy bleomycin; nitrosoureas; chemotherapy recall post-irradiation	Appropriate radiotherapy technique; monitor for early toxicity; avoid known toxic drugs; avoid excessive Po_2
Pneumonitis, chronic	Same as above	Supportive management
Avascular necrosis	Steroid therapy; ? Hodgkin's disease	Anti-inflammatory medication; joint surgery
Growth retardation	Pediatric radiotherapy	Minimize radiotherapy; use symmetric radiotherapy fields
Dental caries	Radiotherapy salivary changes	Maintain good oral hygiene; daily flouride treatments

Adapted from Bookman MA, Longo DL: Concomitant illness in patients treated for Hodgkin's disease. Cancer Treat Rev 13:101, 1986

Hodgkin's disease after radiotherapy. These abnormalities include aortic regurgitation and mitral regurgitation, both of which occur in the setting of myocardial fibrosis.[71,93] Accelerated atherosclerosis has resulted in myocardial infarction in otherwise healthy patients.[94]

Various chemotherapeutic agents have been implicated in cardiac toxicity. The most important agent in the treatment of Hodgkin's disease is doxorubicin. At cumulative doses below 400 mg/m^2, the incidence of cardiomyopathy is less than 2%.[95] In addition to the chronic effects of doxorubicin, patients may experience severe acute side effects such as carditis and arrhythmias.[96] The mortality rate from doxorubicin-induced cardiomyopathy is 50%. Sequential endocardial biopsy may be helpful in predicting whether patients can continue to receive doxorubicin.[71] Previous studies have identified factors associated with cardiomyopathy. Advanced patient age, uncontrolled hypertension, and previous radiotherapy have all been shown to increase the incidence of cardiomyopathy in doxorubicin-treated patients.[95–97] The combination of radiotherapy with doxorubicin has been associated with "radiation recall," which is an inflammatory endothelial reaction. In addition, mitomycin (Mutamycin) and cyclophosphamide may act synergistically with doxorubicin to produce cardiac damage.[98,99]

Pulmonary Complications

The pulmonary system is also subject to the side effects of treatment of Hodgkin's disease. The effects secondary to radiotherapy can be categorized into acute and chronic changes.

Acute radiation pneumonitis is the most common side effect. This phenomenon is related to the total radiation dose, dose rate, and volume of lung treated.[100] Two groups of patients are prone to this side effect: (1) those with mediastinal disease and (2) those who receive total body irradiation for bone marrow transplantation. Acute radiation pneumonitis may present with shortness of breath, cough, fever, pain, and wheezing. Chest x-ray films will most often show paramediastinal densities and interstitial pneumonitis. Pleural effusions may occur.

Some patients require little or no therapy, whereas others may need treatment with corticosteroids.[71] Rapid discontinuation of corticosteroids after MOPP therapy may precipitate acute radiation pneumonitis.[101] There may be synergy of radiotherapy with certain drugs, such as bleomycin, cyclophosphamide, and methotrexate, in producing acute radiation pneumonitis. Doxorubicin, bleomycin, and dactinomycin (Cosmegen) have been implicated in a "radiation recall" phenomenon, characterized by clinical signs and symptoms of chronic restric-

tive fibrosis occurring 9 to 12 months after the completion of therapy, chest x-ray findings consistent with chronic fibrosis, and evidence of restrictive airways disease upon spirometry.[71]

Chemotherapeutic agents associated with pulmonary toxicity include bleomycin and carmustine (BiCNU). Bleomycin toxicity most commonly presents as interstitial pneumonitis; a biopsy may be required to eliminate other causes.[71] Pulmonary fibrosis has been associated with carmustine[102] and hypersensitivity pneumonitis with procarbazine.[103] Increased pulmonary toxicity has also been associated with multiple-agent regimens.[104]

Miscellaneous Complications

Patients with Hodgkin's disease may experience musculoskeletal complications, such as avascular necrosis of bone. The incidence is increased with radiotherapy to bone.[105] Children who receive radiotherapy to bone may experience growth asymmetry secondary to premature closure of the epiphyseal plates.[71] This risk may warrant adjusting or lowering the dose of radiotherapy given. Patients who receive radiation to soft tissue may develop fibrosis with edema, venous thrombosis, and nerve entrapment. Patients treated with mantle or cervical radiotherapy may experience transient or permanent xerostomia, with increased risk of dental caries.[88]

CONCLUSIONS

Hodgkin's disease remains one of the human malignancies most amenable to treatment. A wide range of therapeutic modalities is available, including chemotherapy, radiotherapy, and combinations of the two. Controversies exist among different centers as to the appropriate treatment of this disorder at different stages, but this debate may be resolved with future studies. Finally, the improved outcome of patients with Hodgkin's disease makes it imperative to consider the acute and long-term side effects of treatment and to ameliorate them when possible.

REFERENCES

1. Banks PM: The pathology of Hodgkin's disease. Semin Oncol 17:683, 1990.
2. Maksen JA, Hassan MO, Carter JR: The ultrastructural heterogeneity of the Reed-Sternberg cell and its resemblance to monocyte macrophage differentiation in vivo. Ultrastruct Pathol 4:379, 1983.
3. Hsu S, Jaffe ES: Leu-M1 and peanut agglutinin stain the neoplastic cells of Hodgkin's disease. Am J Clin Pathol 92:29, 1984.
4. Stein H, Uchanska-Ziegler G, Gerdes J, et al: Hodgkin's and Reed-Sternberg cells contain antigens specific to late cells of granulopoiesis. Int J Cancer 29:283, 1982.
5. Carbone A, Gloghini A, Gattei V, et al: Expression of the CD40 receptor on Reed Sternberg cells (RS): A highly reliable tool and a new

clue for understanding the pathophysiology of Hodgkin's disease (HD) (abstract 1261). Proc Am Soc Clin Oncol 13:373, 1994.

6. Hellman S, Jaffe ES, DeVita VT Jr: Hodgkin's disease, in DeVita VT Jr, Hellman S, Rosenberg SA (eds): Cancer: Principles and Practice of Oncology, p 1696. Philadelphia, JB Lippincott, 1989.

7. Hagemeister FB: Controversies in management of Hodgkin's disease, in Freireich EJ, Kantarjian H (eds): Therapy of Hematopoietic Neoplasia, p 249. New York, Marcel Dekker, 1991.

8. Stein H, Hansmann ML, Lennert K, et al: Reed-Sternberg and Hodgkin cells in lymphocyte-predominant Hodgkin's disease of nodular subtype contain J chain. Am J Clin Pathol 86:292–297, 1986.

9. MacLennan KA, Bennett MH, Tu A, et al: Relationship of histopathologic features to survival and relapse in nodular sclerosing Hodgkin's disease. Cancer 64:1686–1693, 1989.

10. Ferry J, Linggood R, Convery K, et al: Hodgkin's disease, nodular sclerosis type. Implications of histologic subclassification. Cancer 71:457–463, 1993.

11. d'Amore ESG, Lee CKK, Aeppli DM, et al: Lack of prognostic value of histopathologic parameters in Hodgkin's disease, nodular sclerosis subtype. Arch Path Lab Med 116:856–861, 1992.

12. Masih AS, Weisenburger DD, Vose JM, et al: Histologic grade does not predict prognosis in optimally treated, advanced-stage nodular sclerosing Hodgkin's disease. Cancer 69:228–232, 1992.

13. Hess JL, Bodis S, Pinkus G, et al: Histopathologic grading of Hodgkin's disease: Lack of prognostic significance in 254 surgically staged patients. Cancer 74:708–714, 1994.

14. Evans AS, Guttensohn NM: A population-based case-control study of EBV and other viral antibodies among persons with Hodgkin's disease and their siblings. Int J Cancer 34:149, 1984.

15. Ree HJ, Strauhen JA, Khan AA, et al: Human immunodeficiency virus-associated Hodgkin's disease: Clinicopathologic studies of 24 cases and preponderance of mixed cellularity type characterized by the occurrence of fibrohistiocytoid stromal cells. Cancer 67:1614, 1991.

16. Jochelson M, Mauch P, Balikian J, et al: The significance of the residual mediastinal mass in treated Hodgkin's disease. J Clin Oncol 3:637–640, 1985.

17. Glatstein E, Guernsey JM, Rosenberg SA, et al: The value of laparotomy and splenectomy in the staging of Hodgkin's disease. Cancer 24:709, 1969.

18. Hagemeister FB, Fuller LM, Martin RG: Staging laparotomy: Findings and applications to treatment decisions, in Fuller LM, Hagemeister FB, Sullivan MP, et al (eds): Hodgkin's Disease and Non-Hodgkin's Lymphoma in Adults and Children, p 170. New York, Raven Press, 1988.

19. Hagemeister FB, Fesus SM, Lamki LM, et al: Role of the gallium scan in Hodgkin's disease. Cancer 65:1090, 1990.

20. Kaplan HS, Rosenberg SA: Current status of clinical trials: Stanford experience, 1962–1972. NCI Monogr 36:363–371, 1973.

21. Rosenberg SA, Kaplan HS: Hodgkin's disease and other malignant lymphomas. Calif Med 113:23, 1970.

22. Rosenberg SA, Kaplan HS: The evolution and summary results of the Stanford randomized clinical trials for the management of Hodgkin's disease 1962-1984. Int J Radiat Oncol Biol Phys 11:5–22, 1985.

23. Farah R, Ultmann J, Griem M, et al: Extended mantle radiation therapy for pathologic stage I and II Hodgkins disease. J Clin Oncol 6:1047–1052, 1988.

24. Carde P, Burgers JMV, Henry AM, et al: Clinical stages I and II Hodgkin's disease: A specifically tailored therapy according to prognostic factors. J Clin Oncol 6:239, 1988.

25. Tubiana M, Henry-Amar M, Carde P, et al: Toward comprehensive management tailored to prognostic factors of patients with clinical stages I and II in Hodgkins disease. The EORTC lymphoma group controlled clinical trial: 1964–1987. Blood 73: 47–56, 1989.

26. Lee CK, Aeppli DM, Bloomfield CD, et al: Hodgkin's disease: A reassessment of prognostic factors following modification of radiotherapy. Int J Radiat Oncol Biol Phys 13:983–991, 1987.

27. Hagemeister FB, Fuller LM, Sullivan JA, et al: Treatment of stage I and II mediastinal Hodgkin's disease: A comparison of involved fields, extended fields, and involved fields followed by MOPP in patients staged by laparotomy. Radiology 141:783, 1981.

28. Anderson H, Deakin DP, Wagstaff J, et al: A randomised study of adjuvant chemotherapy after mantle radiotherapy in supradiaphragmatic Hodgkin's disease PS IA-IIB: A report from the Manchester lymphoma group. Br J Cancer 49:695–702, 1984.

29. Leslie NT, Mauch PM, Hellman S: Stage IA to IIB supradiaphragmatic Hodgkin's disease: Long term survival and relapse frequency. Cancer 55:2072–2078, 1985.

30. Specht L, Nissen LI: Prognostic significance of tumour burden in Hodgkin's disease PS I and II. Scand J Haematol 36:367–375, 1986.

31. Hagemeister FB, Fuller LM, Sullivan JA, et al: Treatment of patients with stages I and II nonmediastinal Hodgkin's disease. Cancer 50:2307–2313, 1982.

32. Zagars G, Rubin P: Laparotomy staged IA versus IIA Hodgkin's disease. A comparative study with evaluation of prognostic factors for stage IIA disease. Cancer 56:864–873, 1985.

33. Tubiana M, Henry-Amar M, Hayat M, et al: Prognostic significance of the number of involved areas in the early stages of Hodgkin's disease. Cancer 54:885–894, 1984.

34. Cimino G, Biti GP, Anselmo AP, et al: MOPP chemotherapy versus extended-field radiotherapy in the management of pathological stages I-IIA Hodgkin's disease. J Clin Oncol 7:732, 1989.

35. Biti GP, Cimino G, Cartoni C, et al: Extended-field radiotherapy is superior to MOPP chemotherapy for the treatment of pathologic stage I-IIA Hodgkin's disease: Eight-year Update of an Italian prospective randomized study. J Clin Oncol 10:378–382, 1992.

36. Longo DL, Glatstein E, Duffey FL, et al: Radiation therapy versus combination chemotherapy in the treatment of early stage Hodgkin's disease: Seven-year results of a prospective randomized trail. J Clin Oncol 9:906–917, 1991.

37. Fuller LM, Hagemeister FB, North LB, et al: The adjuvant role of two cycles of MOPP and low-dose lung irradiation in stage IA through IIB Hodgkin's disease: Preliminary results. Int J Radiat Oncol Biol Phys 14:683–692, 1988.

38. Horning SJ, Hoppe RT, Hancock SL et al: Vinblastine, bleomycin, and methotrexate: An effective adjuvant in favorable Hodgkin's disease. J Clin Oncol 6:1822–1831, 1988.

39. Sutcliffe SB, Gospodarowicz MK, Bergsagel DE, et al: Prognostic groups for management of localized Hodgkin's disease. J Clin Oncol 3:393, 1985.

40. Gospodarowicz MK, Sutcliffe SB, Bergsagel DE, et al: Radiation therapy in clinical stage I and II Hodgkin's disease. Eur J Cancer 28:1841–1846, 1992.

41. Hagemeister FB, Fuller LM, Martin RG: Staging laparotomy: Findings and applications to treatment decisions, in Fuller LM, Hagemeister FB, Sullivan MP, et al (eds): Hodgkin's Disease and Non-Hodgkin's Lymphomas in Adults and Children, pp 203–229. New York, Raven Press, 1988.

42. Pavlovsky S, Maschio M, Santarelli MT, et al: Randomized trial of chemotherapy versus chemotherapy plus radiotherapy for stage I-II Hodgkin's disease. J Natl Cancer Inst 80:1466, 1988.

43. Zittoun R, Audebert A, Hoerni B, et al: Extended versus involved fields combined with MOPP chemotherapy in early clinical stages of Hodgkin's disease. J Clin Oncol 3:207, 1985.

44. Andrieu JM, Montagnon B, Asselain B, et al: Chemotherapy-

radiotherapy association in Hodkgin's disease, clinical stages IA, II$_2$A: Results of a perspective clinical trial with 166 patients. Cancer 46:2126, 1980.

45. Ferme C, Teillet F, d'Ajay MF, et al: Combined modality in Hodgkin's disease: Comparison of six versus three courses of MOPP with clinical and surgical restaging. Cancer 54:2324, 1984.

46. Ferrant A, Hamir V, Binon J, et al: Combined modality therapy for mediastinal Hodgkin's disease: Prognostic significance of constitutional symptoms and size of disease. Cancer 55:317, 1985.

47. Leopold KA, Canellos GP, Rosenthal D, et al: Stage IA-IIB Hodgkin's disease: Staging and treatment of patients with large mediastinal lymphadenopathy. J Clin Oncol 7:1059, 1989.

48. Krikorian J, Portlock C, Mauch P: Hodgkin's disease presenting below the diaphragm: A review. J Clin Oncol 4:1551, 1986.

49. Givens SS, Fuller LM, Hagemeister FB, et al: Treatment of lower torso stages I and II Hodkgin's disease with or without adjuvant MOPP. Cancer 66:69, 1990.

50. Stein RS, Golomb HM, Wiernik PH, et al: Anatomic substages of stage IIIA Hodgkin's disease: Follow-up of a collaborative study. Cancer Treat Rep 66:733, 1982.

51. Hoppe RT, Cox RS, Rosenberg SA, et al: Prognostic factors in pathologic stage III Hodgkin's disease. Cancer Treat Rep 104:145, 1982.

52. Mazza P, Miniaci G, Lauria F, et al: Prognostic significance of lymphography in stage III Hodgkin's disease. Eur J Cancer Clin Oncol 20:1393, 1984.

53. Rogers RW, Fuller LM, Hagemeister FB, et al: Reassessment of prognostic factors in stage IIIA and IIIB Hodgkin's disease treated with MOPP and radiotherapy. Cancer 47:2196, 1985.

54. Mauch P, Goffman T, Rosenthal DS, et al: Stage III Hodgkin's disease: Improved survival with combined modality as compared with radiotherapy alone. J Clin Oncol 3:1166, 1985.

55. Hagemeister FB, Fuller LM, Velasquez WS, et al: Two cycles of MOPP and radiotherapy: Effective treatment for stage IIIA and IIIB Hodgkin's disease. Ann Oncol 2:25, 1990.

56. Henkelman GC, Hagemeister FB, Fuller LM: Two cycles of MOPP and radiotherapy for stage IIIA and stage IIIB Hodgkin's disease. J Clin Oncol 6:1293, 1988.

57. Bonadonna G, Santoro A, Zucoli R, et al: Improved five-year survival in advanced Hodgkin's disease by combined modality approach. Cancer Clin Trials 2:217, 1979.

58. Longo DL, Young RC, Wesley M, et al: Twenty years of MOPP therapy for Hodgkin's disease. J Clin Oncol 4:1295, 1986.

59. DeVita VT Jr, Simon RM, Hubbard SM, et al: Curability of advanced Hodgkin's disease with chemotherapy: Long-term follow-up of MOPP-treated patients at the National Cancer Institute (NCI). Ann Intern Med 92:587, 1980.

60. Pillai G, Hagemeister FB, Velasquez WS, et al: Prognostic factors for stage IV Hodgkin's disease treated with MOPP with or without bleomycin. Cancer 55:691, 1985.

61. Bonadonna G, Valagussa P, Santoro A: Alternating non-cross resistant combination chemotherapy or MOPP in stage IV Hodgkin's disease: A report of eight-year results. Ann Intern Med 104:739, 1986.

62. Canellos GP, Anderson JR, Propert KJ, et al: Chemotherapy of advanced Hodgkin's disease with MOPP, ABVD, or MOPP alternating with ABVD. N Engl J Med 327:1478–1484, 1992.

63. Connors JM, Klimo P: MOPP/ABV hybrid chemotherapy for advanced Hodgkin's disease. Semin Hematol 24:35, 1987.

64. Yahalom J, Ryu J, Straus DJ, et al: Impact of adjuvant radiation on the patterns and rate of relapse in advanced-stage Hodgkin's disease treated with alternating chemotherapy combinations. J Clin Oncol 9:2193, 1991.

65. Fisher RI, DeVita VT Jr, Hubbard SP, et al: Prolonged disease-free survival in Hodgkin's disease with MOPP reinduction after relapse. Ann Intern Med 90:761, 1979.

66. Philip T, Dumont J, Teillet F, et al: High dose chemotherapy and autologous bone marrow transplantation in refractory Hodgkin's disease. Br J Cancer 53:737, 1986.

67. Aisenberg AC: Hodgkin's disease—prognosis, treatment, and etiologic and immunologic considerations. N Engl J Med 270:505, 508, 617, 1964.

68. Kim H, Betti C, Boggs DR: The development of non-Hodgkin's lymphoma following the treatment of Hodgkin's disease. Cancer 46:2596, 1980.

69. Miettinen M, Franssila KO, Saxen E: Hodgkin's disease, lymphocytic predominance nodular: Increased incidence of subsequent non-Hodgkin's lymphoma. Cancer 51:2293, 1983.

70. Glicksman AJ, Pajack TF, Gottlieb A, et al: Second malignant neoplasms in patients successfully treated for Hodgkin's disease: A Cancer and Leukemia Group B study. Cancer Treat Rep 66:1035, 1982.

71. Bookman MA, Longo DL: Concomittant illness in patients treated for Hodgkin's disease. Cancer Treat Rev 13:77, 1986.

72. Halperin EC, Greenberg MS, Suit HD: Sarcoma of bone and soft tissue following treatment of Hodgkin's disease. Cancer 53:232, 1984.

73. List AF, Doll DC, Grew FA: Lung cancer in Hodgkin's disease: Association with previous radiotherapy. J Clin Oncol 3:215, 1985.

74. Wallner KE, Leibel SA, Wara WM: Squamous cell carcinoma of the head and neck after radiation therapy for Hodgkin's disease: A report of two cases and a review of the literature. Cancer 56:1052, 1985.

75. Tucker MA, Misfeldt D, Coleman CN, et al: Cutaneous malignant melanoma after Hodgkin's disease. Ann Intern Med 102:37, 1985.

76. Thar TL, Million RR: Complications of radiation treatment of Hodgkin's disease. Semin Oncol 7:174, 1980.

77. Carey RW, Lingood RM, Wood W, et al: Breast cancer developing in four women cured of Hodgkin's disease. Cancer 54:2234, 1984.

78. Doniach I: Comparison of the carcinogenic effect of X-irradiation with radioactive iodine on the rat's thyroid gland. Br J Cancer 11:67, 1956.

79. Tamura K, Shimaoka K, Friedman M: Thyroid abnormalities associated with treatment of lymphoma. Cancer 47:2704, 1981.

80. Carmosino L, DiBenedetto A, Feffer S: Thymic hyperplasia following successful chemotherapy: A report of two cases and a review of the literature. Cancer 56:1526, 1985.

81. Rowley MJ, Leach DR, Warner GA, et al: Effect of graded doses of ionizing radiation on the human testis. Radiat Res 59:665, 1974.

82. Sieber SM, Correa P, Dalgard DW, et al: Carcinogenic and other adverse effects of procarbazine in nonhuman primates. Cancer Res 38:2125, 1978.

83. daCunha MF, Meistrich ML, Fuller LM, et al: Recovery of spermatogenesis after treatment for Hodgkin's disease: Limiting dose of MOPP chemotherapy. J Clin Oncol 2:571, 1984.

84. Viviani S, Santoro A, Ragni G, et al: Gonadal toxicity after combination chemotherapy for Hodgkin's disease: Comparative results of MOPP versus ABVD. Eur J Cancer Clin Oncol 21:601, 1985.

85. Chapman RM, Sutcliffe SB, Malpes JS: Cytotoxic induced ovarian failure in Hodgkin's disease. JAMA 242:1877, 1979.

86. Schilsky RL, Sherins RJ, Hubbard RJ, et al: Long-term follow-up of ovarian function in women treated with MOPP chemotherapy for Hodgkin's disease. Am J Med 71:552, 1981.

87. Cohn KE, Stewart JR, Fajardo LF, et al: Heart disease following radiation. Medicine 46:281, 1967.

88. Carmel RJ, Kaplan HS: Mantle irradiation in Hodgkin's disease: An analysis of technique, tumor eradication, and complications. Cancer 37:2813, 1976.

89. Byhardt R, Brace K, Ruckdeschl J, et al: Dose and treatment factors in radiation-related pericardial effusion associated with the mantle technique for Hodgkin's disease. Cancer 35:795, 1975.

90. Applefield MM, Cole JF, Pollock SH, et al: The late appearance of chronic pericardial disease in patients treated by radiotherapy for Hodgkin's disease. Ann Intern Med 94:338, 1981.

91. Brosius FC, Waller BF, Roberts WC: Radiation heart disease: Analyses of 16 young (age 15–33) necropsy patients who received over 3,500 rads to the heart. Am J Med 70:519, 1981.

92. Burns RJ, Bar-Shlomo BZ, Druck MN, et al: Detection of radiation cardiomyopathy by gated radionuclide angiography. Am J Med 74:297, 1983.

93. Morton DL, Glancy DL, Joseph WL, et al: Management of patients with radiation-induced pericarditis with effusion: A note on the development of aortic regurgitation in two of them. Chest 64:291, 1973.

94. McReynolds RA, Gold GL, Roberts WC: Coronary heart disease after mediastinal irradiation for Hodgkin's disease. Am J Med 60:39, 1976.

95. Minow RA, Benjamin RS, Gottlieb JA: Adriamycin (NSC-123127) cardiomyopathy: An overview with determination of risk factors. Cancer Chemother Rep 6:195, 1975.

96. Von Hoff DD, Layard MW, Basa P, et al: Risk factors for doxorubicin-induced congestive heart failure. Ann Intern Med 91:710, 1979.

97. Minow RA, Benjamin RS, Lee ET, et al: Adriamycin cardiomyopathy-risk factors. Cancer 39:1397, 1977.

98. Billingham ME, Bristow MR, Glatstein E, et al: Anthracycline cardiotoxicity: Endomyocardial biopsy evidence of enhancement by irradiation. Am J Surg Pathol 1:17, 1977.

99. Weinstein P, Greenwald ES, Grossman J: Unusual cardiac reaction to chemotherapy following mediastinal irradiation in a patient with Hodgkin's disease. Am J Med 60:152, 1976.

100. Hellman S, Mauch P, Goodman RL, et al: The place of radiotherapy in the treatment of Hodgkin's disease. Cancer 42:971, 1978.

101. Castellino RA, Glatstein E, Turbow MM, et al: Latent radiation injury of lungs or heart activated by steroid withdrawal. Ann Intern Med 80:593, 1974.

102. Weiss RB, Poster DJ, Penta JS: The nitrosoureas and pulmonary toxicity. Cancer Treat Rev 8:111, 1981.

103. Cersosimo RJ, Liciardello JT, Matthews SJ, et al: Acute pneumonitis associated with MOPP chemotherapy for Hodgkin's disease. Drug Intell Clin Pharm 18:609, 1984.

104. Levi JA, Wiernik PH, Diggs CH: Combination chemotherapy of advanced previously treated Hodgkin's disease with streptozotocin, CCNU, Adriamycin and bleomycin. Med Radiat Oncol 3:33, 1977.

105. Engel IA, Strauss DJ, Acker M, et al: Osteonecrosis in patients with malignant lymphoma: A review of 25 cases. Cancer 48:1245, 1981.

CHAPTER 8

Multiple Myeloma and Other Plasma-Cell Dyscrasias

Vali Papadimitrakopoulou, MD, *and* Donna M. Weber, MD
Department of Hematology, The University of Texas M. D. Anderson Cancer Center, Houston, Texas

Multiple myeloma is a malignant proliferation of plasma cells that produces a monoclonal globulin. Certain complications, such as anemia, fractures, pain, renal failure, infection, and hypercalcemia, are common. Standard chemotherapies for multiple myeloma include combinations of melphalan (Alkeran)-prednisone or vincristine (Oncovin)-doxorubicin (Adriamycin, Rubex)-dexamethasone (VAD), and the median survival remains 3 years. Recent investigations have focused on more intensive therapies with bone marrow or blood stem-cell support in the hope of producing more marked degrees and longer duration of disease control. Disorders closely related to multiple myeloma, including solitary plasmacytoma of bone, Waldenström's macroglobulinemia, amyloidosis, monoclonal gammopathy of unknown significance, and heavy-chain disease, must be distinguished using clinical and laboratory data. This review focuses on the etiology, diagnosis, clinical features, and therapy for multiple myeloma and other plasma-cell disorders.

MULTIPLE MYELOMA

In 1995, approximately 12,500 new patients will be diagnosed with multiple myeloma in the United States. The annual incidence of this disease per 100,000 population is 4.7 among white men and 3.2 among white women; among African-Americans, the frequency doubles to 10.2 in men and 6.7 in women. This racial difference presumably is due to unknown genetic factors and is not explained by socioeconomic differences. The median age of patients with multiple myeloma is approximately 70 years according to population surveys, but it is approximately 60 years based on reports of treatment trials. The incidence increases with age; the incidence in males at age 70 is almost 70 per 100,000 for African-American and 32 per 100,000 for white populations.[1]

Etiology

No predisposing events appear to be important in the etiology of multiple myeloma. Some events that have been suggested include radiation exposure (in radiologists and radium-dial workers), occupational exposure (in agricultural, chemical, metallurgical, rubber plant, pulp, and paper workers and leather tanners), and chemical exposure to benzene, formaldehyde, epichlorohydrin, hair dyes, paint sprays, and asbestos.[1] Most of these associations have been countered by negative correlations.[1]

Initially, it was reported that survivors of the atomic bombing of Hiroshima had a greater risk of developing myeloma, but longer follow-up data now refute any evidence of increased risk among survivors.[2] Some reports do suggest that a lower level of prolonged radiation exposure over many years may have caused some cases of multiple myeloma among radiologists and radium-dial painters.[3,4] However, no relationship has been shown between the incidence of multiple myeloma and exposure to diagnostic x-rays or therapeutic irradiation.[1,5]

Another factor associated with myeloma may be intense, prolonged exposure to benzene, such as was experienced by unprotected workers in the rubber industry.[6] Whereas the relationship of benzene and its metabolites to the occurrence of leukemia has been accepted by many, benzene's relationship with myeloma remains unproven. With current industrial safeguards, such a relationship may never be shown.

Although myeloma is not an inherited disease, there have been numerous case reports of it in the same family.[1] However, a case-control study revealed no significant increase in myeloma among relatives of patients with multiple myeloma, other hematologic malignancies, or other cancers.[7]

Biology

Multiple myeloma has been the prototype of monoclonal malignancies, in this case, of plasma cells; the disease may result from a mutation of terminally differentiated B cells or even from early but committed B cells that manifest clinically as more differentiated plasma cells.[8–10] The expression of multiple markers of different cell lineages (B and T) by plasma cells supports the possibility of either an aberrant expression of unexpected phenotypes, as in other malignancies, or a stem-cell precursor from which all hematopoietic cells arise.[11]

Multiple studies have described the cytogenetics of myeloma. Although no karyotypic abnormalities are specific, frequent aberrations of chromosomes 1 and 14, the latter containing the heavy-chain immunoglobulin gene, have been noted.[12] In addition, specific translocations have been described, including t(11;14), t(14;18), and t(8;14). Other chromosomal abnormalities include 6q-, 7q-, 5q-, t(9;22), and 17p+. Abnormal expression of the bcl-2 protein has also been noted in patients without a t(14;18) translocation. [12] Mutations of the *ras* oncogene and *p53* gene mutations have been reported, especially in patients with late disease.[13-15] The *ras* mutation correlates with a low treatment response rate,[13] and the *p53* gene mutation has been noted in patients with extramedullary proliferation of plasma cells.[15]

A variety of cytokines stimulate the growth of malignant plasma cells in vitro. Interleukin-6 (IL-6), considered the most important myeloma growth factor, binds to the IL-6 receptor on plasma cells, which is made up of an alpha chain (IL-6R) and a beta-transducer chain (gp130).[16,17] IL-6 acts in concert with an extensive cytokine network (IL-1, IL-3, IL-7, IL-11, 6-colony-stimulating factor [CSF], granulocyte-macrophage colony-stimulating factor [GM-CSF, sargramostim (Leukine)], and tumor-necrosis factor [TNF]) to promote the growth of malignant plasma cells. Other factors (alpha interferon [IFN-α], gamma interferon [IFN-γ], and IL-4) appear to inhibit plasma-cell growth, and some of these cytokines may play a role in therapy.

Recent attention has been focused on the development of the multidrug resistance (*MDR*) phenotype in resistant myeloma, especially after prolonged therapy. The increased expression of p-glycoprotein, the *MDR* gene product, has been noted, particularly after high cumulative doses of vincristine and doxorubicin.[18]

Clinical Features

The clinical presentation of multiple myeloma is quite variable. Bone pain, especially from compression fractures of vertebrae or ribs, is the most common symptom. Findings that suggest a diagnosis of multiple myeloma include lytic bone lesions, anemia, azotemia, hypercalcemia, and recurrent infections. However, approximately 20% of patients with multiple myeloma are free of symptoms and are diagnosed by chance.

Bone Disease: Bone lesions are due to accelerated osteoclast formation with increased resorption of areas infiltrated by plasma cells.[19,20] These changes are mediated by osteoclast-activating factors now known to consist of an extensive network of cytokines.[20] Specifically, IL-1-beta induces and is synergistic with the bone-resorbing activity of IL-6.[20,21] IL-6 increases natural killer-cell activity and appears to play a role in modulating the effects of TNF and IL-1 on bone.[20]

Bone disease is best assessed by a skeletal survey. At diagnosis, nearly 70% of patients with myeloma have lytic bone lesions with or without a pathologic fracture.[22] Nuclear bone imaging is less sensitive, because bone scan isotopes are not taken up by lytic lesions.[23] Magnetic resonance imaging (MRI) provides greater detail of bone disease, paraspinal involvement, and epidural components; abnormalities are noted on MRI even when x-rays are normal,[24] and they appear to be predictive of early disease progression in asymptomatic patients.[25] Painful vertebral compression fractures, with or without cord pressure, require radiation therapy. Decompressive laminectomy is rarely necessary for cord compression, but surgery may be required for radioresistant myeloma, retropulsed bone fragments, or intervertebral disc disease when severe pain and/or disability result. Fractures of the femora or humeri require intramedullary rod fixation. The role of prophylactic bisphosphonate therapy in the reduction of osteoclastic activity and bone mineralization maintenance is under study.[26]

Hypercalcemia: Hypercalcemia (defined as a corrected serum calcium level greater than 11.5 mg/dL) occurs in approximately 20% of patients with newly diagnosed multiple myeloma and results from progressive bone destruction. Treatment includes generous hydration and prompt combination chemotherapy, which should always include a glucocorticoid. Therapy with a regimen of VAD, which produces a rapid response, is most appropriate (Table 1). High-dose pulse dexamethasone remains an alternative, especially for patients who require palliative radiotherapy for the spine. Maximum physical activity should be encouraged, because prolonged immobility exacerbates hypercalcemia. If the aforementioned measures are ineffective, another form of treatment, such as a bisphosphonate, calcitonin, or gallium nitrate, should be considered.

Renal Failure: Approximately 20% of patients with myeloma present with renal insufficiency,[27] and another 20% will develop this complication during the course of their disease.[28] Casts of Bence Jones protein in the distal tubule are the most common cause of renal failure,[29,30] but hypercalcemia, dehydration, and hyperuricemia are also contributing factors.[28] Uncommonly, amyloidosis or light-chain deposition disease may also contribute to renal failure.

Treatment includes hydration, sodium bicarbonate for acidosis, allopurinol for hyperuricemia, and hemodialysis, if necessary. Plasmapheresis has been proposed by some researchers,[28] but controlled studies have not shown that it yields any improvement in survival. In approximately 50% of previously untreated patients with renal

TABLE 1

*Proposed Standard Treatment
of Multiple Myeloma*

Disease or patient status	Treatment approach
Untreated myeloma	
Low-risk disease, age > 70 yr, or major medical problems	Melphalan/prednisone: melphalan, 8 mg/m²/d PO on days 1–4, + prednisone, 100 mg/d PO on days 1–4
High-risk disease, renal failure, or hypercalcemia	VAD: vincristine, 0.4 mg/d IV, + doxorubicin, 9 mg/m²/d IV (both drugs by continuous infusion) on days 1–4, + dexamethasone, 40 mg/d PO on days 1–4, 9–12, and 17–20
With spine radiotherapy	Dexamethasone, 40 mg/d PO on days 1–4, 9–12, and 17–20
Resistant myeloma	
Resistant to melphalan/ prednisone	
Unresponsive	Dexamethasone or VAD (as above)
Relapsing	VAD (as above)
Resistant to VAD or dexamethasone	Cyclophosphamide, 600 mg/m²/d, + etoposide, 180 mg/m²/d IV, on days 1–5, + GM-CSF,ª 0.125 mg/m²/d
Primary refractory disease < 1 yr (high or intermediate tumor mass	Myeloablative therapy + blood or marrow stem-cell transplantation

ª GM-CSF = granulocyte-macrophage colony-stimulating factor
Adapted, with permission, from Weber DM, Alexanian R: Multiple myeloma and other plasma cell dyscrasias, in Pazdur R (ed): Medical Oncology: A Comprehensive Review, p 51. Huntington, NY, PRR Inc, 1993.

failure, the kidney function normalizes with chemotherapy for the myeloma.[30] VAD therapy for myeloma does not require dose adjustments for renal failure, since none of the drugs is metabolized by the kidneys and VAD provides the best chance for rapid disease control.

Anemia: A normocytic, normochromic anemia is present in 60% of patients at diagnosis.[27] Anemia is due primarily to the decreased production of red blood cells secondary to marrow infiltration with plasma cells. Patients with or without renal failure also have decreased levels of erythropoietin, which may worsen the degree of anemia.[31] Recombinant erythropoietin, 4,000 U given subcutaneously three times a week, may be useful if the serum level of erythropoietin is inappropriately low compared with the hematocrit (eg, less than 200 U/L).

Infection: Many patients with myeloma develop bacterial infections that may be quite serious. In the past, gram-positive organisms (eg, *Streptococcus pneumoniae* and *Staphylococcus aureus*) and *Hemophilus influenzae* have been the most common pathogens, although more recently, gram-negative organisms have become an increasing problem.[32] The increased susceptibility of patients with myeloma to bacterial infection has been attributed to impairments in host-defense mechanisms, which include depressed levels of uninvolved immunoglobulins, impaired antibody response,[33] decreased numbers and adherence of polymorphonuclear leukocytes,[34] decreased surface immunoglobulin expression,[35] poor opsonic activity,[36] depressed lysozyme levels,[37] and decreased complement levels.[38]

Diagnosis

A diagnosis of multiple myeloma usually requires the presence of bone marrow plasmacytosis and a monoclonal protein in urine or serum. One class of immunoglobulins is produced in excess, whereas the other immunoglobulin (Ig) classes are depressed. Biclonal elevations of myeloma protein levels occur in less than 1% of cases.[39] The types of monoclonal protein produced are IgG (60%), IgA (20%), IgD (2%), IgE (less than 0.1%), and light-chain kappa or lambda (18%). Fewer than 5% of patients with myeloma are unable to secrete or synthesize light- or heavy-chain immunoglobulins, and their disease is categorized as nonsecretory.[40] The workup should include quantification of both involved and uninvolved immunoglobulins.

After chemotherapy has been instituted, serum and 24-hour urinary measurements of abnormal proteins should be evaluated serially to confirm that the myeloma protein(s) have been reduced markedly in patients who have responded to treatment.

Staging and Prognosis

Different criteria have been used to stage myeloma at different institutions, primarily because of the lack of standard definitions and consistency among investigators (Tables 2 and 3).[41] This results in part from the imprecise quantification of the extent of bone lesions, hypercalcemia (eg, degree of immobility), and factors other than marrow infiltration that cause anemia (eg, renal failure). Our criteria are outlined in Table 3, which also includes a correlation of pretreatment tumor mass and response with survival time. As expected, the short-

TABLE 2

Durie-Salmon Staging System for Multiple Myeloma

Stage	Criteria	Myeloma cell mass (× 10^{12} cells/m²)

I	Hemoglobin > 10 g/dL
	Serum calcium ≤ 12 mg/dL (normal)
	Normal bone or solitary plasmacytoma on x-ray
	Low M-component production rates:
	  IgG < 5 g/dL
	  IgA < 3 g/dL
	  Urine light-chain M-component < 4 g/24 h
		< 0.6 (low)

II	Not fitting stage I or III	0.6–1.20 (intermediate)

III	Hemoglobin < 8.5 g/dL
	Serum calcium > 12 mg/dL
	Multiple lytic bone lesions on x-ray
	High M-component production rates:
	  IgG > 7 g/dL
	  IgA > 5 g/dL
	  Urine light-chain M-component > 12 g/24 h
		> 1.20 (high)

Subclassification	Criterion
A	Normal renal function (serum creatinine level < 2.0 mg/dL)
B	Abnormal renal function (serum creatinine level ≥ 2.0 mg/dL)

Adapted from Durie BG, Salmon SE.[41]

TABLE 3

M. D. Anderson Cancer Center Staging and Survival Data for Multiple Myeloma

Stage	Criteria	Myeloma cell mass
I	Hemoglobin > 10.5 g/dL Corrected serum calcium ≤ 11.5 mg/dL Serum myeloma protein < 4.5 g/dL	Low
II	Not fitting stage I or III	Intermediate
III	Hemoglobin < 8.5 g/dL Corrected serum calcium > 12 mg/dL	High

Tumor response to therapy	Survival by tumor mass (mo)[a]		
	High	Intermediate	Low
Unresponsive	7	17	30
Improved[b]	17	27	32
Responsive	32	50	59

[a] Median value [b] A 50% to 75% reduction of myeloma protein production
Adapted, with permission, from Weber DM, Alexanian R: Multiple myeloma and other plasma cell dyscrasias, in Pazdur R (ed): Medical Oncology: A Comprehensive Review, p 52. Huntington, NY, PRR Inc, 1993.

High serum lactate dehydrogenase (LDH) levels have also been associated with shortened survival (9 months), as well as with drug resistance, in both treated and untreated patients with myeloma.[44,45] Other features associated with an elevated LDH level include lymphoma-like extraosseous disease, plasma-cell leukemia, and plasma-cell hypodiploidy.[44,45]

Shortened survival also has been noted in patients with DNA hypodiploidy,[46] low plasma-cell RNA levels,[47] high plasma-cell labeling indices,[48,49] plasmablastic histology,[50] and the expression of common acute lymphoblastic leukemia antigen (CALLA).[10] Patients with decreased plasma-cell RNA or DNA hypodiploidy are also less likely to respond to chemotherapy.[46,47]

Response Criteria

Because the criteria of response to treatment have varied among institutions, response rates have been difficult to compare. The criteria for partial remission (PR) at M. D. Anderson Cancer Center are a 75% reduction in the rate of myeloma protein production, a 95% reduction in the rate of Bence Jones protein excretion, and less than 5% marrow plasma cells. Bence Jones protein is reduced more rapidly in responders than is serum myeloma protein because of the rapid renal catabolism of light chains. To achieve a complete remission (CR) of disease, there must be disappearance of the

est survival occurs in patients with a high tumor mass that is unresponsive, and the longest survival is observed in patients with a low tumor mass that is responsive.

The level of serum beta-2-microglobulin (β_2M) is an important and convenient prognostic indicator because it reflects the extent of disease in a single measurement. This protein is a catabolic product of the histocompatibility leukocyte antigen that is present on the surface of all nucleated cells and in higher concentration on lymphoid and plasma cells.[42] Because β_2M is excreted by the kidneys, high levels of it are present when renal failure occurs, which complicates the interpretation of a high value. In a study of three staging systems and other variables by Bataille et al, β_2M was the single most important indicator of prognosis.[43]

M-protein by immunofixation and no monoclonal plasma cells in the bone marrow, as assessed by the most sensitive techniques.

Treatment

Concurrent with the management of specific complications, chemotherapy should be instituted promptly to reduce the number of malignant plasma cells. However, despite the development of many different chemotherapeutic regimens, there has been little improvement in outcome during the past 25 years. Only 5% to 10% of patients live longer than 10 years, and there is no hint of a cured subgroup.[51,52] The role of chemotherapy will be addressed here separately for patients with newly diagnosed, responsive, primary resistant, or relapsing disease.

Previously Untreated Patients: Since their introduction in the 1960s, intermittent courses of melphalan and prednisone (MP) have been the standard chemotherapy for multiple myeloma.[53] One schedule for this regimen is shown in Table 1. To standardize the absorption differences of melphalan and to ensure its bioavailability, evidence of adequate myelosuppression should be confirmed 2 to 3 weeks after beginning treatment. If the myeloma is unresponsive, the dose should be increased in 20% increments every 4 to 5 weeks until adequate myelosuppression occurs.[54]

The MP combination has been shown to induce a remission in approximately 40% of previously untreated patients.[55] The median remission for these patients has been approximately 2 years, and the median survival has been approximately 3 years. The low frequency of CR (10%) and the inevitable relapse indicate that inherent drug resistance represents the major impediment to long-term remission or cure.

Many attempts have been made to improve the results of MP with combinations, including multiple alkylating agents, vincristine, a nitrosourea, and/or an anthracycline, but none of these agents has proved superior.[56–63] An exception may be the M2 protocol (carmustine [BiCNU], cyclophosphamide [Cytoxan, Neosar], vincristine [Oncovin], melphalan, and prednisone), which showed a better outcome in two studies,[64,65] but other studies have failed to confirm this finding.[63,66] Virtually all studies have failed to show a superiority in terms of overall survival, and a recent meta-analysis of these studies showed no overall difference in efficacy.[67]

Combination chemotherapy with VAD-based regimens has also been studied. In one study of newly diagnosed patients, the response rate was 55%, and the onset of remission was more rapid, but there was no improvement in survival over standard regimens.[68] The rapid responses may provide some advantage for patients with hypercalcemia, renal failure, or severe bone pain because such complications must be reversed quickly.

In addition to VAD, dexamethasone alone is as effective as MP for newly diagnosed patients, but the response rate is slightly lower than that with VAD.[69] It remains the most active single agent against myeloma and does not contribute to myelosuppression or secondary myelodysplasia.

Interferon (IFN) inhibits plasma-cell growth and has induced responses in 5% to 10% of patients with refractory myeloma and in 15% of patients with newly diagnosed disease.[70,71] Results of studies with IFN and other agents have varied widely. The combination of IFN with standard regimens of alkylating agents plus a glucocorticoid was no more effective than MP in one study,[72] was associated with a higher response rate and similar survival in another study,[73] and showed a high rate of CR with uncertain survival in a third study.[74] Further clarification of the role of IFN in the primary treatment of multiple myeloma is necessary.

Early myeloablative consolidation therapy supported by autologous bone marrow transplantation (ABMT) also has been investigated.[75–77] A controlled study described significant prolongation of remission and survival when myeloablative therapy followed a primary induction program.[78] However, although the CR and PR rates were higher than those with conventional therapy, so was the frequency of treatment-related deaths. Further studies are necessary to determine the role of early myeloablative treatment and to identify the patient groups who are likely to benefit.

Remission Maintenance: The median remission for responding patients is approximately 2 years. Indefinite maintenance therapy with alkylating agents has not shown prolongation of overall remission or survival compared with no maintenance therapy and the resumption of MP when disease relapse occurs.[79] Patients can experience multiple unmaintained remissions that usually become progressively shorter. Continued alkylating agent treatment also exposes approximately 2% of patients to the risk of acute leukemia.[80,81] Also, it has been shown that the residual tumor cells in remission are less proliferative and more resistant to chemotherapy (cytokinetic resistance).[54]

The Italian Myeloma Study Group initially reported a superior response duration (26 vs 14 months) with IFN-α as a remission treatment compared with no maintenance therapy,[82] but in an updated analysis, no survival benefit was shown.[83] Other studies also have shown no gain in survival and divergent results with regard to remission duration.[84–88] After treatment with high-dose melphalan plus total body irradiation and ABMT, maintenance IFN-α was associated with longer remission and survival than no therapy in patients achieving CR.[89] This suggested a possible role for IFN against minimal residual disease (asymptomatic myeloma, solitary plasmacytoma at high risk for progression, or complete remission after chemotherapy). However, IFN is associated with side effects (myalgia, fever, and myelosuppression), is costly, and requires injections. Therefore, further studies are necessary to confirm the role of IFN-α as maintenance therapy, especially in direct comparison with melphalan and prednisone.

Relapsing and Refractory Disease: Approximately one half of patients with newly diagnosed multiple myeloma are unresponsive to chemotherapy. In addition, all patients with an initial response will suffer relapse except for the 2% who die of unrelated diseases. For patients whose disease relapses after an unmaintained remission of longer than 6 months, approximately 50% achieve a second, but shorter, remission with resumption of the original therapy.[90]

VAD is the treatment of choice for patients with disease that relapses despite MP treatment. Approximately 40% of patients with relapsing disease responded to this treatment compared with 25% of patients whose disease was unresponsive to primary therapy.[91] Dexamethasone induced similar results in patients with primary resistant disease but was inferior to VAD in patients with relapsing disease.[92] Patients with hypodiploidy or low RNA content of plasma cells were much less likely to respond to treatment. The median duration of remission was 10 months, and subsequent myeloablative consolidation therapy did not result in improved survival.[93]

Resistance to VAD has been attributed in part to the increased expression of p-glycoprotein, the multidrug resistance gene (*MDR-1*) product that increases the active-transport efflux of certain chemotherapeutic agents (doxorubicin and vincristine) from neoplastic cells.[94,95] Agents that inhibit p-glycoprotein activity, such as verapamil and cyclosporine (Sandimmune), have been combined with chemotherapy in an attempt to circumvent such resistance. Both verapamil and cyclosporine administered with VAD have produced modest response rates, in the face of severe toxicity.[96,97] Further studies of newer analogs, such as PSC-833, are currently underway.

High-dose alkylating agents have also been effective in treating VAD-resistant myeloma. Intravenous melphalan, at a dose of 90 to 100 mg/m^2 (five times the standard dose) has produced responses in one third of such patients but with a very short remission.[98] A combination of high-dose cyclophosphamide (3 g/m^2), etoposide (VePesid,

900 mg/m^2), and GM-CSF was also effective in a similar percentage of patients and induced a median remission of 8 months[99]; high LDH and β$_2$M levels were indicators of a low response rate and short survival times.[100]

Bone Marrow and Stem-Cell Transplantation: All patients younger than 60 years old who have advanced and resistant myeloma should be considered early for intensive therapy supported by bone marrow or blood stem-cell transplantation. Patients should undergo such therapy with minimal delay to prevent disabling complications that could preclude later treatment.

Only 5% of patients with multiple myeloma are candidates for allogeneic transplantation because of the age restriction (younger than 50 years old) and the availability of a matched sibling donor. Treatments consist of either a combination of one or more alkylating agents with total body irradiation or a combination of high-dose busulfan (Myleran)-cyclophosphamide. In the European Bone Marrow Transplant Registry (EBMTR) study, the CR rate was 43% among 90 patients who underwent transplantation and were followed for up to 7 years. The overall survival rate at 5 years was 40%, and the disease-free survival rate was 31%.[101] Similar results have been published by others.[102,103] The sustained disappearance of myeloma protein for more than 5 years has been confirmed in several patients, perhaps due to an additional "graft vs myeloma" effect.[100,101] The available data do not suggest a plateau of disease-free survival, so the potential for curability remains uncertain. Survival was longer for patients who had already responded to treatment prior to the procedure and for patients who had received only one previous regimen. In view of the high mortality rate (approximately 30% to 40% during the first year), this procedure remains a secondary option for selected younger patients with a high benefit/risk ratio.

ABMT in support of myeloablative treatment has been administered more often than allogeneic BMT despite the likelihood of reinfusion of tumor cells with either purged or unpurged marrow.[104] Several investigators showed that high-dose melphalan, either alone or combined with total body irradiation, followed by autologous BMT could produce remission in many patients with recurrent and resistant myeloma.[105] Similar results have been achieved with other intensive regimens, such as a combination of Thiotepa (Thioplex), busulfan, and cyclophosphamide.[106] A sequence of two regimens of high-dose melphalan supported by autologous stem cells has also been used successfully.[107,108]

Patients who appear more likely to benefit from myeloablative therapy supported by autologous cell transplantation have become better defined recently.[109,110]

Survival was markedly improved among patients with primary resistant disease of less than 1 year's duration (survival equals 83 months) in comparison to similar patients who did not undergo transplantation (37 months). Similarly, myeloablative therapy for patients with a longer duration of primary resistant disease, with disease in resistant relapse, or during remission, showed no meaningful benefit compared with control patients.[110,111]

In conclusion, most experts agree that standard myeloablative therapy with autologous bone marrow or blood stem-cell transplantation is not suitable for most patients older than 60 years, with serious or comorbid conditions, or with relapsing disease. The benefit of myeloablative therapy seems most likely in patients with early primary resistant disease, but further studies are necessary to confirm the best treatment groups. Intensive therapy should be administered early before progenitor cells are compromised by prolonged treatment with alkylating agents and before resistance develops.

OTHER PLASMA-CELL DYSCRASIAS

Other plasma-cell dyscrasias include monoclonal gammopathy of unknown significance, solitary plasmacytoma of bone, asymptomatic myeloma, Waldenström's macroglobulinemia, amyloidosis, and immunoglobulin heavy-chain diseases (Table 4).

Monoclonal Gammopathy of Unknown Significance

Monoclonal gammopathy of unknown significance, or benign monoclonal gammopathy, occurs in 1% of normal individuals older than 40 years. The frequency of this disorder rises progressively with age. No specific underlying diseases have been identified.[112] In a study of 241 patients with this disorder, 53 patients (22%) developed multiple myeloma, macroglobulinemia, amyloidosis, or another malignant lymphoproliferative disorder over a span of 19 years.[113] Multiple myeloma developed in 36 patients after a median interval of 9.6 years. The course of the myeloma and the response to therapy were similar to those of other patients treated promptly after diagnosis. This study demonstrates that monoclonal gammopathy of unknown significance usually does not progress to a malignant disorder. The long period of stability supports the value of indefinite periodic observation for such patients.

Solitary Plasmacytoma of Bone

Approximately 5% of patients with myeloma have a solitary plasmacytoma of bone, and approximately one half demonstrate myeloma protein in serum or urine

TABLE 4

Common Laboratory Features of Plasma-Cell Dyscrasias

Multiple myeloma

Marrow plasmacytosis > 15%
Monoclonal immunoglobulin peak (usually > 3.0 g/dL)
Decreased levels of uninvolved immunoglobulins
Bence Jones protein
Lytic bone lesions

Asymptomatic myeloma

Same as multiple myeloma but without symptoms
Hemoglobin > 10.5 g/dL
Normal serum calcium level
Monoclonal immunoglobulin peak < 4.5 g/dL)

Solitary plasmacytoma of bone

Solitary bone lesion due to plasma cell tumor
Negative skeletal survey and spinal MRI
Negative bone marrow
No anemia, hypercalcemia, or renal disease
Preserved levels of uninvolved immunoglobulins

Monoclonal gammopathy of unknown significance (MGUS)

Monoclonal immunoglobulin level < 3.0 g/dL
Bone marrow plasma cells ≤ 10%
No bone lesions
Asymptomatic
Usually preserved levels of uninvolved immunoglobulins

Amyloidosis without myeloma

Same as MGUS + evidence of amyloidosis on biopsy

Adapted, with permission, from Weber DM, Alexanian R: Multiple myeloma and other plasma cell dyscrasias, in Pazdur R (ed): Medical Oncology: A Comprehensive Review, p 55. Huntington, NY, PRR Inc, 1993.

(Table 4).[114] MRI may reveal abnormalities not detected by bone survey and may cause patients who were previously classified as having solitary plasmacytoma to be upstaged to multiple myeloma.[115] Treatment should include radiation therapy of at least 45 Gy. Patients with solitary plasmacytoma of bone often progress to multiple myeloma, with only 20% to 30% of patients remaining free of disease for more than 10 years.[114–116] When disease progression does occur, the median time for its occurrence is 2 years; however, IFN-α may be a useful adjuvant treatment to inhibit the evolution of the disease.

Asymptomatic Myeloma

In approximately 20% of patients, multiple myeloma is diagnosed by chance, during screening examinations that reveal an elevated serum protein concentration in asymptomatic patients. Features of low tumor mass are usually present, with a hemoglobin level greater than 10.5 g/dL; serum myeloma protein level less than 4.5 g/dL; and an absence of renal disease, hypercalcemia, and lytic bone lesions.[117] Chemotherapy should be withheld until there is risk of a complication, except for the few patients who present with more advanced disease, who should receive chemotherapy promptly.

Recent studies have defined the prognostic criteria for groups at high risk for early disease progression: a lytic bone lesion, serum myeloma protein level greater than 3 g/dL, and/or Bence Jones protein level greater than 50 mg/d.[118] The presence of a lytic bone lesion and a second high-risk feature predicts progression within 1 year; the absence of these features has been associated with much slower progression (ie, median longer than 5 years).[118]

The results of a French study revealed similar parameters for early disease progression, such as bone marrow plasmacytosis greater than or equal to 25% and a hemoglobin level less than or equal to 12 g/dL.[119] In one study, a plasma-cell-labeling index of more than 0.4% predicted disease progression within 6 months,[48] and in yet another study, 40% of asymptomatic patients were found to have bone marrow involvement on MRI, a feature that also predicted early progression, despite normal skeletal surveys.[25]

Waldenström's Macroglobulinemia

Waldenström's macroglobulinemia is an uncommon, low-grade lymphoid malignancy composed of mature plasmacytoid lymphocytes with monoclonal IgM production. It usually affects older persons and may cause symptoms due to tumor infiltration (marrow, lymph nodes, and/or spleen), circulating IgM (hyperviscosity, cryoglobulinemia, and/or cold agglutinin anemia); and tissue deposition of IgM (neuropathy, glomerular disease, and/or amyloidosis).[120–122] With hyperviscosity syndrome, patients may have visual disturbances, dizziness, cardiopulmonary symptoms, decreased consciousness, and a bleeding diathesis. Neuropathy usually is caused by an IgM antibody reacting with a myelin-associated glycoprotein (MAG).[123,124]

Therapy for hyperviscosity consists of plasmapheresis followed by chemotherapy to control the malignant proliferation. With alkylating agent-steroid combinations, responses occurred in approximately 50% of previously untreated patients, with a median survival of 5 years.[125–127] Cladribine (Leustatin) has induced a remission of long duration in more than 80% of previously

untreated patients with only two courses of therapy.[128] Cladribine has induced responses in 54% of patients with primary resistant disease and in 83% of patients with relapsing disease occurring while off treatment. Patients whose disease is in resistant relapse are less likely to benefit from such treatment (response rate 18%) and should be considered for more intensive therapies.[122]

Amyloidosis

Amyloidosis (AL) is a plasma-cell proliferative process that results from organ deposition of amyloid fibrils that consist of the NH_2-terminal amino acid residues of the variable portion of the light-chain immunoglobulin molecule. This disease occurs in 10% of patients with multiple myeloma and may produce nephrotic syndrome, cardiomyopathy, hepatomegaly, neuropathy, macroglossia, anemia, carpal tunnel syndrome, and periorbital purpura.[129] Serum immunoelectrophoresis showed a monoclonal immunoglobulin in serum or urine in 89% of patients with amyloidosis.[129] Lambda light chains are more likely than kappa light chains to produce amyloidosis. Diagnosis can be made in many patients by a Congo red-stained sample of subcutaneous fat aspirates or a rectal biopsy that exhibits apple-green birefringence with polarized light.

The median survival is approximately 13 months for all patients, and the presence of congestive heart failure, renal failure, hepatomegaly, and significant weight loss worsens the prognosis.[130,131] An elevated serum creatinine level, the diagnosis of multiple myeloma, the presence of orthostatic hypotension, and a serum M protein had a significant adverse effect on patients who lived 1 year after diagnosis.[130,131] Treatment with colchicine has been ineffective, but approximately 15% of patients appear to benefit from MP chemotherapy, and recent reports suggest an even higher response rate of 30%.[132,133]

Immunoglobulin Heavy-Chain Diseases

Heavy-chain diseases are plasma-cell dyscrasias characterized by the production of heavy-chain immunoglobulin molecules (gamma, alpha, mu) that lack light chains. Alpha-chain disease results from lymphocyte and plasma-cell infiltration of the mesenteric nodes and small bowel and has features of malabsorption, such as diarrhea, weight loss, abdominal pain, edema, and clubbing.[134] The heavy-chain molecule may be detected in serum, jejunal secretions, and urine.

Patients with gamma heavy-chain disease may present with fever, weakness, lymphadenopathy, hepatosplenomegaly, and Waldeyer's ring involvement. Eosinophilia, leukopenia, and thrombocytopenia are common. Treatment with regimens similar to those used for non-Hodgkin's lymphoma may be effective.

Mu heavy-chain disease is seen exclusively in patients with chronic lymphocytic leukemia. Vacuolated plasma cells are common in the marrow, and many patients have lambda light chains in urine. Therapy is similar to that for chronic lymphocytic leukemia.

CONCLUSIONS

There have been many recent advances in the understanding of plasma-cell dyscrasias. The origin of myeloma from a primordial stem cell is suggested by the phenotypic expression of early precursors. Various cytokines are produced that may serve as myeloma cell growth factors or osteoclast-activating factors.

Better understanding of the prognostic factors of myeloma (labeling index), markers of drug resistance, such as LDH; and measures of tumor cell mass, such as β_2M, has helped to identify patients who may benefit from a sequence of VAD followed by the early consideration of myeloablative therapy supported by autologous bone marrow or blood stem-cell transplantation. Melphalan and prednisone appear reasonable for use in older patients and patients with good prognostic features. Certain cytostatic agents, such as IFN-α, must be investigated further as part of primary therapy and for remission maintenance. Waldenström's macroglobulinemia and mu heavy-chain disease have been treated with alkylating agents, but cladribine appears promising for superior long-term results. Further studies are needed to understand the etiology and biology of plasma-cell dyscrasias, to develop more effective agents and regimens for controlling these disorders, and to justify immunologic and other procedures for sustaining long-term control.

The authors wish to acknowledge Dr. Raymond Alexanian for his clinical and scientific advice.

REFERENCES

1. Riedel DA, Pottern LM: The epidemiology of multiple myeloma. Hematol Oncol Clin North Am 6:225–247, 1992.

2. Preston DL, Kusumi S, Tomonaga M, et al: Cancer incidence in atomic bomb survivors. Part III: Leukemia, lymphoma, and multiple myeloma, 1950–1987. Radiat Res 137:568–597, 1994.

3. Lewis EB: Leukemia, multiple myeloma, and aplastic anemia in American radiologists. Science 142:1492–1494, 1963.

4. Stebbings JH, Lucas HF, Stehney AF: Mortality from cancers of major sites in female radium dial workers. Am J Ind Med 5:435–459, 1984.

5. Bofetta P, Stellman SD, Garfinkle L: A case control study of multiple myeloma nested in the American Cancer Society prospective study. Int J Cancer 43:554–559, 1989.

6. Rinsky RA, Smith AB, Hornung R, et al: Benzene and leukemia. N Engl J Med 316:1044–1050, 1987.

7. Bourguet C, Grufferman S, Delzell E, et al: Multiple myeloma

and family history of cancer: A case control study. Cancer 56:2133–2139, 1985.

8. Epstein J, Barlogie B, Katzmann F, et al: Phenotypic heterogeneity in aneuploid multiple myeloma indicates pre-B-cell involvement. Blood 71:861–865, 1988.

9. Epstein J: Myeloma phenotype: Clues to disease origin and manifestation. Hematol Oncol Clin North Am 6:249–256, 1992.

10. Barlogie B, Epstein J, Selvanayagam P, et al: Plasma cell myeloma—new biological insights and advances in therapy. Blood 73:865–879, 1989.

11. Durie BG: The biology of multiple myeloma. Hematol Oncol 6:77–81, 1988.

12. Durie BG: Cellular and molecular genetic features of myeloma and related disorders. Hematol Oncol Clin North Am 6:463–477, 1992.

13. Neri A, Murphy JP, Cro L, et al: Ras oncogene mutation in multiple myeloma. J Exp Med 170:1715–1725, 1989.

14. Portier M, Moles JP, Mazars GR, et al: p53 and Ras gene mutations in multiple myeloma. Oncogene 7:2539–2543, 1992.

15. Neri A, Baldini L, Trecca D, et al: p53 gene mutations in multiple myeloma are associated with advanced forms of the malignancy. Blood 81:128–135, 1993.

16. Gearing DP, Comeau MR, Friend DJ, et al: The IL-6 signal transducer gp130: An oncostatin M receptor and affinity converter for the LIF receptor. Science 255:1434–1437, 1992.

17. Ip NY, Nye SH, Boulton TG, et al: CNTF and LIF act on neuronal cells via shared signaling pathways that involve the IL-6 signal transducing receptor component gp130. Cell 69:1121–1132, 1992.

18. Grogan TM, Spier CM, Salmon SE, et al: P-glycoprotein expression in human plasma cell myeloma: Correlation with prior chemotherapy. Blood 81:490–495, 1993.

19. Bataille R, Chappard D, Marcelli C, et al: Recruitment of new osteoblasts and osteoclasts is the earliest critical event in the pathogenesis of human multiple myeloma. J Clin Invest 88:62–66, 1991.

20. Bataille R, Chappard D, Klein B: Mechanisms of bone lesions in multiple myeloma. Hematol Oncol Clin North Am 6:285–295, 1992.

21. Bataille R, Jourdan M, Zhang X, et al: Serum levels of IL-6, a potent myeloma cell growth factor, as a reflection of disease severity in plasma cell dyscrasias. J Clin Invest 84:2008–2011, 1989.

22. Kyle RA: Multiple myeloma: Review of 869 cases. Mayo Clin Proc 50:29–40, 1975.

23. Woolfenden JM, Pitt MJ, Durie BG, et al: Comparison of bone scintigraphy and radiography in multiple myeloma. Radiology 134:723–728, 1980.

24. Ludwig H, Tscholakoff D, Neuhold A, et al: Magnetic resonance imaging of the spine in multiple myeloma. Lancet II:364–366, 1987.

25. Moulopoulos L, Dimopoulos MA, Smith TL, et al: Prognostic significance of magnetic resonance imaging in patients with asymptomatic multiple myeloma. J Clin Oncol 13:251–256, 1995.

26. Berenson J, Lichtenstein A, Porter L, et al: Pamidronate disodium reduces the occurrence of skeletal related events (SRE) in advanced multiple myeloma (MM) (abstract). Blood 84:386a, 1994.

27. Salmon SE, Cassady JR: Plasma cell neoplasms, in DeVita VT, Hellman S, Rosenberg SA (eds): Cancer: Principles and Practice of Oncology, 3rd ed, pp 1853–1895. Philadelphia, JB Lippincott, 1989.

28. Johnson WJ, Kyle RA, Pineda AA, et al: Treatment of renal failure associated with multiple myeloma: Plasmapheresis, hemodialysis, and chemotherapy. Arch Intern Med 150:863–869, 1990.

29. Rota S, Mougenot B, Baudouin B, et al: Multiple myeloma and severe renal failure: A clinicopathologic study of outcome and prognosis in 34 patients. Medicine 66:126–137, 1987.

30. Alexanian R, Barlogie B, Dixon D: Renal failure in multiple

myeloma: Pathogenesis and prognostic implications. Arch Intern Med 150:1693–1695, 1990.

31. Ludwig H, Fritz E, Kotzmann H, et al: Erythropoietin treatment of anemia associated with multiple myeloma. N Engl J Med 322:1693–1699, 1993.

32. Savage DG, Lindebaum J, Garrett TJ: Biphasic pattern of bacterial infection in multiple myeloma. Ann Intern Med 96:47–50, 1982.

33. Fahey JL, Scoggins R, Utz J: Infection, antibody response, and gamma globulin components in myeloma and macroglobulinemia. Am J Med 35:698–707, 1963.

34. MacGregor RR, Negendank WG, Schreiber AD: Impaired granulocyte adherence in multiple myeloma: Relationship to complement system, granulocyte delivery, and infection. Blood 51:591–599, 1978.

35. Chen Y, Bhoopalam N, Yakulis V, et al: Changes in lymphocyte surface immunoglobulins in myeloma and the effect of an RNA-containing plasma factor. Ann Intern Med 83:625–631, 1975.

36. Cheson BD, Plass RR, Rothstein G: Defective opsonization in multiple myeloma. Blood 55:602–606, 1980.

37. Karle H, Hansen NE, Plesner T: Neutrophil defect in multiple myeloma: Studies on intraneutrophilic lysozyme in multiple myeloma and malignant lymphoma. Scand J Haematol 17:62–70, 1976.

38. Spitler LE, Spath P, Petz N, et al: Phagocytes and C4 in paraproteinemia. Br J Haematol 29:279–292, 1975.

39. Pruzanski W, Ogryzlo MA: Abnormal proteinuria in malignant diseases. Adv Clin Chem 13:335–382, 1970.

40. River GL, Tewksbury DA, Fundenberg HH: 'Nonsecretory' multiple myeloma. Blood 40:204–206, 1972.

41. Durie BG, Salmon SE: A clinical staging system for multiple myeloma: Correlation of measured myeloma cell mass with presenting clinical features, response to treatment, and survival. Cancer 36:842–854, 1975.

42. Alexanian R, Barlogie B, Fritsche H: Beta2-microglobulin in multiple myeloma. Am J Hematol 20:345–351, 1985.

43. Bataille R, Durie BG, Grenier J, et al: Prognostic factors and staging in multiple myeloma: A reappraisal. J Clin Oncol 4:80–87, 1986.

44. Barlogie B, Smallwood L, Smith TL, et al: High serum levels of lactate dehydrogenase identify a high grade lymphoma-like myeloma. Ann Intern Med 110:521–525, 1989.

45. Dimopoulos MA, Barlogie B, Smith TL, et al: High serum lactate dehydrogenase level as a marker for drug resistance and short survival in multiple myeloma. Ann Intern Med 115:931–935, 1991.

46. Smith TL, Barlogie B, Alexanian R: Biclonal and hypodiploid multiple myeloma. Am J Med 80:841–843, 1986.

47. Barlogie B, Alexanian R, Gehan EA, et al: Marrow cytometry and prognosis in myeloma. J Clin Invest 72:853–861, 1983.

48. Greipp PR, Kyle RA: Clinical, morphological, and cell kinetic differences among multiple myeloma, monoclonal gammopathy of undetermined significance, and smoldering multiple myeloma. Blood 62:166–171, 1983.

49. Kyle RA: Prognostic factors in multiple myeloma. Hematol Oncol 6:125–130, 1988.

50. Greipp PR, Raymond NM, Kyle RA, et al: Multiple myeloma: Significance of plasmablastic subtype in morphological classification. Blood 65:305–310, 1985.

51. Alexanian R, Dimopoulos MA: The treatment of multiple myeloma. N Engl J Med 330:484–489, 1994.

52. Alexanian R, Dimopoulos MA: Management of multiple myeloma. Semin Hematol 32:20–30, 1995.

53. Alexanian R, Haut A, Khan A, et al: Treatment for multiple myeloma: Combination chemotherapy with different melphalan dose regimens. JAMA 208:1680–1685, 1969.

54. Boccadoro M, Pileri A: Standard chemotherapy for myelomatosis: An area of great controversy. Hematol Oncol Clin North Am 6:371–382, 1992.

55. McLaughlin P, Alexanian R: Myeloma protein kinetics following chemotherapy. Blood 60:851–855, 1982.

56. Bergsagel DE, Bailey A, Langley G, et al: The chemotherapy of plasma cell myeloma and the incidence of acute leukemia. N Engl J Med 301:743–746, 1979.

57. Salmon SE, Haut A, Bonnet J, et al: Alternating combination chemotherapy and levamisole improves survival in multiple myeloma. J Clin Oncol 1:453–461, 1983.

58. Pavlovsky S, Saslavsky J, Tezanos Pinto M, et al: A randomized trial of melphalan and prednisone versus melphalan, prednisone, cyclophosphamide, meCCNU, and vincristine in untreated multiple myeloma. J Clin Oncol 2:836–840, 1984.

59. Cooper M, McIntyre OR, Propert K, et al: Single, sequential, and multiple alkylating agent therapy for multiple myeloma. J Clin Oncol 4:1331–1339, 1986.

60. Peest D, Deicher H, Coldewe R, et al: Melphalan and prednisone versus vincristine, BCNU, Adriamycin, melphalan, and dexamethasone induction chemotherapy and interferon maintenance treatment in multiple myeloma. Onkologie 13:458–460, 1990.

61. Boccadoro M, Marmont F, Tribalto M, et al: Multiple myeloma: VMCP/VBAP alternating combination chemotherapy is not superior to melphalan and prednisone, even in high risk patients. J Clin Oncol 9:444–448, 1991.

62. MacLennan ICM, Chapman C, Dunn J, et al: Combined chemotherapy with ABCM versus melphalan for treatment of myelomatosis. Lancet 339:200–205, 1992.

63. Oken MM, Tsiatis A, Abramson N: Comparison of standard (MP) with intensive (VBMCP) therapy for the treatment of multiple myeloma (MM) (abstract). Proc Am Soc Clin Oncol 3:270, 1984.

64. Case DC, Lee BJ, Clarkson BD: Improved survival times with melphalan, prednisone, vincristine, and BCNU. Am J Med 63:897–903, 1977.

65. Tirelli U, Crivallari D, Carbone A, et al: Combination chemotherapy for multiple myeloma with melphalan, prednisone, cyclophosphamide, vincristine, and carmustine (BCNU) (M-2 protocol). Cancer Treat Rep 66:1971–1973, 1982.

66. Hansen OP, Clausen NAT, Drivsholm A, et al: Phase III study of intermittent five drug regimen (VBCMP) versus intermittent three drug regimen (VMP) versus intermittent melphalan and prednisone (MP) for myelomatosis. Scand J Haematol 35:518–524, 1985.

67. Gregory WM, Richards MA, Malpas JS: Combination chemotherapy versus melphalan and prednisolone in the treatment of multiple myeloma: An overview of published trials. J Clin Oncol 10:334–342, 1992.

68. Alexanian R, Barlogie B: New treatment strategies for multiple myeloma. Am J Hematol 35:194–198, 1990.

69. Alexanian R, Dimopoulos MA, Delasalle K, et al: Primary dexamethasone treatment in multiple myeloma. Blood 80:887–890, 1992.

70. Mellstedt H, Ahre A, Bjorkholm M, et al: Interferon therapy in myelomatosis. Lancet I:245–247, 1979.

71. Quesada JR, Alexanian R, Hawkins M, et al: Treatment of multiple myeloma with recombinant alpha-interferon. Blood 67:275–278, 1986.

72. Cooper MR, Dear K, McIntyre OR, et al: A randomized clinical trial comparing melphalan/prednisone with or without alpha-2b in newly diagnosed patients with multiple myeloma: A Cancer and Leukemia Group B study. J Clin Oncol 11:155–160, 1993.

73. Osterborg A, Bjorkholm M, Bjoreman M, et al: Natural

interferon-a in combination with melphalan/prednisone in the treatment of multiple myeloma stages II and III: A randomized study from the Myeloma Group of Central Sweden. Blood 81:1428–1434, 1993.

74. Oken MM, Kyle RA, Greipp PR, et al: Complete remission induction with VBMCP and interferon in multiple myeloma (abstract). Proc Am Soc Clin Oncol 8:272, 1989.

75. Attal M, Huguet F, Schlaifer D, et al: Intensive combined therapy for previously untreated aggressive myeloma. Blood 79:1130–1136, 1992.

76. Gore M, Selby P, Viner C, et al: Intensive treatment of multiple myeloma and criteria for complete remission. Lancet II:871–881, 1989.

77. Harousseau J, Milpied N, Laporte J, et al: Double intensive therapy in high risk multiple myeloma. Blood 79:2827–2833, 1992.

78. Attal M, Harousseau J, Stoppa A, et al: High dose therapy in multiple myeloma: A prospective randomized study of the 'Intergroupe Francais du Myelome' (abstract). Blood 82:198a, 1993.

79. Alexanian R, Gehan EA, Haut A, et al: Unmaintained remissions in multiple myeloma. Blood 51:1005–1011, 1978.

80. Bergsagel DE: Chemotherapy of myeloma: Drug combinations versus single agents, an overview, and comments on acute leukemia in myeloma. Hematol Oncol 6:159–166, 1988.

81. Cuzick J, Erskine S, Edelman D, et al: A comparison of the incidence of the myelodysplastic syndrome and acute myeloid leukemia following melphalan and cyclophosphamide treatment for myelomatosis. Br J Cancer 55:523–529, 1987.

82. Mandelli F, Avvisati G, Amadori S, et al: Maintenance treatment with recombinant interferon alpha-2b in patients with multiple myeloma responding to conventional induction therapy. N Engl J Med 322:1430–1434, 1990.

83. Avvisati G, Boccadoro M, Petrucci MT, et al: Interferon alpha as maintenance treatment in multiple myeloma: The Italian experience (abstract), in Program and Abstracts of the IV International Workshop on Multiple Myeloma, pp 87–88. Rochester, Minn, 1993.

84. Westin J: Interferon therapy during the plateau phase of multiple myeloma: An update of a Swedish multicenter study. Semin Oncol 18(suppl 7):37–40, 1991.

85. Brownman GP, Rubin S, Walker I, et al: Interferon alpha 2b maintenance therapy prolongs progression-free and overall survival in plasma cell myeloma: Results of a randomized trial (abstract). Proc Am Soc Clin Oncol 13:408, 1994.

86. Ludwig H, Cohen AM, Huber H, et al: Interferon with VMCP compared to VMCP for induction and IFN compared to control for remission maintenance in multiple myeloma (abstract). Proc Am Soc Clin Oncol 13:408, 1994.

87. Salmon SE, Crowley J: Impact of glucocorticoids and interferon on outcome in multiple myeloma (abstract). Proc Am Soc Clin Oncol 11:316, 1992.

88. Peest D, Bartels H, Bartl R, et al: Melphalan/prednisone versus polychemotherapy for remission induction and interferon A for maintenance treatment in multiple myeloma: A trial of the German Myeloma Treatment Group (abstract), in Program and Abstracts of the IV International Workshop on Multiple Myeloma, p 145. Rochester, Minn, 1993.

89. Cunningham D, Powles R, Malpas JS, et al: A randomized trial of maintenance therapy with Intron-a following high dose melphalan and ABMT in myeloma (abstract). Proc Am Soc Clin Oncol 12:364, 1993.

90. Petrucci MT, Avvisati G, Tribalto M, et al: Intermediate dose (25 mg/m²) intravenous melphalan for patients with multiple myeloma in relapse or refractory to standard treatment. Eur J Haematol 42:233–237, 1989.

91. Barlogie B, Smith TL, Alexanian R: Effective treatment of advanced multiple myeloma refractory to alkylating agents. N Engl J Med 310:1353–1356, 1984.

92. Alexanian R, Barlogie B, Dixon D: High dose glucocorticoid treatment of resistant myeloma. Ann Intern Med 105:8–11, 1986.

93. Alexanian R, Dimopoulos MA, Smith TL, et al: Limited value of myeloablative therapy for late multiple myeloma. Blood 83:512–516, 1994.

94. Riordan J, Ling V: Purification of P-glycoprotein from plasma membrane vesicles of Chinese hamster ovary cell mutants with reduced colchicine permeability. J Biol Chem 254:12701–12705, 1979.

95. Grogan T, Spier C, Salmon S, et al: P-glycoprotein expression in human plasma cell myeloma. Blood 81:490–495, 1993.

96. Sonneveld P, Durie BG, Lokhorst H, et al: Modulation of multidrug-resistant multiple myeloma by cyclosporin. Lancet 340:255–259, 1992.

97. Salmon SE, Dalton WS, Grogan TM, et al: Multidrug resistant myeloma: Laboratory and clinical effects of verapamil as a chemosensitizer. Blood 78:44–50, 1991.

98. Barlogie B, Jagannath S, Dixon D, et al: High-dose melphalan and granulocyte-macrophage colony-stimulating factor for refractory multiple myeloma. Blood 76:677–680, 1990.

99. Dimopoulos MA, Delasalle K, Champlin R, et al: Cyclophosphamide and etoposide therapy with GM-CSF for VAD-resistant multiple myeloma. Br J Haematol 83:240–244, 1993.

100. Dimopoulos MA, Weber D, Hester J, et al: Intensive sequential therapy for VAD-resistant multiple myeloma. Leuk Lymphoma 13:479–484, 1994.

101. Gahrton G, Tura S, Ljungman P, et al: Allogeneic bone marrow transplantation in multiple myeloma. N Engl J Med 325:1267–1273, 1991.

102. Bensinger WI, Buckner CD, Clift RA, et al: A phase I study of busulfan and cyclophosphamide in preparation for allogeneic marrow transplant for patients with multiple myeloma. J Clin Oncol 10:1492, 1992.

103. Cavo M, Tura S, Rosti G, et al: Allogeneic BMT for multiple myeloma (MM): The Italian experience. Bone Marrow Transplant 7(suppl 2):31–32, 1991.

104. Anderson KC, Barut BA, Ritz J, et al: Monoclonal antibody-purged autologous bone marrow transplantation therapy in multiple myeloma. Blood 77:712–720, 1991.

105. Jagannath S, Barlogie B: Autologous bone marrow transplantation for multiple myeloma. Hematol Oncol Clin North Am 6:437, 1992.

106. Dimopoulos MA, Alexanian R, Przepiorka D, et al: Thiotepa, busulfan, and cyclophosphamide: A new preparative regimen for autologous stem cell transplantation in high-risk multiple myeloma. Blood 82:2324–2328, 1993.

107. Jagannath S, Vesole DH, Glenn L, et al: Low-risk intensive therapy for multiple myeloma with combined autologous bone marrow and blood stem cell support. Blood 80:1666–1672, 1992.

108. Vesole DH, Barlogie B, Jagannath S: High-dose therapy for refractory multiple myeloma: Improved prognosis with better supportive care and double transplants. Blood 84:950–956, 1994.

109. Alexanian R, Dimopoulos MA, Hester J, et al: Early myeloablative therapy for multiple myeloma. Blood 84:4278–4282, 1994.

110. Alexanian R, Dimopoulos MA, Hester J, et al: Limited value of myeloablative therapy for late multiple myeloma. Blood 83:512–516, 1994.

111. Attal M, Huynh A, Shlaifer D, et al: Intensive combined therapy for previously untreated aggressive myeloma: Long-term follow-up (abstract). Blood 84:180a, 1994.

112. Kyle RA, Finkelstein S, Elveback LR: Incidence of mono-

clonal proteins in a Minnesota community with a cluster of multiple myeloma. Blood 40:719–724, 1972.

113. Kyle RA: Monoclonal gammopathy of undetermined significance and smoldering multiple myeloma. Eur J Haematol 43(suppl 1):70–75, 1989.

114. Dimopoulos MA, Goldstein J, Fuller L, et al: Curability of solitary bone plasmacytoma. J Clin Oncol 10: 587–590, 1992.

115. Dimopoulos MA, Moulopoulos A, Delasalle K, et al: Solitary plasmacytoma of bone and asymptomatic multiple myeloma. Hematol Oncol Clin North Am 6:359–369, 1992.

116. Chak LY, Cox RS, Bostwick DG, et al: Solitary plasmacytoma of bone: Treatment, progression, and survival. J Clin Oncol 5:1811–1815, 1987.

117. Kyle RA, Greipp PR: Smoldering multiple myeloma. N Engl J Med 302:1347–1349, 1980.

118. Dimopoulos MA, Moulopoulos A, Smith TL, et al: Risk of disease progression in asymptomatic myeloma. Am J Med 94:57–61, 1993.

119. Facon T, Menard JF, Michaux JL, et al: Prognostic factors in low tumor mass asymptomatic multiple myeloma: A report on 91 patients. Am J Hematol 48:71–75, 1995.

120. Waldenström J: Macroglobulinemia. Adv Metab Dis 2:115–158, 1965.

121. Kyle RA, Gahrton JP: The spectrum of monoclonal IgM monoclonal gammopathy in 430 cases. Mayo Clin Proc 62:719–731, 1987.

122. Dimopoulos MA, Alexanian R: Waldenström's macroglobulinemia. Blood 83:1452–1459, 1994.

123. Nobile-Orazio E, Marmiroli P, Baldini L, et al: Peripheral neuropathy in macroglobulinemia: Incidence and antigen-specificity of M proteins. Neurology 37:1506–1514, 1987.

124. Dalakas MC, Engel WK: Polyneuropathy with monoclonal gammopathy. Ann Neurol 10:45, 1981.

125. MacKenzie MR, Fudenberg HH: Macroglobulinemia—An analysis of 40 patients. Blood 39:874–889, 1972.

126. Case DC Jr, Ervin TJ, Boyd MA, et al: Waldenström's macroglobulinemia: Long-term results with the M-2 protocol. Cancer Invest 9:1–7, 1991.

127. Petrucci MT, Avvisati G, Tribalto M, et al: Waldenström's macroglobulinemia—Results in 34 newly diagnosed patients. J Intern Med 226:443–447,1989.

128. Dimopoulos MA, Kantarjian H, Weber D, et al: Primary therapy of Waldenström's macroglobulinemia with 2-chlorodeoxyadenosine. J Clin Oncol 12:2694–2698, 1994.

129. Kyle R, Gertz M: Primary systemic amyloidosis: Clinical and laboratory features in 474 cases. Semin Hematol 32:45–59, 1995.

130. Kyle RA, Greipp PR, O'Fallon M, et al: Primary systemic amyloidosis: Multivariate analysis for prognostic factors in 168 cases. Blood 68:220–224, 1986.

131. Gertz MA, Kyle RA, Greipp PR: Response rates and survival in primary systemic amyloidosis. Blood 77:257–262, 1991.

132. Marinone G, Quaglini S, Bellotti V, et al: AL amyloidosis: Clinical and therapeutic aspects of an Italian study protocol, in Kisilevsky R, Benson MD, Frangione B, et al (eds): Amyloid and Amyloidosis, pp 206–208. Park Ridge, Ill, Parthenon, 1994.

133. Merlini G: Treatment of primary amyloidosis. Semin Hematol 32:60–79, 1995.

134. Matuchansky C, Cogné M, Lemaire M, et al: Nonsecretory alpha-chain disease with immunoproliferative small-intestinal disease. N Engl J Med 320:1534–1539, 1989.

CHAPTER 9

Allogeneic Marrow Transplantation

Paolo Anderlini, MD, *and* Donna Przepiorka, MD, PhD
Department of Hematology, Section of Bone Marrow Transplantation
The University of Texas M. D. Anderson Cancer Center, Houston, Texas

Allogeneic marrow transplantation is used to reconstitute hematopoiesis in patients who have received myeloablative therapy for a hematologic malignancy or in patients with irreversible marrow failure, to reconstitute the immune system in patients with severe immunodeficiency, and to normalize metabolism in patients with select inherited metabolic deficiency disorders.[1]

Because of the intensity and toxicity associated with allogeneic marrow transplantation, this treatment is generally reserved for patients younger than age 55 whose graft is being provided by a human leukocyte antigen (HLA)-matched related donor; However, in younger patients lacking a compatible related donor, partially matched related and unrelated donors are reasonable alternatives. Improvements in supportive care measures have allowed the successful application of allogeneic marrow transplantation in greater numbers of patients. In 1992, approximately 2,500 allogeneic marrow transplants (BMTs) were reported to the International Bone Marrow Transplant Registry.[2]

PREPARATIVE REGIMENS

Standard Regimens

Eradication of the underlying malignancy and successful engraftment of allogeneic marrow require administration of a preparative regimen of high-dose chemotherapy with or without radiation. Two combinations are well established as preparative regimens for leukemia: cyclophosphamide (Cytoxan, Neosar) plus total-body irradiation (TBI) or busulfan (Myleran) plus cyclophosphamide. TBI has been given as a single dose in the past, but a high incidence of complications, especially interstitial pneumonitis, occurred. Fractionated TBI with lung shielding in combination with cyclophosphamide, 60 mg/kg/d intravenously (IV) for 2 days, has been found to provide adequate antileukemic activity with acceptable toxicity.[3] Fractionation schedules vary and may affect the outcome.[4] Hyperfractionation of TBI also has been investigated, with no apparent benefit reported to date.

Busulfan is administered orally at a dose of 1 mg/kg every 6 hours for 16 doses followed by four doses of cyclophosphamide, 50 mg/kg,[5] or two doses at 60 mg/kg.[6] Randomized studies comparing these drug regimens have not been performed, and it is unclear whether either regimen is significantly better than the other with regard to efficacy or toxicity. Busulfan/cyclophosphamide has been compared with cyclophosphamide/TBI in randomized studies, but the results remain controversial.[7,8]

Successful engraftment of allogeneic bone marrow requires both myeloablation and immunosuppression. Although the dose of busulfan used is myeloablative, it is not sufficiently immunosuppressive to allow engraftment. Cyclophosphamide is immunosuppressive but not myeloablative. TBI is both immunosuppressive and myeloablative. Cyclophosphamide, at 50 mg/kg/d IV for 4 days, is the standard preparative regimen for patients with aplastic anemia who do not require myeloablation.[9] To minimize graft rejection, particularly in previously transfused patients, and to avoid the use of TBI, antithymocyte globulin has been successfully added to cyclophosphamide.[10]

Investigational Regimens

To reduce the post-transplant relapse rate, the standard regimens have been intensified or modified. Either cyclophosphamide or TBI is always included to ensure engraftment. At M. D. Anderson Cancer Center, etoposide (VePesid) has been added to the cyclophosphamide/TBI regimen, with a slight reduction in the dose intensity of TBI. The modified combination has been well tolerated by patients with high-risk early leukemia, and the long-term survival rate has been approximately 60%.[11] For patients with advanced hematologic malignancies, thiotepa (Thioplex) has been added to the busulfan/cyclophosphamide combination. The tolerability of the modified regimens is similar to that of the standard regimens,[12] and in initial studies, survival was modestly improved, compared with that reported for etoposide/cyclophosphamide/TBI.[13] The addition of a bone-seeking radionuclide or a radionuclide conjugated to a monoclonal antileukemia antibody are other potential approaches to improve the antileukemic activity of the preparative regimen without increasing the toxic effect to normal organs.[14]

MARROW HARVEST AND PROCESSING

Marrow Transplantation

Marrow is harvested from the posterior iliac crests under general anesthesia. At M. D. Anderson, this procedure is routinely performed on an outpatient basis. With approximately 150 aspirations, 10 to 15 mL/kg of bone marrow is removed (approximately 5% of the total marrow volume). Ideally, this amount should contain 1 to 4 $\times 10^8$ nucleated cells/kg. The procedure is associated with a very low risk of complications. In a review of 1,270 normal donors in whom marrow harvests were performed,[15] all had the expected amount of pain after the aspiration procedure. Six donors (0.5%) experienced life-threatening complications, 10 (0.8%) experienced significant operative-site morbidity (usually transient neuropathies), and 121 (10%) experienced transient postoperative fever. Worldwide, there have been no deaths directly related to this procedure.

If there is no blood group (ABO) incompatibility between the patient and the donor, the marrow is filtered to remove bone particles and infused IV. Day 0 is designated as the day of marrow infusion. If there is ABO incompatibility, the red cells, plasma, or both may need to be removed from the donor marrow to prevent a hemolytic reaction during infusion. ABO incompatibility can also lead to hemolytic reactions at the time of engraftment and to prolonged red cell aplasia caused by circulating red cell antibodies. Transfusion support for ABO-incompatible BMT recipients differs from that for nontransplant patients, and the choice of the appropriate ABO for each component is based on blood typing performed on the patient after the transplant and on prior knowledge of the details of the incompatibility.[16]

Alternative Sources of Hematopoietic Stem Cells

At M. D. Anderson, allogeneic blood stem-cell transplantation has been evaluated as an alternative to allogeneic BMT. The donors receive granulocyte colony-stimulating factor (filgrastim, Neupogen) injections subcutaneously for mobilization, and stem cells are collected by apheresis in a manner similar to that used to collect single-donor platelets. This approach has eliminated the need for general anesthesia and reduced both morbidity and costs for the donor. Despite concerns about the durability of engraftment and the potential adverse effect of infusing large numbers of donor lymphocytes, preliminary results show that engraftment is rapid, and the incidence of graft-vs-host disease (GVHD) is not significantly higher than that in marrow transplant recipients.[17]

Allogeneic cord-blood stem cells have also been utilized for transplantation. The relatively small numbers of cells in cord-blood collections have generally limited this approach to pediatric recipients. Current reports indicate, however, that cord-blood stem-cell engraftment is durable and that the risk of GVHD in histo-incompatible recipients may be reduced using this approach.[18]

TREATMENT-RELATED COMPLICATIONS

Regimen-Related Complications

Nausea, vomiting, stomatitis, enteritis, alopecia, erythema or rash, and diarrhea occur in most graft recipients and can largely be controlled. Phenytoin is routinely given to prevent seizures from high-dose busulfan. More serious complications, which occur in fewer patients, might include idiopathic interstitial pneumonitis, hemorrhagic cystitis, heart failure and/or pericarditis, hepatic veno-occlusive disease (VOD), and, less commonly, pulmonary hemorrhage. Life-threatening or fatal complications occur in less than 20% of patients. For the standard preparative regimens, regimen-related mortality is approximately 5%.[19]

Patients are screened before transplantation for evidence of underlying organ damage that would increase the risk of regimen-related complications. The best studied condition is hepatic VOD, which is seen histologically as occlusion of the central veins of the liver.[20] Toxicity can also lead to centrilobular necrosis without occlusion of the central veins. The VOD liver toxicity syndrome is characterized by fluid retention with weight gain, tender hepatomegaly, ascites, and hyperbilirubinemia. The condition may also result in liver failure.

Risk factors for VOD include a history of hepatitis, an elevated transaminase level at the time of transplantation, use of methotrexate as GVHD prophylaxis, cytoreductive therapy with a high-dose regimen, and mismatched or unrelated marrow grafts. VOD management involves maintaining the intravascular volume to minimize further hepatotoxicity and prevent hepatorenal syndrome. There are no established preventive measures and no specific treatments of advanced VOD other than liver transplantation, although prophylaxis with heparin and the early institution of tissue plasminogen activator have been advocated.[21,22]

Myelosuppression

Engraftment requires a stable absolute neutrophil count of more than 0.5×10^9/L and a platelet count of more than 20×10^9/L, which are usually achieved around 21 to 24 days after transplantation. Fatal bleeding and infection

TABLE I

Timing of Infectious Complications After Allogeneic Marrow Transplantation

Category	0 to 1 month	1 to 3 months	3 to 6 months	6 to 12 months
Bacteria	Gram-positive *cocci* Gram-negative *bacilli*	Gram-positive *cocci* Gram-negative *bacilli*	*Pneumococcus*	*Pneumococcus*
Fungi	*Candida, Aspergillus*	*Aspergillus*	*Aspergillus*	*Aspergillus*
Viruses	Herpes simplex virus Adenovirus	Herpes simplex virus Cytomegalovirus Varicella zoster virus Adenovirus	Cytomegalovirus Varicella zoster virus	Varicella zoster virus
Other		Toxoplasma Pneumocystis	Toxoplasma Pneumocystis	Pneumocystis

can occur in 10% of patients. These conditions can be reduced with standard transfusions and the use of prophylactic and empiric antibiotics, as for any patient with prolonged marrow aplasia. Hematopoietic growth factors have been used to shorten the duration of aplasia without increasing the risk of relapse or GVHD.[23] However, the ability of such growth factors to enhance engraftment is limited when methotrexate is used as GVHD prophylaxis.

Graft Failure

Graft failure occurs in up to 5% of HLA-identical marrow recipients[24] and can be caused by immunologic graft rejection, infection (especially viral), drugs, and insufficient stem cells. An increased risk of graft rejection is associated with a low nucleated marrow cell dose, T-cell depletion, HLA incompatibility, and a positive crossmatch. Under these circumstances, the incidence of graft failure can be as high as 10% to 15%.[24] For patients with aplastic anemia receiving only cyclophosphamide as the preparative regimen, alloimmunization by prior transfusions or pregnancies may also increase the risk of graft rejection.[9]

Infection

Infectious complications result from the profound neutropenia that can occur early after transplantation and from neutrophil dysfunction and cell-mediated immunodeficiencies, which last for as long as 1 year after transplantation.[25] To reduce the potential for fatal infections, significant restrictions are imposed during this period. Changes in the patient's environment and reconstitution of the immune system with time predispose the patient to develop specific opportunistic infections at different times after transplantation (Table 1).

Fluconazole (Diflucan) given prophylactically has reduced the risk of *Candida* infection.[26] Inhalational amphotericin B is also being evaluated as a means to prevent *Aspergillus* pneumonia. Trimethoprim-sulfamethoxazole, twice weekly for 1 year, is given to prevent pneumocystic and pneumococcal infections. For patients who are allergic to sulfas, twice weekly doses of penicillin and pentamidine (NebuPent) can be given by inhalation every 3 weeks.[27] Prophylactic IV immunoglobulin may also prevent infectious complications up to 1 year after transplantation.[28]

Viral infections have posed a significant challenge. Acyclovir, given during the initial period of neutropenia, is reported to reduce the risk of reactivation of herpes simplex virus (HSV) infections. High-dose acyclovir (Zovirax) was shown to decrease cytomegalovirus (CMV) disease reactivation, but prophylactic use of ganciclovir (Cytovene) through day 100 has nearly eliminated the occurrence of CMV disease after transplantation.[29] Use of ganciclovir has been associated with neutropenia and bacteremia, and the incidence of these conditions has not been remedied by reducing the administration of ganciclovir from 5 days per week to 3 days per week.[30] Surveillance using highly sensitive assays such as the antigenemia test[31] with the preemptive administration of ganciclovir to patients with reactivation of CMV should be considered to reduce both the costs and morbidity of prophylaxis. For patients who are CMV seronegative and have CMV-seronegative donors, CMV-seronegative or CMV-filtered blood products and IV immunoglobulin without ganciclovir are effective in preventing primary CMV infections.[32] With the reduction in morbidity and mortality from CMV disease, problems with respiratory viruses are becoming recognized more commonly and are the subjects of intense investigation.[33-35]

Epstein-Barr virus (EBV)-related lymphoproliferative disease (LPD) occurred in 0.6% of patients who received transplants for treatment of leukemia and 0.3%

of patients who received transplants for aplastic anemia. The risk of EBV-related LPD was increased in recipients of anti-CD3 monoclonal antibody (for GVHD therapy) and in recipients of T-cell-depleted and HLA-mismatched marrow who developed GVHD.[36] EBV-related LPD, previously uniformly fatal, has been shown to respond to infusion of peripheral blood donor lymphocytes.[37]

One year after transplantation, patients may need to be reimmunized with diphtheria, measles-mumps-rubella, polio, influenza, and pneumococcal vaccines as warranted. Prior to that time, immunization with live viruses or exposure to children who have recently received live viral vaccines is discouraged. Immunization with live or attenuated virus preparations should not commence until immunocompetence has been demonstrated.

Late Complications

Patients are annually evaluated for evidence of regimen-related organ dysfunction. These evaluations include tests for hypothyroidism (often subclinical), primary gonadal failure, pulmonary fibrosis and obstructive lung disease, growth disturbances, cataracts, and leukoencephalopathy.[38] Late (12 to 18 months) infectious complications are possible, particularly in patients who have received T-cell-depleted grafts, long-term steroids, or both.

Second malignancies have occurred in 4% to 9% of long-term survivors after allogeneic BMT.[39] The most common malignancy has been EBV-associated lymphoma, which occurs particularly in T-cell-depleted graft recipients. Glioblastoma, melanoma, hepatoma, and epithelial tumors in general also have been reported to occur at an incidence slightly higher than that in the general population. However, it is not clear whether the increase in risk occurs as a result of transplant therapy, an underlying predisposition for malignancies, or the effects of the primary therapy prior to referral for transplantation.

With allogeneic BMT, the intensive treatment and prolonged recovery can have a substantial psychosocial effect in the short term. A pretransplant psychosocial evaluation can identify individuals who may require additional intervention after transplantation.[40] Most long-term survivors, however, seem to report good to excellent health and functional ability, with outcomes comparable to those of long-term cancer survivors who receive less intensive treatment.[41]

GRAFT-VS-HOST DISEASE

Immunobiology

GVHD occurs when the donor's immune system reacts against the marrow recipient's tissue. There is evidence that GVHD is mediated by T-cells, natural killer cells, and inflammatory cytokines.[42] The target antigens are thought to include both major and minor histocompatibility antigens.[43] The incidence and severity of GVHD increase as genetic disparity increases. Thus, patients with HLA-matched related donors have the best outcome.

HLA Typing

The HLA system is encoded by a series of genes on chromosome 6. For marrow transplantation, HLA-A, HLA-B and HLA-DR are evaluated. A perfect match requires identity at all three loci on both chromosomes (six antigens). HLA-A and HLA-B (class I antigens) are identified serologically. Identity for the class II antigen regions can be established serologically, molecularly, or by the mixed lymphocyte culture. For related patient-donor pairs, serologic typing and mixed lymphocyte culture results are generally concordant. However, either or both of these tests can be difficult to perform on patients with chronic myeloid leukemia (CML), leukemia in relapse, or lymphocytopenia. Molecular typing for HLA-DR is more reliable under these circumstances.[44] For unrelated patient-donor pairs, different tests for class II typing may not be concordant. As a result, molecular typing is now standard procedure for identifying matched unrelated donors.

Some reagents used for serotyping can distinguish differences in antigens that were previously undetectable. Antigens identified by this method form cross-reactive antigen groups. With these reagents, patients who were previously identified as HLA-A9 can now be split into HLA-A23 and HLA-A24 groups. Typing from different institutions using different reagents should be interpreted carefully to avoid missing potentially identical patient-donor pairs. Antigen-specificity tables should be used to confirm nonidentity (Table 2).[45] Mismatching between cross-reactive antigens is considered a *minor mismatch*, whereas mismatching between non-cross-reactive antigens is considered a *major mismatch*. For related patient-donor pairs, a single minor mismatch may be of no biologic consequence.

Although techniques are available to identify alleles for a number of loci in the HLA-D region, molecular evaluation of the DRβ1 locus is currently considered sufficient for class II testing for BMT. Molecular typing detects nucleotide sequence differences not distinguishable by serologic methods.[45] For example, 16 related alleles identified serologically as HLA-DR11 can be distinguished by high-resolution molecular typing. Each allele is noted by the two-digit serologic identification followed by the molecular designation. Thus, DRβ1*1106

TABLE 2

Complete Listing of Recognized HLA Specificities

A	B		DR
A1	B5	B48	DR1
A2	B7	B49(21)	DR103
A203	B703	B50(21)	DR2
A210	B8	B51(5)	DR3
A9	B12	B5102	DR4
A10	B13	B5103	DR5
A11	B14	B52(5)	DR6
A19	B15	B53	DR7
A23(9) [a]	B16	B54(22)	DR8
A24(9)	B17	B55(22)	DR9
A2403	B18	B56(22)	DR10
A25(10)	B21	B57(17)	DR11(5)
A26(10)	B22	B58(17)	DR12(5)
A28	B27	B59	DR13(6)
A29(19)	B35	B60(40)	DR14(6)
A30(19)	B37	B61(40)	DR1403
A31(19)	B38(16)	B62(15)	DR1404
A32(19)	B39(16)	B63(15)	DR15(2)
A33(19)	B3901	B64(14)	DR16(2)
A34(10)	B3902	B65(14)	DR17(3)
A36	B40	B67	DR18(3)
A43	B4005	B70	
A66(10)	B41	B71(70)	
A68(28)	B42	B72(70)	
A69(28)	B44(12)	B73	
A74(19)	B45(12)	B75(15)	
	B46	B76(15)	
	B47	B77(15)	
		B7801	

HLA = human leukocyte antigen

[a] The numbers in parentheses refer to the broad specificities of the cross-reactive antigens.

Adapted, with permission, from Bodmer JG et al.[45]

refers to an allele of the HLA-DR11 series that is serologically identical to DRβ1*1105 (also HLA-DR11) but with a different nucleotide sequence. This is referred to as a *molecular mismatch*. It has not been firmly established whether molecular mismatches at class II loci affect outcome after unrelated donor marrow transplantation.

Acute GVHD

Patients are monitored for acute GVHD through day 100 after transplantation. Clinical manifestations include skin rash, fever, decreased performance status, nausea, vomiting, diarrhea, and hyperbilirubinemia.[46] These manifestations have been incorporated in a clinical grading system recently reviewed at an international consensus conference[47] (Table 3). Risk factors for acute GVHD include older age, a parous or alloimmunized donor, less intense immunosuppression, and increasing genetic disparity.[48]

The diagnosis of acute GVHD is frequently made at the bedside with histologic confirmation, especially to exclude infection. Histologic grade I GVHD in the skin can be confused with changes caused by radiation or chemotherapy. Apoptosis or individual cell necrosis is more specific in the skin or gut. With advanced disease, there is confluence of necrosis and eventually complete denudation of the epithelium. In the liver, early GVHD may be confused with viral hepatitis.[49]

Prophylaxis: The incidence of acute GVHD in adults varies with the intensity of immunosuppression. Acute GVHD occurs in 100% of patients with no immunosuppression, 40% to 60% of patients with a single agent, and 20% to 30% of patients with a two-drug combination. The combination used most commonly is cyclosporine (Sandimmune) and methotrexate.[50] The former agent prevents the activation of T-cells and the latter inhibits activated T-cells. Methylprednisolone has also been used successfully in combination with cyclosporine,[51] but T-cell-targeted immunotoxins, such as the anti-CD5 ricin A chain immunoconjugate, have not been proven useful in eliminating alloreactive T-cells.[52]

Cyclosporine is a cyclic polypeptide that acts as a peptidylprolyl *cis*-trans isomerase inhibitor and prevents T-cell activation at its earliest stage.[53] The agent inhibits interleukin-2 production and interleukin-2 receptor expression. Side effects include hypertension, nephrotoxicity, hypomagnesemia, seizures, hypertrichosis, gum overgrowth, tremors, nausea, and anorexia. Treatment with cyclosporine at 3 to 5 mg/kg/d IV is initiated 1 to 2 days prior to marrow infusion and is changed to a twice-daily oral dose when possible. Many institutions maintain the cyclosporine whole-blood level in a target range, whereas others change the dose only in response to toxicity. There is evidence of an increase in the risk of acute GVHD when cyclosporine blood concentrations remain below a target level.[51] Metronidazole, fluconazole/ketoconazole (Nizoral), and erythromycin-like antibiotics increase cyclosporine blood concentrations, whereas phenytoin and rifampin (Rifadin, Rimactane) decrease such levels.[53] Cyclosporine is given at full dose for at least 180 days after transplantation and is tapered thereafter. Most patients do not require cyclosporine past 1 year after transplantation.

TABLE 3

Clinical Grading of Acute Graft-vs-Host Disease (Days 1 to 100)

	Extent of Organ Involvement		
	Skin	**Liver**	**Gut**
Stage			
1	Rash on < 25% of skin[a]	Bilirubin 2–3 mg/dL[b]	Diarrhea > 500 mL/d [c] or persistent nausea[d]
2	Rash on 25% to 50% of skin	Bilirubin 3–6 mg/dL	Diarrhea > 1,000 mL/d
3	Rash on > 50% of skin	Bilirubin 6–15 mg/dL	Diarrhea 1,500 mL/d
4	Generalized erythroderma with bullous formation	Bilirubin > 15 mg/dL	Severe abdominal pain with or without ileus
Grade[e]			
I	Stage 1 to 2	None	None
II	Stage 3 **or**	Stage 1 **or**	Stage 1
III	—	Stage 2 to 3 **or**	Stage 2 to 4
IV[f]	Stage 4 **or**	Stage 4	—

a Use the "Rule of Nines" or burn chart to determine the extent of rash.
b Range given as total bilirubin. Downgrade one stage if an additional cause of elevated bilirubin has been documented.
c Volume of diarrhea applies to adults. For pediatric patients, the volume of diarrhea should be based on body surface area. Gut staging criteria for pediatric patients were not discussed at the consensus conference. Downgrade one stage if an additional cause of diarrhea has been documented.
d Persistent nausea with histologic evidence of graft-vs-host disease in the stomach or duodenum.
e Criteria for grading given as the minimum degree of organ involvement required to confer that grade.
f Grade IV may also include lesser organ involvement but with extreme decrease in performance status.
Adapted, with permission, from Przepiorka D et al.[47]

Methotrexate is administered IV at 15 mg/m^2 on day 1 and 10 mg/m^2 on days 3, 6, and 11. This drug increases the severity of regimen-related mucositis and delays engraftment. The toxicity of the drug frequently precludes administration of the full dose as scheduled. At M. D. Anderson, a modification of the combination using "minidose methotrexate" at 5 mg/m^2 on days 1, 3, 6, and 11 in combination with cyclosporine appears to be as effective as the full dose without excess toxicity.[54]

Tacrolimus (Prograf) is a macrolide lactone with a mechanism of action, immunosuppressive activity, spectrum of toxicities, and pharmacologic interactions nearly identical to those of cyclosporine, but it is about 100 times more potent than cyclosporine. At M. D. Anderson and other institutions, tacrolimus has been evaluated for the prevention of acute GVHD on a schedule similar to that of CSA, with initial doses of 0.03 mg/kg/d IV. For adult recipients of HLA-identical BMT using tacrolimus alone as prophylaxis, the incidence of grades II to IV GVHD was 42%.[55] For adult recipients of matched or one-antigen mismatched unrelated donor marrow grafts using tacrolimus with prednisone or methotrexate as prophylaxis, the incidence of grades II to IV GVHD was 48%.[56]

Although these rates are lower than those reported for cyclosporine-based prophylactic regimens, the results of ongoing randomized studies will determine the relative efficacy of tacrolimus.

T-Cell Depletion: Removal of alloreactive T-cells from the marrow prior to infusion has been shown to decrease the incidence and severity of GVHD, but it also leads to an increase in graft rejection, infectious complications, and relapse rates.[57] Overall, recipients of T-cell-depleted HLA-identical BMTs had no improvement in long-term outcome compared with patients who received unmanipulated marrow.[58] Partial T-cell depletion or subset depletion also showed no benefit in the whole group, although in an evaluation at M. D. Anderson, CD8 depletion of marrow appears promising for patients with CML when transplanted during the chronic phase.[59]

Therapy: Grades II to IV acute GVHD is considered moderate-to-severe and warrants treatment. Some investigators recommend treatment for grade-I GVHD in unrelated donor BMT recipients. First-line therapy for established GVHD is methylprednisolone, at a dose of 2 mg/kg/d or more. Antithymocyte globulin (Atgam) is used as second-line therapy. GVHD of the skin is most responsive, and GVHD of the liver is least responsive. Only about half of patients with moderate-to-severe acute GVHD respond to treatment. The case fatality rate for GVHD can be as high as 50%.[60,61]

Chronic GVHD

Chronic GVHD occurs in 20% to 50% of long-term survivors. Risk factors for chronic GVHD include older age, prior acute GVHD, use of donor buffy-coat infusions, and prior HSV infection. Patients are at risk for developing chronic GVHD from about 3 months after transplantation to more than 6 months after discontinuing all immunosuppressive therapy. The most common clinical manifestations include the sicca syndrome, lichen planus-like rash, sclerodermatous skin reactions, esophageal and intestinal fibrosis with dysphagia and malabsorption, obstructive lung disease with or without lymphocytic pneumonitis, and elevated alkaline phosphatase level with or without hyperbilirubinemia.[62] Chronic GVHD resembles an autoimmune disease, and with more rare manifestations alone, it can be difficult to diagnose.

The histologic manifestations of chronic GVHD are best characterized in the skin, lips, and liver.[49,62] It begins with a cellular inflammatory phase and progresses to widespread fibrosis. In the skin, there is acanthosis, dyskeratosis, and hyperkeratosis with a mononuclear infiltrate at the dermal-epidermal junction and in adnexal structures, which progresses to fibrosis of the reticular dermis and epidermal atrophy. Similarly, a mononuclear infiltrate is seen in the salivary glands on lip biopsy. The liver shows a portal mononuclear infiltrate with damage to the bile ducts and eventually ductopenia. The histologic changes of chronic GVHD can be seen in blind biopsies in the absence of clinical manifestations. When study patients were screened routinely at day 100, detection of subclinical GVHD in two or more organs was predictive of the development of clinical GVHD.[63]

Chronic GVHD can present in the absence of ("de novo onset"), following the resolution of ("quiescent onset") prior acute GVHD or following incompletely resolved acute GVHD ("progressive onset"). Limited chronic GVHD (skin, liver, or both) has a good prognosis (60% to 70% long-term survival), whereas clinical extensive chronic GVHD with multiple-organ involvement has a poorer long-term outcome (20% to 30% long-term survival). Other risk factors for poor outcome include progressive onset, thrombocytopenia, hyperbilirubinemia, and lichen planus histology.[62]

Prophylaxis: There are no formal studies of the prevention of chronic GVHD, although it appears that the incidence of chronic GVHD is lower when patients receive full-dose cyclosporine for at least 6 months after transplantation rather than tapering at earlier points in time.[64]

Therapy: High-dose prednisone is the first-line therapy for good-risk chronic GVHD. Therapy continues for at least 9 months before tapering. Patients with poor-risk GVHD have been treated with a combination of prednisone and cyclosporine, and this combination has been advocated for patients with good-risk GVHD as well.[65,66] Preliminary studies show that tacrolimus has activity that is at least comparable to that of cyclosporine and has yielded good results in patients resistant to standard management. The most common cause of death for patients with chronic GVHD is infection. All patients should receive prophylactic trimethoprim-sulfamethoxazole or penicillin/pentamidine with or without intravenous immunoglobulin.

OUTCOME

Relapse

One substantial benefit for allogeneic BMT recipients is the reduction in the relapse rate, compared with the relapse rate following conventional chemotherapy. Relapse rates are clearly higher for patients with advanced leukemia who receive transplants (Table 4). It has become clear that the risk of relapse is markedly lower after allogeneic BMT than after autologous BMT or identical-twin transplants for treatment of leukemia. This is referred to as the graft-vs-leukemia effect.[67] A similar benefit for patients with lymphoma has been reported, although less consistently.[68]

Treatment of leukemia relapse after allogeneic BMT represents a major challenge, although the chimeric state of the lymphohematopoietic system at relapse provides the opportunity for testing innovative strategies.[69] Options include chemotherapy, biologic response modifiers, discontinuation of immunosuppression to amplify a possible graft-vs-leukemia effect, and a second transplant. Interferon has proved successful for treatment of relapse of CML during the chronic phase, but infusion of donor buffy-coat cells with or without interferon has a composite clinical response rate of 83% in this group of patients. However, this form of therapy has been complicated by cytopenia, acute GVHD flare-up, and fatalities in a significant percentage (22%) of the patients.[70] The use of CD8-depleted donor lymphocytes appears to be as effective as interferon, and it causes far fewer adverse effects.[71]

Second HLA-identical sibling transplantations for leukemia recurrence (usually from the same donor) have

TABLE 4

Relapse Rates for HLA-Matched Related Donor Marrow Transplant Recipients Using Conventional Regimens

Acute leukemia in first remission	10% to 30%
Chronic myeloid leukemia (CML) in chronic phase	10% to 20%
Acute leukemia in later remission or CML in accelerated phase	45% to 60%
Acute leukemia in relapse or CML in blast crisis	50% to 75%
Acute leukemia, induction failure	50% to 70%
Myelodysplastic syndrome, excess blasts	45% to 55%
Aplastic anemia	10% to 30%

Based on data from references 2, 7, 9, 72, and 73.

TABLE 5

Long-Term Disease-Free Survival for HLA-Matched Related Donor Marrow Transplant Recipients

Acute myeloid leukemia or acute lymphocytic leukemia, first complete remission	50% to 65%
Acute myeloid leukemia or acute lymphocytic leukemia, > first complete remission	25% to 35%
Acute myeloid leukemia or acute lymphocytic leukemia, relapsed	15% to 30%
Acute myeloid leukemia or acute lymphocytic leukemia, resistant (no complete remission)	15% to 30%
Chronic myeloid leukemia, chronic phase	60% to 80%
Chronic myeloid leukemia, accelerated phase	30% to 45%
Chronic myeloid leukemia, blastic phase	15% to 20%
Myelodysplastic syndromes	30% to 60%
Aplastic anemia	60% to 80%

Based on data from references 2, 7, and 73–80.

been performed in a limited number of patients, and the outcome has been reported to be poorer than after a first BMT.[72] Factors associated with better survival after a second transplantation are a diagnosis of CML or acute myeloid leukemia (AML) in remission, good performance status, and a long duration (more than 6 to 12 months) of initial after-transplantation remission. Sur-

vival is 5% to 20% for patients relapsing less than 6 months after the first transplantation and 20% to 40% for patients relapsing later.[72]

Long-Term Survival

Expected long-term disease-free survival (DFS) rates for HLA-identical BMT recipients vary with disease and disease status (Table 5).[73–80] For patients with early leukemia, the most common causes of treatment failure were GVHD and CMV. For patients with advanced leukemia, relapse made up a large proportion of failures. Using standard supportive measures, treatment-related mortality averaged 30% at 2 years.[81] New measures for enhancement of engraftment, prevention of GVHD, and prevention of infections are being investigated intensely in an effort to reduce early treatment-related mortality and improve long-term outcome.

For patients with AML, the risk of relapse is lower when transplantation is performed in first remission than after first relapse, and long-term DFS is higher in patients who receive transplants during first remission than in patients who receive them later. This must be compared with the outcome of chemotherapy alone when recommending therapy. For patients with CML, the long-term DFS rates are clearly better for patients who receive transplants during the chronic phase than for patients who receive transplants during the accelerated phase or blast crisis. The survival rate appears to be significantly better for patients transplanted within the first year of diagnosis and for patients treated with hydroxyurea as opposed to busulfan.[80]

For patients with chronic lymphocytic leukemia, allogeneic transplantation appears to be superior to autologous transplantation.[82] This finding may be comparable to findings in patients with low-grade lymphoma.[83] Experience with allogeneic transplantation for multiple myeloma is limited, although in selected patients it has provided prolonged DFS and probable cure.[84] The role of allogeneic BMT for relapsed or refractory malignant lymphoma and Hodgkin's disease is currently being evaluated.[85–87]

ALTERNATIVE DONOR MARROW TRANSPLANTATION

Patients for whom there is no fully compatible related donor can be considered for transplantation from a one-antigen mismatched related donor or a matched unrelated donor.[88,89] In view of the high age-related morbidity and mortality from GVHD with alternative donors, this approach is usually limited to patients younger than 45 years. Even in younger patients, however, the DFS rates associated with this procedure are inferior to the rates for

TABLE 6

Long-Term Disease-Free Survival After Alternative Donor Marrow Transplantation

Disease status	Matched mismatch	1-antigen unrelated	2-3 antigen mismatch
Early	40%	40%	15%
Advanced	19%	15%	10%

Based on data from references 88 and 89.

HLA-identical marrow transplant recipients of similar age (Table 6), largely because of the higher incidence of graft failure (primary and secondary) and GVHD-related mortality.[24,88,89]

The use of T-cell depletion of marrow has been shown to be beneficial for alternative donor marrow recipients,[58] and use of the new immunosuppressive agents may also be beneficial in this group.[56,90] With additional refinements in supportive care measures, long-term outcome is likely to improve for these patients.

There are nearly 1.5 million volunteer marrow donors registered with the National Marrow Donor Program. Despite this, the search for an unrelated donor can take 6 months or longer.[88] Currently, only 40% to 50% of searches for Caucasian donors in the United States are successful in locating HLA-A-, HLA-B-, and HLA-DR-matched unrelated donors.[91] Ethnic minorities are underrepresented in the registry, and these patients have a lower probability of success.[92] To utilize this resource most expeditiously, young patients with CML or high-risk acute leukemia should be HLA typed and considered for a preliminary search early in the course of their disease if no HLA-identical sibling is available.

HOW OLD IS TOO OLD?

Patients younger than 20 to 30 years of age are usually considered to have a better outcome after allogeneic BMT,[2,93] and most transplantation programs do not routinely perform transplants in patients older than 50 to 55 years of age. The age-related difference in outcome is usually ascribed to a higher GVHD-related and treatment-related mortality, although relapse rates have been reported to be higher as well.[93] Patient selection is likely to play an important role in this setting, and in selected patients, advancing age does not necessarily have an adverse impact on relapse, mortality, or DFS rates.[94] It has been suggested that the maximum age at which BMT from a fully HLA-matched sibling donor is recommended could be raised to 60 years, at least for patients with CML.[80]

REFERENCES

1. Bortin MM, Horowitz MM, Rimm AA: Increasing utilization of allogeneic bone marrow transplantation. Ann Intern Med 116(6):505, 1992.

2. Bortin MM, Horowitz MM, Rowlings, et al: 1993 progress report from the International Bone Marrow Transplant Registry. Bone Marrow Transplant 12:97, 1993.

3. Thomas ED, Buckner CD, Clift RA, et al: Marrow transplantation for acute nonlymphoblastic leukemia in first remission. N Engl J Med 301:597, 1979.

4. Clift RA, Buckner CD, Appelbaum FR, et al: Allogeneic marrow transplantation in patients with acute myeloid leukemia in first remission: A randomized trial of two irradiation regimens. Blood 76:1867, 1990.

5. Santos GW, Tutschka PJ, Brookmeyer R, et al: Marrow transplantation for acute nonlymphocytic leukemia after treatment with busulfan and cyclophosphamide. N Engl J Med 309:1347, 1983.

6. Tutschka PJ, Copelan EA, Klein JP: Bone marrow transplantation for leukemia following a new busulfan and cyclophosphamide regimen. Blood 70:1382, 1987.

7. Clift RA, Buckner CD, Thomas ED, et al: Marrow transplantation for chronic myeloid leukemia: A randomized study comparing cyclophosphamide and total body irradiation with busulfan and cyclophosphamide. Blood 84:2036, 1994.

8. Blaise D, Maraninchi D, Archimbaud E, et al: Allogeneic bone marrow transplantation for acute myeloid leukemia in first remission: A randomized trial of busulfan-Cytoxan versus Cytoxan-total body irradiation as preparative regimen: A report from the Groupe d'Etudes de la Greffe de Moelle Osseuse. Blood 79:2578, 1992.

9. Storb R, Champlin RE: Bone marrow transplantation for severe aplastic anemia. Bone Marrow Transplant 8:69, 1991.

10. Storb R, Etzioni R, Anasetti C, et al: Cyclophosphamide combined with antithymocyte globulin in preparation for allogeneic marrow transplants in patients with aplastic anemia. Blood 84:941, 1994.

11. Giralt SA, Vriesendorp HM, Andersson B, et al: Etoposide, cyclophosphamide, total body irradiation, and allogeneic bone marrow transplantation: An effective treatment for hematologic malignancies. J Clin Oncol 12:1923, 1994.

12. Przepiorka D, Dimopoulos MA, Smith T, et al: Thiotepa, busulfan, and cyclophosphamide as a preparative regimen for marrow transplantation: Risk factors for early regimen-related toxicities. Ann Hematol 68:183, 1994.

13. Przepiorka D, Ippoliti C, Giralt SA, et al: A phase I/II study of high-dose Thiotepa, busulfan, and cyclophosphamide as a preparative regimen for allogeneic marrow transplantation. Bone Marrow Transplant 14:449, 1994.

14. Champlin RE, Dimopoulos M, Bayouth J, et al: Holmium-166 DOTMP, a bone seeking radiochelate for selective marrow radiotherapy with bone marrow transplantation (BMT) for multiple myeloma. Exp Hematol 21:1117, 1993.

15. Buckner CD, Clift RA, Sanders JE, et al: Marrow harvesting from normal donors. Blood 64:630, 1984.

16. Petz LD: Bone marrow transplantation, in Petz LD, Swisher SN (eds): Clinical Practice of Transfusion Medicine, 2nd ed, p 485. New York, Churchill Livingstone, 1989.

17. Körbling M, Przepiorka D, Engel H, et al: Allogeneic blood stem cell transplantation for refractory leukemia and lymphoma: Potential advantage of blood over marrow allografts. Blood 85:1659, 1995.

18. Bearman SI, Appelbaum FR, Buckner CD, et al: Regimen-related toxicity in patients undergoing bone marrow transplantation. J Clin Oncol 6:1562, 1988.

19. Apperley JF: Umbilical cord blood progenitor cell transplantation. Bone Marrow Transplant 14:187, 1994.

20. Shulman HM, Hinterberger W: Hepatic veno-occlusive disease: Liver toxicity syndrome after bone marrow transplantation. Bone Marrow Transplant 10:197, 1992.

21. Attal M, Huguet F, Rubie H, et al: Prevention of hepatic veno-occlusive disease after bone marrow transplantation by continuous infusion of low-dose heparin: A prospective, randomized trial. Blood 79:2834, 1992.

22. Bearman SI, Shuhart MC, Hinds MS, et al: Recombinant human tissue plasminogen activator for the treatment of established severe veno-occlusive disease of the liver after bone marrow transplantation. Blood 80:2458, 1992.

23. Barge AJ: A review of the efficacy and tolerability of recombinant haematopoietic growth factors in bone marrow transplantation. Bone Marrow Transplant 11(suppl 2):1, 1993.

24. Davies SM, Ramsay NKC, Haake RJ, et al: Comparison of engraftment in recipients of matched sibling or unrelated donor marrow grafts. Bone Marrow Transplant 13:51, 1994.

25. Atkinson K: Reconstruction of the haematopoietic and immune systems after marrow transplantation. Bone Marrow Transplant 5:209, 1990.

26. Goodman JL, Winston DJ, Greenfield RA, et al: A controlled trial of fluconazole to prevent fungal infections in patients undergoing bone marrow transplantation. N Engl J Med 326:845, 1992.

27. Przepiorka D, Selvaggi K, Rosenzweig PQ, et al: Aerosolized pentamidine for prevention of pneumocystis pneumonia after allogeneic marrow transplantation. Bone Marrow Transplant 7:324, 1991.

28. Sullivan KM, Kopecky KJ, Jocom J, et al: Immunomodulatory and antimicrobial efficacy of intravenous immunoglobulin in bone marrow transplantation. N Engl J Med 323:705, 1990.

29. Goodrich JM, Bowden RA, Fisher L, et al: Ganciclovir prophylaxis to prevent cytomegalovirus disease after allogeneic marrow transplant. Ann Intern Med 118:173, 1993.

30. Przepiorka D, Ippoliti C, Panina A, et al: Ganciclovir three times per week is not adequate to prevent cytomegalovirus reactivation after T-cell-depleted marrow transplantation. Bone Marrow Transplant 13:461, 1994.

31. Boeckh M, Bowden RA, Goodrich JM, et al: Cytomegalovirus antigen detection in peripheral blood leukocytes after allogeneic marrow transplantation. Blood 80:1358, 1992.

32. Bowden RA, Sayers M, Flournoy N, et al: Cytomegalovirus immune globulin and seronegative blood products to prevent primary cytomegalovirus infection after marrow transplantation. N Engl J Med 314:1006, 1986.

33. Whimbey E, Vartivarian SE, Champlin RE, et al: Parainfluenza virus infection in adult bone marrow transplant recipients. Eur J Clin Microbiol Infect Dis 12(9):699, 1993.

34. Whimbey E, Elting LS, Couch RB, et al: Influenza A virus infections among hospitalized adult bone marrow transplant recipients. Bone Marrow Transplant 13(4):437, 1994.

35. Whimbey E, Champlin RE, Couch RB, et al: Combination therapy with aerosolized ribavirin and intravenous immunoglobulin for respiratory syncytial virus disease in adult bone marrow transplant recipients. Bone Marrow Transplant, September 1995.

36. Zutter MM, Martin PJ, Sale GE, et al: Epstein-Barr virus lymphoproliferation after bone marrow transplantation. Blood 72: 520, 1988.

37. Papadopoulos EB, Ladanyi M, Emanuel D, et al: Infusions of donor leukocytes to treat Epstein-Barr virus-associated lymphoproliferative disorders after allogeneic bone marrow transplantation. N Engl J Med 330:1185, 1994.

38. Kolb HJ, Bender-Götze C: Late complications after allogeneic

bone marrow transplantation for leukaemia. Bone Marrow Transplant 6:61, 1990.

39. Lowsky R, Lipton J, Fyles G, et al: Secondary malignancies after bone marrow transplantation in adults. J Clin Oncol 12:2187, 1994.

40. Meyers CA, Weitzner M, Byrne K, et al: Evaluation of the neurobehavioral functioning of patients before, during, and after bone marrow transplantation. J Clin Oncol 12:820, 1994.

41. Wingard JR, Curbow B, Baker F, et al: Health, functional status, and employment of adult survivors of bone marrow transplantation. Ann Intern Med 114:113, 1991.

42. Ferrara JLM, Deeg HJ: Graft-versus-host-disease. N Engl J Med 324:667, 1991.

43. Perreault C, Decary F, Brochu S, et al: Minor histocompatibility antigens. Blood 76:1269, 1991.

44. Howell WM, Evans PR, Spellerberg MB, et al: A comparison of serological, cellular, and DNA-RFLP methods for HLA matching in the selection of related bone marrow donors. Bone Marrow Transplant 4:63, 1989.

45. Bodmer JG, Marsh SGE, Albert ED, et al: Nomenclature for factors of the HLA system, 1994. Hum Immunol 41:1, 1994.

46. Vogelsang GB, Hess AD, Santos GW: Acute graft-versus-host disease: Clinical characteristics in the cyclosporine era. Medicine 67:163, 1988.

47. Przepiorka D, Weisdorf D, Martin PJ, et al: Consensus conference on acute GVHD grading. Bone Marrow Transplant 15:825, 1995.

48. Gale RP, Bortin MM, Van Bekkum DW, et al: Risk factors for acute graft-versus-host disease. Br J Haematol 67:397, 1987.

49. Snover DC: Biopsy interpretation in bone marrow transplantation. Pathol Annu 24:63, 1989.

50. Storb R, Deeg HJ, Pepe M, et al: Methotrexate and cyclosporine versus cyclosporine alone for prophylaxis of graft-versus-host disease in patients given HLA-identical marrow grafts for leukemia: Long-term follow-up of a controlled trial. Blood 73:1729, 1989.

51. Przepiorka D, Shapiro S, Schwinghammer TL, et al: Cyclosporine and methylprednisolone after allogeneic marrow transplantation: Association between low cyclosporine concentration and risk of acute graft-versus-host disease. Bone Marrow Transplant 7:461, 1991.

52. Przepiorka D, LeMaistre CF, Huh YO, et al: Evaluation of anti-CD5 ricin A chain immunoconjugate for prevention of acute graft-vs-host disease after HLA-identical marrow transplantation. Ther Immunol 1:77, 1994.

53. Ringden O: Cyclosporine in allogeneic bone marrow transplantation. Transplantation 42:445, 1986.

54. Yau JC, Dimopoulos MA, Huan SD, et al: An effective acute graft-vs-host disease prophylaxis with minidose methotrexate, cyclosporine, and single-dose methylprednisolone. Am J Hematol 38:288, 1991.

55. Fay JW, Weisdorf D, Wingard J, et al: FK506 for prevention of graft versus host disease after allogeneic marrow transplantation (abstract). Blood 80:135a, 1992.

56. Fay JW, Nash RA, Wingard J, et al: FK506-based immunosuppression for prevention of graft-versus-host disease (GVHD) after unrelated marrow donor (UMD) transplantation. Transplant Proc 27:1374, 1995.

57. Marmont AM, Horowitz MM, Gale RP, et al: T-cell depletion of HLA-identical transplants in leukemia. Blood 78:2120, 1991.

58. Passweg JR, Champlin RE, Klein JP, et al: Comparison of techniques for T-cell depletion: Effects on leukemia-free survival. Blood 84(suppl):539a, 1994.

59. Champlin RE, Giralt SA, Przepiorka D, et al: Selective depletion of CD8-positive T-lymphocytes for allogeneic bone marrow transplantation: Engraftment, graft-vs-host disease, and graft-vs-leukemia. Prog Clin Biol Res 377:385, 1992.

60. Hings IM, Severson R, Filipovich AH, et al: Treatment of moderate and severe acute GVHD after allogeneic bone marrow transplantation. Transplantation 58:437, 1994.

61. Martin PJ, Schoch G, Fisher L, et al: A retrospective analysis of therapy for acute graft-versus-host disease: Initial treatment. Blood 76:1464, 1990.

62. Atkinson K: Chronic graft-versus-host disease. Bone Marrow Transplant 5:69, 1990.

63. Loughran TP, Sullivan KM, Morton T, et al: Value of day 100 screening studies for predicting the development of chronic graft-versus-host disease after allogeneic bone marrow transplantation. Blood 76:228, 1990.

64. Bacigalupo A, Van Lint MT, Occhini D, et al: Cyclosporin A and chronic graft-versus-host disease. Bone Marrow Transplant 6: 341, 1990.

65. Sullivan KM, Witherspoon RP, Storb R, et al: Alternating-day cyclosporine and prednisone for treatment of high-risk chronic graft-versus-host disease. Blood 72:555, 1988.

66. Sullivan KM, Gooley T, Nims J, et al: Comparison of cyclosporine (CSP), prednisone (PRED), or alternating-day CSP/PRED in patients with standard and high-risk chronic graft-versus-host-disease (GVHD). Blood 82(suppl):215a, 1993.

67. Horowitz MM, Gale RP, Sondel PM, et al: Graft-vs-leukemia reactions after bone marrow transplantation. Blood 75:555, 1990.

68. Jones RJ, Ambinder RF, Piantadosi S, et al: Evidence of a graft-versus-lymphoma effect associated with allogeneic bone marrow transplantation. Blood 77:649, 1991.

69. Giralt SA, Champlin RE: Leukemia relapse after allogeneic bone marrow transplantation: A review. Blood 84:3603, 1994.

70. Antin JH: Graft-versus-leukemia: No longer an epiphenomenon. Blood 82:2273, 1993.

71. Giralt SA, Hester J, Huh YO, et al: CD8+ depleted donor lymphocyte infusion as treatment for relapsed chronic myelogenous leukemia (CML) after allogeneic bone marrow transplantation (BMT): Graft vs leukemia without graft vs host disease (GVHD). Blood 84(suppl):538a, 1994.

72. Mrsic M, Horowitz MM, Atkinson K, et al: Second HLA-identical sibling transplants for leukemia recurrence. Bone Marrow Transplant 9:269, 1992.

73. Clift RA, Buckner CD, Thomas ED, et al: Marrow transplantation for patients in accelerated phase of chronic myeloid leukemia. Blood 84:4368, 1994.

74. Anderson JE, Appelbaum FR, Fisher LD, et al: Allogeneic bone marrow transplantation for 93 patients with myelodysplastic syndrome. Blood 82:677, 1993.

75. Ljungman P, de Witte T, Verdonck L, et al: Bone marrow transplantation for acute myeloblastic leukaemia: An EBMT Leukaemia Working Party prospective analysis from HLA-typing. Br J Haematol 84:61, 1993.

76. Reiffers J, Gaspard MH, Maraninchi D, et al: Comparison of allogeneic or autologous bone marrow transplantation and chemotherapy in patients with acute myeloid leukaemia in first remission: A prospective controlled trial. Br J Haematol 72:57, 1989.

77. Horowitz MM, Messere D, Hoelzer D, et al: Chemotherapy compared with bone marrow transplantation for adults with acute lymphoblastic leukemia in first remission. Ann Intern Med 115:13, 1991.

78. Sebban C, Lepage E, Vernant JP, et al: Allogeneic bone marrow transplantation in adult acute lymphoblastic leukemia in first complete remission: A comparative study. J Clin Oncol 12: 2580, 1994.

79. Barrett AJ, Horowitz MM, Pollock BH, et al: Bone marrow transplants from HLA-identical siblings as compared with chemotherapy for children with acute lymphoblastic leukemia in a second remission. N Engl J Med 331:1253, 1994.

80. Clift RA, Appelbaum FR, Thomas ED: Treatment of chronic myeloid leukemia by marrow transplantation. Blood 82:1954, 1993.

81. Horowitz MM, Przepiorka D, Champlin RE, et al: Should HLA-identical sibling bone marrow transplants for leukemia be restricted to large centers? Blood 79:2771, 1992.

82. Khouri IF, Keating MJ, Vriesendorp HM, et al: Autologous and allogeneic bone marrow transplantation for chronic lymphocytic leukemia: Preliminary results. J Clin Oncol 12:748, 1994.

83. van Besien K, Khouri IF, Giralt SA, et al: Allogeneic bone marrow transplantation for refractory and recurrent low grade lymphoma: The case for aggressive management. Blood 84(suppl):205a, 1994.

84. Gahrton G, Tura S, Ljungman P, et al: Allogeneic bone marrow transplantation in multiple myeloma. N Engl J Med 325:1267, 1991.

85. Chopra R, Goldstone AH, Pearce R, et al: Autologous versus allogeneic bone marrow transplantation for non-Hodgkin's lymphoma: A case-controlled analysis of the European Bone Marrow Transplant Group Registry Data. J Clin Oncol 10:1690, 1992.

86. Anderson JE, Litzow MR, Appelbaum FR, et al: Allogeneic, syngeneic, and autologous marrow transplantation for Hodgkin's disease: The 21-year Seattle experience. J Clin Oncol 11:2342, 1993.

87. van Besien K, Mehra R, Khouri IE, et al: Double intensification and allogeneic or autologous bone marrow transplantation for poor prognosis lymphoma. Blood 82(suppl):146a, 1993.

88. Kernan NA, Bartsch G, Ash RC, et al: Analysis of 462 transplantations from unrelated donors facilitated by the national marrow donor program. N Engl J Med 328:593, 1993.

89. Anasetti C, Beatty PG, Storb R, et al: Effect of HLA incompatibility on GVHD, relapse, and survival after marrow transplantation for patients with leukemia or lymphoma. Hum Immunol 29:79, 1990.

90. Przepiorka D, von Wolff B, Ippoliti C, et al: Anti-CD5 ricin A chain immunotoxin decreases acute graft-vs-host disease (GVHD) after unrelated donor marrow transplantation (MUD BMT). Exp Hematol 20:709, 1992.

91. Anasetti C, Etzioni R, Petersdorf EW, et al: Unrelated and HLA-partially matched related donor transplants: Advances and controversies in bone marrow transplantation: Keystone symposium on bone marrow transplantation. J Cell Biochem Suppl 18b:48, 1994.

92. Beatty PG, Mori M, Milford E, et al: Racial differences in histocompatibility, implications for unrelated donor BMT: Advances and controversies in bone marrow transplantation: Keystone symposium on bone marrow transplantation. J Cell Biochem Suppl 18b:49, 1994.

93. Gratwohl A, Hermans J, Niederwieser D, et al: Bone marrow transplantation for chronic myeloid leukemia: Long-term results. Bone Marrow Transplant 12:509, 1993.

94. Ringden O, Horowitz MM, Gale RP, et al: Outcome after allogeneic bone marrow transplantation for leukemia in older adults. JAMA 270:57, 1993.

CHAPTER 10

Autologous Transplantation: Basic Concepts and Controversies

Naoto T. Ueno, MD, *and* Richard E. Champlin, MD

Department of Hematology, Section of Bone Marrow Transplantation
The University of Texas M. D. Anderson Cancer Center, Houston, Texas

High-dose chemotherapy (HDCT) with autologous stem-cell is effective against a wide range of malignant diseases. This approach is increasingly used for treating hematologic malignancies and selected solid tumors. Since 1990, the number of autologous transplantations has exceeded the number of allogeneic transplantations.

In this chapter, we review the general procedure of autologous transplantation and its role in the treatment of cancer. Our objectives are to understand the basic concept of autologous transplantation and to build a knowledge to enable an understanding of its future progression.

Autologous transplantation allows patients to receive a high dose of myelosuppressive chemotherapy, followed by infusion of their own hematopoietic cells, to restore marrow function. The hematopoietic cells contain stem cells that proliferate and differentiate into mature blood lineage, such as leukocytes, platelets, and erythrocytes.[1] Stem cells can be collected from bone marrow or peripheral blood.

GENERAL PROCEDURE FOR AUTOLOGOUS TRANSPLANTATION

The general approach to autologous transplantation for malignancies involves the following steps.

Assessment of Patients: Transplantation physicians determine whether patients are appropriate candidates for autologous transplantation by performing a complete history, physical examination, laboratory studies, and staging workup of the neoplastic disease. If a patient is a suitable candidate for autologous transplantation, further tests are performed to evaluate the function of systemic organs, such as the lungs, heart, kidneys, and liver.

Induction Chemotherapy: Standard-dose combination chemotherapy can be given before autologous transplantation to reduce the tumor burden. The long-term outcome of transplantation is better in patients who have a minimum volume of disease that responds to standard-dose chemotherapy.

Stem-Cell Collection: Patients undergo stem-cell collection, cryopreservation, and storage of bone marrow or peripheral-blood progenitor (PBP) cells (blood stem cells and peripheral-blood stem cells). Bone marrow is collected from the posterior superior iliac crests by multiple aspirations while the patient is anesthetized. Marrow collection should occur at a time when the marrow is normally cellular and does not contain malignant cells. With current techniques, marrow cryopreservation can be reliably performed, and the stored cells can remain viable for more than 5 years.[2-4] PBP cells are collected by apheresis, usually by using a large-bore vascular catheter in the subclavian vein. Leukapheresis is repeated by using continuous-flow cell separation.[5,6] To collect an adequate cell dose for transplantation, 8 to 12 daily leukaphereses are required. Circulating progenitor cells are mobilized to a higher level during the recovery phase following cytoreduction and treatment with granulocyte-macrophage colony-stimulating factor (GM-CSF, sargramostim [Leukine]) or granulocyte colony-stimulating factor (G-CSF, filgrastim [Neupogen]).[7,8]

High-Dose Chemotherapy and/or Radiotherapy (Preparative Regimens): The dose of antineoplastic agents or radiation that can be administered clinically is limited by its toxic effects to normal tissues.[9] Bone marrow suppression is the dose-limiting toxicity for most chemotherapeutic agents. The doses of radiation and many drugs can be substantially escalated to more effective levels if followed by transplantation of normal hematopoietic cells, thus rescuing the patient from severe and prolonged myelosuppression. For dose-intensive therapy to be successful, the neoplasm must exhibit a dose-dependent response to chemotherapy and/or irradiation so that one (or possibly several) course of intensive combined-modality treatment can eradicate the malignant cells. Candidate neoplastic diseases are listed in Table 1. The intensity of chemotherapy required varies according to the aggressiveness of the disease, with the need to weigh the benefit-to-risk ratio. The actual preparative regimen involves chemotherapeutic drugs alone or combined with radiotherapy. After the preparative regimens are administered, intense supportive care is required to deal with complications related to prolonged neutropenia and the toxic effects of the preparative regimens.

Reinfusion of Collected Stem Cells: The marrow cells or PBP cells are infused intravenously after completion of the preparative regimens. The cells circulate

TABLE 1

Neoplastic Diseases Treated by Autologous Transplantation

Acute myelogenous leukemia

Acute lymphoblastic leukemia

Chronic myelogenous leukemia

Chronic lymphocytic leukemia

Lymphoma

Hodgkin's disease

Multiple myeloma

Pediatric solid tumors—Ewing's sarcoma, neuroblastoma

Breast carcinoma

Other solid tumors—small-cell lung carcinoma and testicular carcinoma

TABLE 2

Major Controversies in Autologous Transplantation

Autologous vs allogeneic transplantation

Blood-progenitor cells derived from bone marrow vs peripheral blood

Optimal dose-intensive preparation regimen

Integration of autologous transplantation with posttransplantation therapy

Role of purging

Improvement in supportive care

TABLE 3

Comparison of Autologous and Allogeneic Transplantation

	Autologous	**Allogeneic**
HDCT	Yes	Yes
GVHD	No	Yes
Graft failure	Rare	Yes
Relapse	Higher	Lower
Treatment mortality	Less than 10%	10% to 40%
Cost	Lower	Higher

HDCT = high-dose chemotherapy, GVHD = graft-vs-host disease

transiently, and sufficient numbers of stem cells home to the marrow and restore hematopoiesis. Autologous transplantation requires a minimum of approximately 1 to 5 × 10^7 nucleated marrow cells/kg body weight or 0.5 × 10^6 CD34-positive cells/kg to achieve engraftment.[10] Peripheral blood counts are profoundly suppressed as a result of the effects of the conditioning treatment but generally recover within 3 to 4 weeks with marrow transplantation and within 2 to 3 weeks with PBP cell transplantation.

Administration of Colony-Stimulating Factors: Patients generally receive G-CSF, GM-CSF, or other cytokines to accelerate marrow recovery. G-CSF or GM-CSF administration is continued until the absolute neutrophil count is greater than 1,000/mm³.

Restaging of the Neoplastic Diseases: Response to the treatment is assessed after full recovery of the bone marrow.

CONTROVERSIES

The major controversies surrounding autologous transplantation are listed in Table 2.

Autologous vs Allogeneic Transplantation

Autologous transplantation is less likely to produce major side effects than is allogeneic transplantation (Table 3) because the infused cells are not subject to rejection and do not mediate graft-vs-host disease (GVHD) (see chapter on allogeneic transplantation). There is also no immune-mediated graft-vs-tumor effect from the donated cells. Therefore, the most frequent cause of treatment failure is recurrence of the underlying malignancy.

Blood-Progenitor Cells Derived From Bone Marrow vs Peripheral Blood

Transplantation of a relatively small number of stem cells can reconstitute hematopoiesis and immunity in appropriately prepared recipients (Table 4). PBP cells offer an alternative source of hematopoietic cells for transplantation. They are an effective approach for patients who cannot undergo marrow harvest, such as patients who have undergone pelvic radiotherapy. PBP cells are also a potential source for patients with marrow and malignant cell involvement, although it remains to be determined whether the level of contaminating malignant cells is low in the peripheral blood.[11] Transplantation of large numbers of PBP cells results in more rapid recovery of platelets than does marrow transplantation.[7,8] A major area of research involves the development of systems for ex vivo expansion of hematopoietic progenitors from either peripheral blood or marrow.[12,13]

Optimal Dose-Intensive Preparation Regimen

The most frequent cause of failure in autologous transplantation is recurrence of underlying malignant disease; this is due to either inadequate systemic cytoreduction or reinfusion of tumor contaminated marrow or PBP cells. Various approaches have been used to improve the efficacy of HDCT and/or radiotherapy. They include increasing the total delivered dosage of chemotherapeutic agents or radiation, using novel chemotherapeutic agents, and using sequential HDCT. However, although increasing the total dosage may result in increased tumor response, more toxic effects may result without improvement in survival. Different agents have been applied, but a clear-cut difference has not been seen among commonly used preparative regimens. There is interest in selecting high-dose regimens with a decreased potential for regimen-related toxicity. Multiple cycles of HDCT may improve the overall tumor response rate.[14,15] At the University of Texas M. D. Anderson Cancer Center, this approach has recently been applied to metastatic breast cancer (four cycles of HDCT with cyclophosphamide [Cytoxan, Neosar], carboplatin [Paraplatin], and paclitaxel [Taxol] with PBP cell support).

Integration of Autologous Transplantation With Posttransplantation Therapy

Relapse of malignancy is the major problem following autologous transplantation. Posttransplantation therapies using biologic therapies to eradicate minimal residual tumor are currently being studied. In allogeneic transplantation, a lower recurrence of leukemia has been seen among patients with acute and chronic GVHD. It is believed that this antitumor effect is mediated by T-cells. Rarely, a GVHD-like syndrome is seen in patients who have undergone autologous transplantation. Cyclosporine (Sandimmune) may induce this GVHD.[16] Gamma interferon (IFN-γ, Actimmune), which upregulates major histocompatibility complex II expression, enhances this effect and is under evaluation in breast cancer.[17] Interleukin-2 after autologous transplantation in patients with acute leukemia is being evaluated. Also under investigation is alpha interferon (IFN-α) after transplantation in patients with lymphoma and Hodgkin's disease.[18,19]

Role of Purging

A major concern with autologous transplantation is the possibility that the marrow or the PBP cells may be contaminated by malignant cells at the time of collection. Tumor can be detected by immunohistochemical stain-

TABLE 4

The Difference Between Bone Marrow and Peripheral-Blood Progenitor Cells

	Bone marrow	Peripheral-blood progenitor cells
Method of collection	Multiple aspiration of iliac crests	Apheresis via subclavian catheter
General anesthesia	Yes	No
Duration for collection	One day	One to several days
Complication	Pain, anesthesia-related, rare nerve damage	Vascular access-related pneumothorax, infection
Recovery of WBCs to > 500/mL	2 weeks	2 weeks
Platelets > 100,000	4 to 5 weeks	2 to 3 weeks
Tumor contamination	Yes	Yes

WBCs = white blood cells

ing and molecular assays. However, the clinical significance of a positive finding is unknown. A number of investigators are evaluating techniques to detect occult involvement by tumor and approaches to deplete selectively occult malignant cells from the normal marrow cells prior to cryopreservation by ex vivo treatment with antitumor monoclonal antibodies,[20] antibody-toxin conjugates,[21] chemotherapy,[22,23] or physical techniques.[24,25] An alternative method is to select positive hematopoietic stem cells. CD34-positive cells represent less than 1% of the marrow but encompass progenitors capable of reconstituting hematopoiesis.[26] Recently, highly enriched CD34-positive cells have been selected for autologous marrow or blood stem-cell transplantation, resulting in rapid hematologic recovery.[27] The Thy-1 antigen has recently been proposed as a more restricted marker for hematopoietic stem cells.[28]

POTENTIAL COMPLICATIONS OF HIGH-DOSE CHEMOTHERAPY

In autologous transplantation, the major toxic effects are associated with dose escalation of chemotherapy and radiotherapy.[29] The most common effects are infections from granulocytopenia and systemic reactions from the conditioning regimen (Table 5). Fatal complications

TABLE 5

Potential Complications of Autologous Transplantation

Hematologic toxicity from the preparative regimens

Organ toxicity from the preparative regimens

   Posttransplant immunodeficiency

   Posttransplant infections

   Secondary malignancies

generally occur in 10% of patients undergoing autologous transplantation. This rate is lower than that seen with allogeneic transplantation because of the rareness of graft failure and GVHD and because of a more complete immune reconstitution.

Hematologic Toxicity From the Preparative Regimens

HDCT induces profound pancytopenia, lasting approximately 2 to 4 weeks until the stem cells restore hematopoiesis. During the period of granulocytopenia, life-threatening infectious complications may occur. GM-CSF and G-CSF have been shown to accelerate hematopoietic recovery after autologous transplantation[30,31] and to improve hematopoiesis in patients with graft failure.[32] Neither G-CSF nor GM-CSF prevents the nadir of granulocytes, but the granulocytopenic period is shortened by approximately 1 week. Neither factor affects erythrocyte or platelet recovery. Use of these colony-stimulating factors reduces the number of febrile days and shortens the period of hospitalization. Novel growth factors, including interleukin-3, interleukin-6, and interleukin-11, used alone and in combination with other factors to enhance platelet recovery, are being studied.[33,34] Thrombopoietin (c-mpl ligand) has recently been cloned and appears most promising. Clinical trials should begin in 1995.[35,36]

Organ Toxicity From the Preparative Regimens

Preparative regimens may cause severe toxic effects involving the lungs, heart, liver, nervous system, and, rarely, other tissues. Organs affected vary depending on the preparative regimens used. Fatal hepatic veno-occlusive disease occurs in approximately 5% of patients who receive transplants for leukemia.[37] This is more common in older patients, patients with preexisting liver-function abnormalities, patients receiving the most intense condi-

tioning regimens, and patients who have received extensive previous chemotherapy.

Pneumonitis ascribed to the toxicity of the conditioning regimen occurs in 5% to 10% of patients[38]; this is particularly common with carmustine (BiCNU) or alkylating agent-based regimens and in patients who have received transplants following mediastinal radiotherapy.[39,40] This condition is often difficult to distinguish from pneumonitis related to cytomegalovirus or other infections.

Cardiac toxicity is common with high-dose cyclophosphamide regimens, particularly when combined with carmustine or other alkylating agents.[41,42]

Central nervous system complications are relatively uncommon, but dementia or leukoencephalopathy may occur.[43]

Endocrine complications may develop but generally are not life-threatening. Hypothyroidism commonly occurs as a delayed complication 6 months to 2 years following transplantation.[44,45]

Intensive combined-modality therapy typically results in sterility for both men and women, although gonadal endocrine and ejaculation functions usually remain intact.[46–48] Cataracts are a common delayed complication of total-body irradiation (TBI).[49]

Toxic effects to the bladder as a result of high-dose cyclophosphamide chemotherapy is a common problem.[50,51] This is probably mediated by acrolein, a metabolite of 4-hydroxycyclophosphamide that is toxic to transitional epithelium. Hemorrhagic cystitis may develop acutely or as a delayed complication weeks to months later. Concurrent treatment with mesna (Mesnex), a uroprotective agent that binds to acrolein, has been reported to reduce the urinary toxicity of cyclophosphamide in patients with marrow transplants without inhibiting the therapeutic effects of cyclophosphamide.

Posttransplant Immunodeficiency: Recipients of autologous transplants undergo a period of immunodeficiency, but their recovery appears more rapid than after allogeneic transplants, and posttransplant infections are less severe than in allogeneic transplant recipients.[52]

Posttransplant Infections: A number of infectious complications may develop while patients are undergoing autologous transplantation.[53] There are high incidences of bacterial and fungal infections during profound and prolonged granulocytopenia. Mucosal herpes simplex infections also are common during this period but seldom disseminate; prophylactic treatment with acyclovir may decrease their incidence.[54] Patients who have received autologous transplants recover immunity more quickly than do patients who have received allogeneic transplants and have a much lower risk of infection after recovery of peripheral-blood counts. Late infections develop in a small fraction of autograft recipients. *Pneumocystis carinii* infection most frequently occurs in patients with lymphoid malignancies; prophylactic trimethoprim/sulfamethoxazole is indicated. Cytomegalovirus infection may occur in heavily immunocompromised patients.

Secondary Malignancies: HDCT and radiotherapeutic regimens are potentially carcinogenic and may predispose a patient to the development of secondary malignancies. A small number of second malignancies have been reported in long-term survivors of marrow transplantation.[55,56] Several cases of immunoblastic sarcoma arising in donor cells have been reported. Lymphoproliferative disorders related to Epstein-Barr infection may occur,[57,58] particularly in heavily immunosuppressed patients receiving intravenous antithymocyte globulin, anti-T-cell antibody therapy, or human leukocyte antigen (HLA)-mismatched or T-cell-depleted transplantation. The incidence of treatment-induced malignancies may increase with further follow-up, particularly for radiation-induced tumors that may have a long latency, such as thyroid carcinoma. Recently, secondary acute leukemia and myelodysplastic syndrome have developed in recipients of autologous transplants.[59,60] It is unclear whether these conditions are related to the transplantation or are the cumulative effect of previous therapy. It is possible that the proliferative stress after HDCT promotes the evolution of leukemia.

RESULTS OF AUTOLOGOUS TRANSPLANTATION

In this section, we discuss the outcome and current controversies associated with autologous transplantation for various neoplastic diseases (Table 6). The reader is referred to other chapters in this volume on specific diseases for additional discussion of transplantation indications and outcome.

Acute Myelogenous Leukemia

Autologous transplantation has been evaluated for use in patients with acute myelogenous leukemia (AML) who lack an HLA-identical donor.[61-63] Patients undergo collection of marrow or PBP cells while in remission. The major limitation is the likelihood that the remission marrow or PBP cells may be contaminated by small numbers of leukemia cells. The autologous stem cells lack the favorable graft-vs-leukemia effect seen with allograft. For patients receiving autologous transplants while AML is relapsing,[64,65] the major problem has been

TABLE 6

Results of Autologous Transplantation for Treatment of Malignancy

Disease	Benefit of autologous transplantation	Benefit of allogeneic transplantation	Long-term DFS of autologous transplantation
AML	Yes	Yes	30% to 40%
ALL	Yes/No	Yes	30% to 40%
CML	Unknown	Yes	Unknown
CLL	Promising	Yes	Unknown
MDS	No	Yes	Unknown
Lymphoma	Yes	Yes/No	40% to 60%
Hodgkin's disease	Yes	Yes/No	20% to 60%
Breast carcinoma	Promising	Unknown	20%, stage IV 75%, stage II-III

AML = acute myelogenous leukemia, ALL = acute lymphoblastic leukemia, CML = chronic myelogenous leukemia, CLL = chronic lymphocytic leukemia, DFS = disease-free survival, MDS = myelodysplastic syndromes

the rapid relapse of leukemia; the median duration of remission has been 3 to 5 months, and less than 10% of patients survive 1 year. Better results have occurred with autologous transplantation in patients in first or second remission.[62,66–69] Relapse of leukemia remains a major problem, but approximately 20% to 40% of patients who receive transplants in second remission achieve a disease-free survival duration of longer than 2 years. These data indicate that this approach may be successful and that relapse of leukemia may not invariably occur. The timing of transplantation is important. The longer the interval from remission to transplantation, the less likely is leukemic contamination.

A number of purging systems have been explored to deplete occult leukemia cells from the harvested marrow or PBP cells in vitro before cryopreservation. Immunologic approaches using anti-AML monoclonal antibodies,[70,71] hyperthermia,[72] or pharmacologic agents (such as 4-hydroperoxycyclophosphamide or mafosfamide[23,73,74]) have been studied. Although some of the best results are reported in series using purged marrow, no controlled studies have been performed, and the efficacy of purging remains to be determined.

Following autologous transplantation, patients may relapse either from leukemia cells that survive the systemic HDCT or from leukemia cells present in the transplanted marrow. Recent studies in which the autologous marrow was marked in vitro using a retrovirus demonstrated the presence of the marker within leukemia cells after relapse of disease, indicating that malignant cells present in the autologous marrow infusion may contribute to relapse.[75]

Poor prognostic factors include secondary leukemia, short interval of initial remission, and cytogenetics. Neither central nervous system involvement nor FAB classification affects the outcome. Development of effective purging techniques is probably necessary. Novel systemic agents to improve antileukemic efficacy, including the use of etoposide in the preparative regimen, are under evaluation. Use of radionuclide-conjugated antimyeloid monoclonal antibodies or bone-seeking radioconjugates can target the malignant cells or marrow and minimize systemic toxic effects.[76–78]

Acute Lymphoblastic Leukemia

Autologous transplantation has been evaluated in patients with acute lymphoblastic leukemia (ALL).[79–82] Unlike the situation in AML, in ALL, a number of monoclonal antibodies to leukemia-associated antigens that are nonreactive with normal hematopoietic progenitors are available.[20,83,84] They include antibodies to the common ALL antigen (CALLA) or T- or B-cell antigens. A number of patients have received autologous transplants using marrow that was treated ex vivo with one or more of these antibodies and complement.[79,84–87] Although each of these antigens is expressed on subpopulations of normal lymphoid cells, the antigens are not present on hematopoietic progenitors. Engraftment and immunologic recovery have consistently occurred. Limitations of this technique include probable antigenic heterogeneity among neoplastic cells. It is unclear whether leukemia stem cells express these cell-surface antigens. Select patients with ALL in second remission have achieved prolonged remissions after receiving intensive chemotherapy, TBI, and autologous marrow transplantation with anti-CALLA antibody and complement-treated marrow.[79,86] These data are difficult to interpret because many of the successful cases reported involved patients who had a relatively good prognosis with conventional treatment (such as patients whose disease relapsed after a long first remission and in whom maintenance therapy was discontinued. Results in patients with average or poor prognostic features have been much less encouraging.

Chronic Myelogenous Leukemia

Allogeneic transplantation is an effective treatment of chronic myelogenous leukemia (CML). However, because many patients lack a histocompatible donor for transplantation, autologous transplantation has been explored as an alternative approach.[88] Autologous transplantation for CML involves collection and cryopreservation of marrow or PBP cells during the chronic phase of the disease. When the disease progresses to the accelerated phase, patients receive intensive chemotherapy alone or in combination with TBI, followed by reinfusion of cryopreserved autologous cells.[89,90] The objective of this approach is to restore the chronic phase. Because Philadelphia-chromosome-positive cells are reinfused, cure is not possible. Some patients have transiently recovered apparently normal hematopoiesis without the Philadelphia chromosome. However, the Philadelphia-chromosome-positive leukemia cells usually become dominant again within a short interval, and the disease recurs.

A major limitation of autologous transplantation for advanced CML is resistance of acute-phase cells to intensive chemoradiotherapy. Although most patients who receive transplants when their disease is in the accelerated phase or in blast crisis achieve a brief second chronic phase, its median duration is only 4 months, and fewer than 30% of patients survive 1 year. This therapy thus must be considered of marginal benefit and cannot be routinely recommended.

A gene-marking study indicated that tumor contamination of the autograft is one of the reasons for the recurrence of disease.[91] Therefore, attempts have been made to prolong the duration of the chronic phase by performing autologous transplantation in patients whose disease is still in the chronic phase using marrow collected in cytogenetic remission or the early chronic phase. Another recent approach is to collect autologous PBP cells when they contain predominantly diploid cells. PBP cells are collected from patients whose disease is in partial or complete cytogenetic remission after interferon or intensive chemotherapy. The cells may be treated in vitro to separate normal cells from leukemia cells by a variety of developmental approaches, including separation on the basis of HLA-DR expression or treatment in long-term culture.[92–95] Because of the likelihood of residual disease after transplantation, enhanced cytotoxic preparative regimens and posttransplantation biologic therapy, such as that with IFN-α, to eliminate the minimal residual disease are being studied.

Chronic Lymphocytic Leukemia

Recently, autologous transplantation with monoclonal antibody-purged autologous marrow has been evaluated and has produced complete remissions (CRs) in patients with advanced disease.[96] Allogeneic transplantation was more effective in young patients with an HLA-identical donor. Autologous transplantation requires a large-scale study and long-term follow-up to definitely assess its long-term benefits.

Lymphoma

Autologous transplantation has been extensively studied in patients with non-Hodgkin's lymphoma.[97,98] Most of these patients have been treated for high- and intermediate-grade lymphomas that failed to respond or that relapsed after treatment with standard combination chemotherapy. Patients have received either intensive chemotherapy alone, such as with BEAC (carmustine, etoposide [VePesid], cytarabine, and cyclophosphamide) or a cyclophosphamide plus TBI regimen.[98–102] Results have been highly variable. Most patients achieve CR with this treatment, and approximately one third survive in remission for several years.

The best results have been noted in patients treated in second remission or in patients with relapsed disease that is still responsive to chemotherapy.[103] Recently, encouraging results have been reported in patients receiving autologous transplants in partial remission (PR) after initial induction therapy.[104] Toxic reactions have been a major problem, particularly in patients with heavily pretreated disease and in debilitated patients; severe hepatic, cardiac, and pulmonary reactions may occur. Studies have investigated the use of IFN-α as a posttransplantation therapy.[18]

Autologous transplantation in low-grade lymphoma (LGL) has shown encouraging results with high-dose cyclophosphamide plus TBI; 20% to 60% of patients with relapsed LGL survive from 3 to 5 years free of recurrence, depending on prognostic features.[101,102,105] One concern of autologous transplantation for patients with LGL is the propensity of this disease to involve the bone marrow during the course of its natural history and the potential of this disease for late relapse.

Techniques have recently been developed for selectively purging malignant lymphoid cells from normal marrow cells using ex vivo treatment with monoclonal antibodies against lymphoid cell-surface antigens that do not cross-react with normal hematopoietic progenitors. Normal marrow cells can be separated from malignant B-cells by using monoclonal antibody and complement treatment or immunomagnetic beads.[106,107] Many institutions employ ex vivo treatment of the harvested autologous marrow to deplete malignant cells. For clinical marrow harvests, purging techniques generally achieve an approximately 2 to 3 log reduction of malignant cells, and these systems cannot effectively deplete cells from patients with clinically involved marrow. Recently, Gribben et al reported significantly improved disease-free survival in patients receiving autologous transplants that were successfully purged of evidence of residual lymphoma as assessed by *bcl-2* gene rearrangement by polymerase chain reaction.[106–109] The efficacy of purging remains to be definitively established, but the elimination of bone-marrow contamination is likely to be increasingly important with the evolution of effective preparative regimens to eradicate systemic disease successfully.

Hodgkin's Disease

Nearly 30% of patients with Hodgkin's disease fail to achieve a durable CR. Autologous transplantation can produce durable remissions in selected patients with Hodgkin's disease that is chemotherapy sensitive.[110–112] Patients with systemic relapse after receiving combination chemotherapeutic regimens, such as MOPP (mechlorethamine [Mustargen], vincristine [Oncovin], procarbazine [Matulane], and prednisone) and ABVD (doxorubicin [Adriamycin, Rubex], bleomycin [Blenoxane], vinblastine, and dacarbazine), with a first-remission duration of longer than 12 months can be retreated with another round of standard-dose chemotherapy and can achieve a CR rate of more than 90%, although most of these patients ultimately relapse.[113] However, when patients have relapsing disease within 1 year, salvage chemotherapy with MOPP, ABVD, or comparable regimens produces a CR rate of only 29% to 50% and a disease-free survival rate of less than 20% at 5 years.[114,115] Favorable prognostic features include first remission for more than 1 year, good performance status, involvement of a limited number of nodal sites, absence of visceral disease, and absence of B symptoms. For patients in second systemic relapse, long-term disease-free survival with conventional chemotherapy is rare. For patients with recurrent Hodgkin's disease, treatment with HDCT or chemotherapy plus TBI with autologous transplantation results in a CR rate of more than 50% to 80% and a disease-free survival rate of 20% to 60% at 3 to 5 years.[106,116–120] Although no controlled trials have been reported, results in patients with initial remissions of less than 1 year appear superior to those reported with standard-dose salvage chemotherapy.

Controversy remains regarding the selection of patients for autologous transplantation[121] and the definition of the most effective preparative regimen. Initial studies used cyclophosphamide in combination with TBI.[122–124] TBI is not an ideal treatment of Hodgkin's disease; it is not possible to administer whole-body doses greater than 15 Gy in humans, and radiation doses exceeding 40 Gy are necessary to control active sites of Hodgkin's disease when local radiotherapy is used. In addition, patients with Hodgkin's disease frequently receive mediastinal radiotherapy as part of their initial treatment; these patients have a high rate of radiation pneumonitis if they are later treated with TBI. HDCT regimens have been better tolerated. The most commonly used preparative regimens involve therapy with CBV (cyclophosphamide, carmustine, and etoposide).[118,125,126] The doses used have varied widely from institution to institution: 4.5 to 6.0 g/m^2 cyclophosphamide, 300 to 600 mg/m^2 carmustine, and 1,200 to 2,400 mg/m^2 etoposide. With increasing dose, there is an increased rate of extramedullary toxic effects, and treatment-related death rates have ranged from 5% to more than 20%. It is unclear whether the higher-dose regimens result in superior long-term disease-free survival. Other regimens, such as etoposide plus melphalan (Alekeran)[127] and CBV plus cisplatin (Platinol)[128] have been studied, but there is no evidence that any of them is superior to CBV therapy.

Prognostic factors for response and survival after autologous transplantation include age, performance status, disease stage at transplantation, number of extranodal disease sites, number of previous treatment regimens, and response to previous chemo- and radiotherapy. These prognostic factors are similar to those for patients receiving salvage chemotherapy. Patients with all favorable prognostic features have a disease-free survival rate of more than 70% at 4 years, compared with approximately 20% in patients with adverse prognostic factors.[118]

Patient selection and disease-related factors have such a major impact on response and survival rates that it is difficult to compare treatment regimens among institutions or in different subsets of patients in which prognostic features vary or are not well defined. It is also difficult to compare autologous transplantation with salvage chemotherapy because of differences in patient eligibility and selection, time censoring, and prognostic factors. The optimal roles and the interaction of salvage chemotherapy and autologous transplantation are uncertain. Some institutions have performed autologous transplantation as the first treatment of relapsed disease. Others have instituted several courses of a salvage chemotherapy program, such as DHAP with collection of autologous marrow between courses and institution of dose-intensive therapy with autologous transplantation after achieving maximal cytoreduction with the salvage regimen. This latter approach has the advantages of providing treatment immediately after relapse, collecting the marrow between courses, and using the HDCT at the time of minimal tumor burden.

Studies are in progress involving radioimmunoconjugates that localize within the tumor and selectively irradiate the malignancy with minimal systemic toxic effects,[129,130] such as yttrium-90-labeled antiferritin antibodies. High-dose treatment with radioimmunoconjugates often causes severe myelosuppression, which requires autologous marrow or PBP cell infusion for hematologic recovery. Lower doses could potentially be given before or after HDCT as a means of producing additional cytoreduction. PBP cell collection is an effective approach in patients who cannot undergo marrow harvest, such as patients who have received pelvic irradiation or who have extensive bone involvement. It remains to be determined whether the level of contaminating malignant cells is lower in the peripheral blood than in the marrow of these patients; nonetheless, successful transplantation using PBP cells has been reported in patients with marrow involvement.[131]

Multiple Myeloma

Recently, autologous transplantation has been studied in patients up to 65 years of age with multiple myeloma.[132] Favorable results also have been reported with PBP cell transplantation.[133,134] Patients most likely to benefit have primary resistant or responding disease with low beta$_2$-microglobulin and lactate dehydrogenase levels treated within 1 year of diagnosis.[135]

Pediatric Solid Tumors

Autologous transplantation may be useful in the treatment of several pediatric tumors that are highly sensitive to a number of chemotherapeutic agents and radiation yet have a poor prognosis in patients with advanced disease, such as neuroblastoma and Ewing's sarcoma. Patients with highly advanced or recurrent neuroblastoma have a dismal prognosis with standard treatment.[136] Several studies using high-dose combined-modality therapy and allogeneic or autologous transplantation in such patients are currently in progress.[137–139]

Neuroblastoma frequently involves the bone marrow. Monoclonal antibodies to neuroblastoma-related antigens can be used to detect microscopic marrow involvement and to purge metastatic neuroblastoma cells from the marrow prior to cryopreservation.[24] PBP cell transplantation has also been used, although tumor cells may contaminate blood.[11] Gene-marking studies of autologous marrow demonstrate that malignant cells infused in the autotransplant may contribute to relapse.[75] The most encouraging results have been reported with treatment of patients at an earlier point in their disease and with the use of more intensive pretransplant conditioning regimens involving combination chemotherapy plus TBI in addition to either allogeneic or autologous marrow transplantation.

Patients with Ewing's sarcoma are also potential candidates for autologous transplantation. This tumor is responsive to chemotherapy and irradiation and rarely involves the bone marrow. Either high-dose melphalan or cyclophosphamide plus TBI[140] in combination with autologous transplantation can produce a CR in patients with relapsed Ewing's sarcoma, but these responses are usually brief. Intensive chemoradiotherapy with autologous transplantation may be more effective in consolidation treatment as part of first-line therapy.[141]

Breast Cancer

Breast cancer now represents the most common disease treated by autologous transplantation. For metastatic hormone-refractory breast cancer treated with standard-dose combination chemotherapy, such as CMF (cyclophosphamide, methotrexate, and fluorouracil or FAC (fluorouracil, doxorubicin, and cyclophosphamide), increasing the dose intensity improves both CR and PR rates and prolongs the interval to disease progression.[142] Standard-dose chemotherapy produces a CR rate of 15% to 25% and an overall response rate of 50% to 70%. The median response duration is typically 8 to 12 months. The median survival duration ranges from 12 to 18 months, and less than 5% of patients remain disease free at 5 years. The most effective HDCT regimens used with autologous transplantation include combinations of alkylating agents and related drugs, including cyclophosphamide, ifosfamide (Ifex), melphalan, thiotepa (Thioplex), carmustine, cisplatin, or carboplatin.[143,148] The doses of these agents typically can be increased threefold over standard doses when followed by autologous transplantation.

Studies in patients with chemotherapy-responsive metastatic breast cancer have documented that this approach significantly increases the CR rate to more than 50% and that approximately 20% of patients survive longer than 5 years free of recurrent disease. Recently, to improve the efficacy of HDCT, several treatment courses have been evaluated.[149,150] Favorable prognostic factors in these patients include responsiveness to standard-dose chemotherapy, limited tumor bulk and number of disease sites, absence of liver involvement, and good performance status.[146,151] However, this apparent improved outcome may be due to patient selection bias.[152] Randomized prospective studies comparing standard chemotherapy with HDCT currently are underway.

Because dose-intensive therapy is most effective in patients with a minimal burden of chemotherapy-sensitive tumor cells, the optimal use of this approach may be as adjuvant therapy in patients whose local-regional breast cancer is at high risk for relapse.[148,153,154] HDCT and autologous transplantation have recently been evaluated as adjuvant therapy for patients with "high-risk" stage II or III disease (generally defined as stage II disease with 10 or more positive axillary nodes or stage III disease). Five-year disease-free survival rates with standard adjuvant therapy range from 25% to 57%. In preliminary studies, approximately 70% of these high-risk patients survive free of relapse at 5 years after receiving HDCT and autologous transplantation.[148] It is difficult to compare directly the results of HDCT with standard-dose chemotherapy. Patients referred for HDCT must be young (generally younger than age 60), have good organ function and performance status, and must be clinically stable so they can be transferred to the transplantation center. Patients receiving HDCT are thus highly selected, and controlled clinical studies with either case controls or a randomized control group are necessary for definitive analysis.[151,155,156]

Several prospective, randomized studies are ongoing for patients with high-risk local-regional disease to assess the role of HDCT and autologous transplantation in this setting. Dose-intensive therapies must be integrated with other modalities into the overall treatment of breast cancer. This treatment is most likely to be curative if administered at a time of minimal tumor burden and before the evolution of drug resistance. The ideal timing should be as adjuvant therapy in patients with high-risk local-regional disease in whom alternative therapies are likely to fail and in patients with metastatic disease in CR from standard-dose chemotherapy.

Relapse remains a major problem, and the use of biologic or immunologic therapies for minimal residual breast cancer after autologous transplantation is under evaluation. As previously described, autologous GVHD is induced by cyclosporine and interferon is under evaluation.[16,17]

Purged bone marrow with 4-hydroperoxycylcophosphamide[157–159] or CD34-positive selected PBP cells is considered to reduce tumor contamination.[160–163] Controlled trials are needed, however, to demonstrate that purging improves clinical outcome.

Other Solid Tumors

In adults, other chemotherapy-responsive solid tumors, such as ovarian cancer,[164] testicular germ-cell carcinomas,[165–167] small-cell carcinoma of the lungs,[168,169] and melanoma,[170] are under study.

HEALTH-CARE IMPLICATIONS

There is controversy regarding in which clinical settings HDCT and autologous transplantation should be considered as an experimental procedure.[171–174] In experimental therapy, the risks and benefits are unknown. An established treatment is one in which there is sufficient experience to define the risks and the anticipated benefits; unfortunately, established systemic therapies for most advanced cancers are known to have only limited effectiveness. Many insurance carriers exclude coverage for experimental therapy, and some have denied payment for HDCT and autologous transplantation on this basis. This is inappropriate. Thousands of patients have received this therapeutic approach, and the results are consistent and well documented. For the indications previously discussed, nearly every study has determined that the response rate is improved over that with standard-dose alternatives, and a fraction of patients have achieved a prolonged disease-free survival. It is clear, however, that important questions remain regarding the optimal use and role of this form of therapy. Use of autologous transplantation should be restricted to cancer research centers, and patients should be enrolled in ongoing clinical trials.

The cost of HDCT and autologous marrow or PBP cell transplantation is primarily related to the length of hospitalization for supportive care, blood-product transfusions, and antibiotic treatment of granulocytopenic infections. The typical length of hospitalization is 3 to 4 weeks. There has been a recent effort to transfer a major portion of care to outpatient clinics. Well-organized outpatient infusion centers can administer dose-intensive treatment to clinically stable patients, and with the rapid hematologic recovery induced by growth factors and PBP cells, patients may not routinely require admission.

FUTURE DIRECTIONS

The collection of marrow or PBP cells offers the potential for ex vivo genetic therapy to improve treatment results. Transfection of genes for drug resistance, such as *MDR1*, into normal marrow cells may allow better tolerance to subsequent chemotherapy with agents such as doxorubicin, vinca alkaloids, and paclitaxel.[175] Alternative strategies include transfecting cytokine genes into hematopoietic cells or directly into the malignant cells to enhance immune reactivity against the tumor.[176,177] Improvement in the results of autologous transplantation for solid tumors requires the development of more effective treatment regimens that are not excessively toxic to normal tissues. A number of chemotherapeutic agents, including cyclophosphamide, melphalan, busulfan (Myleran), carmustine, lomustine (CCNU), mitomycin (Mutamycin), etoposide, and amsacrine, can be escalated to two to five times their standard dosage in the setting of autologous marrow transplantation. Further phase I and II clinical studies are required to determine the efficacy and nonhematopoietic toxicity of other chemotherapeutic agents in high doses. Candidate drugs should have documented efficacy in standard dosage, should have toxic effects limited primarily to the bone marrow, and should lack substantial nonmarrow toxic effects.

Novel classes of drugs, including anthrapyrazoles, topoisomerase-I inhibitors, and taxanes, have activity against many cancers and may be important components of future high-dose combination chemotherapeutic regimens. Approaches with targeted radiation therapy, such as monoclonal antibody-radionuclide immunoconjugates, are under active evaluation as a means to target radiotherapy to the tumor; this approach results in few systemic toxic effects, other than myelosuppression, which can be ameliorated by autologous marrow or blood stem-cell transplantation.

It may be possible to improve results further using strategies to overcome drug resistance mechanisms, such as the administration of inhibitors to p-glycoprotein or chemoprotectant agents. Kinetic resistance and the presence of poorly vascularized tumor masses are factors that limit the effectiveness of a single course of HDCT. Greater overall dose intensity may be achieved by repeated courses of therapy. The ability to collect large numbers of marrow and peripheral-blood hematopoietic cells allows the administration of two to four courses of treatment.[14,15] Nonhematopoietic toxic effects may be cumulative, and some dose reduction is necessary for multiple-course regimens to achieve optimal cytoreduction with an acceptable level of toxicity.

REFERENCES

1. Quesenberry P, Levitt L: Hematopoietic stem cells. N Engl J Med 307:755–760, 1979.

2. Meagher RC, Herzig RH: Techniques of harvesting and cryopreservation of stem cells. Hematol Oncol Clin North Am 7:501–533, 1993.

3. Areman EM, Sacher RA, Deeg HJ: Processing and storage of human bone marrow: A survey of current practices in North America. Bone Marrow Transplant 6:203–209, 1990.

4. Ahmed T, Wuest D, Ciavarella D, et al: Marrow storage techniques: A clinical comparison of refrigeration versus cryopreservation. Acta Haematol 85:173–178, 1991.

5. Kessinger A: Utilization of peripheral blood stem cells in autotransplantation. Hematol Oncol Clin North Am 7:535–545, 1993.

6. Nademanee A, O'Donnell MR, Snyder DS, et al: High-dose chemotherapy with or without total body irradiation followed by autologous bone marrow and/or peripheral blood stem cell transplan-

tation for patients with relapsed and refractory Hodgkin's disease: Results in 85 patients with analysis of prognostic factors. Blood 85:1381–1390, 1995.

7. Sheridan WP, Begley CG, Juttner CA, et al: Effect of peripheral-blood progenitor cells mobilized by filgrastim (G-CSF) on platelet recovery after high-dose chemotherapy. Lancet 339:640–644, 1992.

8. Peters WP, Rosner G, Ross M, et al: Comparative effects of granulocyte-macrophage colony-stimulating factor (GM-CSF) and granulocyte colony-stimulating factor (G-CSF) on priming peripheral blood progenitor cells for use with autologous bone marrow after high-dose chemotherapy. Blood 81:1709–1719, 1993.

9. Champlin R: Preparative regimens for autologous bone marrow transplantation (editorial). Blood 81:277–280, 1993.

10. Appelbaum FR, Herzig GP, Graw RG: Study of cell dose and storage time on engraftment of cryopreserved autologous bone marrow in canine model. Transplantation 26:245–248, 1978.

11. Moss TJ, Sanders DG, Lasky LC, et al: Contamination of peripheral blood stem cell harvests by circulating neuroblastoma cells. Blood 76:1879–1883, 1990.

12. Brugger W, Möcklin W, Heimfeld S, Berenson RJ, Mertelsmann R, Kanz L: Ex vivo expansion of enriched peripheral blood CD34+ progenitor cells by stem cell factor, interleukin-1 (IL-1), IL-6, IL-3, interferon-gamma, and erythropoietin. Blood 81:2579–2584, 1993.

13. Koller MR, Emerson SG, Palsson BO: Large-scale expansion of human stem and progenitor cells from bone marrow mononuclear cells in continuous perfusion cultures. Blood 82:378–384, 1993.

14. Shea TC, Mason JR, Storniolo AM, et al: Sequential cycles of high-dose carboplatin administered with recombinant human granulocyte-macrophage colony-stimulating factor and repeated infusions of autologous peripheral-blood progenitor cells: A novel and effective method for delivering multiple courses of dose-intensive therapy. J Clin Oncol 10:464–473, 1992.

15. Tepler I, Cannistra SA, Frei E III, et al: Use of peripheral-blood progenitor cells abrogates the myelotoxicity of repetitive outpatient high-dose carboplatin and cyclophosphamide chemotherapy. J Clin Oncol 11:1583–1591, 1993.

16. Kennedy MJ, Vogelsang GB, Beveridge RA, et al: Phase I trial of intravenous cyclosporine to induce graft-versus-host disease in women undergoing autologous bone marrow transplantation for breast cancer. J Clin Oncol 11:478–484, 1993.

17. Kennedy MJ, Vogelsang GB, Jones RJ, et al: Phase I trial of interferon gamma to potentiate cyclosporine-induced graft-versus-host disease in women undergoing autologous bone marrow transplantation for breast cancer (see comments). J Clin Oncol 12:249–257, 1994.

18. Schenkein DP, Dixon P, Desforges JF, et al: Phase I/II study of cyclophosphamide, carboplatin, and etoposide and autologous hematopoietic stem-cell transplantation with posttransplant interferon alfa-2b for patients with lymphoma and Hodgkin's disease. J Clin Oncol 12:2423–2431, 1994.

19. Kennedy MJ. Induced autologous graft-versus-host disease for the treatment of cancer. Cancer Treat Rev 20:97–103, 1994.

20. Bast RC, Ritz J, Lipton JM: Elimination of leukemic cells from human bone marrow using monoclonal antibody and complement. Cancer Res 43:1389–1394, 1983.

21. Vitetta ES, Krolick KA, Miyama-Inaba M, et al: Immunotoxins: A new approach to cancer therapy. Science 219:644–650, 1983.

22. Sharkis SJ, Santos GW, Colvin M: Elimination of acute myelogenous leukemia cells from marrow and tumor suspension in the rat with 4-hydroperoxycylophosphamide. Blood 55:521–523, 1980.

23. Rowley SD, Jones RJ, Piantadosi S, et al: Efficacy of ex vivo purging for autologous bone marrow transplantation in the treatment of acute nonlymphoblastic leukemia. Blood 74:501–506, 1989.

24. Kemshead JT, Heath L, Gibson FM, et al: Magnetic microspheres and monoclonal antibodies for the depletion of neuroblastoma cells from bone marrow. Experience, improvements and observations. Br J Cancer 54:771–778, 1986.

25. Noga SJ, Wagner JE, Rowley SD, et al: Using elutriation to engineer bone marrow allografts. Prog Clin Biol Res 333:345–362, 1990.

26. Civin CI: Identification and positive selection of human progenitor/stem cells for bone marrow transplantation. Prog Clin Biol Res 377:461–473, 1992.

27. Berenson RJ, Bensinger WI, Hill RS, et al: Engraftment after infusion of CD34+ marrow cells in patients with breast cancer or neuroblastoma. Blood 77:1717–1722, 1991.

28. Uchida N, Aguila HL, Fleming WH, et al: Rapid and sustained hematopoietic recovery in lethally irradiated mice transplanted with purified Thy-1.1lo Lin-Sca+ hematopoietic stems cells. Blood 83:3758–3779, 1994.

29. Champlin RE, Gale RP: Early complications of bone marrow transplantation. Semin Hematol 21:101–108, 1984.

30. Nemunaitis J, Rabinowe SN, Singer JW, et al: Recombinant granulocyte-macrophage colony stimulating factor (rhGM-CSF) after autologous bone marrow transplantation for lymphoid cancer. N Engl J Med 324:1773–1778, 1991.

31. Sheridan WP, Morstyn G, Wolf M, et al: Granulocyte colony-stimulating factor and neutrophil recovery after high-dose chemotherapy and autologous bone marrow transplantation. Lancet 2:891–895, 1989.

32. Nemunaitis J, Singer JW, Buckner CD, et al: Use of recombinant human granulocyte-macrophage colony-stimulating factor in graft failure after bone marrow transplantation. Blood 76:245–253, 1990.

33. Nemunaitis J, Appelbaum FR, Singer JW, et al: Phase I trial with recombinant human interleukin-3 in patients with lymphoma undergoing autologous bone marrow transplantation. Blood 82:3273–3278, 1993.

34. van Gameren MM, Willemse PH, Mulder NH, et al: Effects of recombinant human interleukin-6 in cancer patients: A phase I-II study. Blood 84:1434–1441, 1994.

35. Wendling F, Maraskovsky E, Debili N, et al: cMpl ligand is a humoral regulator of megakaryocytopoiesis. Nature 369:571–574, 1994.

36. Kaushansky K, Lok S, Holly RD, et al: Promotion of megakaryocyte progenitor expansion and differentiation by the c-Mpl ligand thrombopoietin. Nature 369:568–571, 1994.

37. McDonald GB, Hinds MS, Fisher LD, et al: Veno-occlusive disease of the liver and multiorgan failure after bone marrow transplantation: A cohort study of 355 patients. Ann Intern Med 118:255–267, 1993.

38. Weiner RS, Bortin MM, Gale RP, et al: Interstitial pneumonitis after bone marrow transplantation. Ann Intern Med 104:168–175, 1986.

39. Jochelson M, Tarbell NJ, Freedman AS, et al: Acute and chronic pulmonary complications following autologous bone marrow transplantation in non-Hodgkin's lymphoma. Bone Marrow Transplant 6:329–331, 1990.

40. Jones RB, Matthes S, Shpall EJ, et al: Acute lung injury following treatment with high-dose cyclophosphamide, cisplatin, and carmustine: Pharmacodynamic evaluation of carmustine. J Natl Cancer Inst 85:640–647, 1993.

41. Ayash LJ, Wright JE, Tretyakov O, et al: Cyclophosphamide pharmacokinetics: Correlation with cardiac toxicity and tumor response. J Clin Oncol 10:995–1000, 1992.

42. Braverman AC, Antin JH, Plappert MT, et al: Cyclophosphamide cardiotoxicity in bone marrow transplantation: A prospective evaluation of new dosing regimens. J Clin Oncol 9:1215–1223, 1991.

43. Thompson CB, Sanders JE, Flournoy N, et al: The risks of central nervous system relapse and leukoencephalopathy in patients receiving marrow transplants for acute leukemia. Blood 67:195–199, 1986.

44. Sklar CA, Kim TH, Ramsay NKC: Thyroid dysfunction among longterm survivors of bone marrow transplantation. Am J Med 73:688–694, 1982.

45. Carlson K, Lonnerholm G, Smedmyr B, et al: Thyroid function after autologous bone marrow transplantation. Bone Marrow Transplant 10:123–127, 1992.

46. Sanders JE, Pritchard S, Mahoney P, et al: Growth and development following marrow transplantation for leukemia. Blood 68:1129–1135, 1986.

47. Sanders JE, Buckner CD, Amos D, et al: Ovarian function following marrow transplantation for aplastic anemia or leukemia. J Clin Oncol 6:813–818, 1988.

48. Sanders JE, Seattle Marrow Transplant Team: The impact of marrow transplant preparative regimens on subsequent growth and development. Semin Hematol 28:244–249, 1991.

49. Deeg HJ, Flournoy N, Sullivan KM, et al: Cataracts after total body irradiation and marrow transplantation: A sparing effect of dose fractionation. Int J Radiat Oncol Biol Phys 10:957–964, 1984.

50. Shepherd JD, Pringle LE, Barnett MJ, et al: Mesna versus hyperhydration for the prevention of cyclophosphamide-induced hemorrhagic cystitis in bone marrow transplantation. J Clin Oncol 9:2016–2020, 1991.

51. Letendre L, Hoagland HC, Gertz MA: Hemorrhagic cystitis complicating bone marrow transplantation. Mayo Clin Proc 67:128–130, 1992.

52. Henon PR, Liang H, Beck-Wirth G, et al: Comparison of hematopoietic and immune recovery after autologous bone marrow or blood stem cell transplants. Bone Marrow Transplant 9:285–291, 1992.

53. Winston DW, Ho WG, Champlin RE, et al: Infectious complications of bone marrow transplantation. Exp Hematol 12:205–215, 1984.

54. Saral R, Burns WH, Laskin OL, et al: Acyclovir prophylaxis of herpes simplex virus infections: A randomized, double blind, controlled trial in bone marrow transplant recipients. N Engl J Med 306:1009–1012, 1981.

55. Socié G, Kolb HJ, Ljungman P: Malignant diseases after allogeneic bone marrow transplantation: The case for assessment of risk factors. Br J Haematol 80:427–430, 1992.

56. Deeg HJ, Witherspoon RP: Risk factors for the development of secondary malignancies after marrow transplantation. Hematol Oncol Clin North Am 7:417–429, 1993.

57. Zutter MM, Martin PJ, Sale GE, et al: Epstein-Barr virus lymphoproliferation after bone marrow transplantation.. Blood 72:520–529, 1988.

58. Waller EK, Ziemianska M, Bangs CD, et al: Characterization of posttransplant lymphomas that express T-cell-associated markers: Immunophenotypes, molecular genetics, cytogenetics, and heterotransplantation in severe combined immunodeficient mice. Blood 82:247–261, 1993.

59. Marolleau JP, Brice P, Morel P, et al: Secondary acute myeloid leukemia after autologous bone marrow transplantation for malignant lymphomas. J Clin Oncol 11:590–591, 1993.

60. Miller JS, Arthur DC, Litz CE, et al: Myelodysplastic syndrome after autologous bone marrow transplantation: An additional late complication of curative cancer therapy. Blood 83:3780–3786, 1994.

61. Labopin M, Gorin NC: Autologous bone marrow transplantation in 2502 patients with acute leukemia in Europe: A retrospective study. Leukemia 6(suppl 4):95–99, 1992.

62. Geller RB: Role of autologous bone marrow transplantation for patients with acute and chronic leukemias. Hematol Oncol Clin North Am 7:547–575, 1993.

63. Busca A, Anasetti C, Anderson G, et al: Unrelated donor or autologous marrow transplantation for treatment of acute leukemia. Blood 83:3077–3084, 1994.

64. Dicke K, Spitzer G: Evaluation of the use of high dose cytoreduction with autologous marrow rescue in various malignancies. Transplantation 41:4–20, 1986.

65. Gorin NC, David R, Strachowiak J, et al: High dose chemotherapy and autologous bone marrow transplantation in acute leukemias, malignant lymphomas and solid tumors. Eur J Cancer 17:557–568, 1981.

66. Rizzoli V, Mangoni L, Carlo-Stella C: Autologous bone marrow transplantation in acute myelogenous leukemia. Leukemia 6:1101–1106, 1992.

67. Keating A, Crump M: High dose etoposide melphalan, total body irradiation and ABMT for acute myeloid leukemia in first remission. Leukemia 6(suppl 4):90–91, 1992.

68. Linker CA, Ries CA, Damon LE, Rugo HS, Wolf JL: Autologous bone marrow transplantation for acute myeloid leukemia using busulfan plus etoposide as a preparative regimen. Blood 81:311–318, 1993.

69. Chao NJ, Stein AS, Long GD, et al: Busulfan/etoposide: Initial experience with a new preparatory regimen for autologous bone marrow transplantation in patients with acute nonlymphoblastic leukemia. Blood 81:319–323, 1993.

70. Ball ED, Mills L, Hurd D, McMillan R, Gingrich R: Autologous bone marrow transplantation for acute myeloid leukemia using monoclonal antibody-purged bone marrow. Prog Clin Biol Res 377:97–111, 1992.

71. Selvaggi KJ, Wilsons JW, Mills LE, et al: Improved outcome for high-risk acute myeloid leukemia patients using autologous bone marrow transplantation and monoclonal antibody-purged bone marrow. Blood 83:1698–1705, 1994.

72. Hermann RP: Prompt haematopoietic reconstitution following hyperthermia purged autologous marrow and peripheral blood stem cell transplantation in acute myeloid leukaemia. Bone Marrow Transplant 10:293–295, 1992.

73. Yeager AM, Kaizer H, Santos GW, et al: Autologous bone marrow transplantation in patients with acute nonlymphocytic leukemia, using ex vivo marrow treatment with 4-hydroperoxycylophosphamide. N Engl J Med 315:141–147, 1986.

74. Gorin NC, Aegerter P, Auvert B, et al: Autologous bone marrow transplantation for acute myelocytic leukemia in first remission: A European survey of the role of marrow purging. Blood 75:1606–1614, 1990.

75. Brenner MK, Rill DR, Moen RC, et al: Gene-marking to trace origin of relapse after autologous bone-marrow transplantation. Lancet 341:85–86, 1993.

76. Matthews DC, Badger CC, Fisher DR, et al: Selective radiation of hematolymphoid tissue delivered by anti-CD45 antibody. Cancer Res 52:1228–1234, 1992.

77. Appelbaum FR, Matthews DC, Eary JF, et al: The use of radiolabeled anti-CD33 antibody to augment marrow irradiation prior to marrow transplantation for acute myelogenous leukemia. Transplantation 54:829–833, 1992.

78. Scheinberg DA, Lovett D, Divgi CR, et al: A phase I trial of monoclonal antibody M195 in acute myelogenous leukemia: Specific bone marrow targeting and internalization of radionuclide. J Clin

Oncol 9:478–490, 1991.

79. Kersey JH: The role of marrow transplantation in acute lymphoblastic leukemia. J Clin Oncol 7:1589–1590, 1989.

80. Ball ED, Rybka WB: Autologous bone marrow transplantation for adult acute leukemia. Hematol Oncol Clin North Am 7:201–131, 1993.

81. Sallan SE, Niemeyer CM, Billett AL, et al: Autologous bone marrow transplantation for acute lymphoblastic leukemia. J Clin Oncol 7:1594–1601, 1989.

82. Ramsay NK, Kersey JH: Indications for marrow transplantation in acute lymphoblastic leukemia. Blood 75:815–818, 1990.

83. Uckun FM, Kersey JH, Gajl-Peczalska KJ, et al: Heterogeneity of cultured leukemic lymphoid progenitor cells from B cell precursor acute lymphoblastic leukemia (ALL) patients. J Clin Invest 80:639–646, 1987.

84. Anderson KC, Soiffer R, DeLage R, et al: T-cell-depleted autologous bone marrow transplantation therapy: Analysis of immune deficiency and late complications. Blood 76:235–244, 1990.

85. Ritz J, Sallan SE, Bast RC, et al: Autologous bone marrow transplantation in CALLA positive acute lymphoblastic leukemia after in vitro treatment with J5 monoclonal antibody and complement. Lancet 2:60–63, 1982.

86. Billett AL, Kornmehl E, Tarbell NJ, et al: Autologous bone marrow transplantation after a long first remission for children with recurrent acute lymphoblastic leukemia. Blood 81:1651–1657, 1993.

87. Körbling M, Knauf W, Funderud S, et al: Autologous transplantation of an immunomagnetic bead purged marrow in patients with relapsed acute lymphoblastic leukemia. Haematologica (Pavia) 76(suppl 1):29–36, 1991.

88. McGlave PB, De Fabritiis P, Deisseroth A, et al: Autologous transplants for chronic myelogenous leukaemia: Results from eight transplant groups. Lancet 343:1486–1488, 1994.

89. Goldman JM, Th'ng KH, Park DS, et al: Collection, cryopreservation and subsequent viability of haematopoietic stem cells intended for treatment of chronic granulocytic leukemia in blast-cell transformation. Br J Haematol 40:185–195, 1978.

90. Goldman JM: Autografting for chronic myeloid leukaemia: Palliation, cure or nothing. Leuk Lymphoma 7(suppl):51–54, 1992.

91. Deisseroth AB, Zu Z, Claxton D, et al: Genetic marking shows that Ph+ cells present in autologous transplants of chronic myelogenous leukemia (CML) contribute to relapse after autologous bone marrow in CML. Blood 83:3068–3076, 1994.

92. Deisseroth AB, Zhang W, Cha Y, et al: New directions in the biology and therapy of chronic myeloid leukemia. Leuk Lymphoma 6:89–95, 1992.

93. McGlave PB, Arthur D, Miller WJ, et al: Autologous transplantation for CML using marrow treated ex vivo with recombinant human interferon gamma. Bone Marrow Transplant 6:115–120, 1990.

94. Barnett MJ, Eaves CJ, Phillips GL, et al: Autografting in chronic myeloid leukemia with cultured marrow. Leukemia 6 (suppl 4):118–119, 1992.

95. Eaves AC, Eaves CJ, Phillips GL, et al: Culture purging in leukemia: Past, present, and future. Leuk Lymphoma 11 (suppl 1):259–263, 1993.

96. Rabinowe SN, Soiffer RJ, Gribben JG, et al: Autologous and allogeneic bone marrow transplantation for poor prognosis patients with B-cell chronic lymphocytic leukemia. Blood 82:1366–1376, 1993.

97. Wheeler C, Strawderman M, Ayash L, et al: Prognostic factors for treatment outcome in autotransplantation of intermediate-grade and high-grade non-Hodgkin's lymphoma with cyclophosphamide, carmustine, and etoposide. J Clin Oncol 11:1085–1091, 1993.

98. Vose JM, Armitage JO: Role of autologous bone marrow transplantation in non-Hodgkin's lymphoma. Hematol Oncol Clin North Am 7:577–590, 1993.

99. Phillips GL, Herzig RH, Lazarus HM, et al: High-dose chemotherapy, fractionated total-body irradiation, and allogeneic marrow transplantation for malignant lymphoma. J Clin Oncol 4:480–488, 1986.

100. Vose JM, Armitage JO, Bierman PJ, et al: Salvage therapy for relapsed or refractory non-Hodgkin's lymphoma utilizing autologous bone marrow transplantation. Am J Med 87:285–288, 1989.

101. Schouten HC, Bierman PJ, Vaughan WP, et al: Autologous bone marrow transplantation in follicular non-Hodgkin's lymphoma before and after histologic transformation. Blood 74:2579–2584, 1989.

102. Freedman AS, Ritz J, Neuberg D, et al: Autologous bone marrow transplantation in 69 patients with a history of low-grade B-cell non-Hodgkin's lymphoma. Blood 77:2524–2529, 1991.

103. Philip T, Armitage JO, Spitzer G, et al: High-dose therapy and autologous bone marrow transplantation after failure of conventional chemotherapy in adults with intermediate grade or high-grade-non-Hodgkin's lymphoma. N Engl J Med 316:1493–1498, 1987.

104. Philip T, Hartman O, Brian P, et al: High dose therapy and autologous bone marrow transplantation in partial remission after first line induction therapy for diffuse non-Hodgkin's lymphoma. J Clin Oncol 8:784–791, 1988.

105. Rohatiner AZS, Lister TA: Myeloablative therapy for follicular lymphoma. Hematol Oncol Clin North Am 5:1003–1012, 1991.

106. Gribben JG, Freedman AS, Neuberg D, et al: Immunologic purging of marrow assessed by PCR before autologous bone marrow transplantation for B-cell lymphoma. N Engl J Med 325:1525–1533, 1991.

107. Gribben JG, Neuberg D, Freedman AS, et al: Detection by polymerase chain reaction with the bcl-2 translocation is associated with increased risk of relapse after autologous bone marrow transplantation for B-cell lymphoma. Blood 81:3449–3457, 1993.

108. Gribben JG, Saporito L, Barber M, et al: Bone marrows of non-Hodgkin's lymphoma patients with a bcl-2 translocation can be purged of polymerase chain reaction-detectable lymphoma cells using monoclonal antibodies and immunomagnetic bead depletion. Blood 80:1083–1089, 1992.

109. Gribben JG, Neuberg D, Barber M, et al: Detection of residual lymphoma cells by polymerase chain reaction in peripheral blood is significantly less predictive for relapse than detection in bone marrow. Blood 83:3800–3807, 1994.

110. Carella AM, Carlier P, Congiu A, et al: Nine years' experience with ABMT in 128 patients with Hodgkin's disease: An Italian study group report. Leukemia 5 (suppl 1) 68–71, 1991.

111. Armitage JO, Bierman PJ, Vose JM, et al: Autologous bone marrow transplantation for patients with relapsed Hodgkin's disease. Am J Med 91:605–611, 1991.

112. Champlin R: Bone marrow transplantation for Hodgkin's disease: Recent advances and current issues. Leuk Lymphoma 10(suppl):103–108, 1993.

113. Longo DL, Duffey PL, Young RC, et al: Conventional-dose salvage combination chemotherapy in patients relapsing with Hodgkin's disease after combination chemotherapy: The low probability for cure. J Clin Oncol 10:210–218, 1992.

114. Bergsagel DE: Salvage treatment for Hodgkin's disease in relapse. J Clin Oncol 10:210–218, 1987.

115. Tannir N, Hagemeister F, Velasquez W, et al: Long-term follow-up with ABDIC salvage chemotherapy of MOPP-resistant Hodgkin's disease. J Clin Oncol 1:432–439, 1983.

116. Philips GL, Reece DE: Clinical studies of autologous bone marrow transplantation in Hodgkin's disease. Clin Hematol 15:155–166, 1986.

117. Chopra R, Linch DC, McMillan AK, et al: Mini-BEAM followed by BEAM and ABMT for very poor risk Hodgkin's disease. Br J Haematol 81:197–202, 1992.

118. Jagannath S, Armitage JO, Dicke KA, et al: Prognostic factors for response and survival after high-dose cyclophosphamide, carmustine, and etoposide with autologous bone marrow transplantation for relapsed Hodgkin's disease. J Clin Oncol 7:179–185, 1989.

119. Vose JM, Armitage JO: Bone marrow transplantation for Hodgkin's disease and lymphoma. Annu Rev Med 44:255–263, 1993.

120. Anderson JE, Litzow MR, Appelbaum FR, et al: Allogeneic, syngeneic, and autologous marrow transplantation for Hodgkin's disease: The 21-year Seattle experience. J Clin Oncol 11:2342–2350, 1993.

121. Desch CE, Lasala MR, Smith TJ, et al: The optimal timing of autologous bone marrow transplantation in Hodgkin's disease patients after a chemotherapy relapse. J Clin Oncol 10:200–209, 1992.

122. Sullivan KM, Appelbaum FR, Horning SJ, et al: Selection of patients with Hodgkin's disease and non-Hodgkin's lymphoma for bone marrow transplantation. Int J Cell Cloning 4:94–106, 1986.

123. Yahalom J, Gulati SC, Toia M, et al: Accelerated hyperfractionated total-lymphoid irradiation, high-dose chemotherapy, and autologous bone marrow transplantation for refractory and relapsing patients with Hodgkin's disease. J Clin Oncol 11:1062–1070, 1993.

124. Phillips GL: Autologous bone marrow transplantation for hematologic cancer. Prog Clin Biol Res 354B:171–184, 1990.

125. Reece DE, Barnett MJ, Connors JM, et al: Intensive chemotherapy with cyclophosphamide, carmustine, and etoposide followed by autologous bone marrow transplantation for relapsed Hodgkin's disease. J Clin Oncol 9:1871–1879, 1991.

126. Wheeler C, Antin JH, Churchill WH, et al: Cyclophosphamide, carmustine, and etoposide with autologous bone marrow transplantation in refractory Hodgkin's disease and non-Hodgkin's lymphoma: A dose-finding study. J Clin Oncol 8:648–656, 1990.

127. Crump M, Smith AM, Brandwein J, et al: High-dose etoposide and melphalan, and autologous bone marrow transplantation for patients with advanced Hodgkin's disease: Importance of disease status at transplant. J Clin Oncol 11:704–711, 1993.

128. Reece DE, Connors JM, Spinelli JJ, et al: Intensive therapy with cyclophosphamide, carmustine, etoposide +/- cisplatin, and autologous bone marrow transplantation for Hodgkin's disese in first relapse after combination therapy. Blood 83:1193–1199, 1994.

129. Vriesendorp HM, Quadri SM, Stinson RL, et al: Selection of reagents for human radioimmunotherapy. Int J Radiat Oncol Biol Phys 22:37–45, 1992.

130. Bierman PJ, Vose JM, Leichner PK, et al: Yttrium 90-labeled antiferritin followed by high-dose chemotherapy and autologous bone marrow transplantation for poor-prognosis Hodgkin's disease. J Clin Oncol 11:698–703, 1993.

131. Kessinger A, Bierman PJ, Vose JM, et al: High-dose cyclophosphamide, carmustine, and etoposide followed by autologous peripheral stem cell transplantation for patients with relapsed Hodgkin's disease. Blood 77:2322–2325, 1991.

132. Barlogie B, Jagannath S: . Autotransplants in myeloma. Bone Marrow Transplant 10(suppl 1):37–44, 1992.

133. Henon P, Beck G, Debecker A, et al: Autograft using peripheral blood stem cells collected after high dose melphalan in high risk multiple myeloma. Br J Haematol 70:254–255, 1988.

134. Fermand J-P, Levy Y, Gerota J, et al: Treatment of aggressive multiple myeloma by high-dose chemotherapy and total body irradiation followed by blood stem cells autologous graft. Blood 73:20–23, 1989.

135. Jagannath S, Barlogie B, Dicke K, et al: Autologous bone marrow transplantation in multiple myeloma: Identification of prognostic factors. Blood 76:1860–1866, 1990.

136. Seeger RC, Siegal SE, Sidell H: Neuroblastoma: Clinical perspectives monoclonal antibodies and retinoic acid. Ann Intern Med 97:873, 1982.

137. August CS, Serota FT, Koch PA, et al: Treatment of advanced neuroblastoma with supralethal chemotherapy, radiation and allogeneic or autologous marrow reconstitution. J Clin Oncol 2:609, 1984.

138. Philip T, Bernard JL, Zucher JM, et al: High dose chemoradiotherapy with bone marrow transplantation as consolidation treatment in neuroblastoma: An unselected group of stage IV patients over one year of age. J Clin Oncol 5:266–271, 1987.

139. Seeger RC, Villablanca JG, Matthay KK, et al: Intensive chemoradiotherapy and autologous bone marrow transplantation for poor prognosis neuroblastoma. Prog Clin Biol Res 366:527–533, 1991.

140. Burdach S, Jürgens H, Peters C, et al: Myeloablative radiochemotherapy and hematopoietic stem-cell rescue in poor-prognosis Ewing's sarcoma. J Clin Oncol 11:1482–1488, 1993.

141. Tepper J, Glaubigger D, Lichter A, et al: Local control of Ewing's sarcoma of bone with radiotherapy and combination chemotherapy. Cancer 46:1969–1973, 1980.

142. Hyrniuk W, Bush H: The importance of dose intensity in chemotherapy of metastatic breast cancer. J Clin Oncol 2:1281–1288, 1984.

143. Frei E III: The modulation of alkylating agents. Semin Hematol 28(suppl 4):22–24, 1991.

144. Antman K, Ayash L, Elias A, et al: A phase II study of high-dose cyclophosphamide, thiotepa, and carboplatin with autologous marrow support in women with measurable advanced breast cancer responding to standard-dose therapy. J Clin Oncol 10:102–110, 1992.

145. Peters WP, Shpall EJ, Jones RB, et al: High dose combination alkylating agents with bone marrow support as initial treatment for metastatic breast cancer. J Clin Oncol 6:1368–1376, 1988.

146. Dunphy FR, Spitzer G, Buzdar AU, et al: Treatment of estrogen receptor-negative or hormonally refractory breast cancer with double high-dose chemotherapy intensification and bone marrow support. J Clin Oncol 8:1207–1216, 1992.

147. Fields KK, Perkins JP, Hiemenz JW, et al: Intensive dose ifosfamide, carboplatin, and etoposide followed by autologous stem cell rescue: Results of a phase I/II study in breast cancer patients. Surg Oncol 2:87–95, 1993.

148. Peters WP, Ross M, Vredenburgh JJ, et al: High-dose chemotherapy and autologous bone marrow support as consolidation after standard-dose adjuvant therapy for high-risk primary breast cancer. J Clin Oncol 11:1132–1143, 1993.

149. Ghalie R, Richman CM, Adler SS, et al: Treatment of metastatic breast cancer with a split-course high-dose chemotherapy regimen and autologous bone marrow transplantation. J Clin Oncol 12:342–346, 1994.

150. Ayash LJ, Elias A, Wheeler C, et al: Double dose-intensive chemotherapy with autologous marrow and peripheral-blood progenitor-cell support for metastatic breast cancer: a feasibility study. J Clin Oncol 12:37–44, 1994.

151. Dunphy FR, Spitzer G, Fornoff JE, et al: Factors predicting long-term survival for metastatic breast cancer patients treated with high-dose chemotherapy and bone marrow support. Cancer 73:2157–2167, 1994.

152. Eddy DM: High-dose chemotherapy with autologous bone marrow transplantation for the treatment of metastatic breast cancer [published erratum appears in J Clin Oncol 10:1655–1658, 1992]. J Clin Oncol 10:657–670, 1992.

153. Abeloff MD: High-dose adjuvant chemotherapy for high-risk breast cancer. Recent Results Cancer Res 127:177–183, 1993.

154. Marks LB, Halperin EC, Prosnitz LR, et al: Post-mastectomy radiotherapy following adjuvant chemotherapy and autologous bone marrow transplantation for breast cancer patients with greater than or equal to 10 positive axillary lymph nodes. Cancer and Leukemia Group B (see comments). Int J Radiat Oncol Biol Phys 23:1021–1026, 1992.

155. Henderson IC, Hayes DF, Gelman R: Dose-response in the treatment of breast cancer: A critical review. J Clin Oncol 5:1501–1510, 1988.

156. Eddy DM, Hillner BE, Smith TJ, et al: High-dose chemotherapy with autologous bone marrow transplantation for metastatic breast cancer. JAMA 268:1536–1537, 1992.

157. Hortobaygyi GN, Dunphy F, Buzdar AU, Spitzer G: Dose intensity studies in breast cancer: Autologous bone marrow transplantation. Prog Clin Biol Res 354B:195–209, 1990.

158. Gonzales Chambers R, Przepiorka D, Shadduck RK, et al: Autologous bone marrow transplantation with 4-hydroperoxycyclophosphamide-purged marrow for acute lymphoblastic leukemia. Med Pediatr Oncol 19:160–164, 1991.

159. Kennedy MJ, Beveridge RA, Rowley SD, et al: High-dose chemotherapy with reinfusion of purged autologous bone marrow following dose-intense induction as initial therapy for metastatic breast cancer (see comments). J Natl Cancer Inst 83:920–926, 1991.

160. Kennedy MJ, Davis J, Passos Coelho J, et al: Administration of human recombinant granulocyte colony-stimulating factor (filgrastim) accelerates granulocyte recovery following high-dose chemotherapy and autologous marrow transplantation with 4-hydroperoxy-cyclophosphamide-purged marrow in women with metastatic breast cancer. Cancer Res 53:5424–5428, 1993.

161. Shpall EJ, Jones RB, Bearman SI, et al: Positive selection of CD34+ hematopoietic progenitor cells for transplantation. Stem Cells (Dayt) 11:48–49, 1993.

162. Shpall EJ, Jones RB, Bearman SI, et al: Transplantation of enriched CD34-positive autologous marrow into breast cancer patients following high-dose chemotherapy: Influence of CD34-positive peripheral-blood progenitors and growth factors on engraftment. J Clin Oncol 12:28–36, 1994.

163. Berenson RJ, Bensinger WI, Hill RS, et al: Engraftment after infusion of CD34+ marrow cells in patients with breast cancer or neuroblastoma. Blood 77:1717–1722, 1991.

164. Broun ER, Belinson JL, Berek JS, et al: Salvage therapy for recurrent and refractory ovarian cancer with high-dose chemotherapy and autologous bone marrow support: A Gynecologic Oncology Group pilot study. Gynecol Oncol 54:142–146, 1994.

165. Broun ER, Nichols CR, Einhorn LH, Tricot GJK: Salvage therapy with high-dose chemotherapy and autologous bone marrow support in the treatment of primary nonseminomatous mediastinal germ cell tumors. Cancer 68:1513–1515, 1991.

166. Broun ER, Nichols CR, Kneebone P, et al: Long-term outcome of patients with relapsed and refractory germ cell tumors treated with high-dose chemotherapy and autologous bone marrow rescue. Ann Intern Med 117:124–128, 1992.

167. Broun ER, Nichols CR, Tricot G, et al: High dose carboplatin/VP-16 plus ifosfamide with autologous bone marrow support in the treatment of refractory germ cell tumors. Bone Marrow Transplant 7:53–56, 1991.

168. Spitzer G, Farha P, Valdivieso M, et al: High-dose intensification therapy with autologous bone marrow support for limited small cell bronchogenic carcinoma. J Clin Oncol 29:359–364, 1986.

169. Humblet Y, Symann M: Small cell lung cancer: High-dose late intensification chemotherapy with autologous bone marrow transplantation. Bone Marrow Transplant 10 (suppl 2):33, 1992.

170. Meisenberg B, Ross M, Vredenburgh J, et al: Randomized trial of high-dose chemotherapy with autologous bone marrow support as adjuvant therapy for high-risk, multi-node-positive malignant melanoma. J Natl Cancer Inst 85:1080–1085, 1993.

171. Hillner BE, Smith TJ, Desch CE: Efficacy and cost-effectiveness of autologous bone marrow transplantation in metastatic breast cancer. Estimates using decision analysis while awaiting clinical trial results (see comments). JAMA 267:2055–2061, 1992.

172. Peters WP, Rogers MC: Variation in approval by insurance companies of coverage for autologous bone marrow transplantation for breast cancer (see comments). N Engl J Med 330:473–477, 1994.

173. Krause KJ: Variations in insurance coverage for autologous bone marrow transplantation for breast cancer (letter). N Engl J Med 331:330–331, 1994.

174. Mahaney FX Jr: Bone marrow transplant for breast cancer: some insurers pay, some insurers don't (news). J Natl Cancer Inst 86:420–421, 1994.

175. Sorrentino BP, Brandt SJ, Bodine D, et al: Selection of drug-resistant bone marrow cells in vivo after retroviral transfer of human MDR1. Science 257:99–103, 1992.

176. Gansbacher B, Zier K, Cronin K, et al: Retroviral gene transfer induced constitutive expression of interleukin-2 or interferon-gamma in irradiated human melanoma cells. Blood 80:2817–2825, 1992.

177. Hock H, Dorsch M, Kunzendorf U, Qin Z, Diamantstein T, Blankenstein T: Mechanisms of rejection induced by tumor cell-targeted gene transfer of interleukin 2, interleukin 4, interleukin 7, tumor necrosis factor, or interferon gamma. Proc Natl Acad Sci USA 90:2774–2778, 1993.

SECTION 2

LUNG CANCER

CHAPTER **11**   Small-Cell Lung Cancer
CHAPTER **12**   Non-Small-Cell Lung Cancer

Small-Cell Lung Cancer

Marcos J. G. de Lima, MD, Issa F. Khouri, MD, *and* Bonnie S. Glisson, MD

Department of Thoracic and Head and Neck Medical Oncology, Division of Medicine
The University of Texas M. D. Anderson Cancer Center, Houston, Texas

Small-cell lung carcinoma (SCLC) accounts for 20% to 25% of all new cases of lung cancer in the United States. It is estimated that approximately 42,000 new cases will occur in the United States in 1995.[1,2] Of the various histologic types of lung cancer, small-cell is the most sensitive to chemotherapy and radiotherapy, yet overall outcome is poor, with only 5% to 10% of patients surviving 5 years from diagnosis. Thus, SCLC has a generally grim prognosis. However, an orderly approach to diagnosis, staging, and treatment based on knowledge of the clinical behavior of the disease allows for the selection of the best curative and palliative therapy for individual patients.

In this review, the epidemiology, etiology, pathology, and natural history of the disease are discussed. In addition, current clinical management is examined.

ETIOLOGY AND EPIDEMIOLOGY

Cigarette smoking remains the major cause of SCLC, with more than 90% of cases in men attributable to tobacco use. The recent increase in SCLC in women is associated with a rise in cigarette smoking among women over the past two to three decades; indeed, SCLC seems to be the most rapidly increasing type of lung cancer in women.[3]

There is a dose-response relationship between the risk of death from SCLC and the total number of cigarettes smoked such that the risk is increased 60- to 70-fold for the smoker with 40 pack-years' exposure compared with the nonsmoker. Conversely, the chance of developing SCLC decreases with cessation of smoking but, especially in the heavy smoker (20 pack-years or more), may never return to the level of risk of the nonsmoker. Among long-term survivors of SCLC, smoking cessation decreases the risk of a second primary (non-small-cell) lung cancer, whereas for patients who continue to smoke, the risk of a second malignancy is increased about 32-fold.[4]

Exposure to industrial or environmental toxins, such as asbestos and radon, in combination with tobacco use synergistically increases the risk of developing SCLC and other lung cancers. Exposure to halogenated ethers also has been associated with an increased risk of SCLC.

In both genders, the majority of SCLC cases occur in the age range of 35 to 75 years, with a peak at age 55 to 65 years.

BIOLOGY

Lung cancer is the final step in a series of morphologic and structural changes that take several years to occur. Multiple genetic changes have been elucidated and likely play a role in field cancerization, through which all the aerodigestive tract epithelium is mutagenized by tobacco and other carcinogens. Genetic lesions may prove useful in the early detection, prevention, and treatment of lung carcinoma in the future.

Tumor-Suppressor Genes

Tumor-supressor gene products are negative growth regulators in the cell cycle. As opposed to classical oncogenes, tumor-suppressor genes are oncogenic through loss of function rather than activation. The first evidence for their existence came from somatic-cell fusion studies that demonstrated the recessive nature of the tumorigenic phenotype. Many years following that first observation, restriction fragment-length polymorphism (RFLP) analysis of tumor and normal tissue from children with retinoblastoma showing loss of heterozygosity (loss of one allele) in tumor tissue provided strong support for loss of putative tumor-suppressor elements as oncogenic. Further studies with retinoblastoma demonstrated that this loss of heterozygosity was correlated with loss of function of both alleles of a single gene, the retinoblastoma (*Rb*) gene on chromosome 13. Application of this methodology to the common solid tumors of adulthood revealed frequent loss of heterozygosity in diverse chromosomal regions known or postulated to be loci for tumor-suppressor genes. This phenomenon is especially common in SCLC.

The *Rb* gene product is a nuclear phosphoprotein involved in cell cycle regulation. Frequent cytogenetic alterations at 13q14, the locus for this gene, in SCLC cell lines and tumors were the catalyst for further study of this area. Analysis of mRNA expression shows that 60% of SCLC cell lines have undetectable transcripts and that the remaining 40% have an abnormal gene product. In addition, evaluation of DNA from 26 SCLC tumors and normal tissues indicated that six of six patients whose normal DNA was heterozygous for an Rb RFLP had lost one of the two alleles in their tumor DNA.[5] These data support the concept of inactivation of the *Rb* gene as a key event in the pathogenesis of SCLC.

Essentially all SCLC tumors and cell lines have deletions of the short arm of chromosome 3 at 3p21 distal-p22.[6–10] Although the precise identity of this gene awaits further investigation, several candidate genes have been studied. These include the genes encoding protein-tyrosine phosphatase-gamma, beta-retinoic acid receptor, and a serine/threonine protein kinase (c-raf-1).[11] However, there is no direct evidence supporting the role of any of these as tumor suppressors in SCLC. Because many other solid tumors also contain deletions in this area of the genome, it remains a fertile area for research.

Mutations in the *p53* tumor-suppressor gene on chromosome 17p are the most commonly identified genetic alteration in human cancers and have been documented in 60% to 100% of SCLC cell lines and in 77% of tumors.[12–14] The normal product of the *p53* locus acts to suppress and control cell division, and its loss may favor unregulated growth.

Proto-Oncogenes

Proto-oncogenes play an important role in normal cell growth. Abnormal expression of these genes by point mutations, translocation, or DNA amplification may confer tumorigenicity. Oncogene products are positive effectors of transformation, superimposing their activity on the cell with a gain in function.

Overall, amplification of the *myc* family of oncogenes (c-*myc*, N-*myc*, and L-*myc*) has been identified in 36 (18%) of 200 tumors and in 38 (31%) of 122 tumor-cell lines from patients with SCLC (see reference 12 for review). Amplification of *Myc* family DNA is more frequent in tumor-cell lines than in tumor specimens and is also more frequent in tumors from previously treated patients. In addition, some studies have suggested that patients with SC/LC histology possessing c-*myc* amplification have a shorter survival, reflecting a more agressive and treatment-resistant tumor.[15–17] However, because these studies used tumor samples from treated patients, the significance of this finding is not clear.

Autocrine Factors

SCLC produces a variety of peptide hormones that act as mitogens and growth factors, eg, insulin-like growth factor-I (IGF-I) and gastrin-releasing peptide.[18] These peptides participate in an autocrine loop resulting in growth of the tumor mass and sustenance of hormone production. This autocrine pathway provides an opportunity for therapy, and in fact, a phase II trial with a murine monoclonal antibody against gastrin-releasing peptide for recurrent SCLC resulted in 1 patient with a complete response and 4 with stable disease among 12 patients.[19]

IGF-I is present in 95% of SCLC tumors and cell lines, and there is a suggestion that it is also an autocrine growth factor. Indeed, somatostatin analogs inhibit the production of IGF-I and are active against SCLC xenografts in rats.[20]

Drug Resistance

The development of drug resistance is one of the most intriguing phenomena in the biology of SCLC. Several events at the cellular level have been described in cell lines made resistant by repeated exposure to cytotoxic agents in vitro.

The best established mechanism for multidrug resistance in cancer cells is overexpression of the multidrug-resistance (*MDR-1*) gene, encoding the multidrug efflux pump termed p-glycoprotein (p for "permeability"). Multidrug resistance to vinca alkaloids, anthracyclines, and epipodophyllotoxins results from the action of the p-glycoprotein in active transport of drug across the cytoplasmic membrane.

The role of *MDR-1* gene expression in SCLC is controversial. No correlation between gene expression and previous exposure to chemotherapy, response to chemotherapy, or in vitro drug sensitivity was found among a panel of six SCLC tumor specimens and 23 SCLC cell lines.[21] However, Poupon et al used tumor samples transplanted into nude mice and correlated responses to treatment in the patients and in the xenografts with *MDR-1* mRNA levels in the xenografts. Two patients who achieved complete responses and long-term survival had a complete xenograft response and no detectable level of *MDR-1* mRNA. Three patients who had recurrences after complete responses had *MDR-1* transcript detected in the pretreatment specimen, and one patient who at the time of recurrence had biopsies before and after chemotherapy had no detectable *MDR-1* mRNA in the first sample but transcripts clearly present in the posttreatment specimen.[22] Although these data are intriguing, the small number of patients studied calls for caution in interpretation.

Given the broad spectrum of drug resistance that characterizes recurrent SCLC, it seems probable that multiple mechanisms are operative simultaneously. Another transporter gene distantly related to *MDR-1* and in the same superfamily of ATP-binding cassette transmembrane transporters encodes a protein termed the multidrug-related protein (MRP). Overexpression of the *MRP* gene has been found in several multidrug-resistant SCLC cell lines selected in vitro.[23,24] A study of 12 fresh tumor samples revealed low expression of the *MRP* gene (relative to the level of sensitive SCLC lines) in 4, increased expression (1.5- to 2-fold) in 5, and 3 with no detectable *MRP* expression.[25] Other investigators analyzed 12 unselected SCLC cell lines and were unable to correlate *MRP* gene expression with chemosensitivity to doxorubicin (Adriamycin, Rubex), etoposide (VePesid), and cisplatin (Platinol).[26]

In multidrug-resistant cells that do not overexpress *MDR-1* or *MRP*, changes in activity or in the amount of topoisomerase I or II may be the basis for the resistance to epipodophyllotoxins and anthracyclines or to camptothecin and its analogs, respectively. Topoisomerases modify the topologic structure of DNA without changing the nucleotide sequence, cutting one (topoisomerase I) or both (topoisomerase II) strands of DNA and allowing strand passage through the transient nick, followed by religation. Topoisomerase-targeted drugs stabilize the usually transient DNA-enzyme complex, the so-called cleavable complex, and in so doing produce aberrations in DNA function that can initiate a process that culminates in cell death. Lower levels of expression or mutations in topoisomerases I and II in cell lines selected in vitro are associated with resistance to drugs that target the respective enzymes.

In addition, topoisomerase II expression has been associated with a multidrug-sensitive phenotype in lung cancer. Levels of topoisomerase II gene expression and sensitivity to doxorubicin, etoposide, teniposide (Vumon), cisplatin, camptothecin, and fluorouracil were directly correlated in a study of eight human lung cancer cell lines.[27] Cell lines expressing this multidrug-sensitivity phenotype were sensitive not only to drugs that directly inhibit topoisomerase II but also to drugs with other clearly defined mechanisms of action, such as camptothecin and cisplatin. Giaccone et al[27] hypothesized that topoisomerase II is a key participant in a final common pathway of cell death initiated by various macromolecular insults.

PATHOLOGY

With the advent of the 1967 World Health Organization (WHO) classification system for SCLC, several subtypes were suggested based on morphologic features (Table 1). However, subtyping SCLC into categories, such as lymphocyte-like, fusiform, and polygonal, was unreliable because judgments varied among observers from case to case and even within individual cases. In

TABLE I

Historical Classifications of Small-Cell Lung Cancer

World Health Organization I (1967)

Fusiform type

Polygonal type

Lymphocyte-like ("oat cell")

Others

World Health Organization II (1977)

Oat cell

Intermediate-cell type

Combined

International Association for the Study of Lung Cancer (1984)

Small cell

Variant (SC/LC)

Combined

Reprinted, with permission, from Khouri IF, Glisson BS: Small-cell lung cancer, in Pazdur R (ed): Medical Oncology: A Comprehensive Review, p 120. Huntington, NY, PRR Inc, 1993.

1977, the second WHO update simplified the SCLC subtyping and designated three categories: oat-cell carcinoma, intermediate small-cell carcinoma, and combined small-cell carcinoma. However, this revised system did not allow for the previously recognized morphologic variant subtype small-cell/large-cell (SC/LC) carcinoma (Table 1).[28] In some studies, this SC/LC subtype correlated with an unfavorable prognosis and appeared to have greater resistance to radiation and chemotherapy. In addition, the second WHO update separated the intermediate-cell subtype from the small-cell subtype, an artificial separation not justified by differences in clinical behavior. As a result, the International Association for the Study of Lung Cancer (IASLC) pathology panel redefined the subtypes of SCLC in an attempt to make them more clinically relevant (Table 1).

Typical SCLC is characterized by hyperchromatic nuclei with a very high nucleus to cytoplasm ratio; a diffuse, finely stippled pattern of chromatin; and indistinct nucleoli. The cells are small, approximately two to three times the size of a lymphocyte. The intermediate-cell subtype shows fusiform or polygonal cells with granular chromatin, inconspicuous nucleoli, and modest amounts of cytoplasm.

Variant-morphology SCLC is marked by distinct clusters of large cells exhibiting vesicular nuclei with finely dispersed chromatin and prominent nucleoli integrally admixed in what would otherwise be a typical SCLC. Because mixed histology in SCLC is not uncommon, especially at autopsy (30%),[29] and in view of in vitro transformation of SCLC to a larger cell type with loss of neuroendocrine features, it has been proposed that initiation of pulmonary carcinogenesis occurs in a pluripotent stem cell capable of differentiation along different pathways.

SCLC expresses several markers of neuroendocrine differentiation, such as chromogranin and gastrin-releasing peptide. A new nomenclature encompassing carcinoids, atypical carcinoids, large-cell neuroendocrine carcinoma, and SCLC and forming a spectrum of neuroendocrine neoplasia has been proposed, with the two ends of this biologic and clinical spectrum occupied by the indolent bronchial carcinoid tumor and the aggressive small-cell anaplastic carcinoma.[30] In addition to the spectrum of pathologic and biologic features, these tumors differ in their sensitivity to cytotoxic agents with response rates increasing as the histology becomes more anaplastic.

No molecular targets specific for SCLC have been completely defined, preventing the use of molecular biology techniques in the diagnosis of SCLC. Deletions in the short arm of chromosome 3, for example, are highly prevalent in SCLC but can be seen in non-small-cell lung cancer and in many other cancers as well.[31–33]

NATURAL HISTORY

The natural history of SCLC is characterized by a relentlessly progressive clinical course and by the early development of metastatic disease. If untreated, this disease is rapidly fatal, with a median survival of 5 to 7 weeks in patients with clinically apparent metastatic disease and 12 weeks in patients with regional thoracic involvement only.[34] Based on the results of an early study, even patients who have seemingly localized disease are presumed to have occult metastatic involvement. In that study, 19 patients with SCLC underwent purportedly curative surgical resection but died within 30 days of non-cancer-related causes. Of those 19 patients, 70% had distant metastatic disease at autopsy.[35] It is not surprising, therefore, that localized forms of treatment used alone fail in the majority of patients. Although radiotherapy was shown to be superior to surgery alone in prolonging median survival in a prospective randomized trial conducted in patients with operable local-regional disease, less than 5% of patients in the study were alive 5 years after treatment with either modality.[36]

In 1969, the Veterans Administration Lung Cancer Study Group (VALCSG) reported that three courses of cyclophosphamide more than doubled the median survival of patients with advanced SCLC.[34] Subsequently, over the past two decades of clinical research, it has become clear that SCLC is fundamentally a systemic, not a localized, disorder and that it is the histologic type of lung cancer most responsive to cytotoxic agents.

CLINICAL PRESENTATION

Compared with patients who have other types of lung cancer, those with SCLC report a shorter duration of symptoms before diagnosis, usually less than 3 months. Because SCLC lesions are usually centrally located, they can induce cough, wheezing, stridor, deep chest pain, hemoptysis, and dyspnea caused by airway obstruction, with or without postobstructive pneumonitis.

Mediastinal involvement, either by direct extension or by lymphatic metastases, is a hallmark of SCLC and can result in a variety of complications. Nerve entrapment can lead to recurrent laryngeal nerve paralysis and hoarseness. Involvement of the phrenic nerve can cause paralysis and elevation of the hemidiaphragm, with resulting dyspnea. Tumor compression of the esophagus can lead to dysphagia. Frequently, a right-sided hilar mass or tumor in the right mediastinal lymph nodes compresses the thin-walled, low-pressure system of the superior vena cava, causing superior vena cava syndrome.[37]

SCLC is particularly notable for producing a variety of paraneoplastic syndromes that can be the first indication of the tumor's presence. Classic examples include hyponatremia caused by production of arginine vasopressin and possibly atrial natriuretic factor[38] and Cushing's syndrome with or without hyperpigmentation caused by excessive production of the precursor peptides of ACTH (pro-opiomelanocortin and pro-ACTH).[39] Also, the development of auto-antibodies to normal neural antigens in patients with SCLC can lead to Eaton-Lambert syndrome, retinal blindness, subacute sensory neuropathy, and subacute cerebellar degeneration. Recently, cognitive dysfunction has been documented in patients with completely responding SCLC prior to elective brain irradiation,[40] and it is hypothesized that this is yet another manifestation of an autoimmune paraneoplastic syndrome.

One of the most distressing syndromes is weight loss and anorexia, which occurs in nearly one third of SCLC patients and for which no causative mechanism is currently known. Experimental models, however, suggest that the actions of various cytokines, including interleukin-1, tumor necrosis factor, and interleukin-6, may be involved in the pathogenesis of this syndrome.

STAGING

The development of a common staging system for malignant diseases has enabled physicians to accurately assess and compare the results of therapy. It has also permitted the elaboration of prognostic factors that can improve the design of future treatments. The American Joint Committee on Cancer has developed a staging system for lung cancer based on the size and extent of the primary tumor (T), the degree of regional lymph-node involvement (N), and the presence or absence of distant metastases (M).[41]

Although this TNM staging system has been shown to be of critical importance in staging non-small-cell lung cancer, TNM stage has been prognostically significant in SCLC. In a series of patients studied in the prechemotherapy era, patients who had no extrathoracic metastases and who were selected to undergo curative resections based on T and N classification survived no longer than did patients whose tumors were deemed unresectable based on the extent of regional disease.[42] Based in part on these data, surgical treatment of SCLC was abandoned. It should be noted, however, that there were very few patients with stage I tumors in that series.

An alternative staging system more clearly prognostic for patients with SCLC was proposed by the VALCSG. This classification divided SCLC into limited disease (LD) and extensive disease (ED), a division based on the clear survival differences observed in earlier studies between patients with regional (or limited) disease and those with distant (or extensive) spread.[34] LD as originally defined included tumors whose total known extent could be covered in one radiotherapy port. This original classification of LD included involvement of ipsilateral and contralateral hilar, mediastinal, and supraclavicular nodes as well as ipsilateral pleural effusion. However, as therapy for LD has evolved and the value of chest radiation has become apparent for a subset of patients, a refined definition of LD excluding contralateral hilar and contralateral supraclavicular nodal involvement as well as pleural effusion is frequently used. This definition identifies patients who are likely to have disease amenable to a combined chemotherapy and radiation (chemoradiation) approach with curative intent and to have disease that will be covered in a tolerable port size. ED denotes tumor beyond these limits and usually accounts for 60% to 70% of patients with SCLC. Long-term follow-up of patients treated with chemotherapy has revealed that survival of more than 3 years occurs almost exclusively in those with LD and that long-term survival in patients with ED remains uncommon.[43] These data indicate that disease classification by the VALCSG staging system is an independent prognostic variable and support its continued use.

The role of TNM classification in identifying patients with SCLC who might benefit from a surgical approach has been reexamined in the past decade. While data from a recent randomized trial show no benefit for adjuvant resection for stage II to III disease, it is fairly clear that patients who present with SCLC at clinical stage I (solitary pulmonary nodule) do very well after initial resection and adjuvant chemotherapy.[44,44a] Thus, TNM staging can be used to define the subset of patients with LD who could benefit from an approach including resection.

PROGNOSTIC FACTORS

Multivariate analyses of large databases have determined that disease extension and performance status are the most important prognostic factors. Female sex correlated with better response rates and survival in one study by the Cancer and Leukemia Group B.[45] Advanced age (older than 60 years), supraclavicular nodal involvement in LD patients, and a large number of metastatic sites also were predictive of a poor outcome. Other poor prognostic signs are low levels of hemoglobin, platelets, sodium, albumin, uric acid, and bicarbonate; elevated levels of leukocytes, lactate dehydrogenase, carcinoembryonic antigens; weight loss; slow response to therapy, and possibly failure to achieve a complete response.[46]

CLINICAL EVALUATION

Although staging is important in assigning prognosis and in locating sites of disease to determine response to therapy, its most critical role is in identifying LD patients who will benefit from an aggressive combined-modality approach with chemoradiation. Since the most important risk factor for treatment-related death appears to be initial performance status, evaluation of the physiologic condition of the patient is required. The initial survey should begin with a complete history and physical examination, chest roentgenography, and hematologic and clinical profile. The usual central location of disease, extensive mediastinal involvement, and postobstructive changes frequently make it difficult to define measurable disease by plain chest films alone. For this reason, computed tomography (CT) scans can aid greatly in the primary staging evaluation, in planning thoracic radiotherapy, and also in evaluating the mediastinal and hilar nodes in patients in whom surgical removal of the primary tumor is being considered.

Involvement of intra-abdominal organs is noted in

30% of patients undergoing initial staging for SCLC,[47] with liver, adrenal gland, pancreas, and intra-abdominal (mesenteric and retroperitoneal) lymph nodes representing the most frequent metastatic sites. CT is probably the best method for defining such intra-abdominal organ involvement. Since normal results of liver function tests, such as levels of serum glutamic-oxaloacetic transaminase (SGOT), lactate dehydrogenase, and alkaline phosphatase, do not exclude liver metastases, a CT scan of the abdomen should be a routine component of the staging evaluation.

Radionuclide bone scans remain the most valuable screening test for detecting early bone metastases, which occur in nearly 30% of patients who present with SCLC. Screening bone scans in asymptomatic patients can yield positive results even when bone pain is absent and alkaline phosphatase levels are normal. Only a small percentage of patients with abnormal findings on bone scans will have positive findings on skeletal radiographs, but radiographs may be useful in excluding benign lesions corresponding to abnormal areas on bone scans.

Bone marrow involvement is present at diagnosis in 20% to 25% of patients with SCLC, and the majority of those have normal peripheral blood findings.[48] Therefore, in the absence of other documented sites of extensive disease, a routine unilateral bone marrow examination is warranted in SCLC. However, bilateral aspirations and biopsies, which would increase the diagnostic yield by 30% but would affect the staging status (and thus alter therapy) in only 5% of cases, are not recommended routinely.[49] The results of bone scans and marrow examinations do not necessarily correlate; rather, the two tests are complementary, each reflecting a separate pattern of disease spread.

The brain is also commonly involved at presentation in SCLC patients. About 10% of patients have symptoms related to cerebral metastases, and another 5% have asymptomatic involvement.[50] Thus, magnetic resonance imaging or CT of the brain is a routine part of complete staging. Carcinomatous leptomeningitis is the second most common form of central nervous system involvement in SCLC but is rarely a problem at presentation (less than 0.5% of patients). For this reason, routine evaluation of cerebrospinal fluid is not indicated in the absence of specific symptoms.

Serum markers as diagnostic tools or as prognostic factors have low positive and negative predictive values. Pretreatment levels of neuron-specific enolase as predictors of disease-free survival have a sensitivity of 65% to 79% and a specificity of 82% to 86%; the overlap between the values for LD and ED prevents the use of this marker as an accurate determinant of disease stage. Serum levels of neuron-specific enolase and carcinoembryonic antigen may correlate with tumor bulk and response to chemotherapy.[51,52]

Expansion of the initial staging evaluation depends on the clinical circumstances. In particular, when patients are not being treated as part of a clinical research protocol, staging can be clinically directed toward obvious sites of metastasis. In this setting, the identification of asymptomatic metastatic disease is unlikely to affect management and outcome. A possible exception is the case of occult brain lesions, for which early radiation may reduce later morbidity from symptomatic brain metastases (see below).

TREATMENT

Approximately two thirds of patients with SCLC present with overt evidence of tumor dissemination beyond the thorax, and most of those with seemingly localized disease are presumed to have occult metastatic involvement.[35] This early metastatic involvement and frequent regional nodal spread support the idea that SCLC is a systemic disease at the time of initial clinical presentation. The systemic nature of the disease and its marked sensitivity to cytotoxic agents have resulted in the establishment of chemotherapy as the foundation for treatment of SCLC.

Single-Agent Chemotherapy

Following the initial VALCSG report showing that treatment with cyclophosphamide (Cytoxan, Neosar) resulted in prolonged survival for SCLC patients, many clinical trials were undertaken in the 1970s to study the efficacy of chemotherapy in this disease. Over the past two decades, many single agents, including cyclophosphamide and ifosfamide (Ifex), doxorubicin and epirubicin (Farmorubicin), etoposide and teniposide, cisplatin and carboplatin (Paraplatin), vincristine (Oncovin), methotrexate, and the nitrosoureas have shown activity against SCLC, with response rates ranging from 15% to 50%.[53–57] Most recently, paclitaxel (Taxol) and the topoisomerase I inhibitors topotecan and irinotecan have also been found active.[58–60]

The activity of the different agents in SCLC appears to be highly dependent on prior therapy. For instance, the early experience with short-course intravenous etoposide showed a response rate of only 9% to 15% when used in patients with treatment-refractory disease[53]; yet when etoposide was administered to previously untreated patients, 40% to 60% had an objective response.[54,56] This has led to the suggestion that phase II trials should be performed in previously untreated patients with ED. While this approach remains somewhat controversial,[61] randomized studies have demonstrated its feasibility and safety provided that effective salvage chemotherapy is administered promptly for progressive disease.[62,63]

The involvement in clinical trials of patients who have had relapses and who have been without treatment for at least 60 to 90 days may be another useful strategy. For example, the response to teniposide was higher in the presence of a drug-free interval longer than 2 months.[56]

Better drugs are still needed, and new agents with novel mechanisms of action, as well as analogs of active drugs, should be tested. In this vein, the identification of paclitaxel and the topoisomerase I inhibitors as active is exciting, and incorporation of these into induction chemotherapy is a current research priority.

Combination Chemotherapy

Overall and complete response rates seen with combination chemotherapy are generally superior to those observed with single agents in previously untreated patients, with the recent exception of oral etoposide in a prolonged schedule (see below). The activity of the cytotoxic agents used, rather than the size of the dose, appears to be the greatest contributor to the therapeutic efficacy of any given combination regimen. Although an early randomized study[64] comparing a low-dose regimen of cyclophosphamide (500 mg/m^2), methotrexate (10 mg/m^2), and lomustine (CeeNu, 50 mg/m^2) (CMC) with a higher-dose regimen (cyclophosphamide, 1,000 mg/m^2; methotrexate, 15 mg/m^2; and lomustine, 100 mg/m^2) showed a dose-response relationship, this was probably because CMC is not a very effective regimen and doses in the low-dose arm were lower than generally accepted as "standard." Further investigation of dose intensity with more effective regimens in the outpatient setting has generally showed no dose-response relationship. A randomized comparison of high-dose versus conventional-dose cyclophosphamide, doxorubicin, and vincristine (CAV)[65] and another trial of high-dose vs standard-dose cisplatin and etoposide (PE)[66] in ED SCLC failed to show any evidence of superior response or prolonged survival with higher doses.

More recent investigations have focused on shortening the interval between treatments as opposed to giving higher doses less frequently. Although data from one study with highly selected ED patients is encouraging,[67] thus far, no randomized trials have been reported that demonstrated an effect on survival for this approach.

In a series of trials investigating dose intensity with regimens requiring autologous marrow rescue, Johnson et al showed that while complete response rates can be increased, this does not translate into a survival benefit for patients with ED.[68] Although more encouraging results with dose-intense regimens as late intensification therapy have been obtained in patients with LD, a randomized trial of this approach failed to produce a survival benefit in the dose-intense arm.[69] However, with the availability of multilineage marrow growth factors and peripheral blood stem-cell support, the issue of dose intensity in SCLC continues to be an area of active research.

Induction Therapy

Many combinations of agents have been used as induction therapy for SCLC with similar results. Prior to the identification of etoposide as an active agent, CAV was one of the most commonly used regimens. However, the cardiac and mucosal toxic effects of doxorubicin caused problems, especially when the drug was combined with thoracic irradiation. Substitution of etoposide for doxorubicin in the CAV combination (CEV) was proven more effective and less toxic in a large randomized trial,[70] and since the early 1980s, etoposide-based regimens have gradually supplanted CAV as induction therapy.

The activity of PE was first identified in refractory/recurrent disease, where it produced a 40% to 50% objective response rate with minimal toxicity.[71] Based on these favorable results, this combination has been tested widely as first-line therapy and found to be at least as effective as other regimens and very well tolerated. Since the full-dose PE regimen lacks significant mucosal toxicity and is effective at minimally myelosuppressive dose levels, it can be safely administered with thoracic radiotherapy. This has increased median and long-term survival for patients with LD SCLC (see below).

Despite the high rate of response to first-line chemotherapy, most patients with SCLC relapse with drug-resistant disease within months. Several approaches have been explored in an attempt to prevent this outcome. Based on treatment strategies for Hodgkin's disease and malignant lymphoma, it was thought that alternating two equally effective non-cross-resistant combinations early in treatment would lead to maximal antitumor effect (Goldie-Coldman principle). Based on the activity of PE in patients with disease refractory to or recurrent after CAV, these two regimens were tested in alternating and sequential strategies in several randomized studies.[72–74] Although one of these trials demonstrated a survival benefit from alternating therapy in a relatively small number of patients with LD,[74] no improvement in outcome was identified for patients with ED. These results are probably due, in part, to the lack of bidirectional non-cross-resistance between CAV and PE.

Based on promising results obtained in a phase II pilot study of ifosfamide added to the base regimen of cisplatin and etoposide (VIP) in patients with ED, a phase III trial of the three-drug regimen vs PE was performed by the Hoosier Oncology Group.[75] Long-term survival in the VIP arm was superior (13% vs 5% at 2 years), although overall and complete remission rates were comparable. In addition, the similar remission durations in both arms raises the issue of an imbalance of unknown prognostic factors contributing to the survival difference.

Most studies addressing the optimal duration of therapy have confirmed the efficacy of relatively short, intensive courses of treatment (4 to 6 months). Data from randomized trials indicate a somewhat longer duration of remission with continued chemotherapy, but without a detriment in survival duration for unmaintained patients if chemotherapy is given at relapse.[76–78]

Salvage Regimens

The activity of PE was first recognized in its use as a salvage regimen in patients with refractory or recurrent disease following initial doxorubicin-based therapy.[71] After extensive evaluation of PE as induction therapy, however, it is clear that the partial non-cross-resistance is not bidirectional, with response rates to CAV of only 10% to 15% in patients failing to respond to or having recurrences after PE.[72,74] It is important to recognize, however, that the likelihood of response to any additional therapy is directly related to the drug-free interval. Patients who have relapses 2 years or more after induction therapy have higher response rates and longer median survivals than do patients who have relapses earlier.[79]

Etoposide given orally over a protracted course produced response rates of 23% and 45% in two studies of relapsed SCLC patients, including those previously treated with intravenous etoposide.[80,81] However, responses were rare in the absence of a 3-month drug-free interval. This same schedule of etoposide as single-agent induction therapy produced response and survival rates similar to those of more toxic combination regimens in patients with ED and represents a reasonable treatment option for elderly or unfit patients.[82–84]

Thoracic Irradiation

After chemotherapy-induced complete remission, the chest remains a significant site of failure in patients with LD. In this context, several randomized trials have documented that the addition of radiotherapy to combination chemotherapy appears to reduce the incidence of relapses in the chest by 10% to 20% and to increase the complete response rate by 10% to 40% and the long-term survival rate by 5% to 15%.[85] Much progress has been made recently in delineating the role of thoracic irradiation in the treatment of LD SCLC. Indeed, recognition of the benefit of thoracic radiotherapy, when properly combined with chemotherapy, can be viewed as one of the major advances in the treatment of this disease in the last decade. It must be recognized that concurrent chemoradiation is given at the expense of higher toxicity that can be prohibitive, especially when doxorubicin-containing regimens are used concomitantly with radiation. To minimize this problem, the minimally myelosuppressive and mucosa-sparing combination of PE has proven very valuable.

The timing of thoracic irradiation in the combined-modality treatment of LD SCLC is crucial. In general, most studies indicate that early administration of radiotherapy is superior to late treatment. In addition, a benefit from radiation has been difficult to demonstrate when it was given following completion of chemotherapy. Radiotherapy's early addition in an alternating or concurrent schedule appears to yield the best results, but it is also critical to maintain the dose intensity of both modalities.[86,87]

Based on promising data using accelerated hyperfractionated radiotherapy in a pilot study, a large, randomized Intergroup trial testing its value vs conventional fractionation (both given concurrently with PE in the first cycle) was conducted. The preliminary results of this trial indicate no significant survival benefit in the hyperfractionated arm, although the duration of remission was approximately 2 months longer.[88] Additionally, the accelerated therapy was associated with a higher incidence of acute esophageal toxic effects.

Nevertheless, the 2-year survival rate of more than 40% in both arms in this large Intergroup trial represents a significant improvement over previous results from large randomized trials in the United States. The favorable long-term outcome and the ability to deliver this regimen safely support the use of four cycles of PE with concurrent (conventional fractionation) thoracic radiotherapy in the first cycle as the standard of care for LD patients with disease amenable to a definitive combined approach.

Radiation to the chest as well as to sites of distant spread, such as the brain and bone, plays an important role in palliation of the patient with ED. Not unexpectedly, radiotherapy is not associated with a survival benefit in this setting.

Elective Brain Irradiation

Central nervous system metastases are an important cause of morbidity and mortality in patients with SCLC. These metastases have been reported in as many as 30% of all patients through the course of the disease and, in some series, in up to 80% of patients surviving 2 years or longer. Central nervous system metastases have occurred despite the use of aggressive combination chemotherapy. This has given rise to the belief that brain micrometastases are protected in a pharmacologic sanctuary. Hence, the concept of using elective brain irradiation to treat occult micrometastatic disease was developed.

Several randomized trials have demonstrated a significant reduction in SCLC relapse rates in the brain, from an average of 22% without elective brain irradiation to an average of 8% (a threefold reduction). Although none of the randomized trials have demonstrated an improvement in overall survival, there have been data that suggest a survival benefit for the subset of patients with a complete response to chemotherapy. The results of a randomized trial by Arriagada et al addressing this issue were recently published.[89] Patients with LD or ED who had achieved a complete remission were randomly assigned to receive elective brain irradiation (24 Gy in 8 fractions) after chemotherapy) or no brain irradiation. The data from this trial of 294 patients reproduce results of earlier trials, demonstrating again a threefold reduction in the incidence of brain metastases in the irradiated group (40% vs 67% in the nonirradiated group at 2 years). Although disease-free survival was improved in the irradiated group, overall survival at 2 years did not differ significantly between the two arms. Similarly, a retrospective review of completely responding patients in one cooperative group's database yielded the same conclusion: a clear reduction in the rate of brain metastasis but no survival benefit with elective brain irradiation.[90]

This absence of impact on survival has been a powerful argument against the use of elective brain irradiation, which is associated with late neurotoxicity, eg, organic brain syndromes, aphonia, hemiparesis, psychomotor retardation, and cerebellar dysfunction. The randomized trial by Arriagada et al is reassuring in that no differences were identified between the groups in neuropsychological function or abnormalities on CT scans, although follow-up is short. It also should be noted that the total dose used in that study was relatively low and that the chemotherapy and radiation were given at different times, two clearly significant variables influencing the risk of late neurotoxicity.

Although there are still no data demonstrating a survival impact for elective brain irradiation and it cannot be recommended routinely, it probably can be done safely, as demonstrated by the Arriagada et al trial. As therapy for SCLC evolves and more long-term survivors face the risk of late isolated brain SCLC recurrence, the question of the efficacy of elective brain irradiation will need to be readdressed.

Surgery

Because of early metastasis to regional nodes and hematogenous dissemination, fewer than 10% of patients with SCLC are eligible for potentially curative surgical resection at the time of presentation. Even among this select subgroup of SCLC patients, surgery alone seldom results in long-term survival, with most major surgical series reporting a 5-year survival rate of 10% or less. However, if surgery is performed before chemotherapy or as an adjuvant treatment, it results in improved local disease control.[91] The patients who appear to benefit most from a surgical approach are those without nodal involvement.[92–94]

In one series,[94] the median survival for patients with T1 or T2N0 tumors was 191 weeks using surgery and CAV chemotherapy, with a projected 5-year survival rate of 48%. On the other hand, the median survival is significantly shorter when nodes are involved, especially in the mediastinum. Because of this, thorough workup, including mediastinoscopy, is indicated for all patients with SCLC before surgical resection is considered.

Chemoprevention of Second Primary Tumors

Similar to patients who survive after treatment of squamous-cell cancer of the head and neck or non-small-cell lung cancer, patients with SCLC who survive longer than 2 years have a very high risk of developing second smoking-related primary tumors. Two recent retrospective analyses identified a 2% to 14% risk per year, with an actuarial cumulative risk of 70% 15 years from the start of treatment.[95,96] Most commonly, second primary tumors occur in the lung, with squamous-cell carcinoma the predominant histology. Unfortunately, very few patients reported in these two series were able to undergo successful surgical resection owing to the extent of tumor and medical contraindications. With the improving survival rates of patients with LD SCLC, second primary tumors are likely to become an increasingly common problem. Chemoprevention is an attractive option given the frequent inability to offer curative resection for the second cancer.

Previous data obtained by Hong et al[97] in patients with squamous-cell cancer of the head and neck and by

Pastorino et al[98] in patients treated surgically for non-small-cell lung cancer indicate that retinoids may have activity in reducing the incidence of second primary cancers. In parallel with ongoing trials in patients treated for early stage head and neck cancers and non-small-cell lung cancers, a National Cancer Institute-sponsored phase III trial of 13-*cis*-retinoic acid vs placebo is in the planning stages for 3-year survivors of SCLC.

REFERENCES

1. Wingo PA, Tong T, Bolden S: Cancer Statistics 1995. CA Cancer J Clin 45:8–30, 1995.

2. Ihde DC: Chemotherapy of lung cancer. N Engl J Med 12:1434–1441, 1992.

3. Richardson GE, Tucker MA, Venzon DJ, et al: Smoking cessation significantly reduces the risk of second primary cancer in long term cancer free survivors of SCLC (abstract). Proc Am Soc Clin Oncol 12:326, 1993.

4. Shaw GL, Hartge P, Schoenberg, et al: Total smoking-related attributable proportion of lung cancer in black and white men and women in New Jersey (abstract). Proc Am Soc Clin Oncol 10:133, 1991.

5. Hensel CH, Hsieh CL, Gazdar AF, et al: Altered structure and expression of the human retinoblastoma susceptibility gene in small cell lung cancer. Cancer Res 50:3067–3072, 1990.

6. Yokota J, Wada M, Shimosato Y, et al: Loss of heterozygosity on chromosomes 3, 13, 17 in small cell lung carcinoma and on chromosome 3 in adenocarcinoma of the lung. Proc Natl Acad Sci USA 84:9252–9256, 1987.

7. Whang-Peng J, Kao-Shen C, Lee EC, et al: Specific chromosomal defect associated with human small cell lung cancer deletion 3p(14-23). Science 215:181–183, 1982.

8. Whang-Peng J, Bunn PA, Kao-Shen C, et al: A non-random chromosomal abnormality del 3p(14–23) in human small cell lung cancer. Cancer Genet Cytogenet 6:119–134, 1982.

9. Naylor L, Johnson BE, Minna JD, et al: Loss of heterozygosity of chromosome 3p markers in small cell lung cancer patients' tumors. Nature 329:451–453, 1987.

10. Albertson DG, Sherrington PD, Rabbitts PH: Localization of polymorphic DNA probes frequently deleted in lung carcinoma. Hum Genet 83:127–132, 1989.

11. Croce CM: Genetic approaches to the study of the molecular basis of human cancer. Cancer Res 51:5015–5018s, 1991.

12. Richardson GE, Johnson BE: The biology of lung cancer. Semin Oncol 20: 105–127, 1993.

13. Takahashi T, Takahashi T, Suzuki H, et al: The p53 gene is very frequently mutated in SCLC with a distinct nucleotide substitution pattern. Oncogene 6:1775–1778, 1991.

14. Hollstein M, Sidranski D, Vogelstein B, et al: p53 mutations in human cancers. Science 253:49–53, 1991.

15. Brennan J, O'Connor T, Makuch RW, et al: myc family DNA amplification in 107 tumors and tumor cell lines from patients with small cell lung cancer treated with different combination chemotherapy regimens. Cancer Res 51:1708–1712, 1991.

16. Noguchi M, Hirohasi S, Hara F: Heterogeneous amplification of myc family oncogenes in small cell lung carcinoma. Cancer 66:2053–2058, 1990.

17. Funa K, Steinholz L, Noe E, et al: Increased expression of N-myc in human small cell lung cancer biopsies predicts lack of response to chemotherapy and poor prognosis. Am J Clin Pathol 88:216–220, 1986.

18. Minna JD, Cuttitta F, Battey J et al: Gastrin-releasing peptide and other autocrine growth factors in lung cancer: Pathogenetic and treatment implications, in DeVita VT Jr, Hellman S, Rosenberg SA (eds): Important Advances in Oncology, pp 55–64. Philadelphia, JB Lippincott, 1988.

19. Kelley MJ, Avis J, Linnoila RI, et al: Complete response in a patient with small cell lung cancer treated in a phase II trial using a murine monoclonal antibody (2A11) directed against gastrin releasing peptide (abstract). Proc Am Soc Clin Oncol 12:330, 1993.

20. Prevost G, Bourgeois Y, Mormont C, et al: Characterization of somatostatin receptors and growth inhibition by the somatostatin analogue BIM23014 in small cell lung carcinoma xenograft SCLC-6. Life Sci 55:155–162, 1994.

21. Lai SL, Goldstein LJ, Gottesman MM, et al: MDR1 gene expression in lung cancer. J Natl Cancer Inst 81:1144–1150, 1989.

22. Poupon MF, Arvelo F, Goguel AF, et al: Response of small cell lung cancer xenografts to chemotherapy: Multidrug resistance and direct clinical correlates. J Natl Cancer Inst 85:2024–2029, 1993.

23. Cole SPC, Bhardwaj G, Gerlach JH, et al: Overexpression of a transporter gene in a multidrug-resistant human lung cancer cell line. Science 258:1650–1654, 1992.

24. Zaman GJR, Versantvoort CHM, Smit JM: Analysis of the expression of MRP, the gene for a new putative transmembrane drug transporter, in human multidrug resistant lung cancer cell lines. Cancer Res 53:1747–1750, 1993.

25. Savaraj N, Wu CJ, Bao JJ, et al: Multidrug resistance associated protein gene expression in small cell and non-small cell lung cancer (abstract). Proc Am Assoc Cancer Res 35:242, 1994.

26. Rubio GJ, Pinedo HM, Gazdar AF, et al: MRP gene assessment in human lung cancer, normal lung, and lung cancer cell lines (abstract). Proc Am Assoc Cancer Res 35:206, 1994.

27. Giaccone G, Gazdar AF, Beck H, et al: Multidrug sensitivity phenotype of human lung cancer cells associated with topoisomerase II expression. Cancer Res 52:1666–1674, 1992.

28. Matthews MJ: Morphologic classification of bronchogenic carcinomas. Cancer Chemother Rep 3:229–302, 1973.

29. Matthews MJ: Effects of therapy on the morphology and behavior of SCLC of the lung: A clinico-pathologic study. Prog Cancer Res Ther 11:155–165, 1979.

30. McCue PA, Finkel GC: SCLC: An evolving histopathological spectrum. Semin Oncol 20:153–162, 1993.

31. Gazdar AF: The molecular and cellular basis of human lung cancer. Anticancer Res 13:261–268, 1994.

32. Warren WH, Faber LP, Gould VE: Neuroendocrine neoplasms of the lung: A clinicopathologic update. J Thorac Cardiovasc Surg 98:321–332, 1989.

33. Haselton PS, Al-Saffar N: The histological spectrum of bronchial carcinoid tumors. Appl Pathol 7:205–218, 1989.

34. Green RA, Humphrey E, Close H, et al: Alkylating agents in bronchogenic carcinoma. Am J Med 46:516–625, 1969.

35. Matthews MJ, Kanhouwa S, Pickren J, et al: Frequency of residual and metastatic tumor in patients undergoing curative surgical resection for lung cancer. Cancer Chemother Rep 4:63–67, 1973.

36. Fox W, Scedding JG: Medical Research Council comparative trial of surgery and radiotherapy for primary treatment of small cell lung carcinoma of bronchus: Ten year follow up. Lancet 2: 63–65, 1973.

37. Cohen MH: Signs and symptoms of bronchogenic carcinoma, in Strauss MJ (ed): Lung Cancer: Clinical Diagnosis and Treatment, pp 85–94. New York, Grune and Stratton, 1977.

38. Bliss DP, Battey JF, Linnoila I, et al: Expression of the atrial natriuretic factor gene in small cell lung cancer tumors and tumor cell lines. J Natl Cancer Inst 82:305–310, 1990.

39. Stewart MF, Crosby SR, Gibson S, et al: Small cell lung cancer cell lines secrete predominantly ACTH precursor peptides not ACTH. Br J Cancer 60:20–24, 1989.

40. Komaki R, Meyers CA, Cox JD: Neuropsychological functioning of patients with small cell lung cancer prior to and shortly following cranial irradiation: Evidence of pre-existing cognitive impairments (abstract). Proc Am Soc Clin Oncol 12:327, 1993.

41. Mountain CF: A new international staging system for lung cancer. Chest 89(suppl 4):225–335, 1986.

42. Mountain CF: Clinical biology of small cell carcinoma: Relationship to surgical therapy. Semin Oncol 5:272–279, 1978.

43. Morstyn G, Ihde DC, Lichter AS, et al: Small cell lung cancer 1973–1983: Early progress and recent obstacles. Int J Radiat Oncol Biol Phys 10:515–539, 1984.

44. Kreisman H, Wolkove N, Quoix EL: Small cell lung cancer presenting as a solitary pulmonary nodule. Chest 101:225–231, 1992.

44a. Ladd T, Piantidosi S, Thomas P, et al: A prospective randomized trial to determine the benefit of surgical resection of residual disease following response of small cell lung cancer to combination chemotherapy. Chest 106:3205–3235, 1994.

45. Skarin AT: Analysis of long term survivors with small cell lung cancer. Chest 103:440–444s, 1993.

46. Leblanc M, Maki E, Feld R: The Consensus Group for Prognostic Factors in SCLC. Verification of a multicenter prognostic model for small cell lung carcinoma. Proc Am Soc Clin Oncol 12:362, 1993 (abstract).

47. Mirvis SE, Whitley NO, Aisner J, et al: Abdominal CT in the staging of small cell carcinoma of the lungs: Incidence of metastases and effect on prognosis. AJR Am J Roentgenol 148:845–847, 1987.

48. Bezwoda WR, Lewis D, Livini N: Bone marrow involvement in aplastic small cell lung cancer: Diagnosis, hematologic features, and prognostic implications. Cancer 58:1762–1765, 1986.

49. Campling B, Quirt I, DeBoer G, et al: Is bone marrow examination in small cell lung cancer really necessary? Ann Intern Med 10:508–512, 1986.

50. Bunn PA Jr, Rosea ST: Central nervous system manifestations of small cell lung cancer, in Aisner J (ed): Contemporary Results in Clinical Oncology: Lung Cancer, pp 287–305. New York, Churchill Livingstone, 1985.

51. Ledermann JA: Serum neuron specific enolase and other neuroendocrine markers in lung cancer. Eur J Cancer 30A:574–576, 1994.

52. Quoix E, Charloux A, Popin E, et al: Inability of serum neuron specific enolase to predict disease extent in small cell lung cancer. Eur J Cancer 8(suppl):49–52, 1993.

53. Asbury RF, Rubins J, Bennet JM: Etoposide in small-cell lung cancer resistant to prior chemotherapy. Cancer Treat Rep 67:951–952, 1983.

54. Pederson AG, Hassen HH: Etoposide (VP-16) in the treatment of lung cancer. Cancer Treat Rev 10:245–264, 1983.

55. Broder LE, Cohen MH, Selawrky OS: Treatment of bronchogenic carcinoma. II. Small cell. Cancer Treat Rev 4:219–260, 1977.

56. Johnson DH: Investigation of new agents in small cell lung cancer. Chest 103:423–425s, 1993.

57. Quoix EA, Giaccone G, Jassem J, et al: Epirubicin in previously untreated patients with small cell lung cancer: A phase II study by the EORTC Lung Cancer Cooperative Group. Eur J Cancer 28A:1667–1670, 1992.

58. Masuda N, Fukuoka M, Kusunaki Y, et al: CPT-11: A new derivative of camptothecin for the treatment of refractory or relapsed small cell lung cancer. J Clin Oncol 10:1225–1229, 1992.

59. Schiller JH, Kim H, Johnson D, for the Eastern Cooperative Oncology Group: Phase II study of topotecan in extensive stage small cell lung cancer (abstract). Proc Am Soc Clin Oncol 13:330, 1994.

60. Ettinger DS, Finkelstein DM, Sarma R, et al: Phase II study of Taxol in patients with extensive-stage small cell lung cancer: An Eastern Cooperative Oncology Group study (abstract). Proc Am Soc Clin Oncol 12:1094, 1993.

61. Grant SC, Gralla RJ, Kris MG, et al: Single agent chemotherapy trials in small cell lung cancer: The case for studies in previously treated patients. J Clin Oncol 10:484–498, 1992.

62. Moore TD, Korn EL: Phase II trial design considerations for small-cell lung cancer. J Natl Cancer Inst 84:150–154, 1992.

63. Ettinger DS, Finkelstein DM, Abeloff MD, et al: Justification for evaluating new anticancer drugs in selected untreated patients with extensive-stage small-call lung cancer: An Eastern Cooperative Oncology Group randomized study. J Natl Cancer Inst 84:1077–1083, 1992.

64. Cohen MH, Creaven PJ, Fossicek BE, et al: Intensive chemotherapy of small cell bronchogenic carcinoma. Cancer Treat Rep 61:349–54, 1977.

65. Johnson DH, Einhorn LH, Birch R, et al: A randomized comparison of high-dose versus conventional-dose cyclophosphamide, doxorubicin, and vincristine for extensive-stage small-cell lung cancer: A phase III trial of the Southeastern Cancer Study Group. J Clin Oncol 5:1731–1738, 1987.

66. Ihde DC, Mulshine JL, Kramer BS, et al: Prospective randomized comparison of high dose and standard dose etoposide and cisplatin chemotherapy in patients with extensive stage small cell lung cancer. J Clin Oncol 12 (10):2022–2034, 1994.

67. Murray N, Shah A, Osoba D, et al: Intensive weekly chemotherapy for the treatment of extensive-stage small-cell lung cancer. J Clin Oncol 9:1632–1638, 1991.

68. Johnson DH, DeLeo MJ, Hande KR, et al: High dose induction chemotherapy with cyclophosphamide, etoposide and cisplatin for extensive stage small cell lung cancer. J Clin Oncol 5:703–709, 1987.

69. Humblet Y, Symann M, Bosly A, et al: Late intensification chemotherapy with autologous bone marrow transplantation in selected small-cell carcinoma of the lung: A randomized study. J Clin Oncol 5:1864–1873, 1987.

70. Hong WK, Nicaise C, Lawson R, et al: Etoposide combined with cyclophosphamide plus vincristine compared with doxorubicin plus cyclophosphamide plus vincristine and with high dose cyclophosphamide plus vincristine in the treatment of small cell carcinoma of the lung: A randomized trial of the Bristol Lung Cancer Study Group. J Clin Oncol 7:450–456, 1989.

71. Evans WK, Osoba D, Feld R, et al: Etoposide (VP-16) and cisplatin: An effective treatment for relapse in small cell lung cancer. J Clin Oncol 3:65–71, 1985.

72. Roth BJ, Johnson DH, Einhorn LH, et al: Randomized study of cyclophosphamide, doxorubicin, and vincristine versus etoposide and cisplatin versus alternation of these two regimens in extensive small-cell lung cancer: Phase III trial of the Southeastern Cancer Study Group. J Clin Oncol 10:282–291, 1992.

73. Evans WK, Feld R, Murray N, et al: Superiority of alternating non-cross-resistant chemotherapy in extensive small cell lung cancer. A multicenter randomized clinical trial by the National Cancer Institute of Canada. Ann Intern Med 107:451–459, 1987.

74. Fukuoka M, Furuse K, Saijo N, et al: Randomized trial of cyclophosphamide, doxorubicin, and vincristine versus cisplatin and etoposide versus alternation of these regimens in small-cell lung cancer. J Natl Cancer Inst 83:855–861, 1991.

75. Ansari R, Loehrer PJ, Conin R, et al: A phase III study of PE alone or PE plus ifosfamide in previously untreated patients with extensive disease small cell lung cancer: A Hoosier Oncology Group Trial (abstract). Proc Am Soc Clin Oncol 13:330 1994.

76. Girling DJ: Controlled trial of twelve versus six courses of chemotherapy in the treatment of small-cell lung cancer. Br J Cancer 59:584–590, 1989.

77. Spiro SG, Souhami RL, Geddes DM, et al: Duration of chemotherapy in small cell lung cancer: A Cancer Research Campaign trial. Br J Cancer 59:578–583, 1989.

78. Giaccone G, Dalesio O, McVie GJ, et al: Maintenance chemotherapy in small-cell lung cancer: Long-term results of a randomized trial. J Clin Oncol 11:1230–1240, 1993.

79. Batist G, Ihde DC, Zabell A, et al: Small cell carcinoma of the lung: Reinduction therapy after late relapse. Ann Intern Med 98:472–474, 1983.

80. Einhorn LH, Pennington K, McClean J: Phase II trial of daily oral VP-16 in refractory small cell lung cancer: A Hoosier Oncology Group study. Semin Oncol 17:32–35, 1990.

81. Johnson DH, Greto FA, Strupp J, et al: Prolonged administration of oral etoposide in patients with relapsed or refractory small cell lung cancer: A phase II trial. J Clin Oncol 8:1613–1617, 1990.

82. Clark P, Cottier B, Joel S, et al: Two prolonged schedules of single-agent oral etoposide of differing duration and dose in patients with untreated small cell lung cancer (SCLC) (abstract). Proc Am Soc Clin Oncol 10:268, 1991.

83. Miller AA, Herndon J, Hollis D, et al: Phase III study of 21 day oral versus 3 day IV etoposide in combination with IV cisplatin in extensive small cell lung cancer: A Cancer and Leukemia Group B study (abstract). Proc Am Soc Clin Oncol 13:326, 1994.

84. Miller D, Johnson D, Garrow G, et al: Brief induction therapy with chronic oral etoposide plus weekly cisplatin in patients with extensive stage small cell lung cancer (abstract). Proc Am Soc Clin Oncol 13:350, 1994.

85. Werde P, Payne D: Does thoracic irradiation improve survival and local control in limited-stage small-cell carcinoma of the lung? A meta-analysis. J Clin Oncol 10:890–895, 1992.

86. McGrackin JD, Janaki LM, Crowley JJ, et al: Concurrent chemotherapy/radiotherapy for limited small cell lung carcinoma: A Southwest Oncology Group study. J Clin Oncol 8:892–893, 1990.

87. Murray N, Coy P, Pater JL, et al: Importance of timing for thoracic irradiation in the combined modality treatment of limited stage small cell lung cancer. J Clin Oncol 11:336–344, 1993.

88. Johnson DH, Kim K, Turrisi AT, et al: Cisplatin and etoposide plus concurrent thoracic radiotherapy administered once versus twice daily for limited stage small cell lung cancer. Preliminary results of an Intergroup Trial (abstract). Proc Am Soc Clin Oncol 13:333, 1994.

89. Arriagada R, LeChevalier T, Borie F, et al: Prophylactic cranial irradiation for patients with small cell lung cancer in complete remission. J Natl Cancer Inst 87:183–190, 1995.

90. Shaw EG, Su JQ, Eagan RT, et al: Prophylactic cranial irradiation in complete responders with small-cell lung cancer: Analysis of the Mayo Clinic and North Central Cancer Treatment Group data bases. J Clin Oncol 12:2327–2332, 1994.

91. Shepherd FA, Ginsberg RJ, Evans WK, et al: Reduction in local recurrence and improved survival in surgically treated patients with small cell lung cancer. J Thorac Cardiovasc Surg 86:498–504, 1983.

92. Mentzer SJ, Reilly JJ, Sugarbaker DJ: Surgical resection in the management of small cell carcinoma of the lung. Chest 103:349–351s, 1993.

93. Davis S, Crino I, Tonato M, et al: A prospective analysis of chemotherapy following surgical resection of clinical stage I-II small cell lung cancer. Am J Clin Oncol 16:93–95, 1993.

94. Shepherd FA, Evans WK, Feld R, et al: Adjuvant chemotherapy following surgical resection for small-cell carcinoma of the lung. J Clin Oncol 6:832–838, 1988.

95. Heyne KH, Lippman SM, Lee JS, et al: The incidence of second primary tumors in long-term survivors of small cell lung cancer. J Clin Oncol 10:1519–1524, 1992.

96. Johnson BE, Linnoila RI, Willimas JP, et al: Risk of second aerodigestive cancers increases in patients who survive free of small cell lung cancer for more than 2 years. J Clin Oncol 13:101–111, 1995.

97. Hong WK, Lippman SM, Itri LM, et al: Prevention of second primary tumors with isotretinoin in squamous cell carcinoma of the head and neck. N Engl J Med 323:795–801, 1990.

98. Pastorino U, Infante M, Maioli M, et al: Adjuvant treatment of stage I lung cancer with high-dose vitamin A. J Clin Oncol 11:1216–1222, 1993.

CHAPTER 12

Non-Small-Cell Lung Cancer

Dimitrios Diamandidis, MD, Martin Huber, MD, *and* Katherine Pisters, MD

Department of Thoracic and Head and Neck Medical Oncology, Division of Medicine
The University of Texas M. D. Anderson Cancer Center, Houston, Texas

Lung cancer has long been the leading cause of cancer-related mortality in men, and beginning in the late 1980s, lung cancer exceeded breast cancer as the leading cause of cancer-related mortality in women. Lung cancer is responsible for one of three cancer-related deaths in men and one of four cancer-related deaths in women (Table 1). An estimated 169,900 new cases of lung cancer will be diagnosed in the United States in 1995.[1] Of these new cases, approximately 80% will be non-small-cell lung cancer (NSCLC). The great majority of cases will occur in current or former cigarette smokers. Over 70% of patients will present with advanced disease at diagnosis, and fewer than 5% of those with metastatic disease will be alive at 5 years. In the United States, 1 of every 14 deaths from any cause is due to lung cancer (Table 2).[1]

Epidemiologic studies have demonstrated a clear correlation between environmental factors—in particular, tobacco exposure—and the development of lung cancer.[2] Increases in lung cancer risk following exposure to carcinogens such as asbestos and radon have also been reported and have an effect independent of cigarette smoking. Other studies have suggested a dietary influence in the development of lung cancer, which has led to investigation of the role of chemoprevention in this disease. Molecular biology studies of lung cancer may give insight into both the pathophysiology and the treatment of this troublesome cancer.

In recent years, several novel chemotherapeutic agents have been identified that have shown activity against NSCLC. Despite this, chemotherapy has had little impact on patients with metastatic disease. Combination chemotherapy has an established role in the combined-modality treatment of patients with locally advanced disease.[3] Surgery remains the treatment of choice for patients with early-stage disease.

EPIDEMIOLOGY

Lung, colorectal, and prostate cancers are the most common cancers in developed countries, whereas cancers of the cervix, liver, and head and neck are the most common cancers in developing countries. Nonetheless, the incidence of lung cancer is beginning to fall in developed countries—which may reflect the efficacy of antismoking campaigns—and rise in developing countries—which may reflect industrialization and the increasing use of tobacco products. Worldwide, lung cancer is the most common cancer in males, accounting for 17.6% of all cancers in men, and the fifth most common cancer in women. The worldwide mortality rate associated with lung cancer is 86%. This rate is exceeded only by the mortality rates of primary tumors of the pancreas, liver, and esophagus.[4]

The incidence of lung cancer has changed over the past four decades. Lung cancer was not common prior to the 1930s. Following the large increase in cigarette smoking during the 1940s, the incidence of lung cancer in men increased dramatically, from 11 per 100,000 in 1940 to 75 per 100,000 in 1985. Over the last decade, the incidence of lung cancer in men has leveled off somewhat, to approximately 70 per 100,000. However, there has been a sharp rise in the incidence of lung cancer in women, from 6 per 100,000 in 1960 to 28 per 100,000 in 1987.[5]

The majority of lung cancer patients are between 35 and 75 years old, with a peak incidence between the ages of 55 and 65 (Table 3).[1] Black males have a 40% higher incidence of lung cancer than do white males; however, the incidence is leveling off in both black and white males in connection with a decrease in cigarette smoking.[6] In addition, the decline in lung cancer is most pronounced in individuals of higher education and appears to correlate with the marked decrease in cigarette consumption among individuals with a college education.[5] While changes in the incidence of lung cancer correlate most closely with changes in the incidence of smoking, there are several other risk factors that appear to contribute to the development of lung cancer (Table 4).

RISK FACTORS/ETIOLOGY

Cigarette Smoking

The most important risk factor for the development of NSCLC is cigarette smoking. Epidemiologic data on smoking and lung cancer demonstrate a causal association. Changes in lung cancer incidence and mortality

TABLE I

Reported Deaths for the Five Leading Cancer Sites by Age, United States, 1991

MALE

All ages	Under 15	15–34	35–54	55–74	75+
All cancer 272,380	**All cancer** 982	**All cancer** 3,699	**All cancer** 27,529	**All cancer** 142,089	**All cancer** 98,607
Lung 91,690	Leukemia 350	Leukemia 661	Lung 8,741	Lung 55,890	Lung 26,896
Prostate 33,564	Brain & CNS 252	Non-Hodgkin's Lymphoma 501	Colon & rectum 2,393	Colon & rectum 13,888	Prostate 20,909
Colon & rectum 28,178	Endocrine 111	Brain & CNS 414	Non-Hodgkin's lymphomas 1,726	Prostate 12,306	Colon & rectum 11,686
Pancreas 12,375	Non-Hodgkin's lymphomas 64	Skin 298	Brain & CNS 1,577	Pancreas 6,730	Pancreas 4,299
Leukemia 10,194	Connective tissue 46	Hodgkin's disease 233	Pancreas 1,298	Esophagus 4,600	Bladder 3,698

FEMALE

All ages	Under 15	15–34	35–54	55–74	75 +
All cancer 242,277	**All cancer** 727	**All cancer** 3,434	**All cancer** 29,302	**All cancer** 111,419	**All cancer** 97,388
Lung 52,068	Leukemia 260	Breast 660	Breast 9,188	Lung 30,154	Lung 16,400
Breast 43,583	Brain & CNS 220	Leukemia 432	Lung 5,372	Breast 19,900	Colon & rectum 15,727
Colon & rectum 29,017	Endocrine 69	Uterus 343	Colon & rectum 1,999	Colon & rectum 11,117	Breast 13,834
Ovary 13,247	Connective tissue 33	Brain & CNS 328	Uterus 1,978	Ovary 6,720	Pancreas 6,637
Pancreas 13,161	Bone 28	Non-Hodgkin's lymphomas 209	Ovary 1,779	Pancreas 5,669	Ovary 4,601

CNS = central nervous system   Adapted, with permission, from Wingo PA, Tong T, Bolden S: Cancer Statistics, 1995. CA Cancer J Clin 45:8–30, 1995.

have paralleled changes in the prevalence of cigarette smoking. The relative risk for lung cancer in current smokers, compared to those who have never smoked, is 13.3. There is also evidence for a dose-response relationship between smoking and lung cancer.[7] In addition, smoking cessation leads to a decrease in lung cancer risk over time.

Chemistry of Carcinogenesis

The *N*-nitrosamines and polycyclic aromatic hydrocarbons are the two major classes of tobacco-related inhaled carcinogens. *N*-Nitrosamines are formed during tobacco processing and pyrosynthesis. They originate from nicotine and the alkaloid arecoline.[8] Chemicals derived from tobacco smoke cause lung tumors in experimental animals. The main nitrosation products of nicotine are NNK (nicotine-derived nitrosamino ketone) and NNN (*N'*-nitrosonornicotine). They are considered very strong lung carcinogens.[9]

The nitrosamines are activated through hydroxylation by the P450 enzyme system and then exert their action through the formation of DNA adducts. The formation of

TABLE 2

Mortality for Leading Causes of Death, United States, 1991

Rank	Cause of death	Number of deaths	Death rate per 100,000 population [a]	Percent of total deaths
	All causes	2,169,518	691.8	100.0
1	Heart diseases	720,862	219.8	33.2
2	Cancer	514,657	173.4	23.7
3	Cerebrovascular diseases	143,481	42.0	6.6
4	Chronic obstructive lung diseases	90,650	28.6	4.2
5	Accidents	89,347	32.1	4.1
6	Pneumonia & influenza	77,860	22.1	3.6
7	Diabetes	48,951	15.8	2.3
8	Suicide	30,810	11.0	1.4
9	HIV infection	29,555	9.5	1.4
10	Homicide	26,513	9.9	1.2
11	Cirrhosis of liver	25,429	9.2	1.2
12	Diseases of arteries	25,055	7.8	1.2
13	Nephritis	21,360	6.4	1.0
14	Septicemia	19,691	6.0	0.9
15	Atherosclerosis	17,420	4.7	0.8
	Other & ill-defined	287,877	93.5	13.3

[a] Age-adjusted to the 1970 US standard population

Adapted, with permission, from Wingo PA, Tong T, Bolden S: Cancer Statistics, 1995. CA Cancer J Clin 45:8–30, 1995.

DNA adducts is directly related to the amount of cigarette consumption.[10] DNA adducts can remain in the system for as long as 5 years without significant change, and in heavy smokers, they may be responsible for as many as 100 mutations per cell genome.

The polycyclic aromatic hydrocarbons benzo[a]pyrene and dimethylbenz[a]anthracene are also significant chemical mutagenic/carcinogenic substances that lead to the formation of DNA adducts.[11]

Passive Smoking

The National Research Council has estimated that the risk of developing lung cancer in nonsmokers exposed to cigarette smoke is approximately 1.35 times the risk of unexposed nonsmokers,[12] although the risk is difficult to estimate. Moreover, according to risk analysis, as many as 40% of lung cancer deaths in nonsmokers may be caused by passive smoking.[13] Indeed, passive smoking has recently been declared a carcinogen by the Environmental Protection Agency on the basis of the correlation between passive exposure to cigarette smoke and the development of lung cancer.

Asbestos

Asbestos exists in many natural forms. The silicate fiber has been implicated in carcinogenesis, is chemically inert, and can remain in a person's lungs for a lifetime. Epidemiologic studies have confirmed the association between asbestos exposure and certain lung diseases such as pulmonary fibrosis, mesothelioma, and lung cancer.[14] Most asbestos exposure occurs in the workplace, for example, among shipyard workers or plumbers. In a study of British asbestos workers, the relative risk of lung cancer was 1.4 to 2.6.[15]

Most likely, asbestos acts as a tumor promoter.[16] As smoking is known to impair bronchial clearance, it is reasonable to assume that smoking prolongs the presence of asbestos in the pulmonary epithelium. When smoking is combined with asbestos exposure, the relative risk of lung cancer is strikingly increased, to 28.8.[17]

TABLE 3

Percentage of Population (Probability) Developing Invasive Cancers at Certain Ages, United States, 1991

		Birth to 39 years	40 to 59 years	60 to 79 years	Ever (birth to death)
All sites	**Male**	1.72 (1 in 58)	7.74 (1 in 13)	34.30 (1 in 3)	44.84 (1 in 2)
	Female	1.92 (1 in 52)	9.33 (1 in 11)	23.22 (1 in 4)	39.26 (1 in 3)
Breast	Female	0.46 (1 in 217)	3.83 (1 in 26)	6.77 (1 in 15)	12.30 (1 in 8)
Colon and rectum	Male	0.06 (1 in 1,667)	0.93 (1 in 108)	4.39 (1 in 23)	6.14 (1 in 16)
	Female	0.05 (1 in 2,000)	0.73 (1 in 137)	3.32 (1 in 30)	5.92 (1 in 17)
Prostate	Male	Less than 1 in 10,000	0.97 (1 in 103)	1.84 (1 in 8)	15.44 (1 in 6)
Lung	Male	0.04 (1 in 2,500)	1.55 (1 in 65)	6.71 (1 in 15)	8.49 (1 in 12)
	Female	0.03 (1 in 3,333)	1.07 (1 in 93)	3.62 (1 in 28)	5.17 (1 in 19)

Adapted, with permission, from Wingo PA, Tong T, Bolden S: Cancer Statistics, 1995. CA Cancer J Clin 45:8–30, 1995.

Radon

Radon is a naturally occurring, chemically inert gas that is a decay product of uranium. Radon decays to products that emit heavy ionizing alpha particles. Radon exposure increases the risk of developing lung cancer as much as 10 times,[18] and lung cancer caused by radon exposure is usually the small-cell type.[19]

Among uranium miners who smoke, the risk of developing lung cancer is 10 times that of their nonsmoking colleagues. Another study estimated that 1,000,000 homes in the United States may be exposed to levels of radon greater than 8 pCi per year, which is similar to or in excess of the level of exposure in uranium miners.[20] Other studies have estimated that as many as 25% of all cases of lung cancer among nonsmokers may be related to radon exposure.[21]

Diet

Diet may also be a risk factor for lung cancer.[22] Of 15 retrospective studies, 14 found an association between increased beta-carotene intake and decreased risk of lung cancer.

A decrease in lung cancer risk was also associated with increased vitamin C intake in four of these studies and with increased fiber intake in two studies. Five of six prospective studies found a decreased risk of lung cancer to be associated with an increased intake of carotenoids. In addition, several studies have demonstrated an inverse correlation between serum beta-carotene levels and the incidence of lung cancer. However, other studies have failed to confirm this correlation.

A recent review of these data suggests that if the general public increased its fruit and vegetable consumption to levels characteristic of the highest 30% of individuals in these studies, the risk of lung cancer in the community might be decreased by 15% to 31%. While the exact agents in the diet that result in a decreased incidence of lung cancer remain unknown, a large body of epidemiologic evidence suggests that increased fruit and vegetable consumption decreases the risk of lung cancer. These data, combined with data on other tumor types, led to the National Cancer Institute's recommendation for the consumption of five or more servings of fruits and vegetables daily.

A surprising result, however, came recently from a randomized, double-blind, placebo-controlled primary prevention trial. The Cancer Prevention Study Group[23] enrolled 29,133 male smokers aged 50 to 69 years, and randomly assigned them to one of four regimens: alpha-tocopherol, 50 mg/d; beta-carotene, 20 mg/d; both alpha-tocopherol and beta-carotene; or placebo. Patients were

TABLE 4

Risk Factors for Lung Cancer

Risk factor	Relative risk	Reference
Cigarette smoking in males	17.4	Garfinkel and Silverberg[5]
Cigarette smoking in females	10.8	Garfinkel and Silverberg[5]
Passive smoking	1.5	Wald et al[12]
Asbestos	1.4–2.6	Hodgson and Jones[15]
Mining	3–8 (lifetime)	Harley et al[18]
Radon (residential, > 8 pCi/yr)	2 (lifetime)	Nero et al[20]

followed up for 5 to 8 years. A total of 876 new cases of lung cancer were diagnosed during the trial, and no reduction in the incidence of lung cancer was observed among the men receiving alpha-tocopherol. Patients receiving beta-carotene had a higher incidence of lung cancer and 8% higher mortality from lung cancer and heart disease than did patients not receiving beta-carotene. The investigators concluded that there was no reduction in the incidence of lung cancer among male smokers after 5 years of dietary supplementation with beta-carotene or alpha-tocopherol and that such supplementation might do as much harm as good.

Genetic Predisposition

It has been estimated that cigarette smoking is responsible for 90% of lung cancers occurring in the United States.[24] However, only a fraction of smokers develop a bronchial malignancy. Passive smoking and occupational exposure to substances such as asbestos, radon, arsenic, nickel, and polycyclic aromatic hydrocarbons are risk factors for lung cancer, but only a portion of individuals exposed to these substances develop cancer. These facts suggest that cancer susceptibility differs among individuals and may have a genetic basis.

Several findings seem to support genetic susceptibility. First, the risk of lung cancer appears to be increased in individuals with chronic obstructive pulmonary disease, even when the degree of cigarette consumption is taken into account. The development of chronic ostructive pulmonary disease appears to have a familial association. Therefore, the increased risk of lung cancer may also involve a genetic risk.[25] Second, recent data have suggested that the predisposition to developing lung cancer at an early age is inherited in a Mendelian codominant fashion.[26]

Third, increased metabolism of the antihypertensive drug debrisoquine has been associated with an increased risk of lung cancer. It has been hypothesized that interindividual variations in the ability to metabolically oxidize substances via the cytochrome P450 system may account, in part, for differences in the susceptibility to cancer. Individuals with increased oxidative activity may be at increased risk of developing cancer because of their increased level of activated carcinogens. Furthermore, the ability to metabolize debrisoquine segregates individuals into different phenotypes. In support of the association between debrisoquine metabolism and lung cancer, individuals with the ability to extensively metabolize debrisoquine showed an increased incidence of lung cancer.[27] This association was further confirmed by a 1990 case-control study, which found that individuals

who could extensively metabolize debrisoquine had an increased risk of lung cancer, with an odds ratio of 6.1.[28]

Familial aggregation of lung cancer has been studied by Tokuhata et al,[29] who conducted a case-control study that examined the frequency of lung cancer among parents and siblings of 270 lung cancer patients. The incidence of lung cancer was twice as great as expected among smokers and four times as great as expected among nonsmokers. Another case-control study conducted by Ooi et al[30] reviewed a population of 336 deceased lung cancer patients from Louisiana. Lung cancer was seen much more commonly in first-degree relatives than in spouses of patients.

Thus, although the genetic risk factors associated with lung cancer are poorly defined, increasing data suggest the existence of a genetic predisposition to the development of lung cancer.

HISTOLOGY

The distinction between non-small-cell lung cancer and small-cell lung cancer is of major clinical import, as it significantly alters treatment options. The histologic types of lung cancer defined by the World Health Organization are listed in Table 5. While specific subtypes of NSCLC do not alter treatment plans overall, certain clinical patterns are associated with specific subtypes, eg, adenocarcinoma, squamous-cell carcinoma, and large-cell carcinoma.

The frequency of the histologic subtypes has changed over the past 20 years. Squamous-cell carcinoma was formerly the most frequent subtype of NSCLC. Recently, however, the incidence of this subtype has decreased while the incidence of adenocarcinoma has increased.

Adenocarcinoma

Adenocarcinoma is the most common subtype of NSCLC in North America and constitutes about 50% of all NSCLC cases in some series. Although adenocarcinoma is associated with smoking, it is especially predominant among women and nonsmokers. Most of these tumors are peripheral and arise from surface epithelium or bronchial mucosal glands and as peripheral scar carcinomas. On histologic examination, adenocarcinoma demonstrates gland formation, papillary structures, or mucin production; on immunohistochemical examination, the tumors stain positive for keratin as well as carcinoembryonic antigen (CEA).

Patients with adenocarcinoma frequently present with metastatic disease prior to the development of symptoms secondary to local disease. Pulmonary adenocarcinoma is associated with hypertrophic osteoarthropathy, Trous-

TABLE 5

WHO Classification of Malignant Pleuropulmonary Neoplasms

I.   Epidermoid carcinoma

II.   Small-cell carcinoma

III.   Adenocarcinoma
   1. Bronchogenic
      a. Acinar
      b. Papillary
   2. Bronchioloalveolar

IV.   Large-cell carcinoma
   1. Solid tumor with mucin
   2. Solid tumor without mucin
   3. Giant cell
   4. Clear cell

V.   Combined epidermoid and adenocarcinomas

VI.   Carcinoid tumors

VII.   Bronchial gland tumors
   1. Cylindromas
   2. Mucoepidermoid tumors

VIII. Papillary tumors of the surface epithelium

IX.   "Mixed" tumors and carcinosarcomas

X.   Sarcomas

XI.   Unclassified

XII.   Melanoma

Reproduced, with permission, from Kreyberg L, Liebow AA, Uehlinger EA: Histological Typing of Lung Tumours, 2nd Ed, pp 19–20. Geneva, World Health Organization, 1981.

seau's syndrome, and cerebellar ataxia. The bronchioalveolar subtype of adenocarcinoma appears to be a distinct clinicopathologic entity. It may present as a solitary peripheral nodule, as multicentric disease, or with rapidly progressing pneumonic involvement. It may occur as early as the second decade of life, and the characteristic clinical presentation is that of multiple pulmonary nodules.

Squamous-Cell Carcinoma

Squamous-cell, or epidermoid, carcinoma, formerly the most common subtype of NSCLC, is now the second most frequent, accounting for roughly 30% of such cancers. This tumor arises most frequently in the proximal bronchi. Because of its central location and the tendency of these cells to exfoliate, squamous-cell carcinoma can be detected on cytologic examination at an early stage. With time, these tumors tend to cause bronchial obstruction and atelectasis or pneumonia. They also tend to remain localized and cavitate.

Of all the subtypes of NSCLC, the squamous-cell variety has the strongest association with smoking. Pathologically, it is characterized by visible keratinization with prominent desmosomes and intercellular bridges. Increased secretion of a parathyroid-like hormone in squamous-cell carcinoma has led to this subtype's association with hypercalcemia.

Large-Cell Carcinoma

The least common subtype of NSCLC, large-cell carcinoma, accounts for approximately 20% of all NSCLC. Refinements in histopathologic techniques have led to the diagnosis of adenocarcinoma or squamous-cell carcinoma in cases previously diagnosed as undifferentiated large-cell carcinoma.

In some cases, the exact histologic subtype of NSCLC cannot be determined; however, as long as NSCLC can be clearly documented, therapeutic plans can proceed.[31]

MOLECULAR BIOLOGY

Advances in our understanding of the biology of lung cancer may lead to progress in the therapy for or prevention of lung cancer. Carcinogenesis of lung cancer appears to evolve through a multiple-step process involving changes in many suppressor genes and oncogenes.[32] Cytogenetic studies of lung cancer have revealed a large number of chromosomal abnormalities, several of which have been found to be nonrandom (Table 6).[33,34]

The most commonly identified deletion involves the short arm of chromosome 3. This event is more frequent in small-cell lung cancer but has been seen in NSCLC as well. Mutations in the tumor-suppressor genes p53 and retinoblastoma (Rb) have been associated with the development of NSCLC. The p53 gene is responsible for the production of a nuclear phosphoprotein that is considered extremely important in DNA repair, growth regulation, cell division, and programmed cell death (apoptosis).[35]

Under normal conditions, the production of p53 protein is increased when DNA damage occurs. Increased amounts of p53 induce G1 arrest, thereby allowing time for DNA repair. Once repair has occurred, the cell is released from the cell-cycle block and proceeds to S-phase and cell division. If the DNA cannot be repaired, the cell is diverted toward programmed death.[36] When a mutation or deletion has occurred in the p53 gene, G1 arrest cannot be achieved. The abnormal cell is allowed to proceed to S-phase, where it divides and further propagates the genetic damage, which may lead to cancer.

Inherited lesions of p53 have been found in the Li-Fraumeni syndrome, which is associated with an increased incidence of brain cancer, breast cancer, and

TABLE 6

Frequently Involved Dominant and Recessive Oncogenes in Human Lung Cancer

Dominant oncogenes

c-*myc*,N-*myc*, L-*myc* (deregulated expression)
K-*ras*, H-*ras*, N-*ras* (activating mutation)
Her-2/neu (deregulated expression)

Recessive oncogenes ("Tumor-suppressor" Genes)

3p14 (U2020 deletion)
3p21.3 (region of the *Gnai-2* gene)
3p24-25 (region of the Von Hippel Lindau gene)
5q (*FAP, MCC* gene cluster)
9p (interferon gene cluster)
11p15, ~ 11p13
13q14 (retinoblastoma gene, *rb*)
17p13 (*p53* gene)

Adapted, with permission, from Minni J, Bader S, Bansel A, et al: Molecular genetics of lung cancer, in Motta G (ed): Proceedings of the International Meeting: Lung Cancer, Frontiers in Science and Treatment, p 27. Genoa, Italy, 1994.

soft-tissue sarcomas. Lung cancer also is frequently found in families with this syndrome. Although mutations of the *p53* gene have been found in about 50% of NSCLC,[37] correlation of *p53* mutations with prior smoking, tumor histology, and survival has not been elucidated.

The *Rb* gene codes for a nuclear phosphoprotein that appears to be involved in the cell cycle. Mutations of the *Rb* gene are very common in patients with small-cell lung cancer. However, only 20% of tumor specimens from NSCLC contain an *Rb* mutation.[38]

The dominant oncogene *ras* codes for a 21-kDa protein that has structural homology to the G proteins and mediates signal transduction pathways between cell-surface receptors and intracellular molecules. Transfection of a mutated *ras* gene into small-cell lung cancer cell lines results in a phenotype consistent with NSCLC.[39] Mutations of codon 12 of the K-*ras* gene are commonly found in NSCLC adenocarcinomas.[39] The presence of the K-*ras* codon-12 mutation is an adverse prognostic factor for survival in patients with resected adenocarcinoma of the lung and may be associated with early metastatic disease.[41] The *myc* oncogene family appears to play a role in the pathogenesis of small-cell lung cancer.

The cell surface expresses a variety of molecules that play a role in cell-cell and cell-matrix communication. It has been found that various human cancers lose the cell-surface expression of blood-group determinants.[42] In NSCLC, patients whose tumors do not express ABO blood group antigen have shorter survival than do pa-

tients whose tumors maintain blood group antigen A and AB expression.[43] Enhanced expression of H/Ley/Leb antigens, which is associated with the absence of A and B group antigens, is also associated with decreased survival.[44]

Autocrine production of peptides and inappropriate production of hormones or hormone-like substances have been associated with tumor growth in many malignancies. In NSCLC, epidermal growth factor binds to the epidermal growth factor receptor and stimulates the growth of the tumor.[45] This receptor is present in approximately two thirds of NSCLC.[46] Monoclonal antibodies blocking the action of epidermal growth factor are being tested in clinical trials.[47]

Activation of opioid receptors on the surface of human lung cancer cells results in inhibition of tumor growth. Nicotine has been found to reverse this inhibition.[48] Methadone in low doses is able to inhibit the growth of lung cancer cells, presumably through diversion of the cells to programmed cell death.[49]

Advances in the understanding of the molecular biology of lung cancer may improve the diagnosis, staging, and even treatment of patients with this disease. In addition, understanding of molecular markers may allow identification of individuals at increased risk for the development or recurrence of lung cancer and selection of those individuals for chemoprevention or adjuvant therapy studies.

CLINICAL PRESENTATION

The signs and symptoms of lung cancer are related to the location of the disease and the occurrence of paraneoplastic syndromes.[31,50] Many patients present asymptomatically with a coin lesion discovered on a routine chest roentgenogram. The symptoms of centrally located lesions include cough, hemoptysis, wheezing, stridor, dyspnea, and postobstructive pneumonia. Peripheral lesions may result in pain from pleural or chest wall invasion, cough, or restrictive dyspnea.

A lesion involving the intrathoracic nerves may result in one of several syndromes. Pancoast's syndrome, which is characterized by shoulder pain radiating to the arm in an ulnar distribution, is caused by tumor invasion of the eighth cervical and first thoracic nerves in the superior sulcus. Horner's syndrome, which consists of enophthalmos, ptosis, meiosis, and ipsilateral dyshidrosis, may be caused by extension of the tumor into the paravertebral sympathetic nerves. Because the left recurrent laryngeal nerve passes through the aortic pulmonary window, it is susceptible to injury secondary to mediastinal node involvement. Such injury causes vocal cord paralysis with

TABLE 7

Most Common Sites of Lung Cancer Metastases

Hilar and mediastinal lymph nodes

Pleura

Opposite lung

Liver

Adrenal glands

Bone

Central nervous system

Other (kidney, abdominal lymph nodes, pancreas, esophagus)

subsequent hoarseness. Elevation of the hemidiaphragm secondary to phrenic nerve paralysis may be caused by tumor invasion into the mediastinum. Other symptoms also occur commonly with mediastinal involvement. For instance, malignant pleural effusions may result in dyspnea. Cardiac symptoms may result from malignant pericardial effusions secondary to pericardial invasion. Superior vena cava syndrome may result from either right-sided tumors or mediastinal nodal involvement. Dysphagia may result from compression of the esophagus.

Non-small-cell lung cancer is frequently metastatic, and symptoms secondary to the site of metastases are common. The most common sites of metastases in descending order of frequency are listed in Table 7. Bone metastases may be associated with pain, pathologic fractures, or spinal cord compression. Liver metastases may be associated with pain. Central nervous system metastasis may be indicated by seizures, headache, nausea, vomiting, altered mental status, or focal neurologic signs.

Finally, the clinical observation of weight loss and tumor related cachexia has been found to be an independent adverse prognostic factor.

Paraneoplastic Syndromes

The production of ectopic hormones or hormone-like substances is not uncommon in lung cancer and results in paraneoplastic syndromes, which have been described most commonly with small-cell carcinoma. Nonetheless, a significant number of patients with NSCLC develop a paraneoplastic syndrome during the course of the disease.

Hypercalcemia, caused by bone metastases or ectopic production of a parothyroid hormone-related peptide, is the most frequent paraneoplastic syndrome in NSCLC.

Hypercalcemia is most commonly associated with the squamous-cell subtype.

Hypertrophic pulmonary osteoarthropathy characterized by painful periostitis of the long bones and clubbing of the fingers and toes is usually seen with adenocarcinoma. Radionuclide bone scans and plain roentgenograms are usually helpful in establishing this diagnosis. Trousseau's syndrome or migratory thrombophlebitis, leukocytosis, and thrombocytosis have also been observed in lung cancer patients.

DIAGNOSIS

Obtaining a pathologic diagnosis is essential to the management of lung cancer, because NSCLC is managed differently than small-cell lung cancer. A complete history, physical examination, and chest roentgenograms may reveal sites of disease, such as cervical or supraclavicular lymph nodes, skin nodules, or pleural effusions. This initial survey may establish whether the tumor is operable.

Sputum cytology is an appropriate first diagnostic study, especially in the case of a central lesion, since this will allow for a noninvasive diagnosis in some patients. If an easily biopsied lesion is not found and the sputum cytology is negative, the next step is usually flexible fiberoptic bronchoscopy. For lesions that can be visualized endoscopically, diagnoses are made in 97% of tumors with the combination of biopsies, bronchial washings, and bronchial brushings.[51] Only 55% of cases can be diagnosed with bronchial brushings and washings when the lesion is peripheral and cannot be visualized.[31]

In the absence of a histologic diagnosis following broncoscopy, the clinical setting will dictate the next appropriate step. Percutaneous transthoracic fine-needle aspiration of pulmonary nodules can be useful in some clinical settings. It is usually performed under fluoroscopic or computed tomographic (CT) guidance. Negative results on fine-needle aspiration biopsy are frequent and must be considered indeterminate until the diagnosis is established by another method. Supraclavicular adenopathy, pleural effusions, or metastasis to liver, bone, or adrenal glands may be confirmed using the fine-needle aspiration technique. Finally, if a diagnosis still cannot be established using the above studies, mediastinoscopy with biopsy may be used. If the mediastinal nodes are negative, resection of the nodule will lead to a definitive diagnosis.

Solitary Pulmonary Nodule

The solitary pulmonary nodule represents a unique diagnostic dilemma. A solitary pulmonary nodule is a single mass, usually found incidentally on chest x-ray examination, that is surrounded by lung, is well circumscribed, and does not show evidence of mediastinal or hilar adenopathy. A review of an old chest x-ray film is the single most important step in evaluating a solitary pulmonary nodule. Age less than 40 years, nonsmoker status, a history of exposure to tuberculosis, or residence in an area endemic for histoplasmosis are other factors suggestive of a benign lesion.

If old chest x-ray films are not available and the patient has none of the risk factors described above, surgical resection for diagnosis and therapy is indicated following a staging workup. Radiologic evaluation may also be useful in the presence of factors such as distinct margins, certain calcification patterns (diffuse, central core bull's eye [granuloma], "popcorn ball" [hamartoma], or concentric layers) or high density on CT scans, all of which suggest a benign lesion. However, radiologic tests alone are not sufficient to conclusively rule out malignancy.[31]

STAGING

Once the histologic diagnosis of NSCLC has been established, the extent of disease must be evaluated to guide appropriate therapy. A complete history and physical examination often suggests sites of extrathoracic spread, which should be confirmed with appropriate imaging studies. A laboratory evaluation, including a complete blood count and routine electrolyte and blood chemistry tests (with liver enzyme studies), should be performed. Any patient who is being considered for surgery should have pulmonary function tests.

A CT scan of the chest and upper abdomen (to include the adrenal glands) is done in the vast majority of patients treated in the United States because the liver and adrenal glands are frequent sites of metastatic involvement. This test permits evaluation of the mediastinum and the contralateral lung and can detect pleural effusions. Patients with abnormal biochemistry values, including elevations in serum calcium or alkaline phosphatase, and patients with pain should have radionuclide bone scans performed to document metastatic disease. The routine use of CT scanning or magnetic resonance imaging of the brain in asymptomatic patients remains controversial, but it is probably not cost effective. Mediastinoscopy can reveal the occasional patient with unsuspected mediastinal lymph-node spread and, thereby, avoid unnecessary thoracotomy and resection. Its routine use in patients with normal imaging of the mediastinum on CT scanning is controversial.

Clinical staging often underestimates the true disease extent. To most accurately predict prognosis, surgical/pathologic staging should be considered. Following the completion of a staging workup, the disease is assigned a TNM stage (outlined in Tables 8 and 9 on p 193).[52] Schematic interpretation of the TNM system is given in Figures 1 to 9 (pp 190–192).[53]

TREATMENT

Stages I and II Disease

Patients with stage I or II lung cancer should undergo surgical resection if possible. Despite thorough investigation prior to surgery, many patients are found to have more extensive disease at thoracotomy. The 5-year survival rate for those who have pathologically proven stage I disease (T1-2N0) is 65%.[54] For the subset of patients with completely resected T1N0M0 disease, the 5-year survival rate approaches 75%. For patients with pathologically proven stage II disease (T1N1 or T2N1)—about 10% of all NSCLC patients—the overall 5-year disease-free survival rate is 39%.[55]

Surgery is the standard treatment for stages I and II disease, and radiotherapy is indicated for patients who cannot undergo surgery. Several studies have reported 5-year survival rates of 15% to 20% when potentially curative radiotherapy is used in patients with inoperable disease. The decreased survival is probably due, in part, to the lack of pathologic staging in this population as well as to concomitant medical illnesses.[56]

The major causes of mortality in patients with stage I and II disease are distant metastatic disease[57] and second primary tumors. In a trial by the Lung Cancer Study Group, the rate of second cancers (not lung primaries) was 1.8% per year, and the rate of new lung cancers was 1.6% per year.[58] A series of nearly 600 stage I NSCLC patients with mature follow-up from Memorial Sloan-Kettering Cancer Center revealed an overall incidence of recurrence of 27% (local or regional, 7%; systemic, 20%) and an incidence of second primary tumors of 34%.[59] This has led to current studies aimed at identifying prognostic factors that may indicate those patients at risk for relapse and to trials of chemoprophylaxis. An ongoing intergroup clinical trial is evaluating the role of 13-*cis*-retinoic acid as a chemopreventive agent for patients who have undergone resection of stage I disease.[60]

Adjuvant chemotherapy has been explored in early-stage NSCLC, and the results have been mixed. Most studies have not documented a survival benefit. A recently reported study of combination chemotherapy with cyclophosphamide (Cytoxan, Neosar), doxorubicin (Adriamycin, Rubex), and cisplatin (Platinol) as adjuvant treatment vs no further therapy was conducted in patients with completely resected stage I NSCLC. No

FIGURE 1

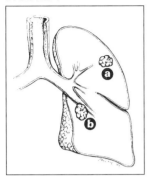

FIGURE 2

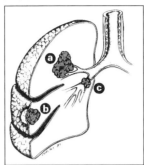

Diagram of T2 disease. A tumor that is (a) more than 3 cm in greatest dimension, or a tumor of any size that (b) invades the visceral pleura; (c) the proximal extent of the tumor must be within a lobar bronchus or at least 2 cm distal to the carina. Increasing size, > 3 cm, and invasiveness are characteristics of T2 disease.

Diagram of T1 disease. A tumor that is (a) 3 cm or less in greatest dimension surrounded by lung or visceral pleura. (b) no evidence of invasion proximal to a lobar bronchus at bronchoscopy.

FIGURE 3

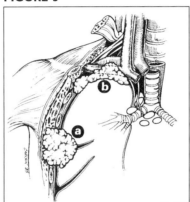

Diagram of T3 disease. A tumor of any size with direct extension into the (a) chest wall, including (b) superior sulcus tumors, or the diaphragm, mediastinal pleura or pericardium, without involving the heart, great vessels, trachea, esophagus or vertebral body, or a tumor in the main bronchus within 2 cm of the carina without involving the carina.

FIGURE 4

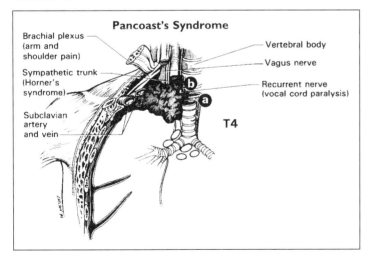

Pancoast's Syndrome

Brachial plexus (arm and shoulder pain)

Sympathetic trunk (Horner's syndrome)

Subclavian artery and vein

Vertebral body

Vagus nerve

Recurrent nerve (vocal cord paralysis)

T4

FIGURE 5

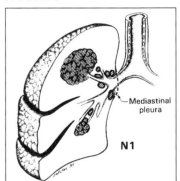

Mediastinal pleura

N1

Diagram of N1 disease. Metastasis to the lymph nodes in the peribronchial or the ipsilateral hilar region or both, including direct extension, is classified as N1.

Diagram of T4 disease. A tumor of any size with invasion of the mediastinum, or involving heart, great vessels, trachea, (a) esophagus, (b) vertebral body or carina or presence of malignant pleural effusion.

FIGURE 6

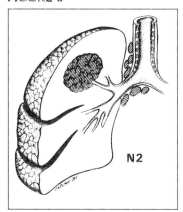

Diagram of N2 disease. Enlarged ipsilateral mediastinal lymph nodes indicate and are classified clinically as N2. However, because all enlarged lymph nodes do not contain metastasis, objective assessment of the nodes is advised to confirm N2 disease in patients who may be candidates for surgery.

FIGURE 7

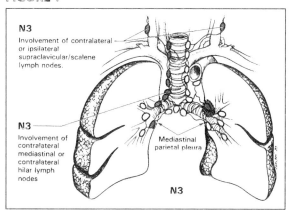

N3
Involvement of contralateral or ipsilateral supraclavicular/scalene lymph nodes.

N3
Involvement of contralateral mediastinal or contralateral hilar lymph nodes

Mediastinal parietal pleura

N3

Diagram of N3 disease. About 7% of patients with lung cancer present with supraclavicular lymph-node metastasis. Clinical judgment regarding involvement of these nodes is remarkably accurate, and routine biopsy of the nodes usually is not warranted for clinical staging.

FIGURE 8

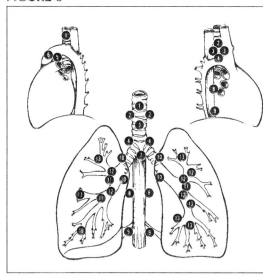

N2 Nodes

Superior mediastinal nodes
1. Highest mediastinal
2. Upper paratracheal
3. Pre- and retrotracheal
4. Lower paratracheal
   (including Azygos nodes)

Aortic nodes
5. Subaortic (aortic window)
6. Para-aortic (ascending aorta or phrenic)

Inferior mediastinal nodes
7. Subcarinal
8. Paraesophageal (below carina)
9. Pulmonary ligament

N1 Nodes
10. Hilar
11. Interlobar
12. Lobar
13. Segmental

Lymph-node classification nomenclature. Single-digit numbers are assigned to the mediastinal, N2, lymph nodes and double-digit numbers to the peribronchial and hilar, N1, lymph nodes.

differences in time to recurrence or overall survival were found.[61] In contrast, a study from Finland did find improvements in disease-free survival among patients randomly assigned to receive postresection chemotherapy.[62] At present, adjuvant chemotherapy or radiotherapy in patients with stage I or II NSCLC should be administered only within the context of a well-designed clinical trial. As these patients are at increased risk for second primary tumors and recurrence of their disease, close follow-up is indicated.[63]

Stage III Disease

The use of combined-modality therapy in stage III NSCLC is an area of considerable investigation.[64] Intensive research has led, in turn, to the subdivision of stage III disease into stage IIIa (potentially resectable) and stage IIIb (not resectable) based on the difference in outcomes following surgical resection. Stage IIIa patients have a 5-year survival rate approaching 15% with

surgery, whereas stage IIIb patients have a 5-year survival rate of less than 5%.[55] However, as the current staging system has been in place only since 1986, much of the literature classifies all locally advanced disease into one category. In addition, under the old staging system in use prior to 1986, distant metastasis was included in the stage III category. Therefore, interpretation of much of the past literature is difficult.[64]

Surgery: The efficacy of surgery varies with the subset of stage III disease. For instance, patients with T3N0 disease have a favorable outcome. A 5-year survival rate of 54% was reported from the Mayo Clinic[65] in T3N0M0 patients whose T3 designation was based on chest wall involvement. Patients whose stage III classification is based on N2 disease have a less favorable outcome.

In a large series of patients at Memorial Sloan-Kettering Cancer Center,[66] the 5-year survival rate for patients with N2 disease was 30%. The majority of survivors, however, were patients whose disease was clinically

FIGURE 9

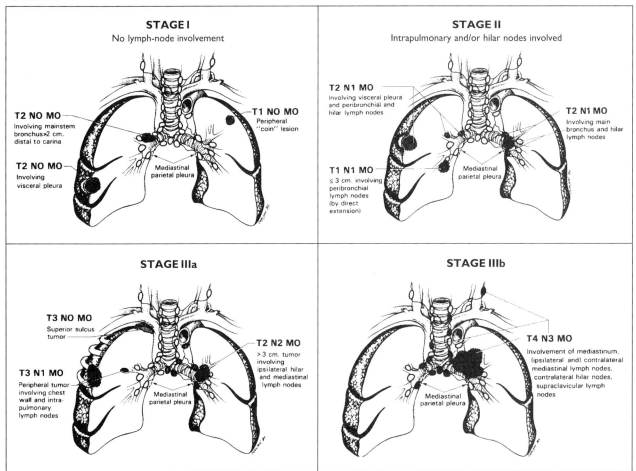

Diagrams of staging. Reprinted, with permission, from Mountain CF, Libshitz HI, Hermes KE: Lung Cancer: A Handbook for Staging and Imaging. Houston, 1992.

TABLE 8
TNM Classification of Non-Small-Cell Lung Cancer

Primary tumor (T)

Tx: tumor proven by the presence of malignant cells in bronchopulmonary secretions but not visualized radiographically or bronchoscopically, or any tumor that cannot be assessed (as in a retreatment staging)

T0: no evidence of primary tumor

Tis: carcinoma in situ

T1: a tumor ≤ 3.0 cm in greatest dimension, surrounded by lung or visceral pleura and with no evidence of invasion proximal to a lobar bronchus at bronchoscopy[a]

T2: a tumor > 3.0 cm in greatest dimension, or a tumor of any size that either invades the visceral pleura or has associated atelectasis or obstructive pneumonitis extending to the hilar region; at bronchoscopy, the proximal extent of demonstrable tumor must be within a lobar bronchus or at least 2.0 cm distal to the carina; any associated atelectasis or obstructive pneumonitis must involve less than an entire lung

T3: a tumor of any size with direct extension into the chest wall (including superior sulcus tumors), diaphragm, or the mediastinal pleura or pericardium without involving the heart, great vesssels, trachea, esophagus, or vertebral body, or a tumor in the main bronchus within 2 cm of the carina without involving the carina

T4: a tumor of any size with invasion of the mediastinum or involving the heart, great vessels, trachea, esophagus, vertebral body, or carina, or presence of a malignant pleural effusion[b]

Nodal involvement (N)

N0: no demonstrable metastasis to regional lymph nodes

N1: metastasis to lymph nodes in the peribronchial or the ipsilateral hilar region, or both, including direct extension

N2: metastasis to ipsilateral mediastinal lymph nodes and subcarinal lymph nodes

N3: metastasis to contralateral mediastinal lymph nodes, contralateral hilar lymph nodes, ipsilateral or contralateral scalene or supraclavicular lymph nodes

Distant metastasis (M)

M0: no (known) distant metastasis

M1: distant metastasis present (specify site[s])

---

[a] Uncommon superficial tumors of any size with an invasive component limited to the bronchial wall and possibly extending proximal to the main bronchus are classified as T1.

[b] Most peural effusions associated with lung cancer are due to the presence of a tumor. There are, however, a few patients in whom cytopathologic examination of pleural fluid (on more than one specimen) is negative for tumor, the fluid is nonbloody, and it is not an exudate. In such cases, where these elements and clinical judgment dictate that the effusion is not related to the tumor, patients should be staged T1, T2, or T3, excluding effusion as a staging element.

Adapted, with permission, from Mountain CF: Chest 89:225–233s, 1986.

TABLE 9
Stage Grouping of TNM Subsets

Stage grouping	T	N	M
Occult carcinoma	Tx	N0	M0
Stage 0	Tis	Carcinoma in situ	
Stage I	T1	N0	M0
	T2	N0	M0
Stage II	T1	N1	M0
	T2	N1	M0
Stage IIIa	T3	N0	M0
	T3	N1	M0
	T1–3	N2	M0
Stage IIIb	Any T	N3	M0
	T4	Any N	M0
Stage IV	Any T	Any N	M1

Adapted, with permission, from Mountain CF: Chest 89:225–233s, 1986

defined as N0 or N1 and were found to have N2 disease at surgery. Among those patients with clinically evident N2 disease, the 5-year survival rate was 9%. Because the majority of these patients were evaluated between 1974 and 1984, it is unlikely that CT scans of the chest were done routinely.

At present, surgery in stage III disease should be reserved for patients with certain clinical presentations of stage IIIa disease and should not be considered as primary therapy for patients with stage IIIb disease.

Radiotherapy: Radiotherapy has been considered a routine measure for patients with inoperable, locally advanced disease. The standard therapy is 50 to 60 Gy in 200-Gy fractions five times weekly for 5 to 6 weeks. This regimen is based on a Radiation Therapy Oncology Group (RTOG) trial[67] that found improved local control and a nonsignificant trend toward improved survival at 2 years in patients receiving 50 to 60 Gy vs 40 Gy (19% survival vs 11% survival).

To study the relationship between radiotherapy and survival in detail, a study performed by the Southeastern Oncology Group[68] randomly assigned patients with locally advanced, unresectable NSCLC to one of three treatments: (1) 60 Gy of radiotherapy over 6 weeks; (2) vindesine, 3 mg/m²; or (3) a combination of radiotherapy and vindesine. Median survival durations with the three treatment regimens were 8.6, 10.1, and 9.4 months, respectively. The study concluded that radiotherapy did not improve survival in patients with locally advanced NSCLC.

There are two major criticisms of this study. First, treatment with the single agent vindesine at 3 mg/m^2 is currently considered suboptimal chemotherapy and would not be expected to have a significant impact on survival. Thus, as the response rate was only 11%, this arm represents more a control arm than a chemotherapy arm. Second, the vindesine-only patients were crossed over to radiotherapy if they became symptomatic, which occurred in 37% of patients initially assigned to vindesine only. Therefore, a conclusion of this study may be that early radiotherapy has no benefit over late thoracic radiotherapy.

In a recent retrospective analysis[69] of a randomized phase I/II trial of 120 cGy twice daily escalating to 60 to 79.2 Gy, the RTOG reported that in a subset of patients with locally advanced, unresectable stage III disease who had good performance status, no supraclavicular lymph-node involvement, and less than 6% weight loss, survival increased with increased radiation dose. Patients in this subset who received 69.6 Gy or more had a median survival of 13 months, with 29% of patients alive at 2 years. In contrast, similar patients receiving 60.0 Gy had a median survival of 10 months and a 2-year survival rate of 18% ($P = .02$). The improved median survival seen with high doses of radiotherapy may demonstrate that improved survival in locally advanced disease is possible with improvements in local therapy. Because the overall survival of stage III patients remains poor after radiotherapy or surgery alone, the role of multimodality therapy has become an area of intensive investigation.

Adjuvant Chemotherapy: The role of adjuvant chemotherapy in NSCLC is unclear. The Lung Cancer Study Group[70] randomly assigned patients with stage II or III adenocarcinoma or large-cell carcinoma to receive either cyclophosphamide, doxorubicin, and cisplatin (CAP) or a regimen of bacillus Calmette-Guérin (BCG) and levamisole (Ergamisol). Disease-free survival was increased by 7 months ($P < .05$) in the group receiving chemotherapy, and overall survival increased by 7 months.

Furthermore, in another Lung Cancer Study Group trial of squamous-cell carcinoma patients with positive margins or involved high paratracheal nodes,[71] patients who received concurrent chemotherapy (CAP) and radiotherapy showed improved disease-free survival compared with those who received radiotherapy alone (14 vs 8 months, $P \leq .004$). However, overall survival was not significantly improved. Concerns about these studies include the use of doxorubicin and cyclophosphamide, which do not have major single-agent activity in NSCLC, and the very low dose of cisplatin.

Memorial Sloan-Kettering Cancer Center conducted a prospective, randomized study of adjuvant radiation with or without vindesine and cisplatin in stage III (T1-3N2M0) NSCLC patients. No difference in time to progression or overall survival was found.[72] A similar study conducted in Japan randomly assigned stage III patients whose disease had been completely resected to receive no further treatment or adjuvant vindesine and cisplatin chemotherapy. Again, no difference in disease-free or overall survival was found.[73] In summary, cisplatin-based postoperative chemotherapy for stage III NSCLC has not resulted in significantly prolonged survival. The use of such therapy should not be recommended outside the context of a clinical trial.

Neoadjuvant Chemotherapy: The use of chemotherapy prior to surgery in patients with stage IIIa disease has been extensively investigated. Several studies have demonstrated response rates of 50% to 70% and long-term disease-free survival rates of 20% to 30% in patients treated with neoadjuvant chemotherapy. Two randomized trials have confirmed these results (Table 10).

In one study, 60 patients with stage IIIa NSCLC were randomly assigned to receive either surgery alone or three courses of mitomycin (Mutamycin), ifosfamide (Ifex), and cisplatin given at 3-week intervals followed by surgery.[74] Mediastinal radiotherapy was given to all patients after surgery. The median overall and disease-free survivals were 26 and 20 months, respectively, for the chemotherapy-plus-surgery group vs 8 and 5 months, respectively, for the surgery-only group.

A second study conducted at the University of Texas M. D. Anderson Cancer Center[75] randomly assigned 60 patients with previously untreated, potentially operable stage IIIa disease to six cycles of perioperative chemotherapy (cyclophosphamide, etoposide [VePesid], and cisplatin) and surgery or surgery alone. The major response rate to the preoperative chemotherapy was 35%. Patients treated with perioperative chemotherapy and surgery had an estimated median survival of 64 months, compared with 11 months for patients who had surgery alone. The estimated 2- and 3-year survival rates, respectively, were 60% and 56% for the perioperative chemotherapy patients and 25% and 15% for those who had surgery alone.

Adjuvant Radiotherapy: Several retrospective trials of radiotherapy following resection of stage II or III lung cancer have demonstrated an improvement in overall survival.[76-78] However, a large randomized trial conducted by the Lung Cancer Study Group[79] failed to confirm an overall survival benefit of postoperative radiotherapy in patients with resected stage II or III squamous-cell lung carcinoma. A significant decrease in local recurrence

TABLE 10

Results of Preoperative Chemotherapy Trials for Non-Small-Cell Lung Cancer

Reference	Number of patients	Chemotherapy	Schedule	Median survival (months)	Survival rate
Roth et at[75]	28	Etoposide, 100 mg/m^2 × 3 + cyclophosphamide, 500 mg/m^2 + cisplatin, 100 mg/m^2	Chemotherapy for 3 cycles preoperatively	64	2 yr / 60%
	32	None	Surgery alone	11	2 yr / 25%
Rosell et al[74]	30	Mitomycin, 6 mg/m^2 + ifosfamide, 3 g/m^2 + cisplatin, 50 mg/m^2	Chemotherapy for 3 cycles preoperatively	26	1 yr / 75%
	30	None	Surgery alone	8	1 yr / 20%

was found, however, and in patients with N2 disease, the overall recurrence rate was decreased, though survival was not improved.

Preoperative Radiotherapy for stage III disease has been investigated in two large randomized trials,[80,81] neither of which showed a benefit of this approach. However, both trials included patients with small-cell lung carcinoma, and neither provided adequate preoperative staging by current protocol standards. The use of CT scans, now standard practice, would likely have revealed metastatic disease in some of these patients.

Superior sulcus tumors may represent a unique subset of stage III tumors. Some small uncontrolled series[82,83] demonstrated improved survival in patients with superior sulcus tumors who received preoperative radiotherapy, compared with historical controls. Randomized trials, however, will be necessary to confirm this finding.

Chemoradiotherapy: The combination of chemotherapy and radiotherapy in the treatment of locally advanced, surgically unresectable NSCLC is an active area of research. Of the large randomized trials performed to date, trials conducted by four groups—Dillman et al,[84] LeChevalier et al,[85,86] Schaake-Koning et al,[87] and more recently, the RTOG (RTOG 88-08) and Eastern Cooperative Oncology Group (ECOG 4588)[88]—have shown improvement in survival, albeit modest, in patients receiving chemotherapy plus radiotherapy. However, these trials have used two different approaches to the combination of chemotherapy and radiotherapy: sequential and concurrent.

The sequential chemoradiotherapy and radiotherapy trials listed in Table 11 used systemic doses of chemotherapy prior to and sometimes following radiotherapy. Mattson et al[89] found no benefit of chemotherapy alternating with radiotherapy vs radiotherapy alone; however,

the chemotherapy was given during the interval between two courses of radiotherapy. The presence of a gap during radiotherapy may be considered to be suboptimal in radiotherapy-only trials but has not been found to result in decreased survival in phase III trials. In addition, if only the M0 patients are evaluated, a strong trend toward improved survival is found in the chemotherapy-plus-radiotherapy arm. Morton et al[90] also failed to demonstrate a benefit for chemotherapy, but cisplatin was not included in the chemotherapy arm.

The studies reported by Le Chevalier et al [85,86] and Dillman et al[84] both involved cisplatin-based chemotherapy (three and two cycles, respectively) prior to radiotherapy. In both of these trials, the patients receiving chemotherapy had a significant survival advantage. Of particular interest, Le Chevalier et al[85,86] found significantly fewer failures secondary to metastatic disease in patients given chemotherapy. Dillman et al [84] found no difference in the pattern of relapse, but formal staging was not performed at the time of failure. Furthermore, a higher number of unexpected deaths than expected[90] were found among the patients who received radiotherapy only, compared with only four deaths in the chemoradiotherapy group.

In the study by Van Houtte et al,[91] there was no distinction between stages IIIa and IIIb, which could have led to bias. The study failed to show an advantage in median survival with a cisplatin-containing combination. However, this trial involved far fewer patients than did the other studies. Also, a trend toward a survival advantage was identified at 2 years.

Mira et al[92] and Trovo et al[93] also failed to demonstrate improved survival with chemotherapy, although both trials used suboptimal chemotherapy. Furthermore, Trovo et al[93] utilized suboptimal radiation therapy, with only

45 Gy in both treatment arms. Finally, the RTOG and ECOG study[88] confirmed that cisplatin-based induction chemotherapy followed by radiotherapy was superior to hyperfractionated radiotherapy or standard radiotherapy alone in terms of 1-year survival rates and median survival durations (60% and 13.8 months; 51% and 12.3 months; and 46% and 11.4 months, respectively). The patients in this study had stages II, IIIa, and IIIb disease, had good performance status, and were considered clinically to have unresectable disease.

Another group of studies, summarized in Table 12, involved the use of concurrent chemoradiotherapy to take advantage of the radiosensitizing effects of cisplatin in patients with inoperable tumors. Soresi et al[94] found a trend toward improved survival in a group of patients receiving cisplatin, 15 mg m²/wk, in addition to radio-

therapy. A significant decrease in the rate of intrathoracic relapses was noted in the chemoradiotherapy arm, compared with the radiotherapy-only arm (48% vs 59%).

A second study of radiotherapy vs concurrent chemoradiotherapy for inoperable patients by Schaake-Koning et al[87] revealed a statistically significant survival advantage for the groups receiving daily cisplatin (6 mg/m²) plus radiotherapy, compared with the patients who received radiotherapy alone. Daily cisplatin appeared to have an advantage over weekly cisplatin, but not a statistically significant one. As in the trial by Soresi et al,[94] this study showed a decrease in local recurrence with the combination of chemotherapy and radiotherapy. A major criticism of both of these studies is that they gave relatively low doses of split-course radiotherapy.

In a third large randomized trial by Ansari et al,[95]

TABLE 11

Sequential Chemoradiotherapy for Locally Advanced Non-Small-Cell Lung Cancer

Reference	Number of patients	Radiation dose (Gy)	Chemotherapy	Schedule	Survival, 1 yr/2 yr (median in months)
Morton et al[87]	56	60	Methotrexate + doxorubicin + cyclophosphamide + lomustine	Chemotherapy × 2, radiotherapy	46%/21% (10.5)
	58	60	None	Radiotherapy	45%/16% (10.5)
Mattson et al[86]	119	55	Cyclophosphamide + doxorubicin + cisplatin	Chemotherapy × 2, radiotherapy, chemotherapy × 6	42%/19% (10.5)
	119	55	None	Radiotherapy	41%/17% (9)
LeChevalier et al[82,83]	176	65	Cisplatin + cyclophosphamide + vindesine + lomustine	Chemotherapy × 3, radiotherapy	50%/21% (12)
	177	65	None		41%/14% (10)
Dillman et al[81]	78	60	Cisplatin + vinblastine	Chemotherapy × 2, radiotherapy	55%/26% (13.8)
	77	60	None	Radiotherapy	40%/13% (9.7)
van Houtte et al[88]	27	55	Cisplatin + etoposide + vindesine	Chemotherapy × 3, radiotherapy	40%/18% (11)
	32	55	None	Radiotherapy	42%/7% (11)
Mira et al[89]	109	58	Cisplatin + cyclophosphamide + doxorubicin + fluorouracil + vincristine + mitomycin	Chemotherapy, radiotherapy + chemotherapy	(9.1)
	117	58	None	Radiotherapy	(9.2)
Trovo et al[93]	62	45	Cyclophosphamide + doxorubicin + methotrexate	Radiotherapy, chemotherapy × 12	(11.7)
	49	45	None	Radiotherapy	(10.0)
Sause et al[85]	151	60	Cisplatin + vinblastine	Chemotherapy × 1, radiotherapy	60%/13.8
	152	69.6	None	Hyperfractionated radiotherapy	51% (12.3)
	149	60	None	Radiotherapy	46% (11.4)

TABLE 12

Concurrent Chemoradiotherapy for Locally Advanced Non-Small-Cell Lung Cancer

Reference	Number of patients	Radiation dose (Gy)	Chemotherapy	Schedule	Survival, 1 yr/2 yr
Soresi et al[91]	45	50.4	Cisplatin	Chemotherapy weekly + radiotherapy	75%/40%[a]
	50	50.4	None	Radiotherapy	70%/30%[a]
Schaake-Koning et al[84]	110	55	Cisplatin	Chemotherapy weekly + radiotherapy	44%/19%
	107	55	Cisplatin	Chemotherapy daily + radiotherapy	54%/26%
	114	55	None	Radiotherapy	46%/13%
Ansari et al[92]	90	60	Cisplatin	Chemotherapy every 3rd week + radiotherapy	35%/15%
	93	60	None	Radiotherapy	40%/9%
Trovo et al[93]	87	45	Cisplatin	Chemotherapy daily + radiotherapy	— /17%
	89	45	None	Radiotherapy	— /20%

[a] Estimated from survival curves in actuarial life tables

reported in abstract form only, patients with inoperable stage III disease received 60 Gy of radiotherapy without interruption or the same radiation dose with cisplatin (70 mg/m² every 3 weeks). The survival rate at 2 years was slightly better in patients who received chemotherapy plus radiotherapy, but the difference between the two groups did not approach statistical significance. Data on patterns of failure were not included. The failure to demonstrate a benefit from the addition of cisplatin may be due to the lack of radiosensitization resulting from the infrequent cisplatin administration.

While these three studies together suggest a benefit for the addition of chemotherapy to radiotherapy, the combination should not be considered standard therapy for stage III NSCLC at present. Finally, an abstract published by Trovo et al[96] reported no survival advantage for daily cisplatin combined with radiotherapy, compared with radiotherapy alone. However, one fourth of the patients in this study could not be evaluated, and only 45 Gy was administered, both to patients receiving radiotherapy and chemotherapy and to those receiving radiotherapy alone.

Stage IV Disease

Chemotherapy: The presence of metastatic spread (ie, stage IV disease) is an ominous finding in NSCLC. While many trials have been performed using various chemotherapy regimens to combat metastases, it has been difficult to determine whether patients receiving chemotherapy have improved survival. The most active single agents are listed in Table 13. No single agent has been demonstrated to significantly prolong survival. The combination of active agents has been shown to increase response rates to as high as 50% in phase II trials. Unfortunately, it has been difficult to demonstrate signif-

icant improvements in survival with such combinations in randomized trials.

As cisplatin appears to be one of the most active and best studied single agents, multiple trials have attempted to demonstrate that combinations containing cisplatin are superior to regimens that do not include this agent. Despite improved response rates for cisplatin-based combinations in most of the major trials,[55] only one of six trials comparing cisplatin-containing regimens with regimens not containing cisplatin has demonstrated a significant survival advantage for cisplatin-based therapy.[97] This is not unexpected, as these regimens rarely result in major response rates exceeding 30%. Further attempts have been made to improve response rates by giving cisplatin

TABLE 13

Chemotheraputic Agents for Non-Small-Cell Lung Cancer

> 15% Response rates

Cisplatin
Ifosfamide
Mitomycin
Vinblastine
Vindesine
Vinorelbine
Paclitaxel
Oral etoposide

Investigational agents

Edatrexate
Gemcitabine
Docetaxel
CPT-11

TABLE 14

Cisplatin-Based Chemotherapy vs Supportive Care

Reference	Number of patients	Chemotherapy	Median survival
Cellerino et al[96]	62	Cyclophosphamide + epirubicin + cisplatin	34.3 wk
	61	None	21.1 wk
Rapp et al[97]	44	Vindesine + cisplatin	32.6 wk
	43	Cyclophosphamide + doxorubin + cisplatin	24.7 wk
	50	None	17.0 wk
Woods et al[98]	97	Vindesine + cisplatin	6 mo
	91	None	4 mo
Ganz et al[99]	31	Vinblastine + cisplatin	4.8 mo
	32	None	3.2 mo
Quoix et al[100]	24	Vindesine + cisplatin	199 d
	22	None	73 d

in escalated doses, but this has resulted in an increase in toxicity with no increase in the response rate.[98]

In view of the finding that NSCLC is not sensitive to chemotherapy, the appropriateness of using chemotherapy for NSCLC has been questioned. Five large randomized trials, summarized in Table 14,[99–103] have compared best supportive care with cisplatin-based chemotherapy. All five trials demonstrated an improved median survival in patients receiving chemotherapy; however, this difference attained statistical significance in only two studies.[100,103] In a study by Rapp et al,[100] chemotherapy was found to be cost-effective and to improve quality of life, compared with best supportive care.

A study conducted at Memorial Sloan-Kettering Cancer Center[104] attempted to identify prechemotherapy characteristics of NSCLC patients that are important prognostic factors and predictive of chemotherapy response. According to this study, pretreatment characteristics associated with a good response to cisplatin-based chemotherapy were Karnofsky performance status greater than or equal to 80, no bone or liver metastases, normal lactate dehydrogenase levels, female gender, less than one site of metastasis, no prior chemotherapy, and weight loss of less than 5%.

Investigational Agents: Several new agents are currently being evaluated in phase II trials. Oral etoposide, paclitaxel (Taxol), and vinorelbine (Navelbine) are relatively recent additions to the list of active chemotherapy agents for the treatment of NSCLC.

Etoposide, when given orally as a single agent over short intervals (less than 5 days), produces responses in approximately 15% of patients, but prolonged (14 to 21 days), low-dose oral administration has produced response rates in excess of 20%.[102]

Paclitaxel has also been found to have a response rate in excess of 20% in phase II trials.[106,107] Further studies exploring paclixatel in combination with cisplatin and carboplatin (Paraplatin) are ongoing.

Vinorelbine is a semisynthetic vinca alkaloid recently approved by the Food and Drug Administration for the treatment of inoperable NSCLC. Phase II trials of vinorelbine have been conducted mainly in Europe in patients with NSCLC, breast cancer, ovarian cancer, and Hodgkin's disease. The biologic effect is exerted by inhibition of the microtubule assembly, which results in mitosis blockade. A randomized trial comparing single-agent vinorelbine with the combination of fluorouracil and leucovorin was conducted in NSCLC patients. The median survival was significantly improved for patients receiving vinorelbine (30 vs 22 weeks).[108] Another study conducted in France compared vinorelbine with vinorelbine plus cisplatin in patients with advanced NSCLC.[109] This trial found the vinorelbine-cisplatin combination to be superior to the other treatment regimens in terms of response rates and overall survival. Further trials exploring the role of vinorelbine in the treatment of NSCLC are currently under way in several cancer centers.

Docetaxel (Taxotere) is a semisynthetic taxoid compound related to paclitaxel that has been evaluated in phase II studies. Response rates of 33% to 38% have been reported in previously untreated NSCLC patients.[110,111]

Edatrexate has been shown to be active in phase II trials.[112,113] Kris et al explored a combination of edatrexate, mitomycin, and vinblastine in patients with stage III or IV NSCLC. In this study, the major response rate was 58% and median survival time, 13.6 months.[114] Based on these results, a large phase III trial enrolling over 600 patients was performed comparing the three-drug regimen of edatrexate, mitomycin, and vinblastine with the combination of mitomycin plus vinblastine. No significant improvement in survival was found.[115] Although the use of second-line chemotherapy was not reported, it is noteworty that median survival was 8 months in both arms in this multi-institutional study.

Gemcitabine, a new antimetabolite with an excellent toxicity profile[116] that has been evaluated in both phase I and phase II studies, has produced single-agent response rates of approximately 20%.[117]

Topoisomerase inhibitors are currently being investigated. One such agent, CPT-11, was associated with a response rate exceeding 30% in one phase II trial.[118] Topotecan, another drug in this class, is also being studied.

Other Therapies: Although chemotherapy may be used in most patients with metastatic disease, radiotherapy and surgery may be helpful in managing disease in selected patients with stage IV NSCLC. Radiotherapy is indicated for palliation of symptomatic lesions in this population. Radiotherapy to the chest may help relieve pain, hemoptysis, or obstructive symptoms. Furthermore, radiotherapy of bone metastases may help prevent pathologic fractures and relieve pain.

Surgery may be helpful in selected patients with metastatic disease, even though surgical debulking of the primary tumor has not been found to benefit patients with stage IV disease. In patients with a metachronous solitary brain metastasis, surgical resection of the metastatic lesion may improve survival in those patients whose primary lesion is adequately controlled.[119]

Finally, proximal bronchial obstructive lesions may be relieved with bronchoscopic Rd/YAG laser treatment or with brachytherapy, both of which are highly effective as short-term (2 to 4 months) palliative measures, even in patients who have had previous radiotherapy.[120]

Screening and Prevention: Because advanced-stage NSCLC has a poor prognosis, two strategies—screening and chemoprevention—have been studied for their potential benefits before or early in the course of the disease. Unfortunately, however, large randomized trials conducted over the past 20 years suggest that screening strategies have had little impact.

Whether screening for lung cancer could alter survival in men who smoked heavily was examined in three large studies (Table 15).[121] A study performed at the Mayo Clinic compared sputum cytology and chest x-ray films vs no scheduled screening. Although the screened population was found to have twice as many pathologic stage I tumors as the unscreened group, there was no difference in overall lung cancer mortality. The other two trials were primarily tests of the screening capabilities of sputum cytologies, as both the control and test groups were followed with chest x-ray films. Neither study showed a reduction in rates of lung cancer mortality among patients who underwent routine sputum cytologies.

Current efforts at developing effective screening programs are based on the development of molecular markers of the early onset of lung cancer. For example, the use of monoclonal antibodies to screen sputum specimens preserved from the Johns Hopkins screening trial was very effective in detecting patients destined to develop lung cancer.[122]

The second approach to early intervention is chemoprevention. Several lines of evidence suggest that such intervention may be effective. First, NSCLC is a multistep process characterized by premalignant changes, such as bronchial metaplasia and dysplasia, in heavy smokers. These changes may permit identification of high-risk individuals who are candidates for early intervention.

Second, dietary evidence presented earlier in this

TABLE 15

Randomized Screening Studies for Lung Cancer

Trial	Number of patients	Screening procedure	Lung cancer mortality per year
Mayo Clinic	9,211	Chest x-ray + sputum cytology None	3.2/1,000 3.0/1,000
Johns Hopkins	10,386	Chest x-ray + sputum cytology Annual chest x-ray	3.4/1,000 3.8/1,000
Memorial Sloan-Kettering	10,040	Chest x-ray + sputum cytology Annual chest x-ray	No difference

review suggests that substances such as beta-carotene or retinoids may help prevent lung cancer.[22] Several studies have been undertaken to demonstrate the benefits of various retinoids in preventing lung cancer. In a randomized trial of patients who had undergone resection of primary head and neck cancers (a group at very high risk for lung cancer),[123] patients randomized to receive 13-cis-retinoic acid had a significantly lower incidence of second primary tumors than did a placebo group. In addition, no lung cancers developed in the cis-retinoic acid group, whereas three lung cancers developed in the placebo group.

A large intergroup trial is currently being planned to determine whether 13-cis-retinoic acid can prevent second primary tumors in patients with pathologic stage I disease. In view of the continued lack of effective therapy for advanced NSCLC, ongoing efforts to determine effective screening and chemoprevention programs have assumed the utmost importance.

CONCLUSIONS

Non-small-cell lung cancer remains one of the most devastating illnesses in the United States in terms of the number of patients and overall mortality. Surgery offers the potential for significant long-term survival in those patients who have pathologically staged early, local disease. Unfortunately, 70% of all NSCLC patients have regional, nodal, or metastatic involvement at the time of presentation.

Although current efforts to develop multimodality therapies may offer some hope of improved survival for the patient with locally advanced disease, current therapies are simply ineffective for patients with metastatic disease. Therefore, one of the oncologist's most important roles must be to promote primary prevention, with an emphasis on advising patients to stop smoking, as this will affect lung cancer mortality. In addition, further attempts to improve screening strategies and to develop effective chemoprevention regimens are essential.

REFERENCES

1. Wingo PA, Tong T, Bolden S: Cancer statistics, 1995. CA Cancer J Clin 45:8–30, 1995.

2. US Department of Health and Human Services: The health consequences of smoking: A report of the Surgeon General 1982. DHHS publication no 82-50179, Washington, DC, 1982.

3. Souquet PJ, Chauvin F, Boissel JP, et al: Polychemotherapy in advanced non small cell lung cancer: A meta-analysis. Lancet 342:19–21, 1993.

4. Parkin DM, Pisani P, Ferlay J: Estimates of the worldwide incidence of eighteen major cancers in 1985. Int J Cancer 54: 594–606, 1993.

5. Garfinkel L, Silverberg E: Lung cancer and smoking trends in the United States over the past 25 years. CA Cancer J Clin 41:137–146, 1991.

6. Boring CC, Squires TS, Heath CW: Cancer statistics for African Americans. CA Cancer J Clin 42:7–19, 1992.

7. Shopland DR, Eyre HJ, Pechacek TF: Smoking-attributable cancer mortality in 1991: Is lung cancer now the leading cause of death among smokers in the U.S.? J Natl Cancer Inst 83:1142–1148, 1991.

8. Hoffmann D, Heath S: Nicotine derived N-nitrosamines and tobacco related cancer: Current status and future directions. Cancer Res 45:935–944, 1985.

9. Hecht S, Hoffmann D: Tobacco-specific nitrosamines, an important group of carcinogens in tobacco and tobacco smoke. Carcinogenesis 9:87, 1988.

10. Phillips DH, Hewer A, Martin CN, et al: Correlation of DNA adduct levels in human lung with cigarette smoking. Nature 336: 790–797, 1988.

11. King HW, Osborne MR, Brookes P: The in-vitro and in-vivo reaction at the N7-position of guanine of the ultimate carcinogen derived from benzolalpyrene. Chem Biol Interact 24:345–353, 1979.

12. Wald NJ, Nanchahal K, Thompson SG, et al: Does breathing other people's tobacco smoke cause lung cancer? Br Med J 293:1217–1222, 1986.

13. National Cancer Institute: Respiratory Health Effects of Passive Smoking: Lung Cancer and Other Disorders. The report of the U.S. Environmental Protection Agency. Smoking and Tobacco Control Monograph No. 4. NIH publication no. 93-3605, Bethesda, Maryland, 1993.

14. Mossman B, Bignon J, Corn M, et al: Asbestos: Scientific developments and implications for public policy. Science 247: 294–301, 1990.

15. Hodgson JT, Jones RD: Mortality of asbsestos workers in England and Wales, 1971–1981. Br J Ind Med 43:1158–1164, 1986.

16. Marsh J, Mossman B: Mechanisms of induction of ornithine decarboxylase activity in tracheal epithelial cells by asbestiform minerals. Cancer Res 48:709–714, 1988.

17. Kjuss H, Skjaerven R, Langard S, et al: A case-referent study of lung cancer, occupational exposures and smoking. II. Role of asbestos exposure. Scand J Work Environ Health 12:203–209, 1986.

18. Harley N, Samet J, Cross F, et al: Contribution of radon and radon daughters to respiratory cancer. Environ Health Perspect 70:17–21, 1986.

19. Samet J: Radon and Lung Cancer. J Natl Cancer Inst 81: 745–757, 1989.

20. Nero AV, Schwehr MB, Nazaroff WW, et al: Distribution of airborne radon-222 concentrations in US homes. Science 234:992–997, 1986.

21. Radford E: Potential health effects of indoor radon exposure. Environ Health Perspect 62:281–287, 1985.

22. Ziegler RG, Subar AF, Craft NE, et al: Does beta-carotene explain why reduced cancer risk is associated with vegetable and fruit intake? Cancer Res 52(suppl 7):2060s–2066s, 1992.

23. The alpha-tocopherol, beta-carotene cancer prevention study group. The effect of vitamin E and beta-carotene on the incidence of lung cancer and other cancers in male smokers. N Engl J Med 330:1029–1035, 1994.

24. US Department of Health and Human Services: The health benefits of smoking cessation. DHHS publication no. (CDC) 90-8416. US Department of Health and Human Services, Public Health Service, Centers for Disease Control, Center for Chronic Disease Prevention and Health Promotion, Office of Smoking and Health, 1990.

25. Minna JD, Pass H, Glatstein E, et al: Cancer of the lung, in DeVita VT, Hellman S, Rosenberg S (eds): Cancer: Principles and Practice of Oncology, pp 591–705. Philadelphia, JB Lippincot, 1991.

26. Sellers TA, Bailey-Wilson JE, Elston RC, et al: Evidence for Mendelian inheritance in the pathogenesis of lung cancer. J Natl Cancer Inst 82:1272–1279, 1990.

27. Ayesh R, Idle JR, Ritchie JC, et al: Metabolic oxidation phenotypes as markers for susceptibility to lung cancer. Nature 312:169–170, 1984.

28. Caporaso NE, Tucker MA, Hoover RN, et al: Lung cancer and the debrisoquine metabolic phenotype. J Natl Cancer Inst 82:1264–1272, 1990.

29. Tokuhata GK, Lilienfeld AM: Familial aggregation of lung cancer in humans. J Natl Cancer Inst 30:249–253, 1963.

30. Ooi WL, Elston RC, Chen VW, et al: Increased familial risk for lung cancer. J Natl Cancer Inst 76:217–222, 1986.

31. Ihde DC: Non-small-cell lung cancer: I. Biology, diagnosis and staging. Curr Probl Cancer 15:65–103, 1991.

32. Minna J: The molecular biology of lung cancer pathogenesis. Chest 103:449, 1993.

33. Wang-Peng J, Knutsen T, Gazdar A, et al: Nonrandom structural and numerical chromosome changes in non-small cell lung cancer. Genes Chromosom Cancer 3:168–188, 1991.

34. Minni J, Bader S, Bansel A, et al: Molecular genetics of lung cancer, in Motta G (ed): Proceedings of the International Meeting: Lung Cancer, Frontiers in Science and Treatment, p 27. Genoa, Italy, 1994.

35. Kastan MB, Plunkett BS, Kuerbitz SJ: p53 protein is a cell cycle checkpoint following DNA damage. AACR proceedings 33:169, 1992.

36. Fisher DE: Apoptosis in cancer therapy: Crossing the threshold. Cell 78:539–542, 1994.

37. Chiba I, Takahashi T, Nau MM, et al: Mutations in the p53 gene are frequent in primary, resected non small cell lung cancer. Oncogene 5:1603–1610, 1990.

38. Reissmann PT, Koga H, Takahashi R, et al: Inactivation of the retinoblastoma susceptibility gene in non-small cell lung cancer. Oncogene 8:1913–1919, 1993.

39. Doyle LA, Marby M, Stahel RA, et al: Modulation of neuroendocrine surface antigens in oncogene-activated small cell lung cancer lines. Br J Cancer Suppl 14:39–42, 1991.

40. Rondenhuis S, Slebos RJC, Boot AJM, et al: Incidence and possible clinical significance of K-ras oncogene activation in adenocarcinoma of the human lung. Cancer Res 48:5738–5741, 1988.

41. Slebos RJC, Kibbelaar RE, Dallesio O, et al: K-ras oncogene activation as a prognostic marker in adenocarcinoma of the lung. N Engl J Med 323:561–565, 1990.

42. Davidsohn I: Early immunologic diagnosis and prognosis of carcinoma. Am J Clin Pathol 57:715–730, 1972.

43. Lee JS, Ro JY, Sahin AA, et al: Expression of blood group antigen A: A favorable prognostic factor in non-small cell lung cancer. N Engl J Med 324:1084–1090, 1991.

44. Miyake M, Taki T, Hitomi S, et al: Correlation of expression of H/Le(y) Le(b) antigens with survival in patients with carcinoma of the lung. N Engl J Med 327:14–18, 1992.

45. Hwang DL, Tay YC, Lin SS, et al: Expression of epidermal growth factor receptors in lung tumors. Cancer 58:2260–2263, 1986.

46. Berger MS, Gullick WJ, Greenfield C, et al: Epidermal growth factor receptors in tumors. J Pathol 152:297–307, 1987.

47. Perez-Soler R, Donato NJ, Shin DM, et al: Tumor epidermal growth factor receptor studies in patients with non-small cell lung cancer or head and neck cancer treated with monoclonal antibody RG83852. J Clin Oncol 12:730–739, 1994.

48. Maneckjee R, Minna JD: Opioid and nicotine receptors affect growth regulation of human lung cancer cell lines. Proc Natl Acad Sci USA 87:3294–3298, 1990.

49. Maneckjee R, Minna JD: Nonconventional opioid binding sites mediate growth inhibitory effects of methadone on human lung cancer cell lines. Proc Natl Acad Sci USA 89:1169–1173, 1991.

50. DeVita VT, Hellman S, Rosenberg SA (eds): Cancer: Principles and Practice of Oncology, 4th edition, pp [AUS?]. Philadelphia, JB Lippincott, 1994.

51. Popp W, Rauscher H, Ritschka L, et al: Diagnostic sensitivity of different techniques in the diagnosis of lung tumors with the flexible fiberoptic bronchoscope. Cancer 67:72–75, 1991.

52. Mountain CF: A new international staging system for lung cancer. Chest 89(suppl 4):225–233s, 1986.

53. Mountain C, Libshitz HI, Hermes KE: Lung Cancer: A handbook for staging and imaging. Houston, The University of Texas M. D. Anderson Cancer Center, 1992.

54. Williams DE, Pairolero PC, Davis CS, et al: Survival of patients surgically treated for stage I lung cancer. J Thorac Cardiovasc Surg 82:70–76, 1981.

55. Martini N, Burt ME, Bains MS, et al: Survival after resection of stage II non-small cell lung cancer. Ann Thorac Surg 54:460–466, 1992.

56. Ihde DC, Minna JD: Non-small-cell lung cancer. II: Treatment. Curr Probl Cancer 15:107–154, 1991.

57. Martini N, Beattie EJ: Results of surgical treatment in stage I lung cancer. J Thorac Cardiovasc Surg 74:499–505, 1977.

58. Thomas P, Rubinstein L: Cancer recurrence after resection: T1N0M0 non small cell lung cancer: Lung Cancer Study Group. Ann Thorac Surg 49:242–246, 1990.

59. Martini N, Bains M, Burt M, et al: Incidence of local recurrence and second primary tumors in resected stage I lung cancer. J Thorac Cardiovasc Surg 109:120–129, 1995.

60. Lippman SM: The University of Texas M. D. Anderson Cancer Center: Phase III, double blind, randomized trial of 13-CRA vs placebo to prevent second primary tumors in patients with totally resected stage I NSCLC, MDA-ID-91025.

61. Feld R, Rubinstein L, Thomas PA, et al: Adjuvant chemotherapy with cyclophosphamide, doxorubicin, and cisplatin in patients with completely resected stage I non-small cell lung cancer. J Natl Cancer Inst 85; 299–306, 1993.

62. Niiranen A, Niitamo-Korhonen S, Kouri M, et al: Adjuvant chemotherapy after radical surgery for non small cell lung cancer: A randomized study. J Clin Oncol 10: 1927–1932, 1992.

63. Feld R, Rubinstein L, Weisenberger T, et al: Sites of recurrence in resected stage I non-small-cell lung cancer: A guide for future studies. J Clin Oncol 2:1352–1358, 1984.

64. Strauss GM, Langer MP, Elias AD, et al: Multimodality treatment of stage IIIa non-small-cell lung carcinoma: A critical review of the literature and strategies for future research. J Clin Oncol 10:829–838, 1992.

65. Piehler JM, Pairolero PC, Weiland LH, et al: Bronchogenic carcinoma with chest wall invasion: Factors affecting survival following en bloc resection. Ann Thorac Surg 34:684–691, 1982.

66. Burt ME, Pomerantz AH, Bains MS, et al: Results of surgical treatment of stage III lung cancer invading the mediastinum. Surg Clin North Am 67:987–999, 1987.

67. Perez CA, Stanley K, Grundy G, et al: Impact of irradiation technique and tumor extent in tumor control and survival of patients with unresectable non-oat-cell carcinoma of the lung. Cancer 50:1091–1099, 1982.

68. Johnson DH, Einhorn LH, Bartolucci A, et al: Thoracic radiotherapy does not prolong survival in patients with locally advanced unresectable non-small-cell lung cancer. Ann Intern Med 113:33–38, 1990.

69. Cox JD, Azarnia N, Byhardt RW, et al: A randomized phase I/

II trial of hyperfractionated radiation therapy with total doses of 60.0 Gy to 79.2 Gy: Possible survival benefit with 69.6 Gy in favorable patients with stage III non-small-cell lung carcinoma: Report of Radiation Therapy Oncology Group 83-11. J Clin Oncol 8:1543–1555, 1990.

70. Holmes E, Gail M, for the Lung Cancer Study Group: Surgical adjuvant therapy stage II and III adenocarcinoma and large-cell undifferentiated carcinoma. J Clin Oncol 4:710–715, 1986.

71. Lad T, Rubinstein L, Sadagh A, et al: The benefit of adjuvant treatment for resected locally advanced non-small-cell lung cancer. J Clin Oncol 6:9–17, 1988.

72. Pisters KM, Kris MG, Gralla RJ, et al: Randomized trial comparing postoperative chemotherapy with vindesine and cisplatin plus thoracic irradiation with irradiation alone in stage III (N2) non small cell lung cancer. J Surg Oncol 56:236–241, 1994.

73. Ohta M, Tsuchiya R, Shimoyama M, et al: Adjuvant chemotherapy for completely resected stage III and non-small-cell lung cancer: Results of a randomized prospective study. J Thorac Cardiovasc Surg 106:703–708, 1993.

74. Rosell R, Codina JG, Camps C, et al: A randomized trial comparing preoperative chemotherapy plus surgery with surgery alone in patients with NSCLC. N Engl J Med 330:153–158, 1994.

75. Roth JA, Fossella F, Komaki R, et al: A randomized trial comparing perioperative chemotherapy and surgery with surgery alone in resectable stage IIIa non small cell lung cancer. J Natl Cancer Inst 86:673–680, 1994.

76. Green N, Kurohara SS, George FW, et al: Postresection irradiation for primary lung cancer. Radiology 116:405–407, 1975.

77. Kirsch MM, Roman H, Argenta L, et al: Carcinoma of the lung: Results of treatment over ten years. Ann Thorac Surg 21:371–377, 1976.

78. Choi NCH, Grillo HC, Gardiello M, et al: Basis of new strategies in postoperative radiotherapy of bronchogenic carcinoma. Int J Radiat Oncol Biol Phys 6:31–35, 1980.

79. Weisenburger TH, Gail M, for the The Lung Cancer Study Group: Effects of postoperative mediastinal radiation on completely resected stage II and stage III epidermoid cancer of the lung. N Engl J Med 315:1377–1381, 1986.

80. Shields TW: Preoperative radiation therapy in the treatment of bronchial carcinoma. Cancer 30:1388–1394, 1972.

81. Warram J: Preoperative irradiation of cancer of the lung: Final report of a therapeutic trial: A collaborative study. Cancer 36:914–925, 1975.

82. Paulson DL: Carcinoma in the superior pulmonary sulcus. J Thorac Cardiovasc Surg 70:1095–1097, 1975.

83. Miller JI, Mansour KA, Hatcher CR: Carcinoma of the superior pulmonary sulcus tumor. Ann Thorac Surg 28:44–46, 1979.

84. Dillman RO, Seagren SL, Propert KJ, et al: A randomized trial of induction chemotherapy plus high-dose radiation versus radiation alone in stage III non-small-cell lung cancer. N Engl J Med 323:940–945, 1990.

85. Le Chevalier T, Arriagada R, Quoix E, et al: Radiotherapy alone versus combined chemotherapy and radiotherapy in non-resectable non-small-cell lung cancer: First analysis of a randomized trial in 353 patients. J Natl Cancer Inst 83:417–423, 1991.

86. Le Chevalier T, Arriagada R, Tarayre M, et al: Significant effect of adjuvant chemotherapy on survival in locally advanced non-small-cell lung carcinoma (letter). J Natl Cancer Inst 84:58, 1992.

87. Schaake-Koning C, van den Bogaert W, Dalesio O, et al: Effects of concomitant cisplatin and radiotherapy on inoperable non-small-cell lung cancer. N Engl J Med 326:524–530, 1992,

88. Sause WT et al : Radiation Therapy Oncology Group (RTOG 88-08) and Eastern Cooperative Oncology Group (ECOG 4588):

Preliminary results of a phase III trial in regionally advanced unresectable non-small cell lung cancer. J Natl Cancer Inst 87: 198–205, 1995.

89. Mattson K, Holsti LR, Holsti P, et al: Inoperable non-small-cell lung cancer: Radiation with or without chemotherapy. Eur J Cancer Clin Oncol 24:477–482, 1988.

90. Morton RF, Jett JR, McGinnis WL, et al: Thoracic radiation therapy alone compared with combined chemoradiotherapy for locally unresectable non-small-cell lung cancer. Ann Intern Med 115:681–687, 1991.

91. Van Houtte P, Klastersky J, Renaud A, et al: Induction chemotherapy with cisplatin, etoposide, and vindesine before radiation therapy for non-small-cell lung cancer. Antibiot Chemother 41:131–137, 1988.

92. Mira JG, Miller TP, Crowley JJ: Chest irradiation (RT) vs chest RT and chemotherapy with prophylactic brain RT in localized non-small-cell lung cancer: A Southwest Oncology Group randomized study. Int J Radiat Oncol Biol Phys 19(suppl):145, 1990.

93. Trovo MG, Minatel E, Veronesi A, et al: Combined radiotherapy and chemotherapy vs radiotherapy alone in locally advanced bronchogenic carcinoma: A randomized study. Cancer 65:400–404, 1990.

94. Soresi E, Clerici M, Grilli R, et al: A randomized clinical trial comparing radiation therapy v radiation therapy plus cis-dichlorodiammine platinum (II) in the treatment of locally advanced non-small-cell lung cancer. Semin Oncol 15(suppl 7):20–25, 1988.

95. Ansari R, Tokars R, Fisher W, et al: A phase III study of thoracic irradiation with or without concomitant cisplatin in locoregional unresectable non small cell lung cancer (NSCLC): A Hoosier Oncology Group (H.O.G.) protocol (abstract). Proc Am Soc Clin Oncol 10:241, 1991.

96. Trovo MG, Minatel E, Franchin G, et al: Radiotherapy (RT) versus RT enhanced by cisplatin (CDDP) in stage III non-small-cell lung cancer (NSCLC): Randomized cooperative study. Lung Cancer 7(suppl):158, 1991.

97. Elliott J, Ahmedzal S, Hole D, et al: Vindesine and cisplatin combination chemotherapy compared with vindesine as a single agent in the management of non-small-cell lung cancer: A randomized study. Eur J Cancer 20:1025–1032, 1984.

98. Klastersky J, Sculier J, Ravez P, et al: A randomized study comparing a high and a standard dose of cisplatin in combination with etoposide in the treatment of advanced non-small cell lung carcinoma. J Clin Oncol 4:1780–1786, 1986.

99. Cellerino R, Tummarello D, Guidi F, et al: A randomized trial of alternating chemotherapy versus best supportive care in advanced non-small-cell lung cancer. J Clin Oncol 9:1453–1461, 1991.

100. Rapp E, Pater J, Willan A, et al: Chemotherapy can prolong survival in patients with advanced non-small-cell lung cancer: Report of a Canadian multicenter randomized trial. J Clin Oncol 6:633–641, 1988.

101. Woods R, Williams C, Levi J, et al: A randomized trial of cisplatin and vindesine versus supportive care only in advanced non-small-cell lung cancer. Br J Cancer 61:608–611, 1990.

102. Ganz P, Figlin R, Haskell C, et al: Supportive care versus supportive care and combination chemotherapy in metastatic non-small-cell lung cancer. Cancer 63:1271–1278, 1989.

103. Quoix E, Dietrman A, Charbonneau J, et al: Is cisplatin-based chemotherapy useful in disseminated non-small-cell lung cancer? Report of a French multicenter randomized trial. Bull Cancer (Paris) 78:344–346, 1991.

104. O'Connell JP, Kris MG, Gralla RJ, et al: Frequency and prognostic importance of pretreatment clinical characteristics in patients with advanced NSCLC treated with combination chemotherapy. J Clin Oncol 4:1604–1614, 1986.

105. Waits TM, Johnson DH, Hainsworth JD, et al: Prolonged administration of oral etoposide in non-small-cell lung cancer: A phase II trial. J Clin Oncol 10:292–296, 1992.

106. Murphy WK, Fossella FV, Winn RJ, et al: Phase II study of Taxol in patients with untreated advanced non-small cell lung cancer. J Natl Cancer Inst 85:384–388, 1993.

107. Chang AY, Kim K, Glick J, et al: Phase II study of Taxol, merbarone and piraxantrone in stage IV NSCLC: The Eastern Cooperative Oncology Group results. J Natl Cancer Inst 85:388–394, 1993.

108. O'Rourke M, Crawford J, Schiller J, et al: Survival advantage for patients with stage IV NSCLC treated with single agent Navelbine in a randomized control trial. Proc Am Soc Clin Oncol 12:343, 1993.

109. Le Chevalier T, Brisgand D, Douillard JY, et al: Results of a phase III randomized study of vinorelbine vs vinorelbine-cisplatin in NSCLC. J Clin Oncol 12:360–367, 1994.

110. Fossella FV, Lee JS, Murphy WK, et al: Phase II study of docetaxel for recurrent or metastatic NSCLC. J Clin Oncol 12: 1238–1244, 1994.

111. Francis PA, Rigas JR, Kris MG, et al: Phase II trial of docetaxel in patients with stage III and IV NSCLC. J Clin Oncol 12(6):1232–1237, 1994.

112. Lee JS, Libsitz H, Murphy W, et al: Phase II study of 10EdAM for stage III or IV NSCLC. Invest New Drugs 8:299–304, 1990.

113. Shum KY, Kris MG, Gralla RJ, et al: Phase II study of 10-ethyl-10deaza- Aminopterin in patients with stage III and IV NSCLC. J Clin Oncol 6:446–450, 1990.

114. Kris MG, Gralla RJ, Potanovich LM, et al: Assessment of pretreatment symptoms and improvement after EDAM+ mitomycin+vinblastine (EMV) in patients with inoperable non small cell lung cancer (abstract). Proc Am Soc Clin Oncol 1990.

115. Comis R et al: Multicenter randomized trials in 673 patients comparing the combination of edatrexate, mitomycin, and vinblastine with mitomycin and vinblastine in patients with stage III and IV non small lung cancer (abstract 455). Lung Cancer 1994.

116. Anderson H, Lund B, Bach F, et al: Single agent activity weekly gemcitabine in advanced NSCLC: A phase II study. J Clin Oncol 12:1821–1826, 1994.

117. Abratt RP, Bezwoda WR, Falkson G, et al: Efficacy and safety profile of gemcitabine in non small cell lung cancer: A phase II study. J Clin Oncol 12:1535–1540, 1994.

118. Fukuoka M, Niitani H, Suzuki A, et al: A phase II study of CPT-11, a new derivative of camptothecin, for previously untreated non-small-cell lung cancer. J Clin Oncol 10:16–20, 1992.

119. Patchell R, Tibbs P, Walsh J, et al: A randomized trial of surgery in the treatment of single metastases to the brain. N Engl J Med 322:494–500, 1990.

120. Miller JI Jr, Phillips TW: Neodymium:YAG laser and brachytherapy in the management of inoperable bronchogenic carcinoma. Ann Thorac Surg 50:190–196, 1990.

121. Miller AB: Lung cancer screening. Chest 89(suppl 4):324–326s, 1986.

122. Tockman MS, Gupla PK, Myers JD, et al: Sensitive and specific monoclonal antibody recognition of human lung cancer antigen on preserved sputum cells: A new approach to early lung cancer detection. J Clin Oncol 6:1685–1693, 1988.

123. Hong WK, Lippman SM, Itri LM, et al: Prevention of second primary tumors with isotretinoin in squamous-cell carcinoma of the head and neck. N Engl J Med 323:795–801, 1990.

SECTION 3

HEAD & NECK CANCER

CHAPTER **13**   **Head & Neck Cancer**

Head and Neck Cancer

Edgardo J. Rodriguez-Monge, MD, Dong M. Shin, MD, *and* Scott M. Lippman, MD

Division of Medicine, The University of Texas M. D. Anderson Cancer Center, Houston, Texas

Head and neck cancers are a diverse group of diseases, each with its own distinct epidemiologic, anatomic, and pathologic features, natural history, and treatment considerations. Despite improvements in diagnosis and local management, long-term survival rates for patients with this disease have not increased significantly over the past 30 years and are among the lowest for the major cancers. In this chapter we will review the major aspects of the epidemiology, biology, diagnosis, chemoprevention, and therapy for head and neck cancer. Because squamous-cell carcinoma accounts for almost 95% of the neoplasms in this region, the discussion will refer mainly to this histopathologic subtype.

EPIDEMIOLOGY

In the United States, head and neck cancers account for 3.2% (39,750) of all new cancers and 2.2% (12,460) of cancer deaths.[1] The disease is more common in many developing countries, with a worldwide annual incidence of more than 500,000. The incidence of head and neck cancer increases with age; most patients are older than age 50. Mainly because of the increasing use of tobacco among women, the male-to-female ratio has decreased from 4 to 5:1 to approximately 3:1 over the past 5 to 10 years. Furthermore, some studies have reported a higher risk for women at each successive pack-year stratum of smoking,[2] a finding not shown for alcohol.[3] From 1973 to 1989, the incidence of oral and pharyngeal carcinomas decreased in white men of all ages, whereas the African-American population experienced a significant increase.[4]

The greatest risk factor is tobacco use. Although alcohol use produces a modest independent risk, it exponentially potentiates tobacco risk. A recent review showed heavy smokers to have a 5- to 25-fold higher risk of head and neck cancer than nonsmokers. Smoking unfiltered cigarettes, rather than filtered cigarettes, lowered the risk only minimally. Although the risk of developing head and neck carcinoma is lowered substantially by smoking cessation, the relative risk of former heavy smokers never reaches that of nonsmokers.

The use of smokeless tobacco, particularly prevalent among teenagers as they attempt to emulate sports personalities, is strongly associated with the formation of premalignant oral lesions (hyperkeratosis, epithelial dysplasia), at rates ranging from 16% to 60%.[5,6] Smoking of marijuana, cigars, and pipes is also associated with head and neck neoplasia, especially in the oral cavity.[7,8]

Genetic susceptibility to environmental carcinogens may explain the fact that only a fraction of carcinogen (eg, tobacco)-exposed individuals develop these cancers. The best recent support for the importance of inherent susceptibility to carcinogens in the development of head and neck cancer comes from an assay of sensitivity of peripheral blood lymphocytes to mutagen-induced chromosomal damage. Mutagen sensitivity (eg, to bleomycin [Blenoxane]) has been shown to be a strong independent risk factor for the development of head and neck cancer and seems to have a multiplicative interaction with smoking. Mutagen-induced chromosome sensitivity also has been reported to correlate with the prospective development of second primary tumors.[9,10]

Dietary factors also seem to play a prominent role in the risk of oral and pharyngeal cancers. Numerous epidemiologic studies have shown an increased risk of cancer in individuals whose diets lack sufficient quantities of nutrients. Other risk factors are listed in Table 1.

Certain viruses may contribute to the development of head and neck cancer.[4,11] The best-described agent is the Epstein-Barr virus (EBV), which is associated with nasopharyngeal carcinoma (NPC), an uncommon form of head and neck cancer in the United States but a common form in some north African and Asian countries. Most patients with NPC show evidence of an elevated serum titer of immunoglobulin (Ig)G and IgA antibodies against viral capsid antigen, and EBV viral genome has been found in NPC tissue.[12,13] The association of NPC and EBV (in antibody and DNA) is particularly strong in patients with endemic undifferentiated carcinoma.[11] In China, multiple other risk factors for NPC have been reported, including ingestion of salted fish and inhalation of smoke from cooking fires. In certain parts of China, the rate of NPC is as high as 54.7 in 100,000 persons, compared with fewer than 1 in 100,000 in the United States, where NPC has been linked to tobacco use.[14] Human papillomavirus, especially types 16 and 18, and herpes simplex virus type

TABLE 1

Risk Factors for Head and Neck Cancer

Tobacco
Smoked (cigarettes, cigars, pipes, marijuana)
Smokeless

Alcohol

Viruses
Epstein-Barr virus (nasopharyngeal)
Other (herpes simplex virus, human papillomavirus)

Betel nut, inverted smoking

Industrial (nasal cavity/peripheral nervous system)
Metals (nickel, chromium)
Wood dust, textiles, furniture, leather

Asbestos

Diet
Vitamin A deficiency

Prior radiotherapy (to salivary gland, thyroid, skin)

Iron deficiency (Plummer-Vinson syndrome)

Mutagen-induced chromosome fragility

I have been detected in the sera and neoplastic tissues of patients with head and neck cancer, but no risk vs prevalence relationship has been found.[15,16]

BIOLOGY

The mucosal surfaces of the upper aerodigestive tract, lungs, and esophagus are repeatedly exposed to the same carcinogens (eg, tobacco, alcohol). Therefore, multiple independent neoplastic lesions may arise and progress in the same patient, either simultaneously or sequentially, in a process known as "field cancerization."[17] Metachronous second primary tumors develop at a constant rate of 4% to 7%, are generally of squamous pathology, are not treatment-related, and occur in the carcinogen-exposed regions of the aerodigestive tract.[18,19]

Tumorigenesis in the aerodigestive tract is a multistep process believed to be driven by genetic damage caused by continuous exposure to carcinogens.[20] Specific genetic alterations linked with head and neck cancer include the activation of oncogenes (eg, *cyclin D1*), the inactivation or mutation of tumor-suppressor genes (eg, *p53*), and the amplification of growth factors and their receptors (eg, epidermal growth factor, epidermal growth factor receptor [EGFR], and transforming growth factor). These specific gene alterations may result in phenotypic changes in cell differentiation or proliferation or both (Table 2).

Multiple allelic abnormalities (eg, 3p, 9p, 11q, 13q,

and 17p) have been documented, and in some studies they appear to have prognostic value.[21,22] The *cyclin D1* gene, also known as *PRAD-1*, *bcl*-1, or *CCND*-1, has been the focus of several recent studies.[23-25] This oncogene, located on chromosome 11q13, is amplified in 30% to 50% of patients with head and neck cancers. Overexpression and amplification of *cyclin D1* has been associated with more advanced disease, more rapid and frequent recurrence of disease, and shortened survival.[24] Alterations in the expression of other genes on 11q13 (eg, *int*-2, *hst*-1, and *ems*-1) are also under active study in the head and neck.

The tumor-suppressor gene *p53*, located on the short arm of chromosome 17, is the most thoroughly studied gene in head and neck neoplasia and many other cancers. Mutations and overexpression of *p53* occur in 40% to 60% of cancer patients and have been associated with a poor prognosis.[26] Brachman et al[27] reported that tumors with *p53* mutations recurred at a median time of 6 months, compared with a median time to recurrence of 17.4 months for tumors without mutations. The introduction of sensitive molecular techniques has made it possible to detect neoplastic changes in tissue "free of disease" by routine cytology. Brennan et al[28] recently reported that 13 of 25 patients who appeared to have complete tumor resection according to histopathologic assessment had *p53* mutations in at least one tumor margin. Thirty-eight percent of the patients with *p53*-positive margins relapsed, compared with none of the 12 patients found by polymerase chain reaction (PCR) to have all tumor margins free of *p53* mutations. This method may prove useful for identifying patients who are prone to local tumor recurrence and, therefore, in need of adjuvant therapy.

Mutations of *p53* have been associated with tobacco and alcohol use. A recent study showed *p53* mutations in 58% of tumors of cigarette smokers who also used alcohol. Among patients who smoked but did not drink

TABLE 2

Genetic Alterations in Head and Neck Cancer

Oncogenes
c-erbB-1
11q13 (cylin D1, int-2, hst-1, ems-1)
Other: c-myc, ras, HER-2/neu

Tumor-suppressor genes
p53, p16, p21
9p, 3p, 13q

alcohol, 33% had mutations, whereas only 17% of the patients who neither smoked nor drank alcohol showed mutations of the *p53* gene. Furthermore, the number of types of *p53* base-pair mutations was highest in patients who smoked and drank and lowest in patients who did neither. These findings provided molecular evidence that tobacco may play a role in the molecular progression of squamous-cell carcinoma of the head and neck.[29]

EGFR is a cellular oncogene likely to play a role in head and neck tumorigenesis. Its gene amplification and overexpression have been demonstrated in preinvasive and invasive lesions, with high expression associated with an increased sensitivity to cytotoxic therapy.[30] The finding that anti-EGFR monoclonal antibodies upregulate EGFR may prove useful in enhancing chemotherapeutic efficacy. As a recent study demonstrated, in patients who smoked or drank alcohol or did both, increased expression of EGFR is found in histologically normal tissue surrounding cancers, compared with levels in controls never exposed to tobacco or alcohol.[31] These findings supported the theory of field cancerization in which epithelia exposed to carcinogenic insult may express early premalignant features.

Proliferating cell nuclear antigen (PCNA) is a nuclear protein whose expression is associated with DNA synthesis and cell proliferation. Shin et al[32] analyzed PCNA expression in squamous-cell carcinoma tissue samples and surrounding premalignant and normal tissues; PCNA expression sequentially increased 4- to 10-fold as tissue progressed from adjacent normal epithelium to squamous-cell carcinoma. Similarly high expression of TGF-alpha was also documented to be a strong mitogenic factor capable of inducing epithelial proliferation.[32]

ANATOMY

Cancers of the head and neck include a great variety of neoplasms, specifically those involving the upper aerodigestive tract. Tumors of the central nervous system, eye, skin, and thyroid, as well as tumors of lymphatic origin, are usually excluded.

Head and neck cancers originate in the area under the base of the skull to just below the larynx in a cephalocaudal orientation and by the anterior nasal cavity and the vermilion border of the lips anteriorly to the pharynx posteriorly (Figure 1). These boundaries enclose the nasal cavity, pharynx, larynx, and salivary glands. The oral cavity encompasses the oral mucosa, anterior two thirds of the tongue, and floor of the mouth. The oropharynx (which includes the posterior one third of the tongue), hypopharynx, and nasopharynx are subdivisions of the pharynx.

DIAGNOSIS AND STAGING

Optimal therapy and survival depend on the proper identification of the primary tumor as well as the local, regional, and distant extent of disease. Patients with early-stage disease may present with vague symptoms and minimal physical findings, which is why a high index of suspicion is needed, especially if the patients use tobacco. Most patients will present with signs and symptoms of locally advanced disease that vary according to the subsite in the head and neck. Sinusitis, unilateral nasal airway obstruction, and epistaxis may be early symptoms of cancer of the nasal cavity and paranasal sinus. Persistent hoarseness demands visualization of the larynx. Otitis media that remains unresponsive to antibiotics may indicate a nasopharyngeal neoplasm. Chronic dysphagia or odynophagia (lasting 6 weeks or more) may be the presenting symptom of oropharyngeal or hypopharyngeal cancer. Supraglottic laryngeal neoplasms rarely present early symptoms; in some patients, a neck mass will be the presenting sign. Detailed examination of lymph nodes in the facial, cervical, or supraclavicular regions is important because the location of adenopathy provides clues to the specific subsite of a head and neck primary tumor, as shown in Figure 2. Subdigastric adenopathy, for example, suggests primary cancer of the oral tongue or oropharynx, and posterior cervical adenopathy is a frequent result of regional spread of a nasopharyngeal tumor.

Physical examination should include careful inspection of all mucosal surfaces, bimanual palpation of the floor of the mouth, and palpation of the neck. Leukoplakia (white mucosal patches that cannot be removed by scraping) and higher risk erythroplakia (red or mixed red-white patches) are the most common premalignant lesions in the head and neck. Up to 40% of cases of dysplastic oral leukoplakia transform into invasive carcinoma. Any suspicious surface in the oral mucosa (eg, erythroplakia) should undergo biopsy to rule out cancer.[33]

Three-dimensional imaging with computerized tomography (CT), magnetic resonance imaging (MRI), and ultrasonography may be used to evaluate the extent of disease and to stage the neoplasm. These techniques are also helpful in evaluating a patient's response to therapy. Because the lungs are the most common site of distant metastasis, a chest x-ray should be performed as well.[34] Circulating tumor markers that would be useful for identifying squamous-cell carcinoma of the head and neck have not been discovered. Epstein-Barr virus DNA is found in nasopharyngeal carcinoma but not in other types of upper aerodigestive tract neoplasms. In patients

FIGURE I

Structures encompassed by the "head and neck" area, bounded by the base of the skull, the inferior border of the laryngeal cartilage, the anterior nasal cavity and vermilion border of the lip, and the posterior pharyngeal wall

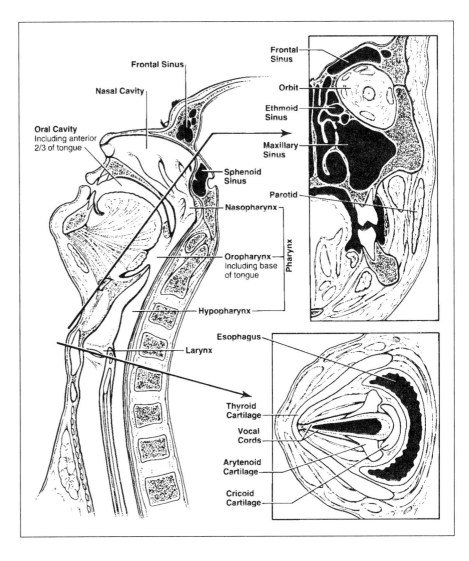

with cervical lymphadenopathy and no obvious primary tumor, identification of EBV DNA in the lymph node may suggest a tumor of nasopharyngeal origin.[35]

Patients who present with a suspicious neck mass and no obvious lesion in the oral cavity should undergo a flexible fiberoptic nasopharyngoscopy or indirect laryngoscopy to search for the primary tumor. A panendoscopy (direct laryngoscopy, bronchoscopy, esophagoscopy), performed while the patient is under anesthesia, is the definitive diagnostic and staging procedure, and it should be performed for all patients except those whose lesions originate in the oral cavity. Multiple biopsies of any visualized abnormality, or "blind biopsies" of random areas, are performed to define the extent of disease and to identify synchronous second primary tumors. If no obvious primary site is found, fine-needle aspiration of the lymph node is performed to establish the diagnosis. Open biopsy is a last resort, after fine-needle aspiration

or panendoscopy fail to reveal the specific site and histopathology. In patients whose neck is surgically violated by open biopsy, subsequent curative therapy may be compromised.

Staging criteria for head and neck cancers are based on the tumor-nodes-metastasis (TNM) staging system, which classifies tumors according to anatomic site and extent of disease.[36] Head and neck primary (T) tumor staging is complex, varying with each primary subsite in the head and neck region. Classifications for lymph-node (N) and distant metastases (M) are uniform for all sites (Table 3).

THERAPY

Surgery and radiation therapy have been the standard of care for most patients with head and neck neoplasms. Traditionally, chemotherapy has been used only for patients with recurrent or metastatic disease. More recently, chemotherapy has had an important role in the

FIGURE 2

*Possible sites of lymphadeno-
pathy in the facial, cervical,
and supraclavicular areas,
which may reflect the specific
location of a primary tumor*

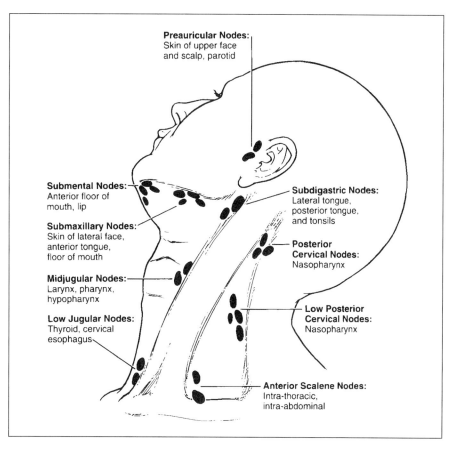

Preauricular Nodes:
Skin of upper face
and scalp, parotid

Submental Nodes:
Anterior floor of
mouth, lip

Submaxillary Nodes:
Skin of lateral face,
anterior tongue,
floor of mouth

Midjugular Nodes:
Larynx, pharynx,
hypopharynx

Low Jugular Nodes:
Thyroid, cervical
esophagus

Subdigastric Nodes:
Lateral tongue,
posterior tongue,
and tonsils

**Posterior
Cervical Nodes:**
Nasopharynx

**Low Posterior
Cervical Nodes:**
Nasopharynx

Anterior Scalene Nodes:
Intra-thoracic,
intra-abdominal

primary treatment of most patients with locally advanced resectable laryngeal cancer, in whom induction chemotherapy followed by radiotherapy may be used to avoid the need for total laryngectomy.

More than two thirds of patients with head and neck cancer will present with stage III or IV disease. For patients with early-stage disease (I or II), surgery or radiotherapy is used with curative intent, and more than 80% of patients with stage I disease and more than 60% with stage II disease achieve this goal. In patients with stage III disease and most patients with stage IV disease, surgery followed by radiation therapy is considered standard care unless the patient is unable to undergo surgery or the lesion is unresectable. In many cases, this curative treatment, especially for patients with disease at an advanced stage, is accompanied by severe cosmetic and psychological problems and long-term loss of organ function. Despite optimal local therapy, more than 50% of patients with stage III and IV disease will develop local or regional recurrence, and nearly 30% will develop distant metastases. The need to improve survival rates and decrease treatment-related morbidity has encouraged the investigation of new approaches. Chemotherapy is under intense study in locally advanced disease,

with promising results. In this section we will review standard and new approaches to treating patients with head and neck cancer.

Nasopharynx: The three histopathologic subtypes of nasopharyngeal carcinoma are type 1, differentiated squamous-cell carcinoma; type 2, nonkeratinizing squamous-cell carcinoma; and type 3, undifferentiated or lymphoepithelioma.[37] About 50% to 75% of NPCs in the United States are type 1 or 2, whereas in Asian and African areas, type 3 NPC predominates. NPC is an aggressive neoplasm involving cervical lymphadenopathy in 60% to 90% of patients.[38] Because of the tumor's unique anatomic, biologic, and clinical characteristics, therapy for NPC is different from that of other head and neck cancers. Radiation is the therapeutic mainstay. Pilot studies of intracavitary radiotherapy for NPC have reported excellent palliation. The anatomic location of the nasopharynx limits the role of surgery to obtaining the initial biopsy and to resecting residual lymphadenopathy after radiotherapy. The lymphoepitheliomas (type 3) are the most chemoradiosensitive.

Five-year survival rates range from 30% to 65% depending on tumor stage, the radiation technique employed, and the percentage of patients with lymphoepi-

TABLE 3

Staging System for Head and Neck Cancer

Tumor-node metastasis (TNM) system

TX   Primary tumor cannot be assessed

T0   No evidence of primary tumor

Tis Carcinoma in situ

T1   Tumor < 2 cm in greatest dimension

T2   Tumor > 2 cm but < 4 cm

T3   Tumor > 4 cm

T4   Tumor invades adjacent structures (eg, cortical bone, deep muscle of tongue, maxillary sinus, skin)

NX   Regional lymph nodes cannot be assessed

N0   No regional node metastases

N1   Metastasis to a single ipsilateral lymph node (≥ 3 cm)

N2   Metastasis to a single ipsilateral lymph node (> 3 cm but ≤ 6 cm), to multiple ipsilateral lymph nodes (none > 6 cm), or to bilateral or contralateral lymph nodes (none > 6 cm)

  a   Metastasis to a single ipsilateral lymph node (> 3 cm but ≤ 6 cm)

  b   Metastases to multiple ipsilateral lymph nodes (none > 6 cm)

  c   Metastases to bilateral or contralateral lymph nodes (none > 6 cm)

N3   Metastasis to a lymph node > 6 cm

MX   Presence of distant metastasis cannot be assessed

M0   No evidence of distant metastasis

M1   Distant metastasis

Clinical stage

0   Tis N0 M0

I   T1 N0 M0

II   T2 N0 M0

III T3 N0 M0; T1 N0 M0

IV   T4 N0–1 M0; any T N2–3 M0; any T and N M1

theliomas.[38] Patients with N0 disease have a 5-year survival rate of approximately 65%, whereas patients with cervical node involvement have a significantly worse prognosis.[39]

Oral Cavity: The majority of oral-cavity neoplasms occur in the anterior two thirds of the tongue (oral tongue) and the floor of the mouth. Radiation or surgery, or both, are the main therapeutic methods. Treatment-related morbidity, especially with respect to speech and swallowing, are major issues in managing these patients; the treatment decision is also complicated by the high rate of regional metastases.

For most early-stage cancers (T1 and T2) that arise in the floor of the mouth, comparable results are obtained with either surgery or radiation therapy alone. Small, superficial lesions may be excised with little morbidity.[40] For T2 lesions that are deeply invasive, radiation therapy offers the advantage of simultaneously treating the bilateral neck lymph nodes, which have a 30% to 40% rate of involvement.[18] Interstitial radiotherapy is used in select cases and achieves higher control rates than external radiation alone. With either surgery or radiation, survival rates of patients with stage I and II tumors are 80% to 90% and 50% to 80%, respectively.[41]

Oral-tongue cancers commonly arise on the lateral and ventral surfaces of the anterior part of the tongue. They are so aggressive that 40% of patients present with clinically evident lymph nodes and 35% with occult node metastasis. Bilateral node involvement is not uncommon. For T1 lesions, radiotherapy or surgery has a similar result, and both achieve good preservation of organ function. For infiltrative T2 lesions, surgery usually includes hemiglossectomy and selective nodal dissection, which achieve excellent control at the expense of compromising oral function. Brachytherapy combined with external radiotherapy may be as effective as surgery at this stage. More than 90% of patients with early recurrence after radiation may be salvaged by surgical intervention.

For patients with more advanced disease (T3, T4), surgery followed by radiation therapy is the most widely accepted approach. Neck dissection is usually performed when patients have cervical lymphadenopathy or are at high risk for occult metastasis. Radiation therapy alone has a failure rate of 80% to 90% in patients with advanced disease, compared with a failure rate of less than 30% for the combined modality of surgery and radiotherapy.[42] Survival rates for patients with advanced oral-cavity cancer are between 18% and 42%.[18]

Oropharynx: The most common cancers of the oropharynx are of the base of the tongue and tonsils. Early tonsillar lesions (T1 and T2) may be treated with radiotherapy or surgery, with good results. The tendency is to irradiate the lesions, because local control rates of 90% for T1 lesions and 80% for T2 lesions have been obtained, and regional lymph nodes may be treated concurrently.[43] Intraoral wide local excision is possible for small, superficial lesions, with comparable results. For larger or deeper T1 or T2 lesions, radiation therapy is preferred to surgery because of the latter's higher morbidity (disfigurement and loss of oral function).[44] For T3 tumors without clinical evidence of nodal involvement (N0), radiation therapy alone has resulted in a 5-year survival rate of 82%. Some studies have shown increased local control for combined-modality approaches.[45] For patients with T4 lesions, combined surgery and irradiation have achieved increased survival rates at the expense of a substantial decline in the quality of life.

Cancer at the base of the tongue presents a more difficult situation than tonsillar cancer because of its anatomic location, late diagnosis, and common metastasis. At presentation, 75% of patients have stage III or IV disease. For patients with T1 and T2 disease, surgery with or without neck dissection has shown a local control rate of 75% to 80%, whereas radiation therapy with or without brachytherapy has yielded local control rates of 70% to 100%.[46] Radiotherapy is preferred because of the preservation of oral function. The major prognostic determinant is lymph node involvement. For patients with N0 disease, the 5-year survival rate is higher than 60%, but for N1 to N3 patients it is lower than 30%.[47]

Hypopharynx: With 75% of lesions occurring in the piriform sinus, carcinoma of the hypopharynx is relatively uncommon but highly lethal. At presentation, more than 80% of patients have advanced disease (T3 and T4), and more than 20% have distant metastases.[48] The rare patient with a T1 lesion is usually treated with radiation therapy; those with T2 to T4 lesions are mainly treated with total laryngectomy and partial pharyngectomy, radical neck dissection, and postoperative radiotherapy. The overall 5-year survival rate is lower than 25%. For early lesions CO_2 laser surgery has been used with encouraging results and with preservation of more pharyngeal function than is possible with other surgical techniques.[49] A recent phase III trial showed that laryngeal preservation with sequential chemoradiotherapy is a feasible alternative to radical surgery.[50]

Larynx: The most widely used treatment of T1 and T2 cancers of the larynx is radiotherapy, which has demonstrated 5-year survival rates of 96% to 98% for patients with T1 disease and 80% to 94% for those with T2 disease.[51] At early tumor stages, endoscopic laser surgery has shown local control rates of up to 90%, but the patients' voice quality was poor.[52] For early-stage carcinomas of the supraglottic larynx, supraglottic laryngectomy has resulted in excellent local control; an alternative is radiation therapy, for which rates of local control range from 50% to 90% in T1 or T2 disease. For fixed vocal

cords (T3 disease) radiotherapy has produced local control rates of between 30% and 60%. In cases of localized recurrence, laryngectomy has achieved a cure rate of up to 80%.[53] For most patients with T3 lesions, and virtually all patients with T4 lesions, total laryngectomy with postoperative radiation had been the standard treatment. Chemotherapy now has a more prominent role in the treatment of these cancers; most patients with locally advanced laryngeal carcinoma can now be offered the option of sequential chemoradiotherapy in an attempt to preserve the larynx (see Organ Preservation).

Cervical Nodes: Management of the neck should be integrated with management of the primary tumor.[40] In patients with clinically negative nodes (N0) the decision to treat the neck electively depends mainly on the T stage and site of the primary tumor. Because of the relatively high incidence of nodal involvement in early stages, some authors have recommended treating the neck for N0 cancer in the nasopharynx, hypopharynx, oropharynx, and supraglottic larynx. For stage I or II glottic laryngeal carcinoma, however, the rate of nodal involvement is less than 5%, and neck treatment is not usually performed.[52]

When surgery is the treatment chosen for a primary tumor with N0 disease, conservative nodal dissection could achieve good control in more than 90% of cases.[54] Similarly, when irradiation is the primary treatment, it may be applied to both sides of the neck.

When nodes are clinically present, combined-modality surgery and radiation may be used, depending on the primary treatment results. If radiation is primary, surgery is reserved for residual disease. For patients with advanced nodal disease (N2, N3) treated with surgery, irradiation is added (including to the contralateral nodes) to increase local control.

Salivary Glands: Tumors of the salivary glands (mucoepidermoid carcinoma, adenoid cystic carcinoma, adenocarcinoma, malignant mixed tumor, acinic-cell carcinoma, and epidermoid carcinoma) are considered different from other head and neck cancers because of their diverse histology (fewer than 3% are squamous carcinomas) and high percentage of benign lesions, compared with tumors at other sites. Benign lesions account for 80% of tumors arising in the parotid gland, 50% of tumors arising in the submandibular glands, and 25% of tumors arising in minor salivary glands. The most common malignant tumor of the major salivary glands is mucoepidermoid; its most common subsite is the parotid gland. Adenoid cystic carcinomas, which make up nearly 25% of malignant salivary gland tumors, are the most common type encountered in the minor salivary glands. This subtype is considered unique because of its prolonged natural history (10 to 15 years) and its resistance to radiation and chemotherapy. For this reason, chemotherapy and radiotherapy are not indicated unless the tumor is growing rapidly, is symptomatic, is causing local problems, or is associated with extrapulmonary metastatic visceral disease. Cranial nerve involvement is common and associated with poor local control and survival. Surgery and postoperative radiotherapy remain the major treatments for patients with cancer limited to the primary site and regional lymph nodes. Chemotherapy has been used mainly as palliation; trials of chemotherapy have been limited by the rarity of the disease. Doxorubicin (Adriamycin, Rubex) and cisplatin (Platinol) seem to be the most active agents. Their combination with cyclophosphamide (Cytoxan, Neosar) in CAP, the regimen studied most frequently, has shown response rates of from 22% to 100% and complete response rates of 0% to 40%. However, these responses lasted only 5 to 9 months.[18,55]

Chemotherapy for Metastatic or Recurrent Disease

Patients with metastatic or recurrent disease who are undergoing chemotherapy, the standard treatment of diseases at these stages, have a median overall survival of 4 to 6 months. The role of chemotherapy is palliative; its goal is to improve quality of life while reducing disease symptoms. The single agents active in head and neck cancer—with response rates between 15% and 40%—include methotrexate, cisplatin, carboplatin (Paraplatin), fluorouracil, ifosfamide (Ifex), bleomycin, paclitaxel (Taxol), and docetaxel. There is no evidence that methotrexate or cisplatin has a dose-response effect; they are the only agents that have undergone phase III studies regarding this issue. Methotrexate, administered weekly at 40 to 60 mg/m^2, has been the standard chemotherapeutic approach because of low cost, low toxicity, and easy administration for outpatients. Attempts to improve methotrexate's therapeutic index, including the use of high-dose methotrexate with leucovorin rescue, sequential methotrexate–fluorouracil, and analog development, have been unsuccessful. A phase III, head-to-head comparison of methotrexate and the methotrexate analog edatrexate showed the analog to produce similar response and survival results but increased toxicity.[56]

Paclitaxel and docetaxel are new agents active in head and neck neoplasms. In a multicenter Eastern Cooperative Oncology Group (ECOG) phase II trial, 28 patients had a 40% response rate to paclitaxel with a 9.2-month median survival, which exceeds the 15% to 30% response rate and 5- to 6-month survival observed with

other agents used in this setting.[57] Paclitaxel was also found to have radiosensitizing activity and is under study with concomitant radiation.[58] Docetaxel, studied in a group of previously treated and untreated patients,[59] showed a 32% response rate. Studies of these drugs in combination with other agents are currently under way. Two new promising agents being ivestigated in patients with head and neck cancer are topotecan and gemcitabine (Gemzar).

Randomized trials in patients with recurrent disease have failed to demonstrate the superiority of combination therapy over single-agent therapy in terms of overall survival, despite the combinations' higher overall and complete response rates. Cisplatin plus infusional fluorouracil, the combination most frequently studied, has produced overall response rates ranging from 11% to 79% and complete response rates ranging from 0% to 27%.[60] A randomized study in which this combination was compared with either cisplatin or infusional fluorouracil alone showed that with the combined drugs, the overall response rate, and time to disease progression were better. No significant difference in median survival was found, but of the patients treated with the combination, 40% were alive after 9 months of follow-up, compared with 24% of patients treated with cisplatin and 27% of patients treated with fluorouracil.[61]

Another study of combined treatment with cisplatin and fluorouracil showed a significantly higher response rate but similar survival rate compared with results using methotrexate alone.[62] At present, treatment with methotrexate, cisplatin, carboplatin, or infusional fluorouracil as single agents or with the combination of cisplatin and infusional fluorouracil may represent acceptable palliative therapy. In choosing the most appropriate therapeutic option for a patient with recurrent or metastatic disease, a careful risk and benefit assessment should be made to determine what level of treatment will improve the patient's quality of life and not affect his remaining time adversely.

COMBINED MODALITY THERAPY FOR LOCAL OR REGIONAL ADVANCED DISEASE

In patients with untreated locally advanced disease, combination chemotherapy achieves a higher response rate (70% to 90%) compared with the rate of less than 40% in previously treated patients.[63] By adding chemotherapy to the standard surgery and/or irradiation regimen, we pursue two major objectives: to decrease the morbidity associated with standard therapy, minimizing the need for radical resection (ie, organ preservation), and to increase overall survival. The three approaches to the use of primary chemotherapy are neoadjuvant chemotherapy, which is designed to reduce the patient's tumor burden before definitive local and regional treatment begins; adjuvant chemotherapy, which attempts to eradicate microscopic disease left after primary treatment; and concomitant chemoradiotherapy, which attempts to enhance the cytotoxic effect of radiation on resectable and unresectable tumor while increasing local control and decreasing systemic disease.

Neoadjuvant Chemotherapy

Neoadjuvant and adjuvant chemotherapy have been studied for 20 years. In the initial induction trials of patients with head and neck cancer, single-agent therapy consisted of methotrexate, cisplatin, or bleomycin. Patients receiving these drugs had response rates of between 10% and 40% and complete response rates of 0% to 5%. These early efforts evolved into trials of drug combinations, which yielded a significant increase in response rates. The most thoroughly studied combination active in locally advanced disease was cisplatin plus fluorouracil, with an overall response rate of approximately 80% and a complete response rate of 30% to 40%, but a 5-year survival rate of less than 25%.[64]

The Head and Neck Contract Program[65] conducted the first major randomized trial of the neoadjuvant approach. It included three arms: induction chemotherapy followed by standard local therapy; induction chemotherapy followed by standard local therapy and then adjuvant chemotherapy; and standard local therapy alone. Only one cycle of induction chemotherapy (cisplatin-bleomycin) was administered. Overall survival and disease-free survival did not differ significantly among the three arms, but a significant decrease in distant metastases was seen in the group who received adjuvant chemotherapy.

In a recent randomized study of patients with operable and inoperable disease, the effects of four cycles of neoadjuvant chemotherapy followed by radiation therapy were compared with the effects of radiotherapy alone.[66] The only significant finding in the overall analysis was a decrease in the rate of distant metastases in patients in the chemotherapy-radiotherapy arm. However, a subset analysis of patients with inoperable disease revealed a significant improvement at 3 years in disease-free survival (34% vs 26%), time to distant metastasis (24% vs 42%) and overall survival (24% vs 10%) in the patients who had received neoadjuvant chemotherapy. A larger randomized trial involving only patients with inoperable disease is needed to support these results.

Chemotherapy for Organ Preservation: Although advances in surgical techniques have had some influence on morbidity, primary chemotherapy is being investigated as an alternative to the surgical component of current standard therapy, especially in the larynx, to preserve organ function. Several pilot trials using induction chemotherapy have suggested that surgery could be omitted without compromising survival in patients who respond to chemotherapy.[67–69] These organ preservation trials culminated in 1991 with the report of the Veteran's Administration Laryngeal Cancer Study Group.[70,71] In this trial, induction chemotherapy with cisplatin and infusional fluorouracil plus sequential definitive radiotherapy were compared with treatment with standard surgery (total laryngectomy) and postoperative radiotherapy. Patients who achieved at least a partial response after two cycles of cisplatin and fluorouracil entered a third cycle, which was followed by definitive radiotherapy, then by direct laryngoscopy and primary tumor-site biopsy to determine pathologic response. In these patients, surgery was reserved for later salvage of persistent or recurrent disease. Nonresponders to two cycles of induction chemotherapy underwent immediate surgery followed by radiotherapy.

After two cycles of induction chemotherapy, 85% of patients achieved a major response at the primary tumor site (31% complete response). After three cycles of chemotherapy, the overall response rate was 98% (49% complete), and 64% of patients had a pathologically complete response. At a median follow-up of 60 months, estimated 3-year survival rates were 56% (48% to 64%) for the surgery-radiotherapy group and 53% (45% to 61%) for the chemotherapy-radiotherapy group. Survival for the subset of patients with T4 disease was significantly worse (ie, shorter) in the chemotherapy arm than in the surgery arm.

The study also indicated that the short delay in definitive surgery in the nonresponders to chemotherapy was not detrimental (ie, survival in this subgroup was not significantly different from that of the standard arm). In 64% of all patients in the chemotherapy arm, the larynx was preserved. Given these rates of survival and larynx preservation, most patients with locally advanced laryngeal cancer now have the option of preserving their voice without risking shorter survival.

Early phase III results from two other large, multicenter chemotherapy-radiotherapy studies, including a large French study of all cancer sites and a European Organization for Research and Treatment of Cancer (EORTC) trial of patients with hypopharyngeal disease, seemed to confirm the Veterans Administration (VA) trial results and suggested a role for this approach for other locally advanced resectable head and neck cancer sites (Table 4). The French study design was similar to that of the VA trial, except that carboplatin was substituted for cisplatin.[72] The EORTC experimental arm design differed from that of the other two phase III studies in that only patients in complete remission after two cycles of cisplatin-fluorouracil were treated with sequential radiotherapy (70 Gy). Patients with a less than a complete response underwent the standard surgery and radiation.[50]

Nasopharyngeal Carcinoma: Two randomized trials of neoadjuvant chemotherapy for patients with advanced NPC (N2, N3), WHO histopathology, have produced differing results. One was an international trial that included 399 patients and had a median follow-up of 24 months. A regimen of cisplatin, epirubicin, and bleomycin, administered for three cycles followed by radiotherapy, was compared with standard radiotherapy alone. Patients so treated achieved increases in 3-year disease-free survival (47% vs 31%, $P < .02$) and overall survival ($P = NS$).[73] In the other randomized trial, neoadjuvant cisplatin-fluorouracil (two cycles), followed by adjuvant therapy (four cycles) with the same agents, was compared to standard radiotherapy. This study included 77 patients and had a median follow-up of 29 months. Two-year overall survival (80% vs 81%) and disease-free survival (68% vs 72%) rates for the experimental arm and standard radiotherapy arm were similar, and there were no differences in patterns of treatment failure.[74]

Adjuvant Chemotherapy

To date, seven phase III trials of adjuvant (maintenance) chemotherapy have been reported, but only one small trial (33 patients) has reported a significant increase in overall survival.[75] Another adjuvant trial of cisplatin plus concomitant radiotherapy with positive results is discussed in the section on concomitant chemotherapy.[76] From two recent, large phase III trials come reports of a decrease in the rate of distant metastases in patients in the chemotherapy arm.[77,78]

Concomitant Chemoradiotherapy

Simultaneous chemoradiotherapy seems to be the most promising approach to prolong the survival of patients with locally advanced disease. The independent local activity of radiotherapy in combination with the systemic activity of chemotherapy has several advantages over the results achievable with sequential therapy, including the avoidance of a 2- to 3-month delay in initiating definitive local therapy.[79]

Among the two different schedules used are the standard radiotherapy schedules to which low- or moderate-dose single-agent chemotherapy is added. Single agents with radiosensitizing effects as shown in preclinical studies are bleomycin, infusional fluorouracil, mitomycin (Mutamycin), hydroxyurea (Hydrea), methotrexate, cisplatin, carboplatin, and paclitaxel.[80]

Of nine phase III trials of concomitant bleomycin and radiation, one demonstrated a significant improvement in disease-free survival, and another showed significant improvement in disease-free and overall survivals. Four phase III concomitant trials of fluorouracil[81–83] demonstrated significant increases in disease-free survival (three trials) and in disease-free and overall survival (two trials). Among two phase III trials of cisplatin and radiation, one was a study of primary therapy for locally advanced disease and reported negative results,[84] the other was a trial of adjuvant therapy in patients with stage III to IV disease with extracapsular spread, and the findings were positive.[76] Results of the other phase III

TABLE 4

Phase III Trials of Neoadjuvant Chemotherapy for Organ Preservation in Head and Neck Neoplasms

Author	Study arms	Number of patients	Responses Overall	Responses Complete	Overall survival	Organ preservation
VACSP[70] (larynx)	Cisplatin, fluorouracil, RT	166	81%	31%	53% (3 yr)	64%
	surgery, RT	166	—	—	56%	12%
Martin et al[72] (all sites)	Carboplatin-fluorouracil, LRT	152	56%	31%	49% (4 yr)	48%
	LRT	154	—		38%	20%
EORTC[50] (hypopharynx)	Cisplatin-fluorouracil, RT	100	—		47% (3 yr)	28%
	surgery, RT	97	—		44%	—

EORTC = European Organization for Research and Treatment of Cancer, LRT = local-regional treatment, RT = radiotherapy, VACSP = Veterans Affairs Cooperative Study Program   Adapted, with permission, from Chemotherapy and chemoprevention, in Myers E, Suen JY (eds): Cancer of the Head and Neck, 3rd ed. Philadelphia, WB Saunders, in press.

TABLE 5

Randomized Studies of Concomitant vs Sequential Chemoradiotherapy

Author	Number of patients	Chemotherapy	Radiotherapy arms (Gy)	Disease-free/ progression- free survival	Overall survival	Toxicity
SECOG[85]	267	Vinblastine, bleomycin, methotrexate × 4 2 × 2 (factorial)	Alt (60) Seq (60 pre/postop)	37% 28%	37% (3 yr) 36%	Alt > seq
Merlano et al[86]	116[a]	Vinblastine, bleomycin, methotrexate × 4	Alt (60) Seq (65–75)	22% 14%	22% (4 yr) 10%	Alt > seq
Adelstein et al[87]	48	Cisplatin, fluorouracil (2 preop, 2 postop) (3 preop)	Sim (60, split) Seq (60)	60%[b] 39%	68% (3 yr) 43%	Sim > seq
Pinnaro et al[88]	93	Cisplatin × 3 Cisplatin, fluorouracil × 3	Sim (65–70) Seq (65–70)	20% 16%	16% (5 yr) 11%	Sim > seq (heme)
Taylor et al[89]	214 [a]	Cisplatin, fluorouracil × 7 Cisplatin, fluorouracil × 3	Sim (65) Seq (65)	17 mo[c] 13 mo[c]	20 mo[c] 20 mo[c]	Sim > seq

Alt = alternating, SECOG = South England Cooperative Oncology Group, Sim = simultaneous, Seq = sequential   [a] Unresectable   [b] $P < .05$ [c] Median   Adapted, with permission, from Chemotherapy and chemoprevention, in Myers E, Suen JY (eds): Cancer of the Head and Neck, 3rd ed. Philadelphia, WB Saunders, in press.

trials (of methotrexate, hydroxyurea, and mitomycin) were mostly negative. In most of these studies, increased toxic reactions (mucositis) were found in the concomitant-therapy group compared with the radiation alone group.

In the second approach, chemotherapy at full dosage is combined with radiotherapy. Because toxicity is substantially increased with this approach, patients require regularly scheduled interruptions of one or both treatment modalities to allow them to recover from normal tissue toxicity. A variation of the second approach is to alternate chemotherapy and radiation therapy. The detrimental effect of interrupted radiotherapy when used alone has been documented.[80] Despite this reservation, several studies have shown favorable long-term and overall survivals compared with those of standard radiotherapy. Five trials compared combination chemotherapy plus concomitant radiotherapy with induction chemotherapy followed by radiation therapy. All reported increased disease-free or overall survival in the concomitant-treatment group (Table 5).[85–89]

In four phase III trials, concomitant therapy was compared with radiotherapy alone, with improved survival in the concomitant arms found in three (statistically significant in two) trials (Table 6).[90–93] From a recent study in which patients with advanced head and neck cancer were randomized to receive cisplatin and fluorouracil alternating with radiotherapy or radiotherapy alone, the investigators reported a rate of complete remissions

in 53% of the concomitant-therapy group compared with a rate of 26% in the radiation-alone group. Overall survivals at 3 years in the two groups were 41% in the combined-therapy group and 23% in the radiotherapy group ($P < .05$).[92]

CHEMOPREVENTION

Chemoprevention is defined as a pharmacologic strategy to block or reverse carcinogenesis before the development of invasive cancer.[94] This approach has been studied in patients with premalignant lesions as well as patients in the adjuvant setting to prevent second primary tumors. In patients who are cured by radiation, surgery, or both, second primary tumors remain a major threat to long-term survival.[95,96] For this group, chemoprevention may be important in the long-term control of neoplasia of the upper aerodigestive airway.

Retinoids, including natural vitamin A and synthetic analogs, are the most thoroughly studied compounds for chemoprevention. In vitro, retinoids modulate tumor-cell differentiation, proliferation, and apoptosis and also affect other important functions, such as cell adhesion and invasion.[97] Retinoid activity in reversing premalignant lesions has been established in several clinical trials. Hong et al studied isotretinoin (13-*cis*-retinoic acid [13cRA]) at high doses in 44 patients with oral leukoplakia. Major responses occurred in 67% of patients treated with isotretinoin compared with 10% of patients in the placebo group. Within 3 months of cessation of therapy,

TABLE 6

Randomized Studies of Concomitant Chemotherapy vs Radiotherapy-Only Control Arms

Author	Number of patients	Chemotherapy	Study arms (Gy)	Overall survival (median)	Toxicity
Bezwoda et al[90]	58	7 drugs	Sim (~ 70) RT (~ 70)	36 wk [a] 18 wk	Sim > RT
Keegan et al[91]	51	Cisplatin, fluorouracil	Sim (60 bid, split) RT (same)	97/38 wk [b] 93/26 wk	Sim > RT
Merlano et al[92]	157 (unresectable)	Cisplatin, fluorouracil	Alt (60) RT (70)	16.5 wk/41% (3 yr) [a] 11.7 wk/23% (3 yr)	Alt > RT (heme only)
Keane et al[93]	212 (larynx, hypopharynx)	Mitomycin, fluorouracil	Sim (50, split) RT (50)	2.7 yr 2.7	Sim = RT

Sim = simultaneous, RT = radiotherapy, Alt = alternating   [a] $P < .05$ [b] Resectable/unresectable
Adapted, with permission, from Chemotherapy and chemoprevention, in Myers E, Suen JY (eds): Cancer of the Head and Neck, 3rd ed. Philadelphia, WB Saunders, in press.

however, the lesions recurred in more than 50% of the patients, and they experienced substantial dose-related side effects; the major effects were cheilitis, conjunctivitis, and hypertriglyceridemia.[98] These results indicated the need for a less toxic dose and a longer period of treatment with isotretinoin.

In a subsequent randomized study of patients whose lesions responded or remained stable after high-dose isotretinoin, participants received maintenance therapy with either low-dose isotretinoin or beta-carotene. Only 8% of the lesions in the isotretinoin group progressed, compared with 55% in the beta-carotene group ($P < .001$). Low-dose isotretinoin was relatively well tolerated.[99]

Another retinoid (fenretinide) has been studied for maintenance in an adjuvant setting, with results similar to those for isotretinoin.[100] Two other randomized trials of retinoid induction documented significant activity in reversing oral premalignant lesions.[101,102] Furthermore, beta-carotene and alpha-tocopherol (vitamin E) have been reported to have activity in patients in several nonrandomized trials.[103,104]

In view of the suboptimal ability of adjuvant therapy to prevent primary disease recurrence and lower the risk of second cancer development, Hong et al designed an adjuvant chemoprevention trial of high-dose 13cRA.[105] In this phase III study, 103 patients with stage I to IV head and neck cancer were randomly assigned to receive either placebo or 13cRA for 1 year. Patients were eligible for the study after definitive local therapy with surgery and/or radiotherapy. At a median follow-up of 32 months, only two of the 51 patients in the 13cRA arm had developed a second primary tumor, compared with 12 of the 49 patients in the placebo group ($P = .005$). A recent update of this trial, at a median follow-up of 55 months, reported that 14% of patients who received 13cRA developed a second primary tumor, compared to 31% of the placebo group ($P = .04$).[106]

In a recent placebo-controlled trial in France, the synthetic retinoid etretinate was tested in the adjuvant setting. The study included patients with stage I to III squamous-cell cancer of the oral cavity and/or oropharynx after definitive local therapy. At a median follow-up of 24 months, the occurrence of second primary lesions and primary recurrence rates were similar in the two arms.[107]

CONCLUSIONS

Although relatively uncommon in the United States, head and neck cancer continues to be a devastating disease with high mortality and morbidity. Management of this tumor requires a multidisciplinary approach, with surgery and radiotherapy being the mainstays. New combined-modality approaches with chemotherapy are starting to show promising results in overall survival and quality of life, especially in patients with locally advanced disease. Because organ preservation, particularly in the larynx, has shown encouraging results, other areas are being studied. Molecular biology has evolved, enabling a better understanding of tumorigenesis of the head and neck. Chemoprevention has been shown to reduce the incidence of second primary tumors and to reverse premalignant lesions; continuing trials will define its role in the management of head and neck neoplasia. Knowing that this disease is, for the most part, preventable, we must continue to support research efforts to decrease the rate of tobacco use.

REFERENCES

1. Wingo P, Tony T, Bolden S: Cancer Statistics 1995. CA Cancer J Clin 45:8–30, 1995.

2. Spitz, MR, Fueger JT, Goepfert H, et al: Squamous cell carcinoma of the upper aerodigestive tract: A case comparison analysis. Cancer 61:203–208, 1988.

3. Fracerchi S, Bidoli E, Negri E, et al: Alcohol and cancer of the upper aerodigestive tract in men and women. Cancer Epidemiol Biomarkers Prev 3:299–304, 1994.

4. Spitz MR: Epidemiology and risk factors for head and neck cancer. Semin Oncol 21:281–288, 1994.

5. Khugars GE, Riley WT, Brandt RB, et al: The prevalence of oral lesions in smokers, tobacco users and an evaluation of risk factors. Cancer 70:2579–2585, 1992.

6. Wray A, McGuire WF: Smokeless tobacco usage associated with oral carcinoma, incidence and treatment outcome. Arch Otolaryngol Head Neck Surg 119:929–933, 1993.

7. International Agency for Research on Cancer: Evaluation of the carcinogenic risk of chemicals to humans: Tobacco smoking. WHO IARC Monogr 38:1–421, 1986.

8. Caplan GA, Brigham BA: Marijuana smoking and carcinoma of the tongue: Is there an association? Cancer 66:1005–1006, 1990.

9. Spitz MR, Foeger JI, Bedding NA, et al: Chromosome sensitivity to bleomycin-indued mutagenesis, an independent risk factor for upper aerodigestive tract cancer. Cancer Res 49:4626–4628, 1989.

10. Schantz SP, Hsu TC, Ainslie N, et al: Young adults with head and neck cancers express increased susceptibility to mutagen-induced chromosomal damage. JAMA 262:3313–3315, 1989.

11. Liebowitz D: Nasopharyngeal carcinoma. The Epstein-Barr Virus Association. Semin Oncol 21:376–381, 1994.

12. Henle G, Henle W: Epstein-Barr virus specific IgA serum antibodies as an outstanding feature of nasopharyngeal carcinoma. J Natl Cancer Inst 17:1–7, 1976.

13. Hadar T, Rahima M, Kahan E, et al: Significance of specific Epstein-Barr virus IgA and elevated IgG antibodies to vital capsid antigens in nasopharyngeal carcinoma patients. J Med Virol 20:329–339, 1986.

14. Ho JHC: An epidemiologic study of nasopharyngeal carcinoma. Int J Radiat Oncol Biol Phys 4:183–197, 1978.

15. Watts SL, Brewer EE, Paz TL: Human papillomavirus DNA types in squamous cell carcinoma of the head and neck. Oral Surg Oral Med Oral Pathol 71:701–707, 1991.

16. Shillitoe EJ, Greenspan D, Greenspan JS, et al: Antibody to early and late antigens of herpes simplex virus type I in patients with oral cancer. Cancer 54:266–273, 1984.

17. Slaughter DL, Southwick HW, Smejkal W: "Field cancerization" in oral stratified squamous epithelium: Clinical implication of multicentric origin. Cancer 6:963–968, 1953.

18. Wolf G, Lippman SM, Laramore G, et al: Head and neck cancer, in Holland JF, Frei E, Bast RC Jr, et al (eds): Cancer Medicine, 3rd ed, pp 1211–1278. Philadelphia, Lea & Febiger, 1993.

19. Cooper JS, Pajak TF, Rubin P, et al: Second malignancies in patients who have head and neck cancer: Incidence, effect on survival and implications based on the RTOG experience. Int J Radiat Oncol Biol Phys 17:449–456, 1989.

20. Farber E: The multistep nature of cancer development. Cancer Res 44:4217–4223, 1984.

21. Li X, Lee NK, Ye YW, et al: Allelic loss at chromosomes 3p, 8p, 13q, and 17p associated with poor prognosis in head and neck cancers. J Natl Cancer Inst 86:1524–1529, 1994.

22. Nawroz H, van der Riet P, Hruban RH, et al: Allelotype of head and neck squamous cell carcinoma. Cancer Res 54:1152–1155, 1994.

23. Jares P, Fernandez PL, Campo E, et al: PRAD-1/cyclin D1 gene amplification correlates with messenger RNA overexpression and tumor progression in human laryngeal carcinomas. Cancer Res 54:4813–4817, 1994.

24. Michalides R, van Veelen N, Hart A, et al: Overexpression of cyclin D1 correlates with recurrence in a group of forty-seven operable squamous cell carcinomas of the head and neck. Cancer Res 55:975–978, 1995.

25. Bartkova J, Lukas J, Muller H, et al: Abnormal pattern of D-type cyclin expression and G1 regulation in human head and neck cancer. Cancer Res 55:949–956, 1995.

26. Brachman DG: Molecular biology of head and neck cancer. Semin Oncol 21:320–329, 1994.

27. Brachman DG, Grover D, Voker E, et al: Occurrence of p53 gene deletions and human papilloma virus infection in human head and neck cancer. Cancer Res 62:4832–4836, 1992.

28. Brennan JA, Mao L, Hauban RH, et al: Molecular assessment of histopathologic staging. N Engl J Med 332:429–443, 1995.

29. Brennan JA, Boyle JO, Koch WM: Association between cigarette smoking and mutation of the p53 gene in squamous-cell carcinoma of the head and neck. N Engl J Med 332:712–717, 1995.

30. Kwok TT, Sotherland RM: Enhancement of sensitivity of human squamous carcinoma cells to radiation by epidermal growth factor receptor. J Natl Cancer Inst 81:1020–1024, 1989.

31. Shin DM, Ro JY, Hong WK, et al: Dysregulation of epidermal growth factor receptor in premalignant lesion during head and neck tumorigenesis. Cancer Res 54:3153–3159, 1994.

32. Shin DM, Voravud N, Ro JY, et al: Sequential increases in proliferation of cell nuclear antigen expression in head and neck tumorigenesis: A potential biomarker. J Natl Cancer Inst 85:971–978, 1993.

33. Vokes EE, Weichselbaum RR, Lippman SM, et al: Head and neck cancer. N Engl J Med 328:184–194, 1993.

34. Calhoun KH, Fulmer P, Weiss R, et al: Distant metastases from head and neck squamous cell carcinomas. Laryngoscope 104(10):1199–1205, 1994.

35. Feinmesser R, Miyasaki I, Cheung R, et al: Diagnosis of nasopharyngeal carcinoma by DNA amplification of tissue obtained by fine-needle aspiration. N Engl J Med 326: 17–21, 1992.

36. American Joint Committee on Cancer: Manual for Staging of Cancer, 3rd ed. Philadelphia, J B Lippincott, 1988.

37. Peters LJ, Batsakis JG, Goepfert H, et al: The diagnosis and management of nasopharyngeal cancer in Caucasians, in Williams CJ, Krikoniau JG, Green MR, et al (eds): Textbook of Uncommon Cancer, pp 975–1006. Chichester, England, John Wiley & Sons, 1988.

38. Perez CA: Carcinoma of the nasopharynx, in Brady LW, Peser C (eds): Principles and Practice of Radiation Oncology, 2nd ed, pp 617–644. Philadelphia, J B Lippincott, 1992.

39. Gasmi J, Bachouch M, Costkauic E, et al: Nasopharyngeal carcinoma, a medical oncology viewpoint: The Gustave Roussy experience. Ann Oncol 1:245–253, 1990.

40. Sweeney PJ, Harvaf DJ, Vokes EE, et al: Radiation therapy in head and neck cancer: Indication and limitations. Semin Oncol 21:296–303, 1994.

41. Mazeron JJ, Grimard L, Raynal M, et al: Iridium-192 curietherapy for T1 and T2 epidermoid carcinomas of the floor of the mouth. Int J Radiat Oncol Biol Phys 18: 1299–1309, 1990.

42. Wallner PE, Hansk GE, Kramer S, et al. Pattern of care study: Analysis of outcome survey data—Anterior two-thirds of tongue and floor of the mouth. Am J Clin Oncol 9:50–57, 1986.

43. Lusinchi A, Wibaust P, Marandas P, et al: Exclusive radiation therapy: The treatment of early tonsillar tumors. Int J Radiat Oncol Biol Phys 17:273–277, 1989.

44. Perez CA, Carmichael T, Devineni VR, et al : Carcinoma of the tonsillar fossa: A nonrandomized comparison of irradiation alone or combined with surgery: Long-term results. Head Neck 13:282–290, 1991.

45. Amornarn R, Prempre T, Jainitama J, et al: Radiation management of carcinoma of the tonsillar region. Cancer 54:1293, 1984.

46. Foore RL, Parsons JT, Mendenhor WM, et al: Is interstitial implantation essential for successful radiotherapeutic treatment of the base of the tongue carcinoma? Int J Radiation Oncol Biol Phys 18:1293–1298, 1990.

47. Wever RS, Gidley P, Morrison WH, et al: Treatment selection for carcinoma of the base of the tongue. Am J Surg 160:415, 1990.

48. Van den Bronck C, Eschwege F, De La Rochefordicere A, et al: Squamous cell carcinoma of the pyriform sinus: Retrospective study of 351 cases treated at the Institut Gustave Roussy. Head Neck Surg 10:4, 1987.

49. Steiner W: Results of curative laser microsurgery of laryngeal carcinoma. Am J Otolaryngol 14:116–121, 1993.

50. Lefebvre JL, Sahmoud T, for the EORTC Head and Neck Cancer Cooperative Group: Larynx preservation in hypopharynx squamous cell carcinoma: Preliminary results of a randomized study (EORTC 24891). Proc Am Soc Clin Oncol 13:283, 1995.

51. Horaf DJ, Weichselbaum RR: Treatment selection in T1 and T2 vocal cord carcinoma. Oncology 2(10):41–50, 1988.

52. Mendenhall WM, Parson JT, Stringer SP, et al: T1-T2 vocal cord carcinoma: A basis for comparing the results of radiotherapy and surgery. Head Neck Surg 10:373–377, 1988.

53. Mendenhall WM, Parsons JT, Stringer SP, et al: Stage T3 squamous cell carcinoma of the glottic larynx: A comparison of laryngectomy and irradiation. Int J Radiat Oncol Biol Phys 23:725–732, 1992.

54. Medina JE, Byers RM: Supraomokyoid neck dissection: Rationale, indication and surgical techniques. Head Neck 11:111–112, 1989.

55. Creagan E, Woods J, Rubin J: Cisplatin-based chemotherapy for neoplasms arising from salivary glands and contiguous structures in the head and neck. Cancer 62:2313–2319, 1988.

56. Schornagel JH, Verweij J, de Mulder P, et al: Randomized phase III trial of edatrexate versus methotrexate in patients with metastatic and/or recurrent squamous cell carcinoma of the head and neck: A European Organization for Research and Treatment of Cancer, Head and Neck Cancer Cooperative Group Study. J Clin Oncol 13:1649–1655, 1995.

57. Forastiere AA, Neuberg D, Taylor SG, et al: Phase II evaluation of Taxol in advanced head and neck cancer: Eastern Cooperative Oncology Group trial. Monogr Natl Cancer Inst 15:181–184, 1993.

58. Forastiere AA: Paclitaxel (Taxol) for the treatment of head and neck cancer. Semin Oncol 21:49–52, 1994.

59. Catimel G, Verweij J, Mattijssen V, et al: Docetaxel (Taxotere): An active drug for the treatment of patients with advanced squamous cell carcinoma of the head and neck. EORTC Early Clinical Group. Ann Oncol 5: 533–537, 1994.

60. Urba SG, Forastiere AA: Systemic therapy of head and neck cancer: Most effective agents, areas of promise. Oncology 3(4):79–88, 1989.

61. Jacobs C, Lyman G, Velez-Garcia E, et al: A phase III randomized study comparing cisplatin and fluorouracil as single agents and in combination for advanced squamous cell carcinoma of the head and neck. J Clin Oncol 10:257–263, 1992.

62. Forastiere AA, Metch B, Schuller DE, et al: Randomized comparison of cisplatin plus fluorouracil and carboplatin plus fluorouracil versus methotrexate in advanced squamous cell carcinoma of the head and neck: A Southwest Oncology Group study. J Clin Oncol 10:1245–1251, 1992.

63. Vokes EE, Weichselbaum RR: Chemoradiotherapy for head and neck cancer. Principal Practice in Oncology Updates 7:1–8, 1993.

64. Forastiere AA: Randomized trials of induction chemotherapy: A critical review. Hematol Oncol Clin North Am 5:725–736, 1991.

65. Jacobs C, Makosh R: Efficacy of adjuvant chemotherapy for patients with resectable head and neck cancer: A subset analysis of the head and neck cancer. A subset analysis of the head and neck contract program. J Clin Oncol 8:838–847, 1990.

66. Paccagnella A, Olando A, Marchiori C, et al: Phase III trial of initial chemotherapy in stage III or IV head and neck cancer: A study by the Gruppo di Studio sui Tumori della Testa e del Collo. J Natl Cancer Inst 86:265–272, 1994.

67. Jacobs C, Goffinet DR, Goffinet L, et al: Chemotherapy as a substitute for surgery in the treatment of resectable head and neck cancer: A report from the Northern California Oncology Group. Cancer 60:1178–1183, 1987.

68. Pfister DG, Stong E, Harrison L, et al: Larynx preservation with combined chemotherapy and radiation therapy in advanced but resectable head and neck cancer. J Clin Oncol 9:850–859, 1991.

69. Hong WK, Lippman SM, Wolf GT: Recent advances in head and neck cancer—Larynx preservation and cancer chemoprevention: The Seventeenth Annual Richard and Hinda Rosenthal Foundation Award Lecture. Cancer Res 53:5113–5120, 1993.

70. The Department of Veterans Affairs Laryngeal Cancer Study Group: Induction chemotherapy plus radiation compared with surgery plus radiation in patients with advanced laryngeal cancer. N Engl J Med 324:1685–1690, 1991.

71. Spaulding MB, Fischer SG, Wolf GT, et al: Tumor response, toxicity and survival after neoadjuvant organ-preserving chemotherapy for advanced laryngeal carcinoma. J Clin Oncol 12:1592–1599, 1994.

72. Martin M, Lelievre G, Gehanno P, et al: Induction carboplatin (CBDCA) and 5-fluorouracil (5FU) treatment versus no chemotherapy before locoregional treatment for oro- and pharyngeal cancers: Preliminary results of a randomized study. Proc Am Soc Clin Oncol 11:240, 1992.

73. Cvitkovic E, for the International Nasopharynx Study Group, Institut G.-Roussy-La Grange-Savigny le Temple (France): Neoadjuvant chemotherapy (NACT) with epirubicin (EPI), cisplatin (CDDP), bleomycin (BLEO) (BEC) in undifferentiated nasopharyngeal cancer (UCNT): Preliminary results of an international (INT) phase (PH) III trial. Proc Am Soc Clin Oncol 14:283, 1994.

74. Chan ATC, Te PML, Leung WT, et al: Chemotherapy adjunctive to definitive radiotherapy in locoregionally advanced nasopharyngeal carcinoma (NPC): Results of a prospective randomized trial using cisplatin and 5-fluorouracil (5-FU) (abstract). Proc Am Soc Clin Oncol 14:299, 1995.

75. Bitter K: Postoperative chemotherapy versus postoperative cobalt 60 radiation in patients with advanced oral carcinoma: report on a randomized study. Head Neck Surg 3:264, 1981.

76. Bachaad JM, David JM, Boussin G, et al: Combined postoperative radiotherapy and weekly cisplatin infusion for locally advanced squamous cell carcinoma of the head and neck: Preliminary report of a randomized trial. Int J Radiat Oncol Biol Phys 20:243–246, 1991.

77. Laramore GE, Scott CB, al-Sarraf M, et al: Adjuvant chemotherapy for resectable squamous cell carcinomas of the head and neck: Report on Intergroup Study 0034. Int J Radiat Oncol Biol Phys 23:705–713, 1992.

78. Horuchi M, Inuyana Y, Miyake H: Efficacy of surgical adjuvant with tegafur and uracil (UFT) in resectable head and neck cancer: A prospective randomized study. Proc Am Soc Clin Oncol 13:284, 1994.

79. Vokes EE, Weichselbaum RR: Concomitant radiotherapy: rationale and clinical experience in patients with solid tumors. J Clin

Oncol 8:911–934, 1990.

80. Stupp R, Weichselbaum RR, Vokes EE: Combined modality therapy of head and neck cancer. Semin Oncol 21:349–358, 1994.

81. Shigmatsu Y, Sakai S, Fuchihata H: Recent trials in the treatment of maxillary sinus carcinoma with special reference to the chemical potentiation of radiation therapy. Acta Otolaryngol (Stockh) 71:63, 1971.

82. Lo TC, Wiley AL Jr, Ansfield FJ, et al: Combined radiation therapy and 5 fluorouracil for advanced squamous cell carcinoma of the oral cavity and oropharynx: A randomized study. Am J Roentgenol 126:229–235, 1976.

83. Browman GP, Cripps C, Hodson DI, et al: Placebo-controlled randomized trial of infusional fluorouracil during standard radiotherapy in locally advanced head and neck cancer. J Clin Oncol 12:2648–2653, 1994.

84. Haselow RE, Warshaw MG, Oken MK: Radiation alone versus radiation with weekly low-dose cisplatin in unresectable cancer of the head and neck, in Strong EW, Ward PH Jr, (eds): Head and Neck Cancer, pp 279–281. Philadelphia, BC Decker, 1990.

85. A randomized trial of combined multi-drug chemotherapy and radiotherapy in advanced squamous cell carcinoma of the head and neck: an interim report from the SECOG participants. Eur J Surg Oncol 12:289–295, 1986.

86. Merlano M, Corvo R, Margarino G, et al: Combined chemotherapy and radiation therapy in advanced inoperable squamous cell carcinoma of the head and neck: The final report of a randomized trial. Cancer 67:915–921, 1991.

87. Adelstein DJ, Shanan VM, Earle S, et al: Simultaneous versus sequential combined technique therapy for squamous cell head and neck cancer. Cancer 65:1685–1691, 1990.

88. Pinnaro P, Cercato MC, Giannarelli D, et al: A randomized phase II study comparing sequential versus simultaneous chemo-radiotherapy in patients with unresectable locally advanced squamous cell cancer of the head and neck. Ann Oncol 5:513–519, 1994.

89. Taylor SG, Murthy AK, Vannetzel JM, et al: Randomized comparison of neoadjuvant cisplatin and fluorouracil infusion followed by radiation versus concomitant treatment in advanced head and neck cancer. J Clin Oncol 12:385–395, 1994.

90. Bezwoda WE, de Moor NG, Deman DP: Treatment of advanced head and neck cancer by means of radiation therapy plus chemotherapy: a randomized trial. Med Pediatr Oncol 6:353, 1979.

91. Keegan P, Pillsbury HC, Weissler M, et al: Hyperfractionated radiotherapy with or without simultaneous cisplatin and fluorouracil (5-FU) in the treatment of advanced head and neck cancer. Proc Am Soc Clin Oncol 9:172, 1990.

92. Merlano M, Vitale V, Rosso R, et al: Treatment of advanced squamous cell carcinoma of the head and neck with alternating chemotherapy and radiotherapy. N Engl J Med 327:1115–1121, 1992.

93. Keane TJ, Harwood AR, Danjoux C: Results of a randomized trial of radiation compared to radiation and chemotherapy for advanced laryngeal and hypopharyngeal squamous carcinoma. Proc Second Intl Conf Head Neck Cancer (abstract 55). Boston, MA, 1988.

94. Sporn MB, Dunlap NM, Newton DL, et al: Prevention of chemical carcinogenesis by vitamin A and its synthetic analogs (retinoids). Fed Proc 35:1332–1338, 1976.

95. Vikram B: Changing patterns of failure in advanced head and neck cancer. Arch Otolaryngol 110:564–565, 1984.

96. Cooper JS, Pajak TF, Rubin P, et al: Second malignancies in patients who have head and neck cancers: incidence, effect on survival and implications for chemoprevention based on the RTOG experience. Int J Radiat Oncol Biol Phys 17:449–456, 1989.

97. Fontillas G: Retinoids in the management of head and neck cancer: An update. J Chemother 6(2):127–138, 1994.

98. Hong WK, Endicott J, Itri LM, et al: 13-*cis* retinoic acid in the treatment of oral leukoplakia. N Engl J Med 315:1501–1505, 1986.

99. Lippman SM, Batsakis JG, Toth BB, et al: Comparison of low-dose isotretinoin with beta carotene to prevent oral carcinogenesis. N Engl J Med 328:15–20, 1993.

100. Chiesa F, Tradat N, Marraza M, et al: Prevention of local relapses and new localization with the synthetic retinoid fenretinide (4-HPR): Preliminary results. Eur J Cancer 28:97–102, 1992.

101. Stich HF, Hornby AP, Mathew B, et al: Response of oral leukoplakias to the administration of vitamin A. Cancer Lett 40:93–101, 1988.

102. Han J, Lu Y, Sun Z, et al: Evaluation of N-4-(hydroxycarbopenyl) retinamide as a cancer prevention agent and as a cancer chemotherapeutic agent. In Vivo 4:153–160, 1990.

103. Garewal HS, Pitcock J, Friedman S, et al: Beta-carotene in oral leukoplakia. Proc Am Soc Clin Oncol 11:141, 1992.

104. Benner SE, Winn RJ, Lippman SM, et al: Regression of oral leukoplasia with alpha-tocopherol: A community clinical oncology program study. J Natl Cancer Inst 85(1):44–47, 1993.

105. Hong WK, Lippman SM, Itri LM, et al: Prevention of secondary primary tumors with isotretinoin in squamous cell carcinoma of the head and neck. N Engl J Med 323:795–801, 1990.

106. Benner SE, Pajak TF, Lippman SM, et al: Prevention of secondary primary tumors with isotretinoin in squamous cell carcinoma of the head and neck: Long-term follow up. J Natl Cancer Inst 86:140–141, 1994.

107. Bolla M, Lefur R, Ton Van J, et al: Prevention of second primary tumors with etretinate in squamous cell carcinoma of the oral cavity and oropharynx: Results of a multicentric double-blind randomized study. Eur J Cancer 6:767–772, 1994.

SECTION 4

GASTRO-INTESTINAL CARCINOMAS

CHAPTER **14** **Carcinoma of the Esophagus**

CHAPTER **15** **Gastric Carcinoma**

CHAPTER **16** **Pancreatic, Hepatic, and Biliary Carcinomas**

CHAPTER **17** **Colorectal Cancer: Diagnosis and Management**

CHAPTER **18** **Neuroendocrine Tumors of the Gastrointestinal Tract**

Carcinoma of the Esophagus

Philip Agop Philip, MB, ChB, PhD, MRCP, *and* Jaffer Ajani, MD

Department of Gastrointestinal Medical Oncology and Digestive Diseases
The University of Texas M. D. Anderson Cancer Center, Houston, Texas

Carcinoma of the esophagus or the gastroesophageal junction is uncommon, accounting for approximately 1% of all malignancies in the United States.[1] An estimated 12,100 new cases and 10,900 deaths will occur in 1995.[1] The diagnosis of esophageal cancer is often made late in the course of the disease in Western countries. Thus, according to the tumor-node-metastasis (TNM) system of staging, T3 or T4 and N-positive lesions are observed frequently. In fact, nearly 50% of patients have advanced incurable disease at the time of diagnosis. Therefore, the prognosis of patients with carcinoma of the esophagus remains poor, and the overall 5-year survival rates are still less than 10%.[1]

The incidence of adenocarcinoma of the esophagus and proximal stomach in the Western world and especially in white males has increased in the past 15 years.[2,3] The proportion of adenocarcinomas has increased from the traditionally reported rate of 5% to 10% to 20% to 40% of all esophageal tumors.[2] It is our estimation that currently in the United States, adenocarcinoma occurs more frequently than does squamous-cell carcinoma.

Squamous-cell carcinoma of the esophagus has the greatest variation in geographical distribution, a fact that provides insight into its pathogenesis. Geographic variations in the incidence often exist within the same country. Unlike squamous-cell carcinoma, for which alcohol and tobacco (among other factors) have been implicated as risk factors, the risk factors for adenocarcinoma remain elusive. Coexistence of Barrett's esophagus does not yet explain this phenomenal rise in the frequency of adenocarcinoma.

PATHOGENESIS

A number of predisposing conditions have been identified in the pathogenesis of squamous-cell carcinoma of the esophagus. These conditions include achalasia, caustic injury, and esophageal diverticula and webs. Esophageal cancer may also develop as second primary tumors in patients with other primary tumors of the upper aerodigestive tract that are associated with tobacco consumption. In Barrett's esophagus, the normal stratified squamous epithelium of the esophagus is replaced by metaplastic columnar epithelium. It develops as a result of chronic gastroesophageal reflux and can lead to the development of adenocarcinoma through a multistep process characterized by a progression from metaplasia, to indefinite or low-grade dysplasia, to high-grade dysplasia, and ultimately to invasive cancer.[4]

Over the past several years, intensive research into the molecular changes in carcinoma of the esophagus, pre-malignant lesions, and normal mucosa have identified a number of genetic events that play a major role in the pathogenesis of esophageal cancer. Both the loss of heterozygosity and replication errors have been identified as genetic alterations in esophageal cancer. Allelic losses at frequencies of at least 30% were observed at loci on chromosomal arms 3p, 3q, 5q, 9p, 9q, 10p, 13q, 17p, 17q, 18q, 19q, and 21q,[5,6] suggesting that several putative tumor-suppressor genes may be associated with the development and/or progression of esophageal cancer.

MTS-1 (CDKN2) is a candidate tumor-suppressor gene on chromosome 9p21-22. This region is frequently observed to have a loss of heterozygosity in patients with esophageal squamous-cell carcinomas and adenocarcinomas,[7] and there is evidence of mutations of this gene in esophageal tumors.[8] It has been shown that 67% of esophageal squamous-cell carcinoma cell lines have deletions of both exons 1 and 2 of the *MTS-1* gene, suggesting that it has a role in the pathogenesis of esophageal cancer.[9]

Mutations in the *p53* gene may be detected in a high proportion of esophageal squamous-cell carcinomas[10,11] and adenocarcinomas.[11] However, the overexpression of the *p53* gene product did not correlate with either the TNM stage or the prognosis in these patients. These results suggest that *p53* mutations occur early in the course of esophageal carcinogenesis. A recent study described the expression of *p53* in 28 esophageal specimens that all contained Barrett's mucosa and a spectrum of low- to high-grade dysplasia and intramucosal and submucosal cancer.[12] Immunoreactivity to *p53* was not detected in any of the Barrett's mucosa or low-grade dysplasia specimens. However, it was present in specimens of high-grade dysplasia, intramucosal cancer, and submucosal cancer. The conclusion of this study was that *p53* mutations occurred late in the metaplasia-dysplasia-carcinoma sequence, during the transition to high-grade dysplasia.

It has also been proposed that *p53* expression may potentially be utilized as an intermediate biomarker in Barrett's esophagus.[13] In addition to *p53* mutations that may be induced by environmental chemical carcinogens, viruses such as the papillomavirus may inactivate the normal *p53* function by the binding of the E6 protein to the p53 protein.[14] The tumor-suppressor gene *APC* is infrequently mutated in esophageal cancer[15] despite the high frequency of allelic losses at the 5q locus,[5] which suggests that other tumor-suppressor genes exist at this locus.

Activation of oncogenes probably play an important role in the pathogenesis of esophageal cancer. Expression of growth factors and growth factor receptors facilitates autocrine or paracrine growth stimulation and may be important in the pathogenesis of esophageal cancers.[16] Epidermal growth factor receptor (EGFR) overexpression was detected in 71% of primary squamous-cell carcinomas of the esophagus and 88% of the lymph node metastases and was associated with a tendency for worse prognosis.[17] EGFR overexpression correlates with the degree of dysplasia and the frequency of lymph node metastases.[18] Overexpression of both epidermal growth factor and transforming growth factor-alpha, which are the normal ligands of EGFR, has been demonstrated in esophageal cancers.[16]

Amplification of c-*myc* has been frequently observed in esophageal cancer cell lines.[19] *HER-2/neu* gene overexpression is observed in approximately 20% of esophageal adenocarcinomas and is an independent indicator of poor prognosis.[20] The *hst-1* gene is also amplified in 30% of primary esophageal carcinomas but is without any prognostic significance.[21] However, *ras* mutations that are common in several gastrointestinal tumors are infrequently found in esophageal cancers.[22]

Genes involved in cell-cycle control have also been investigated in esophageal cancer.[23] In one report, amplification of the cyclin *D1* gene was present in 32% of primary tumors and in two of four cell lines. Seventeen percent of tumor samples had no expression of the retinoblastoma (Rb) gene product. It was also noted that there was a correlation between *D1* gene amplification and normal Rb protein levels, and by contrast absent expression of Rb correlated with the expression of low levels of cyclin D1 protein.

PROGNOSTIC FACTORS

Earlier studies have indicated that the length of the primary tumor predicted the duration of patients' survival.[24,25] Recently, however, the depth of wall penetration has been accepted as a better prognostic indicator than the length. Thus, T3 or T4 lesions impart a poorer prognosis than T1 or T2 lesions, irrespective of the length of the primary tumor. Patients with lymph node metastases have a poorer prognosis than those without lymph node metastases. Additionally, pretreatment weight loss of more than 10% carries a poor prognosis. At present, there are no molecular markers to reliably predict accurately the clinical behavior of esophageal carcinoma.

STAGING

Accurate staging is required in validating and comparing the results of studies of multimodality therapy for esophageal cancer. The revised TNM system (1987)[25a] for staging esophageal cancer is determined by the depth of wall penetration by the primary tumor, metastases to the regional lymph nodes, and distant metastases (Table 1).

The staging process should include a complete history and physical examination, a chest radiograph, pulmonary function studies, histologic confirmation, bronchoscopy in patients with lesions at or above the carina, blood tests to define hematology and organ functions, and computed tomographic scans of the chest and abdomen.

Improvements in staging techniques have been achieved with endoscopic ultrasonography (EUS), which is superior to computed tomography or magnetic resonance imaging in staging the primary tumor and in detecting small lesions (less than 5 mm in diameter).[26] In patients with biopsy-proven esophageal cancer, local staging was 77% to 86% accurate for the T stage and 55% to 90% accurate for the N stage.[27] Nevertheless, limitations of this method have been recognized: EUS displays lymph nodes with high resolution but cannot distinguish inflammatory nodal changes from malignant adenopathy. Furthermore, EUS cannot be performed in patients with significant stenosis. Whether EUS will affect the outcome in patients with esophageal tumor is unclear, but accurate tumor staging and response to treatment is a critical part of any therapeutic protocol.

TREATMENT

Single-Modality Therapy

Surgery: Surgical resection is considered the standard approach for patients with stages I and II and even stage III carcinomas. Curative resection is feasible in only about 50% of patients because often the lesions are more extensive than judged by the routine clinical staging. A high rate of local relapse following resection has been reported in some series, and the median survival of patients with resected tumors is approximately 11 months.

TABLE I

TNM Classification and Staging

Primary Tumor (T)

TX	Primary tumor cannot be assessed
T0	No evidence of primary tumor
Tis	Carcinoma in situ
TI	Tumor invades lamina propria or submucosa
T2	Tumor invades muscularis propria
T3	Tumor invades adventitia
T4	Tumor invades adjacent structures

Regional Lymph Nodes (N)

NX	Regional lymph nodes cannot be assessed
N0	No regional lymph node metastasis
NI	Regional lymph node metastasis

Distant Metastasis (M)

MX	Presence of distant metastasis cannot be assessed
M0	No distant metastasis
MI	Distant metastasis

Stage Grouping

Stage 0	Tis	N0	M0
Stage I	TI	N0	M0
Stage IIA	T2	N0	M0
	T3	N0	M0
Stage IIB	TI	NI	M0
	T2	NI	M0
Stage III	T3	NI	M0
	T4	Any N	M0
Stage IV	Any T	Any N	MI

Adapted, with permission, from Beahrs OH et al (eds): Handbook for Staging of Cancer: American Joint Committee on Cancer. Philadelphia, JB Lippincott, 1993.

Over the past 10 years, surgical mortality has declined substantially and is well below 10% at centers where the procedure is frequently performed. Type of surgical resection does not seem to alter the long-term outcome of these patients.

Radiation Therapy: Long-term results seen with radiation therapy as a single modality have been as disappointing as the results with surgery. However, irradiation as primary therapy is often used for patients who are medically unfit for operation or whose tumors are tech-

nically unresectable. Overall survival after radiation therapy is approximately 18% at 1 year and 6% after 5 years.[28] Radiation therapy might be equally effective against squamous-cell carcinoma and adenocarcinoma of the esophagus.[29]

Most surgical series have reported better long-term results than have radiation therapy-only series.[30] However, such comparisons have limitations; for example, in some studies, patients with unresected tumors are not accounted for. Prospective randomized trials in accurately staged and stratified patients will be necessary to compare surgery with irradiation (or chemoradiation). Two such trials were launched—one in Europe[31] and another in the United States—but both trials were aborted, because of poor patient accrual. This problem was the result of reluctance on the part of physicians and patients to accept randomization. Thus, this issue poses a significant challenge and will require an enormous effort to resolve.

At present, there is no evidence that radiation therapy alone can achieve local control similar to that afforded by surgery. By some estimates, surgery offers more durable palliation of dysphagia than does irradiation.[32] However, contradictory statements have been made in the literature. Potential benefits of brachytherapy are being investigated at present.[33,34]

Chemotherapy: Chemotherapy is not effective as a single modality in the treatment of locoregional esophageal carcinoma.

Multimodality Therapy

Rationale: Locoregional esophageal carcinoma, limited to the esophageal bed and regional lymph nodes, continues to be the dominant cause of morbidity in many patients. However, the natural history suggests that it is a systemic disease at the outset in the majority of patients. If locoregional disease can be effectively controlled, most patients eventually succumb to the metastatic disease.[35] Multimodality therapy has emerged as a result of the failures of single modalities against esophageal carcinoma.

Despite improving methods of clinical investigation, limitations are encountered, including small numbers of patients accrued in many studies, small proportions of patients with adenocarcinoma in some trials, the use of different chemotherapy regimens, and varying schedules and doses of chemotherapy and radiation therapy. Moreover, many studies have required several years to complete accrual.

When discussing multimodality therapy of esophageal carcinoma, the following issues warrant consideration: (1) radiation therapy alone vs chemoradiation therapy to improve local control, (2) impact of chemotherapy on distant metastases, and (3) cost of therapy, which continues to gain importance.

Chemotherapy: Systemic therapy is an important cornerstone of multimodality therapy because more than 75% of the patients harbor occult metastases at presentation.[36,37] Sixteen cytotoxic drugs have been investigated in depth in phase II trials in patients with metastatic disease,[38] and the majority of these agents have been evaluated in patients with the squamous-cell carcinoma histologic subtype.

Cisplatin (Platinol) is one of the most active agents, with a single-agent response rate that is consistently around 20%.[39] With cisplatin-based combination chemotherapy, superior response rates of 30% to 50% have been reported but only a few complete responses.[39–42] Furthermore, responses are typically brief (usually less than 4 months).

Although it has been predominantly investigated in squamous-cell carcinomas, cisplatin continues to form the backbone of combination therapy for both histologic subtypes.[43] Pilot studies suggest that adenocarcinoma would probably respond to chemotherapy with a frequency similar to that of squamous-cell carcinoma.[35,44]

Extensively studied cisplatin-based chemotherapy regimens have included bleomycin (Blenoxane), the investigational agent vindesine (Eldisine), and fluorouracil in various combinations. The most popular combination has been infusional fluorouracil and cisplatin. Fractionating the dose of cisplatin over several days can result in less nausea and vomiting than occurs with a single total dose. Bleomycin, once a popular component of combination chemotherapy regimens, has now been dropped because of the significant perioperative pulmonary morbidity associated with its use.

The optimum duration and dose intensity of chemotherapy in esophageal carcinoma has not been determined. It is logical to assume that more than two treatment cycles are required, based on the results achieved in sensitive tumor types (eg, germ-cell tumors and lymphomas). The age range of patients who develop carcinoma of the esophagus (60 years and older) often limits the cumulative cisplatin dose to approximately 500 mg/m^2 because of neurotoxic and ototoxic effects. Dose-intensive chemotherapy has not demonstrated an advantage.

Ajani et al[45] reported a pilot study in 26 patients who received high doses of etoposide (VePesid), doxorubicin (Adriamycin, Rubex), and cisplatin, with granulocyte-macrophage colony-stimulating factor (GM-CSF, sargramostim [Leukine]). Fifty percent of the patients achieved a major response, and 65% of the patients were able to undergo curative resection for their tumors. None of the patients had a pathologically complete response, and significant toxicity was associated with this regimen. Therefore, higher doses result in poor patient tolerance.

Preoperative Radiation Therapy: Preoperative radiation therapy can potentially increase the resectability rate and local control. The majority of pilot studies using preoperative radiation therapy have reported a decent rate of pathologically complete responses, curative resections, and survival, but only in comparison with historical parameters.[46] Another weakness is the influence of patient selection in some of these studies.

Several prospective randomized trials have investigated survival duration following preoperative radiation therapy. Launois et al[47] compared patients who underwent irradiation preoperatively with those who did not and found no difference in the rate or duration of survival between the groups. Gignoux et al[48] reported a trial involving 192 patients who were randomized to receive preoperative radiation therapy (33 Gy) or immediate surgery. Here again, no survival benefit was observed, but in the irradiated group there was a longer median time to recurrence as well as fewer local recurrences than in the control group.

Wang et al[49] investigated 206 patients with tumors less than 8 cm in length who had a good performance status and dysphagia only to solid foods. The dose of preoperative radiation was 40 Gy. The 5-year survival durations were similar in both arms of the study. Another reported randomized study showed no benefit of low-dose (20 Gy) radiation therapy in prolonging the survival duration of patients with squamous-cell carcinoma or adenocarcinoma of the esophagus.[50]

It would appear that despite 60% to 70% "response rates," including up to 25% pathologically complete responses in some studies, there has not been a statistically significant survival advantage with the use of preoperative radiation therapy.[51] Thus, preoperative radiation therapy alone cannot be recommended for routine use.

Postoperative Radiation Therapy: Postoperative radiation therapy is aimed at improving local control. In addition, better delivery of radiotherapy may be possible if the surgical bed is demarcated by clips. Occasional limitations may be attributed to the distorted anatomy and enhanced toxicity to the stomach, when it is used for reconstruction.

When resection is incomplete, postoperative radiation therapy is usually recommended to prevent morbidity from locoregional disease.[52,53] Results of a randomized study that involved 221 patients who had curative resection of esophageal carcinoma showed only a slight reduction (85% vs 70% at 5 years) in local relapse among patients who received postoperative radiation therapy.[54] A statistically significant difference in local relapse was achieved only in node-negative patients, but there was no survival advantage. Thus, postoperative radiation therapy alone does not alter the natural history of the disease even if the surgical margins contain tumor.

Preoperative Chemotherapy (Neoadjuvant): According to the Goldie and Coldman hypothesis, chemotherapy early in the natural history of a malignancy potentially delays the emergence of drug-resistant malignant clones.[55] The benefit of preoperative chemotherapy in the eradication of micrometastatic disease is also supported by data from studies in animal tumor models.[56,57] With preoperative chemotherapy, optimum drug delivery may be achieved because of the intact vasculature. In addition, preoperative chemotherapy allows an assessment of in vivo chemosensitivity and can guide postoperative therapy.

A number of pilot studies have reported 40% to 60% response rates, but few have shown pathologically complete responses.[58,59] Roth et al[60] reported on a small prospective study in which patients were randomized to undergo either immediate surgery (20 patients) or to receive two cycles of cisplatin, vindesine, and bleomycin preoperatively (19 patients). Major responses were achieved in 47% of the patients but with only one pathologically complete response. Resectability and survival were similar regardless of whether patients received preoperative chemotherapy.

A second prospectively randomized study compared the effectiveness of preoperative chemotherapy (cisplatin, vindesine, and bleomycin) with preoperative radiation therapy (55 Gy).[61] Ninety-six patients with resectable squamous-cell carcinoma of the esophagus were enrolled. Postoperatively, patients with positive lymph nodes were crossed over (to receive either radiation therapy or chemotherapy). Response rates, survival duration (limited by the crossover design), resectability, and surgical morbidity were similar.[61]

Earlier trials used only one or two courses of systemic chemotherapy in the combined-modality setting, but it is possible to administer five cycles of chemotherapy.[35,45,62] In the current Intergroup trial, a total of five courses of chemotherapy are being administered to patients before and after surgery, and the results will be compared with those of patients receiving surgery alone. The value of preoperative chemotherapy in patients with carcinoma of the esophagus remains unproved; the current trial may help to define the role of this strategy.

Postoperative Chemotherapy: The role of adjuvant chemotherapy after resection has not been investigated adequately. Currently there is no evidence that it is useful, and thus, it cannot be recommended as a routine clinical practice.

Concurrent Chemotherapy and Radiation Therapy Followed by Surgery: In terms of design, the earliest trials of chemotherapy with radiation therapy in esophageal cancer[63] were based on the successes in treating anal cancer. The goal has been to control local and systemic disease simultaneously, with a greater emphasis on the local disease. Drugs such as fluorouracil, cisplatin, and mitomycin (Mutamycin) are also radiation enhancers and may potentially improve local tumor control.

Several pilot studies with small numbers of selected patients have reported clinical response rates up to 70% and a pathologically complete response rate of up to 37%.[64,65] Poplin et al[66] from the Southwest Oncology Group reported a study of 113 patients who received fluorouracil plus cisplatin and radiation therapy followed by esophagectomy. Median survival duration was 12 months, with a 2-year survival rate of 28% and an operative mortality rate of 11%. The median survival duration was 32 months for those attaining a pathologically complete response.[66]

Mercke et al[67] reported the use of preoperative fluorouracil plus cisplatin followed by radiation therapy in 60 patients, which resulted in effective palliation in 50% of patients and a pathologically complete response rate of 15%. In another study, 43 patients received concurrent hyperfractionated radiation therapy (37.5 to 45 Gy) and an intensive 21-day inpatient course of cisplatin, vinblastine, and fluorouracil before undergoing trans-hiatal esophagectomy.[68] Thirty-six (84%) patients had a curative surgical resection and 10 (24%) had a pathologically complete response. Myelosuppression and severe esophagitis were the major toxic effects. Two patients died of treatment-related causes before undergoing surgery. The median survival time was 29 months; 34% of patients are alive at 5 years. The best survival results were observed in 6 of the 10 patients who achieved the pathologically complete response. A follow-up study is comparing concurrent preoperative chemoradiotherapy plus surgery with surgery alone and will be most helpful in evaluating the role of intensive chemoradiotherapy.

Naunheim et al[44] investigated 47 patients, with either histologic subtype of esophageal cancer, treated simultaneously with radiation therapy (30 to 36 Gy) and cisplatin plus fluorouracil. Of the 39 patients taken to surgery, 83% (or 66% of the entire group) had a curative resection. Eight patients (21%) had a pathologically complete response. Siewart et al[69] reported a significant improvement in survival compared with their historical controls in 58 patients with adenocarcinoma treated concurrently with cisplatin, fluorouracil, and leucovorin (folinic acid) and radiation therapy (76% of patients remain alive at 24 months).[69]

Gill et al[70] compared the patterns of failure after preoperative (fluorouracil plus cisplatin and 36-Gy radiation) with those of chemotherapy and radiation therapy (54 to 60 Gy) without surgery and found the local failure rates to be similar (17% vs 12%) whether or not surgery was performed. Distant metastases were the predominant sites of failure. In addition, there was a higher rate of complete durable relief of dysphagia in patients receiving radiation therapy and chemotherapy than in those who also had surgery.

Concurrent radiation therapy and chemotherapy results in substantial morbidity and up to a 15% therapy-related mortality rate,[44,68,71] with the respiratory distress syndrome being a major complication.[72] This strategy might prove highly effective in the future, but more cmphasis is required on the development of less toxic combinations with newer radiation enhancers. The other important option to consider is sequential chemotherapy and radiation therapy.

The role of preoperative concurrent chemotherapy and radiation therapy remains to be defined, but this strategy seems to result in a higher rate of pathologically complete responses than does preoperative chemotherapy alone.

Definitive Radiation Therapy and Chemotherapy: Promising pilot study results with concurrent chemotherapy and radiation therapy[73-76] prompted prospectively randomized trials. The Eastern Cooperative Oncology Group studied 130 patients who had unresectable squamous-cell carcinomas treated with radiation therapy (40 Gy) with or without fluorouracil and mitomycin.[77]

A survival advantage was observed in patients who received the combined-modality therapy (14.9 vs 9 months). To some extent, however, the results might have been influenced by the surgical salvage accomplished in some patients. This study has not yet been published.

Araujo et al[78] compared radiation therapy with a combination of fluorouracil, mitomycin, and bleomycin plus radiation therapy in a small number of patients and found no differences in statistical survival between the two arms. Hatlevoll et al[79] also compared radiation therapy alone with two sequential courses of bleomycin and cisplatin followed by radiation therapy in 97 patients with squamous-cell carcinoma and demonstrated no statistically significant survival advantage with either treatment.

A study conducted by the Radiation Therapy Oncology Group[80] demonstrated a statistically significant but modest survival advantage (12.5 vs 8.9 months) favoring combined-modality treatment over radiation therapy alone in patients who had unresectable tumors or were medically unfit for surgery. Sixty patients were randomized to receive radiation therapy (50 Gy) alone and 61 patients to receive combined-modality therapy consisting of four courses of fluorouracil and cisplatin given concurrently with radiation therapy (45 Gy).

In this trial, 40% of patients receiving radiation therapy alone had persistent local disease; an additional 24% developed local relapse after a short median follow-up. In contrast, the combined-modality arm had a 43% local failure rate ($P = .005$). However, the local failure rate at longer follow-up will be more meaningful. The modest improvement in survival among patients who received chemotherapy and radiation therapy was associated with substantial morbidity because of severe myelosuppression and mucositis. In addition, less than 60% of the patients completed the planned combined-modality therapy.

The combination of chemotherapy and radiation therapy suggests benefit for both local control and, albeit modest, overall survival. This approach may be appropriate for patients with either unresectable squamous-cell carcinoma or those who are medically unfit to undergo surgery.[81] A relatively high local failure rate remains a concern, as does patient compliance and morbidity. Overall, there seems to be increasing interest in studying concurrent chemotherapy and radiation therapy, either as preoperative therapy or definitive therapy. Patients with adenocarcinoma histology have not yet been adequately studied.

The challenges lie ahead for investigators to develop less toxic chemoradiotherapy regimens. In addition, there is growing momentum to develop strategies to compare the effectiveness of chemoradiotherapy with that of surgery in patients with locoregional carcinoma of the esophagus.

Palliative Therapy

Surgical bypass to alleviate dysphagia is no longer recommended on a routine basis. There are a number of appropriate palliative approaches, but discussion of these is beyond the scope of this chapter. Significant palliation for a limited time may be obtained with radiation therapy in approximately 50% of patients.[80] In addition, the use of concurrent fluorouracil with less than 45 Gy of radiation therapy might produce the most effective palliation without prohibitive morbidity.[81]

Cost

The cost of cancer therapy is a growing concern in the current milieu of health-care reform. Treatment cost for patients with carcinoma of the esophagus is high, and long-term benefits have not yet been demonstrated. There will be increasing scrutiny of our standard treatment and research approaches as related to the cost of care. At the present time, available information is scanty and remains to be validated, but more data are likely to appear in the next 2 years.

CURRENT OPTIONS, FUTURE DIRECTIONS

Significant advances have been made in the management of patients with carcinoma of the esophagus. Improvements in short-term outcome have resulted from advances in all disciplines. Combined-modality therapeutic approaches have taken the central stage in the management of carcinoma of the esophagus. The major limitations at present include the lack of more effective cytotoxic therapy and less toxic chemoradiotherapy. Substantial efforts are underway to improve combined-modality therapy for carcinoma of the esophagus.

With regard to the current therapeutic options for locoregional carcinoma of the esophagus:

(1) For severe dysplasia with or without Barrett's esophagus and with or without aneuploidy, consider chemoprevention protocols, frequent close observations, or surgical resection as a last resort.

(2) For the above conditions with carcinoma in situ (with or without invasion), consider surgical resection.

(3) For a T1 or T2 primary tumor with N0 and M0 status, consider surgical resection or chemoradiotherapy for patients medically unfit for surgery.

(4) For a T2 or T3 primary tumor with N1 and M0 status, consider investigational studies, surgical resection, or chemoradiotherapy for the medically unfit.

(5) For a T4 primary tumor with any N and M0 status, consider chemoradiotherapy or investigational studies and other palliative options as appropriate.

The aim of preoperative therapy must be to increase the rate of pathologically complete responses. Hyperfractionated radiation therapy, the search for new radiation enhancers, and sequential therapy must also be investigated. Nevertheless, the combined-modality therapy has demonstrated short-term benefit for patients with locoregional carcinoma of the esophagus, and we remain optimistic that further research efforts will translate into long-term benefits for our patients.

The search must continue for novel therapeutic agents, novel approaches, and exploitation of the unique biologic features of precancerous and cancerous tissues. Analyses of molecular events underlying the development of esophageal cancer may yield new strategies for diagnosis, prevention, and therapy.

REFERENCES

1. Wingo PA, Tong T, Bolden S: Cancer statistics, 1995. CA Cancer J Clin 45:8–30, 1995.

2. Blot WJ, Devesa SS, Kneller RW, et al: Rising incidence of adenocarcinoma of the esophagus and gastric cardia. JAMA 265:1287–1289, 1991.

3. Reed PI: Changing pattern of esophageal cancer. Lancet 338:178, 1991.

4. Neshat K, Sanchez CA, Galipeau PC, et al: Barrett's esophagus: The biology of neoplastic progression. Gastroenterol Clin Biol 18:D71–76, 1994.

5. Avoki T, Mori T, Du X, et al: Allelotype study of esophageal carcinoma. Gene Chromosom Cancer 10:177–182, 1994.

6. Mori T, Avoki T, Matsubara T, et al: Frequent loss of heterozygosity in the region including BRCA1 on chromosome 17q in squamous cell carcinomas of the esophagus. Cancer Res 54:1638–1640, 1994.

7. Zhou X, Tarmin L, Yin J, et al: The MTSI gene is frequently mutated in primary human esophageal tumors. Oncogene 9:3737–3741, 1994.

8. Tarmin L, Yin J, Zhou X, et al: Frequent loss of heterozygosity on chromosome 9 in adenocarcinoma and squamous cell carcinoma of the esophagus. Cancer Res 54:6094–6096, 1994.

9. Liu Q, Yan YX, McClure M, et al: MTS-1 (CDKN2) tumor suppressor gene deletions are a frequent event in esophagus squamous cancer and pancreatic adenocarcinoma cell lines. Oncogene 10:619–622, 1995.

10. Sarbia M, Porschen R, Borchard F, et al: p53 protein expression and prognosis in squamous cell carcinoma of the esophagus. Cancer 74:2218–2223, 1994.

11. Vijeyasingam R, Darnton SJ, Jenner K, et al: Expression of p53 protein in oesophageal carcinoma. Br J Surg 81:1623–1626, 1994.

12. Rice TW, Goldblum JR, Falk GW, et al: p53 immunoreactivity in Barrett's metaplasia, dysplasia, and carcinoma. J Thorac Cardiovasc Surg 108:1132–1137, 1994.

13. Jones DR, Davidson AG, Summers CL, et al: Potential application of p53 as an intermediate biomarker in Barrett's esophagus. Ann Thorac Surg 57:598–603, 1994.

14. Huibregtse JM, Scheffner M, Howley PM: A cellular protein mediates association of p53 with the E6 oncoprotein of human papillomavirus types 16 or 18. EMBO J 10:4129–4135, 1991.

15. Powell SM, Papadoupoulos N, Kinzler KW, et al: APC gene mutations in the mutation cluster region are rare in esophageal cancers. Gastroenterology 107:1759–1763, 1994.

16. Stemmermann G, Heffelfinger SC, Noffsinger A, et al: The molecular biology of esophageal and gastric cancer and their precursors: Oncogenes, tumor suppressor genes, and growth factors. Hum Pathol 25:968–981, 1994.

17. Itakura Y, Sasano H, Shiga C, et al: Epidermal growth factor receptor overexpression in esophageal carcinoma. An immunohistochemical study correlated with clinicopathologic findings and DNA amplification. Cancer 74:795–804, 1994.

18. Iihara K, Shiozaki H, Tahara H, et al: Prognostic significance of transforming growth factor-alpha in human esophageal carcinoma: Implications for the autocrine proliferation. Cancer 71:2902–2909, 1993.

19. Kanda Y, Nishiyama Y, Shimada Y, et al: Analysis of gene

amplification and overexpression in human esophageal-carcinoma cell lines. Int J Cancer 58:291–297, 1994.

20. Nakamura T, Nekarda H, Hoelscher AH, et al: Prognostic value of DNA ploidy and c-erb-2 oncoprotein overexpression in adenocarcinoma of Barrett's esophagus. Cancer 73:1785–1794, 1994.

21. Shiga C, Shiga K, Hirayama K, et al: Prognostic significance of hst-1 gene amplification in primary esophageal carcinomas and its relationship to other prognostic factors. Anticancer Res 14: 651–656, 1994.

22. Galiana C, Fusco C, Martel N, et al: Possible role of activated ras genes in human esophageal carcinogenesis. Int J Cancer 54:978–982, 1993.

23. Jiang W, Zhang YJ, Kahn SM, et al: Altered expression of the cyclin D1 and retinoblastoma genes in human esophageal cancer. Proc Natl Acad Sci USA 90:9026–9030, 1993.

24. Beatty JD, DeBoer G, Rider WD: Carcinoma of the esophagus: Pretreatment assessent, correlation of radiation treatment parameters with survival, and identification and management of radiation treatment failure. Cancer 43:2254–2267, 1979.

25. Shao LF, Gao ZG, Yang NP, et al: Results of surgical treatment in 6,123 cases of carcinoma of the esophagus and gastric cardia. J Surg Oncol 42:170–174, 1989.

25a. Sobin LH, Hermanek P, Hutter RVP: TNM classification of malignant tumors: A comparison between the new (1987) and the old editions. Cancer 6:2310–2314, 1988.

26. Tio T, Cohen P, Coene P, et al: Endosonography and computed tomography of esophageal carcinoma. Gastroenterology 96:1478–1486, 1989.

27. Rusch VW, Levine DS, Haggitt R, et al: The management of high grade dysplasia and early cancer in Barrett's esophagus. Cancer 74:1225–1229, 1994.

28. Earlam R, Cunha-Melo JR: Oesophageal squamous cell carcinoma: II. A critical review of radiotherapy. Br J Surg 67:457–461, 1980.

29. Caspers RJ, Welvaart K, Verkes RJ, et al: The effect of radiotherapy on dysphagia and survival in patients with esophageal cancer. Radiother Oncol 12:15–23, 1988.

30. Harrison LB, Fogel TD, Picone JR, et al: Radiation therapy for squamous cell carcinoma of the esophagus. J Surg Oncol 37:40–43, 1988.

31. Earlam R: An MRC prospective randomized trial of radiotherapy versus surgery for operable squamous cell carcinoma of the esophagus. Ann R Coll Surg Engl 73:8–12, 1991.

32. Cooper JD, Jamieson WR, Blair N, et al: The palliative value of surgical resection for carcinoma of the esophagus. Can J Surg 24:145–147, 1981.

33. Pakisch B, Kohek P, Poier E, et al: Iridium-192 high dose rate brachytherapy combined with external beam irradiation in non-resectable oesophageal cancer. Clin Oncol 5:154–158, 1993.

34. Caspers RJ, Zwinderman AH, Griffioen G, et al: Combined external beam and low dose rate intraluminal radiotherapy in oesophageal cancer. Radiother Oncol 27:7–12, 1993.

35. Ajani JA, Roth JA, Ryan MB, et al: Evaluation of pre- and postoperative chemotherapy for resectable adenocarcinoma of the esophagus or gastroesophageal junction. J Clin Oncol 8:1231–1238, 1990.

36. Anderson LL, Lad TE: Autopsy findings in squamous-cell carcinoma of the esophagus. Cancer 50:1587–1590, 1982.

37. Bosch A, Frias Z, Caldwell WL, et al: Autopsy findings in carcinoma of the esophagus. Acta Radiol Oncol 18:103–112, 1979.

38. Wittes RE, Adrianza ME, Parsons R, et al: Compilation of phase II results with single antineoplastic agents. Cancer Treat Symposia 4:91–130, 1985.

39. Kelsen D: Treatment of advanced esophageal cancer. Cancer 50:2576–2581, 1982.

40. Panettiere F, Leichman L, O'Bryan, et al: Cisdiamminedichloride platinum (II), an effective agent in treatment of epidermoid carcinoma of the esophagus. Cancer Clin Trials 76:643–654, 1981.

41. Vogl SE, Greenwald E, Kaplan BH: Effective chemotherapy for esophageal cancer with methotrexate, bleomycin, and cis-diamminedichloroplatinum II. Cancer 48:2555–2558, 1981.

42. Iizuka T, Kakegawa T, Ide H, et al: Phase II evaluation of cisplatin and 5-fluorouracil in advanced squamous cell carcinoma of the esophagus: A Japanese Esophageal Oncology Group Trial. Jpn J Clin Oncol 22:172–176, 1992.

43. Leichman L, Berry BT: Experience with cisplatin in treatment regimens for esophageal cancer. Semin Oncol 18:64–72, 1991.

44. Naunheim KS, Petruska PJ, Roy TS, et al: Preoperative chemotherapy and radiotherapy for esophageal carcinoma. J Thorac Cardiovasc Surg 103:887–895, 1992.

45. Ajani JA, Roth JA, Ryan MB, et al: Intensive preoperative chemotherapy with colony-stimulating factor for resectable adenocarcinoma of the esophagus or gastroesophageal junction. J Clin Oncol 11:22–28, 1993.

46. Wilson SE, Hiatt JR, Stabile BE, et al: Cancer of the distal esophagus and cardia: Preoperative irradiation prolongs survival. Am J Surg 150:114–121, 1985.

47. Launois B, Delarue D, Campion JP, et al: Preoperative radiotherapy for carcinoma of the esophagus. Surg Gynecol Obstet 153:690–692, 1981.

48. Gignoux M, Buyse M, Segol P, et al: Radiotherapie preoperatoire du cancer de l'oesophage: Chu Cote de nacre et centre francois baclesse et centre henri becquerel. Acta Chirurgica Belgica 81:373–379, 1982.

49. Wang M, Gu XZ, Huang GJ, et al: Randomized clinical trial on the combination of preoperative irradiation and surgery in the treatment of esophageal carcinoma: Report on 206 patients. Int J Radiat Oncol Biol Phys 16:325–327, 1989.

50. Arnott SJ, Duncan W, Kerr GR, et al: Low dose preoperative radiotherapy for carcinoma of the oesophagus: Results of a randomized clinical trial. Radiotherapy Oncol 24:108–113, 1992.

51. Diehl LF: Radiation and chemotherapy in the treatment of esophageal cancer. Gastroenterol Clin North Am 20:765–774, 1991.

52. Kasai M, Mori S, Watanabe T: Follow-up results after resection of thoracic esophageal carcinoma. World J Surg 2:543–551, 1980.

53. Fok M, Sham JS, Choy D, et al: Postoperative radiotherapy for carcinoma of the esophagus: A prospective, randomized controlled study. Surgery 113:138–147, 1993.

54. Teniere P, Hay J-M, Fingerhut A, et al: Postoperative radiation therapy does not increase survival after curative resection for squamous cell carcinoma of the middle and lower esophagus as shown by a multicenter controlled trial. Surg Gyn Obstet 173:123–130, 1991.

55. Goldie J, Coldman A: The genetic origin of drug resistance in neoplasms: Implications for systemic therapy. Cancer Res 44:3643–3653, 1984.

56. Fisher B, Gunduz N, Coyle J, et al: Presence of a growth-stimulating factor in serum following primary tumor removal in mice. Cancer Res 49:1996–2001, 1989.

57. Fisher B, Saffer E, Rudock C, et al: Effect of local or systemic treatment prior to primary tumor removal on the production of and response to a serum growth-stimulating factor in mice. Cancer Res 49:2002–2004, 1989.

58. Kelsen DP: Chemotherapy for local-regional and advanced esophageal cancer, in Devita VT Jr, Hellman S, Rosenberg SA (eds): Cancer, Principles and Practices of Oncology, vol 2, 3rd ed. Philadelpha, JB Lippincott, 1989.

59. Wilke H, Stahl M, Preusser P, et al: Phase II trials of 5-FU, folinic acid, etoposide and cisplatin ± surgery in advanced esophageal cancer. Proc Am Soc Clin Oncol 11:170, 1992.

60. Roth JA, Pass HI, Flanagan MM, et al: Randomized clinical trial of preoperative and postoperative chemotherapy with cisplatin, vindesine, and bleomycin for carcinoma of the esophagus. J Thorac Cardiovasc Surg 96:242–248, 1988.

61. Kelsen D, Minsky B, Smith M, et al: Preoperative therapy for esophageal cancer: A randomized comparison of chemotherapy versus radiation therapy. J Clin Oncol 8:1352–1361, 1990.

62. Ajani JA, Ryan B, Rich TA, et al: Prolonged chemotherapy for localized squamous cell carcinoma of the esophagus. Eur J Cancer 28:880–884, 1992.

63. Franklin R, Steiger Z, Vaishampayan G, et al: Combined modality therapy for esophageal squamous carcinoma. Cancer 51:1062–1071, 1983.

64. Steiger Z, Franklin R, Wilson RF, et al: Eradication and palliation of squamous cell carcinoma of the esophagus with chemotherapy, radiotherapy and surgical therapy. J Thorac Cardiovasc Surg 82:713–719, 1981.

65. Denham JW, Gill PG, Jamieson GG, et al: Preliminary experience with a combined-modality approach to the management of oesophageal cancer. Med J Aust 148:9–13, 1988.

66. Poplin E, Fleming T, Leichman L, et al: Combined therapies for squamous cell carcinoma of the esophagus, a Southwest Oncology Group Study (SWOG-8037). J Clin Oncol 5:622–628, 1987.

67. Mercke C, Albertsson M, Hambraeus G, et al: Cisplatin and 5-FU combined with radiotherapy and surgery in the treatment of squamous cell carcinoma of the esophagus. Acta Oncol 30:617–622, 1991.

68. Forastiere AA, Orringer MB, Perez-Tamayo C, et al: Preoperative chemoradiation followed by transhiatal esophagectomy for carcinoma of the esophagus: Final report. J Clin Oncol 11:1118–1123, 1993.

69. Siewart JR, Hoff SJ, Merrill MS, et al: Improved survival with neoadjuvant therapy and resection for adenocarcinoma of the esophagus. Ann Surg 218:571-576, 1993.

70. Gill PG, Denham JW, Jamieson GG, et al: Patterns of treatment failure and prognostic factors associated with the treatment of esophageal carcinoma with chemotherapy and radiotherapy either as sole treatment or followed by surgery. J Clin Oncol 10:1037–1043, 1992.

71. Urba SG, Orringer MB, Perez-Tamamyo C, et al: Concurrent preoperative chemotherapy and radiation therapy in localized esophageal adenocarcinoma. Cancer 69:285–291, 1992.

72. Scholz J, Steinhofel U, Durig M, et al: Postoperative pulmonary complications in patients with esophageal cancer. Clin Invest 71:294–298, 1993.

73. Keane TJ, Harwood AR, Elhakim T, et al. Radical radiation therapy with 5-fluorouracil infusion and mitomycin C for oesophageal squamous carcinoma. Radiother Oncol 4:205–210, 1985.

74. Coia LR, Engstrom PF, Paul A: Nonsurgical management of esophageal cancer: Report of a study of combined radiotherapy and chemotherapy. J Clin Oncol 5:1783–1790, 1987.

75. Coia LR, Paul AR, Engstrom PF: Combined radiation and chemotherapy as primary management of adenocarcinoma of the esophagus and gastroesophageal junction. Cancer 61:643–649, 1988.

76. Coia LR, Engstrom PF, Paul A, et al: Long-term results of infusional 5FU mitomycin-C and radiation as primary management of esophageal carcinoma. Int J Radiat Oncol Biol Phys 2029–2036, 1991.

77. Sischy B, Haller D, Smith T, et al: Interim report of EST 1282 phase II protocol for the evaluation of combined modalities in the treatment of patients with carcinoma of the esophagus, stage I and II. Proc Am Soc Clin Oncol 9:105, 1990.

78. Araujo CM, Souhami L, Gil RA, et al: A randomised trial comparing radiation therapy versus concomitant radiation therapy and chemotherapy in carcinoma of the thoracic esophagus. Cancer 67:2258–2261, 1991.

79. Hatlevoll R, Hagen S, Hansen HS, et al: Bleomycin/cisplatin as neoadjuvant chemotherapy before radical radiotherapy in localized, inoperable carcinoma of the esophagus: A prospective randomized multicentre study: The second Scandinavian trial in esophageal cancer. Radiother Oncol 24:114–116, 1992.

80. Herskovic A, Martz K, Al-Sarraf M, et al: Combined chemotherapy and radiotherapy compared with radiotherapy alone in patients with cancer of the esophagus. N Engl J Med 326:1593–1598, 1992.

81. Haller DG: Treatments for esophageal cancer. N Engl J Med 326:1629–1630, 1992.

CHAPTER 15

Gastric Carcinoma

Philip Agop Philip, MB, ChB, PhD, MRCP, *and* Jaffer A. Ajani, MD

Department of Gastrointestinal Medical Oncology and Digestive Diseases
The University of Texas M. D. Anderson Cancer Center, Houston, Texas

Despite an overall rise in the incidence of gastro-intestinal malignancies in the United States, there has been a significant decrease in the incidence of adenocarcinoma of the stomach over the past few decades. Nevertheless, gastric carcinoma remains the eighth leading cause of cancer death in the United States.[1] In 1995, an estimated 22,800 new cases of gastric cancer will occur in the United States, 14,000 of which will occur in men, and approximately 14,700 patients will die of this disease. Unfortunately, only a small fraction of patients with gastric carcinoma present with localized disease.[2] The 5-year survival rate of less than 20%[1] has not changed significantly during the past 30 to 40 years.

EPIDEMIOLOGY

The incidence of gastric carcinoma varies widely throughout the world. Countries such as Japan and Chile have incidence rates as high as 78/10,000 and 70/100,000 population, respectively.[3] In contrast, in the United States, the rate is only 10/100,000 persons.[4] In addition, studies among migrants have shown that emigrants from high-incidence countries to low-incidence locations often experience a decreased risk of developing gastric carcinoma. This reduction in the risk was seen in subsequent generations and to a lesser degree in the first generation.[5] Such findings strongly suggest that environmental factors play an important role in the etiology of gastric cancer and that exposure to risk factors occurs early in life.

Over the past 30 years, the incidence of gastric carcinoma in the United States has decreased by approximately 20%, whereas the mortality rate has decreased by 30%.[6] Although the reason for the decline in incidence is not entirely known, it probably is related to changes in dietary habits and food preservation.

Predisposing Factors and Premalignant Disease

Chemical carcinogens have been thought to represent a major environmental etiologic factor in the pathogenesis of gastric cancer. Sugimura and Fujimura[7] reported that N-nitroso compounds formed by the interaction of dietary nitrite and amide compounds could induce gastric carcinogenesis in experimental animals. However, other studies have shown that increased consumption of processed, smoked, or salted meat and fish, which are high sources of N-nitroso compounds, is not consistently associated with an increased risk of gastric carcinoma.[8] Diets low in vegetables, fruits, milk, and vitamin A and high in fried food, processed meat, and fish and alcohol have been associated with an increased risk of gastric carcinoma in several cohort studies.[9] Diets low in citrus fruit show the strongest association with gastric carcinoma. The protection afforded by vegetables and fruits is most likely related to their vitamin C content, which is thought to reduce the formation of carcinogenic N-nitroso compounds inside the stomach. Cooked vegetables, however, do not show the same protective effect as uncooked vegetables.[10]

There is also evidence that fiber-rich foods[11] can decrease the formation of N-nitroso compounds. Calcium and vitamin A are postulated to protect the gastric mucosa against carcinogenesis by chemicals. Although no consistent association has been found between alcohol and tobacco consumption and an increased risk of gastric carcinoma,[10] a number of prospective studies have linked cigarette smoking with an increased risk of this cancer.[12]

Gastric resection also has been implicated as a predisposing factor for gastric carcinoma. Giarelli et al[13] reviewed autopsy results of 480 patients who had undergone gastric resections for benign disease and found that 31 (6.5%) of these patients had gastric-stump carcinomas. The mechanism is believed to be related to duodeno gastric bile reflux.[14] Other epidemiologic studies of patients who underwent gastric operations for benign disease[15,16] suggest that the achlorhydria and atrophic gastritis that often occur after such procedures induce premalignant changes. However, the drawback to these studies is the absence of complete matching between the study and control groups for other environmental and life-style factors besides gastric surgery.

At least two premalignant conditions—intestinal metaplasia and pernicious anemia—may lead to gastric carcinoma. Intestinal metaplasia has a higher incidence in countries with a higher incidence of gastric carcinoma,[17] and the former has been shown to precede gastric carcinoma.[18] The estimated risk of developing gastric carcinoma in a patient with pernicious anemia is 20 times higher than the risk in age-matched controls.[19]

The role of chronic *Helicobacter pylori* infection in gastric carcinogenesis remains controversial. Current evidence shows an association between serologic positivity for *Helicobacter* infection and the subsequent risk of developing gastric cancer.[20] It is hypothesized that early life acquisition of *H pylori* increases the risk of developing both gastric cancer and gastric ulcer.[21]

PATHOLOGY AND PROGNOSIS

More than 95% of malignant gastric neoplasms are adenocarcinomas; the remaining 5% consist of lymphomas, leiomyosarcomas, and, infrequently, carcinoid tumors, carcinosarcomas, and squamous-cell carcinomas.[22] Gastric cancer in humans is characterized by two histopathologic patterns that have demonstrated value in terms of epidemiologic parameters of demographic distribution and survival. The most common variant in populations at high risk for such cancer is the so-called intestinal type, in which malignant cells are united with each other to form glandular structures that somewhat resemble the glands of the gastrointestinal tract. The overriding etiologic factors in this type are of an environmental nature and are related to diet and infection. Diffuse carcinomas are relatively more common in populations at low risk of developing gastric cancer. Environmental factors appear to be of less etiologic significance than genetic influences are in diffuse carcinomas.[22a]

Gastric carcinoma tends to invade through the gastric wall early and can involve adjacent structures, such as the transverse colon, pancreas, greater and lesser omentum, biliary tract, liver, and peritoneal ligaments. Even if gastric tumors do not involve adjacent structures, it is not uncommon for a T3 lesion to shed in the peritoneal cavity.[23]

A common site of involvement in peritoneal seeding is Blumer's rectal shelf. In addition to regional spread, metastases can spread through the submucosal and subserosal lymphatic channels into the regional lymph nodes. The more commonly involved lymph nodes include those in the gastrohepatic ligament, celiac, and gastroduodenal region. The liver is the most common site of hematogenous metastasis,[24] followed by the lungs and bones.

Tumor penetration, nodal metastases, location in the stomach, multicentricity, and distant metastases (TNM stage) have been the most important guides to prognosis in patients with gastric cancer.[22] Certain pathologic features of gastric carcinoma, such as the gross appearance of the tumor have prognostic significance. More than one third of stomach carcinomas present as ulcers and show extensive submucosal infiltration that often involves the serosa.[25] One fourth of tumors are scirrhous, with diffuse infiltration of the stomach wall leading to a marked fibrotic reaction. The 5-year survival rate for patients with scirrhous gastric carcinoma after gastric resection is only 2%,[26] whereas the mucosal or polypoidal type is associated with a better prognosis.

The location of the tumor in the stomach also affects prognosis. A Gastrointestinal Tract Study Group (GITSG) study showed that lesions that occur in the cardia or esophagogastric junction have a poorer prognosis than do more distal lesions.[27] Of note, cancer incidence data show a rise in the incidence of cardia carcinomas,[28] which currently account for one-half of all gastric carcinomas. The reasons for this rise in incidence, however, is unknown. Speculation is that the decrease in distal gastric carcinomas might be linked to a decrease in the rate of *H pylori* gastritis.

The histologic grade of gastric cancer provides no additional prognostic information to the TNM stage. Recently, however, the Goseki histologic grading system was evaluated and showed good correlation with the pattern of tumor spread at necropsy.[29] This grading system, which relies on tubular differentiation and mucous production, also identifies subgroups of patients who have a poorer prognosis than is predicted by TNM staging alone.

MOLECULAR BIOLOGY OF GASTRIC CANCER

The majority of gastric cancers are thought to be caused by environmental factors that result in damage to the mucosa and that inhibits its ability to repair itself.[29a] This response is regulated, in part, by inhibitory and stimulatory factors that are products of proto-oncogenes and tumor-suppressor genes.[30] The molecular basis of the progression of normal gastric epithelial cells through invasive cancer has been slowly emerging in recent years.[31] The development of proper biomarkers associated with specific stages of multistep carcinogenesis as an intermediate study endpoint is strongly needed.

Up to now, the chromosomal changes found in gastrointestinal tumors remain poorly defined, and traditional cytogenetic techniques have been limited by the low number of mitotic cells obtained directly from the tumor and by the degree of karyotypic complexity observed in such mitoses.

Similar to colonic carcinogenesis, multiple genetic aberrations have been shown to involve both oncogenes and tumor-suppressor genes. The latter involve the loss of heterozygosities of several chromosomal loci and mutations in *p53*[32] and *DCC* genes.[33] These mutations, the most common in human malignancies, appear at a variable frequency in patients with gastric cancer.[32] Histologic type, stage, and study size and methodology account for the majority of these variations among the different studies. Some investigators have demonstrated a positive correlation between *p53* mutations and the depth of tumor invasion, lymph-node metastases, and poor clinical outcome.[34] *APC* gene mutations were identified in adenomatous precursors of gastric lesions, which suggests that such mutations play a role in early carcinogenesis.[35]

Epidermal growth factor (EGF), its related peptide transforming growth factor-alpha, and their common receptor epidermal growth factor receptor (EGFR) have been implicated in the control of cell proliferation and differentiation in the gastrointestinal epithelium and may play an important role in gastric carcinogenesis.[36] The coexpression of this receptor together with its ligand EGF in the same tumor correlates with a poor prognosis.[37] Abnormalities of EGFR, EGF, and *HER-2/neu* also have been demonstrated in precursor lesions, which suggests that all have a role in early carcinogenesis.[36] Overexpression of the *HER-2/neu* oncogene has been demonstrated in a significant proportion of gastric cancers with preferential amplification in well-differentiated cancers[38] and independent of EGFR expression.[39] In general, *HER-2/neu* expression is associated with large tumors, lymphatic invasion, metastases, and shorter survival after curative resection.[40,41] In contrast to other gastrointestinal tumors, most studies have found that mutations in K-*ras* and c-*myc* are rare in gastric cancers.[38]

Microsatellite instability and the development of the mutator phenotype are represented by alterations in DNA repeats and are detected in up to one third of gastric cancers, especially in poorly differentiated tumors. They were much more common in advanced-stage disease and were associated with chromosomal losses at 5q and 17p loci but not with tumor-suppressor gene mutations.[42]

The diffuse growth patterns of gastric cancer have been associated with mutations in the E-cadherin gene, which encodes a cell-surface adhesion molecule.[43] Preliminary evidence shows that gastric cancer cells express basic fibroblast growth factor and angiogenin, which function as angiogenic factors during the process of neovascularization.[44]

DIAGNOSIS AND STAGING

Previously, the keystone of diagnosis of gastric carcinoma was an upper gastrointestinal barium study or x-ray. However, a study comparing radiographic findings with endoscopic biopsy results suggested that 9% to 40% of endoscopically positive lesions may be missed by barium studies.[45] Endoscopy and biopsy of all lesions should be mandatory, even for lesions that appear to be benign on radiographic examination. The success rate of a single endoscopic biopsy in correctly identifying malignant gastric carcinoma has been reported to vary widely.[46] Factors affecting the outcome include the tumor's gross appearance, size, and location, as well as the number of biopsies. The more biopsies performed, the higher the yield. In difficult situations, brush cytology may improve the diagnostic yield,[47] and when combined with biopsy, it increases the sensitivity to 96.2%.[48] In ulcerative, infiltrative, and submucosal lesions, fine-needle aspiration enables sampling of submucosal tissues. The biopsy may not be positive in patients with linitis plastica.

In addition to the aforementioned diagnostic tools, endoscopic sonography also may be used in the diagnostic workup and staging of patients. Lightdale et al[49] demonstrated that endoscopic sonography provided a more accurate assessment of the depth of tumor invasion and the spread to regional nodes than did chemotherapy. Serum tumor markers, such as carcinoembryonic antigen and CA19-9, have not proved useful for diagnosing gastric carcinoma because of their low specificity.

The most commonly used system for staging gastric cancer is the TNM system, which is based on postgastrectomy pathologic staging. A recent modification of this system defined a T4 lesion as any tumor invading adjacent structures and eliminated the N3 category. Table 1 lists the American Joint Committee on Cancer's TNM staging of gastric cancer.

TREATMENT

The management of gastric carcinoma is determined primarily by the extent of the disease and ranges from surgical resection to surgery plus adjuvant radiotherapy and chemotherapy for patients with resectable disease to palliative therapy for patients with advanced carcinomas.

Resectable Gastric Carcinoma

Surgery: Surgical resection of gastric cancer is only feasible for tumors below stage T4. Curative resection, which involves removal of the primary tumor and regional lymph nodes with free margins, is useful only in patients with stage T1-2N0M0 tumors. Only 40% of patients who undergo exploratory laparotomy have a curative resection,[50,51] and the majority of these patients eventually develop distant metastases. Even when curative resection is technically feasible, local and regional

TABLE I

TNM Classification of Gastric Cancer

Primary tumor (T)

TX: primary tumor cannot be assessed

T0: no evidence of primary tumor

Tis: carcinoma in situ

T1: tumor invades lamina propria or submucosa

T2: tumor invades the muscularis or the subserosa[a]

T3: tumor invades muscularis propria

T4: tumor invades adjacent structures

Regional lymph nodes (N)

NX: regional lymph node(s) cannot be assessed

N0: no regional lymph-node metastasis

N1: metastasis in perigastric lymph node(s) within 3 cm of the edge of the primary tumor

N2: metastasis in perigastric lymph node(s) more than 3 cm from the edge of the primary tumor or in lymph nodes along the left gastric, common hepatic, splenic, or celiac arteries

Distant metastasis (M)

MX: presence of distant metastasis cannot be assessed

M0: no distant metastasis

M1: distant metastasis

Stage grouping	T	N	M
Stage 0	Tis	N0	M0
Stage IA	T1	N0	M0
Stage IB	T1	N1	M0
	T2	N0	M0
Stage II	T1	N2	M0
	T2	N1	M0
	T3	N0	M0
Stage IIIA	T2	N2	M0
	T3	N1	M0
	T4	N0	M0
Stage IIIB	T3	N2	M0
	T4	N1	M0
Stage IV	T4	N2	M0
	Any T	Any N	M1

Reprinted, with permission, from Soh LT, Ajani JA: Gastric carcinoma, in Pazdur R (ed): Medical Oncology: A Comprehensive Review, p 167. Huntington, NY, PRR Inc, 1993.

treatment failures are common. The median survival of patients who undergo curative resection for gastric cancer is 24 months, and the 5-year survival rate varies from 20% to 30%.[52,53] A study of recurrence patterns in patients with resected gastric carcinoma emphasized the high local-regional failure rate for this disease.[54]

Planning the extent of surgical resection in gastric cancer remains an area of controversy because improved outcome has not been linked conclusively with more radical surgery.[55] A new system designates gastric resections as D-0, D-1, or D-2, depending on the extent of nodal resection. D-0 refers to gastrectomy with incomplete resection of N1 nodes; D-1 and D-2 indicate complete resection of the regional lymph nodes in and outside the perigastric region, respectively. In addition, D-2 resection may also involve resections of other organs, which increases the operative risk.

In Western countries, D-1 resection is the most common operation performed in patients with gastric cancer. In Japan, a systematic approach has been developed to guide the extent of lymph-node dissection. Lymph nodes are classified as N1 through N4, depending on their relation to the primary tumor. N1 and N2 nodes represent regional disease, and N3 and N4 nodes are distant nodal metastases. An improvement in the survival rate (from 33% to 58%) was noted in a large series,[56] as the extent of resection increased from D-1 to D-3. However, the significance of this study was limited by its retrospective nature. In contrast, a review[57] focusing on patients with gastric carcinoma treated between 1936 and 1963 found that survival rates decreased and operative mortality rates increased during the period when extended lymph-node dissection was being performed.

The prognostic relevance of systematic lymph-node dissection was evaluated in a prospective multicenter study of 2,394 patients in Germany.[58] Radical dissection, defined as dissection of 26 or more lymph glands, was compared with standard dissection of fewer than 26 lymph nodes. Multivariate analysis identified radical dissection as an independent prognostic factor in the subgroups of patients with tumor stages II and IIIA as designated by the International Union Against Cancer (UICC). There was no survival advantage in patients with pN2 tumors. There was a significant difference in morbidity and mortality rates between radical and standard lymph-node dissection.[58]

Recently, Bunt et al[59] investigated the effect of the extent of lymph-node resection on the pathologic TNM stage in 473 patients who underwent curative resection for gastric cancer. Tumor upstaging with D-2 resections occurred in 30% of patients. The extent of resection (D-2) together with the diligence of the surgeon in the number of nodes examined accounted, at least partially, for the superior stage-specific survival rates after D-2 resections compared with D-1 resections, without a real survival benefit in individual patients. Bonenkamp et al[60] reported a prospective trial comparing D-1 with D-2 dissections in 996 Dutch patients with gastric cancer. D-2 patients had a higher operative mortality rate than D-1 patients (10% vs 4%, $P = .004$) and experienced increased complications (43% vs 25%; $P < .001$). D-2 patients also had longer postoperative hospital stays (median, 25 vs 18 days). Two prospective randomized studies comparing D-1 with D-2 resections have been completed. Accrual and results currently are pending.

An important issue regarding resection of gastric carcinomas and potential for cure is that of resection-line involvement with the cancer, which also may determine whether additional postoperative therapy is indicated. Data from the British Stomach Cancer Group[61] indicate that of the operations considered potentially curable, 13% involved one or both resection lines, rendering the surgery palliative. Only 9% of patients with stages I to III disease who had resection-line involvement survived beyond 5 years compared with 27% of patients with clear lines.

Adjuvant Therapy: The high incidence of local and distant tumor recurrence after curative surgery for gastric cancer[54] stimulated interest in adjuvant (postoperative) therapy in the hope of improving the long-term outcome for these patients.

Adjuvant Radiotherapy: Radiation treatment alone has been shown to have curative potential in only a small percentage of patients who have residual disease following surgery or in patients with localized unresectable disease.[62] However, available data suggest that radiotherapy might be effective in reducing local-regional recurrence rates and increasing the recurrence-free survival rates.[63] The drawback of external-beam radiotherapy is the sensitivity of the gastric bed to radiation treatment, which limits the radiation dose to between 45 and 50 Gy. To achieve a greater effect from irradiation, fluorouracil has been given concurrently as a radiosensitizer. Sixty-two patients with resectable gastric carcinoma but a poor prognosis were treated with adjuvant fluorouracil (given as three 15-mg/kg intravenous boluses) plus radiation (3,750 cGy over 24 fractions) initiated 3 to 6 weeks after surgery. The 5-year survival rate was superior in the treated group (23%) to that in patients treated with surgery alone (4%).[64]

Another nonrandomized trial conducted by the Eastern Cooperative Oncology Group (ECOG) also showed improvement in survival with postoperative adjuvant chemotherapy and radiotherapy.[65] The current Intergroup protocol addresses the issue of postoperative radiation treatment and chemotherapy in a randomized design. Patients undergoing curative resection of a stomach tumor are randomized to receive either four cycles of fluorouracil and leucovorin (folinic acid) or follow-up without any therapy. Radiotherapy is administered concurrently with the second cycle of chemotherapy. The projected accrual is 550 patients, of whom 350 patients have been enrolled so far.

Adjuvant Chemotherapy. Several controlled adjuvant chemotherapy studies have been conducted in patients with gastric carcinoma.[27,66-73] Of all randomized adjuvant chemotherapy trials, only two have shown a survival benefit for the treated patients. The findings of the two positive trials[27,73] have not been confirmed by another European or North American study. In the GITSG study,[27] 142 patients were randomized to receive postoperative fluorouracil plus semustine (MeCCNU) or surgery alone. The chemotherapy group showed an improved 5-year survival rate (47% vs 33%). Grau et al[73] showed a survival advantage for patients treated with adjuvant mitomycin (Mutamycin), 20 mg/m^2, compared with patients treated with surgery alone.

The use of fluorouracil, doxorubicin (Adriamycin, Rubex), and mitomycin, or FAM, was evaluated by the International Collaborative Cancer Group in 281 patients who were randomized to either adjuvant FAM or no treatment.[70] Although the treated patients showed no improvement in survival, there was a statistically significant difference in the survival rate (41.4% vs 22.8%; $P < .04$) favoring treated patients with T3-4 disease. In another study of gastric carcinoma patients with stages IB, IC, II, and III disease conducted by the Southwest Oncology Group, adjuvant treatment with FAM did not improve survival over the rate achieved without adjuvant treatment.[71] FAM2, which is FAM modified by increasing the drug doses and reducing the interval between treatment cycles, was studied by the European Organization for Research and Treatment of Cancer (EORTC) as an adjuvant therapy.[74] Although the control group had a higher gastric cancer recurrence rate, there was no statistically significant difference in recurrence rates between the treated and untreated groups. The British Stomach Cancer Group trial of surgery alone vs either adjuvant chemotherapy (FAM) or radiotherapy in 436 patients showed no survival advantage at 5 years for patients receiving either form of adjuvant therapy compared with those undergoing surgery alone.[75]

Since the late 1950s, adjuvant chemotherapy has been incorporated routinely into postoperative therapy for patients with gastric carcinoma in Japan. The drug most commonly used in the Japanese regimens is mitomycin. In a randomized study of 2,000 patients followed up for more than 10 years, only the group treated with a medium dose of mitomycin showed a significant survival advantage at 8 years compared with controls (73.6% vs 53.9%).[76] When only patients with stage II disease were considered, the difference in survival rates between the treated and control groups was even greater (75% vs 42%). In contrast, four other randomized studies[77–80] using mitomycin combined with fluoropyrimidine or cytarabine showed no survival benefits except in subgroups with positive lymph nodes and serosal involvement.

A meta-analysis of randomized trials of adjuvant chemotherapy for gastric cancer confirms the finding that adjuvant chemotherapy regimens, although effective in phase II studies, do not significantly improve survival.[81] At present, postoperative chemotherapy cannot be considered standard therapy in patients with curatively resected gastric cancer. New trials of adjuvant treatment of gastric cancer must include a nonchemotherapy control arm unless testing a potentially very active chemotherapy regimen.

Adjuvant Chemoimmunotherapy: Randomized trials of adjuvant chemoimmunotherapy in the management of gastric carcinoma have been reported. Several immunostimulators have been used in patients with gastric cancer. They include bacterial extracts from *Schizophyllum commune*,[82] *Nocardia rubra*,[83,84] *Streptococcus* species[85,86] fungal extracts such as *Streptomyces olivoreticuli*[87] and *Coriolus versicolor*,[86,88] chemicals such as levamisole,[89,90] and protein-bound polysaccharide.[91] Only five of these trials, however, were randomized, and all treated groups showed a survival benefit.[84,86,91–93] Immunotherapy not only improved survival but also decreased the infection rate associated with chemotherapy. Patients with advanced disease who had undergone curative and even noncurative resections benefited most from chemoimmunotherapy, whereas patients who underwent early curative resection or late palliative resection benefited least. Thus, the results obtained to date with chemoimmunotherapy appear more encouraging than those achieved with other adjuvant systemic therapies.

Newer Approaches in Adjuvant Therapy: A newer approach in adjuvant therapy includes the use of intraperitoneal treatment in an attempt to improve local relapse rates. Atiq et al[94] reported results of adjuvant intraperitoneal and systemic therapy after curative resection for T2N1-2M0 or T3-4 any N M0 in 35 patients. Adjuvant intraperitoneal cisplatin (Platinol), 25 mg/m[2], and fluorouracil, 750 mg, were administered daily for 4 days with simultaneous intravenous fluorouracil, 750 mg/m[2], as a continuous intravenous infusion for 24 hours. Five cycles were repeated at monthly intervals. Seven (25%) of 28 patients had disease recurrence; after a median follow-up of 24 months, 51% of patients remained alive and free of disease. Of 16 patients who had recurrence, 13 had an intra-abdominal component. The major two toxic effects were neutropenia and peritoneal fibrosis. The latter was treated with surgical lysis of adhesions.

A more recent study using postoperative intraperitoneal cisplatin showed a pattern of relapse and survival similar to that expected from a comparable population with gastric cancer.[95] Sautner et al[96] reported a randomized study on patients with advanced gastric cancer (stages III and IV) who received intraperitoneal cisplatin postoperatively. No survival advantage was noted; median disease-free survival was 12.7 months compared with 9.7 months in patients treated with surgery alone. Intraperitoneal therapy did not influence the pattern of disease recurrence.

Localized Unresectable Gastric Carcinoma

Approximately two thirds of locally confined gastric tumors are considered to be locally advanced. Such tumors have a poor prognosis, particularly when they are bulky (> T3), located in the cardia, or involve localregional lymph nodes. The aim of initial therapy is either to downstage the tumor to facilitate resection or to reduce the tumor size for palliative purposes.

External-Beam Radiotherapy: Moderate-dose (35 to 40 Gy) external-beam irradiation as a single modality has value in pain palliation but does not improve survival.[97] However, when used concurrently with chemotherapy, it may prolong survival. Moertel et al[98] compared fluorouracil plus radiotherapy at 3,500 to 4,000 cGy with radiotherapy alone in the treatment of patients with locally unresectable gastric carcinoma. There was a 6-month survival advantage favoring patients who received both chemotherapy and radiotherapy. In another study, the GITSG randomized 90 patients with locally advanced gastric carcinoma either to combination chemotherapy, consisting of fluorouracil plus semustine, or to splitcourse radiotherapy, with an intravenous infusion of fluorouracil given during the first 3 days of two radiation courses of 25,000 cGy, separated by a 2-week break, followed by maintenance therapy with fluorouracil plus semustine. In the first 26 weeks, mortality was higher in the combined-modality group. At 3 years, the probability of survival plateaued in the combined-modality arm but continued to fall in the chemotherapy-alone arm.[99]

Intraoperative Radiotherapy: Intraoperative irradiation may be used to deliver effective doses safely to unresectable lesions by moving the sensitive viscera from the radiation field. However, intraoperative irradiation has some disadvantages, which include uncertainty about the dose that can be given as a single fraction and the inability to sterilize bulky tumors with a single treatment.

Abe et al[100] and Abe and Takahashi[101] reported a nonrandomized study in which survival was improved in 194 patients with locally advanced gastric carcinoma treated with single-fraction (2,800 to 4,000 cGy) intraoperative radiation in addition to gastric resection.[101] A prospective, randomized, three-arm study compared surgical resection plus intraoperative radiotherapy with gastrectomy alone in patients with stage I or II disease. The third arm included patients with disease that extended beyond the gastric wall (stages III and IV) who received postoperative external-beam radiotherapy to the upper abdomen. In this small study of 100 patients, there was a significant reduction in the local failure rate in patients who received intraoperative radiotherapy.[102] Further studies are needed to determine the role of intraoperative radiotherapy in the management of unresectable gastric cancer.

Preoperative Chemotherapy: Trials utilizing preoperative chemotherapy aim not only to increase resectability rates but also to improve survival rates and to reduce relapse rates in patients with gastric cancer that can be resected surgically. However, there have been few mature reports of neoadjuvant therapy in patients with gastric cancer, and most of the early reports included patients whose tumors were initially unresectable. Stephens[103] reported that 11 of 27 patients were disease free 1 to 5 years after preoperative FAM plus carmustine (BiCNU) given intra-arterially. Wilke et al[104] reported on 34 patients with locally advanced, unresectable disease established by initial laparotomy who were treated with etoposide (VePesid), doxorubicin, and cisplatin (EAP).[104] Twenty-three (70%) of 33 patients demonstrated a major response after EAP, with 21% having a clinically complete response. Nineteen of the 23 responders subsequently underwent gastric resection. Five clinically complete responses were pathologically confirmed; 10 patients with clinically partial responses were rendered free of disease after resection. After a median follow-up of 20 months, the relapse rate was 60% in patients who were pathologically free of disease. The median survival time for the entire group of patients was 18 months and for disease-free patients was 24 months. Another two-institution trial treated 48 patients with three cycles of EAP chemotherapy followed by surgery and two additional postoperative cycles.[105] Of 48 patients, 6 achieved a clinically complete response preoperatively, and 9 had partial responses. No pathologically complete responses were noted at the time of resection. Seventy-seven percent of the group achieved a curative resection. The median survival of this group was 15.5 months.

Two recent studies combined preoperative chemotherapy and postoperative intraperitoneal adjuvant therapy. In one study, 38 patients with resectable gastric cancer received neoadjuvant fluorouracil by protracted continuous infusion with cisplatin and weekly leucovorin over 4 weeks.[106] Thirty-five (92%) patients underwent laparotomy, 33 (87%) of whom had gastric resection, with 76% (29) having a total resection with disease-negative margins. Twenty-six (68%) of 38 patients received postoperative intraperitoneal therapy. Four (14%) of 29 patients have had recurrence at a median follow-up of 19 months. The median survival has not been reached at more than 17 months.

Investigators at Memorial Sloan-Kettering Cancer Center reported on 29 patients with high-risk gastric cancer (T3-4 any N M0).[107] The patients were treated with three preoperative cycles of fluorouracil, doxorubicin, and methotrexate (FAMTX) followed by surgical resection and postoperative intraperitoneal and intravenous fluorouracil-based therapy. Of 23 patients who completed therapy, tumors in 18 (78%) patients were operable and tumors in 16 (70%) patients were resectable. Thirteen of 23 patients had curative resections with disease-negative margins. At 6-month median follow-up, 9 (39%) patients remained disease free.

A phase II trial of preoperative chemotherapy recently was reported combining continuous intravenous infusion of fluorouracil (1,000 mg/m^2 for 5 days) and cisplatin (100 mg/m^2 on day 2) repeated every 4 weeks.[108] Thirty patients with locally advanced gastric cancer were entered into this study. One patient achieved a complete response and 14 a partial response. D-0 resections were feasible in 60% of patients, mainly after objective response. No pathologically complete responses were seen in this study.

It should be noted that the rate of complete pathologic responses remains very low in the studies previously described. As such, the impact on survival is limited. No standard preoperative therapy exists for patients with locally advanced or unresectable gastric cancer, and the search for new therapies, possibly with newer agents, should continue. Preoperative chemotherapy also appears to be an attractive tool for clinical investigations in patients with earlier stages of gastric cancer.

Newer Approaches: Preoperative radiotherapy with local microwave hyperthermia has been evaluated in patients with locally advanced gastric cancer.[109] A randomized trial of three groups has been reported of 293 patients who received surgery alone, surgery preceded by preoperative irradiation, or surgery followed by preoperative irradiation and hyperthermia treatment. Preoperative radiotherapy (20 Gy) did not improve the 3- or 5-year survival rate in gastric cancer patients compared with patients who received surgery alone. Local hyperthermia in combination with radiotherapy followed by surgery produced a statistically significant improvement in both the 3- and 5-year survival rates (22.1% and 21.3%, respectively).

Metastatic Gastric Cancer

Advanced gastric cancer encompasses patients with metastatic disease who are not curable with any of the current treatment modalities. Included in this category are patients with localized disease associated with extensive local-regional metastases.

Chemotherapy: As with other gastrointestinal tumors, gastric carcinoma responds to fluorouracil, but with an objective single-agent response of less than 20%.[110] Other agents that achieve approximately a 20% response rate when used as single agents include the anthracyclines,[45] mitomycin,[110] etoposide,[111] and cisplatin.[112] However, most objective responses to these agents are partial and short-lived and have no survival benefit. In general, better responses are seen in patients who have a small tumor volume and a good performance status and in patients who have not been pretreated with other forms of chemotherapy.

Active drugs with nonoverlapping toxic effects can be combined to improve efficacy at tolerable toxicity levels. To date, however, few combination regimens have been shown to be effective against gastric carcinoma. The FAM regimen was reported first for inpatients with advanced gastric carcinoma.[113] The response rate in that study was 42% (all partial responses), and the median duration of survival was 9 months. Subsequent studies using FAM have yielded varied results, with response rates ranging from 17% to 55%, but no complete responses were achieved.[114] A phase III study by the North Central Cancer Therapy Group compared FAM with fluorouracil alone and with fluorouracil plus doxorubicin and found no significant survival difference among the three regimens.[115] These findings suggest that combination chemotherapy may be superior to single-agent fluorouracil.

The FAMTX regimen was based on the in vitro evidence for synergy between fluorouracil and methotrexate. Use of this regimen in the treatment of 187 patients with metastatic gastric carcinoma was reported first by Klein et al.[116] The overall response rate was 43%, with complete responses in 11% of patients. In a study reported by the EORTC,[117] FAMTX achieved an objective response rate of 33% and a complete response rate of 13.4% in 71 patients with advanced gastric cancer; median survival in these patients was 6 months. However, toxicity in the EORTC study was significant, and there were four deaths,

three of which were due to protocol violation. In an EORTC phase III trial comparing FAM with FAMTX,[118] the FAMTX-treated group showed a superior response rate (41% vs 9%) and a superior median survival (40 vs 29 weeks). FAMTX, however, is a complex and expensive regimen with a 50% incidence of severe neutropenia, and therefore it has been abandoned.

The fluorouracil, doxorubicin, and cisplatin regimen has been evaluated by several investigators.[119–121] In these studies, response rates varied between 29% and 55%, but there were no complete responses. The median survival ranged from 4 to 12 months.

Interest in the EAP combination chemotherapy regimen was triggered by reports of possible synergism between cisplatin and etoposide[122,123] and by the reported synergism between cisplatin and doxorubicin.[124] EAP originally was reported to yield an objective response rate of 64%, including a 21% clinically complete response rate when used in the treatment of 67 patients with locally advanced or metastatic gastric carcinoma.[125] In the 12 patients who had advanced local-regional disease, 5 had pathologically complete responses and 7 had partial responses. In the patients with metastatic disease, the objective response rate was 56%, including a 15% complete response rate. The median survival of the entire group was 9 months, but among the complete responders, the median survival was 17 months.

In another series by Wilke et al,[104] 33 patients with locally advanced gastric carcinoma treated with EAP had a response rate of 70%, with a 21% complete response rate (15% pathologically complete responses). In yet another series of patients treated with EAP,[126] the response rate was only 33% (including an 8% clinically complete response rate) but with significant myelotoxicity and an unacceptably high treatment-related mortality rate of 11%. In a prospective, randomized comparison of FAMTX and EAP performed by investigators at Memorial Sloan-Kettering Cancer Center,[127] response rates and median survival durations were similar in the two arms. However, toxicity was more severe in the EAP arm, with four treatment-related deaths. Use of EAP has been abandoned largely because of lower-than-expected response rates and unacceptably high levels of toxicity.

The combination of etoposide, leucovorin, and fluorouracil also has been tested in patients with advanced gastric cancer.[128,129] Reported objective response rates were 48% to 49%, including a 6% to 12% complete response rate. Median survival was 11 to 12.4 months and toxicity was acceptable. This regimen is easier to administer, and results of an EORTC-sponsored study comparing it with fluorouracil and FAMTX are awaited.

Modification of the schedule of fluorouracil administration has been used to improve the efficacy of chemotherapy. A continuous infusion of fluorouracil in combination with other agents has been used in a number of small trials. Response rates have varied from 8% to 66%.[130-132] Furthermore, the predominant toxic effect associated with these continuous infusion regimens was more severe mucositis but less myelosuppression and toxicity to other organs.

Despite all the foregoing attempts to devise an effective chemotherapeutic approach to gastric cancer, there is at present no standard chemotherapy regimen.

Palliative Procedures: Surgery has been used in the palliation of advanced unresectable gastric carcinoma. However, a surgical procedure would be justified only in selected cases of advanced disease. Fujimoto et al[133] treated 30 patients with advanced gastric carcinoma with debulking surgery followed by intraperitoneal hyperthermic perfusion. The catheter for infusion of the perfusate was inserted into the Douglas pouch and upper abdominal cavity during surgical treatment. The perfusate contained mitomycin, and special attention was paid to the effect on cardiorespiratory function. Temperatures at the inflow point and at the Douglas pouch were maintained at 45.0 to 46.3°C and 43.5 to 45.1°C, respectively. The temperature at the pulmonary artery was measured using a Swan-Ganz catheter and was kept below 41°C. Following such treatment, Fujimoto et al reported 2-year survival rates of 45% in the group with intraperitoneal seeding and 56.5% in the group without peritoneal seeding.

Future Directions

The failure pattern after curative resection suggests that there is a high rate of micrometastases before surgery and, thus, a need for adjuvant therapy. However, at present there is no effective chemotherapeutic regimen with tolerable toxicities available for the treatment of metastatic disease. There is a need, in particular, to develop treatment strategies that consistently will result in high complete response rates to alter significantly the natural history of the disease. The type of adjuvant chemotherapy, its timing and scheduling, and route of administration should be considered systematically in future trials if an assumed therapeutic gain is to be demonstrated by adjuvant treatment of gastric cancer.

The plateau reached in treating patients with advanced gastric cancer underscores the need to develop new drugs in the treatment of this disease. Improvements in our understanding of the molecular events that initiate early gastric carcinogenesis and the cellular changes with disease progression will provide potential targets for the development of new treatment strategies. Examples of such approaches include gene therapy to introduce tumor-suppressor genes or to block the expression of oncogenes. Other strategies include targeting critical biochemical steps in tumor cells with antibody- or ligand-guided therapies. Circumventing cytotoxic-drug resistance in tumor cells may be one approach to improve the response to currently available cytotoxic drugs. For example, recent evidence suggests that overexpression of glutathione transferase-π may significantly alter sensitivity to cisplatin and may therefore provide a rational target for biochemical modulation.

Another important issue in the treatment of gastric cancer relates to primary and secondary prevention of the disease. The role of *H pylori* infection is currently under intense investigation. Screening for early premalignant and malignant lesions has been undertaken successfully in Japan and has resulted in significant reduction in the incidence of the disease and marked downstaging of the tumor at presentation.[134] The economic value of such an approach should be determined in Western societies that have seen a significant drop in the incidence of gastric cancer over the past several decades.

REFERENCES

1. Wingo PA, Tong T, Bolden S: Cancer statistics. CA Cancer J Clin 45:8–30, 1995.
2. Dupont BJ Jr, Cohn I Jr: Gastric adenocarcinoma. Curr Probl Cancer 4:25–42, 1980.
3. Dunham LJ, Bailar JC III: World maps of cancer mortality rates and frequency ratios. J Natl Cancer Inst 41:155–203, 1968.
4. Ries LAG, Hankey BF, Miller BA, et al: Cancer Statistics Review, 1973–1988 (NIH publication no. 91-2789). Bethesda, National Institutes of Health, 1988.
5. Haenszel W: Migrant studies, in Schottenfeld D, Fraumeni JF (eds): Cancer Epidemiology and Prevention, pp 194–207. Philadelphia, WB Saunders, 1982.
6. Gloeckler LA, Hankey BF, Miller BA, et al: Cancer Statistics Review, 1973–1988 (NIH Publ 91-2789). Bethesda, National Institutes of Health, 1988.
7. Sugimura T, Fujimura S: Tumor production in glandular stomach of rat by N-methyl-N-nitro-N-nitrosoguanidine. Nature 216:943–944, 1967.
8. Hall CN, Darkin D, Brimblecombe R, et al: Evaluation of the nitrosamine hypothesis of gastric carcinogenesis in precancerous conditions. Gut 27:491–498, 1986.
9. Graham S, Haughey B, Marshall J, et al: Diet in the epidemiology of gastric cancer. Nutr Cancer 13:19–34, 1990.
10. Buiatti E, Palli D, Decarli A, et al: A case-control study of gastric cancer and diet in Italy. Int J Cancer 44:611–616, 1989.
11. Moller ME, Dahl R, Bockman OC: A possible role of the dietary fiber product, wheat bran, as a nitrite scavenger. Food Chem Toxicol 26:841–845, 1988.
12. Hammond EC: Smoking in relation to the death rates of 1 million men and women. Natl Cancer Inst Monogr 19:127–204, 1966.
13. Giarelli L, Melato M, Stanta G: Gastric resection. Cancer 52:1113–1116, 1983.

14. Weiman TJ, Max MH, Volges CR, et al: Diversion of duodenal contents: Its effect on the production of experimental gastric cancer. Arch Surg 115:959–961, 1980.

15. Viste A, Opheim P, Thunold J, et al: Risk of carcinoma following gastric operation for benign disease. Lancet 2:502–505, 1986.

16. Offerhaus GJA, Tersmette AC, Huibregtse K, et al: Mortality caused by stomach cancer after remote partial gastrectomy for benign conditions: Forty years of follow-up of an Amsterdam cohort of 2,633 postgastrectomy patients. Gut 29:1588–1590, 1988.

17. Correa P, Cuello C, Duque E, et al: Carcinoma and intestinal metaplasia of the stomach in Columbian migrants. J Natl Cancer Inst 44:297–305, 1970.

18. Sasajima K, Kawachi T, Matsukura N, et al: Intestinal metaplasia and adenocarcinoma induced in the stomach of rats by *N*-propyl-*N*-nitro-*N*-nitrosoguanidine. J Cancer Res Clin Oncol 94:201–206, 1979.

19. Hitchcock CR, Schneiner SL: Early diagnosis of gastric cancer. Surg Gynecol Obstet 113:655, 1961.

20. Munoz N. Is *Helicobacter pylori* a cause of gastric cancer? An appraisal of the seroepidemiological evidence. Cancer Epidemiol Biomarkers Prev 3:445–451, 1994.

21. Blaser MJ, Chyou PH, Nomura A. Age at establishment of *Helicobacter pylori* infection and gastric carcinoma, gastric ulcer, and duodenal ulcer risk. Cancer Res 55:562–565, 1995.

22. Coit DG, Brennan MF: Gastric neoplasms. In: Moody FG, Carey LC, Jones RS, Kelly KA, Nahrwold DL, Skinner DB, eds, Surgical Treatment of Digestive Disease, pp 212–235. Chicago, Year Book Medical Publishers, 1990.

22a. Aird I, Bentall HH: A relationship between cancer of the stomach and the ABO blood groups. Br Med J 1:799–801, 1953.

23. Sugarbaker PH: Gastric cancer: Therapeutic implications of new concepts of gastric tumor biology. Cancer Treat Res 55:19–25, 1991.

24. Warren S: Studies on tumor metastases: IV. Metastases of cancer of stomach. N Engl J Med 209:825, 1933.

25. Ming SC: Classification of gastric cancer, in Filipi MI, Jass JR (eds): Gastric Carcinoma, pp 297–300. Edinburgh, Churchill Livingstone, 1986.

26. Higgins Ga, Serlin O, Amadeo JH, et al: Gastric cancer factors in survival. Surg Gastrointest 10:393, 1976.

27. Gastrointestinal Tumor Study Group: Controlled trial of adjuvant chemotherapy following curative resection for gastric cancer. Cancer 49:1116–1122, 1982.

28. Blot WJ, Devesa SS, Kneller RW, et al: Rising incidence of adenocarcinoma of the esophagus and gastric cardia. JAMA 265:1287–1289, 1991.

29. Martin IG, Dixon MF, Sue-Ling H, et al. Goseki histological grading of gastric cancer is an important predictor of outcome. Gut 35:758–763, 1994.

29a. Hotz J, Goebell H: Epidemiology and pathogenesis of gastric carcinoma, in Meyer HJ, Schmoll HJ, Hotz J (eds): Gastric Carcinoma, pp 3–15. New York, Springer-Verlag, 1989.

30. Tahara E: Molecular mechanism of stomach carcinogenesis. J Cancer Res Clin Oncol 119:265–272, 1993.

31. Stemmermann G, Heffelfinger SC, Hoffsinger A, et al: The molecular biology of esophageal and gastric cancer and their precursors; Oncogenes, tumor suppressor genes, and growth factors. Hum Pathol 25:968–981, 1994.

32. Hong SI, Hong WS, Jang JJ, et al: Alterations of *p53* gene in primary gastric cancer tissues. Anticancer Res 14:1251–1255, 1994.

33. Barletta C, Scillato F, Sega FM, et al: Genetic alteration in gastrointestinal cancer. A molecular and cytogenetic study. Anticancer Res 13:2325–2330, 1993.

34. Kakeji Y, Korenaga D, Tsujitani S, et al: Gastric cancer with p53 overexpression has high potential for metastasising to lymph nodes. Br J Cancer 67:589–593, 1993.

35. Tamura G, Maesawa C, Suzuki Y, et al. Mutations of the *APC* gene occur during early stages of gastric adenoma development. Cancer Res 54:1149–1151, 1994.

36. Filipe MI, Osborn M, Linehan J, et al. Expression of transforming growth factor alpha, epidermal growth factor receptor, and epidermal growth factor in precursor lesions to gastric carcinoma. Br J Cancer 71:30–36, 1995.

37. Yonemura Y, Takamura H, Ninomiya I, et al: Interrelationship between transforming growth factor alpha and epidermal growth factor receptor in advanced gastric cancer. Oncology 49:157–161, 1992.

38. Yoshida T, Sakamoto H, Terada M: Amplified genes in cancer in upper digestive tract. Semin Cancer Biol 4:33–40, 1993.

39. Lee EY, Cibull ML, Strodel WE, et al: Expression of HER-2/neu oncoprotein and epidermal growth factor receptor and prognosis in gastric carcinoma. Arch Pathol Lab Med 118:235–239, 1994.

40. Uchino S, Tsuda H, Maruyama K, et al: Overexpression of c-erbB-2 protein in gastric cancer. Cancer 72:3179–3184, 1993.

41. Motojima K, Furui J, Kohara N, et al: erbB-2 Expression in well-differentiated adenocarcinoma of the stomach predicts shorter survival after curative resection. Surgery 115:349–354, 1994.

42. Mironov NM, Aguelon MA, Potapova GI, et al: Alterations of (CA)n DNA and tumor suppressor genes in human gastric cancer. Cancer Res 54:41–44, 1994.

43. Becker KF, Atkinson MJ, Reich U, et al: E-cadherin gene mutations provide clues to diffuse type gastric carcinoma. Cancer Res 54:3845–3852, 1994.

44. Li D, Bell J, Brown A, et al: The observation of angiogenin and basic fibroblast growth factor gene expression in human colonic adenocarcinomas, gastric adenocarcinomas, and hepatocellular carcinomas. J Pathol 172:171–175, 1994.

45. Laufer I: Double contrast radiology in the diagnosis of gastrointestinal cancer, in Glass J (ed): Progress in Gastroenterology, pp 643–669. New York, Grune & Stratton, 1977.

46. Moertel CG: The stomach, in Holland JH, Frei E III (eds): Cancer Medicine, pp 1527–1541. Philadelphia, Lea & Febiger, 1973.

47. Winawer SJ, Melamed M, Sherlock P: Potential of endoscopy, biopsy, and cytology in diagnosis and management of patients with cancer. Clin Gastroenterol 5:575, 1976.

48. Monico S, Glansanti M, Fugiani P: Cytodiagnosis of gastric cancer by brushing: 1978–1983. Tumori 73:147–150, 1987.

49. Lightdale C, Botet J, Brennan M, et al: Endoscopic ultrasonography compared to computerized tomography for preoperative staging of gastric cancer. Gastrointest Endosc 35:154, 1989.

50. Bizer LS: Adenocarcinoma of the stomach: Current results of treatment. Cancer 51:743–745, 1983.

51. Lawrence WT, Lawrence W Jr: Gastric cancer: The surgeon's viewpoint. Semin Oncol 7:400–417, 1980.

52. Adashek K, Sanger J, Longmire WP: Cancer of the stomach: Review of consecutive ten-year intervals. Ann Surg 189:6–10, 1979.

53. Weed TE, Nuessle W, Ochsner A: Carcinoma of the stomach: Why are we failing to improve survival? Ann Surg 193:407–413, 1981.

54. Gunderson L, Sosin H: Adenocarcinoma of the stomach: Areas of failure in a reoperation series (second or symptomatic look): Clinicopathologic correlation and implications for adjuvant therapy. Int J Radiat Oncol Biol Phys 8:1–11, 1982.

55. Dalton RR, Eisenberg BL: Rationale for the current surgical management of gastric adenocarcinoma. Oncology 8:99–107, 1994.

56. Kodama Y, Sugimachi K, Soejima K, et al: Evaluation of extensive lymph node dissection for carcinoma of the stomach. World J Surg 5:241, 1981.

57. Gilbertson VA: Results of treatment of stomach cancer: An appraisal of efforts for more extensive surgery and a report of 1,983 cases. Cancer 23:1305–1308, 1969.

58. Siewert JR, Bottcher K, Roder JD, et al: Prognostic relevance of systematic lymph node dissection in gastric carcinoma. Br J Surg 80:1015–1018, 1993.

59. Bunt AMG, Hermans J, Smit VTHBM, et al: Surgical/pathologic-stage migration confounds comparisons of gastric cancer survival rates between Japan and Western countries. J Clin Oncol 13:19–25, 1995.

60. Bonenkamp JJ, Songun I, Hermans J, et al: Randomized comparison of morbidity after D1 and D2 dissection for gastric cancer in 996 Dutch patients. Lancet 345:745–748, 1995.

61. Hallissey MT, Jewkes AJ, Dunn JA, et al: Resection-line involvement in gastric cancer: A continuing problem. Br J Surg 80:1418–1420, 1993.

62. Takahashi T: Studies on preoperative and postoperative telecobalt therapy in gastric cancer. Nippon Acta Radiol 24:129, 1964.

63. Budach VG: The role of radiation therapy in the management of gastric cancer. Ann Oncol 5(suppl):37–48, 1994.

64. Moertel CG, Childs DS, O'Fallon JR, et al: Combined 5-FU and radiation therapy as a surgical adjuvant for poor prognosis gastric carcinoma. J Clin Oncol 2:1249–1254, 1984.

65. Horvath W, Pipoly G, Krupp K: Improved survival in 35 gastric cancer patients treated with postoperative chemoradiotherapy. Proc Ann Meet Am Soc Clin Oncol 9:A428, 1990.

66. Dixon W, Longmire W, Holden W: Use of triethylenethiophosphoramide as an adjuvant to the surgical treatment of gastric and colorectal carcinoma. Ann Surg 173:26–39, 1971.

67. Serlin O, Wokoff J, Amadeo J, et al: Use of 5-fluorodeoxyuridine (FUDR) as an adjuvant to the surgical management of carcinoma of the stomach. Cancer 24:223–228, 1969.

68. The Veterans Administration Surgical Oncology Group: Efficacy of prolonged intermittent therapy with combined 5-FU and methyl-CCNU following resection for gastric carcinoma. Cancer 52:1105–1112, 1983.

69. The Eastern Cooperative Oncology Group: Postoperative adjuvant 5-FU plus methyl-CCNU therapy for gastric cancer patients. Cancer 55:1868–1873, 1985.

70. Coombes R, Schein P, Chivers C: A randomized trial of adjuvant fluorouracil, doxorubicin, and mitomycin with no treatment in operable gastric cancer. J Clin Oncol 8:1362–1369, 1990.

71. MacDonald JS, Gagliano R, Fleming T, et al: A phase III trial of FAM (5-fluorouracil, Adriamycin, mitomycin-C) chemotherapy vs. control as adjuvant treatment for resected gastric cancer: A Southwest Oncology Group trial—SWOG 7804. Proc Am Soc Clin Oncol 11:168, 1992.

72. Krook JE, O'Connell MJ, Wiend HS: Surgical adjuvant therapy of gastric cancer with doxorubicin and 5-fluorouracil: A joint May/North Central Cancer Treatment Group Study. Proc Am Soc Clin Oncol 7:93, 1988.

73. Grau JJ, Estape J, Alcobendas F, et al: Positive results of adjuvant mitomycin-C in resected gastric cancer: A randomized trial on 134 patients. Eur J Cancer 29A:340–342, 1993.

74. Lise M, Nitti D, Buyse M, et al: Results of adjuvant FAM2 regimen in resectable gastric cancer (EORTC Gastrointestinal Tract Cancer Cooperative Group) (GITSG). 92e Congres Français de Chirurgie, Paris, Abstract Book 1:394, 1990.

75. Hallissey MT, Dunn JA, Ward LC, et al: The second British Stomach Cancer Group trial of adjuvant radiotherapy or chemotherapy in resectable gastric cancer: Five-year follow-up. Lancet 343:1309–1312, 1994.

76. Imanaga H, Nakazato H: Results of surgery for gastric cancer and effect of adjuvant mitomycin C on cancer recurrence. World J Surg

1:213–221, 1977.

77. Inokuchi K, Hattori T, Taguchi T, et al: Postoperative adjuvant chemotherapy for gastric cancer. Cancer 53:2393–2397, 1984.

78. Nakajima T, Takahashi T, Takagi K, et al: Comparison of 5-fluorouracil and ftorafur in adjuvant chemotherapies with combined inducive and maintenance therapies for gastric cancer. J Clin Oncol 2:1366–1371, 1984.

79. Hattori T, Inokuchi K, Taguchi T, et al: Postoperative adjuvant chemotherapy for gastric cancer: The second report: Analysis of data on 2,873 patients followed for five years. Jpn J Surg 16:175–180, 1986.

80. Yammura Y, Nakajima T, Iwanaga T, et al: Multidrug adjuvant chemotherapy for gastric cancer performed by the Exploratory Study Group (ESAC) in Japan and Chile. Proc Am Soc Clin Oncol 8:115, 1989.

81. Hermans J, Bonenkamp JJ, Boon MC, et al: Adjuvant therapy after curative resection for gastric cancer: Meta-analysis of randomized trials. J Clin Oncol 11:1441–1447, 1993.

82. Fujimoto S, Furue H, Kimura T, et al: Clinical evaluation of schizophylian adjuvant immunochemotherapy for patients with resectable gastric cancer: A randomized controlled trial. Jpn J Surg 14:286–292, 1984.

83. Ochiai T, Sato H, Hayashi R, et al: Randomly controlled study of chemotherapy versus chemoimmunotherapy in postoperative gastric cancer patients. Cancer Res 43:3001–3007, 1983.

84. Koyama S, Ozaki A, Iwasaki Y, et al: Randomized controlled study of postoperative adjuvant immunochemotherapy with *Nocardia rubra* cell wall skeleton (N-CWS) and Tegafur for gastric carcinoma. Cancer Immunol Immunother 22:148–154, 1986.

85. Kim JP: The concept of immunochemosurgery in gastric cancer. World J Surg 11:645–672, 1987.

86. Hattori T, Nakajima T, Nakazato H, et al: Postoperative adjuvant immunochemotherapy with mitomycin-C, Tegafur, PSK, and/or OK-432 for gastric cancer, with special reference to the change in stimulation index after gastrectomy. Jpn J Surg 20:127–136, 1990.

87. Niimoto M, Saeki T, Toi M, et al: Prospective randomized study on Bestatin in resectable gastric cancer: Third report. Jpn J Surg 20:186–191, 1990.

88. Hattori T, Niimoto M, Koh T, et al: Postoperative long-term adjuvant immunochemotherapy with mitomycin-C, PSK, and FT-207 in gastric cancer patients. Jpn J Surg 13:480–485, 1983.

89. Hattori T, Niimoto M, Toge T, et al: Effects of levamisole in adjuvant immunochemotherapy for gastric cancer: A prospective randomized controlled study. Jpn J Surg 13:480–485, 1983.

90. Niimoto M, Hattori T, Ito I, et al: Levamisole in postoperative adjuvant immunochemotherapy for gastric cancer: A randomized controlled study of the MMC and Tegafur regimen with or without levamisole, Report 1. Cancer Immunol Immunother 18:13–18, 1984.

91. Nakazato H, Koike A, Saji S, et al: Efficacy of immunochemotherapy as adjuvant treatment after curative resection of gastric cancer. Study group of immunochemotherapy with PSK for gastric cancer. Lancet 343:1122–1126, 1994.

92. Niimoto M, Hattori T, Tamada R, et al: Prospective adjuvant immunochemotherapy with mitomycin-C, Futraful, and PSK for gastric cancer: An analysis of data on 579 patients followed for 5 years. Jpn J Surg 18:681–686, 1988.

93. Maehara Y, Moriguchi S, Sakaguchi Y, et al: Adjuvant chemotherapy enhances long-term survival of patients with advanced gastric cancer following curative resection. J Surg Oncol 45:169–172, 1990.

94. Atiq OT, Kelsen DP, Shiu MH, et al: Phase II study of postoperative adjuvant intraperitoneal cisplatin and fluorouracil and systemic fluorouracil chemotherapy in patients with resected gastric cancer. J Clin Oncol 11:425–433, 1993.

95. Jones AL, Trott P, Cunningham D, et al: A pilot study of

intraperitoneal cisplatin in the management of gastric cancer. Ann Oncol 5:123–126, 1994.

96. Sautner T, Hofbauer F, Depisch D, et al: Adjuvant intraperitoneal cisplatin chemotherapy does not improve long-term survival after surgery for advanced gastric cancer. J Clin Oncol 12:970–974, 1994.

97. Wieland C, Hymmen U: Megavoltage therapy for malignant gastric tumors. Strahlentheronkol 140:20–26, 1970.

98. Moertel C, Childs D, Reitemeier R, et al: Combined 5-fluorouracil and supervoltage radiation therapy for locally unresectable gastrointestinal cancer. Lancet 2:865–867, 1969.

99. The Gastrointestinal Study Group: The concept of locally advanced gastric cancer: Effect of treatment on outcome. Cancer 66:2324–2330, 1990.

100. Abe M, Shibamoto Y, Ono K, et al: Intraoperative radiation therapy for carcinoma of the stomach and pancreas. Front Radiat Ther Oncol 25:258–269, 1991.

101. Abe M, Takahashi M: Intraoperative radiotherapy: The Japanese experience. Int J Radiat Oncol Biol Phys 7:863–868, 1981.

102. Sindelar WF, Kinsella TJ, Tepper JE, et al: Randomized trial of intraoperative radiotherapy in carcinoma of the stomach. Am J Surg 165:178–186, 1993.

103. Stephens FO: The role of regional chemotherapy in gastric cancer. Eur J Surg Oncol 20:187–188, 1994.

104. Wilke H, Preusser P, Fink U, et al: Preoperative chemotherapy in locally advanced and nonresectable gastric cancer: A phase II study with etoposide, doxorubicin, and cisplatin. J Clin Oncol 7:1318–1326, 1989.

105. Ajani JA, Roth JA, Bernadette Ryan M, et al: Intensive preoperative chemotherapy with colony-stimulating factor for resectable adenocarcinoma of the esophagus or gastroesophageal junction. J Clin Oncol 11:22–28, 1993.

106. Leichman L, Silberman H, Leichman CG, et al: Preoperative systemic chemotherapy followed by adjuvant postoperative intraperitoneal therapy for gastric cancer. J Clin Oncol 10: 1933–1942, 1992.

107. Schwartz G, Kelsen D, Christman K, et al: A phase II study of neoadjuvant FAMTX and postoperative intraperitoneal 5-FU and cisplatin in high-risk patients with gastric cancer. Proc Am Soc Clin Oncol, A572, 1993.

108. Rougier P, Mahjoub M, Lasser P, et al: Neoadjuvant chemotherapy in locally advanced gastric carcinoma: A phase II trial with combined continuous intravenous 5-fluorouracil and bolus cisplatinum. Eur J Cancer 30A(9):1269–1275, 1994.

109. Shchepotin IB, Evans SR, Chorny V, et al: Intensive preoperative radiotherapy with local hyperthermia for the treatment of gastric carcinoma. Surg Oncol 3:37–44, 1994.

110. Comis S: Integration of chemotherapy into combined modality treatment of solid tumors. Cancer Treat Rev 1:221–238, 1974.

111. Kelsen DP, Magill G, Cheng E, et al: Phase II trial of etoposide (VP-16) in the treatment of upper gastrointestinal malignancies. Proc Am Soc Clin Oncol 1:96, 1982.

112. Lacave A, Izarzugaza I, Aparicio L, et al: Phase II clinical trial of cisdichlorodiommineplatinum in gastric cancer. Am J Clin Oncol 6:35–38, 1983.

113. MacDonald JS, Philip SS, Woolley PV, et al: 5-Fluorouracil, doxorubicin, and mitomycin (FAM) combination chemotherapy for advanced gastric cancer. Ann Intern Med 93:533–536, 1980.

114. Gohmann JJ, MacDonald JS: Chemotherapy of gastric cancer. Cancer Invest 7:39–52, 1980.

115. Cullinan SA, Moertel CG, Fleming TR, et al: A comparison of three chemotherapeutic regimens in the treatment of advanced pancreatic and gastric carcinoma: Fluorouracil vs. fluorouracil and doxorubicin vs. fluorouracil, doxorubicin, and mitomycin. JAMA 253:2061–2067, 1985.

116. Klein HO, Wickramanayake PD, Farrakh GR: 5-Fluorouracil, Adriamycin, and methotrexate: A combination protocol (FAMTX) for treatment of metastasized stomach cancer. Proc Am Soc Clin Oncol 5:84, 1986.

117. Wils J, Bleiberg H, Otilia D, et al: An EORTC Gastrointestinal Group evaluation of the combination of sequential methotrexate and 5-fluorouracil combined with Adriamycin in advanced measurable gastric cancer. J Clin Oncol 4:1799–1803, 1986.

118. Wils JA, Klein HO, Wagener DJ, et al: FAMTX (5-FU, Adriamycin, and methotrexate): A step ahead in the treatment of advanced gastric cancer: A Trial of the European Organization for Research and Treatment of Cancer of the Gastrointestinal Tract Cooperative Group. J Clin Oncol 9:827–831, 1991.

119. Cazap EL, Gisselbrecht Ch, Smith FP, et al: Phase II trials of 5-FU, doxorubicin, and cisplatin in advanced measurable adenocarcinoma of the lung and stomach. Cancer Treat Rep 70:781–783, 1986.

120. Moertel CG, Rubin J, O'Connell MJ, et al: A phase II study of combined 5-fluorouracil, doxorubicin, and cisplatin in the treatment of advanced upper gastrointestinal adenocarcinoma. J Clin Oncol 4:1053–1057, 1986.

121. Wagener DJTH, Yap SH, Wobbes T, et al: Phase II trial of 5-fluorouracil, Adriamycin, and cisplatin (FAP protocol) in advanced gastric cancer. Cancer Chemother Pharmacol 15:86–87, 1985.

122. Mabel JA, Little AD: Therapeutic synergism in murine tumors for combinations of cis-dichlorodiamineplatinum with VP-16-213 or BCNU (abstract). Proc Am Assoc Cancer Res 20:230, 1979.

123. Schabel FM Jr, Trader MW, Laster WR Jr, et al: Cis-dichlorodiamineplatinum (II): Combination chemotherapy and cross-resistance studies with tumors of mice. Cancer Treat Rep 63:1459–1473, 1979.

124. Schabel FM Jr, Skipper HE, Trader MW, et al: Establishment of cross-resistance profiles for new agents. Cancer Treat Rep 42:905–922, 1983.

125. Preusser PH, Wilke H, Achterrath W, et al: Phase II study with the combination of etoposide, doxorubicin, and cisplatin in advanced measurable gastric cancer. J Clin Oncol 7:1310–1317, 1989.

126. Lerner A, Gonin R, Steele GD, et al: Etoposide, doxorubicin, cisplatin (EAP) chemotherapy for advanced gastric adenocarcinoma: Results of a phase II trial. J Clin Oncol 10:536–540, 1992.

127. Kelsen D, Atiq OT, Saltz L, et al: FAMTX versus etoposide, doxorubicin, and cisplatin: A random assignment trial in gastric cancer. J Clin Oncol 10:541–548, 1992.

128. Wilke H, Preusser P, Fink U, et al: High-dose folinic acid/etoposide/5-fluorouracil in advanced gastric cancer: A phase II study in elderly patients or patients with cardiac risk. Invest New Drugs 8:65–70, 1990.

129. Neri B, Gemelli MT, Pantalone D, et al: Epidoxorubicin and high-dose leucovorin plus 5-fluorouracil in advanced gastric cancer: A phase II study. Anticancer Drugs 4:323–326, 1993.

130. Berenberg JL, Goodman PJ, Oishi N, et al: 5-Fluorouracil (5-FU) and folinic acid (FA): For the treatment of metastatic gastric cancer. Proc Am Soc Clin Oncol 8:101, 1989.

131. Lacave AJ, Esteban E, Fernandez-Hidal O, et al: Phase II clinical trial with cisplatin and 5-fluorouracil in gastric cancer: Final results. Proc Am Soc Clin Oncol 7:106, 1988.

132. Kim R, Kim C: Chemotherapy of advanced gastric cancer with mitomycin-C, BCNU, cisplatin, and 5-fluorouracil in combination. Proc Am Soc Clin Oncol 5:78, 1986.

133. Fujimoto S, Shrestha RD, Kokubun M, et al: Positive results of combined therapy of surgery and intraperitoneal hyperthermic perfusion for far-advanced gastric cancer. Ann Surg 212:592–596, 1989.

134. Oshima A, Hirata N, Ubukata T, et al: Evaluation of a mass screening program for stomach cancer with a case-control study design. Int J Cancer 38:829–833, 1986.

CHAPTER 16

Pancreatic, Hepatic, and Biliary Carcinomas

Edgardo Rivera, MD, *and* James L. Abbruzzese, MD

Division of Medicine, The University of Texas M. D. Anderson Cancer Center, Houston, Texas

Pancreatic, hepatic, and biliary carcinomas in adults represent three of the most challenging malignancies facing the oncologist. Although groups at high risk for these malignancies are recognized, screening and early-detection strategies have not been successful. For each neoplasm, surgery represents the only practical curative treatment option. Radiation and chemotherapy have been helpful only in selected clinical circumstances. Hopefully, our evolving understanding of the molecular biology and cellular biochemistry of these neoplasms will provide new approaches for early detection and therapy. This chapter will review the current approaches to management of these three gastrointestinal malignancies.

PANCREATIC CANCER

Pancreatic cancer is the second most common gastrointestinal cancer and the fourth leading cause of cancer death in the United States. The incidence of pancreatic cancer is exceeded only by that of lung, colorectal, skin, prostate, and breast cancers. It is estimated that 24,000 new cases of pancreatic cancer will be diagnosed in the United States during 1995.[1] The median survival of patients with this disease is 3 to 4 months, and the 5-year survival rate is only 3%.[2] One reason for the dismal prognosis is that the initial symptoms of this disease are nonspecific and, thus, the disease is usually advanced with obvious or occult metastases established before a diagnosis is ever made. Currently, most clinical efforts are diagnostic and palliative. The development of successful treatment strategies will be based on the evolving understanding of the molecular events involved in cellular transformation, tumor progression, and regulation of neoplastic growth.

Epidemiology and Etiology

The incidence of cancer of the pancreas increases with age. Risk increases after age 30 years, with most cases ocurring between the ages of 65 and 79. However, the disease has also been reported in younger individuals, including children.[1]

The ratio of males to females affected differs according to age, varying from 2:1 for patients younger than 40 years of age to 1:1 for patients older than 80 years. The slight male predominance prevails in both whites and nonwhites. Pancreatic cancer is more common in Hispanic and African-American than in white populations. The incidence in blacks is 14.9 per 100,000, as compared with 8.7 per 100,000 in whites.[2]

A variation in incidence and mortality among different religious groups has also been observed. There is an increased incidence of pancreatic cancer among Jews in New York City and in Israel and a lower mortality rate is lower among Mormons.[3]

The incidence in countries of origin and in first- and second-generation immigrants to the United States has been examined. The rate in the first-generation immigrants rapidly increases to the rate of US whites.

The cause of pancreatic carcinoma remains uncertain, but several factors have been implicated. Cigarette smoking has been associated with an increased risk of pancreatic carcinoma.[4,5] A study from Veterans Administration hospitals showed almost twice the rate of pancreatic carcinoma for heavy cigarette smokers (ie, at least two packs daily) as for nonsmokers. The risk increases as the level of cigarette smoking increases, and the excess risk levels off 10 to 15 years after cessation of smoking.[6]

Dietary factors also appear to play a role in the development of this disease. In animal studies, dietary fat enhances the experimental production of azaserine-induced pancreatic tumors.[7] Although coffee consumption was believed to be a strong etiologic factor,[8] more recent studies have failed to support this observation.[9] Alcohol has not been conclusively associated with pancreatic cancer.[5]

A third factor possibly involved in the development of pancreatic carcinoma is prior gastrectomy[10] for benign conditions, which may increase the risk of developing pancreatic cancer by two- to fivefold. It has been postulated that the postgastrectomy achlorhydric environment favors the colonization of bacteria that reduce nitrate-containing compounds to *N*-nitroso compounds. The latter are believed to be carcinogenic.[11] Another explanation for the correlation between gastrectomy and pancreatic cancer is the increased plasma cholecystokinin (CCK) levels associated with prior gastrectomy. CCK stimulates the growth of normal pancreatic cells and, in animal models, is believed to mediate the growth stimulus in carcinogenesis.[12] Inhibition of pancreatic cancer by a CCK antagonist has also been observed in experimental studies.[13]

Besides smoking, diet, and prior gastrectomy, certain disease states, including chronic pancreatitis and diabetes mellitus, also have been associated with pancreatic carcinoma. Calcifications associated with chronic pancreatitis have been found in 3% of patients with documented pancreatic carcinoma.[14] About 15% of pancreatic carcinoma patients are diabetics, and in more than half, the onset of clinical diabetes precedes the diagnosis of pancreatic carcinoma by less than 3 months.[15]

Finally, occupational exposure to solvents, petroleum compounds, beta-naphthylamine, and benzidine has been found to be associated with pancreatic cancer.[16,17] The nitrosamines are recognized as potent pancreatic carcinogens in hamsters.[11] Azaserine has produced pancreatic tumors in rats.[18] Indeed, exposure to these industrial chemicals for 10 years or more may increase the risk of pancreatic carcinoma fivefold.[16]

Pathology

Pancreatic cancer arises from both the exocrine and endocrine parenchyma of the pancreas.[19] Approximately 95% of pancreatic cancers occur within the exocrine portion of the pancreas and may arise from ductal epithelium, acinar cells, connective tissue, or lymphatic deposits. The most common pancreatic cancer is a ductal adenocarcinoma, which accounts for about 80% of all pancreatic cancers.[20] Most carcinomas arise in the proximal portion of the pancreas, which includes the head, neck, and uncinate process. Only 20% of pancreatic carcinomas arise in the body, and only 5% to 10% in the tail.[21]

The majority of patients with pancreatic carcinoma present with advanced disease. At presentation, 85% of patients have clinically obvious metastases or micrometastases. The usual breakdown of patients after staging is: disease apparently confined to the pancreas, 20%; locally advanced disease, 40%; and visceral metastases, 40%. The most common sites of metastases are the liver, peritoneum, lymph nodes, and lung.

Clinical Features

The initial symptoms, which include anorexia, weight loss, abdominal pain, and jaundice, are generally vague and nonspecific. As a result, two thirds of patients experience symptoms for at least 2 months before the diagnosis is made. Weight loss, often gradual and progressive,

is one of the earliest and most frequently unappreciated symptoms. A typical patient with pancreatic carcinoma has lost more than 10% of his or her body weight by the time of diagnosis. Abdominal pain, the most common symptom, is present in 70% to 80% of patients. The pain is due to local tumor infiltration into the retroperitoneum and splanchnic nerve plexus. Severe pain is often considered a sign that the tumor is not resectable.

Jaundice secondary to biliary obstruction can present as either an early or a late symptom depending upon the tumor location. Associated symptoms of dark urine and pale stools occur. Gastric outlet obstruction and duodenal obstruction can occur in as many as 25% of pancreatic head cancers and are usually secondary to local tumor invasion and motility problems from infiltration of the splanchnic nerves.

Other occasional findings include a palpable gallbladder at presentation (Courvoisier's sign),[22] splenomegaly, depression, and a higher frequency of venous thrombosis and migratory thrombophlebitis (Trousseau's sign).[14]

Diagnosis

Computed tomography (CT), ultrasonography, endoscopic retrograde cholangiopancreatography, and fine-needle aspiration biopsy have all been used successfully to diagnose pancreatic cancer. However, CT of the abdomen is the most useful procedure for diagnosis and staging. The advantages of CT scanning are that it is not operator dependent, it is not limited by stomach or bowel gas, and it will demonstrate liver metastases as small as 2 cm, involvement of peripancreatic lymph nodes, perivascular invasion, and lymphadenopathy.[23] It can also reveal dilation of the pancreatic duct and the site of obstruction in 88% to 97% of instances. However, CT has certain limitations, as not all pancreatic carcinomas are observed as masses and not all masses are pancreatic carcinomas. Nevertheless, a review of 100 cases of pancreatic carcinoma showed a false-negative rate for CT of only 5%.[24]

Unlike CT, ultrasonography does not involve ionizing radiation. For the patient presenting with jaundice, ultrasonography is more accurate than CT in distinguishing obstructive from nonobstructive jaundice.[25] However, the efficacy of ultrasonography decreases with obesity and excessive bowel gas.[26,27]

Although endoscopic retrograde cholangiopancreatography and fine-needle aspiration biopsy are invasive procedures, they do offer certain advantages. Endoscopic retrograde cholangiopancreatography (ERCP) has high sensitivity in diagnosing pancreatic carcinoma (94%).[28] It can localize the tumor and detect the site of ductal obstruction. Furthermore, endoscopic retrograde cholangiopancreatography permits the aspiration of pancreatic secretions for cytologic examination. Access to bile also allows measurement of other cancer-derived factors such as the K-*ras* oncogene. As reported in one series,[29] the false-negative rate for ERCP is only 3%. Although the radiographic diagnosis of pancreatic cancer can generally be made using a combination of CT, ultrasonography, and endoscopic retrograde cholangiopancreatography, fine-needle aspiration biopsy, which has a sensitivity of 86%,[30] can provide a histologic diagnosis.

Serologic Markers

The search for a specific tumor marker for pancreatic cancer that might aid in screening and early diagnosis has not yet been successful, although several serologic markers are helpful in managing the disease. Carcinoembryonic antigen (CEA), a high-molecular-weight glycoprotein normally found in fetal tissue, has been studied most extensively. It is elevated (greater than 2.5 mg/mL) in only 40% to 50% of patients with pancreatic cancer. It can be elevated in pancreatitis as well as in many other benign intestinal disorders and in biliary, gastric, hepatocellular, and colorectal carcinomas.

Other serologic markers associated with pancreatic carcinoma include CA 19-9 and the ratio of testosterone to dihydrotestosterone. CA 19-9 is a mucinous glycoprotein with a half-life of less than 1 day that is associated with a variety of malignancies (pancreatic, hepatobiliary, gastric, and colorectal). The sensitivity of CA 19-9 for pancreatic cancer has been found to range from 67.6% to 92% (37 U/mL is the upper limit of normal).[31] In general, the level of CA 19-9 increases with more advanced disease stage; the CA 19-9 level in patients with stage I or II disease is usually within the normal range. Hence, the sensitivity of this marker in diagnosing early, resectable pancreatic tumors is lower.[31,32] When 37 U/mL is used as the cutoff point, the CA 19-9 level is also elevated in 4.3% to 28% of patients with chronic pancreatitis and in 21% to 35% of those with extrapancreatic gastrointestinal cancers.[31,32] Raising the cutoff level improves the specificity of CA 19-9 for pancreatic carcinoma.

Another serologic marker that can be analyzed is the ratio of testosterone to dihydrotestosterone, which has been shown to be less than 5 in 67% of men with pancreatic cancer.[33] This is related to the increased level of 5-alpha-reductase associated with pancreatic cancer.[34] Compared with CA 19-9, the ratio of testosterone to dihydrotestosterone is less sensitive but more specific for pancreatic cancer.[33]

Two other antibodies, DU-PAN-2 and SPAN-1, have been screened in patients with pancreatic carcinoma. Both were raised against human pancreatic cancer cell lines. The specificity of these newer markers in patients with pancreatic cancer is comparable to that of CA 19-9.[35,36] However, the antibodies are reactive against several other types of cancer, principally gastrointestinal neoplasms, and against many other benign conditions.

Hence, no single marker alone is sufficiently sensitive or specific to be used as a screening test, but combining these markers can help to confirm the diagnosis of pancreatic carcinoma.

Staging

Staging is useful in choosing treatment, assessing prognosis, and comparing the results of different treatment programs. The most commonly used staging system for pancreatic cancer is the tumor-node-metastasis (TNM) classification devised in 1981 by the American Joint Committee for Cancer Staging and End Results Reporting (Table 1).

In the TNM system, the primary tumor status is defined by extension through the pancreatic capsule; nodal status is defined by the presence of regional pancreatic lymph-node involvement; and metastatic disease status is defined by the presence of distal lymph node, peritoneal, or visceral disease. Only stage I disease, which is localized within the pancreatic capsule, is amenable to resection.

Treatment

The approach to therapy differs in patients with pancreatic carcinoma depending on the stage of their disease at presentation.

Resectable Disease: As mentioned, only patients with T1-2N0M0 disease are considered to have resectable disease, and surgery is the only potentially curative modality. In general, curative surgery is feasible only in patients with cancer of the pancreatic head, since patients with cancer of the pancreatic tail or body invariably present with advanced disease. Even among those patients whose disease is resectable, 90% die of tumor recurrence within 1 to 2 years.[19,37] The median survival after curative resection is 12 to 18 months.

The site of recurrence is often local. In one study, local recurrence was the sole site of failure in 27% of patients who underwent resection and was a component of failure in 70%.[38] Whipple resection or pancreatoduodenectomy is considered the standard surgical procedure for cancer of the head of the pancreas.[39]

Adjuvant Radiotherapy: Most patients who undergo curative resection subsequently die of recurrent disease,

TABLE I

AJCC Staging System
for Pancreatic Carcinoma

Primary tumor (T)

TX: Primary tumor cannot be assessed

T0: No evidence of primary tumor

T1: Tumor limited to pancreas
    T1a: Tumor ≤ 2 cm in greatest dimension
    T1b: Tumor > 2 cm in greatest dimension

T2: Tumor extends directly to the duodenum, bile duct, or peripancreatic tissues

T3: Tumor extends directly to the stomach, spleen, colon, or adjacent large vessels

Regional lymph nodes (N)

NX: Regional lymph nodes cannot be assessed

N0: No regional lymph-node metastasis

N1: Regional lymph-node metastasis

Distant metastasis (M)

MX: Presence of distant metastasis cannot be assessed

M0: No distant metastasis

M1: Distant metastasis

Stage grouping	T	N	M
Stage I	T1	N0	M0
	T2	N0	M0
Stage II	T3	N0	M0
Stage III	Any T	N1	M0
Stage IV	Any T	Any N	M1

AJCC = American Joint Committee for Cancer Staging and End Results Reporting

Adapted, with permission, from Soh LT, Ajani JA: Pancreatic carcinoma, in Pazdur R (ed): Medical Oncology. A Comprehensive Review, p 179. Huntington NY, PRR Inc, 1993.

which indicates the need for effective postoperative adjuvant therapy. In 1974, the Gastrointestinal Tumor Study Group (GITSG)[40] evaluated the role of adjuvant radiation and chemotherapy following curative resection. A total of 43 patients were randomized to either a control arm for observation or a treatment arm in which 40 Gy of radiation was given in a split course, with intravenous fluorouracil administered for the first 3 days of each radiation course and on a weekly basis beginning 1 month after the completion of radiotherapy and continuing for 2 years thereafter. Survival was longer in the treatment group than in the observation group (21 vs 10.9 months). Because of the small size of the study, 30 additional patients[41] with better performance status were subsequently registered, and the results again showed improved survival for patients in the treatment arm. Although the statistical power in these two trials is weak and subject to criticism, this treatment approach has become common practice.

Adjuvant Chemotherapy: Whereas combined postoperative radiation and chemotherapy for pancreatic carcinoma has been systematically evaluated, adjuvant chemotherapy alone has not. However, before effective adjuvant therapy strategies can be developed, it is necessary to find an effective regimen for the treatment of advanced pancreatic cancer. No such regimen is known at the present time.

Unresectable Disease: Patients with unresectable disease are treated palliatively. Biliary obstruction in the presence of unresectable disease is relieved by endoscopic placement of a stent. Percutaneous biliary drainage is best avoided in a patient in whom no further therapy is planned, because it results in recurrent infections. Duodenal obstruction, which is uncommon, can be relieved with bypass surgery or with recently developed laparascopic techniques.

Chemotherapy: As mentioned earlier, the results of chemotherapy for pancreatic carcinoma have been disappointing. This disease is sensitive to only a few agents. Table 2 shows those drugs that have produced measurable responses in at least 10% of patients in phase II studies.

Fluorouracil offers the best response rate: 28% in a collective series,[42] with a range of 0% to 67%. The wide range is probably due to patient selection rather than to differences in scheduling or response criteria. However, the numbers of patients in these mostly uncontrolled trials are small.

Another agent with low-level activity against pancreatic cancer is mitomycin (Mutamycin), for which response rates range from 10% to 38%, with an average response rate of 21%.[43] Responses with streptozocin (Zanosar) and doxorubicin (Adriamycin, Rubex) have been reported to be 11%[44] and 13%,[43] respectively. However, the responses seen with all of these single agents are rarely complete, and the response durations are usually short. Complete responses have been reported with ifosfamide (Ifex), although the rates differed widely in the two studies reported so far: A trial involving 25 patients reported a response rate of 60% (with 4% complete responses) to ifosfamide,[45] whereas another trial involving 29 patients reported a response rate of 22% (with 3.5% complete responses).[46]

Since fluorouracil and mitomycin are the most effective single agents for pancreatic carcinoma, most combination chemotherapy regimens have included these two agents. In one of the earliest studies, FAM (fluorouracil, doxorubicin, and mitomycin) produced a response rate of 37%.[47] Thirty-nine patients with advanced pancreatic cancer were treated with fluorouracil, 600 mg/m^2 intravenously (IV) on days 1, 8, 29, and 36; doxorubicin, 30 mg/m^2 IV on days 1 and 29; and mitomycin, 10 mg/m^2 IV on day 1. The cycle was repeated every 8 weeks. No complete responses were observed, and the median survival of the responders was 12 months. However, a subsequent study by the North Central Cancer Treatment Group comparing fluorouracil alone vs fluorouracil plus doxorubicin vs FAM failed to detect a survival advantage for combination chemotherapy over single-agent fluorouracil.[48]

Another chemotherapeutic combination, SMF (fluorouracil, mitomycin, and streptozocin), was originally reported by Wiggans et al[49] to yield a response rate of 43%. In this study, 23 patients with advanced pancreatic cancer were treated with streptozocin, 1 g/m^2 IV on days 1, 8, 29, and 36; mitomycin, 10 mg/m^2 IV on day 1; and fluorouracil, 600 mg/m^2 IV on days 1, 8, 29, and 36. The cycle was repeated every 8 weeks. A subsequent study by the GITSG[50] comparing the efficacy of FAM with that of SMF failed, however, to reproduce those promising initial results. The responses for the two regimens were 13% and 15%, respectively.

Other attempts to improve the results of chemotherapy have centered on modifying the dosing schedule. In general, the drug whose schedule is modified has been fluorouracil, which may be given either in a bolus or as a continuous infusion. Based on the rationale that fluorouracil is a cell cycle-specific drug with a short half-life, it should be more effective if given as an infusion. Nevertheless, response rates in trials where this drug was administered by continuous infusion varied from 0% to 39%. The trials were limited by their small sample sizes.[51]

Modulations of fluorouracil by leucovorin (folinic acid)[52,53] and N-phosphonacetyl-L-aspartate (PALA)[54] in the treatment of pancreatic cancer have also been tried. Leucovorin increases the intracellular concentration of 5, 10-methyltetrahydrofolic acid, which results in prolonged inhibition of thymidylate synthetase by the fluorouracil metabolite FdUMP. However, results with high-dose leucovorin and fluorouracil in patients with advanced pancreatic carcinoma have been poor.[52,53]

PALA inhibits the enzyme aspartate transcarbamylase, resulting in a reduction in the pool of uridine triphosphate and cytosine triphosphate, an effect that

TABLE 2

Effectiveness of Single Chemotherapeutic Agents for Pancreatic Carcinoma

Drug	Number of patients	Response (%)
Fluorouracil	212	28
Streptozotocin	27	11
Mitomycin	53	20.8
Ifosfamide	54	22–60
Doxorubicin	15	13

Adapted, with permission, from Soh LT, Ajani JA: Pancreatic carcinoma, in Pazdur R (ed): Medical Oncology. A Comprehensive Review, p 180. Huntington NY, PRR Inc, 1993.

could enhance the therapeutic index of fluorouracil. However, a study by the Southwest Oncology Group (SWOG) reported a response rate of only 5% when PALA was given with high-dose fluorouracil as a short-term infusion.[55]

Only a few trials have utilized intra-arterial chemotherapy. In those that did, results were disappointing and did not show a survival benefit.[56,57]

Finally, new compounds continue to be elevated. Gemcitabine (2,2'-difluorodeoxycytidine) is a novel pyrimidine antimetabolite that demonstrated preclinical antitumor activity in murine solid tumor models and responses in patients with pancreatic cancer during phase I evaluation. A phase II trial by Casper et al was performed in chemo-naive patients with adenocarcinoma of the pancreas.[57a] Gemcitabine, 800 mg/m^2, was administered intravenously weekly for 3 consecutive weeks every 28 days. A response rate of 11% was observed (all partial responses). Despite these marginal response rates, interesting improvements in pain and performance status were frequently observed. Based on these observations, a randomized trial of gemcitabine vs fluorouracil was conducted, which demonstrated significant improvements in symptom control and survival with gemcitabine.[57b] Thus, gemcitabine should be considered for the front-line management of symptomatic patients with advanced pancreatic adenocarcinoma.

Hormonal Therapy: Hormonal therapy also has potential as palliative treatment for pancreatic carcinoma. Results with experimental models have suggested that pancreatic cancer is a hormone-dependent tumor.[58,59] Theve et al[60] treated 14 patients with advanced pancreatic carcinoma with tamoxifen and reported that median survival was prolonged to 8.5 months (3 patients survived for 22 months). In another study of tamoxifen, however, Miller and Benz[61] did not achieve such promising results.

Reports that somatostatin (octreotide) inhibits pancreatic carcinoma growth in animals[62] suggest that it may have potential use in treating pancreatic cancer. CCK and secretin stimulate the growth of the exocrine pancreas in animals. Although the role of these hormones in human tumorigenesis is uncertain, CCK can stimulate the growth of a human pancreatic adenocarcinoma cell line.[63] Among the actions of somatostatin and its analogs is the inhibition of the secretion or action of gastrointestinal hormones, including CCK. In two human pancreatic adenocarcinoma cell lines, growth inhibition was seen with somatostatin. Direct inhibitors of CCK have also been evaluated recently, but no effect on disease progression or quality of life has been documented.[64]

Radiotherapy: Palliative radiotherapy has been used to control pain in patients with pancreatic carcinoma. Radiotherapy by itself does not improve survival but, when combined with fluorouracil, does.[65] In a GITSG study comparing 6,000 cGy alone with fluorouracil plus 4,000 or 6,000 cGy, in patients with locally unresectable pancreatic cancer, median survival was longer in both chemoradiation treatment arms than in the radiotherapy alone arm (10 vs 5.5 months).

Other investigational radiotherapy techniques have been used in attempts to improve the management of pancreatic cancer, with mixed results. One of these, intraoperative radiotherapy, has been reported to enable a higher dose of radiation to be delivered to the disease site without injuring neighboring tissues.[66] In a study at the Mayo Clinic,[67] 159 patients were randomly assigned to either intraoperative radiotherapy plus external-beam radiation, or with external-beam radiation alone. Although local control was superior in the intraoperative radiotherapy group, this improved local control did not translate into improved survival. Finally, other attempts to improve survival in pancreatic cancer, such as ultrasonically guided percutaneous implantation of iodine-125 seeds, have not yielded significant results.

Biologic Therapy: There has been considerable interest in the use of monoclonal antibodies to treat patients with pancreatic cancer. Monoclonal antibodies are believed to kill the tumor target either indirectly, by interaction with cells that affect antibody-dependent cell-mediated cytotoxicity (ADCC) and natural killer cell activity, or directly by complement-dependent cytolysis.[68,69] Two monoclonal antibodies, MoAb 494/32 and MoAb CO 17-1A, show strong reactivity against pancreatic cancer.

MoAb 494/32 is a murine antibody of the immuno-globulin (Ig) G1 isotype that binds strongly to human pancreatic cancer cells and mediates ADCC. A partial response was seen in a patient with pancreatic cancer during phase I-II evaluation of this antibody. In a prospective, randomized trial in patients who had undergone pancreatic resection, median survival of the 29 patients who received postoperative MoAb 494/32 was 14.2 months, not significantly different from the 12.9-month median survival of the 32 control patients.[70]

Another important monoclonal antibody is MoAb 17-1A, which is a murine IgG2a that targets a 37-kd glycoprotein on the surface of a variety of human gastrointestinal adenocarcinomas.[71] It does not mediate complement-dependent lysis of tumor cells, but it does participate in ADCC. In preliminary clinical studies of MoAb 17-1A, some responses were seen in patients with pancreatic carcinoma.[69] Another opportunity for therapeutic intervention would be using antibodies against the epidermal growth factor receptor. It has been found that pancreatic cancer cells overexpress the epidermal growth factor receptor.[72] This receptor is a transmembrane glycoprotein expressed by a variety of normal and malignant cells.

Future Targets: As molecular biologists and biochemists develop better understanding of pancreatic cancer, new targets for therapy will emerge. One such target is the K-ras oncogene. It has been found that at least 80% of pancreatic adenocarcinomas contain a mutated K-ras gene.[73] This oncogene plays an important role in the development and progression of pancreatic cancer and is a target for new therapeutic approaches.

Pain Control: Pain is a symptom experienced by virtually all patients with pancreatic carcinoma at some time in the course of their disease. It is often what motivates the patient to seek medical attention. Pain may arise when the tumor infiltrates into the retroperitoneum or the splanchnic nerve plexus. It is typically burning and severe, and if there is nerve compression, it may be accompanied by dysesthesia and hyperesthesia in the area of innervation. Anticonvulsants and tricyclic antidepressants are useful in treating this type of pain.[74,75] In addition, steroids can reduce the edema associated with pancreatic cancer and lessen the compression and pain.

Pain may also be due to gastric or small bowel obstruction or bile duct dilatation, which leads to intense muscular spasm. This, in turn, leads to ischemia with cellular breakdown and liberation of pain-producing substances. This type of pain is diffuse and poorly localized and is referred to the dermatomes that share the same innervation as the affected viscus.

Treatment for such pain involves the generous use of

narcotics, which can be given in two ways. The oral route is preferred, as it is painless and convenient. The use of long-acting narcotics, such as controlled-release morphine, usually achieves better pain control. In general, the required dose is titrated with a short-acting morphine preparation given every 4 hours. If oral administration fails to control the pain, parenteral administration can be used. Under these circumstances, the drug is preferably given via a continuous infusion pump, since the pump can be programmed to administer the drug at a background infusion rate and allow for a boost dose to be given on demand by the patient.

In patients with intractable pain, more radical procedures, such as a celiac axis block, can be carried out under fluoroscopic guidance. The celiac plexus is a dense network of nerves between the two large ganglia formed by the splanchnic nerves. The splanchnic nerves and sympathetic trunks are the sole mediators of pain arising from the pancreas and the extrahepatic biliary ducts. Therefore, by blocking the celiac axis, pain can be blocked. Pain relief with this procedure is greater than 90% in most reported series.[76–78]

Radiotherapy also has been used to control pain.[65] Usually administered with a radiosensitizer, the radiation acts by shrinking the tumor and relieving compression of nerves. The disadvantage of radiotherapy treatment is delayed relief. Nevertheless, this method is quite effective when it is well coordinated.

HEPATOCELLULAR CARCINOMA

Hepatocellular carcinoma (HCC) is one of the most common malignancies; it causes an estimated 1,250,000 deaths every year worldwide. The distribution of HCC shows striking geographic variations. Countries and populations are grouped according to incidence rates, ie, high (20 or more per 100,000 males per year) in China, Southeast Asia, Western and Southern Africa, and in Chinese populations in Singapore, Taiwan, and Hong Kong; intermediate (6 to 19 per 100,000 males per year) in Japan, Bulgaria, Poland, France, Hungary, Yugoslavia, Czechoslovakia, Belgium, and Austria and among New Zealand Maoris and Hawaiians and Chinese living in the United States; and low (fewer than 5 cases per 100,000 males per year) in the United Kingdom, the United States, Canada, Australia, Israel, Scandinavia, Latin America, India, and New Zealand.[79]

Worldwide, HCC occurs in approximatley three times as many males as females. The incidence increases with age independent of risk until it levels off in the elderly. In high-incidence regions, there is a marked shift toward increased incidence in the younger age group.

Risk Factors

HCC is almost always associated with chronic underlying liver disease, principally hepatitis B and hepatitis C. There is a positive correlation between the geographic pattern of hepatitis B surface antigen (HBsAG) and the incidence of HCC. Molecular biologic studies have shown integrated hepatitis B virus DNA in the livers of patients with chronic hepatitis and hepatocellular carcinoma.[80]

Aflatoxin, a mycotoxin resulting from *Aspergillus* fungi, appears to be an important cocarcinogen in rural Africans. Aflatoxin-contaminated food has been reported to produce liver tumors in trout, rats, and rhesus monkeys fed aflatoxin B1 over a long period of time.[81]

In the West, HCC generally occurs in the setting of cirrhosis. Eighty to 90% of cases are related to ethanol-induced cirrhosis. Other risk factors include hemochromatosis and parasitic infections of the liver.

Pathology

HCC occurs in two gross patterns, a diffuse form and a nodular form. The diffuse form may evolve from a unicentric lesion.[82]

Of all the histologic patterns of HCC, only the fibrolamellar variant is of importance in treatment and clinical behavior. This variant is more frequent in females, occurs at an earlier age, is not associated with cirrhosis, and tends to be solitary and, thus, more amenable to surgical resection. These fibrolamellar carcinomas, characterized histologically by eosinophilic polygonal-shaped cells separated by lamellar fibrosis, have better prognosis than do the other histologic types of HCC.[82]

Invasion of the portal vein has been found in 14% of resected HCC specimens when the lesion was smaller than 2.0 cm and in 71% of specimens when the lesion was larger than 5.1 cm. These thrombi may involve the hepatic vein, vena cava, and portal vein.[83]

Clinical Features

The most common symptoms in patients with HCC are abdominal pain (91%), ascites (43%), weight loss (35%), weakness (31%), fullness and anorexia (27%), vomiting (8%), and jaundice (7%). About one third of patients are asymptomatic. Metastatic disease can present as malignant ascites, skeletal pain, dyspnea with pulmonary involvement, and neurologic abnormalities due to brain metastases.[84]

Ascites may occur as a consequence of underlying chronic liver disease or may be due to a rapidly expanding tumor. Other less common symptoms include fever of unknown origin, intra-abdominal hemorrhage, upper gastrointestinal bleeding, bone pain, coma secondary to hepatic failure, hypercalcemia, and respiratory symptoms. Jaundice occurs infrequently and usually is secondary to the underlying liver disease.

Among the physical signs present in patients with HCC, hepatomegaly is the most frequent, ocurring in 50% to 90% of patients. Signs of cirrhosis such as spider angiomas and gynecomastia are common. Abdominal bruits can arise from the HCC, presumably secondary to the increased vascularity. Ascites can occur as part of the underlying liver disease, caused by a hemoperitoneum, or as malignant ascites. Splenomegaly may occur as a result of associated portal hypertension from the underlying liver disease. Weight loss and fever are also common, particularly with rapidly growing or large tumors. The Budd-Chiari syndrome, Virchows or Trosier's nodes, and cutaneous metastases have also been reported.

A number of paraneoplastic syndromes have been reported in association with HCC. The most important ones include hypoglycemia (also caused by end-stage liver failure), erythrocytosis, hypercalcemia, hypercholesterolemia, dysfibrinogenemia, carcinoid syndrome, increased thyroxine-binding globulin, sexual changes, and porphyria cutanea tarda.

The changes in laboratory values with HCC are very similar to those with cirrhosis; they include elevated levels of alkaline phosphatase, transaminases, and bilirubin. These changes are usually present in about 50% of patients and predict a short survival.[85]

Alpha fetoprotein (AFP) and alpha-1-globulin are the tumor markers usually associated with HCC.[86] In humans, they are normally detected in the embryo beginning 6 weeks after fertilization and disappear a few weeks after birth. Although AFP levels are also elevated in germ-cell tumors and during pregnancy, the immunoassay will still detect between 70% and 90% of all HCCs. Reports have associated normal levels of AFP with improved survival. Postresection AFP levels are used in monitoring clinical progress.

Diagnosis

Hepatocellular carcinomas are best visualized on CT scans. CT can demonstrate primary lesions larger than 1 cm and may also identify compression or invasion of the portal or hepatic veins and extrahepatic metastatic disease, particularly to the hepatoduodenal ligament and lungs.[87]

Ultrasonography is inexpensive and noninvasive, but the hyperechoic appearance of HCC may lead to confusion with benign as well as metastatic tumors. HCC may show as a focal form that appears on ultrasound as a rounded or lobular mass lesion, often multiple, with high- and low-level echoes. Ultrasound may show both hepatic veins and portal veins and occasionally demonstrates intravascular tumor. HCC may also present as a diffuse form with changes that may be subtle and indistinguishable from the diffuse changes seen with cirrhosis and chronic active hepatitis.

Magnetic resonance imaging has not as yet been demonstrated to be more useful than CT scanning in the liver. The most sensitive tests are CT portography and lipoidol CT scanning. These are considered mandatory if resection is contemplated since they pick up small lesions in the apparently normal residual lobe and are reported to be capable of diagnosing 50% more lesions than can be diagnosed with CT scanning alone.

Laparoscopy is more invasive, but it provides direct visualization of the liver, peritoneal cavity, and viscera and allows for a percutaneous needle biopsy under direct vision. It may result in more accurate staging and the avoidance of unnecessary laparotomies.

Percutaneous biopsy techniques include fine-needle aspiration cytology and core-needle biopsy. Needle biopsy may be performed directed by ultrasound or CT, blindly, or, as already mentioned, under direct vision using the laparoscope.

Staging

The staging system for hepatic tumors was developed by the Union Internationale Contre le Cancer (UICC), and it essentially follows the TNM system (Table 3).

Stage I solitary tumors smaller than 2 cm in diameter without vascular invasion have the best prognosis. Multiple tumors, vascular invasion, either microscopic or macroscopic, and lymph-node spread are considered adverse prognostic factors.

Treatment

Surgery: Surgery is the only curative modality for HCC, but its use depends mainly on tumor size and location and the condition of the uninvolved liver. Small, encapsulated HCCs may be cured with resection 50% of the time, but these tumors are rare. Patients with clinical stage I or II tumors should be considered for resection.

As mentioned, another limiting factor for many patients with HCC is the hepatic reserve available. Diffuse HCC and advanced cirrhosis are generally considered unresectable. The goal in patients with cirrhosis is to preserve as much functioning liver tissue as possible to avoid postoperative liver failure.[88] Subsegmental or segmental resections are preferable in patients with small

TABLE 3

Staging System for Liver Tumors

Primary tumor (T)

TX: Primary tumor cannot be assessed

T0: No evidence of primary tumor

T1: Solitary tumor ≤ 2 cm in greatest dimension without vascular invasion

T2: Solitary tumor ≤ 2 cm in greatest dimension with vascular invasion, or
Multiple tumors limited to one lobe, none > 2 cm in greatest dimension without vascular invasion, or
A solitary tumor > 2 cm in greatest dimension without vascular invasion

T3: Solitary tumor > 2 cm in greatest dimension with vascular invasion, or
Multiple tumors limited to one lobe, none > 2 cm in greatest dimension, with vascular invasion, or
Multiple tumors limited to one lobe, any > 2 cm in greatest dimension, with or without vascular invasion

T4: Multiple tumors in more than one lobe or tumor(s) involving a major branch of portal or hepatic vein(s)

Lymph node (N)

NX: Regional lymph nodes cannot be assessed

N0: No regional lymph-node metastasis

N1: Regional lymph-node metastasis

Distant metastasis (M)

MX: Presence of distant metastasis cannot be assessed

M0: No distant metastasis

M1: Distant metastasis

Stage grouping	T	N	M
Stage I	T1	N0	M0
Stage II	T2	N0	M0
Stage III	T1	N1	M0
	T2	N1	M0
	T3	N0	M0
	T3	N1	M0
Stage IVA	T4	Any N	M0
Stage IVB	Any T	Any N	M1

lesions and cirrhosis. Intraoperative hepatic ultrasound can help detect satellite or metastatic tumors and allow exact localization and ligation of segmental portal and hepatic veins during minimal resections.

Operative mortality increases with the extent of resec-tion and with a decrease in the degree of function of the remaining liver tissue and has been reported to range from 5% to 33%.[89] The type and extent of tumor and the coexistence of cirrhosis or hepatitis will determine the long-term survival. One-year survival rates have been reported to be about 80%, with 5-year survival rates ranging from 30% to 46%.

There is no role for adjuvant chemotherapy or radio-therapy following curative resection.

Cryosurgery: Cryosurgery involves the in situ de-struction of tumor by the application of subzero temper-atures. With the use of liquid nitrogen, temperatures less than –20°C can be achieved. This procedure will lead to the death of both tumor and nontumor tissue either immediately or during the thawing period. Multiple freeze-thaw cycles are used to increase the percentage of tumor tissues destroyed.

Theoretically, cryosurgery should be an ideal modal-ity for the treatment of patients with cirrhosis who have inadequate hepatic reserve and multifocal tumor. In-stead, the complications associated with this procedure and the very low survival reported in the literature have shown that cryosurgery offers no clear improvement over standard surgery and that its use should be limited to the research setting.[90]

Chemotherapy: Most patients with HCC are not can-didates for curative surgery, so chemotherapy is their only option. Unfortunately, currently there is no very effective chemotherapy for HCC.[91] Doxorubicin, still considered the single-agent standard for HCC, has only a 20% response rate. No other single agent has yet demonstrated a higher rate. Combination chemotherapy has been found to increase toxicity with no improvement in survival. Interferon alfa-2a (Roferon-A) also has been used in HCC with no impact on patient survival.[92,93]

Another approach to the treatment of HCC is hepatic intra-arterial infusion, in which high concentrations of chemotherapy are delivered directly to the liver. Hepatic intra-arterial infusion of agents such as floxuridine (FUDR), mitomycin, and interferon have produced re-ported response rates as high as 50%.[94,95] Unfortunately, these responses are not usually durable. Another draw-back of this method is that these treatments require either long-term percutaneous catheterization of the hepatic artery or laparotomy for the placement of an infusion device, which tends to be costly and prone to complica-tions. Hepatic intra-arterial infusion is currently not recommended as standard practice.

Chemoembolization, the administration of chemo-therapy concomitant with percutaneous hepatic artery embolization, is yet another approach to treating HCC.

The major blood supply to HCC is derived from the hepatic artery, while normal liver parenchyma is supplied primarily by the portal vein. Thus, occlusion of the hepatic artery can accomplish relatively selective tumor ischemia.

Gelatin sponge is the most widely used vaso-occlusive material, although, other substances such as starch, polyvinyl alcohol, collagen, chemotherapy microspheres, and autologous blood clot have also been tried. The different sizes of these particles predict for a different level of arterial blockage, and their differing degrees of degradability predict for differences in the duration of blockade. The optimal material has yet to be determined.

Chemoembolization for HCC produces partial responses in approximately 50% of patients. Nonetheless, no definitive study has demonstrated a superiority of chemoembolization over hepatic intra-arterial infusion, other palliative therapies, or the state-of-the-art supportive care for HCC.

Radiotherapy: External-beam radiotherapy has a role in the palliative management of HCC, but this role has been limited by the total organ dose tolerance of radiation therapy. Radiation hepatitis with subsequent fibrosis is one of the possible complications seen when doses of 3 to 30 Gy are delivered. Conformal radiotherapy ports can be used to minimize the beam scatter and allow the delivery of therapeutic doses of radiation to solitary lesions.

A new technique being used is radiation-labeled antibodies to ferritin. Ferritin is not only found in normal tissues but also synthesized and secreted by HCC. Use of the ^{131}I polyclonal antiferritin antibody[96] has produced a 48% remission rate in phase I and II studies. It has also downstaged a small percentage of inoperable cancers to resectable ones. When a radiolabeled antibody-chemotherapy regimen was compared with chemotherapy alone, no survival advantage was found with the combination therapy.[97] Attempts were made to substitute the iodine isotope for a beta-emitting ^{90}Y antiferritin isotope, but it was found that the antiferritin moeity was no longer selective for HCC. Current investigation is focused on the use of a human monoclonal antiferritin antibody.

Liver Transplantation: Liver transplantation has been used as an alternative to resection in patients with advanced bilobar HCC or HCC in the presence of advanced cirrhosis.[98] The results of this strategy, however, have been discouraging, with 3-year survival rates amounting to less than 50% and long-term survival rates of approximately 20%.[99]

GALLBLADDER CARCINOMA

Carcinoma of the gallbladder was first described by Maximilian de Stoll in 1777.[100] It is now the fourth most common tumor of the gastrointestinal tract. Together with liver cancer, carcinoma of the gallbladder will account for an estimated 18,500 new cancers and 14,200 estimated US deaths in 1995.[1] Gallbladder carcinoma is an aggressive disease, and the prognosis for patients is dismal, with an overall 5-year survival rate of less than 5% and a median survival of 6 months.[101,102]

Epidemiology and Etiology

Carcinoma of the gallbladder is a disease of older people. Incidence peaks in the seventh decade, with three times as many women as men affected. There is no difference in the age of onset between males and females.[103] The incidence is higher in white women than in black women and 10 times higher in Mexicans, American Indians, and Alaskan natives, suggesting a genetic basis of susceptibility.[4,104]

The female predominance in this disease has suggested an association between benign and malignant gallbladder disease. Silk et al[102] reviewed their 22-year experience with gallbladder carcinoma at Roswell Park Cancer Institute and found that cholelithiasis was present in 48 (68%) of 69 patients. A calcified (porcelain) gallbladder was found in seven patients (10%). Another study by Paraskevopoulos et al[105] found gallstones in 18 (86%) of 21 patients with histologically proven carcinoma. Other authors have emphasized the occurrence of carcinoma in porcelain gallbladders,[106] but because some of the patients with porcelain gallbladders also have gallstones, it is difficult to attribute an exact role to each of these factors. Cholecystitis has also been considered one of the contributing factors in this disease. Silk et al found acute and/or chronic cholecystitis in 54 (76%) of the 69 patients in their series.

Other possible contributing factors for this disease include chemical carcinogens, especially nitrosamines and methylcholanthrene, and inflammatory processes like ulcerative colitis in which there is a strong association with carcinoma of the gallbladder.

Pathology

Overall, 80% to 85% of gallbladder carcinomas are adenocarcinomas, and most are of the scirrhous type. The anaplastic, squamous-cell, and adenoacanthoma types are rare. In the series from Roswell Park,[102] 67 (94%) of the patients had adenocarcinoma, and 4 (6%) had squamous-cell carcinoma. In a series by Yamaguchi et al,[107]

TABLE 4

TNM Staging System for Gallbladder Carcinoma

Tis: Carcinoma in situ

T1: Confined to mucosal or muscular layer
   T1a: Limited to mucosa
   T1b: Invades muscular layer

T2: Invades perimuscular connective tissue

T3: Invades serosa and/or one organ, liver < 2 cm

T4: Invades two or more organs, or liver > 2 cm

N1A: Hepatoduodenal ligament nodes: cystic duct, pericholedocal, or hilar

N1B: Other regional nodes: peripancreatic (head only), periportal celiac, or superior mesenteric

Stage grouping	T	N	M
Stage 0	Tis	N0	M0
Stage I	T1	N0	M0
Stage II	T2	N0	M0
Stage III	T1	N1	M0
	T2	N1	M0
	T3	Any N	M0
Stage IV	T4	Any N	M0
	Any T	Any N	M1

29 patients had adenocarcinoma and 2 patients had adenosquamous carcinoma. Carcinoma was limited to the fundus in 21 patients, to the body in 1 patient, to the neck in 2 patients, and involved the entire organ in 6 patients.

Natural History

Gallbladder carcinoma is usually detected at an advanced stage, when the prognosis is poor. Many gallbladder carcinomas are discovered by pathologists as an incidental finding after the removal of the gallbladder for chronic cholecystitis. In some patients, the cancer is diagnosed at autopsy.

Gallbladder cancer can be found as a polypoid projection into the lumen of the gallbladder or as a diffuse thickening of the wall of the organ, with or without extension into the liver and other adjacent organs. The liver and the regional lymph nodes are the most common sites of involvement, followed by peritoneal carcinomatosis.

Cancer invasion of the liver is usually by direct extension of the disease, by spread via the lymph channels or Luschka's ducts, or by a combination of these processes.[108] Liver metastases far from the gallbladder bed are seen in half of patients.

Invasion of the local lymph nodes by the tumor tends to occur early. The lymphatic drainage is to the lymph nodes along the cystic and common bile ducts and then through the pancreaticoduodenal nodes to the paraaortic nodes. The cystic node is invaded in 42% to 79% of cases. Almost half of patients have an extension of the tumor to the common bile duct. However, invasion to the colon, pancreas, and stomach is seen in only 10% to 20% of patients.[109]

Clinical Features

Patients with gallbladder carcinoma may be asymptomatic or may present with abdominal pain, jaundice, weight loss, anorexia, or nausea and vomiting. Others may present with a right upper quadrant mass or complications such as gastrointestinal hemorrhage. Some of these symptoms and signs make distinguishing between carcinoma and benign disease a difficult task.

Serum chemistries are not always very helpful because serum bilirubin levels are often normal. An elevated alkaline phosphatase level often accompanies a normal serum bilirubin level in this disease.[103]

Diagnosis

Ultrasonography of the gallbladder can be helpful in the diagnosis of gallbladder cancer. It may show a localized thickening or a mass. Unfortunately, the appearance of gallbladder carcinoma or ultrasound is difficult or impossible to differentiate from the wide spectrum of appearances associated with gallstones.[105] In the series from Paraskevopoulos,[105] 21 of 3,197 patients who had routine cholecystectomies were found to have carcinoma of the gallbladder at operation. The correct preoperative diagnosis was made in only two patients despite the fact that all but one had ultrasound examination, which revealed gallstones in 18.

CT scanning can also demonstrate gallbladder abnormalities. It can aid by identifying irregular thickening of the gallbladder wall, masses in the gallbladder region, and intraluminal masses.[110] Endoscopic retrograde cholangiopancreatography may demonstrate filling defects in the gallbladder or evidence of infiltration of the common bile duct.

Angiography can demonstrate irregularities and tumor vessels arising from the cystic artery. However, it is not considered a screening procedure since by the time the diagnosis is made, the tumor is incurable.[110]

Another method used to diagnose gallbladder carcinoma, is an upper gastrointestinal contrast study, which may show displacement of stomach and duodenum when extensive disease is present; however, findings are not specific.

Staging

There are two commonly used staging systems for gallbladder carcinoma: the TNM staging system of the International Union Against Cancer and the Nevin staging system (Table 4).[101]

In the classification system of Nevin and Moran, stage I tumors are localized to the mucosa; stage II tumors penetrate the muscularis; stage III tumors involve all three layers; stage IV disease involves metastases in the cystic duct lymph nodes; and stage V disease involves invasion of metastases to liver or adjacent or distant organs.

The management of gallbladder carcinoma largely depends upon the stage of disease at presentation. In the series of Silk et al,[102] stage of disease was the only factor that consistently influenced survival.

Treatment

Surgery: Surgical resection is the primary treatment modality for carcinoma of the gallbladder. Cholecystectomy may be all that is required for stage I and II disease. It is generally effective in those cases in which the carcinoma is an incidental finding on histopathologic examination of a gallbladder removed for symptomatic benign disease. Shieh[111] reported a 66.6% 5-year survival rate for patients whose tumors were confined in the wall of the gallbladder and were found incidentally by the examining pathologist.

Some authors believe that patients with gallbladder carcinoma invading beyond the mucosal layer may benefit from more radical procedures such as extended cholecystectomy with regional lymph-node dissection and resection of the gallbladder bed. Once the lesion invades the gallbladder serosa it is considered incurable. After cholecystectomy or radical surgery the 5-year survival rate is 10% to 30%, with locoregional recurrences seen in about 80% of the cases.[109] Pancreaticoduodenectomy has also been recommended when lymphadenopathy posterior to the pancreas or duodenal invasion is present.

Radiotherapy: The role of radiation as either primary or adjuvant therapy for this disease has been difficult to evaluate because of small series and the difficulty in assessing tumor response. Nevertheless available data thus far have suggested an important role for radiation as palliative and adjuvant therapy for gallbladder cancer.

Vaittinen[103] reported on 24 patients treated with surgery alone and 7 patients treated with surgery and postoperative external irradiation and found the average survivals of 29 and 63 months, respectively. Hanna and Rider[112] reported on 51 patients with cancer of the gallbladder, of whom 35 received radiation therapy. Irradiation increased the total survivals of patients treated curatively and palliatively. Bosset[109] reported five of seven gallbladder cancer patients free of disease at 5, 9, 11, 31, and 58 months after complete resection and postoperative radiotherapy to 5,400 cGy in 30 fractions. Todoroki[113] reported on 17 patients with stage IV gallbladder carcinomas who received 2,000 to 3,000 cGy of intraoperative radiotherapy; 10 of the patients also received 3,600 cGy of external-beam irradiation. The 3-year survival rate for the radiation-treated group was 10%, whereas none of nine stage IV patients treated with resection alone were alive at 3 years.

These results suggest an increased benefit in terms of survival and palliation in patients receiving postoperative radiation as either palliative or adjuvant therapy.

Chemotherapy: Chemotherapy provides little benefit in advanced gallbladder cancer or as an adjuvant treatment after surgical resection. Fluorouracil, considered the most active single agent in the treatment of advanced gallbladder disease, produces only transient responses in about 20% of patients. Other agents that have been used include mitomycin and doxorubicin. For patients with localized disease, postoperative radiotherapy combined with fluorouracil may offer some benefit. Smoron[114] observed one patient with a survival of 6 years after external postoperative irradiation and chemotheraphy with fluorouracil.

Newer drugs and alternate routes of delivery are essential if there is to be any success with this line of treatment.

REFERENCES

1. American Cancer Society: Cancer Statistics—1995. J Am Cancer Society 45:8–30, 1995.

2. Gloeckler LA, Hankey BF, Miller BA, et al: Cancer Statistics Review, 1973–1988 (NIH Publ 91-2789). Bethesda, National Institutes of Health, 1988.

3. Enstrom JE: Cancer and total mortality among active Mormons. Cancer 42:1943–1951, 1978.

4. Krain L: The rising incidence of carcinoma of the pancreas: An epidemiologic appraisal. Am J Gastroenterol 54:500, 1970.

5. Wynder E et al: An epidemiologic evaluation of the causes of cancer of the pancreas. Cancer Res 35:2228, 1975.

6. Kahn H: The Dorn study of smoking and mortality among US veterans: Report on eight and one-half years of observation. NCI

Monogr 19:1, 1966.

7. Roebuck BD, Yager JD Jr, Longnecker DS, et al: Promotion by unsaturated fat of asazerine-induced pancreatic carcinogenesis in the rat. Cancer Res 41: 3961–3966, 1981.

8. MacMahon B, Yen S, Trichopoulos D, et al: Coffee and cancer of the pancreas. N Engl J Med 304:630–633, 1981.

9. Goldskin HR: No association between coffee and cancer of the pancreas (letter). N Engl J Med 306:997, 1982.

10. Offerhaus GJA, Tersmette AC, Tersmette KWF, et al: Gastric, pancreatic and colorectal carcinogenesis following remote peptic ulcer surgery. Mod Pathol 1: 352–356, 1988.

11. Pour P, Althoff J, Kruger F, et al: The effect of N-nitrosobis-(2-oxopropyl)-almine after oral administration to hamsters. Cancer Lett 2:323, 1977.

12. Pour P, Lawson T, Helgeson S, et al: Effect of cholecystokinin on pancreatic carcinogenesis in the hamster model. Carcinogenesis 9:5197–5201, 1988.

13. Nio Y, Tsubono M, Morimoto H, et al: Loxiglumide (CR1505), a cholecystokinin antagonist, specifically inhibits the growth of human pancreatic cancer cell lines xenografted into nude mice. Cancer 72:3599–3606, 1993.

14. Robin A, Scott J, Rosenfeld D: The ocurrence of carcinoma of the pancreas in chronic pancreatitis. Radiology 94:289, 1970.

15. Karmody A, Kyle J: The association between carcinoma of the pancreas and diabetes mellitus. Br J Surg 56:362, 1969.

16. Brooks J: Cancer of the pancreas, in Brooks JR (ed): Surgery of the Pancreas, p 263. Philadelphia, WB Saunders, 1983.

17. Mancuso T, El-Attar A: Cohort study of workers exposed to betanaphthylamine and benzidine. J Occup Med 9:277–285, 1967.

18. Longnecker D, Curphey T: Adenocarcinoma of the pancreas in asazerine-treated rats. Cancer Res 35:2249, 1975.

19. Cubilla AL, Fitzgerald PJ: Surgical pathology of tumors of the exocrine pancreas in Moosa AR (ed): Tumors of the Pancreas, pp 159–193. Baltimore, Williams & Wilkins, 1980.

20. Legg MA: Pathology of the pancreas, in Brooks JR (ed): Surgery of the Pancreas pp 41–77. Philadelphia, WB Saunders, 1983.

21. Howard JM, Jordan GL: Cancer of the pancreas. Curr Probl Cancer 2–1, 1977.

22. Moertel CG: Exocrine pancreas, in Holland JF (ed): Cancer Medicine, pp 1792–1804. Philadelphia, Lea & Febiger, 1982.

23. Hessel SJ, Siegelman SS, McNeil BJ, et al: Prospective evaluation of computed tomography and ultrasound of the pancreas. Radiology 143:129–133, 1982.

24. Ward EM, Stephens DH, Sheedy PR: Computed tomographic characteristics of pancreatic carcinoma: An analysis of 100 cases. Radiographics 3:547, 1983.

25. Taylor KJW, Rosenfield AT: Grey scale ultrasonography in the diagnosis of jaundice. Arch Surg 112: 820–825, 1977.

26. Lees WR: Pancreatic ultrasonography. Clin Gastroenterol 13:763–789, 1984.

27. Rosch T, Lightdale CJ, Botet JF, et al: Localization of pancreatic endocrine tumors by endoscopic ultrasonography. N Engl J Med 326:1721–1726, 1992.

28. Freeny PC, Ball TJ: Endoscopic retrograde cholangiopancreatography (ERCP) and percutaneous transhepatic cholangiography (PTC) in the evaluation of suspected pancreatic carcinoma: Diagnostic limitations and contemporary roles. Cancer 47:1666–1678, 1981.

29. Freeny PC, Lawson TL: Radiology of the Pancreas, p 457. New York, Springer-Verlag, 1982.

30. Mitty H, Efremidis S, Yeh HC: Impact of fine-needle biopsy on the management of patients with carcinoma of the pancreas. Am J Roentgenol 137:119–121, 1981.

31. Pasquali C, Sperti C, Alfano D, et al: Evaluation of carbohydrate antigens 19-9 and CA-125 in patients with pancreatic cancer. Pancreas 2:34–37, 1987.

32. Malesci A, Tommasini MA, Bonato C, et al: Determination of CA 19-9 antigen in serum and pancreatic juice for differential diagnosis of pancreatic adenocarcinoma from chronic pancreatitis. Gastroenterol 92:60–67, 1987.

33. Robles-Diaz G, Diaz-Sanchez V, Fernandez-del Castillo C, et al: Serum testosterone:Dihydrotestosterone ratio and CA 19-9 in the diagnosis of pancreatic cancer. Am J Gastroenterol 86:591–594, 1991.

34. Igbal MJ, Greenway B, Wilkinson ML, et al: Sex steroid enzymes aromatase and 5 alpha reductase in the pancreas: A comparison of normal adult, fetal, and malignant tissue. Clin Sci (Lolch) 65:71–75, 1983.

35. Kiriyama S, Hayakewa T, Kondo T, et al: Usefulness of a new tumor marker, SPAN-1, for the diagnosis of pancreatic cancer. Cancer 65:1557–1561, 1990.

36. Mahvi DM, Meyers WC, Bast RC, et al: Therapeutic efficacy as defined by a serodiagnostic test utilizing a monoclonal antibody in carcinoma of the pancreas. Ann Surg 202:440, 1985.

37. Romond EH, Mendelsohn LA, MacDonald JS: Adjuvant therapy of gastrointestinal cancer. Cancer Treat Res 33:273–295, 1987.

38. Griffin JF, Smalley SR, Jewell W, et al: Patterns of failure after curative resection of pancreatic carcinoma. Cancer 66:56–61, 1990.

39. Whipple AO, Parsons WB, Mullins CR: Treatment of carcinoma of the ampulla of Vater. Ann Surg 102:763, 1935.

40. Gastrointestinal Tumor Study Group: Pancreatic cancer: Adjuvant combined radiation and chemotherapy following curative resection. Arch Surg 120:899–903, 1985.

41. Gastrointestinal Tumor Study Group: Further evidence of effective adjuvant combined radiation and chemotherapy following curative resection of pancreatic cancer. Cancer 59:2006–2010, 1987.

42. Carter SK, Connis RL: Adenocarcinoma of the pancreas: Current therapeutic approaches, prognostic variables and criteria of response, in Staquet MJ (ed): Cancer Therapy: Prognostic Factors and Criteria of Response, pp 235–237. New York, Raven Press, 1975.

43. Crooke ST, Bradner WT: Mitomycin C: A review. Cancer Treat Rev 3:121–139, 1976.

44. Smith FP, Schein PS: Chemotherapy of pancreatic cancer. Semin Oncol 6:368–377, 1979.

45. Mawla NGE: Ifosfamide in advanced pancreatic cancer. Cancer Chemother Pharmacol 18(suppl 2):55–56, 1986.

46. Loehrer PJ, Williams SD, Einhorn L, et al: Ifosfamide: An active drug in the treatment of adenocarcinoma of the pancreas. J Clin Oncol 3:367–372, 1985.

47. Frederick PS et al: 5-Fluorouracil, adriamycin and mitomycin C (FAM) chemotherapy for advanced adenocarcinoma of the pancreas. Cancer 46:2014–2018, 1980.

48. Cullinan SA et al: A comparison of three chemotherapeutic regimens in the treatment of advanced pancreatic and gastric carcinoma. JAMA 253:2061–2067, 1985.

49. Wiggans G, Woolley PV, Macdonald JS, et al: Phase II trial of streptozotocin, mitomycin and 5-fluorouracil (SMF) in the treatment of advanced pancreatic cancer. Cancer 41:387–391, 1978.

50. Gastrointestinal Tumor Study Group: Phase II studies of drug combinations in advanced pancreatic carcinoma: Fluorouracil plus doxorubicin plus mitomycin C and two regimens of streptozotocin plus mitomycin C plus fluorouracil. J Clin Oncol 4:1794–1798, 1986.

51. Hansen RM: Gastric and pancreatic carcinomas, in Lokich JJ (ed): Cancer Chemotheraphy by Infusion, 2nd ed, pp 340–357. Chicago, Precept Press, 1990.

52. Crown J, Casper ES, Botet J, et al: Lack of efficacy of high-dose leucovorin and fluorouracil in patients with advanced pancreatic adenocarcinoma. J Clin Oncol 9: 1682–1686, 1991.

53. Decaprio JA, Mayer RJ, Gonin R, et al: Fluorouracil and high-dose leucovorin in previously untreated patients with advanced adenocarcinoma of the pancreas: Results of a phase II trial. J Clin Oncol 9:2128–2133, 1991.

54. Ardalan B, Glazer RI, Kenle TW, et al: Synergistic effect of 5-fluorouracil and N-(phosphonacetyl)-1-aspartate on cell growth and ribonucleic acid synthesis in a human mammary carcinoma. Biochem Pharmacol 30:2045–2049, 1981.

55. Morrell LM, Bach A, Richman SP, et al: A phase II multiinstitutional trial of low dose N-(phosphonacetyl)-1-aspartate and high dose 5-fluorouracil as a short term infusion in the treatment of adenocarcinoma of the pancreas: A Southwest Oncology Group Study. Cancer 67:363–366, 1991.

56. Bengmark S, Andren-Sandberg A: Infusion chemotheraphy in inoperable pancreatic carcinoma: Recent results. Cancer Res 86:13–14, 1983.

57. Theodors A, Bukowski R, Hewlett J, et al: Intermittent regional infusion of chemotherapy for pancreatic adenocarcinoma. Am J Clin Oncol 5:555–558, 1982.

57a. Casper ES, Green MR, Kelsen DP, et al: Phase II trial of gemcitabine (2,2′-difluorodeoxycytidine) in patients with adenocarcinoma of the pancreas. Invest New Drugs 12(1):29–34, 1994.

57b. Moore M, Andersen J, Burris H, et al: A randomized trial of gemcitabine vs 5-FU as first-line therapy in advanced pancreatic cancer (abstract). Proc Am Soc Clin Oncol 14:199, 1995.

58. Benz C, Hollander C, Miller B: Endocrine-responsive pancreatic carcinoma: Steroid binding and cytotoxicity studies in human tumor cell lines. Cancer Res 46:2276–2281, 1986.

59. Benz C, Wiznitzer I: Steroid binding and cytotoxicity in cultured human pancreatic carcinomas (abstract). J Steroid Biochem Mol Biol 19(suppl):125S, 1983.

60. Theve NO, Pousette A, Carlstrom K: Adenocarcinoma of the pancreas—a hormone sensitive tumor? A preliminary report on Nolvadex treatment. Clin Oncol (R Coll Radiol) 9:193, 1983.

61. Miller B, Benz C: Endocrine treatment of pancreatic carcinoma (abstract). Proc Am Soc Clin Oncol 4:90, 1985.

62. Upp JR, Olson D, Poston GJ, et al: Inhibition of growth of two human pancreatic adenocarcinomas in vivo by somatostatin analog SMS 201–995. Am J Surg 142:308–311, 1988.

63. Smith JP, Solomon TE, Baghari S, Kramer S: Cholecystokinin stimulates growth of human pancreatic adenocarcinoma SW-1990. Dig Dis Sci 35:1377–1384, 1990.

64. Abbruzzese JL, Gholson CF, Daugherty K, et al: A pilot trial of the cholecystokinin receptor antagonist ML-329 in patients with advanced pancreatic cancer. Pancreas 7:165–171, 1992.

65. Moertel CG et al: Therapy of locally unresectable pancreatic cancer: A randomised comparison of high-dose (6000 R) radiation alone, moderate dose radiation (4000 R plus 5-fluorouracil) and high-dose radiation plus 5-fluorouracil: The Gastrointestinal Tumor Study Group. Cancer 48:1705–1710, 1981.

66. Shibamoto Y, Manabe T, Baba N, et al: High dose external beam and intraoperative radiotherapy in the treatment of resectable and unresectable pancreatic cancer. Int J Radiat Oncol Biol Phys 19:605–611, 1990.

67. Roldan GE, et al: External beam versus intraoperative and external beam irradiation for locally advanced pancreatic cancer. Cancer 61:1110–1116, 1988.

68. Bosslet K, Kern HF, Kanzy A, et al: A monoclonal antibody with binding and inhibitory activity towards human pancreatic carcinoma cells. Cancer Immunol Immunother 23:185–191, 1986.

69. Herlyn DM, Koprowski H: IgG 2a monoclonal antibodies inhibit human tumor growth through interaction with effector cells. Proc Natl Acad Sci USA 79:4761–4795, 1982.

70. Buchler M, Friess H, Schultheiss HK, et al: A randomized controlled trial of adjuvant immunotheraphy (murine monoclonal antibody 494/32) in resectable pancreatic cancer. Cancer 68:1507–1512, 1991.

71. Gottlinger H, Funke I, Johnson J P, et al: The epithelial cell surface antigen 17-1A, a target for antibody mediated tumor therapy: Its biochemical nature, tissue distribution and recognition by different monoclonal antibodies. Int J Cancer 38:47–53, 1986.

72. Korz M, Meltzer P, Trent J: Enhanced expression of epidermal growth factor receptor correlates with alterations of chromosome 7 in human pancreatic cancer. Proc Natl Acad Sci USA 83:5141–5144, 1986.

73. Almoquera C, Shibata D, Forrester K, et al: Most human carcinomas of the exocrine pancreas contain mutant c-k-ras genes. Cell 53:49, 1988.

74. Budd K: Psychotropic drugs in the treatment of chronic pain. Anaesthesia 33:531, 1978.

75. Serdlow M: The treatment of shooting pain. Postgrad Med J 56:159–161, 1980.

76. Ischia S, Luzzani A, Ischia A, et al: A new approach to the neurolytic block of the coeliac plexus: The transaortic technique. Pain 16:333–341, 1983.

77. Leung JWC, Bowen-Wright M, Aveling W, et al: Coeliac plexus block for pain in pancreatic cancer and chronic pancreatitis. Br J Surg 70:730–732, 1983.

78. Thompson GE, Moore DC, Bridenbaugh LD, et al: Abdominal pain and alcohol coeliac plexus block. Anaesthesia Analgesia 56:1–5, 1977.

79. International Union Against Cancer: Workshop on Biology of Human Cancer. Rep. 17: Hepatocellular carcinoma. Geneva, 1982.

80. Beasley RP et al: Prevention of perinatally transmitted hepatitis B virus infections with hepatitis B immune globulin and hepatitis B vaccine. Lancet 2:1099–1122, 1983.

81. Adamson RC, Corree P, et al: Carcinogenicity of aflatoxin B1 in rhesus monkeys: Two additional cases of primary liver cancer. J Natl Cancer Inst 57:67–78, 1976.

82. Beazley R, Cohn I Jr: Tumors of the pancreas, gallbladder, and extrahepatic ducts. ACS Textbook of Clin Onc 16:219–231, 1994.

83. Okuda K, Ryu M, Takayoshi T: Surgical management of hepatoma: The Japanese experience, in Wanebo JH (ed): Hepatic and Biliary Surgery, pp 219–238. New York, Marcel Dekker, 1987.

84. Okuda K, Obata H, et al: Prognosis of primary hepatocellular carcinoma. Hepatology 4:3–6S, 1984.

85. Chin H, Cheng E, Gellar N: Hepatocellular carcinoma: Statistical analysis of 78 consecutive patients (abstract). Proc Am Soc Clin Oncol 3:6, 1984.

86. Buamah PK, Cornell C, James OFW, et al: Serial Serum AFP heterogeneity changes in patients with hepatocellular carcinoma during chemotherapy. Cancer Chemother Pharmacol 17:182–184, 1986.

87. Hosoki T, Chatani M, Mori S: Dynamic computerized tomography of hepatocellular carcinoma. Am J Radiol 139:1099–1106, 1982.

88. Tsuzuki T, Ogata Y, et al: Hepatic resection in 125 patients. Arch Surg 119:1025–1032, 1984.

89. Adson MA: Primary hepatocellular cancers: Western experience in Blumgart LH (eds): Surgery of the Liver and Biliary Tract, p 1155. New York, Churchill-Livingstone.

90. Zhou XD, Tang ZY, Yu YQ, et al: Clinical evaluation of cryosurgery in the treatment of primary liver cancer. Cancer 61:1889–1892, 1988.

91. Lewis BJ, Friedman MA: Current status of chemotheraphy for hepatoma, in Ogawa M (ed): Chemotherapy of Hepatic Tumors, pp 63–

74. Princeton, NJ, Excerpta Medica, 1984.

92. Gastrointestinal Tumor Study Group: A prospective trial of recombinant human interferon alpha 2B in previously untreated patients with hepatocellular carcinoma. Cancer 66:135–139, 1990.

93. Kardinal CG, Moertel CG, et al: Combined doxorubicin and alpha-interferon therapy of advanced hepatocellular carcinoma. Cancer 71:2187–2190, 1993.

94. Atiq OT, Kemeny N, Niedzwiecki D, et al: Treatment of unresectable primary liver with intrahepatic fluorodeoxyuridine and mitomycin C through an implanted pump. Cancer 69:920–924, 1992.

95. Yodono H, Sasaki T, et al: Arterial infusion chemotherapy for advanced hepatocellular carcinoma with EPF and EAP therapies. Cancer Chemother Pharmacol 31:S89–92, 1992.

96. Order SE, Stillwagon GB, Klein JL, et al: Iodine 131 antiferritin, a new treatment modality in hepatoma: An RTOG study. J Clin Oncol 3:1573–1582, 1985.

97. Order SE, Pajak T, et al: A randomized prospective trial comparing full dose chemotheraphy to 131 I antiferritin: An RTOG study. Int J Radiat Oncol Biol Phys 20:953–963, 1991.

98. Iwatsuki S, Starzl TE, Sheahan DG, et al: Hepatic resection versus transplantation for hepatocellular carcinoma. Ann Surg 214:221–229, 1991.

99. Penn I: Hepatic transplantation for primary and metastatic cancers of the liver. Surgery 110:726–735, 1991.

100. de Stoll M: Rationis Mendendi in Nosocomio practico vendobonensi. Part I Lugduni Batavorium, Haak et Socios et A et J. Honkoop, 1788.

101. Nevin JE, Moran TJ: Carcinoma of the gallbladder: Staging, treatment and prognosis. Cancer 37:141–148, 1976.

102. Silk YN et al: Carcinoma of the gallbladder: The Roswell Park experience. Ann Surg 210:751–757, 1989.

103. Vaittinen E: Carcinoma of the gallbladder: A study of 390 cases diagnosed in Finland 1953–1967. Ann Chir Gynaecol 168(suppl):1–18, 1970.

104. Krain LS: Gallbladder and extrahepatic bile duct carcinoma: Analysis of 1808 cases. Geriatrics 27: 1111–1117, 1972.

105. Paraskevopoulos JA, et al: Primary carcinoma of the gallbladder: A 10-year experience. Ann R Coll Surg Engl 74:222–224, 1992.

106. Polk HC: Carcinoma in the calcified gallbladder. Gastroenterology 50:582, 1966.

107. Yamaguchi K, Tsuneyoshi M: Subclinical gallbladder carcinoma. Am J Surg 163: 382–386, 1992.

108. Fahim RB, McDonald JR, Richard JC, et al: Carcinoma of the gallbladder: A study of its modes of spread. Ann Surg 156:114–124, 1962.

109. Bosset JF et al: Primary carcinoma of the gallbladder: Adjuvant postoperative external irradiation. Cancer 64:1843–1847, 1989.

110. Itai Y, Araki K, et al: Computed tomography of gallbladder carcinoma. Radiology 137:713–718, 1980.

111. Shieh CJ, Dunn E, Standard JE: Primary cancer of the gallbladder: A review of a 16-year experience at the Waterbury Hospital Health Center. Cancer 47:996–1004, 1981.

112. Hanna SS, Rider WD: Carcinoma of the gallbladder or extrahepatic bile ducts: The role of radiotherapy. Can Med Assoc J 118:59–61, 1978.

113. Todoroki T et al: Intraoperative radiotherapy for advanced carcinoma of the biliary system. Cancer 46: 2179–2184, 1980.

114. Smoron GL: Radiation therapy of carcinoma of the gallbladder and biliary tract. Cancer 40:1422–1424, 1977.

CHAPTER 17

Colorectal Cancer: Diagnosis and Management

Enrique A. Diaz-Canton, MD, *and* Richard Pazdur, MD

Department of Gastrointestinal Medical Oncology and Digestive Diseases
The University of Texas M.D. Anderson Cancer Center, Houston, Texas

In the United States, cancer of the large bowel is the second most common cause of cancer deaths after cancer of the lung.[1] 1995 estimates place large bowel cancer as the third most common malignancy, behind lung and prostate carcinomas in men and behind lung and breast cancers in women. For unknown reasons, overall incidence and mortality rates for colorectal cancer have begun to drop.[2-4] This may be related, at least in part, to better public and professional health education, better primary prevention, including improved diet, and possibly to excision of large bowel adenomas.[5] Mortality rates have begun to decline in whites, remained stable in black women, and risen in black men.[6] Among blacks and Hispanics, there is a trend toward later-stage colorectal cancers at presentation; moreover, these ethnic groups had the worst survival rates at each stage of disease,[7] and this trend increased with age. In the United States, the lifetime risk of developing a colorectal cancer is roughly 1 in 20.[8]

The overall incidence of this malignancy is nearly identical in men and women; colon tumors occur slightly more often in women and rectal carcinomas are seen slightly more frequently in men. The risk of developing colorectal cancer usually begins in the fourth decade of life and increases with age; only about 3% of these cancers develop in persons under the age of 40.[9] The mean patient age at presentation is 60 to 65 years. For persons under 65, the incidence of colorectal cancer is 19.2 per 100,000, and for those 65 or older, 337.1 per 100,000.[3]

The natural history of colorectal carcinoma has changed over the last 3 decades. Colon carcinomas now constitute approximately 70% of all cancers in the large bowel, with the right side of the proximal colon the most common site.[10] This finding may be the result of more frequent use of sigmoidoscopy and polypectomy, which may have lessened the relative incidence of cancers of the rectum and sigmoid colon. The incidence of colon carcinomas in blacks has increased by 30% since 1973 and is now higher than in whites.[3] The reasons for these changes are not known, but dietary and environmental factors may be responsible. Five-year survival rates for patients with Dukes' A, B, and C colon carcinoma (TNM stages I, II,

and III, respectively) have improved in recent years (Table 1). This improvement may be due to the wider surgical dissections performed, modern anesthetic techniques and supportive care, better pathologic examination of resected specimens, and preoperative staging and abdominal exploration, which reveal clinically occult disease.

In this review, we will discuss the molecular genetics and biology, etiology and risk factors, pathology, clinical presentation, screening and diagnosis, staging and prognostic factors, and management of carcinomas of the colon and rectum.

MOLECULAR GENETICS AND BIOLOGY

Several articles have been published recently on the molecular biology of tumors of the large bowel. Research in genetic epidemiology found that roughly 10% of large bowel tumors may arise in persons with a genetic susceptibility to them.[11] Molecular genetic information now can be used to screen high-risk populations more aggressively and in the future may have therapeutic applications.

The best characterized conditions that predispose to large bowel cancer are dominantly inherited diseases that can be categorized into one of two groups depending on the presence or absence of a polyposis phenotype. These conditions are the familial adenomatous polyposis (FAP)

TABLE I

Surgical Stage and Postoperative Prognosis of Colorectal Cancer

Surgical stage[a]	Five-year survival (%)	
	1940s to 1950s	1960s to 1970s
Dukes'-Kirklin A	80	> 90
Dukes'-Kirklin B1	60	85
Dukes'-Kirklin B2	45	70–75
Dukes' C	15–30	45–60
Dukes' D	< 5	< 5

[a] A = disease limited to mucosa; B1 = disease extends to muscularis propria; B2 = disease extends beyond the muscularis propria into serosa; C = positive regional lymph nodes; D = distant metastases

syndrome and the hereditary nonpolyposis colorectal cancer (HNPCC) syndrome, both described below in more detail. The FAP syndrome appears to be due to defects in a single gene, whereas defects in the HPNCC syndrome seem genetically heterogeneous.[11]

In 1954, Armitage et al[12] suggested that several types of cancers develop secondary to an accumulation of as many as seven events. Today it is believed that genes are the molecular targets of those events. Colorectal cancer appears to arise as a result of the mutational activation of oncogenes combined with the mutational inactivation of tumor supressor genes, with the latter a predominant action, and a newly described class of mutations, replication errors (RERs).[10]

Activation of Oncogenes: To contribute to carcinogenesis, oncogenes must be activated by mutational changes, which can involve either point mutation or overexpression. Alteration of only one allele is needed to induce malignant changes, an effect called transdominance.[13] The most commonly affected oncogenes in the genesis of large bowel tumors are c-*myc* and c-Ki-*ras*; those less frequently affected include c-*src*, c-*myb*, and c-*erb-b2*.[14-16]

The c-Ki-*ras* oncogene is responsible for synthesis of a protein involved in the transduction of mitogenic messages across the plasmatic membrane of the cell.[17] Point mutations on this oncogene were detected in 39% to 71% of colorectal cancers and in 42% of adenomatous polyps.[18-20] Interestingly, the c-Ki-*ras* mutation was encountered in more than 40% of the cases involving adenomas larger than 1 cm in diameter, whereas only 10% of adenomas smaller than 1 cm had that mutation. As noted in Figure 1, the mutation of the ras oncogene seems to be involved in the pass from small adenoma to large adenoma, with the latter more likely to progress to cancer than the former.[21] In a study by Sidransky et al[22] of patients whose benign and malignant large bowel tumors contained c-*ras* mutations, 8 of 9 mutations were found in DNA from stools.[22]

The c-*myc* oncogene is activated by its overexpression in colorectal tumors. This oncogene is believed to encode a nuclear phosphoprotein that may be necessary for DNA synthesis.[23,24] In studies of adenoma and colorectal cancer patients, c-*myc* levels in RNA were increased in 60% to 70% of the cases[25-28] and c-*myc* expression was greater in tumors from the descending colon than in other tumors.

Inactivation of Tumor-Suppressor Genes: In contrast to the transdominant activity of oncogenes, tumor-suppressor genes exhibit a recessive activity pattern, ie, inactivation of both alleles is necessary, whether by point mutation, deletion, or both.[13] These genes seem to have great importance in the pathogenesis of colorectal tumors.

The FAP syndrome, which confers a susceptibility to large bowel tumors, is the result of point mutations in the adenomatous polyposis coli (*APC*) tumor-suppressor gene. The *APC* gene is inherited through the germ line (the first mutational event; cancer develops when the second copy of the gene is deleted or mutated in the somatic tissue) and is localized to chromosome 5 (5q21). This gene encodes a protein whose function is at present poorly understood but that may interact with beta and perhaps alpha catenins. Those proteins together with E-cadherin may be implicated in tumor progression through alteration of the cytoskeleton and cell adhesion systems.[29-33] Disease manifestation depends on the type of mutation occurring in the *APC* gene; with some types of *APC* gene mutations (after exon 9), ophthalmologic manifestations of the FAP syndrome are evident, leading to a patchy hyperpigmentation of the retina.[34] Additionally, some types of mutations (in the 5′ region) are associated with attenuated forms of the disease[35-36] rather than with the more virulent form. Inactivation of the *APC* gene seems to play an important role in sporadic and FAP tumorigenesis and has been detected in 36% to 79% of patients with colorectal tumors and adenomas.[37-38]

Deletions and point mutations have been identified in a second gene on the long arm of chromosome 5—the mutated in colon carcinoma (*MCC*) gene[39-40]; up to 55% of colorectal cancer patients showed deletions involving this gene. *MCC* function is unknown, but this gene might interact with the *APC* gene to form a biologically active complex that regulates proliferation and differentiation.

The deleted in colorectal cancer (*DCC*) gene, a candidate tumor-suppressor gene located on chromosome 18,[41] is activated in 73% of colorectal cancers but in only 11% of adenomas.[19] Preliminary studies suggested that the *DCC* gene product resembles a cell adhesion molecule and may therefore regulate the interaction of the cell with its enviroment.[13] The loss of chromosome 18q could thus lead to impaired contact between cells and thereby contribute to tumor growth and invasion.[42] Jen et al showed that the status of chromosome 18q has strong prognostic value in patients with stage II colon cancer; the prognosis in patients with stage II disease and 18q allelic loss is similar to that in patients with stage III colon cancer, who are thought to benefit from adjuvant therapy. In contrast, patients with stage II disease who do not have 18q allelic loss in their tumors have a survival rate similar to that of patients with stage I disease and may not require additional therapy.

A deletion on the short arm of the chromosome 17 was

FIGURE I

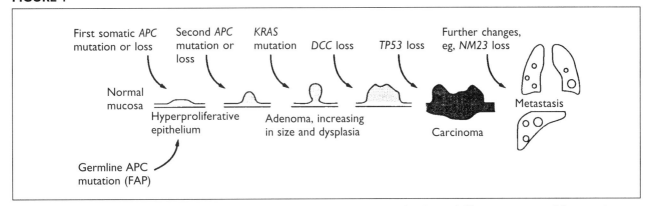

Colorectal carcinogenesis: This model is adapted from Fearon and Vogelstein and illustrates a possible genetic pathway for the development of colorectal carcinoma from normal mucosa. Reprinted, with permission, from Bishop OT, Hall NR: The genetics of colorectal cancer. Eur J Cancer 30A: 1946-1956, 1994.

associated with point mutations in the *p53* allele on the homologous chromosome.[43] In several patients the 17p loss was associated with progression from adenoma to carcinoma and also with poor prognosis. The 17p deletion was observed in 75% to 95% of the colorectal cancers and less commonly in adenomas.[44] Other allelic losses include those from chromosomes 1p, 8q (which also may be associated with poor prognosis), 13q, and 22q.[13]

Replication Errors: A newly described class of mutations, called replication errors (RERs) or microsatellite instability, has been described recently.[11] Cells with this phenotype are characterized by genomic instability at simple repeated sequences in DNA.[45] This instability, produced by slippage of DNA strands in the moment of replication, may be secondary to a mutation of genes committed to reparation and/or replication of DNA. Thus, cells with this genetic abnormality accumulate deletions and insertions at repeated sequences.[46] Microsatellite loci are small regions of the genome characterized by mono-, di-, or trinucleotide repetitive sequences and are in general noncoding. The two best-known are (A)n and (CA)n, where n = 10–30. Of interest, colorectal tumors having this abnormality are more often located on the right side of the colon, appear to be associated with a good clinical outcome, and may serve as a marker for HNPCC.[11] A candidate for the HNPCC gene has been identified on chromosome 2. This gene, called *MSH-2*, appears to regulate RERs and is a homolog of the bacterial missmatch repair gene *MUT-S*.[47–48] Aaltonen et al[49] found RERs in 78% of tumors from patients with HNPCC; RERs also were found in sporadic tumors.[42] The candidate gene on chromosome 2 appears to regulate HNPCC type II (site nonspecific), whereas another gene, on

chromosome 3, seems to be involved in HNPCC type I (site specific).[50-51] The latter gene, *hMLH-1*, encodes a protein homologous to the bacterial DNA missmatch protein MutL.[52] Recently, two more genes that regulate RERs were discovered: *hPMS-1* (homologous to the bacterial *PMS-1*) on chromosome 2 and *hPMS-2* (homologous to the bacterial *PMS-2*) on chromosome 7.[53]

Adenoma-Carcinoma Sequence

Several trials have suggested that most colorectal tumors arise from adenomas.[54] Tumorigenesis has long been thought to be a multistep process.[55] Recently, the molecular events that underlie tumoral initiation and progression have been identified.[56, 56a] Comparison of the frequency with which tumor-suppressor genes and oncogenes are altered in adenomas and carcinomas suggests that there is a preferred order for the occurence of these genes in the adenoma-carcinoma sequence (Figure 1). Fearon et al[21] pointed out, however, that it is the accumulation rather than the order of these mutational events that is essential for carcinogenesis.

ETIOLOGY AND RISK FACTORS

The specific causes of colorectal carcinoma are unknown, but environmental, nutritional, genetic, and familial factors and preexisting diseases have been found to be associated with this cancer. The incidence of colorectal carcinoma is higher in industrialized regions, such as the United States, northern and western Europe, New Zealand, Australia, and Canada, whereas a lower rate is observed in Asia, Africa (among blacks), and South America (except Argentina and Uruguay).[57] Immigrants from low-risk areas assume the colon cancer risk of their adopted country, suggesting the importance of environmental factors.[58–59] Nevertheless, differences in diet within high- or low-risk regions could lead to distinct results. For instance, within the United States, a country with a very high colon cancer risk, a significantly lower risk is noted among Mormons and Seventh Day Adventists, whose diet avoids meat and consists mainly of vegetables, fruits, and whole-grain cereals.[60]

Dietary Factors: Diets rich in fat and cholesterol have been linked to an increased risk of tumors of the colon and rectum.[8] The effects of animal fat appear independent of total calorie intake.[61] A sedentary lifestyle[62] and obesity, both linked with dietary fat, also correlate with the incidence of colorectal cancer.[63–64] Dietary fat increases the endogenous production, bacterial degradation, and excretion of bile acids and neutral steroids, which are carcinogens, thereby promoting colonic carcinogenesis.[65] Excess lipids in the colon may lead to an increase in the concentration of secondary bile acids, which may stimulate protein kinase C (PKC), a major cellular communication pathway, resulting in the promotion of cancer.[66] Some authors[67–68] suggested that in colorectal cancer PKC may inhibit growth, while in normal mucosa it may stimulate growth through the action of bile acids. A diet high in fat could lead to a predominance of anaerobic bacteria in the intestinal microflora, and the enzymes in such bacteria may activate carcinogens.[69–71] Nonetheless, prospective trials in Israel, Japan, and the United States failed to find a link between either fat or meat intake and large bowel cancer.[72–73] Interestingly, a protective effect has been suggested for a diet containing fiber and yellow and green vegetables.[74] However, some authors believe that cereal fiber, although beneficial, is not as important as fiber from fresh fruits and vegetables.[75] Possible effects of fiber on colorectal carcinogenesis may include decreased fecal transit time through the bowel, resulting in decreased exposure to fecal carcinogens; reduced carcinogenic microflora in the bowel; and decreased fecal pH, with a consequent decrease in bacterial enzymatic activity and a dilution of carcinogens via an increase in stool bulk.[76–78] In addition, a higher incidence of rectosigmoid tumors in men has been associated with alcohol consumption. A protective role has been ascribed to calcium salts and calcium-rich foods because of their capacity to decrease colon cell turnover rates and reduce the colon cancer-promoting effects of bile and fatty acids.[79] Other diet compounds that may decrease large bowel carcinogenesis are selenium; vitamins C, D, and E; indoles; and beta-carotene.[80–82]

Nonsteroidal Anti-Inflammatory Drugs (NSAIDs): NSAIDs are known to inhibit the synthesis of prostaglandins. Human tumors have been shown to produce large amounts of prostaglandins, particularly E, which has been implicated in blocking natural killer (NK) cell cytotoxicity.[83] Recent trials suggested that inhibition of prostaglandin synthesis by the NSAID sulindac decreases the development of colonic polyps.[84] Sulindac causes regression of rectal polyps in FAP.[84–85] A phase III randomized trial is planned comparing fluorouracil, levamisole (Ergamisol), and sulindac with fluorouracil and levamisole as adjuvant therapy in patients with resected stage III colon cancer.[86] NSAIDs also may have antiangiogenic effects[87] and may reduce the synthesis of certain growth factors.[88]

An American Cancer Society study[89] suggested that aspirin confers a protective effect against colon cancer. In this prospective study in 424 adults, mortality rates from large bowel cancer decreased in both sexes with more frequent aspirin use. Whether this was an overall decrease in colon cancer incidence or just a decrease in the number of deaths from colon cancer was not noted.[89]

Familial Factors: Several genetic premalignant polyposis syndromes have been described, including familial adenomatous polyposis (FAP) coli, Gardner syndrome, Oldfield syndrome, Turcot syndrome, Peutz-Jeghers syndrome, juvenile polyposis, and hereditary non-polyposis colorectal cancer (HNPCC).

Even if none of these syndromes is present, patients with family histories of colorectal carcinomas still have an increased risk for the disease.[90] Fuchs et al[91] confirmed this in the first prospective study of 32,085 men and 87,031 women who were first-degree relatives with colorectal cancer and pointed out that the risk was more evident in younger people.[91]

Few colon cancer patients have FAP coli (US incidence, 1/6,850).[92] FAP is inherited as an autosomal dominant trait with more than 90% penetrance. Patients with this disorder develop pancolonic and rectal adenomatous polyposis in the mid-teenage years and may develop colorectal carcinoma if prophylactic total colectomy is not done. The risk of colorectal carcinoma is almost 100% if the patient lives long enough. As stated above, a gene predisposing to FAP was identified; this gene, *APC*, is linked to a region on the long arm of chromosome 5 (band 5q21).[93–94] One or more genes on chromosome 5 are involved in the inheritance of FAP as well as in the development of more common sporadic colorectal tumors. This finding may allow genetic identification of FAP family members who will develop colorectal tumors and open the door for studies of genetic events associated with the development of sporadic colorectal cancer.

Gardner syndrome, which occurs 50% less frequently than FAP, is inherited as an autosomal dominant trait.[95]

The whole large and small bowel may be affected by adenomatous polyps that may degenerate into cancer. This is accompanied by desmoid tumors of the mesentery and abdominal wall,[96] sebaceous cysts, lipomas, fibromas, and osteomas.

Oldfield syndrome, which is related to Gardner syndrome, consists of multiple sebaceous cysts accompanied by polyposis that may degenerate into colorectal carcinoma.[97]

Turcot syndrome occurs less frequently than the other syndromes and is possibly inherited as an autosomal recessive condition. This syndrome involves premalignant polyposis of the colon associated with central nervous system tumors.[98]

Peutz-Jeghers and juvenile polyposis syndromes are characterized by hamartomatous polyps of the bowel associated with hyperpigmentation of the oral mucosa and skin (in Peutz-Jeghers).[91] These syndromes carry only a small risk of malignancy (2% to 3%).[99-100]

Some families without a history of adenomatous polyps in the large intestine also have a higher risk of developing colorectal tumors.[101-102] The familial aggregation of these tumors is HNPCC. The cancers that arise from this syndrome differ from the sporadic form by an earlier age of onset (median, 44 years), an increased frequency of right-sided tumors (60% to 70%), an excess of metachronous and synchronous large bowel cancers,[103] and an increased frequency of mucinous and poorly differentiated tumors.[103]

The clinical diagnosis of HNPCC is made by the Amsterdam Criteria.[104-105] The patient must have (1) three or more relatives with histologically confirmed colorectal cancer, one of whom is a first-degree relative of the other two; (2) familial colorectal cancer affecting at least two generations; and (3) one or more familial colorectal cancer cases diagnosed before age 50. HNPCC is inherited as an autosomal dominant trait with more than 90% penetrance.[101] The two types of HNPCC are A and B, which together currently account for 5% to 15% of all colorectal cancers.[106-107] HNPCC type A, formerly called "Lynch syndrome I," is a site-specific familial nonpolyposis colon cancer. This syndrome is associated with colon tumors only and with a tumor predilection for the right side. In HNPCC type B, formerly "Lynch syndrome II," nonpolyposis colon cancer occurs in association with other cancers, such as breast, endometrial, gastric, small bowel, pancreatic, bile duct, urothelial, kidney, and ovarian carcinomas.

Inflammatory Bowel Disease: Patients with inflammatory bowel disease (ulcerative colitis and Crohn's disease) have a higher-than-normal (up to 30-fold) incidence of colorectal carcinoma. The risk of carcinoma in ulcerative colitis patients is associated with the duration of active disease, extent of colitis, development of mucosal dysplasia, and continuity of symptoms.[108-111] The risk of carcinoma increases exponentially with increasing duration of colitis; it is estimated to be approximately 3% in the first decade of disease, 20% in the second decade, and more than 30% in the third decade.[112-113] The risk of developing colorectal cancer also is increased in patients with Crohn's disease, although to a lesser extent than in patients with ulcerative colitis.

Polyps: Colorectal tumors develop more often in patients who have had adenomatous polyps than in those without polyps. There is an approximate 5% probability that carcinoma will be present in an adenoma; the risk correlates with the histology and size of the polyp. The potential for malignant transformation is higher for villous and tubulovillous adenomas than for tubular adenomas.[114] Adenomatous polyps smaller than 1 cm have a less than 1% chance of being malignant compared with adenomas larger than 2 cm, which have up to a 40% likelihood of malignant transformation.[114] In 1993, the National Polyp Study Workgroup concluded that colonoscopy-guided polypectomy lowered the incidence of unexpected colorectal cancer, supporting the view that colorectal adenomas progress to carcinomas.[115]

Cancer History: Patients with a history of colorectal carcinoma are at increased risk of developing a second primary colon cancer or other malignancy.[116] Women with a history of breast, endometrial, or ovarian carcinoma also have an increased chance of developing colorectal carcinoma.[117] An increased incidence of colon cancer at or near the suture line following ureterosigmoidostomy has been reported.[118] Cholecystectomy also has been associated with colon cancer in some studies, but others have found no relationship between this procedure and colon cancer.[119]

Other Predisposing Factors: Finally, sedentary occupations,[120] no or low parity,[121] a history of pelvic irradiation for gynecologic cancer,[121] and a diet poor in vegetables and grains[122] all have been linked to a higher risk of colon carcinoma.

PATHOLOGY

In colorectal carcinoma, the tumor's gross appearance is ulcerating and/or stenosing in about 75% of the cases (left-sided) and fungating in the remaining 25%, which are more frequently located on the right side.[123]

With regard to histologic type, adenocarcinomas make up between 90% and 95% of all large bowel neoplasms.[124-125] These tumors consist of cuboidal or columnar epithelium with multiple degrees of differentiation and variable amounts of mucin. Mucinous adenocarcinoma is a histologic variant characterized by huge amounts of extracellular mucus in the tumor; this tumor variant occurs more often in males and is more frequently diagnosed when the disease is advanced.[126–127] Signet-ring-cell carcinoma is another variant, containing large quantities of intracellular mucin elements that cause the cytoplasm to displace the nucleus. This variant is more common in young females, is frequently diagnosed when the disease is advanced (stage III to IV), and thus tends to have a particularly poor prognosis.[127] Signet-ring-cell tumors tend to spread diffusely through the bowel wall, with relative sparing of the mucosa, producing an appearance of linitis plastica, which could be oligosymptomatic and result in disease-negative biopsies.[128] This tumor shows very little evidence of an association with adenomas.[129] Squamous-cell carcinomas, carcinoid tumors, and adenosquamous and undifferentiated carcinomas all have been reported as colon and rectal cancers.[130] Nonepithelial tumors such as sarcomas[131] and lymphomas[125] are exceedingly rare histologic types in colorectal carcinoma.

Broders and Dukes pioneered the classification of colorectal carcinomas based on their degree of differentiation.[132–133] Broders' system has four grades. Dukes' system, currently the most widely used, considers the arrangement of the cells rather than the percentage of differentiated cells. This system has three grades, with grade 1 the most differentiated tumors and grade 3 the least differentiated.[134–135]

Colorectal carcinoma has a tendency for local invasion by circumferential growth (with this type more important in rectal than colon tumors) and for lymphatic, hematogenous, transperitoneal, and perineural spread.[136] The most common site of extralymphatic involvement is the liver, with the lungs the most frequently affected extra-abdominal organ.[130] Other sites of hematogenous spread include the bones, kidneys, adrenal glands, and brain.

CLINICAL PRESENTATION

Symptoms of colorectal tumors vary depending on the anatomic region involved. During the early stages, patients may be asymptomatic or may complain of vague abdominal pain and flatulence, which may be attributed to gallbladder or peptic ulcer disease. Minor changes in bowel movements with or without rectal bleeding also are seen, but these are frequently ignored and/or attributed to hemorrhoids or other benign disorders. Cancers occurring on the left side of the colon generally cause constipation alternating with diarrhea; abdominal pain; a decrease in the caliber of the stools (pencil stools); and obstructive symptoms such as nausea and vomiting. Right-side colon lesions produce vague abdominal aching (unlike the colicky pain seen with obstructive left-side lesions) and also may present as palpable abdominal masses on the physical exam. Anemia resulting from chronic blood loss, weakness, weight loss, and an abdominal mass also may accompany right-side colon carcinoma. Patients with cancer of the rectum may have a change in bowel movements, rectal fullness, urgency, bleeding, and tenesmus. Pelvic pain is seen at later stages of the disease and usually indicates local extension of the tumor to the pelvic nerves.

Many trials tried to identify preoperative clinical findings that will predict patient prognosis. One such finding is rectal bleeding as a presenting symptom. Those patients might have more localized lesions and therefore a better prognosis than the patients who do not bleed.[137–138] Patients presenting with acute symptoms such as obstruction and perforation have a poorer prognosis.[139–140] Age has been implicated as a prognostic factor in very young patients (younger than 20 years old) because of the poor workup usually done in these patients and their high incidence of signet-ring-cell carcinomas[141] and also in very old patients because of their higher incidence of surgical complications. Some authors point out that older patients may have slower-growing tumors than do younger patients.[142]

SCREENING AND DIAGNOSIS

Average-Risk Individuals: Currently available screening techniques for populations not at high risk for the development of colorectal cancer are far from ideal.

Many fecal occult blood tests (FOBTs) use guaiac, which detects the peroxidase-like capacity of hemoglobin. Although these guaiac-based FOBTs are inexpensive, easy to perform, and carry no risk for the patient, they have been associated with many false-positive and -negative results. Almost all colonic polyps and more than half of all colorectal carcinomas are undetected by this test because they are not bleeding at the time of testing; the test requires more than 20 mL of blood per day to yield a positive result.[143] The newer FOBTs, including a guaiac-based product called Hemoccult SENSA (Smith-Kline Diagnostics), immunochemical tests for hemoglobin (HemeSelect; Smith Kline Diagnostics), and Hemo-Quant (a heme-porphyrin assay specific for fecal heme) appear to have better sensitivity than the older tests without sacrificing specificity.[144] Several trials of FOBTs in Europe and the United States, with a total enrollment of 309,000 patients, failed to conclusively demonstrate a reduction in colorectal cancer mortality, although Winawer et al[145] reported a nonstatistically significant decrease and one European trial reported a trend toward a decrease.[146–150] The latter trial found that when FOBT was done once a year, colorectal cancer mortality decreased by 33%, the first significant reduction in mortality reported. Of note, in this trial testing was done after rehydration of the stool sample.

Digital rectal examination is simple and can detect lesions up to 7 cm from the anal verge. Currently, the American Cancer Society recommends that this procedure be performed annually to screen for rectal and prostate cancers in average-risk populations after age 40.

Flexible proctosigmoidoscopy is safe and more comfortable than examination using a rigid proctoscope. In addition, almost 50% of all colorectal neoplasms are within the reach of a 60-cm sigmoidoscope. Two recent case-control studies support the use of sigmoidoscopy for colorectal screening in average-risk populations after age 50.[151–152]

Colonoscopy provides information on the mucosa of the entire colon, and its sensitivity in detecting tumors is extremely high. Colonoscopy can be used to obtain biopsy specimens of adenomas and carcinomas and allows excision of adenomatous polyps. Limitations of colonoscopy include its inability to detect some polyps and small lesions because of blind corners and mucosal folds and the fact that with colonoscopy the cecum sometimes cannot be reached.[153] Today, most clinical trials use colonoscopy for definitive diagnosis after positive screening tests. Also, colonoscopy may significantly reduce colorectal cancer mortality in high-risk populations.[154]

Barium enemas are also accurate in detecting colorectal carcinoma, although double-contrast barium enemas have a false-negative rate of 2% to 18% owing to misreading, poor preparation, and difficulties in detecting smaller lesions.[136] A barium enema should be viewed as complementary to colonoscopy.

The American Cancer Society has recommended that asymptomatic patients with no risk factors should have a digital rectal examination annually beginning at age 40 and should have fecal occult blood tests yearly and flexible sigmoidoscopy every 3 to 5 years starting at age 50.[155] An analysis of combinations of screening methods found fecal occult blood testing and flexible sigmoidoscopy to be the most cost-effective strategy for reducing mortality from cancer of the rectum and distal colon.

High-Risk Patients: There is no proven screening recommendation for patients at high risk for colorectal cancer, but it is not unreasonable to start screening family members of patients with familial polyposis with annual flexible sigmoidoscopy between the ages of 10 and 12 years.[156] Patients with one or more first-degree relatives who developed colorectal cancer at age 55 years or younger should have an annual FOBT and either a colonoscopy or double-contrast barium enema every 5 years beginning at age 35 to 40 years.[155] Members of families with a history of HNPCC require earlier and more frequent examination with colonoscopy. For patients with a single or several adenomas over 1 cm and/or adenomas with villous changes, surveillance of the entire remaining large intestine has been recommended 1 year after resection and if the initial findings are normal, every 3 to 5 years thereafter. The timing of follow-up colonoscopic examinations after polyp removal has been questioned recently. Winawer and associates of Memorial Sloan-Kettering Cancer Center found that a follow-up colonoscopic examination 3 years after a polypectomy was as effective as were follow-ups at 1 and 3 years. These investigators recommend first follow-up colonoscopy no sooner than 3 years after all polyps are removed.[157] In addition, other investigators have noted that follow-up colonoscopic examinations are warranted in patients with tubulovillous, villous, or large (1 cm) adenomas in the rectosigmoid, particularly if the adenomas are multiple; however, in patients having only a single, small tubular adenoma, surveillance colonoscopy may not have value because the risk of cancer is low.[158] Patients with a longer-than-8-year history of ulcerative colitis with pancolitis who have not undergone proctocolectomy require colonoscopy with multiple random biopsies every 1 to 2 years to detect dysplasia.[156] Individuals with a personal history of colorectal cancer are also at high risk for developing another colorectal cancer and need surveillance of the large bowel as well as regular follow-up for metastatic disease.

Better screening methods for colorectal cancer are needed for both average- and high-risk patients. Stool DNA analysis for mutations of the K-*ras* gene and other genetic abnormalities may be utilized in the future for early detection of colorectal tumors.[159]

Initial Diagnostic Workup: The initial diagnostic workup for patients suspected of having colorectal tumors should include digital rectal examination or an FOBT. An air-contrast barium enema and/or colonoscopy with biopsy of any detected lesions also should be performed prior to surgery in order to detect synchronous polyps or carcinomas. Endoscopic ultrasonography has markedly improved the accuracy of preoperative tumor and node staging in rectal cancers.[160] A chest x-ray, computed

TABLE 2

Comparison of Staging Systems for Colorectal Adenocarcinoma

Dukes'	TNM		TNM[a]		Modified Astler-Coller
A	I	Tis	N0	M0	A
		T1T2	N0	M0	B1
B	II	T3T4a	N0	M0	B2
		T4b	N0	M0	B3
C	III	T1T2	N1N2N3[b]	M0	C1
		T3T4a	N1N2N3	M0	C2
		T4b	N1N2N3	M0	C3
D	IV	Any T	Any N	M1	D

[a] Tis: Carcinoma in situ; T1: Tumor invades submucosa; T2; Tumor invades muscularis propria; T3: Tumor invades through the muscularis propria into the subserosa, or into nonperitonealized pericolic or perirectal tissues; T4a: Tumor perforates the visceral peritoneum; T4b: Tumor (is adherent to or) directly invades other organs or structures (surgical or pathological definition). N0: No regional lymph node metastasis; N1: Metastasis in 1-3 pericolic or perirectal lymph nodes; N2: Metastasis in ≥ 4 pericolic or perirectal lymph nodes; N3: Metastasis in any lymph node along the course of a named trunk; M0: No distant metastasis; M1: Distant metastasis

Note: T4 is substaged and information in parentheses added to more clearly define patients with differential failure risks.

[b] Lymph nodes beyond those encompassed by standard resection of the primary tumor and regional lymphatics (eg, retroperitoneal nodes) are considered distant metastasis.

From O'Connell MJ and Gunderson LL, World J Surg 16:510-515, 1992. Source: Am Society Clinical Oncology Educational Book, 1994.

tomography (CT) scan of the abdomen and pelvis, complete blood count, platelet count, liver and renal function tests, urinalysis, and preoperative measurement of carcinoembryonic antigen (CEA) level also should be done for adequate staging prior to surgical intervention. Magnetic resonance imaging is under investigation but is not routinely used in the staging of large bowel carcinoma. A CT scan of the abdomen is useful to detect liver metastases larger than 2 cm, but its diagnostic yield drops when the metastases are smaller than 2 cm. Improvement in the detection of liver metastases less than 2 cm in size has been noted using CT arterial portography, which involves insertion of a catheter in the superior mesenteric artery followed by CT scanning of the liver while contrast material is delivered into the artery. This procedure is used in patients with liver metastases from colorectal cancer who may be candidates for surgical resection of the liver.[161–162]

Satumomab pendetide (Oncoscint CR/OV) was recently approved as a diagnostic imaging agent indicated for determining the extent and location of extrahepatic malignant disease in colorectal cancer patients.[163–164] This agent is an immunoconjugate of monoclonal antibody B72.3 that has been radiolabeled with [111]In. In a study of 92 patients, these antibody scans were able to detect occult lesions in 11 patients with surgically confirmed adenocarcinoma, and the scans may be particu-

larly useful in detecting extrahepatic disease. In a study of 155 patients with colorectal carcinoma, immunoscintigraphy and CT demonstrated similar sensitivities (69% and 68%, respectively) and specificity (77%). Although CT was able to detect a greater proportion of liver metastases (84% vs 41%), immunoscintigraphy showed greater sensitivity in detecting pelvic tumors and extrahepatic abdominal metastases (84% vs 41%, $P < .001$).[164]

STAGING AND PROGNOSTIC FACTORS

The three main staging systems for colorectal cancer are the Dukes, TNM, and modified Astler-Coller (MAC) systems (Table 2).[165] In the United States, the most widely used clinical and pathologic staging system for colorectal tumors is the modified Astler-Coller Dukes' system, which is based on the depth of tumor invasion into and through the intestinal wall, on the number of regional lymph nodes involved, and on the presence or absence of distant metastases. The 1990 NIH Consensus Conference statement urged a more standard use of the TNM system.

Pathologic stage is the single most important prognostic factor following surgical resection of colorectal tumors.[130] The prognosis for early stages (I and II) is favorable overall, in contrast to the prognosis for advanced stages (III and IV) (Table 1).

Other, less powerful prognostic factors include the following:

(1) When adjusted for other factors, age has never been proven an independent prognostic factor for colorectal carcinoma in young people[166]; however, a delay in diagnosis and a higher incidence of mucin-producing tumors may be related to a higher disease stage at presentation. Old patients are prone to have slower-growing tumors, but the incidence of surgical complications in these patients is higher than in younger ones.

(2) Patients without symptoms tend to have better prognoses, independent of disease stage.[130] However, rectal bleeding has been associated with better survival.[167]

(3) Obstruction and perforation are related to poor prognosis independent of disease stage.[168]

(4) With regard to tumor location, rectal tumors have a poorer prognosis than colon tumors.

(5) DNA content is an independent factor for survival.[130] The 18q chromosome deletion has been associated with a poorer prognosis (see above).

(6) Histologic grade also is correlated with survival. Five-year survival rates of 56% to 100%, 33% to 80%, and 11% to 58% have been reported for grades 1, 2, and 3 colorectal tumors, respectively.[130]

Other prognostic factors, such as preoperative CEA level, sex, tumor histologic features, perioperative blood transfusions,[169] perineural invasion, venous or lymphatic invasion, and S-phase fraction, have not consistently been correlated with overall disease recurrence and survival.[159] Furthermore, the size of the primary lesion has had no influence on survival.[170–172]

TREATMENT

Curative management of colorectal carcinoma relies primarily on surgical resection, possibly accompanied by adjuvant systemic or local chemotherapy and immunotherapy. In rectal cancer, radiation therapy also is used. Palliative treatment is field-of-surgery radiation therapy and chemotherapy, when indicated.

Surgery

Primary Tumor: The primary therapy for adenocarcinoma of the colon and rectum is surgical extirpation of the bowel segment containing the tumor, the adjacent mesentery, and draining lymph nodes. The type of surgical resection depends on the tumor's anatomic location. Right or left hemicolectomy is the surgical treatment of choice in patients with right- or left-side colonic tumors, respectively. Tumors in the sigmoid colon may be treated by wide sigmoid resection.[130]

For rectal carcinoma, abdominoperineal resection and permanent colostomy should be performed if the tumor is located in the distal 5 cm of the rectum.[173] However, this treatment sacrifices the rectum and may be associated with urologic dysfunction and impotence. If the tumor is located proximally between 6 and 10 cm, a lower anterior resection with end-to-end anastomosis may be performed. Local excision alone may be indicated for selected rectal cancer patients who have small (less than 3 to 4 cm),[174] exophytic,[175] and well-differentiated to moderately differentiated tumors confined to the submucosa and for which a disease-free surgical margin can be achieved.[176] Adam et al showed the importance of the circumferential margin in local recurrence of rectal cancer, reporting a significantly higher recurrence in patients with tumor involvement of the circumferential margin than in those without such involvement.[177]

Patients who have low-lying rectal adenocarcinomas and are not candidates for local excision and postoperative radiotherapy may be managed with preoperative radiotherapy (40 to 50 Gy) or preoperative chemoradiotherapy followed by surgery to preserve the sphincter and control local tumor.[178–179] The advantages of this approach include downstaging of the tumor with chemoradiation or radiation, which may allow an adequate surgical margin and sphincter-sparing surgery.

Metastases: Surgical excision is the standard of care in patients with resectable liver and pulmonary metastases from colorectal carcinoma owing to the potential for long-term survival after complete resection in these cases and to the fact that without surgery, such disease remains incurable at present.

Only a small number of patients with large bowel cancer present with lung metastases as the first site of recurrence. One large series demonstrated a 5-year survival rate of 31%.[180] The presence of more than one lung metastasis and an elevated CEA level prior to surgery have been noted as poor-prognosis factors after resection.[130]

Twenty-five percent of colorectal cancer patients present with liver metastases (synchronous); about 50% of colorectal cancer patients develop liver metastases after surgical resection of the primary tumor (metachronous).[181] In six series with more than 100 patients each, 5-year survival rates of from 25% to 39% and a median survival of longer than 2 years were reported after resection of liver metastases.[182–187] In multivariate analyses, the most consistent predictors of long-term survival were stage of the primary tumor, percentage of tumor involvement[185] (with fewer than three metastases and small tumors conferring a better prognosis),[188–189] and disease-negative surgical margins.[190]

Of interest, Nordlinger et al concluded that selected patients with liver metastases from colorectal carcinoma can undergo subsequent resection if needed and that a percentage of these patients enjoy long-term survival; this finding emphasizes the need for careful follow-up after hepatectomy for liver metastases.[191]

Nonhepatic intra-abdominal recurrence of colon carcinoma frequently is found in patients who have disseminated disease; however, in the presence of localized disease or as treatment of symptomatic disease, surgical resection should be considered with the expectation that some patients will enjoy long-term survival and that many with unresectable disease will be palliated.[192]

Adjuvant Therapy for Colon Carcinoma

Approximately 75% of all patients with colorectal carcinoma will present at a stage when all gross carcinoma can be surgically resected.[193] Nevertheless, despite the high resectability rate, almost half of all patients with colorectal adenocarcinoma die of metastatic disease,[1] primarily because of residual disease that is not apparent at the time of surgery. These individuals are candidates for adjuvant local or systemic therapies.

The natural history and patterns of failure following "curative" resection for colon cancer differ from those for rectal carcinomas. Local-regional failure as the only or major site of recurrence is common in rectal cancer, whereas colon cancer tends to recur in the peritoneum, liver, and other distant sites, with a lower rate of local failure. As a result, a local therapy such as radiation may have a significant role in the treatment of rectal tumors but is not routinely used for colon cancers. Nonetheless, investigators from Harvard pointed out that certain patients with colon carcinoma, such as those with B3 and C3 lesions (MAC), tumors associated with abscess or fistula formation, and residual disease after subtotal resection, may benefit from postoperative radiotherapy in addition to systemic therapy.[194] Systemic chemotherapy plus levamisole is the principal adjuvant therapy for colon cancer.

Systemic Therapy: The administration of either fluorouracil or floxuridine (FUDR) to patients with Dukes' stage II and III colon tumors following surgical resection has failed to produce a survival advantage over postsurgical observation,[195] and a recent meta-analysis did not show any benefit from adjuvant fluorouracil.[196–197] Five trials compared the combination of semustine (methyl-CCNU), vincristine (Oncovin), and fluorouracil with no adjuvant treatment, immunotherapy with bacillus Calmette-Guerin (BCG) or its methanol extraction residue (MER), and fluorouracil alone. Four of these trials, with a total of almost 2,500 patients, failed to demonstrate any effect of adjuvant therapy on overall survival.[198–201] Initial

analysis of the fifth trial, which included 1,166 patients and was conducted by the National Surgical Adjuvant Breast and Bowel Project (NSABP), showed an improvement in disease-free and overall survivals in patients who received combination chemotherapy compared with those in the control arm.[202] Sixty-seven percent of patients treated with adjuvant chemotherapy and 59% of those treated with surgery alone survived for 5 years (P = .05). A recent update of this trial, however, failed to show any survival advantage for the chemotherapy arm, at least from the statistical viewpoint (P = .06).[203] It is inappropriate to conclude that a regimen containing methyl-CCNU is effective adjuvant therapy, as final analysis of these five trials failed to show any benefit. Furthermore, methyl-CCNU is leukemogenic and nephrotoxic, which may negate the small survival benefit seen in one trial.

Levamisole is an anthelmintic agent with nonspecific immunostimulating properties in patients with cancer. It enhances fluorouracil's toxicity to human colon cancer cell lines in a dose-dependent manner. This may be caused by levamisole's inhibition of tyrosine phosphatases in tumor cells. Levamisole may also enhance natural-killer lymphocyte activity and may induce expression of HLA-1 molecules in cancer cell membranes.[204] Windle and associates first reported the effectiveness of levamisole plus fluorouracil as adjuvant therapy for colorectal cancer.[205] The North Central Cancer Treatment Group (NCCTG) and Mayo Clinic researchers randomly assigned 401 patients with resectable Dukes' stage II and III colon cancer to receive postsurgical observation alone or postsurgical adjuvant therapy with levamisole alone or levamisole plus fluorouracil for 1 year.[206–207] Levamisole plus fluorouracil significantly reduced the recurrence rate compared with no adjuvant therapy (P = .003), and a benefit from levamisole alone was also suggested (P = .05). In addition, survival advantages were observed in stage III patients treated with levamisole plus fluorouracil (P = .03).

A confirmatory national intergroup trial was implemented using essentially the same methodology, except that patients with stage II tumors were randomly assigned to one of two arms (postsurgical observation or postsurgical levamisole plus fluorouracil) and patients with stage III disease were randomly assigned to one of three arms (observation, levamisole alone, or fluorouracil plus levamisole).[208] A total of 1,269 patients with resected colon cancer were included in the trial. Among the 929 evaluable patients with stage III tumors, therapy with levamisole plus fluorouracil reduced the risk of cancer recurrence by 41% and the overall death rate by 33%. The 3-year overall survival rate for the levamisole plus fluororuracil arm was estimated at 71% vs 55% for the observation arm ($P = .0064$). Levamisole alone did not produce a disease-free survival advantage over observation alone. Follow-up of patients with stage II tumors is insufficient to allow analysis at this time. As mentioned previously, stage II colon cancer patients whose tumors have aneuploidy; a high cell-proliferation index on DNA flow cytometric examination; complication by intestinal perforation or colon obstruction; invasion or adherence to adjacent structures; and the 18q chromosome abnormality are noted to have a higher risk of tumor relapse and should be considered for adjuvant therapy. The intergroup trial updated its data on patients with stage III colon carcinoma in 1992, and the final report was published recently.[209] With all 929 stage III colon cancer patients receiving follow-up for 5 years or more (median, 6.5 years), levamisole plus fluorouracil was found to reduce the risk of cancer recurrence by 40% ($P < .0001$) and the death rate by 33% ($P < .0007$). Levamisole alone produced no benefit in patients with stage III colon carcinoma. The reported toxicity was mild with no late side effects noted.

Levamisole plus fluorouracil is now considered the standard adjuvant therapy against which future treatments for stage III colon cancer should be compared and the nonprotocol adjuvant therapy of choice for patients with stage III colon cancer when formal clinical trials are not available. However, this opinion is not universally accepted by other investigators for several reasons: levamisole's claimed immunomodulatory effects have been difficult to substantiate, this effect appears more significant at higher doses than those used, single-agent levamisole appears to have no antitumor activity, and the possibility exists of long-term adverse effects such as multifocal leukoencephalopathy. Also, European study findings have raised suspicions about an increase (in a small number of patients) in cancer- and non-cancer-related deaths. Finally, the NCCTG-Intergroup trials lacked a single-agent fluorouracil study arm. In fact, these trials compared the efficacy of fluorouracil plus levamisole with results in historical controls using different doses, schedules, and patient compliance.[210]

Based on the encouraging antitumor activity in patients with advanced disease, several investigators reported their results using the combination of fluorouracil and leucovorin in the adjuvant setting. Results of a NSABP C-03 adjuvant colon cancer trial comparing fluorouracil plus leucovorin to MOF (semustine, vincristine, and fluorouracil) suggest that postoperative fluorouracil plus leucovorin results in a 30% reduction in the risk of developing treatment failure and a 32% reduction in mortality compared with patients treated with MOF.[211] This combination also significantly prolongs disease-free and overall survivals[211] based on results 3 years after surgery.

Preliminary results from other studies have also suggested benefits of fluorouracil plus leucovorin in the adjuvant treatment of colon carcinomas.[211–213] Recently, The International Multicentre Pooled Analysis of Colon Cancer Trials (IMPACT) investigators analyzed the role of adjuvant fluorouracil plus leucovorin for stage II and stage III colon cancer compared with surgery only.[213] These investigators independently undertook three randomized trials done in Italy, Canada, and France and pooled the data for analysis. The dosage was 370 to 400 mg/m^2 fluorouracil plus 200 mg/m^2 folinic acid intravenously for 5 days every 28 days for a total of 6 cycles. A total of 1,493 patients were eligible for analysis. The treatment arm showed significant reductions in mortality (by 22%; 95% CI, 3–38; $P = .029$) and relapse (by 35%; 95% CI, 22–46; $P = .0001$). The 3-year relapse-free survival and overall survival rates increased from 62% to 71% and from 78% to 83%, respectively. Toxicity was mild, with less than 3% of the patients experiencing grade 4 toxicity.

Future adjuvant therapy trials for colorectal cancer should determine whether perioperative chemotherapy has a positive effect on survival, the optimal duration of treatment (6 vs 12 months), better chemo-inmunotherapy (ie, the role of alpha interferon [IFN-α], high-dose levamisole, leucovorin, combination fluorouracil-leucovorin-levamisole), and the role of adjuvant treatment in stage II disease (Table 3). Currently active cooperative group trials are comparing various combinations of fluorouracil, folinic acid, levamisole, and IFN.[214]

Portal Vein Infusion: The liver is the sole site of recurrence in 25% of patients who ultimately develop metastatic colorectal carcinoma. Micrometastatic hepatic disease derives its vascular supply from the portal vein, and delivery of chemotherapeutic agents directly by this route is being investigated. Taylor and associates randomized 244 patients to receive portal vein infusion of fluorouracil and heparin or observation immediately after resection of Dukes' stage A, B, or C colon or rectal tumors.[215–216] The mean duration of follow-up was more than 4 years, and a significant survival advantage and decrease in incidence of liver metastases were observed in treated patients with stage B colon and stage C rectal carcinomas. The 5-year overall survival rates were 77.8% and 57.5% for the treatment and control arms, respectively ($P = .002$). In a study by the Swiss Group for Clinical Cancer Research (SAKK), 469 patients with Dukes' stage A, B, or C colon or rectal carcinoma were randomly assigned to receive portal vein infusion with fluorouracil, mitomycin (Mutamycin), and heparin or observation following curative resection.[217–218] With a median follow-up of 8 years, the adjuvant therapy arm had a 21% reduction in the risk of recurrence (hazards ratio, .79; 95% CI, .62–1) and a 26% reduction in the risk of death (hazards ratio, .74; 95% CI .57–.97; P = .026). The authors concluded that part of the benefit might result from the systemic effects of the intraportal chemotherapy; in fact, disease recurrence was reduced not only in the liver but also in extrahepatic sites. In contrast, randomized trials conducted by the NCCTG and Mayo Clinic failed to observe a benefit from portal vein infusion of fluorouracil and heparin.[219] These trials included 224 patients with Dukes' stage B2 or C colorectal cancer. The median follow-up was 5.5 years, and the incidence of liver metastases was similar in each group. The 5-year overall survival rate was identical in the treatment and control arms (68%, P = .61).

An NSABP trial randomized 901 eligible Dukes' stage A, B, or C colon cancer patients to receive either portal vein administration of fluorouracil and heparin or no adjuvant therapy.[220] There was a disease-free survival advantage at 4 years for the treatment group (74% vs 64%, P = .02). However, the trial failed to show a reduction in hepatic metastases as the first recurrence in the treated patients. The 4-year overall survival rates were 81% and 73% for the treatment and control arms, respectively (P = .07).

Fielding et al randomized 398 colorectal cancer patients to receive portal vein infusion of fluorouracil and heparin, heparin alone during curative resection and for 7 days thereafter, or resection alone.[221] They found neither reduction in the incidence of liver metastasis nor an increase in overall survival in either active treatment arm. Patients who underwent resection of Dukes' stage C colon tumors and received intraportal infusion of fluorouracil plus heparin demonstrated a significant (P < .03) survival advantage of approximately 16% compared with surgery-only controls.

Results of clinical trials of adjuvant portal vein infusion of chemotherapy for colorectal tumors thus have not consistently shown a benefit for this approach, and it is not recommended outside of clinical research trials.

Hepatic Arterial Infusion (HAI): Adjuvant HAI was evaluated in a single phase II study to administer three courses of floxuridine and mitomycin. Of 38 patients, 50% were alive and free of disease 8 years later.[222] However, HAI has not been compared with less toxic and less expensive delivery approaches such as systemic treatment and should not be recommended outside the context of a clinical trial.

Tumor Vaccine: Autologous and surrogate vaccines also have been utilized as adjuvant therapy for colorectal tumors. Hoover and coworkers randomly assigned 80 patients with Dukes' stage B2 or C colon or rectal carcinomas to receive either vaccination with BCG plus irradiated autologous tumor cells or observation.[223–224] Survival benefits were initially observed in immunized patients,[223] but a recent analysis of the control arm has shown similar survival.[224] Further follow-up is needed to reach conclusions about disease-free or overall survival. An Eastern Cooperative Oncology Group (ECOG) trial is currently accruing patients for this purpose.

The major concerns about this treatment modality are that patients must be identified prospectively and that fresh tumor cells must be processed according to specific stringent laboratory guidelines.

Monoclonal Antibodies (MoAbs): A German group[225] evaluated the effect of MoAbs used as adjuvant therapy for resected colorectal cancer in 189 patients with stage III disease who were randomly assigned to either a MoAb treatment arm or a control arm. The MoAb used was 17-1 A, a murine Ig G2A against a cell-surface glycoprotein (adhesion molecule) expressed in malignant and normal epithelial cells. With a median follow-up of 5 years, MoAb therapy reduced the death rate by 30% (P = .05) and the recurrence rate by 27% (P = .05). The toxicity was mild (gastrointestinal and constitutional symptoms).

Adjuvant Therapy for Rectal Cancer

Although some of the factors and issues involved in adjuvant therapy for colon cancer apply also to such therapy for rectal cancer, there are some differences. (a) Attaining a tumor-free surgical margin is more difficult in rectal cancers, leading to a higher incidence of local-regional relapses. (b) Radiation therapy is a mainstay of treatment in rectal cancer but not in colon cancer. (c) Adjuvant therapy for rectal tumors has produced an advantage in stage II and III disease, while such therapy for colon tumors has been advantageous only in stage III disease. (d) The standard adjuvant therapy for rectal cancer is fluorouracil given intravenously (IV) by bolus in 2 monthly cycles before and 2 after the radiation therapy (sandwich schedule). Protracted-infusion fluorouracil is given during pelvic irradiation.[226–227]

Local recurrence alone or in combination with distant metastases has occurred in 20% to 87% of rectal carcinoma patients in various trials.[228–232] The presence of nodal metastases and deep bowel wall penetration are significant risk factors for local-regional failure. In the absence of nodal metastases, the rate of local recurrence may be

TABLE 3

Findings in Clinical Trials of Adjuvant Therapy for Rectal Cancer

Treatment	Number of patients	Results	Group
Surgery alone vs chemotherapy (fluorouracil + methyl-CCNU) alone vs radiotherapy alone vs fluorouracil + methyl-CCNU + radiotherapy	202	Chemotherapy plus radiotherapy superior to surgery alone in disease-free (P = .009) and overall (P = .05) survival	GITSG
Postop radiotherapy vs fluorouracil + methyl-CCNU + radiotherapy followed by fluorouracil + methyl-CCNU	200	Combined modality superior to radiotherapy alone in disease-free (P = .001) and overall (P = .025) survival	NCCTG
Surgery alone vs postop radiotherapy vs fluorouracil + methyl-CCNU + vincristine	555	Chemotherapy superior to surgery in disease-free (P = .006) and overall (P = .05) survival; benefit in males only	NSABP
Bolus vs continuous-infusion fluorouracil during radiotherapy; all patients received 2 monthly cycles of fluorouracil before and after radiotherapy with or without semustine	660	Continuous infusion of fluorouracil with radiotherapy resulted in increased time to relapse (P = .01) and improvement in survival (P = .05); no benefit was noted with the addition of semustine	NCCTG

Adapted from Macdonald JS: Oncology 3(6):87–98, 1989

as low as 5% to 10% for stage I rectal cancer and 25% to 30% for stage II tumors. In stage III disease, the incidence of pelvic failure increases to 50% or more.

Adjuvant radiation therapy has been used to control the local-regional recurrence of rectal tumors. Preoperative radiation therapy has been demonstrated to reduce local tumor recurrence, albeit without affecting overall survival, in patients with stage II or III rectal cancer.[233–234] An improvement in local control also was observed with postoperative irradiation, but again no benefit with regard to disease-free or overall survival was demonstrated.[235]

Chemotherapy, alone or combined with radiation therapy, has been prospectively compared with surgical resection alone and with radiation therapy alone in patients with stage II or III rectal cancer (Table 3). The Gastrointestinal Tumor Study Group (GITSG)[231,236] and NCCTG[99] trials have demonstrated that the postsurgical combination of fluorouracil-based chemotherapy and pelvic irradiation reduces local-regional failures[231,237] and increases disease-free[231,237] and overall survivals[236–237] compared with pelvic irradiation or postsurgical chemotherapy alone or with observation following surgery. The NSABP trial of 555 patients with stage II or III rectal carcinoma randomly assigned patients to receive chemotherapy (fluorouracil, methyl-CCNU, and vincristine), irradiation, or observation following curative resection.[232] Disease-free (P = .006) and overall (P = .05) survival advantages were reported in the group that received chemotherapy compared with the group treated by sur-

gery alone. However, this benefit was observed only in men younger than 65 years of age. The rate of local-regional recurrence also was lower in the group that received postoperative radiation than in the control group (16% vs 25%, P = .06).

A combination of fluorouracil chemotherapy and radiation appears to be the best adjuvant therapy for patients with stage II or III rectal cancer.[226] O'Connell et al randomly assigned 660 stage II and III rectal cancer patients to receive bolus injections or protracted venous infusions of fluorouracil during postoperative radiation therapy to the pelvis. The patients also received semustine plus fluorouracil or fluorouracil alone at a higher dose both before and after the radiation. Patients who received the protracted fluorouracil treatment had a significantly increased time to relapse (P = .01) and improvement in survival (P = .005). No benefit was noted with the addition of semustine.[226]

The most effective combination of drug, particularly the role of the leucovorin and/or levamisole added to fluorouracil, the optimal mode of administration, and the sequence of radiation and chemotherapy still need to be determined. Ongoing multi-institutional trials of therapy for rectal cancer should help clarify some of these issues.[238–240]

Therapy for Advanced Colorectal Cancer

The most effective single agent in the management of advanced colorectal carcinoma is fluorouracil. Recent trials have reported a 10% to 15% objective response rate

TABLE 4

Controlled Trials of Fluorouracil/Folinic Acid Chemotherapy for Advanced Colorectal Cancer

Institution	Number of patients	Fluorouracil schedule	Folinic acid Duration	Dose (mg/m²)	Tumor response [a]
Roswell Park	52	Weekly	2 h	500	Yes
GITSG	343	Weekly	10 min	25	No
		Weekly	2 h	500	Yes
Italian	95	Weekly	2 h	500	Yes
City of Hope	68	Loading	24 h	500	Yes
Princess Margaret	130	Loading	Push	200	Yes
Mayo/North Central	251	Loading	Push	200	Yes [b]
			Push	20	Yes [b]
Northern California Oncology Group	162	Loading	Push	200	No
Mayo/North Central	372	Randomized loading	Push	20	Yes [c]
		Randomized weekly	2 h	600	Yes [c]

[a] Statistically significant improvement in response rate for fluorouracil/folinic acid regimen compared with fluorouracil alone
[b] Statistically significant prolongation of survival for patients with metastatic disease
[c] Intensive-course fluorouracil + low-dose leucovorin showed therapeutic index superior to that of weekly fluorouracil + high-dose leucovorin

Adapted from Mayer R, O'Connell MJ: ASCO Educational Booklet No. 8, pp 95–104, 1989

with standard intermittent intravenous administration of fluorouracil for metastatic colorectal disease.[240–242] Fluorouracil has been administered using various dosage schedules and methods, including both bolus and short-term, continuous intravenous infusion and protracted intravenous infusion via portable, ambulatory infusion pumps. Response rates have increased with increasing doses of fluorouracil[243] and prolonged infusion,[244] but fluorouracil alone has failed to improve survival rates in patients with metastatic colorectal disease.

Chloroethylnitrosoureas, mitomycin, and the newly identified agents tauromustine,[245] doxifluridine,[246] aminothiadiazole,[247] 4-deoxydoxorubicin,[248] nimustine,[249] CPT-11, UFT (uracil-ftorafur),[251] oxaliplatin,[250] and Tomudex (ZD 1694) also have shown some activity against advanced colorectal tumors.

CPT-11(Irinotecan),[251a] a semisynthetic derivative of camptothecin that is converted by cellular carboxylesterases to its principal metabolite (SN-38), has powerful topoisomerase I-inhibitory activity[107] and shows promise, particularly in patients with fluorouracil-refractory stage IV disease. Shimada et al showed that 25% of previously treated patients and 36% of patients without prior therapy responded to this drug.[252] The 25% response rate has been reproduced by investigators at San Antonio,[253] although other investigators have reported lower response rates (eg, 16%).[254] CPT-11 also has been eval-

uated as first-line therapy for patients with advanced colorectal cancer and achieved a response rate of 33% (all partial responses) (The Upjohn Company, unpublished data, 1994).

Given its good activity in this setting, CPT-11 is being evaluated in combination with fluorouracil and leucovorin in patients with advanced colorectal cancer. A recently reported study from Japan[255] discouraged to some extent the simultaneous administration of fluorouracil and CPT-11. As stated above, for optimal antitumor action, CPT-11 needs to be converted to its metabolite SN-38 by the enzyme carboxylestearase. SN-38 is almost 1,000 times more effective in inhibiting topoisomerase I than CPT-11 is. The Japanese investigators suggested that a metabolite of fluorouracil may inhibit carboxylestearase and, therefore, reduce the area under the curve of SN-38. An ongoing multicentric study is evaluating the combination of fluorouracil plus folinic acid with CPT-11 given in an alternating schedule.

UFT, an oral combination of uracil and ftorafur, also has shown some activity against advanced colorectal cancer. Ftorafur is converted to fluorouracil in the liver, and this may lead to a slow but sustained level of fluorouracil in tumor cells. Uracil seems to inhibit the catabolism of fluorouracil, allowing higher fluorouracil levels in the tissues. Pazdur et al tested UFT plus oral leucovorin in stage IV colorectal cancer patients and reported a response rate of 42%.[246] A phase III trial comparing UFT plus oral leucovorin with fluorouracil plus folinic acid has recently begun.

Tomudex (ZD 1694) is a quinazoline folate analog that acts as a pure thymidylate synthase inhibitor. A European phase II trial of this drug reported a 26% response rate in stage IV colorectal cancer patients. The advantage of ZD 1694 over fluorouracil plus leucovorin is the more convenient schedule of the former (one intravenous dose every 21 days compared with a daily × 5 schedule every 28 days for fluorouracil and folinic acid) and possibly its decreased incidence of severe toxicity.[257] Two phase III studies (one in Europe and one in the United States) comparing Tomudex with fluorouracil plus folinic acid in patients with stage IV colorectal cancer recently have been completed.

Oxaliplatin showed a 10% response rate in patients who failed to respond to fluorouracil and folinic acid.[250]

Doxorubicin, epirubicin, etoposide, carboplatin, cyclophosphamide, methotrexate, topotecan, CI 980, paclitaxel, docetaxel, and cisplatin are inactive against colorectal adenocarcinomas.

Various combination chemotherapy regimens, including fluorouracil, methyl-CCNU, and vincristine (MOF),[258]; MOF plus streptozocin[259]; cisplatin plus fluorouracil[260]; and methotrexate[261] or N-phosphonacetyl-L-aspartate (PALA)[259] followed by fluorouracil have failed to provide a survival advantage over single-agent fluorouracil.

The combination of folinic acid plus fluorouracil, in various dosages and treatment schedules, has produced higher response rates than fluorouracil alone in previously untreated patients with advanced colorectal cancers (Table 4). Although survival benefits were originally observed in two of these trials,[262-263] a recent update of one of these trials comparing fluorouracil plus leucovorin with fluorouracil alone in advanced colorectal carcinoma showed that the survival advantages initially seen were not maintained.[263] The advanced colorectal cancer meta-analysis project included nine randomized trials that compare fluorouracil alone with fluorouracil plus intravenous leucovorin.[264] The investigators observed a highly significant benefit favoring fluorouracil plus leucovorin over single-agent fluorouracil in terms of tumor response rate but no improvement in overall survival. Gastrointestinal effects such as diarrhea and mucositis, rather than myelosuppression, are the dose-limiting toxicities of folinic acid and fluorouracil combinations.[265]

In a prospective randomized trial, Buroker et al showed that a regimen of fluorouracil, 425 mg/m^2, plus folinic acid, 20 mg/m^2, daily × 5 every 4 to 5 weeks is therapeutically equally effective and has a superior therapeutic index compared with weekly fluorouracil, 600 mg/m^2, plus folinic acid, 500 mg/m^2, weekly for 6 weeks with courses repeated every 8 weeks.[266]

Although the modulation of fluorouracil by folinic acid has been suggested as a standard of care for patients with metastatic colorectal carcinoma, a recently published Southwest Oncology Group (SWOG) study has noted lower response rates for this combination than had previously been reported.[267] A study to assess the efficacy and toxicity of seven fluorouracil regimens randomized more than 600 stage IV colorectal cancer patients to receive one of the following: fluorouracil IV push; fluorouracil IV push plus low-dose leucovorin; fluorouracil IV push plus high-dose leucovorin; fluorouracil continuous infusion; fluorouracil continuous infusion plus low-dose leucovorin; fluorouracil 24-hour infusion; or fluorouracil 24-hour infusion plus PALA. No regimen produced a higher response rate and/or survival rate than fluorouracil alone. Response rates ranged between 15% and 29%, with a median survival for the entire group of 14 months. Survival ratios showed a positive trend favoring the unmodulated infusion regimens; meanwhile, high-grade toxic effects (neutropenia and diarrhea) were more frequently observed in the fluorouracil bolus arms. The single-agent infusion regimens demonstrated the best results, with a favorable toxicity profile and a 2-month longer survival duration than fluorouracil given by bolus.[267]

Fluorouracil in conjunction with recombinant IFN-α has also been utilized in the treatment of advanced colorectal carcinoma. The initial trial of this combination suggested an overall response rate in excess of 50%,[268] but subsequent phase II and III studies have reported lower response rates ranging from 19% to 30%.[269-272] A recent multinational randomized trial by the Corfu-A Study Group compared fluorouracil plus IFN-α with fluorouracil plus leucovorin in 496 patients with advanced colorectal cancer and reported respective response rates of 21% and 18%.[270] The overall median survival was around 11 months in both treatment arms, but the toxicity profiles differed. Constitutional symptoms and neutropenia were more frequent and severe in the fluorouracil plus IFN-α arm, and gastrointestinal toxicity was worse with the fluorouracil plus leucovorin combination. Remarkably, more patients interrupted treatment because of toxicity with fluorouracil plus IFN-α than with fluorouracil plus leucovorin.[270] Similar results were reported in another recently published phase III study by the Royal Marsden Hospital comparing fluorouracil plus leucovorin with fluorouracil plus IFN-α in advanced colorectal cancer patients.[272]

Renewed interest in regional delivery of floxuridine into the liver has followed the introduction of effective implantable infusion pumps. These pumps allow delivery of higher concentrations of chemotherapeutic agents directly into the hepatic artery, the blood supply of most hepatic metastases. Using this delivery method, these higher concentrations of drug (floxuridine is the most frequently used) result in more frequent responses in the liver than achieved with systemic chemotherapy,[273–277] although toxicity (occasionally irreversible) to the liver and bile ducts is common and gastrointestinal bleeding is possible.[278] Investigators from Memorial Sloan-Kettering Cancer Center studied 62 patients with liver metastases from colorectal cancer, of whom 33 had received prior chemotherapy. In this study, patients were treated with hepatic arterial floxuridine, leucovorin, and dexamethasone, which produced a response rate of 78%; the addition of dexamethasone significantly reduced the incidence of biliary toxicity.[279] Only two randomized trials compared systemic chemotherapy with intrahepatic arterial infusion of chemotherapy, and no differences in survival between the two treatment groups were observed.[276–277] Moreover, hepatic chemotherapy is costly, cumbersome, and associated with gastroduodenal mucosal ulceration hepatitis and sclerosing cholangitis. Thus, there is so far no evidence that this method results in survival improvement in patients with liver metastases from colorectal cancer, and this delivery method should not be used outside the context of a clinical trial.

Laser photoablation also is gaining popularity for the temporary relief of obstructive rectal cancer, especially in the presence of distant metastases or when colostomy is not feasible because of comorbidity.

CONCLUSIONS

Fluorouracil and levamisole have produced disease-free and overall survival advantages in patients with stage III colon carcinoma. Chemotherapy combined with pelvic irradiation also has proven beneficial in stage II and III rectal carcinoma patients. Nevertheless, the development of new chemotherapeutic agents or new combinations of existing ones is necessary to further reduce the mortality from colorectal cancer.

REFERENCES

1. Wingo PA, Tong T, Bolden S: Cancer Statistics, 1995. CA 45:8–30, 1995.

2. Cady B, Persson AV, Monson DO, et al: Changing patterns of colorectal cancer. Cancer 33:433–436, 1974.

3. Boring CC, Squires TS, Heath CW Jr: Cancer statistics for African Americans. CA Cancer J Clin 42:7–17, 1992.

4. Hoel DG, Davis DL, Miller AB, et al: Trends in cancer mortality in 15 industrialized countries, 1969–1986. J Natl Cancer Inst 84:313–320, 1992.

5. De Cosse JJ, Tsioulias GJ, Jacobson JS: Colorectal cancer: Detection, treatment and rehabilitation. CA Cancer J Clin 44:27–42, 1994.

6. Devesa SS, Silverman DT, Young JL Jr, et al: Cancer incidence and mortality trends among whites in the United States, 1947–84. J Natl Cancer Inst 79:701–770, 1987.

7. Seidman H, Mushinski MH, Gelb SK, et al: Probabilities of eventually developing or dying of cancer:United States, 1985. CA 35:36–56, 1985.

8. Steele GD Jr: The national cancer data base report on colorectal cancer. Cancer 74:1979–1989, 1994

9. Griffin PM, Liff JM, Greenberg RS, et al: Adenocarcinomas of the colon and rectum in persons under 40 years old: A population-based study. Gastroenterology 100:1033–1040, 1991.

10. Miller BA, Ries LAG, Hankey BF, et al: Cancer Statistics Review 1973–1989. National Cancer Institute, NIH Publication N 92-2789, 1992.

11. Giller T: Advances in genetics and molecular biology of colorectal tumors. Curr Opin Oncol 6:406–412, 1994.

12. Armitage P, Doll R: The age distribution of cancer and a multistage theory of carcinogenesis. Br J Cancer 8:1–13, 1954.

13. Scott N, Quirke P: Molecular biology of colorectal neoplasia. Gut 34:289–292, 1993.

14. Meltzer SJ, Ahnen DJ, Battifora H, et al: Proto-oncogene abnormalities in colon cancers and adenomatous polyps. Gastroenterology 92:1174–1180, 1987.

15. Cartwright CA, Kamps MP, Meister AI, et al: pp60 C-src activation in human colon carcinoma. J Clin Invest 83:2025–2032, 1989.

16. Tal M, Wetzler M, Josefberg Z, et al: Sporadic amplification of the Her2/neu proto-oncogene in adenocarcinoma of various tissues. Cancer Res 48:1517–1520, 1988.

17. Barbacid M: Ras genes. Ann Rev Biochem 56:779–827, 1987.

18. Forrester K, Almoguera C, Han K, et al: Detection of high incidence of K-ras oncogenes during human tumorogenesis. Nature 327:298–303, 1987.

19. Vogelstein B, Fearon ER, Hamilton SR, et al: Genetic alterations during colorectal developement. N Engl J Med 319:525–532, 1988.

20. Benhattar J, Lossiu L, Roncucci L, et al: Stability of K-Ras mutations throughout the natural history of human colorectal cancer. Gut 33:S46, 1992.

21. Fearon ER, Vogelstein B: A genetic model for colorectal tumorogenesis. Cell, 61:759–767, 1990.

22. Sidransky D, Tokino T, Hamilton SR, et al: Identification of ras oncogene mutations in the stool of patients with curable colorectal tumors. Science 256:102–104, 1992.

23. Kelly K, Siebenlist U: The role of c-myc in the proliferation of normal and neoplastic cells. J Clin Immunol 5:65–77, 1985.

24. Studzinski GP, Brelvi ZS, Feldman SC, et al: Participation of c-myc protein in DNA synthesis of human cells. Science 234:467–469, 1986.

25. Erisman MD, Rothberg PG, Diehl RE, et al: Deregulation of c-myc gene expression in human colon carcinoma is not accompained by amplification or rearrangement of the gene. Mol Cell Biol 5:1969–1976, 1985.

26. Finley GG, Schulz NT, Hill SA, et al: Expression of the myc gene family in different stages of human colorectal cancer. Oncogene 4:963–971, 1989.

27. Rothberg PG, Spandorfer HM, Erisman MD, et al: Evidence that c-myc expression defines two genetically distinct forms of colorectal

adenocarcinoma. Br J Cancer 52:629–632, 1985.

28. Stewart J, Evan G, Watson J, et al: Detection of the c-myc oncogene product in colonic polyps and carcinomas. Br J Cancer 53:1–6, 1986.

29. Bodmer WF, Bailey GJ, Bodmer J, et al: Localisation of the gene for familial adenomatous polyposis on chromosome 5. Nature 328:614–616, 1986.

30. Leppert M, Dobbs M, Scambler P, et al: The gene for familial polyposis colimaps to the long arm of chromosome 5. Science 238:1411–1413, 1987.

31. Kinzler KW, Nilbert MC, Su L, et al: Identification of FAP locus genes from chromosome 5q21. Science 253:661–665, 1991.

32. Rubinfeld B, Souza B, Albert I, et al: Association of the APC gene product with beta-catenin. Science 262:1731–1734, 1993.

33. Su LK, Vogelstein B, Kinzler KW: Association of the APC tumor suppressor protein with catenins. Science 262:1734–1737, 1993.

34. Olschwang S, Tiret E, Laurent-Puig P, et al: Restriction of ocular fundus lesions to a specific subgroup of APC mutations in adenomatous polyposis coli patients. Cell 75:959–968, 1993.

35. Spirio L, Otterud B, Stauffer D, et al: Linkage of a variant attenuated form of adenomatous polyposis coli to the adenomatous polyposis coli (APC) locus. Am J Hum Genet 51:92–100, 1992.

36. Spirio L, Olschwang S, Groden J, et al: Alleles of the APC gene: An attenuated form of familial polyposis. Cell 75:951–957, 1993.

37. Vogelstein B, Eng N, Okamoto M, et al: Loss of constitutional heterozygosity in colon carcinoma from patients with familial polyposis coli. Nature 331:273–277, 1988.

38. Miyoshi Y, Ando H, Nagase H, et al: Germ-line mutations of the APC gene in 53 familial adenomatous polyposis patients. Proc Natl Acad Sci 89:4452–4456, 1992.

39. Kinzler KW, Nilbert MC, Vogelstein B, et al: Identification of a gene located at chromosome 5q21 that is mutaterd in colorectal cancers. Science 251:1366–1369, 1991.

40. Miki Y, Nishisho I, Miyoshi Y, et al: Frequent loss of heterozygosity at the MCC locus on chromosome 5q21-22 in sporadic colorectal carcinomas. Jpn J Cancer Res 82:1003–1007, 1991.

41. Fearon ER, Cho KR, Nigro JM, et al: Identification of a chromosome 18q gene that is altered in colorectal cancers. Science 247 49–56, 1990.

42. Jen J, Kim H, Piantadosi S, et al: Allelic loss of chromosome 18q and prognosis in colorectal cancer. N Engl J Med 331(4):213–221, 1994.

43. Baker SJ, Fearon ER, Nigro JM, et al: Chromosome 17 deletions and p53 gene mutations in colorectal carcinomas. Science 244:217–221, 1989.

44. Baker SJ, Presinger AC, Jessup JM, et al: p53 gene mutations occur in combination with 17p allelic deletions as late events in colorectal tumorogenesis. Cancer Res 50:7712–7717, 1990.

45. Ionov J, Peinado MA, Malkhosyan S, et al: Ubiquitous somatic mutations in simple repeated sequences reveal a new mechanism for colonic carcinogenesis. Nature 363:558–561, 1993.

46. Guillem JG, Paty PB, Rosen N: Molecular biology of colorectal cancer, in Cohen AM, Winawer SJ, Friedman MA, et al, (eds): Cancer of the Colon, Rectum and Anus, pp 149–156. New York, McGraw Hill, 1995.

47. Leach FS, Nicolaides NC, Papadoupolous N, et al: Mutations of a muts homolog in hereditary nonpolyposis colorectal cancer. Cell 75:1215–1225, 1993.

48. Fishel R, Lescoe MK, Rao MRS, et al: The human mutation gene homolog MSH2 and its association with hereditary non polyposis colon cancer. Cell 75:1027–1038, 1993.

49. Aaltonen LA, Peltomaki P, Leach FS, et al: Clues to the pathogenesis of familial colorectal cancer. Science 260:812–816, 1993.

50. Peltomaki P, Aaltonen LA, Sistonen P, et al: Genetic mapping of a locus predisposing to human colorectal cancer Science 260:810–812, 1993.

51. Lindblom A, Tannergard P, Werelius B, et al: Genetic mapping of a second locus predisposing to hereditary non poliposis colon cancer. Nature Genet 5:279–282, 1993.

52. Bronner CE, Baker SM, Morrison PT, et al: Mutation in the DNA mismatch gene homologue hMLH1 is associated with hereditary non polyposis colon cancer. Nature 994,368:258–261, 1994.

53. Nicolaides NC, Papadopoulos N, Liu B, et al: Mutations of 2 PMS homologues in hereditary non-polyposis colorectal cancer. Nature 371(6492):75–80, 1994.

54. Sugarbaker JP, Gunderson LL, Witter RE: Colorectal cancer, in de Vita VT, Hellman S, Rosenberg SA (eds): Cancer: Principles and Practice of Oncology, pp 800–803. Philadelphia, JB Lippincott, 1985.

55. Foulds L: The natural history of cancer. J Chronic Dis 8:2–37, 1958.

56. Bishop JM: The molecular genetics of cancer. Science 235:305–311, 1987.

56a. Weinberg RA: Oncogenes, antioncogenes, and the molecular basis of multistep carcinogenesis. Cancer Res 49:3713–3721, 1989.

57. Ziegler RG, Devesa SS, Fraumeni JF Jr: Epidemiology pattern of colorectal cancer, in Devita VT Jr, Hellman S, Rosenberg SA (eds): Important Advances in Oncology, pp 209–232. Philadelphia, JB Lippincott, 1986.

58. McMichael AJ, McCall MG, Hartshorne JM, et al: Patterns of gastrointestinal cancer in European migrants to Australia: The role of dietary change. Int J Cancer 25:431–437, 1980.

59. Locke FB, King H: Cancer mortality risk among Japanese in the United States. J Natl Cancer Inst 65:1149–1156, 1981.

60. Burkitt DP: Dietology and prevention of colorectal cancer. Hosp Pract 19:67, 1984.

61. Maclennan R, Jenson OM: Dietary fibre, transit time, faecal bacteria, steroids, and colon cancer in two Scandinavian populations: Reports from the International Agency for Research in Cancer Intestinal Microecology Group. Lancet 2:207–211, 1977.

62. Lee IM, Paffenbarger RS Jr, Hsieh C: Physical activity and risk of developing colorectal cancer among college alumni. J Natl Cancer Inst 83:1324–1329, 1991.

63. West DW, Slattery ML, Robinson LM, et al: Dietary intake and colon cancer: Sex and anatomin site-specific associations. Am J Epidemiol 130:883–894, 1989.

64. Kune GA, Kune S, Watson LF: Body weight and physical activity as predictors of colorectal cancer risk. Nutr Cancer 13:9–17, 1990.

65. Calabresi P, Schein PS, Canellos GP: Medical Oncology, 2nd ed, pp 749–782. New York, McGraw Hill, 1993.

66. Morotomi M, Guillem JG, LoGerfo P, et al: Production of diacylglycerol, an activator of protein kinase C, by human intestinal microflora. Cancer Res 50:3595–3500, 1990.

67. Levy MF, Poscidio J, Guillem JG, et al: Decreased levels of protein kinase C (PKC) enzyme activity and PKC mRNA in primary human colon tumors. Dis Colon Rectum 36:913–921, 1993.

68. Choi P, Tchou-Wong KM, Weinstein IB: Overexpression of protein kinase C in HT29 colon cancer cells causes growth inhibition and tumor supression. Mol Cell Biol 10:4650–4657, 1990.

69. Reddy BS, Narisawa T, Weisburger JH, et al: Promoting effect of sodium deoxycholate on adenocarcinomas in germ free rats. J Natl Cancer Inst 56:441, 1976.

70. Nigro ND, Singh DV, Campbell RL, et al: Effect of dietary beef fat on intestinal tumor formation by azoxymethane in rats. J Natl Cancer Inst 54:439, 1975.

71. Wargovich MJ, Felkner IC: Metabolic activation of DMH by colonic microsomes: A process influenced by type of dietary fat. Nutr Cancer 4:146, 1983.

72. Bjelke E: Dietary factors and the epidemiology of cancer of the stomach and large bowel. Akt Ernaerhungsmed Klin Prax 2(suppl):10, 1978.

73. Stemmerman GN, Nomura AMY, Heilburn LK: Dietary fat and the risk of colorectal cancer. Cancer Res 44:4633, 1984.

74. Weisburger JH: Causes, relevant mechanisms, and prevention of large bowel cancer. Semin Oncol 18:316–336, 1991.

75. Wargovich MJ, Mastromarino AJ: Dietary factors in the etiology and prevention of colon cancer. Cancer Bull 46:303–308, 1994.

76. Burkitt DP, Walker ARP, Painter NS: Dietary fiber and disease. JAMA 229:1068, 1974.

77. Cummings JH, Bingham SA: Dietary fiber, fermentation and large bowel cancer. Cancer Surv 6:61, 1987.

78. Walker AR, Walker BF, Walker AJ: Fecal ph, dietary fiber intake, and proneness to colon cancer in four South American populations. Br J Cancer 53(4):489, 1986.

79. Newmark HL, Wargovich MJ, Bruce WR: Colon cancer and dietary fat, phosphate, and calcium. J Natl Cancer Inst 72:1323–1325, 1984.

80. Schober SE: Vitamin A, vitamin E, selenium and colon cancer risk. Diss Abstr Int (Sci) 46(11):3808, 1986.

81. Potter JD, McMichael AJ: Diet and cancer of the colon and rectum: A case control study. J Natl Cancer Inst 76(4):557, 1986.

82. Wargovich MJ, Baer AR, Hu PJ, et al: Dietary factors and colorectal cancer. Gastroenterol Clin North Am 17(4):727, 1988.

83. Wiltrout RH, Herbermann RB, Zhang SR, et al: Role of organ-associated NK ells in decreased formation of experimental metastases in lung and liver. J Immunol 134:4267–4275, 1985.

84. Labayle D, Fischer D, Vielh P, et al: Sulindac causes regression of rectal polyps in familial adenomatous polyposis. Gastroenterology 101:635, 1991.

85. Jaffe BM: Prostaglandins and cancer: An update. Prostaglandins 6:453–461, 1991.

86. Sinicrope FA, Sugarman SM: Adjuvant therapy for colon carcinoma: Current status and future directions. Cancer Bull 46:344–351, 1994.

87. Ziche M, Jones J, Guillino PM: Role of prostaglandin E1 and copper in antiangiogenesis. J Natl Cancer Inst 69:475–482, 1982.

88. Levine L: Effects of tumor promoters on arachidonic acid metabolism by cells in culture. Carcinogenesis 7:477–494, 1982.

89. Thun MJ, Mamboodiri MM, Heath CW: Aspirin use and reduced risk of fatal colon cancer. N Engl J Med 325:1593, 1991.

90. Macklin MT: Inheritance of cancer of the stomach and large intestine in man. J Natl Cancer Inst 24:551–571, 1960.

91. Fuchs CS, Giovanucci EL, Colditz GA,et al: A prospective study of family history and the risk of colorectal cancer. N Engl J Med 331(25):1669–1674, 1994.

92. Lipkin M, Sherlock P, De Cosse JJ: Risk factors and preventive measures in the control of cancer of the large intestine. Curr Probl Cancer 4:1057, 1980.

93. Groden J, Thilveria A, Samowitz W, et al: Identification and characterization of the familial adenomatous polyposis coli gene. Cell 66:589–600, 1991.

94. Nishisho I, Nakamura Y, Miyoshi Y, et al: Mutations of chromosome 5q21 genes in FAP and colorectal cancer patients. Science 253:665–669, 1991.

95. McKusic VA: Genetics and large bowel cancer. Am J Dig Dis 19:954–957, 1974.

96. Arvanitis ML, Jagelman DG, Fazio VW, et al: Mortality in patients with familial adenomatous polyposis. Dis Colon Rectum 33:639–642, 1990.

97. Oldfield MC: The association of familial polyposis of the colon with multiple sebaceous cysts. Br J Surg 41:534–541, 1954.

98. Turcot J, Depres JP, St Pierre F: Malignant tumors of the central nervous system associated with familial polyposis of the colon: Report of two cases. Dis Colon Rectum 2:465–468, 1959.

99. Reid JD: Intestinal carcinoma in the Peutz-Jeghers syndrome. JAMA 229:833–834, 1974.

100. Kussin SZ, Lipkin M, Winawer S: Inherited colon cancer: Clinical implications. Am J Gastroenterol 72:443–457, 1979.

101. Lynch HT, Lynch PM: Heredity and gastrointestinal tract cancer, in Lipkin M, Good RA (eds): Gastrointestinal Tract Cancer. New York, Plenum Press, 1978.

102. Lynch HT, Albano WA, Lynch JF, et al: Recognition of the cancer family syndrome. Gastroenterology 84:672–673, 1983.

103. Vasen HFA: What is hereditary nonpolyposis colorectal cancer (HNPCC). Anticancer Res 14:1613–1616, 1994

104. Vasen HF, Mecklin JP, Meera Khan P et al: The international collaborative group on hereditary non-polyposis colorectal cancer. Dis Colon Rectum 34:424–425, 1991.

105. Vasen HFA, Mecklin JP, Meera Khan Pet al: Hereditary non-polyposis colorectal cancer. Lancet 338:877, 1991.

106. Lynch HT, Lynch J: Genetic predictability and minimal cancer clues in Lynch syndrome II. Dis Colon Rectum 30:243–246, 1987.

107. Rustgi AK: Hereditary gastrointestinal polyposis and non polyposis syndromes. N Engl J Med 331(25):1694–1702, 1994

108. Lee EC, Truelove SC: Proctocolectomy for ulcerative colitis. World J Surg 4:195–201, 1980.

109. Butt JH, Morson BC: Dysplasia and cancer in inflammatory bowel disease. Gastroenterology 80:865–868, 1981.

110. Edwards FC, Truelove SC: The course and prognosis of ulcerative colitis. Gut 5:1–22, 1964.

111. Morson BC: Cancer and ulcerative colitis. Gut 7:425–426, 1966.

112. Leonard-Jones JE, Morson BC, Ritchie JR, et al: Cancer in colitis: Assessment of the individual risk of clinical and histological criteria. Gastroenterology 73:1280–1289, 1977.

113. Kewenter J, Ahlman H, Hulten L: Cancer risk in extensive ulcerative colitis. Ann Surg 188:824–828, 1978.

114. Muto T, Bussey HJ, Morson BC: The evolution of cancer of the colon and rectum. Cancer 36:2251–2260, 1975.

115. Winawer SJ, Zauber AG, Ho MN, et al and the National Polyp Study Workgroup: Prevention of colorectal cancer by colonoscopic polypectomy. The National Polyp Study Workgroup. N Engl J Med 329:1977–1981, 1993.

116. Schottenfield D, Berg J, Vitsky B: Incidence of multiple primary cancer: II. Index cancers arising in the stomach and lower digestive system. J Natl Cancer Inst 43:77–86, 1969.

117. McGregor RA, Bacon HE: Multiple cancers in colon surgery: Report of 162 cases. Surgery 44:828–833, 1958.

118. Bristol JB, Williamson RC: Ureterosigmoidostomy and colon carcinogenesis. Science 214:351, 1981.

119. Weisburger JH: Colorectal cancer: Etiologic factors and their mode of action as an effective approach to prevention, in Kirsner JB, Shorter RG (eds): Diseases of the Colon, Rectum, and Anal Canal. Baltimore, Williams & Wilkins, 1988.

120. Ballard-Barbash R, Schatzkin A, Albanes D, et al: Physical activity and risk of large bowel cancer in the Framingham study. Cancer Res 50:3610–3613, 1990.

121. Weiss NS, Daling JR, Chow WH: Incidence of cancer of the large bowel in women in relation to reproductive and hormonal factors. J Natl Cancer Inst 67:57–60, 1981.

122. Thun MJ, Calle EE, Namboodiri MM, et al: Risk factors for fatal colon cancer in a large prospective study. J Natl Cancer Inst 84:1491–1500, 1992.

123. American Joint Committee on Cancer. Manual for Staging of

Cancer, 2nd ed. Philadelphia, JB Lippincott, 1983.

124. Hermanek P: Evolution and pathology of rectal cancer. World J Surg 6:502–509, 1982.

125. Spjut HJ: Pathology of neoplasms, in Spratt JS (ed): Neoplasms of the Colon, Rectum, and Anus: Mucosal and Epithelial. Philadelphia, WB Saunders, 1984.

126. Symonds DA, Vickery AL: Mucinous carcinoma of the colon and rectum. Cancer 37:1891–1900, 1976.

127. Secco GB, Fardelli R, Campora E,et al: Primary mucinous adenocarcinomas and signet-ring cell carcinomas of the colon and rectum. Oncology 51:30–34, 1994.

128. Bonello JC, Quan SH, Sternberg SS: Primary linitis plastica of the rectum. Dis Colon Rectum 23:337–342, 1980.

129. Kirkham N: Colorectal signet ring cell carcinoma in young people. J Pathol 155:93–94, 1988.

130. De Vita V Jr, Hellman S, Rosenberg SA: Cancer: Principles and Practice of Oncology, 4th ed, 929–977. Philadelphia, JB Lippincott, 1993.

131. Evans HL: Smooth muscle tumors of the gastrointestinal tract: A study of 56 cases followed for a minimum of 10 years. Cancer 56:2242–2250, 1985.

132. Broders AC: The grading of carcinoma. Minn Med 8:726–730, 1925.

133. Dukes CE: The classification of cancer of the rectum. J Pathol 35:323–332, 1932.

134. Hermanek P: Evolution and pathology of rectal cancer. World J Surg 6:502–509, 1982.

135. Qizilbash AH: Pathologic studies in colorectal cancer: A guide to the surgical pathology examination of colorectal specimens and review of features of prognostic significance. Pathol Annu 17:1–46, 1982.

136. Takahashi T, Mori T, Moosa AR: Tumors of the colon and rectum: Clinical features and surgical management, in Moosa AR, Schimpff SC, Robson MC (eds): Comprehensive Textbook of Oncology, 2nd ed, pp 904–933. Baltimore, Williams & Wilkins, 1991.

137. Wiggers T, Arends JW, Volovics A: Regression analysis of prognostic factors in colorectal cancer after curative resections. Dis Colon Rectum 31(1):33, 1988.

138. Steinberg SM, Barkin JS, Kaplan RS, et al: Prognostic indicators of colon tumors. Cancer 57:1866, 1986.

139. Cohen A, Willett C, Tepper JE, et al: Obstructive and perforative colonic carcinoma: Patterns of failure. J Clin Oncol 3:379, 1985.

140. Chapuis PH, Dent OF, Fisher R, et al: A multivariate analysis of clinical and pathologic variables in prognosis after resection of large bowel cancer. Br J Surg 72:698, 1985.

141. Odone V, Chang L, Caces J, et al: The natural history of colorectal carcinoma in adolescents. Cancer 49:1716, 1982.

142. Block GE, Enker WE: Survival after operations for rectal carcinomas in patients over 70 years of age. Ann Surg 174:521, 1971.

143. Songster CL, Barrows GH, Jarrett DD: Immunochemical detection of fecal occult blood: The fecal smear punch-disc test: A new non-invasive screening test for colorectal cancer. Cancer 45:1099–1102, 1980.

144. St. John DJB: Screening tests for colorectal neoplasia. J Gastroenterol Hepatol 6:538–544, 1991.

145. Winawer SJ, Schottenfeld D, Flehinger BJ: Colorectal cancer screening. J Natl Cancer Inst 83:243–253, 1991.

146. Kronborg O, Fenger C, Worm J, et al: Causes of death during the first 5 years of a randomized trial of mass screening for colorectal cancer with fecal occult blood test. Scand J Gastroenterol 27:47–52, 1992.

147. Ahlquist DA, Wieand HS, Moertel CG, et al: Accuracy of fecal occult screening for colorectal neoplasia: A prospective study using Hemoccult and HemoQuant tests. JAMA 268:1262–1267, 1993.

148. Flehinger BJ, Herbert E, Winawer SJ, et al: Screening for colorectal cancer with fecal occult blood test and sigmoidoscopy: Preliminary report of the colon project of Memorial Sloan-Kettering Cancer Center and PMI-Strang Clinic, in Chamberlain J, Miller AB, (eds): Screening for Gastrointestinal Cancer, pp 9–19. Toronto, Hans Huber, 1988.

149. Kewenter J, Bjork S, Haglind E,Set al: Screening and re-screening for colorectal cancer: A controlled trial of fecal occult blood testing in 27,700 subjects. Cancer 62:645–651, 1988.

150. Mandel JS, Bond JH, Church TR, et al: Reducing mortality from colorectal cencer by screening for fecal occult blood. N Engl J Med 328:1365–1371, 1993.

151. Selby JV, Friedman GD, Quesenbery CP Jr, et al: A case-control study of screening sigmoidoscopy and mortality from colorectal cancer. N Engl J Med 326:653, 1992.

152. Newcomb PA, Norfleet RG, Storer BE, et al: Screening sigmoidoscopy and colorectal cancer mortality. J Natl Cancer Inst 84:1572, 1992.

153. Miller RE, Lehman G: Polypoid colonic lesions undetected by endoscopy. Radiology 129:295–297, 1978.

154. Eddy DM, Nugent FW, Eddy JF, et al: Screening for colorectal cancer in a high-risk population: Results of a mathematical model. Gastroenterology 92:682–692, 1987.

155. Levin B, Murphy GP: Revision in American Cancer Society recommendations for the early detection of colorectal cancer. CA Cancer J Clin 42:296–299, 1992.

156. Winawer SJ, Schottenfeld D, Flehinger BJ: Colorectal cancer screening. J Natl Cancer Inst 83:243–253, 1991.

157. Winawer SJ, Zauber AG, O Brien MJ, et al: Randomized comparison of surveillance intervals after colonoscopic removal of newly diagnosed adenomatous polyps. N Engl J Med 328:901–906, 1993.

158. Atkin WS, Morson BC, Cuzick J: Long-term risk of colorectal cancer after excision of rectosigmoid adenomas. N Engl J Med 326:658–662, 1992.

159. Sidransky D, Tokino T, Hamilton S, et al: Identification of ras oncogene mutations in the stool of patients with curable colorectal tumors. Science 256:102–105, 1992.

160. Roubein LD, Charnsangavej C: Preoperative staging of colorectal cancer. Cancer Bull 46(4):309–314, 1994

161. Heiken JP, Weyman PJ, Lee JKT, et al: Detection of focal hepatic masses: Prospective evaluation with CT, delayed CT, CT during arterial portography and MR imaging. Radiology 171:47–51, 1989.

162. Oudkerk M, Ooijen BV, Mali SPM, et al: Liver metastases from colorectal carcinoma: Detection with continuous CT angiography. Radiology 185:157–161, 1992.

163. Doerr RJ, Abdel-Nabi H, Krag D, et al: Radiolabeled antibody imaging in the management of colorectal cancer. Ann Surg 214:118–124, 1991.

164. Collier BD, Abdel-Nabi H, Doerr RJ: Immunoscintigraphy performed with IN-111-labeled CYT-103 in the management of colorectal cancer: Comparison with CT. Radiology 185:179–186, 1992.

165. O'Connell MJ, Gunderson LL: Comparision of staging systems for colorectal adenocarcinoma. World J Surg 16:510–515, 1992.

166. Odone-Umpleby HC, Williamson RCM: Carcinoma of the large bowel in the first four decades. Br J Surg 71:272–277, 1984.

167. Steinberg SM, Barkin JS, Kaplan RS, et al: Prognostic indications of colon tumors: The Gastrintestinal Tumor Group Experience. Cancer 57:1866–1870, 1986.

168. Wolmark K, Wieand HS, Rockette HE, et al: The prognostic significance of tumor and location and bowel obstruction in Dukes B and C colorectal cancer: Findings from the NSABP clinical trials. Ann

Surg 198:743–752, 1983.

169. Sibbering DM, Locker AP, Hardcastle JD, et al: Blood transfusion and survival in colorectal cancer.Dis Colon Rectum, pp 358–363, 1994.

170. Wolmark N, Cruz I, Redmond CD, et al: Tumor size and regional lymph node metastasis in colorectal cancer: A preliminary analysis from the NSABP clinical trials. Cancer 51:1315–1322, 1983.

171. Rao AR, Kagan AR, Chan PM, et al: Patterns of recurrence following curative resection alone for adenocarcinoma of the rectum and sigmoid colon. Cancer 48:1492–1495, 1981.

172. Chapuis PH, Dent OF, Fisher R, et al: A multivariate analysis of clinical and pathological variables in prognosis after resection of large bowel cancer. Br J Surg 72:698–702, 1985.

173. Enker WE, Laffer VT, Block GE: Enhanced survival of patients with colon and rectal cancer is based upon wide anatomic resection. Ann Surg 190:350–357, 1979.

174. Mason AY: The place of local resection in the treatment of rectal carcinoma. Proc R Soc Med 63:1250–1262, 1970.

175. Stearns MW Jr, Sternberg SS, DeCosse JJ: Treatment alternatives: Localized rectal cancer. Cancer 54:2691–2694, 1984.

176. Morson BC: Factors influencing the prognosis of early cancer of the rectum. Proc R Soc Med 59:607–608, 1966.

177. Adam IJ, Mohamdee MO, Martin IG, et al: Role of circumferential margin involvement in the local recurrence of rectal cancer. Lancet (344):707–711, 1994.

178. Minsky BD, Cohen AM, Kemeny N, et al: Enhancement of radiation-induced downstaging of rectal cancer by fluorouracil and high-dose leucovorin chemotherapy. J Clin Oncol 10:79–84, 1982.

179. Skibber JM: New approaches to rectal cancer. Cancer Bull 44:282–285, 1992.

180. Mc Affe MK, Allen MS, Trastek VP: Colorectal lung metastases: Results of surgical excision. Ann Thorac Surg 53:780–786, 1992.

181. Fong Y, Blumgart LH, Cohen AM: Surgical management of colorectal metastases to the liver. CA Cancer J Clin 45:50–62, 1995.

182. Adson MA, van Heerden JA, Adson MH, et al: Resection of hepatic metastases from colorectal cancer. Arch Surg 119:647–651, 1984.

183. Hughes KS, Simon R, Songhorabodi S, et al: Resection of the liver for colorectal carcinoma metastases. A multiinstitutional study of patterns of reccurrrence. Surgery 100:278–284, 1986.

184. Schlag P, Hohenberger P, Herfarth C: Resection of liver metastases in colorectal cancer: Competitive analyses of treatment results in synchronous versus methachronous metastases. Eur J Surg Oncol 16:360–365, 1990.

185. Doci R, Gennari L, Bignami P, et al: One hundred patients with hepatic metastases from colorectal cancer treated by resection: Analyses of prognostic determinants. Br J Surg 78:797–801, 1991.

186. Scheele J, Stangl R, Altendorf-Hoffmann A, et al:Indicators of prognosis after hepatic resection for colorectal carcinoma. Ann Surg 11:541–547, 1987.

187. Rosen CB, Nagorney DM, Taswell HF, et al: Perioperative blood transfusion and determinants of survival after resection of metastatic colorectal carcinoma. Ann Surg 216:493–504, 1992.

188. Ekberg H, Tranberg KH, Andersson R, et al: Pattern of reccurence in liver resection for colorectal secondaries. World J Surg 11:541–547, 1987.

189. Hughes KH, Simons R, Songhorabodi S, et al: Resection of the liver for colorectal carcinoma metastases: A multi-institutional study of indications for resection. Surgery 103:278–288, 1988.

190. Cortner JG, Silva JS, Cox EB, et al: Multivariate analyses of a personal series of 247 consecutive patients with liver metastases from colorectal cancer. Ann Surg 199(3):317–324, 1984.

191. Nordlinger B, Vaillant JC, Guiguet M, et al, for the Association Francaise of Chirurgie: Survival benefit of repeat liver resections for recurrent colorectal metastases: 143 cases. J Clin Oncol 12(7):1491–1496, 1994.

192. Gwin JL, Sigurdson ER: Surgical considerations in nonhepatic intra-abdominal recurrence of carcinoma of the colon. Semin Oncology 20(5):520–527, 1993.

193. Kewenter J, Bjork S, Haglind E, et al: Screening and rescreening for colorectal cancer: A controlled trial of fecal occult blood testing in 27,700 subjects. Cancer 62:645–651, 1988.

194. Willet CG, Fung CY, Kaufman DS,et al: Postoperative radiation therapy for high-risk colon carcinoma. J Clin Oncol 11:1112–1117, 1993.

195. Douglass HO Jr: Adjuvant treatment in colorectal cancer: An update. World J Surg 11:478–492, 1987.

196. Buyse M, Zeleniuch-Jacquotte A, Chalmers TC: Adjuvant therapy of colorectal cancer: Why we still don't know. JAMA 259:3571–3578, 1988.

197. Levin B, O Connell MC: Colorectal cancer chemotherapy: Meta-analysis of large scale trials. JAMA 159:3611, 1988.

198. Gastrointestinal Tumor Study Group: Adjuvant therapy of colon cancer: Results of a prospectively randomized trial. N Engl J Med 310:737–743, 1984.

199. Panetierre FJ, Goodman PJ, Constanzi JJ, et al: Adjuvant therapy in large bowel adenocarcinoma: Long-term results of a Southwest Oncology Group study. J Clin Oncol 6:947–954, 1988.

200. Higgins GA Jr, Amadio JH, McElhenney J, et al: Efficiency of prolonged intermittent therapy with combined 5-FU and methyl-CCNU following resection for carcinoma of the large bowel. Cancer 53:1–8, 1984.

201. Abdi E, Harbora D, Hanson J, et al: Adjuvant chemoimmuno- and immunotherapy in stage B2 and C colorectal cancer (abstract). Proc Am Soc Clin Oncol 6:93, 1987.

202. Wolmark N, Fisher B, Rockette H, et al: Postoperative adjuvant chemotherapy or BCG for colon cancer: Results from NSABP protocol C-01. J Natl Cancer Inst 80:30–36, 1988.

203. Kane MJ: Adjuvant systemic treatment for carcinoma of the colon and rectum. Semin Oncol 18:421–442, 1991.

204. Abdalla EE, Blair E, Jones RA, et al: Mechanism of synergy of levamisole and fluorouracil: Induction of human leucocyte antigen class I in a colorectal cancer cell line. J Natl Cancer Inst 87:472–489, 1995.

205. Windle R, Bell P, Shaw D: Five year results of a randomized trial of adjuvant 5-FU and levamisole in colorectal cancer. Br J Surg 74:569–572, 1984.

206. Laurie JA, Moertel CG, Fleming TR, et al: Surgical adjuvant therapy of poor prognosis colorectal cancer with levamisole alone or combined levamisole and 5-FU: A North Central Cancer Treatment Group and Mayo Clinic study (abstract). Proc Am Soc Clin Oncol 5:81, 1986.

207. Laurie JA, Moertel CG, Fleming TR, et al: Surgical adjuvant therapy of large bowel carcinoma: An evaluation of levamisole and the combination of levamisole and 5-fluorouracil. J Clin Oncol 7:1447–1456, 1989.

208. Moertel CG, Fleming TR, MacDonald JS, et al: Levamisole and fluorouracil for adjuvant therapy of resected colon carcinoma. N Engl J Med 322:352–358, 1990.

209. Moertel CG, Fleming TR, Macdonald JS, et al: Fluorouracil plus levamisole as effective adjuvant therapy after resection of stage III colon carcinoma: A final report. Ann Intern Med 122:321–326, 1995.

210. Cassidy J: Adjuvant 5-fluorouracil plus levamisole in colon cancer: The plot thickens? (editorial). Br J Cancer. 69:986–987, 1994.

211. Wolmark N, Rockette H, Fisher B, et al: The benefit of leucovorin-modulated fluorouracil as postoperative adjuvant therapy

for primary colon cancer: Results from National Surgical Adjuvant Breast and Bowel Project C-03.J Clin Oncol 11:1879–1887, 1993.

212. Zaniboni A, Erlichman C, Seitz JF, et al: FUFA increases disease-free survival in resected B2-C colon cancer: Results of a prospective pooled analysis of three randomized trials (abstract). Proc Am Soc Clin Oncol 12:191, 1993.

213. The International Multicentre Pooled Analysis of Colon Cancer Trials (IMPACT) Investigators: Efficacy of adjuvant fluorouracil and folinic acid in colon cancer. Lancet 345:939–943, 1995.

214. Haller DG, MacDonald JS, Mayer RJ: Eastern Cooperative Oncology Group, Southwest Oncology Group, Cancer and Leukemia Group B, NCI High Priority Clinical Trial: Phase III randomized comparison of adjuvant low-dose CF/5-FU vs high-dose CF/5-FU vs low-dose CF/5-FU/LEV vs 5-FU/LEV following curative resection in selected patients with Dukes B2 and C carcinoma of the colon (summary last modified 03/92). EST-2288; SWOG-8899; CLB- 8896, clinical trial, active 08/22/88.

215. Taylor I, Brooman P, Rowling JT: Adjuvant liver perfusion in colorectal cancer: Initial results of a clinical trial. Br Med J 2:1320–1322, 1977.

216. Taylor I, Machin D, Mulee M, et al: A randomized controlled trial of adjuvant portal vein cytotoxic perfusion in colorectal cancer. Br J Surg 72:359–363, 1985.

217. Mayer RJ, Stablein DM: Adjuvant colon cancer trials of the Gastrointestinal Tumor Study Group, in Hamilton JM, Elliott JM (eds): NIH Consensus Development Conference: Adjuvant Therapy for Patients with Colon and Rectum Cancer. NIH Consensus Conference Proceedings (abstract). Bethesda, MD, National Institutes of Health, 1990.

218. Swiss Group for Clinical Cancer Research (SAAK): Long-term results of a single-course adjuvant intraportal chemotherapy for colorectal cancer. Lancet 345:349–353, 1995.

219. Beart RW, Moertel CG, Wieand HS, et al: Adjuvant therapy for resectable colorectal carcinoma with fluorouracil administered by portal vein infusion. Arch Surg 125:897–901, 1990.

220. Wolmark N, Rockette H, Wickerham DL, et al: Adjuvant therapy of Dukes A, B, and C adenocarcinoma of the colon with portal vein fluorouracil hepatic infusion: Preliminary results of National Surgical Adjuvant Breast and Bowel Project Protocol C-02. J Clin Oncol 8:1466–1475, 1990.

221. Fielding LP, Hittinger R, Grace RH, et al: Randomised controlled trial of adjuvant chemotherapy by portal-vein perfusion after curative resection for colorectal adenocarcinoma. Lancet 340:502–506, 1992.

222. Patt YZ, Mavligt G: Arterial chemotherapy in the management of colorectal cancer: An overview. Semin Oncol 18:478–490, 1991.

223. Hoover HC, Surdyke MG, Dangel RB: Prospectively randomized trial of adjuvant active- specific immunotherapy for human colorectal cancer. Cancer 55:1236–1243, 1985.

224. Hoover HC, Surdyke MG, Brandhorst JS, et al: Five-year follow-up of a controlled trial of active specific immunotherapy in colorectal cancer (abstract). Proc Am Soc Clin Oncol 9:106, 1990.

225. Riethmuller G, Schneider-Gadicke E, Schlimok G, et al: Randomised trial of monoclonal antibody for adjuvant therapy of resected Dukes' C colorectal carcinoma. Lancet 343:1177–1183, 1994.

226. O'Connell MJ, Martenson JA, Wieand HS, et al: Improving adjuvant therapy for rectal cancer by combining protracted infusion fluorouracil with radiation therapy after curative surgery. N Engl J Med 331:502–507, 1994.

227. Moertel CG, Gunderson LL, Mailliard JA, et al, for the North Central Cancer Treatment Group: Early evaluation of combined fluorouracil and leucovorin as a radiation enhancer for locally unresectable, residual, or recurrent gastrointestinal carcinoma. J Clin Oncol 12:21–27, 1994

228. Gunderson LL, Sosin H: Areas of failure at reoperation (second or symptomatic look) following "curative surgery" for adenocarcinoma of the rectum. Cancer 34:1278–1292, 1974.

229. Cass AW, Million RR, Pfaff WW: Patterns of recurrence following surgery alone for adenocarcinoma of the colon and rectum. Cancer 37:2861–2865, 1976.

230. McDermott FT, Hughes ESR, Johnson WR, et al: Local recurrence after potentially curative resection for rectal cancer in a series of 1008 patients. Br J Surg 72:34–37, 1985.

231. Gastrointestinal Tumor Study Group: Prolongation of the disease-free interval in surgically treated rectal carcinoma. N Engl J Med 312:1465–1472, 1985.

232. Fisher B, Wolmark N, Rockette H, et al: Postoperative adjuvant chemotherapy or radiation therapy for rectal cancer: Results from NSABP protocol R-01. J Natl Cancer Inst 80:21–29, 1988.

233. Gerrard A, Buyse M, Nordlinger B, et al: Preoperative radiotherapy as adjuvant treatment in rectal cancer: Final results of a randomized trial of the European Organization for Research and Treatment of Cancer. Ann Surg 208:606–614, 1988.

234. Higgins GA, Humphrey EW, Dwight RW, et al: Preoperative radiation and surgery for cancer of the rectum: Veterans Administration Surgical Oncology Group Trial II. Cancer 58:352–354, 1986.

235. Hoskins RB, Gunderson LL, Dosoretz DE, et al: Adjuvant post-operative radiotherapy in carcinoma of the rectum and rectosigmoid. Cancer 55:61–71, 1985.

236. Douglass HO Jr, Moertel CG, Mayer RJ, et al: Survival after post-operative combination treatment of rectal cancer. N Engl J Med 315:1294–1295, 1986.

237. Krook J, Moertel CG, Gunderson LL, et al: Effective surgical adjuvant therapy for high risk rectal carcinoma. N Engl J Med 324:709–715, 1991.

238. Hamilton JM, Sznol M, Friedman MA: 5-fluorouracil plus levamisole: Effective adjuvant treatment for cancer, in Devita VT Jr, Hellman S, Rosenberg SA (eds): Important Advances in Oncology, pp 115–130. Philadelphia, JB Lippincott, 1990.

239. Mohiuddin M, Marks G: Adjuvant radiation therapy for colon and rectal cancer. Semin Oncol 18:411–420, 1991.

240. Erlichman G, Fine S, Wong A, et al: A randomized trial of fluorouracil and folinic acid in patients with metastatic colorectal carcinoma. J Clin Oncol 6:469–475, 1988.

241. Petrelli N, Herrera C, Rustum Y, et al: A prospective randomized trial of 5-fluorouracil versus 5-fluorouracil and high-dose leucovorin versus 5-fluorouracil and methotrexate in previously untreated patients with advanced colorectal carcinoma. J Clin Oncol 5:1559–1565, 1987.

242. Kemeny N: Role of chemotherapy in the treatment of colorectal carcinoma. Semin Surg Oncol 3:190–214, 1987.

243. Ansfield F, Klotz J, Nealon T, et al: A phase III study comparing the clinical utility of four regimens of 5-fluorouracil. Cancer 39:34–40, 1977.

244. Lokich J, Ahlgren J, Gullo J, et al: A prospective randomized comparison of continuous infusion fluorouracil with a conventional bolus schedule in metastatic colorectal carcinoma: A Mid-Atlantic Oncology Program. J Clin Oncol 7:425–432, 1989.

245. Gunderson S, Brutsch U, Cavalli F, et al: Phase II trial with tauromustine (TCNU, LS2667) in patients with advanced colorectal cancer (abstract). Proc Am Soc Clin Oncol 7:109, 1988.

246. Alberto P, Mermillod B, Germano G, et al: A randomized comparison of doxifluridine and fluorouracil in colorectal carcinoma. Eur J Cancer Clin Oncol 24:559–563, 1988.

247. Asbury RF, Kramar A, Haller DG: Aminothiadiazole (NSC #4728) in patients with advanced colon cancer: A phase II study of the Eastern Cooperative Oncology Group. Am J Clin Oncol 10:380–382,

1987.

248. Ferrari L, Ross A, Brambilla C, et al: Phase I study with 4-deoxydoxorubicin. Invest New Drugs 2:287–295, 1984.

249. Fiebig HH, Wellens W, Peukert M, et al: Phase II study of the water-soluble nitrosourea compound ACNU in advanced colorectal carcinomas. Onkologie 7:370–377, 1984.

250. Levi F, Perpoint B, Garuti C, et al: Oxaliplatin activity against metastatic colorectal cancer. A phase II study of 5-day continuous venous infusion at circadian rhythm modulated rate. Eur J Cancer 29A:1658–1663, 1993.

251. Dorr RT, Von Hoff DD (eds): CPT-11, in Cancer Chemotherapy Handbook, 2nd ed, pp 314–316. East Norwalk, Connecticut, Appleton and Lange, 1994.

251a. Rothenberg ML, Kuhn J, Burris HA, et al: A phase I and pharmacokinetics trial of CPT-11 in patients with refractory solid tumors (abstract). Proc Am Soc Clin Oncol 11:273, 1992.

252. Shimada Y, Yoshino M, Wakui A,et al for the CPT-11 Gastrointestinal Cancer Study Group: Phase III study of CPT-11,a new campothecin derivative in metastatic colorectal cancer. J Clin Oncol 11:909–913, 1993.

253. Rothenberg ML, Eckardt JR, Burris HA III, et al: Irinotecan (CPT-11) as second-line therapy for patinets with 5-FU refractory colorectal cancer. Proc Am Soc Clin Oncol 13(578):198, 1994.

254. Bugat R, Rougier P, Douillard JY, et al: Efficacy of irinotecan HCL (CPT-11) in patients with metastatic colorectal cancer after progression while receiving a 5-FU-based chemotherapy. Proc Am Soc Clin Oncol (abstract) 567:222, 1995.

255. Sasaki Y, Ohtsu A, Shimada Y, et al: Simultaneous administration of CPT-11 and fluorouracil: Alteration of the pharmacokinetics of CPT-11 and SN-38 in patients with advanced colorectal cancer. J Natl Cancer Inst 86:1096–1097, 1994.

256. Pazdur R, Lassere Y, Rhodes V, et al: Phase II trial of UFT plus oral leucovorin: An effective oral regimen in the treatment of metastatic colorectal carcinoma. J Clin Oncol 12(11):2296–2300, 1994.

257. The International Medical Function Tomudex (ZD1694), a Thymidylate Synthase Inhibitor. Zeneca Pharmaceuticals, Clinical Investigators Manual, 1994.

258. Engstrom P, MacIntyre J, Douglass H Jr, et al: Combination chemotherapy of advanced bowel cancer (abstract). Proc Am Assoc Cancer Res 19:384, 1978.

259. Buroker TR, Moertel CG, Fleming TR, et al: A controlled evaluation of recent approaches to biochemical modulation or enhancement of 5-fluorouracil therapy in colorectal carcinoma. J Clin Oncol 3:1624–1631, 1985.

260. LoRusso P, Pazdur R, Redman S, et al: Low-dose continuous infusion 5-fluorouracil and cisplatin: Phase II evaluation in advanced colorectal carcinoma. Am J Clin Oncol 12:486–490, 1989.

261. Hermann R, Spehn J, Beyer J, et al: Sequential methotrexate and 5-fluorouracil: Improved response rate in metastatic colorectal cancer. J Clin Oncol 2:591–594, 1984.

262. Poon MA, O'Connell MJ, Wieand HS, et al: Biochemical modulation of fluorouracil with leucovorin: Confirmatory evidence of improved therapeutic efficacy in advanced colorectal cancer. J Clin Oncol 9:1967–1972, 1991.

263. Erlichman C: Fluorouracil/leucovorin study update. J Clin Oncol 9:2076, 1991.

264. The Advanced Colorectal Cancer Meta-analysis Project: Modulation of fluorouracil by leucovorin in patients with advanced colorectal cancer: Evidence in terms of response rate. J Clin Oncol 10:896–903, 1992.

265. The Advanced Colorectal Cancer Meta-Analysis Project: Meta-Analysis of randomized trials testing the biochemical modulation of fluorouracil by methotrexate in colorectal cancer. J Clin Oncol, 12(5):960–969, 1994.

266. Buroker TR, O'Connell MJ, Wieand HS, et al: Randomized comparision of two schedules of fluorouracil and leucoovorin in the treatment of advanced colorectal cancer. J Clin Oncol 12:14–20, 1994.

267. Leichman CG, Fleming TR, Muggia FM, et al: Phase II study of fluorouracil and its modulation in advanced colorectal cancer: A Southwest Oncology Group Study. J Clin Oncol 13:1303–1311, 1995.

268. Wadler S, Schwartz E, Goldman M, et al: Fluorouracil and recombinant alfa-2a interferon: An active regimen against advanced colorectal carcinoma. J Clin Oncol 7:1769–1775, 1989.

269. Pazdur R, Ajani J, Patt Y, et al: Phase II study of fluorouracil and recombinant alfa-2a- interferon in previously untreated advanced colorectal carcinoma. J Clin Oncol 8:2027–2031, 1990.

270. Corfu-A Study Group: Phase III randomized study of two fluorouracil combinations with either interferon alfa-2a or leucovorin for advanced colorectal cancer. J Clin Oncol 13:921–928, 1995.

271. York M, Greco FA, Figlin RA, et al: A randomized phase III trial comparing 5-FU with or without interferon alfa-2a for advanced colorectal cancer (abstract). Proc Am Soc Clin Oncol 12:200, 1993.

272. Hill M, Norman A, Cunningham D, et al: Royal Marsden phase III trial of fluorouracil with or without interferon alfa-2b in advanced colorectal cancer. J Clin Oncol 13:1297–1302, 1995.

273. Hohn DC, Stagg RJ, Friedman MA, et al: A randomized trial of continuous intravenous versus hepatic intraarterial fluoxiuridine in patients with colorectal cancer metastatic to the liver: The Northern California Oncology Group trial. J Clin Oncol 7:1646–1654, 1987.

274. Kemeny N, Daly J, Reichman B,et al: Intrahepatic or systemic infusion of fluoro deoxyuridine in patients with liver metastases from colorectal carcinoma. A randomized trial. Ann Intern Med 107:459–465, 1987.

275. Rougier P, Laplanche A, Huguier M, et al: Hepatic arterial infusion of floxuridine in patients with liver metastases from colorectal carcinoma: Long term results of a prospective randomized trial. J Clin Oncol 10:1112–1118, 1992.

276. Chang AE, Schneider PD, Sugarbaker PH,et al: A prospective randomized trial of regional versus systemic continuous 5-fluorodeoxyuridine chemotherapy in the treatment of colorectal liver metastases. Ann Surg 206:685–693, 1987.

277. Martin JK Jr, O'Connell MJ, Wieand HS, et al: Intra-arterial floxuridine vs systemic fluorouracil for hepatic metastases from colorectal cancer: A randomized trial. Arch Surg 125:1022–1027, 1990.

278. Moertel CG: Chemotherapy for colorectal cancer. N Engl J Med 330(16):1136–1142, 1994.

279. Kemeny N, Conti JA, Cohen A, et al: Phase II study of hepatic arterial floxuridine, leucovorin, and dexamethasone for unresectable liver metastases from colorectal carcinoma. J Clin Oncol 12(11):2288–2295, 1994.

Neuroendocrine Tumors of the Gastrointestinal Tract

Nikolaos Touroutoglou, MD, PhD, Anthony Arcenas, MD, *and* Jaffer A. Ajani, MD

Department of Gastrointestinal Oncology and Digestive Diseases
The University of Texas M. D. Anderson Cancer Center, Houston, Texas

Neuroendocrine tumors manifest in the gastrointestinal tract mainly as carcinoid and pancreatic islet-cell tumors. They comprise an interesting group of rare neoplasms that are derived from neuroendocrine cells interspersed within the gastrointestinal system amd throughout the body. Neuroendocrine tumors are well known for producing various hormonal syndromes and for their indolent clinical course in most patients, although some of these tumors do not produce hormones of clinical significance. Patients may have symptoms for many years before the diagnosis is suspected and confirmed. Therefore, the index of suspicion must be high in order to diagnose these tumors in a timely fashion.

Symptoms are caused by hormonal excess, local tumor growth, or metastatic spread. Therapy should be dictated by the severity of symptoms and the pace of the disease. Surgical extirpation remains the only curative modality for localized disease, but palliation of hormone-related symptoms can be achieved with the somatostatin analog octreotide (Sandostatin) in a significant proportion of patients. Combination chemotherapy, biologic response modifiers, vascular occlusion treatment, and newer somatostatin analogs are being used for the treatment of metastatic disease.

EPIDEMIOLOGY

Neuroendocrine tumors constitute approximately 2% of all malignant tumors of the gastrointestinal system.[1] These tumors are particularly rare in pediatric patients. It is estimated that fewer than 2,000 new cases are diagnosed yearly in the United States.

Carcinoid tumors are more common than pancreatic islet-cell carcinomas (65:35 incidence). Although approximately 600 new cases of small-intestine carcinoids are seen yearly in the United States, autopsy data from the Mayo Clinic indicate that the incidence of these tumors may be approximately 650 cases per 100,000 people.[1] Of the noncarcinoid tumors, insulinomas and gastrinomas have the highest incidence, whereas other types are extremely rare. A center in Belfast has established a registry for tumors of the gastroenteropancreatic endocrine system[2]; these investigators have reported incidences of 0.9 and 0.4 cases per million individuals per year for insulinomas and gastrinomas, respectively.

ETIOLOGY

The precise etiology of neuroendocrine tumors is not well understood. Some insight into the molecular biology of these tumors can be gained by studying a subset of tumors that occurs as part of the multiple endocrine neoplasia type I (MEN I) syndrome. In 1954, Wermer recognized that a neoplastic disorder involving the anterior pituitary gland, parathyroids, and pancreatic islet cells was familial and transmitted in an autosomal dominant fashion.[3]

More recently, Larsson et al reported linkage of the *MEN I* gene to the muscle phosphorylase locus on chromosome 11q13.[4] Using another gene known to be localized to 11q13 (INT2), Bale et al found similar linkage of the *MEN I* gene with this gene locus.[5] Radford et al investigated DNA isolated from tumors and somatic tissues in 12 patients with *MEN I* and found loss of heterozygosity markers mapped to chromosome band 11q13 in 9 (82%) of 11 informative tumors.[6] There was no allelic loss from other chromosomes. Such a high incidence of chromosomal deletion involving 11q13 suggests that this region is important in the oncogenesis of neuroendocrine tumors. The same deletion on chromosome 11q13 (PYGM locus) was subsequently demonstrated in sporadic islet-cell tumors, pituitary tumors, and parathyroid tumors.[7,8] Preliminary data suggest that the candidate *MEN I* gene may be a tumor-suppressor gene and that deletions or mutations of this gene may play a major role in the development of neuroendocrine tumors.[9]

PATHOLOGY

The Neuroendocrine Concept

Advances in the fields of histochemistry, electron microscopy, and immunocytochemistry have influenced which cells can be classified as neuroendocrine. Neuroendocrine tumors originate from cells that are capable of amine precursor (such as dopa and 5-hydroxytryptophan) uptake and decarboxylation (APUD cells).[10] As a result, these tumors have high intracellular levels of carboxyl groups and nonspecific esterase. The latter is used as a neuroendocrine marker.

As the name suggests, neuroendocrine cells were previously considered to be derived from the neural crest, from which they subsequently migrate throughout the body. However, extensive embryologic investigations have shown that while certain APUD cells are, indeed, derived from the neural crest, the neuroendocrine cells of the digestive tract cannot be traced back to the neural ectoderm.[11] It is now clear that similar cell phenotypes can arise from different germ layers, and the search for a common origin of neuroendocrine cells has become less important as more phenotypic characteristics (markers) of these cells are identified by new immunocytochemical methods.[11] Regardless of embryonic origin, these cells have a common genetic program for the expression of several biochemical markers of neuroendocrine function.[12]

Thus, the term "neuroendocrine" is used to define cells by their secretory products and cytoplasmic proteins rather than by their localization and embryologic derivation. The neuroendocrine cell system, therefore, includes all neuronal and endocrine cells that share a common phenotypic program characterized by simultaneous expression of certain marker proteins (general neuroendocrine markers) and cell type–specific hormonal products. These peptides are contained within membrane-bound vesicles from which they are released by a process of regulated exocytosis in response to external stimuli.

Neuroendocrine cells differ from neurons in that axons and specialized nerve terminals are absent in the former, and consequently, their mode of transmission is endocrine or paracrine rather than synaptic. The neuroendocrine cells normally form either small organs, distinct cell clusters within other tissues, or a network of cells dispersed in the lung and gut mucosa.[11,13] In addition to carcinoids and islet-cell neoplasms, other tumors that arise from these cells include small-cell carcinoma (of pulmonary and extrapulmonary origin), medullary carcinoma of the thyroid gland, neuroblastoma, and Merkel-cell tumors of the skin.

Diagnostic Pathologic Features

Gross Histology: Carcinoid tumors may show any of a variety of architectural patterns that have been referred to as insular, trabecular, glandular, mixed, or undifferentiated.[14,15] Typically, there is extensive necrosis of both sheets of cells and individual cells. In some tumors, such as midgut carcinoids, there is extensive stromal fibrosis surrounding tumor islets. However, other aspects of tumor cell appearance are uniform: a pale pink or granular cytoplasm and a round to oval nucleus with stippled chromatin. There is minimal mitotic activity, cytologic atypia, or nuclear pleomorphism, except in undifferentiated tumors, and secretory granules can be demonstrated under the electron microscope.

Such histologic features are inadequate to distinguish pancreatic endocrine tumors from carcinoids and malignant from benign neuroendocrine tumors. The actual clinical behavior, such as infiltration of adjacent organs or structures and metastases to regional lymph nodes or the liver, is what usually substantiates the malignant nature of the tumor. However, multivariate analysis has demonstrated that histologic type and primary site have independent prognostic significance. (Patients with glandular and undifferentiated histology and foregut or hindgut tumor location have a worse outcome.)[16,17]

Further Diagnostic Techniques

For tumors that show the classic morphologic properties described above, use of special techniques merely confirms the diagnosis. Frequently, however, a pathologist will need to confirm the morphologic impression with standard histochemical, electron microscopic, or immunohistochemical analysis.

Standard Histochemical Analysis: This relatively old staining procedure relies on the ability of well-differentiated neuroendocrine tumors to stain positively with silver in the presence of endogenous cellular reducing agents (argentaffin cells) or with the addition of exogenous reducing reagents (argyrophilic cells). This silver stain rarely is positive in poorly differentiated lesions.

Electron microscopy reveals the neurosecretory or dense core granules of the neuroendocrine cells. In this setting, however, use of this method is uncommon, as it is limited by substantial cost, the extensive tissue preparation required, and the small number of cells that can be examined.

Immunohistochemical Markers: During the past 15 years, identification of a number of components of neuronal and neuroendocrine cells by immunohistochemical methods has markedly affected the classification of tumors as neuroendocrine. These methods provide reliable information at low cost, require relatively simple tissue preparation, and have a rapid turnaround time. Several general neuroendocrine markers associated with cytoplasmic proteins, small secretory vesicles, or dense-core secretory granules have thus been established.[18–20]

Cytoplasmic Constituents: Neuron-specific enolase, a glycolytic enzyme found in the cytosol, is the best known marker of cells with neuroendocrine differentiation. However, this marker is nonspecific, as it stains positive on fibroadenomas of the breast, renal-cell carcinoma, and certain malignant lymphomas. Its positivity is therefore not considered to be diagnostic, and consequently, this reagent is also known as nonspecific esterase.[13]

Secretory Vesicle Membrane Constituents: Synaptophysin is an integral membrane glycoprotein that is involved in calcium binding and occurs in presynaptic vesicles of neurons and small vesicles of normal and neoplastic neuroendocrine cells.[19]

Granule Contents: Chromogranins A, B, and C are acidic proteins that serve as powerful universal markers for neuroendocrine tissues and tumors. Chromogranins are a family of soluble proteins located in large (dense-core) secretory granules. The most frequently used antibody is against chromogranin A.[20]

Plasma membrane constituents include receptors for peptides or neurotransmitters (somatostatin, glutamate, and gamma-aminobutyric acid), and neural cell adhesion molecules (NCAMs), the most important of which appear to be NCAM and L-1.[11] Somatostatin receptors are present in 82% of carcinoid tumors and in 67% to 100% of islet-cell tumors.[21] Moreover, most metastases of primary somatostatin receptor–positive tumors are also positive for this peptide. Somatostatin inhibits peptide hormone secretion of most neuroendocrine cells by a mechanism that involves the suppression of secetory pathways that are dependent on cyclic adenosine monophosphate and the disruption of the second messenger function of intracellular calcium.[22]

Somatostatin receptor status correlates highly with the ability of long-acting somatostatin analogs, such as octreotide, to inhibit in vivo hormone secretion.[23] The presence of these receptors enables in vivo imaging of tumors using ^{111}In-labeled octreotide. Somatostatin analogs are thus used in both imaging and treatment of neuroendocrine tumors.

Growth Factors and Nuclear Antigens: The expression of growth factors and the presence of nuclear antigens, although not unique to neuroendocrine tumors, are of particular interest. Ki-67 is a monoclonal antibody against a nuclear antigen present in proliferating cells.[24] Patients who have tumors with a high index for Ki-67 were found to have a significantly shorter survival than those whose tumors are low in Ki-67 content.[25]

Various growth factors have been studied, including platelet-derived growth factors, transforming growth factors-alpha and -beta (TGF-alpha and -beta), fibroblast growth factors, and epidermal growth factors, and the data suggest that platelet-derived growth factors may be involved in the autocrine stimulation of neuroendocrine tumor cells and stimulation of stromal cell growth through paracrine or autocrine mechanisms.[26,27] Moreover, the TGF family known for its fibroblast-stimulating ability (TGF-beta) may play a role in the proliferation of fibroblasts and their production of matrix in the fibrotic lesions associated with carcinoids.[28] In endocrine pancreatic tumors, expression of CD44 correlates with the tumor's ability to give rise to lymph node metastases, and may play a vital role in determining the fate of metastasizing cells.[29]

Different types of neuroendocrine cells share many specific properties and express several proteins in common, but the expression of any one marker protein is not an absolute criterion. Thus, there is no "universal" marker. In addition to the above substances that serve as general markers, immunoperoxidase staining has shown that tumors can synthesize numerous biogenic amines and peptides. These include 5-hydroxytryptamine, 5-hydroxytryptophan, serotonin, insulin, glucagon, somatostatin, vasoactive intestinal polypeptide, growth hormone, corticotropin melanocyte-stimulating hormone, gastrin, pancreatic polypeptide, calcitonin, and substance P. Clinical signs of hormone hyperfunction may therefore be correlated to their precise source.[30] Tumors are named primarily according to the predominant peptide secreted that can be related to the clinical features.

NATURAL HISTORY AND DIAGNOSIS

Neuroendocrine tumor cells can synthesize and secrete a variety of physiologically active peptides that generate disabling symptoms. However, some tumors produce peptides only after a prolonged period of inactivity.[1] In the case of islet-cell carcinoma, the dominant hormone and hormonal syndrome can also change.[31]

Patients with nonsecreting tumors usually present with a large tumor burden but may lack any of the cancer-associated cachexia or morbidity that may be associated with smaller, peptide-secreting tumors. Thus, some patients with nonsecreting tumors are diagnosed with a large pancreatic mass or enlarged liver during a routine physical examination, whereas others with small but hormonally active tumors can have significant debilitating symptoms that require prompt diagnostic evaluation. In a study of 154 patients with gastrointestinal carcinoid tumor, 60% of tumors found at surgery were asymptomatic and 40% were symptomatic.[32]

Because of their rarity, a specific staging system for neuroendocrine tumors of the gastrointestinal system is not required, but as is the case with many other tumors, involvement of lymph nodes and size of the primary tumor are the two most important prognostic factors.

Carcinoid Tumors

Carcinoid tumors are the most common neuroendocrine tumors. They arise from neuroendocrine cells located primarily in the submucosa of the intestine but can also arise in the main bronchi. Between 1981 and 1989, a shift in the anatomic origin of these tumors was noted, with an increase in the percentage of carcinoids of the bronchus from 10% to 30% and a decrease in the number of tumors of the jejunoileum and rectum.[33] Moertel has reported that the majority of carcinoid tumors arise from the appendix (45%), small intestine (30%), and rectum (15%).[1]

In 1 of every 200 to 300 appendectomies, usually in young adults, a carcinoid tumor is found incidentally. In patients with appendiceal tumors 1 cm in diameter, surgical cure is possible in 95% of cases, whereas patients with tumors between 1 and 2 cm in diameter remain at more than 50% risk of having established metastases that eventually manifest. A right hemicolectomy should be considered for patients with tumors > 2 cm in diameter, younger patients, and those with vascular invasion, as these patients have nearly a 95% risk of developing overt metastatic disease.[34]

Rectal carcinoids occur more frequently in middle-aged adults. These tumors are found incidentally in approximately 1 in 2,500 proctoscopies as a small yellow-gray submucosal nodule in the anterior and lateral walls of the rectum. They seldom bleed.[1] Unlike other carcinoid tumors, rectal carcinoids may not take up silver stain and histochemically may not show evidence of serotonin production. The majority of rectal carcinoids are < 1 cm in diameter and do not metastasize; fulguration can be adequate treatment for these small lesions. Tumors larger than 2 cm almost always will metastasize. Patients with aneuploid rectal carcinoids appear to have a poor prognosis, as do those with other carcinoid tumors of the gastrointestinal tract.[35]

Small intestinal carcinoid tumors are the carcinoids most frequently associated with clinical symptoms, are usually found in the distal ileum within 60 cm of the ileocecal valve, and tend to be multiple. The likelihood of spread is associated with the size and location of the primary tumor; primaries in the small bowel are more likely to metastasize than are those in the rectum or the appendix.[15]

A fibroblastic reaction can be stimulated in the mesentery and retroperitoneum, leading to complications (recurrent, intermittent partial or acute complete intestinal obstruction), with intermittent obstruction and abdominal pain being the most common clinical presentation. Recently, it was shown that platelet-derived growth factor is involved in this fibroblastic reaction by stimulating stromal cell growth through paracrine and possibly autocrine mechanisms.[26] Metastases from mesenteric and iliac lymph nodes can result, though rarely, in progressive encasement of the mesenteric artery, followed by bowel ischemia and infarction.

Carcinoid metastatic deposits in the liver tend to grow slowly. Thus, a patient with large masses in a grossly enlarged liver can be fully active and productive, with minimal symptoms and normal or nearly normal liver function test results.

Carcinoid Syndrome: The most common systemic syndrome caused by carcinoid tumors is the carcinoid syndrome. It occurs when hormonal tumor products reach the systemic circulation. This usually implies the presence of disease that has venous drainage in the systemic circulation in such a way as to circumvent the liver and its "first-pass" effect. Such is the case with metastatic disease in the liver itself or primary disease in the bronchi. During the "first pass," the liver is able to remove from the bloodstream even large amounts of a primary tumor's hormonal products before they reach the systemic circulation. Hepatic metastasis is the most frequently associated condition in patients with carcinoid syndrome. Because tumors of the jejunum, ileum, appendix, and ascending colon are the most common and frequently metastasize, they account for about 80% of the carcinoids that cause the carcinoid syndrome.[35] The syndrome also occurs in association with gastric, pancreatic, appendiceal, cecal, colonic, and, in rare instances, rectal carcinoids.

Carcinoid syndrome is characterized by paroxysmal flushing, watery diarrhea, abdominal cramping, telangiectasia of the face, episodes of asthma or wheezing, endocardial fibrosis and valvular heart disease, and pellagra-like lesions of the skin and oral mucosa.[15] The distinction between the carcinoid syndrome and malignant carcinoid syndrome (or carcinoid crisis) is based on the severity of symptoms.[36] Progressive, relentless symptoms (namely, symptomatic carcinoid heart disease, severe diarrhea, and episodes of hypotension or hypertension) constitute the malignant version of the syndrome. This may be precipitated by stressful interventions, such as anesthesia induction or hepatic arterial occlusion.

Several peptides have been implicated as a cause of the carcinoid syndrome. The principal agent appears to be serotonin, although other peptides, such as substance P, histamine, bradykinin, kallikrein, and perhaps prostaglandins, may play a minor contributory role. In the tumor, tryptophan is converted to 5-hydroxytryptophan, which is then converted to serotonin by L-dopa decarboxylase and is stored in the neurosecretory tumor granules or is released in the systemic circulation. Most of the serotonin is converted by monoamine oxidase to 5-hydroxyindole acetic acid (5-HIAA), which appears in increased amounts in the urine.

The severity of the syndrome appears to be related to tumor bulk, the level of urinary excretion of 5-HIAA, and the degree of liver dysfunction caused by metastatic disease.[37] Hepatic metastases frequently reach sizes several times that of the primary tumor and can produce large amounts of serotonin and 5-hydroxytryptophan. Urinary 5-HIAA can serve as a useful marker in monitoring the course of the disease and the effectiveness of treatment.[1]

The exact etiology of flushing remains unexplained. Histamine, kinins, and prostaglandins, but not serotonin, have been implicated in various situations. Flushing is present in as few as 25% of patients initially but in as many as 75% at some time during the disease course.[38] It consists of a sudden onset of violaceous erythema of the face and neck and is often associated with diarrhea and an unpleasant feeling of warmth. Sometimes it is accompanied by itching, palpitations, and facial edema.

Serotonin is considered responsible for diarrhea, which is seen in up to 84% of patients during the course of their disease,[38] and is manifested by frequent, profuse, watery stools often associated with abdominal cramps.

About one third of patients with carcinoid syndrome die of carcinoid heart disease and not of tumor growth.[38] Carcinoid heart disease is not due to direct involvement of the heart by the tumor, but rather, to fibrosis that primarily affects the endocardium of the right heart and is most commonly seen on the ventricular aspect of the tricuspid valve. This leads to tricuspid regurgitation; evidence of heart failure is seen in 80% of patients with such heart lesions.[39] Transforming growth factor-beta likely plays a major role in fibroblast proliferation and matrix production in carcinoid heart lesions, as well as in other locations of stromal fibrosis associated with carcinoids.[28]

The laboratory diagnostic test most frequently used to detect carcinoid syndrome is the quantitative measurement of 5-HIAA levels in a 24-hour urine sample (normal range, 2 to 8 mg/24 h). False-positive results occur with consumption of serotonin-rich foods and medications that affect urinary 5-HIAA levels, such as guaifenesin, acetaminophen, and salicylates. The test may be false-negative in patients with carcinoids of the stomach,

pancreas, and proximal duodenum, as these often do not produce significant levels of serotonin (and therefore of 5-HIAA). Urinary 5-HIAA levels correlate well with tumor mass and can be used as a marker for the extent of disease.[1]

Imaging Studies: Rectal, colonic, and gastric carcinoids are most frequently localized by endoscopic methods. Some tumors can be localized by angiography, computed tomography (CT), or magnetic resonance imaging (MRI). In a recent study of patients with pancreatic carcinoid tumors, the primary tumor was detected on CT and MRI scans in 79% and 88% of cases, respectively. While CT is the standard imaging procedure for staging the disease, angiography is the most sensitive method for detecting liver metastases and for defining vascular supply to the tumor before surgery or embolization.

Somatostatin receptor scintigraphy has markedly improved the visualization of neuroendocrine tumors. ^{111}In-labeled diethylenetriamine penta-acetic acid (DTPA) octreotide currently is widely available, and indium 111 is the most commonly applied isotope for this test. The sensitivity of a scintiscan is 80% to 90%. This method successfully revealed additional metastases that had not appeared on conventional imaging scans in about one third of patients with various neuroendocrine tumors.[40] In addition, scintiscans revealed carcinoids in about one third of patients in whom there was a strong clinical suspicion of insulinoma or gastrinoma but in whom conventional scans were negative.[40]

One of the most recent imaging developments is based on the fact that in serotonin-producing tumors, the precursor 5-hydroxytryptophan can be labeled with carbon 11 and subsequently traced by means of positron emission tomography (PET). With this method, tumors can be localized and their metabolic activity (and thus, response to treatment) followed with repeat scans.[41]

Survival Rates: The most common sites of metastases from carcinoids include regional lymph nodes, liver, lung, bones, and the peritoneal cavity. Frequent causes of death among individuals with these tumors include liver failure (most common) and cardiac failure (10% to 30% of patients), although up to 50% of patients may have cardiac involvement.[36,38] Rates of 5-year survival correlate with the site and extent of disease. Reported rates are highest (92% to 99%) in patients with carcinoids of the appendix and vary between 76% and 100% in patients with rectal carcinoids and between 42% and 71% in those with carcinoids of the small intestines.[35] In one study,[42] 10-year disease-specific survival rates were correlated with Dukes' classification and were found to be 100% for Dukes' stage A, 80% for stage B, 55% for stage C, and

10% for stage D carcinoid tumors. The presence of carcinoid syndrome is associated with decreased survival, with median survival durations ranging between 2 and 8.5 years from the onset of symptoms.[38,41,43]

Gastrinomas

The presence of jejunal ulceration is almost pathognomonic of gastrinoma. Recurrent peptic ulceration after adequate surgery or multiple ulcers should raise the suspicion of a gastrinoma. Patients with both peptic ulcers and diarrhea, patients whose ulceration persists with use of H_2-receptor blockers or recurs frequently after their discontinuation, and patients in whom endoscopy and barium meals reveal hypertrophied gastric mucosal folds also warrant investigation for the presence of a gastrin-secreting tumor.

The Zollinger-Ellison syndrome, which occurs in 1 of 1,000 patients with peptic ulcer disease, is the classic syndrome associated with gastrinoma. Its hallmark is the hypersecretion of gastrin, which results in significant hyperacidity, abdominal pain, diarrhea, and multiple recurrent peptic ulcers.[44] This syndrome is more common in males (60%) than in females; the mean age at diagnosis is 45 to 50 years.[44,45]

Gastrinomas are malignant in 60% of cases, and 50% of patients with these tumors have established metastases at diagnosis.[46,47] Most gastrinomas are located in the gastrinoma triangle, defined by the junction of the second and third portions of the duodenum and the junction of the neck and body of the pancreas.[48] Multiple tumors have been reported in approximately half of patients.[49]

Most gastrinomas are indolent, and long-term survival, even with metastatic disease, is not uncommon. Median survival in patients with gastrinomas is between 3 and 6 years.[50] In patients in whom no tumor was found at laparotomy (tumor microscopic in size) or in whom complete resection was possible, 5- and 10-year survival rates were 70% to 100%.[51–53] It appears that duodenal tumors have a higher recurrence rate and metastatic potential than pancreatic tumors.[35,52,54]

Approximately 20% of cases of Zollinger-Ellison syndrome occur as part of the MEN I syndrome. A patient with both duodenal ulcer and hypercalcemia should be suspected of having MEN I with a gastrinoma. The most commonly associated tumor is a parathyroid adenoma. There also appears to be an increased incidence of gastric argyrophil carcinoidosis in these patients.[55] Patients in this subset have a much higher incidence of multiple gastrinomas than patients with the sporadic Zollinger-Ellison syndrome. The survival rate of patients with MEN I is not adversely affected by the presence of

adenomas in multiple organs.[50] The presence of MEN I in patients with Zollinger-Ellison syndrome is associated with improved survival.[52]

An elevated concentration of gastrin in a blood sample from a fasting patient and increased basal gastric acid output (> 15 mEq/h in patients who have not undergone prior acid-reducing surgery) suggest the presence of gastrinoma. However, gastrin levels may also rise as a result of hypochlorhydria, chronic renal failure, vagotomy, short gut syndrome, retained gastric antrum, pyloric stenosis, and antral G-cell hyperplasia. A gastrin-provocative test is required to differentiate gastrinomas from these other causes of gastrin elevation. The secretin test has become the provocative test of choice because it is easy to perform, highly sensitive and specific, and not associated with side effects.

Localization Techniques: Gastrinomas are small submucosal tumors and can easily be missed during routine upper gastrointestinal endoscopy even in areas such as the duodenum. In 40% to 60% of patients, no gastrinoma is identified during surgery,[56,57] and as stated above, 50% of patients with gastrinomas have metastases at the time of diagnosis. Localization of gastrinomas by imaging studies or other techniques is imperative, as it could avert surgery in metastatic disease or increase the number of tumors identified and removed by carefully planned surgery. In addition to external ultrasonography, CT, and MRI, currently used localization studies include intraoperative ultrasonography (used mostly to identify pancreatic gastrinomas), selective injection of secretin into abdominal arteries with collection of venous samples from the hepatic arteries and assessment of gastrin levels, ^{111}In-octreotide scan (as a single diagnostic test, this method identified 77% of all gastrinomas in one study[40]),and angiography.

Insulinomas

Insulinomas are the most common type of islet-cell tumor. Generally, these tumors are benign (90%), intrapancreatic (nearly 100%), solitary, and small (< 2 cm). The peak incidence of insulinomas occurs in patients between 30 and 60 years of age, more frequently women. Because of hyperinsulinism, most patients are overweight. Children younger than 15 years old are rarely affected. Islet-cell dysplasia in children may lead to hypoglycemic episodes because of the autonomous secretion of insulin. In one report, DNA ploidy analysis was not a useful prognostic factor for patients with insulinomas.[58] About 5% of these tumors are associated with the MEN I syndrome; consequently, family members of index cases need to be screened periodically.[59]

Patients with insulinomas may present with neurologic or psychiatric disturbances. An important feature is that symptoms tend to occur at night or early in the morning. The diagnosis is made by demonstrating inappropriately high concentrations of both insulin and C-peptide in the blood and a blood glucose level of less than 50 mg/dL together with the clinical picture of a hypoglycemic episode (confusion, altered consciousness, visual disturbances, weakness, sweating, tremulousness, and less commonly, seizures). Provocative testing with a 48-hour fast can be done in a hospital setting. Frequent measurements of the blood glucose concentration should be made during the fast. Only when a low value is recorded should a sample be taken to provide serum for insulin and C-peptide assay.

Computed tomography, ultrasonography, and selective arteriography fail to localize an insulinoma in about 40% of cases. Moreover, because these tumors have no predilection for a particular area within the pancreas, blind partial pancreatectomy is not warranted. As most insulinomas are solitary and benign, surgical resection is curative in the majority of cases. Thus, it is important to use additional tumor localization procedures (portal venous sampling, ^{111}In-octreotide scanning) in cases in which the tumor cannot be visualized by conventional methods. If these additional studies are negative, the patient should undergo surgical exploration and intraoperative ultrasonography.

Recent reports demonstrated intraoperative ultrasonography to be a highly sensitive and specific procedure for localization of pancreatic endocrine tumors.[60,61] Rosch et al studied 37 patients in whom transabdominal ultrasonography and CT scans were negative but who were later shown to have 39 endocrine tumors of the pancreas.[60] Using endoscopic ultrasonography, these investigators were able to localize 32 of the 39 tumors; no tumor was incorrectly localized. Among the 22 patients who underwent both angiography and endoscopic ultrasonography, the latter was significantly more sensitive for tumor localization. Among 19 control patients without pancreatic endocrine tumors, endoscopic ultrasonography was negative in 18. These authors recommend this modality for preoperative localization of pancreatic endocrine tumors once the clinical and laboratory diagnosis has been established.[60]

Glucagonoma

Glucagonomas are rare alpha-cell tumors of the pancreas that occur in people between 50 and 70 years old. These tumors are mostly malignant, with metastases present at diagnosis in 50% to 80% of patients.[12] The primary tumor is located within the pancreas, and the liver is the most common site of metastasis.[62] Symptoms may not appear until the tumor is quite large. The tumors are usually > 5 cm in diameter, penetrate the pancreatic capsule, and invade the regional lymph nodes. Glucagon levels are usually quite elevated (> 1,000 pg/mL; normal range, 150 to 200 pg/mL) at diagnosis.

Mild glucose intolerance, a characteristic rash called necrolytic erythema migrans, psychiatric disturbances, anemia, and thromboembolic disease with venous thrombosis or pulmonary emboli are the salient clinical features in patients with a glucagonoma.[63] Mild glucose intolerance is the most common feature and is usually the first symptom to be recognized in the majority (> 90%) of patients. Plasma concentrations of amino acids, particularly the glucogenic amino acids, are usually severely depressed in patients with this tumor. Plasma amino acid concentrations vary with the extent of disease and rise to normal levels following tumor resection.

Necrolytic migratory erythema is probably the most characteristic clinical feature of the glucagonoma syndrome. This skin lesion may precede the diagnosis by at least 5 years.[12] The initial lesion consists of red papules or pale brown macules on the face, abdomen, groin, perineum, or extremities. The erythematous areas form superficial bullae that eventually break down and become encrusted. The pathogenesis of the rash is unknown. Hyperglucagonemia, zinc deficiency, and hypoaminoacidemia have been proposed as contributory causes.

Somatostatinoma

Approximately 50 somatostatin-secreting tumors have been reported to date, the majority of which are found in the pancreas or duodenum.[64,65] These tumors are generally malignant. Patients with a somatostinoma present with diabetes mellitus, cholelithiasis, diarrhea, steatorrhea, hypochlorhydria, anemia, and weight loss. Disease is usually diagnosed late in its course, and metastases to lymph nodes, liver, and bone are found at diagnosis.

Vipomas

In 1958, Verner and Morrison described a patient with watery diarrhea, hypokalemia, and achlorhydria.[66] These symptoms appeared to be mediated by a hormone called vasoactive intestinal polypeptide (VIP) and other peptides secreted by malignant islet-cell tumors in adults and by benign ganglioneuroblastomas in children.[12] In adults, vipomas are located in the pancreas and are usually large and solitary, whereas in children, these tumors are extrapancreatic. The tumor is usually solitary and large and is already metastatic in 80% of patients at diagnosis.[12]

The major presenting abnormality of patients with a vipoma is a large volume of secretory diarrhea, generally more than 3 L/d. The stool is essentially isotonic, and the diarrhea persists even during fasting with nasogastric secretion. Large amounts of potassium and bicarbonate are lost in the stool, leading to hypokalemia and metabolic acidosis. Diagnosis rests on the typical clinical presentation, the findings of a pancreatic mass, and elevation of plasma VIP levels.

Pancreatic Polypeptideoma

In the normal adult, pancreatic polypeptide (PP) is located primarily within the pancreas, where it is synthesized and released from PP cells. Little is known about the physiologic actions of PP. Fasting plasma levels increase with age, prolonged fasting, exercise, chronic renal failure, and pancreatic disorders.[12] A recent review found 21 patients with pancreatic polypeptideomas reported in the literature.[64,67] From 50% to 75% of nonfunctioning endocrine tumors can be classified as pancreatic polypeptideomas because they are associated with elevated fasting plasma PP concentrations.

Patients with pancreatic polypeptideoma range in age from 20 to 74 years (mean, 51 years).[12] The clinical picture of pancreatic polypeptideoma is complicated by the finding that many functioning islet-cell tumors are multihormonal. Patients with high plasma PP levels have been reported as having watery diarrhea, chronic duodenal ulcer, PP cell hyperplasia, nesidioblastosis, and multiple endocrine tumors. Other symptoms seen in these patients include diarrhea, hypochlorhydria, and weight loss. Pancreatic polypeptideomas are often found unexpectedly in patients with symptoms produced by metastases to the liver.

TREATMENT

Whenever possible, a localized tumor should be completely resected, as this is the only treatment modality that is potentially curative.[52] Surgical resection can cure more than 90% of patients with carcinoid tumors up to 1 cm in diameter and approximately 20% to 25% of patients with lymph node metastases.[1] In symptomatic patients, partial resection of tumors has a definite and occasionally sustained palliative effect.[68]

Patients with gastrinoma who undergo complete resection have an excellent prognosis. Gastric acid hypersecretion and its complications are adequately managed by medical treatment, but it is the tumor and its potential malignant behavior that determine survival. For this reason, all patients with the Zollinger-Ellison syndrome should be considered for surgical resection.

In patients with advanced islet-cell tumors, debulking surgery should be considered when all other treatment options are exhausted, as it may significantly improve the degree of symptoms and success of medical therapy by decreasing tumor load.[69] Data also suggest that debulking may prolong survival.[53] Surgery can be particularly challenging if multiple islet-cell tumors or extrapancreatic (usually duodenal) gastrinomas are present. Both preoperative and intraoperative tumor localization strategies are thus important for a successful outcome. If surgery is not possible or feasible, symptomatic localized disease may be treated with radiotherapy in some cases.[70] However, unresectable cancer remains incurable.

Knowledge of the natural history of neuroendocrine tumors should be the basis for the treatment of unresectable (advanced) neuroendocrine tumors.[36] In view of the indolent course of these tumors, it is prudent to withhold specific therapy in asymptomatic or mildly symptomatic patients (in whom symptoms do not interfere with daily routine activities). This group of patients should be monitored every 3 months. Only symptomatic patients or those with impending organ failure should be treated. Treatment usually entails a multidisciplinary effort aimed at addressing problems related to hormone hypersecretion and tumor expansion.

Management of Hormonal Excess

Octreotide is a long-acting somatostatin analog that can provide effective amelioration of carcinoid syndrome and diarrhea associated with vipomas.[71–74] The parent hormone, native somatostatin, contributes to the inhibition of the secretion of virtually every known endocrine and exocrine hormone.[75] It affects autonomic processes, gut motility, mucosal-cell proliferation, vascular smooth muscle tone, and intestinal absorption of nutrients. Native somatostatin effectively reduces the symptoms of carcinoid syndrome, but its general use is severely limited by a short half-life (1 to 2 minutes). The synthetic analog has a longer half-life (90 to 120 minutes), allowing for more practical management of patients.

The efficacy of octreotide, like that of the parent compound, is based on its ability to inhibit the synthesis and release of various peptides by neuroendocrine cells. Response to octreotide correlates largely with the presence of somatostatin receptors in the tumor tissue.[76,77] Using radiolabeled octreotide, Lamberts et al showed that a positive scan can predict that octreotide will control symptoms of hormonal hypersecretion.[76,78]

Kvols et al studied the effects of octreotide (500 μg given subcutaneously three times daily) in 25 patients with metastatic carcinoid tumors and carcinoid syndrome.[71] Of these patients, 72% achieved a significant biochemical response (greater than 50% reduction in 5-HIAA levels). Seven patients obtained complete relief of flushing, and four had complete relief of diarrhea. After a median treatment period of 5 months, the severity of symptoms seemed to reach pretreatment levels in five patients, suggesting that the initial effectiveness of octreotide is excellent. Overall, the median duration of symptomatic improvement was approximately 12 months.

The recommended starting dose of octreotide is 50 µg injected subcutaneously every 8 hours. Patients need to be assessed every 2 to 3 weeks to determine whether the dose must be increased. The dose is titrated to a level that achieves the most ideal symptom control without producing major steatorrhea. In some patients, doses up to 500 µg every 8 hours may be required to obtain maximum effects. The estimated median duration of response for all responding patients is more than 1 year, with more than one third estimated to remain responsive for 2 years or more.

Although octreotide is well tolerated for prolonged periods, it may be associated with side effects, including steatorrhea and fat malabsorption, glucose intolerance, nausea and vomiting, pain at the injection site, and fluid retention. Rarely, long-term use of this compound can result in biliary sludge or cholelithiasis.

Anthony et al studied the dose-limiting toxic effects and potential antitumor efficacy of octreotide in 12 patients with the carcinoid syndrome.[79] The highest dose escalation was 2,000 µg every 8 hours. They observed two partial responses by CT scans; generally, 5-HIAA excretion was maximally suppressed at 150 µg every 8 hours and did not decrease further with increasing octreotide doses. In seven patients, symptoms such as flushing were better controlled at doses above 150 µg every 8 hours. Toxic effects did not increase as the dose was escalated above 150 µg every 8 hours. The investigators concluded that octreotide is well tolerated at higher doses, and the maximum tolerated dose has yet to be achieved.

Octreotide is also indicated for tumors that produce VIP, which causes watery diarrhea, hypokalemia, hypochlorhydria, hypophosphatemia, and, sometimes, hypercalcemia.[80] Most patients respond to this drug with a reduction in diarrhea. Other investigators have demonstrated a beneficial effect of octreotide in patients with gastrinomas; in such cases, the drug can lower the gastrin concentration and gastric acid secretion.[73] However, the greater proportion of patients with islet-cell tumors have only transitory responses that are frequently not of substantive benefit; the median duration of response is 2.5 months.[1]

The efficacy of octreotide correlates with the presence of somatostatin receptors on tumor cells. Receptors are found in great number on vipomas and gastrinomas but less frequently on insulinoma cells. Still, an overall improvement in hypoglycemic symptoms has been observed in about 50% of patients with insulinoma in one study.[81] However, this treatment also may reduce compensating factors, such as growth hormone and glucagon, relatively more than insulin and thus worsen hypoglycemia. For this reason, patients given octreotide should be monitored in a hospital setting during the initiation of treatment.

The use of octreotide truly represents a dramatic development in the management of endocrine pancreatic tumors and carcinoid tumors. The hypersecretion of hormones, such as VIP, gastrin, and glucagon, as well as the secretory products of carcinoid tumors (eg, 5-hydroxytryptamine and tachykinins) and their clinical effects may be blocked successfully.[73] This drug provides excellent palliation of such tumors and often affords patients a better quality of life. Eventually, a decrease in (and finally, an absence of) clinical effectiveness occurs, however, despite the reintroduction of other treatment modalities.[82]

Omeprazole (Prilosec) is another significant new drug for the management of gastric hypersecretion in patients with the Zollinger-Ellison syndrome.[83] This benzimidazole analog blocks the hydrogen-ion pump of the parietal cell and can practically abolish acid secretion. The drug has a long duration of action and is easily administered (on a once-daily basis). A reasonable starting dosage is 60 mg/d, which may be increased to 120 mg/d.

Omeprazole is more effective than H_2-receptor antagonists in providing symptomatic relief and mucosal healing and does not cause significant toxic effects.[84,85] There are reports of gastric carcinoids developing in patients who had received omeprazole, but these patients also had MEN I syndrome, suggesting that the presence of the latter condition per se may be important in the pathogenesis of gastric carcinoids.[55,86]

Other Therapies: Other symptoms produced by hormonal excess can be managed appropriately.[12] Recurrent hypoglycemia may be prevented by frequent carbohydrate-rich meals and diazoxide, a drug that inhibits the release of stored insulin in both normal and tumor islet cells. Patients with the glucagonoma syndrome may benefit from the empiric use of a high-protein diet, oral and topical zinc preparations, and amino acid infusions. Insulin may be administered to counteract the catabolic effects of glucagon. Oral anticoagulation protects against the development of venous thrombosis in patients with glucagon excess. Loperamide and codeine can supplement the antidiarrheal management in patients with vipomas.

Biologic Therapy

Interferons are produced by T-cells in response to various stimuli, such as viruses, bacteria, toxic drugs, and certain cytokines.[87] These substances mediate a wide range of biologic responses, including antiviral effects, antiproliferative effects, immunomodulation, gene activation, and differentiation. A possible mechanism of action of interferon is a direct inhibitory action on tumor-cell proliferation and hormone synthesis. Interferon may also inhibit tumor-derived hormones that serve as autocrine growth factors.[88]

Öberg et al were the first to demonstrate the favorable biochemical effects of interferon in patients with the carcinoid syndrome.[89] Among seven patients treated with human leukocyte inteferon, the majority had a significant biochemical response (ie, a decline in tumor marker levels). Subsequently, in a larger number of patients, Öberg et al presented further evidence that various interferon preparations yield antitumor as well as biochemical responses in patients with carcinoids.[90]

Moertel et al treated 27 patients who had carcinoid tumors with recombinant leukocyte interferon at a daily dose between 6 and 24×10^6 U/m² given three times a week.[91] In many patients, severe toxic effects resulting from high starting doses of interferon led to frequent dose reductions. Of these patients, 20% experienced an objective tumor response and 39% had a biochemical response. However, the durations of responses and treatments were brief.

A recent report also questioned the efficacy of interferon in the treatment of patients with metastatic carcinoids.[92] The combination of octreotide and alpha interferon (IFN-α) was used to treat patients with carcinoid malignancies resistant to either octreotide or interferon alone. Biochemical responses (complete in 4 of 22 patients) were observed in 77% of patients, with a median response duration of 15 months.[42]

Interferon also has been investigated in patients with advanced islet-cell tumors. In one study,[88] 22 patients were given human leukocyte inteferon at an intravenous dose of 3 to 6×10^6 U/m²/d. Partial responses were noted in 16 of 20 assessable patients. The median duration of response was 8.5 months, and the therapy was tolerated by the patients. These results need to be confirmed.

Chemotherapy and Biochemotherapy

Carcinoid Tumors: Chemotherapy may be palliative in patients with carcinoid syndrome who are suffering from dominant symptomatic metastases and who are no longer responsive to octreotide therapy. In general, carcinoids are relatively resistant to chemotherapy.[36] Because of the general refractoriness of the tumor to cytotoxic drugs, there is no standard systemic chemotherapy for patients with metastatic carcinoid tumors. Fluorouracil and doxorubicin (Adriamycin, Rubex) are considered the most active chemotherapeutic agents.[93] In contrast, streptozotocin (Zanosar) and dacarbazine are relatively inactive against carcinoid tumors.[93–95]

In general, single-agent response rates have varied between 10% and 25%; durations of responses have been short (usually less than 6 months), and complete remissions have been rare.[94] Doxorubicin-based combinations have resulted in response rates of up to 35%.[96] The combination of streptozotocin and fluorouracil has been reported to have a response rate of 33%.[1] The current status of combination chemotherapy for patients with carcinoids is characterized by low response rates (less than 35%), short durations of response (< 9 months), and rare complete remissions.[36] Anaplastic variants of carcinoids may be more responsive to combined etoposide (VePesid) and cisplatin (Platinol).[97]

On the basis of preclinical data suggesting that synergistic cytolytic activity occurs when doxorubicin is combined with IFN-α, Ajani et al studied the effect of the combination of doxorubicin (40 mg/m² given over 72 hours) and IFN-α (5×10^6 U/m² given subcutaneously on days 1 through 14, with the courses repeated every 28 days).[98] Among 12 patients with carcinoids, one complete and two partial responses were observed. The biochemical response of the tumors was also significant.

Islet-cell carcinomas are relatively more sensitive to chemotherapy than are carcinoid tumors. Active drugs include streptozotocin, fluorouracil, chlorozotocin, doxorubicin, and dacarbazine.[99,100] Streptozotocin is a glucosamine- nitrosourea compound originally isolated from a culture of *Streptomyces achromogenes*. Broder and Carter reported an objective tumor regression in 50% of 52 patients with metastatic islet-cell tumors treated with this drug.[101] The median duration of response was more than 12 months.

The major toxic effects of streptozotocin are nausea, vomiting, myelosuppression, and renal impairment. Moertel et al studied 84 patients with islet-cell carcinomas in a randomized prospective trial of streptozotocin vs fluorouracil plus streptozotocin. Of 42 patients who received streptozotocin alone, 14 (33%) responded, as compared with 36% of those receiving the combination.[102] Complete remission rates were 12% in the study arm that received streptozotocin alone and 33% in the arm that received the combination. Patient survival was significantly greater among those who received combination chemotherapy than in those treated with streptozotocin alone. This study was the basis for recommending the combination of fluorouracil and streptozotocin as standard chemotherapy for patients with advanced symptomatic islet-cell tumors.

However, more recently, Moertel et al reported the results of a prospective, multicenter trial of 106 patients with advanced islet-cell tumors randomized to three treatment arms: chlorozotocin alone, streptozotocin plus doxorubicin, and fluorouracil plus streptozotocin (the standard arm).[103] Chlorozotocin was given as a single intravenous injection (150 mg/m^2), which was repeated every 7 weeks. For the combination regimens, streptozotocin was given by intravenous injection at a dosage of 500 mg/m^2/d for 5 consecutive days every 6 weeks. Fluorouracil was given by intravenous injection at a dosage of 400 mg/m^2/d for 5 days concurrently with streptozotocin. Doxorubicin was given along with streptozotocin by intravenous injection at a dose of 50 mg/m^2 on days 1 and 22 of each 6-week treatment, with a maximum total dose of 500 mg/m^2.

The combination of streptozotocin plus doxorubicin was superior to streptozotocin plus fluorouracil in terms of the rate of tumor regression (69% vs 45%, $P = .05$) and the length of time to tumor progression (median, 20 vs 6.9 months; $P = .001$). Streptozotocin plus doxorubicin also had a significant advantage in terms of survival (median, 2.2 vs 1.4 years; $P = .004$). Monotherapy with chlorozotocin, a relatively new drug that is structurally similar to streptozotocin, produced a response rate similar to that of standard therapy. The major toxic effect of chlorozotocin was hematologic depression. Compared with streptozotocin, the new drug caused less nausea and vomiting. The investigators concluded that the combination of streptozotocin and doxorubicin is superior to standard therapy and that chlorozotocin needs to be studied further as a constituent of combination drug regimens.

Despite these advances, curative chemotherapy has not been developed for neuroendocrine tumors. Novel agents and combinations of biologic and cytotoxic therapy still need to be identified. Preclinical data from studies using neuroendocrine tumor-cell lines may be helpful in this regard.[104]

Local-Regional Therapy With Hepatic Arterial Embolization

Metastatic neuroendocrine tumors are hypervascular, and vascular occlusion can result in significant deprivation of the blood supply to the liver. Hepatic metastases receive most of their vascular supply from the hepatic arterial circulation, whereas normal liver parenchyma receives the majority of its blood supply from the portal vein and only 30% from the hepatic artery. Hepatic arterial embolization is an invasive procedure that involves the use of inert material, such as Ivalon particles or gel foam, to occlude the blood vessels. If feasible, this procedure is recommended for cases of carcinoid syndrome that are unresponsive or partially responsive to octreotide therapy and in patients with advanced islet-cell tumors suffering from dominant symptomatic metastases; the technique can provide effective palliation in these patients. Hepatic arterial embolization can also deliver chemotherapeutic agents intra-arterially, thereby delivering a large amount of drug into the tumor.[105–107]

Carrasco et al reported the results of microembolization treatment in 25 patients with carcinoid syndrome.[108] The majority of patients achieved both a biochemical and objective response to therapy. The average duration of effective palliation was more than 11 months. Ajani et al also reported effective palliation using this technique in 22 symptomatic patients with islet-cell tumors.[109] Of 20 evaluable patients, 12 had a partial remission. The patients developed marked abnormalities in hepatic enzyme levels, which returned to baseline a few weeks later during the recovery period.

After the microembolization procedure, patients frequently experience abdominal pain, nausea, vomiting, and fever. Complications can be severe and may include death from hepatic failure or hepatorenal syndrome. Careful patient selection is therefore mandatory.[108] Patients who have jaundice, poor performance status (Zubrod 3 or 4), or a liver largely replaced by tumor (> 75%) are ineligible for this therapy. This modality is available only in major cancer centers and requires a team effort and skilled interventional radiologists. Its impact on the survival of patients with metastatic disease remains to be determined.

Future Directions

New agents are desperately needed for patients with neuroendocrine tumors. However, due either to the absence of new exciting agents or a lack of initiative on the part of sponsors to pursue investigation in rare diseases, no new agents have been demonstrated to be active in these diseases for some time. Moreover, research efforts focused on these relatively rare tumors are relatively few compared with endeavors dealing with more common malignancies. Nevertheless, efforts are being made in clinical and preclinical areas.

Various somatostatin analogs are now under investigation to assess whether they can control carcinoid syndrome more effectively than does octreotide and can produce a higher rate of objective regression. In addition, encapsulation of these agents for intramuscular injection results in sustained therapeutic blood levels for approximately 6 weeks. If found effective in controlling carcinoid syndrome, this approach would result in a dramatic advancement for patients who must now receive subcutaneous injections of the drug two to three times per day. In addition, the new analogs purportedly have a higher affinity for somatostatin receptors. If this is true, one can expect better imaging techniques and higher efficacy in therapeutic targeting than is possible today.

Investigational therapeutic approaches using somatostatin-receptor antibodies attached to radioactive isotopes such as indium 111 make use of the overexpression of somatostatin receptors in neuroendocrine tumors. Such approaches could selectively deliver relatively higher doses of radioactivity to tumor tissue and potentially ablate the tumor.

In the arena of vascular occlusion, encapsulation of various drugs in capsules in the range of 100 μm is being pursued. In addition, these capsules may be more effectively targeted by coating the surface with octreotide analogs. Such ideas are preliminary and must await confirmation in the preclinical setting. Because metastases from neuroendocerine tumors are often highly vascular, it may be useful to study angiogenesis inhibitors in patients with these diseases.

REFERENCES

1. Moertel CG: An odyssey in the land of small tumors. J Clin Oncol 5:1503–1522, 1987.

2. Buchanan KD, Johnston CF, O'Hare MMT: Neuroendocrine tumors. Am J Med 81:14, 1986.

3. Wermer P: Genetic aspects of adenomatosis of endocrine glands. Am J Med 116:363–371, 1954.

4. Larsson C, Shogseid B, Öberg K, et al: MEN-1 gene maps to chromosome 11 and is lost in insulinoma. Nature 332:85–87, 1988.

5. Bale S, Bale AE, Stewart S: Linkage analysis of multiple endocrine neoplasia type 1 with INT2 and other markers on chromosome 11. Genomics 4:320–322, 1989.

6. Radford DM, Ashley SW, Wells JA, et al: Loss of heterozygosity of markers on chromosome 11 in tumors from patients with multiple endocrine neoplasia syndrome type 1. Cancer Res 50:6529–6533, 1990.

7. Friedman EL, DeMarco PV, Gejman PV, et al: Allelic loss from chromosome 11 in parathyroid tumors. Cancer Res 52:6804–6809, 1992.

8. Thakker RV, Bouloux C, Wooding C, et al: Association of parathyroid tumors in multiple endocrine neoplasia type 1 with loss of alleles on chromosome 11. N Engl J Med 321:218–224, 1989.

9. Öberg K: Expressions of growth factors and their receptors in neuroendocrine gut and pancreatic tumors, and prognostic factors for survival. Ann NY Acad Sci 46–55, 1994.

10. Pearse AGE: The diffuse neuroendocrine system and the APUD concept: Related endocrine peptides in brain, intestine, pituitary,

placenta and anuran cutaneous glands. Med Biol 55:115–125, 1977.

11. Langley K: The neuroendocrine concept today. Ann NY Acad Sci 733:1–17, 1994.

12. Gower WR, Fabri PJ: Endocrine neoplasms (nongastrin) of the pancreas. Semin Surg Oncol 6:98–109, 1990.

13. Klöppel G, Heitz P: Classification of normal and neoplastic neuroendocrine cells. Ann NY Acad Sci 733:18–23, 1994.

14. Wilander E: Diagnostic pathology of gastrointestinal pancreatic neuroendocrine tumors. Acta Oncol 288:363–369, 1989.

15. Cotran RS, Kumar V, Robbins SL: Robbins' Pathologic Basis of Disease, pp 818–820. Philadelphia, WB Saunders, 1994.

16. Moertel CG, Hanley JA: Combination chemotherapy trials in metastatic carcinoid and malignant carcinoid syndrome. Cancer Clin Trials 2:327, 1979.

17. Johnson LA, Lavin PT, Moertel CG, et al: Carcinoids: The prognostic effect of primary site histologic type variations. J Surg Oncol 33:81–83, 1986.

18. Polak JM: Diagnostic histopathology of neuroendocrine tumours, pp 1–39. Edinburgh, Churchill Livingstone, 1993.

19. Wiedenmann B, Huttner W: Synaptophysin and chromogranins/secretograninsd: Widespread constituents of distinct types of neuroendocrine vesicles and new tools in tumor diagnosis. Virchows Arch B Cell Pathol 58:95–121, 1989.

20. Klöppel G, Veld PI: Neural and endocrine markers as diagnostic tools in pancreatic and gastrointestinal endocrine tumors. Acta Histochem XXXVIII(suppl):93–98, 1990.

21. Reubi JC, Laissue J, Waser B, et al: Expression of somatostatin receptors in normal, inflamed and neoplastic human gastrointestinal tissues. Ann NY Acad Sci 733:122–137, 1994.

22. Scherubl H, Hescheler J, Riecken EO: Molecular mechanisms of somatostatin's inhibition of hormone release: Participation of voltage-gated calcium channels and G-proteins. Horm Metab Res 27(suppl):1–4, 1993.

23. Reubi JC, Kvols LK, Waser B, et al: Detection of somatostatin receptors in surgical and percutaneous needle biopsy samples of carcinoids and islet cell carcinomas. Cancer Res 50:5969–5977, 1990.

24. Gerdes J, Schwab H, Lenke H, et al: Production of mouse monoclonal antibody reacting with a human nuclear antigen associated with proliferation. Int J Cancer 31:13–20, 1983.

25. Chaudhry A, Öberg K, Wilander E: A study of biological behavior based on the expression of a proliferating antigen in neuroendocrine tumors of the digestive system. Tumor Biol 13:27–35, 1992.

26. Chaudhry A, Funa K, Öberg K, et al: Expression of growth factor peptides and their receptors in neuroendocrine tumors of the digestive system. Acta Oncol 32:107–114, 1993.

27. Chaudhry A, Papanicolau V, Öberg K, et al: Expression of platelet-derived growth factor and its receptors in neuroendocrine tumors of the digestive system. Cancer Res 52:1006–1012, 1992.

28. Waltenberger J, Lundin L, Öberg K, et al: Involvement of transforming growth factor-beta in the formation of fibrotic lesions in carcinoid heart disease. Am J Pathol 142:71–78, 1993.

29. Chaudhry A, Gobl A, Eriksson B, et al: Different splice variants of CD44 are expressed in gastrinomas but not in other subtypes of endocrine pancreatic tumors. Cancer Res 54:981–986, 1994.

30. Solcia E, Capella C, Fiocca R, et al: The gastro-pancreatic endocrine system and related tumors. Gastroenterol Clin North Am 4:671–693, 1989.

31. Wynick D, Williams SJ, Bloom SR: Symptomatic secondary hormone syndromes in patients with established malignant pancreatic endocrine tumors. N Engl J Med 319:605–607, 1988.

32. Thompson GB, van Heerden JA, Martin JK, et al: Carcinoid tumors of the gastrointestinal tract: Presentation, management and prognosis. Surgery 98:1054, 1985.

33. Vinik AI, McLeod MK, Fig LM, et al: Clinical features,

diagnosis, and localization of carcinoid tumors and their management. Gastroenterol Clin North Am 18:865, 1989.

34. Moertel CG, Weiland LH, Nagorney DM, et al: Carcinoid tumor of the appendix: Treatment and prognosis. N Engl J Med 317:1699–1701, 1987.

35. Norton J, Levin B, Jensen R: Cancer of the endocrine system, in DeVita VT, Hellman S, Rosenberg SA (eds): Cancer: Principles and Practice of Oncology, pp 1371–1435. Philadelphia, JB Lippincott, 1993.

36. Ajani JA, Carrasco H, Samaan NA, et al: Therapeutic options in patients with advanced islet cell and carcinoid tumors. Reg Cancer Treat 3:235–242, 1991.

37. Moertel CG: Treatment of carcinoid tumors and the malignant carcinoid syndrome. J Clin Oncol 1:727–740, 1983.

38. Norheim I, Öberg K, Theodorsson-Norheim E, et al: Malignant carcinoid tumors. Ann Surg 206:115, 1987.

39. Lundin L: Carcinoid heart disease. Acta Oncol 30:499, 1991.

40. Krenning EP, Kwekkeboom DJ, Oei HY, et al: Somatostatin-receptor scintigraphy in gastroenteropancreatic tumors. Ann NY Acad Sci 733:416–424, 1994.

41. Öberg K: Treatment of neuroendocrine tumors. Cancer Treat Rev 20:331–355, 1994.

42. Agranovich AL, Anderson GH, Manji M, et al: Carcinoid tumor of the gastrointestinal tract: Prognostic factors and disease outcome. J Surg Oncol 47(1):45–52, 1991.

43. Davis Z, Moertel CG, McIlrath DC: The malignant carcinoid syndrome. Surg Gynecol Obstet 137:637, 1973.

44. Zollinger RM, Ellison EH: Primary peptic ulcerations of the jejunum associated with islet cell tumors of the pancreas. Ann Surg 142:709–129, 1955.

45. Jensen RT, Gardner JD: Zollinger-Ellison syndrome: Clinical presentation, pathology, diagnosis and treatment, in Dannenberg A, Zakim D (eds): Peptic Ulcer and Other Acid-Related Diseases, p 117. New York, Academic Research Association, 1991.

46. Townsend CM, Lewis BG, Gourley WK, et al: Gastrinoma. Curr Prob Cancer 7:1–33, 1982.

47. Townsend CM, Thompson JC: Gastrinoma. Semin Surg Oncol 6:91–97, 1990.

48. Stabile BE, Morrow DJ, Passaro E: The gastrinoma triangle: Operative implications. Am J Surg 147:25–31, 1984.

49. Fox PS, Hofman JW, Wilson SD, et al: Surgical management of the Zollinger Ellison syndrome. Surg Clin North Am 54:394, 1974.

50. Thompson JC, Terris BG, Wiener I, et al: The role of surgery in the Zollinger-Ellison syndrome. Ann Surg 197:590–607, 1983.

51. Malagelada JR, Edis AJ, Adson MA, et al: Medical and surgical options in the management of patients with gastrinoma. Gastroenterology 84:1524–1532, 1983.

52. Norton JA, Dopppman JL, Jensen RT: Curative resection in Zollinger-Ellison syndrome: Results of a 10 year prospective study. Ann Surg 215:8, 1992.

53. Ellison EC, Carey LC, Sparks J, et al: Early surgical treatment of gastrinoma. Am J Med 82:17, 1987.

54. Thom AK, Norton JA, Axiotis CA, et al: Location, incidence and malignant potential of duodenal gastrinomas. Surgery 110:1086, 1991.

55. Solcia E, Capella C, Fiocca R, et al: Gastric argyrophil carcinoidosis in patients with Zollinger-Ellison syndrome due to type 1 MEN: A newly recognized association. Am J Surg Pathol 14:503–508, 1990.

56. Deveney CW, Deveney K E, Stark D, et al: Resection of gastrinomas. Ann Surg 198:546, 1983.

57. McCarthy DM: The place of surgery in the Zollinger-Ellison syndrome. N Engl J Med 302:1344, 1980.

58. Graeme CF, Bell DA, Flotte TJ: Aneuploidy in pancreatic insulinomas does not predict malignancy. Cancer 66:2365–2368, 1990.

59. Jadoul M, Koppenshaar HP, Box MA, et al: Insulinomas in MEN-1 patients early detection and treatment of insulinomas in patients with MEN-1 syndrome. Neth J Med 37:95–102, 1990.

60. Rosch T, Lighdale CJ, Botit JF, et al: Localization of pancreatic endocrine tumors by endoscopic ultrasonography. N Engl J Med 326:1721–1726, 1992.

61. Doppmann J: Pancreatic endocrine tumors—the search goes on (editorial). N Engl J Med 326:1770–1772, 1992.

62. Stacpoole PW: The glucagonoma syndrome: Clinical features, diagnosis, and treatment. Endocrin Rev 2:347, 1981.

63. Bloom SR, Polak JM: Glucagonoma syndrome. Am J Med 82:25–36, 1987.

64. Vinik AI, Strodel WE, Eckhauser FE, et al: Somatostatinomas, PPomas, neurotensinomas. Semin Oncol 14:263–281, 1987.

65. Krejs GJ, Orci L, Conlon M, et al: Somatostatinoma syndrome (biochemical, morphological and clinical features). N Engl J Med 301:289–292, 1979.

66. Verner JV, Morrison AB: Islet cell tumor and a syndrome of refractory watery diarrhea and hypokalemia. Am J Med 25:375–380, 1958.

67. Adrian TE, Uttenthal LO, Williams SJ, et al: Secretion of pancreatic polypeptide in patients with pancreatic endocrine tumors. N Engl J Med 315:287–291, 1986.

68. Wilson H: Carcinoid syndrome. Curr Prob Surg 11:36–41, 1970.

69. Thompson NW, Eckhauser FE: Malignant islet cell tumors of the pancreas. World J Surg 8:940–951, 1984.

70. Rich TA: Radiation therapy for pancreatic cancer: Eleven year experience in the JCRT. Int J Radiat Oncol Biol Phys 11:759–763, 1985

71. Kvols LK, Moertel CG, O'Connell MJ, et al: Treatment of the malignant carcinoid syndrome: Evaluation of a long-acting somatostatin analogue. N Engl J Med 315:663–666, 1986.

72. Garden P, Comi RJ, Maton PN, et al: NIH conference: Somatostatin and somatostatin analogue (SMS 201-995) in treatment of hormone-secreting tumors of the pituitary and gastrointestinal tract and non-neoplastic disease of the gut. Ann Intern Med 110:350–354, 1989.

73. Wynick D, Bloom SR: Clinical review: The use of the long-acting somatostatin analog octreotide in the treatment of gut neuroendocrine tumors. J Clin Endocrinol Metab 73:1–3, 1991.

74. Öberg K, Norheim I, Theodorsson E: Treatment of malignant midgut carcinoid tumors with a long-acting somatostatin analogue octreotide. Acta Oncol 30:503–507, 1991.

75. Reichlin S: Somatostatin. N Engl J Med 309:1495–1501, 1983.

76. Lamberts SW, Bakker WA, Renbi JC, et al: Treatment with Sandostatin and in-vivo localization of tumors with radiolabeled somatostatin analogues. Metabolism 39:1525, 1990.

77. Reubi JC, Koals LK, Waser B, et al: Detection of somatostatin receptors in surgical and percutaneous needle biopsy samples of carcinoids and islet cell carcinomas. Cancer Res 50:5969–5972, 1990.

78. Kvols L, Reubi JC, Moertel C, et al: Somatostatin receptors may predict responsiveness of malignant neuroendocrine syndromes to therapy with somatostatin analogue (SMS 201-995, Sandostatin) (abstract 389). Proc Am Soc Clin Oncol 8:101, 1989.

79. Anthony LB, Winn SD, Krozely MG, et al: Relationship of octreotide dose to its efficacy and toxicity in carcinoid syndrome (abstract). Proc Am Soc Clin Oncol 10:387, 1991.

80. Kvols LK, Buck M, Moertel CG, et al: Treatment of metastatic islet cell carcinoma with a somatostatin analogue (SMS 201 995). Ann

Intern Med 107:162–168, 1987.

81. Dunne MJ, Elton R, Fletcher T, et al: Sandostatin and gastro-enteropancreatic endocrine tumors-therapeutic characteristics, in O'Dorisio TM (ed): Somatostatin in the Treatment of GEP Endocrine Tumors, pp 93–113. Berlin, Springer Verlag, 1989.

82. Öberg K, Erikson B: Medical treatment of neuroendocrine gut and pancreatic tumors. Acta Oncol 28:425–431, 1989.

83. Maton PN: Role of acid suppressants in patients with Zollinger-Ellison syndrome. Aliment Pharmacol Ther 5:25–35, 1991.

84. Solvell L: The clinical safety of omeprazole. Digestion 47:59–63, 1990.

85. Frucht H, Maton PN, Jensen RT: The use of omeprazole in patients with Zollinger-Ellison syndrome. Dig Dis Sci 36:394–404, 1991.

86. Maton PN, Lack EE, Collin MJ, et al: The effect of ZES and omeprazole therapy on gastric oxyntic endocrine cells. Gastroenterology 94:943–50, 1990.

87. Rosenberg SA, Longo DL, Litze MT: Principles and applications of biologic therapy in cancer, in DeVita VT, Hellman S, Rosenberg SA (eds): Cancer: Principles and Practice of Oncology, 3rd Ed. Philadelphia, JB Lippincott, 1989.

88. Eriksson B, Öberg K, Alm G: Treatment of malignant endocrine pancreatic tumors with human leukocyte interferon. Lancet 2:1307–1308, 1986.

89. Öberg K, Funa K, Alm G: Effects of leukocyte interferon on clinical symptoms and hormonal levels in patients with midgut carcinoid tumors and the carcinoid syndromes. N Engl J Med 309:129–133, 1983.

90. Öberg K, Norheim I, Lind E, et al: Treatment of malignant carcinoid tumors with human leukocyte interferon. Long term results. Cancer Treat Rep 70:1297–1304, 1986.

91. Moertel CG, Rubin J Kvols L: Therapy of metastatic carcinoid tumor and the malignant carcinoid syndrome with recombinant leukocyte A interferon. J Clin Oncol 7:865–868, 1989.

92. Valimaki M, Jarvinen H, Salmella P, et al: Is the treatment of metastatic carcinoid tumor with interferon not as successful as suggested? Cancer 67:547–549, 1991.

93. Legha SS, Valdivieso M, Nelson RS, et al: Chemotherapy for metastatic carcinoid tumors: Experience with 32 patients and a review of the literature. Cancer Treat Rep 61:1699–1703, 1977.

94. Stolinsky DC, Sadoff L, Braunwald J, et al: Streptozotocin in the treatment of cancer: Phase II study. 30:61–67, 1972.

95. Kissinger A, Foley FJ, Lemon HJ: Use of DTIC (dacarbazine) in the malignant carcinoid tumors. Cancer Treat Rep 61:101–102, 1977.

96. Ajani JA, Legha SS, Karlin DA, et al: Combination chemotherapy of metastatic carcinoid tumors with 5-FU, adriamycin, and cytoxan (FAC) and 5-FU, adriamycin, mitomycin-C, and methyl CCNU (FAMMe) (abstract). Proc Am Soc Clin Oncol 2:124, 1983.

97. Moertel CG, Kvols LK, O'Connell MJ, et al: Treatment of neuroendocrine carcinomas with combined etoposide and cisplatin: Evidence of major therapeutic activity in the anaplastic variants of these neoplasms. Cancer 68:227–232, 1991.

98. Ajani JA, Kavanagh J, Patt Y, et al: Roferon and doxorubicin combinations active against advanced islet cell or carcinoid tumors. Proc Am Assoc Cancer Res 30:293, 1989.

99. Haller I, Schutt A, Sayal Y, et al: Chemotherapy for metastatic carcinoid tumors: An ECOG phase II-III trial (abstract). Proc Am Soc Clin Oncol 9:395, 1990.

100. Hahn RG, Cnaan A, Kissinger A, et al: A phase II study of DTIC in the treatment of non-resectable islet cell carcinoma: An ECOG treatment protocol (abstract). Proc Am Soc Clin Oncol 9:417, 1990.

101. Broder LE, Carter SK: Pancreatic islet cell tumors with streptozotocin. Ann Intern Med 79:108, 1973.

102. Moertel CG, Hahnley JA, Johnsson LA: Streptozocin alone compared with streptozocin plus fluorouracil in the treatment of advanced islet cell carcinoma. N Engl J Med 303:1189, 1980.

103. Moertel CG, Lefkopoulos M, Lipsitz S, et al: Streptozocin-doxorubicin, streptozocin-fluorouracil or chlorozotocin in the treatment of advanced islet cell carcinoma. N Engl J Med 326:519–523, 1992.

104. Evers BM, Halbut SC, Tyring SK, et al: Novel therapy for the treatment of human carcinoid. Ann Surg 213:411–416, 1991.

105. Vallete J, Souquet JC: Pancreatic islet cell tumors metastatic to the liver: Treatment by hepatic arterial chemo-embolization. Horm Res 32:77–79, 1989.

106. Mavligit G, Pollack R: Islet cell carcinoma of the pancreas: Prospective (neoadjuvant) chemoembolization infusion in patients with concomitant primary lesions and liver metastases (meeting abstract). 3rd International Congress on Neo-Adjuvant Chemotherapy. Paris, France, February 1991.

107. Venook A, Stagg R, Frye J, et al: Chemoembolization of patient with liver metastases from carcinoid and islet cell tumors (abstract). Proc Am Soc Clin Oncol 10:386, 1991.

108. Carrasco CH, Charnsangavej C, Ajani JA: The carcinoid syndrome: Palliation by hepatic artery embolization. Am J Roentgenol 147:149–154, 1986.

109. Ajani JA, Carrasco CH, Charnsangavej C, et al: Islet cell tumors metastatic to liver: Effective palliation by sequential hepatic artery embolization. Ann Intern Med 108:340–344, 1988.

SECTION 5

BREAST CANCER

CHAPTER **19**   **Early-Stage Breast Cancer
and Adjuvant Therapy**

CHAPTER **20**   **Metastatic Breast Cancer**

CHAPTER **21**   **Special Issues in Breast Cancer
Management**

Early-Stage Breast Cancer and Adjuvant Therapy

Juan Herrada, MD, Pamela Hughes, MD, *and* Aman Buzdar, MD

Department of Breast and Gynecologic Medical Oncology

The University of Texas M. D. Anderson Cancer Center, Houston, Texas

Carcinoma of the breast is the most common cancer in women in the United States and is second only to lung cancer as a cause of cancer death in women. The incidence of breast cancer has risen steadily over the past decade, with the most dramatic increase seen in smaller primary breast tumors, partly because widespread use of screening mammography permits earlier detection.[1]

Approximately 183,000 new cases of breast cancer will be diagnosed in 1995.[2] Adjuvant therapy can significantly reduce the risk of recurrence and death in patients with breast cancer. However, many patients with early-stage breast cancer are cured by local therapy (surgery and radiotherapy) alone, and these patients should be spared the risks and costs of adjuvant therapy.

The challenge for the clinican is to determine which patients have the highest risk of recurrence and, thus, are most likely to benefit from adjuvant therapy. In this chapter, we will detail the prognostic factors that affect whether adjuvant therapy is indicated and then describe the various adjuvant treatments that are available.

PROGNOSTIC FACTORS

Breast carcinoma is characterized by a long natural history and by wide variation in its clinical course. The spread of primary cancer occurs by direct infiltration into the breast parenchyma, along the mammary ducts, and through the breast lymphatics. The most frequent site of regional involvement of breast cancer is the axillary lymph-node region. Patients with axillary node involvement have a worse prognosis than do patients with negative axillary nodes. In fact, prognosis progressively worsens as the number of disease-positive lymph nodes increases.

Nemoto et al[3] found a direct relationship between the number of involved nodes and the 5-year disease-free survival rate, with rates of 62% for one to three positive axillary lymph nodes, 58% for four to nine positive nodes, and 29% for 10 or more positive axillary nodes. The Consensus Development Council now recommends that patients with positive axillary nodes be divided into the four groups Nemoto and colleagues used.[4]

Intensive efforts have been made over the last several years to identify patients who are at high risk for recurrence and would benefit from adjuvant therapy. Gasparini et al[5] recently reported that in patients with operable node-positive breast cancer, the expression of the bcl-2 protein in the primary tumor predicts for benefit of adjuvant treatment (chemotherapy or tamoxifen [Nolvadex]). Although patients with node-negative breast cancer have a relatively low risk of recurrence, it is well established that despite the best local treatment, up to 20% to 30% of these women will die of metastatic disease.[6,7] Because adjuvant therapy has been shown to reduce the risk of relapse and to improve overall survival in patients with breast cancer regardless of their lymph-node status,[8] it is important to characterize the subset of node-negative patients who are at high risk for relapse and, thus, could benefit from adjuvant therapy.

The prognostic factors evaluated to identify node-negative patients at high risk for recurrence are summarized in Table 1. The standard prognostic factors commonly used today are tumor size, nuclear/histologic

TABLE 1

Prognostic Factors in Node-Negative Breast Cancer

Prognostic factors widely accepted

Tumor size
Nuclear/histologic grade
Estrogen- and progesterone-receptor expression
Ploidy and S-phase fraction

Prognostic factors currently under investigation

HER-2/neu oncogene
Angiogenesis markers
Histologic subtype
Lymphatic invasion
Epidermal growth factor receptor
Ki-67
pS2
Stress response proteins
Type IV collagenases
nm23
p53
Plasminogen activators

grade, estrogen-receptor (ER) and progesterone-receptor (PR) expression, and DNA flow cytometry-derived ploidy and S-phase fraction.

Tumor Size

There is a strong, direct correlation between tumor size and risk of recurrence, whether disease is node-positive or node-negative. Two studies have confirmed the prognostic importance of primary tumor size in axillary node-negative patients. The Surveillance, Epidemiology, and End Results (SEER) study correlated tumor diameter with survival in more than 13,000 patients and found that the relative overall 5-year survival rate was almost 99% in patients with tumors less than 1 cm in diameter, approximately 91% in patients with tumors of 1 to 3 cm, and 85% in patients with tumors of more than 3 cm.[8] The other important study revealed that node-negative patients with tumors less than or equal to 1 cm in diameter had a 20-year recurrence rate of 14%, while patients with tumors of 1.1 to 2.0 cm had a 20-year recurrence rate of 31%.[9,10]

Nuclear/Histologic Grade

Nuclear, or histologic, grade describes the degree of tumor differentiation and is based on the pathologist's assessment of nuclear size and shape, number of mitoses, and degree of tubule formation. Tumors of low malignancy are designated grade 1 and are associated with the best prognosis; grade 3 tumors are associated with the worst prognosis. At one center, only 10% of all patients with node-negative breast cancer had well-differentiated tumors, but this small subset of patients had a 5-year disease-free survival rate of more than 90%.[11] Since studies have demonstrated significant interobserver variability in nuclear grading, the grading should be done by experienced pathologists so that results are reliable.

Hormone-Receptor Status

Estrogen- and progesterone-receptor positivity correlate with prolonged disease-free and overall survival. However, the importance of hormone-receptor status has been documented more consistently in node-positive than in node-negative disease. McGuire found a difference of only 8% to 10% in disease-free survival between women with node-negative breast cancer who were ER positive and those who were ER negative.[12] Measurement of hormone-receptor level is valuable in both node-negative and node-positive patients for identifing patients likely to benefit from adjuvant endocrine therapy.

S-Phase Fraction and DNA Ploidy

The degree of cellular proliferation in breast cancer specimens has shown a strong correlation with outcome. Flow cytometry simultaneously measures both DNA ploidy (DNA content) and S-phase fraction (the fraction of cells actively cycling or synthesizing DNA). Aneuploid tumors with a high percentage of cells in S-phase are more likely to recur than are tumors with a low S-phase fraction. Clark et al studied S-phase fraction in node-negative patients with small (less than 3 cm), ER-positive tumors. Patients with a low S-phase fraction had a higher disease-free survival rate than did those with a high S-phase fraction, whether their tumors were diploid or aneuploid.[13]

Published data suggest a relationship between tumor cell kinetics and response to chemotherapy. Remvikos et al found that patients with an S-phase fraction greater than 10% had significantly higher response rates to chemotherapy than did those with an S-phase fraction less than 5%.[14] It is important to note that the cutoff points separating low from high S-phase fractions may differ between laboratories and, therefore, may affect the validity of comparisons.

Other Factors

Other potentially important prognostic factors currently being studied include cathepsin D level, *HER-2/neu* oncogene expression, angiogenesis markers, histologic subtype, lymphatic invasion, epidermal growth factor receptor,[15] Ki-67,[16,17] pS2(18), stress response (heat shock) proteins,[19] type IV collagenases,[20] nm23,[21] p53,[22,23] and plasminogen activators.[24]

Cathepsin D Level: Cathepsin D is a lysosomal protein that is synthesized in normal tissues but is overexpressed and secreted in breast cancers. Cathepsin D may play a role in invasion and metastasis. Although data from a group of node-negative patients with aneuploid tumors revealed a 5-year recurrence rate of 60% in patients with high levels of cathepsin D,[25] other studies were unable to confirm this finding.[26] Cathepsin D was once considered to be an important predictor of recurrence and survival in node-negative patients, but further work has failed to show its prognostic value in clinical practice.[27]

HER-2/neu (c-erbB-2) Expression: Overexpression of the *HER-2/neu* oncogene reflects an increase in the proliferative activity of a tumor. Overexpression has been demonstrated in 15% to 30% of patients with breast cancer and has been found by most investigators to be associated with shorter survival.[28,29] However in a report from the Cancer and Leukemia Group B (CALGB),[30]

HER-2/neu overexpression was associated with significantly longer disease-free and overall survival in breast cancer patients who received higher doses of anthracycline-containing adjuvant chemotherapy. Although the above data suggest a role of *HER-2/neu* in predicting sensitivity to chemotherapy, further studies are needed before this marker can be used in making clinical decisions.

Angiogenesis Markers: Experimental evidence has shown that angiogenesis plays a key role in tumor growth, invasiveness, and progression.[31] Tumor angiogenesis as manifested by microvessel density within the invasive primary carcinoma has been shown in preliminary studies[32,33] to be a reliable prognostic marker in node-negative breast cancer patients.

Histologic Subtypes: Rosen and colleagues found that in addition to ductal carcinoma in situ, the pure tubular, papillary, and typical medullary histologic subtypes had long-term recurrence rates of less than 10%.[5] Another study found that the recurrence rate in patients with ductal carcinoma in situ and microinvasion was only 9% at 7 years.[34]

Lymphatic Invasion: Lymphatic invasion, which refers to the presence of tumor emboli in breast lymphatics, is seen in approximately 25% of breast tumors. It is associated with a lower likelihood of survival.[35]

Application

In summary, factors associated with a low risk of tumor recurrence include ductal carcinoma in situ, the pure tubular, papillary, and typical medullary histologic types, tumor size smaller than 1 cm, tumors of nuclear grade 1, diploidy low S-phase fraction, the presence of hormone receptors, and intermediate tumor size in the absence of other high-risk features. Factors associated with a high risk of recurrence include tumor size larger than 3 cm, high nuclear grade, aneuploidy, high S-phase fraction, and the absence of hormone receptors.

Estimating the risk of recurrence in an individual patient remains a difficult issue. For patients with tumors less than 1 cm in diameter, the chance of recurrence is less than 10% at 10 years. Therefore, it may be reasonable not to offer these patients systemic adjuvant therapy.[1] With larger tumors, other prognostic factors can be considered when deciding whether to use adjuvant therapy.

ADJUVANT THERAPY

Node-Negative Disease: There is increasing evidence that systemic adjuvant therapy can lead to improved disease-free and overall survival in node-negative breast cancer patients. The Early Breast Cancer Trialists' Collaborative Group is a worldwide collaboration to obtain information on mortality and recurrence for each patient entered in a randomized trial of systemic adjuvant therapy for early-stage breast cancer before 1985. Data are now available on 75,000 women in 133 randomized trials. The majority of women in these trials were node positive, but about 31% were node negative.

The percentage reduction in recurrence and mortality in node-negative patients is summarized in Table 2. A total of 12,910 node-negative patients were treated with tamoxifen, with a 26% ± 4% (SD) reduction in recurrence and a 17% ± 5% reduction in mortality. A total of 2,710 node-negative patients were treated with combination chemotherapy, with a 26% ± 7% reduction in the recurrence rate and an 18% ± 8% reduction in the mortality rate.[8]

Node-Positive Disease: The benefit of systemic adjuvant therapy in node-positive breast cancer patients is established. The greatest benefit has been seen in patients with one to three positive nodes, with more modest benefit seen in patients with four or more involved nodes. Most trials have not included patients with 10 or more positive nodes, the majority of whom will have disease recurrence within 5 years if they are treated with local therapy alone.

At M. D. Anderson Cancer Center, 283 patients with 10 or more positive nodes were included in a prospective trial that examined adjuvant doxorubicin (Adriamycin, Rubex)-containing regimens. The 5-year disease-free survival rate in these patients was about 41%.[36] Patients with 10 or more positive nodes are currently being entered into randomized trials with high-dose chemotherapy and autologous bone-marrow rescue because of the high failure rate with conventional adjuvant therapies.

Tamoxifen Therapy: The Early Breast Cancer Trialists' Collaborative Group reviewed data on 30,000 women with breast cancer in 42 randomized tamoxifen trials. Results were broken down by age group, nodal status,

TABLE 2

Effects of Systemic Adjuvant Therapy in Node-Negative Breast Cancer Patients

	Number of patients	Percent reduction[a] in Recurrence	Mortality
Tamoxifen	12,910	26 ± 4	17 ± 5
Chemotherapy	2,710	26 ± 7	18 ± 8

[a] Percent reduction in annual risk of recurrence or mortality during the first 10 years; observed value ± standard deviation

Adapted from Early Breast Cancer Trialists' Collaborative Group.[8]

TABLE 3

Effects of Tamoxifen Therapy on Breast Cancer

| Duration of therapy | Number of patients | | Percent reduction [a] in | |
	Tamoxifen	Control [b]	Recurrence	Mortality
< 2 years	4,088	4,122	16 ± 3	11 ± 4
2 years (mean)	7,732	7,736	27 ± 2	18 ± 3
> 2 years (mean)	3,202	3,196	38 ± 4	24 ± 6
Total	15,022	15,054	25 ± 2	17 ± 2

[a] Percent reduction in annual risk of recurrence or mortality during first 10 years; observed value ± standard deviation
[b] No tamoxifen

Adapted from Early Breast Cancer Trialists' Collaborative Group. [8]

TABLE 4

Effects of Ovarian Ablation in Breast Cancer Patients Under Age 50

| Treatment | Number of patients | | Percent reduction [a] in | |
	Treatment	Control [b]	Recurrence	Mortality
Ovarian ablation alone	456	422	30 ± 9	28 ± 9
Ovarian ablation + chemotherapy	478	461	21 ± 9	19 ± 11
Total	934	883	26 ± 6	25 ± 7

[a] Percent reduction in annual risk of recurrence or mortality during first 10 years; observed value ± standard deviation
[b] No ovarian ablation

Adapted from Early Breast Cancer Trialists' Collaborative Group. [8]

and ER status. A meta-analysis of these trials is summarized in Table 3. Overall, there was a significant, 25% ± 2% reduction in the risk of recurrence with adjuvant tamoxifen at 10 years. Tamoxifen also significantly reduced mortality overall (by 17% ± 2%). There was a statistically significant reduction in the risk of recurrence in all age groups, but the improvement in the survival rate was statistically significant only in patients 50 years of age and older.

The duration of tamoxifen therapy in the majority of these trials was 1 to 2 years. Although data from direct randomized comparisons of different durations of tamoxifen therapy (usually 5 years vs 1 or 2 years) suggested that a longer duration was associated with longer survival, the differences were not significant (7% ± 11% reduction in mortality).[8]

Contralateral breast cancer was reported in 2% of controls vs 1.3% of tamoxifen-treated patients, a statistically significant difference.[8] Treatment with adjuvant chemotherapy had no effect on the development of a second breast cancer.[8]

Ovarian Ablation: Ovarian ablation can be accomplished by surgery, irradiation, or hormone therapy. This mode of adjuvant therapy has been evaluated in 10 randomized trials involving 3,000 women, 1,746 of whom were younger than 50 years. A meta-analysis of these data performed by the Early Breast Cancer Trialists' Collaborative Group is summarized in Table 4. For women older than 50, ovarian ablation produced no significant effect on recurrence-free or overall survival. For women younger than 50, ovarian ablation produced a significant, 26% ± 6% improvement in recurrence-free survival and a 25% ± 7% improvement in overall survival. It appeared that ovarian ablation produced less improvement among patients given chemotherapy, but the difference was not statistically significant. The improvements in recurrence-free and overall survival were statistically significant only for node-positive patients, although the same trend was suggested in node-negative patients. All of these trials were done prior to the availability of ER and PR assays.[8]

The luteinizing hormone-releasing hormone (LHRH) agonist allows for the suppression of ovarian function with minimum morbidity. Ongoing trials of the effect of an LHRH agonist and other means of ovarian ablation in patients with ER/PR-positive tumors are underway. More data are necessary to determine the effect of ovarian ablation on survival.

Other Endocrine Agents: Other endocrine agents that have been used in the adjuvant setting include progestins, antiadrenal drugs, and prednisone. Prednisone, which is thought to suppress adrenal estrogen synthesis, has been used in combination with other cytotoxic drugs in the adjuvant setting. In most randomized studies, however, it provided no additional benefit. There was some improvement in disease-free and overall survival in one trial in which prednisone was used together with ovarian ablation.[37]

Aminoglutethimide (Cytadren), an aromatase inhibitor, resulted in improved disease-free but not overall survival in one adjuvant trial.[38] In a study by Tally and colleagues, progestin significantly improved disease-free and overall survival in post- and premenopausal patients with more than three positive nodes, when compared with matched historical controls.[39] These drugs have significant toxicity, and none offer any advantage over tamoxifen according to available data. Newer hormonal agents that may prove more useful are the aromatase inhibitors and the antiprogestins.

ADJUVANT CHEMOTHERAPY

The early adjuvant chemotherapy trials compared one course of perioperative, single-agent chemotherapy (cyclophosphamide [Cytoxan, Neosar], melphalan [Alkeran], or thiotepa) with surgery alone and showed only minimal improvement in disease-free survival. These studies were important in establishing a role for adjuvant therapy and in leading to trials comparing single-agent and combination chemotherapy.

Combination Chemotherapy: Studies comparing single-agent and combination chemotherapy consistently show the superiority of combination regimens in terms of recurrence-free and overall survival (Table 5). In fact, single-agent chemotherapy is no longer used as an adjuvant treatment. In a review by the Early Breast Cancer Trialists' Collaborative Group of 11,041 patients randomized in 31 trials of long-term combination chemotherapy vs no chemotherapy, combination chemotherapy was clearly associated with significantly improved recurrence-free and overall survival. Indeed, with adjuvant combination chemotherapy, there were significant reductions in both risk of recurrence and mortality (28% ± 3% and 16% ± 3%, respectively) at 10 years. The improvements in recurrence-free and overall survival were greater in node-positive than in node-negative women but were statistically significant for both groups. Also, with regard to recurrence-free and overall survival, there was a trend toward greater effects among younger women.[8]

Duration of Therapy: In most of the early adjuvant chemotheray trials, therapy was continued for 1 to 2 years. Subsequent studies were designed to evaluate the efficacy of shorter durations of chemotherapy. Studies showed that there was no improvement in disease-free or overall survival when chemotherapy was continued beyond six cycles. Limited data suggest that to achieve the maximum effect, therapy must be continued for more than 3 months. In a retrospective study from M. D. Anderson Cancer Center, patients who received less than six cycles of combination chemotherapy had decreased disease-free survival, compared with those who received six or more cycles of the same regimen.[40]

Regimens With and Without Anthracycline: Anthracycline-containing regimens have been compared to non-anthracycline-containing regimens in several stud-

TABLE 5

Effects of Combination Chemotherapy on Breast Cancer in All Age Groups

Chemotherapy regimen	Number of patients		Percent reduction [a] in	
	Chemotherapy	Control [b]	Recurrence	Mortality
Cyclophosphamide + methotrexate + fluorouracil (CMF)	2,098	2,078	32 ± 4	22 ± 5
CMF with additional chemotherapeutic agents	1,298	1,277	23 ± 6	10 ± 7 [c]
Other chemotherapeutic agents	2,344	2,355	25 ± 5	12 ± 6
Total	5,740	5,710	28 ± 3	16 ± 3

[a] Percent reduction in annual risk of recurrence or mortality during first 10 years; observed value ± standard deviation
[b] No chemotherapy
[c] Difference not statistically significant

Adapted from Early Breast Cancer Trialists' Collaborative Group. [8]

TABLE 6

Randomized Clinical Trials of Anthracycline- vs Non-Anthracycline-Containing Adjuvant Chemotherapy Regimens

Trial	Regimen[a]	Number of patients	Follow-up (mo)	Disease-free survival with anthracycline (%)	Disease-free survival without anthracycline (%)	P value
Onco, France[41]	AVCF CMF	325	120	54	43	.04
Institut Curie[42]	mMAC mMFC	121	96	–	–	–
ICCG[43]	FEC CMF	636	37	–	–	.22
SECSG[44]	CAF CMF	527	42	–	–	–
Milan[45] (1–3+ nodes)	CMF × 12 CMF × 8 → A × 4	433	61	74	72	.73
ECOG[46]	CMFPT × 12 CMFPTH/vATHT × 12	533	61	63	70	.04
CALGB[47]	CMFVP CMFVP → vATH	897	23	–	–	.01
Milan[48] (≥ 4 nodes)	A × 4 → CMF × 8 CMF/A × 12	359	72	56	38	.0007
NSABP-11[49]	pF pAF	697	88	38	46	.01
NSABP-12[49]	pFT pAFT	1,093	87	56	58	.36
NSABP-15[49]	CMF AC	1,473	44	64	64	.5
SWOG[50]	FACM CMFVP	532	38	52	52	NS

[a] A = doxorubicin, C = cyclophosphamide, E = epirubicin, F = fluorouracil, H = fluoxymesterone, M = methotrexate, m = mitomycin, P = prednisone, p = melphalan, T = tamoxifen, V = vincristine, v = vinblastine

Adapted, with permission, from Hughes P, Buzdar A: Early stage breast cancer and adjuvant therapy, in Pazdur R (ed): Medical Oncology: A Comprehensive Review, p 206. Huntington, NY, PRR Inc, 1993.

ies (Table 6).[41-50] Even though some studies had a relatively small number of patients and short follow-up, data suggest that anthracycline-containing regimens may be associated with better disease-free survival. However, only 3 of the 12 studies showed a statistically significant improvement in overall survival with the addition of an anthracycline.

Ten-year results from a randomized prospective French trial were published in 1992: Among 249 node-positive breast cancer patients given either cyclophosphamide, methotrexate, and fluorouracil (CMF) or an anthracycline-containing regimen, the addition of doxorubicin reduced the risk of relapse by one third and the risk of death by one half in premenopausal patients.[51]

Non-Cross-Resistant Therapies: Tumor cell heterogeneity and the presence of subsets of cells resistant to certain drugs provide the rationale for treatment with multiple non-cross-resistant drugs. The Milan group reported updated results from a study in which pre- and postmenopausal patients with more than three positive axillary nodes were randomized to four courses of doxorubicin followed by eight courses of CMF (sequential chemotherapy) or two courses of CMF alternated with one course of doxorubicin for a total of 12 courses (alternating chemotherapy). Relapse-free and overall survival rates were significantly superior in the sequential chemotherapy group and appeared superior to those obtained with CMF alone.[48]

The CALGB reported a higher disease-free and overall survival across all nodal subgroups in patients treated with CMF plus vincristine (Oncovin) and prednisone (CMFVP) than in those who received vinblastine, doxorubicin, thiotepa, and fluoxymesterone (VATH).[47] An M. D. Anderson Cancer Center study showed that the addition of methotrexate and vinblastine after FACVP (fluorouracil, doxorubicin, cyclophosphamide, vincristine, and prednisone) significantly prolonged disease-free survival but not overall survival in ER-positive patients.[52] These preliminary data support the use of sequential, non-cross-resistant chemotherapy, although further studies are needed to confirm these observations.

Chemohormonal Combinations: The addition of tamoxifen to adjuvant chemotherapy has been evaluated in several clinical trials. Earlier reports from these trials suggested that adding tamoxifen resulted in no definite advantage. However, more recent data suggest a potential benefit, particularly in postmenopausal patients. One study randomized postmenopausal patients to receive CFP (cyclophosphamide, fluorouracil, and prednisone) alone, CFP plus tamoxifen, or no treatment. At 7 years median follow-up, both the chemotherapy-alone and chemotherapy-plus-tamoxifen groups had a significantly better disease-free survival than the control group had. There was also a trend toward on improved overall survival rate in the chemotherapy-plus-tamoxifen group.[53]

The National Surgical Adjuvant Breast and Bowel Project B-16 study randomized node-positive, ER-positive patients to receive doxorubicin, cyclophosphamide, and tamoxifen; melphalan, fluorouracil, doxorubicin, and tamoxifen; or tamoxifen alone. This study found a superior 5-year disease-free survival rate in the chemotherapy-plus-tamoxifen groups.[54] An Eastern Cooperative Oncology Group (ECOG) study in postmenopausal, node-positive patients found a delayed time to recurrence among patient groups given chemotherapy plus tamoxifen, as compared with groups given chemotherapy alone.[55]

Biological Therapies: Several different biological agents (bacillus Calmette Guérin [BCG], levamisole [Ergamisol], polyA-polyU, *Corynebacterium parvum*, Azimexon, Basidio.p.p., interferon) have been evaluated in a total of 24 randomized trials involving 6,300 women. There has been no consistent improvement in either disease-free or overall survival with the use of these agents as adjuvant therapy for early-stage breast cancer.[8]

Dose-Intensive Chemotherapy: In general, retrospective studies support the concept that higher dose intensity correlates with a better response.[56–58] CALGB conducted a study in which breast cancer patients with stage II,

node-positive disease were randomized to one of three FAC (fluorouracil, doxorubicin, and cyclophosphamide) dose-intensity arms, all within the standard dose range.[59] After a median follow-up of 3.4 years, there was a significant improvement in disease-free and overall survival in the high-dose arm as compared with the low-dose arm. This study suggests that doses that were 50% lower than the standard dose produced inferior outcomes. What remains to be determined is whether doses higher than the standard dose would further improve the efficacy of adjuvant therapy. Preliminary results of a randomized trial to assess the efficacy of high-dose adjuvant chemotherapy with doxorubicin and cyclophosphamide failed to support a benefit of dose increase for cyclophosphamide above the standard range.[60]

Experience with high-dose chemotherapy has largely been focused on breast cancer patients with 10 or more positive axillary lymph nodes. Peters et al conducted a study of stage II or III breast cancer patients with 10 or more positive axillary nodes.[61] Patients were treated with four cycles of FAC postoperatively followed by high-dose cyclophosphamide, cisplatin, and carmustine (BiCNU) with autologous bone marrow rescue. For the 85 evaluable patients, the therapy-related mortality rate was 12% and the estimated event-free survival rate was 72% at a median follow-up of 2.5 years. This is a significant improvement in event-free survival compared with historical controls (38% to 52%). However, comparison to historical populations is subject to many potential biases (eg, differences in patient selection, extent of pre-study staging evaluation).

In a study by Lyding et al,[62] 13 patients with high-risk, stage II or III breast cancer were treated with high-dose chemotherapy (cyclophosphamide, mitoxantrone [Novantrone], and thiotepa) and autologous bone-marrow or peripheral-stem-cell rescue. All 13 patients remained in complete remission at a median follow-up of 7 months.

Whether high-dose chemotherapy offers advantages to high-risk patients remains to be determined. Patients from several centers with 10 or more positive axillary nodes are currently being entered into randomized clinical trials involving high-dose chemotherapy with autologous stem-cell support vs standard adjuvant therapy.

CARCINOMA OF THE MALE BREAST

Breast carcinoma in men accounts for 0.5% of all breast cancers in the United States, and it is estimated that 1,400 new cases will be diagnosed in 1995.[2] The epidemiology, prognostic factors, survival by stage, pattern of metastasis, and response to treatment are similar in men and women with breast carcinoma. The data suggest, however, that breast cancer in men is more likely to respond to hormonal manipulation.[63]

FUTURE PERSPECTIVES

Randomized trials addressing the issues described above are presently underway. Future adjuvant studies will include new cytotoxic agents such as paclitaxel (Taxol), docetaxel (Taxotere), and vinorelbine (Navelbine), all of which have shown encouraging results in advanced breast cancer.[64–66] Novel therapeutic approaches include ongoing trials using monoclonal antibodies targeted against growth factors or oncoproteins.[67]

Current knowledge of the adjuvant treatment of breast cancer has emerged from controlled randomized trials. Because there are still many controversies, it remains of paramount importance to continue pursuing clinical and basic research in this field.

REFERENCES

1. Consensus Development Panel: Consensus statement: Treatment of early-stage breast cancer, in Early Stage Breast Cancer, pp 1–5. National Cancer Institute monograph no 11. Washington, DC, US Government Printing Office, 1992.

2. Wingo PA, Tong T, Bolden S: Cancer Statistics, 1995. CA Cancer J Clin 45:8–30, 1995.

3. Nemoto T, Vana J, Bedwani RN, et al: Management and survival of female breast cancer: Results of a national survey by the American College of Surgeons. Cancer 45:2917–2924, 1980.

4. Consensus Conference: Adjuvant chemotherapy for breast cancer. JAMA 254:3461–3463, 1985.

5. Gasparini G, Barbareschi M, Doglioni C, et al: Expression of bcl-2 protein predicts efficacy of adjuvant treatments in operable node-positive breast cancer. Clin Cancer Research 1:189–198, 1995.

6. Carter CL, Allen C, Henson DE: Relation of tumor size, lymph node status, and survival in 24,740 breast cancer cases. Cancer 63:181–187, 1989.

7. Fisher B, Bauer M, Margolese R, et al: Five-year results of a randomized clinical trial comparing total mastectomy and segmental mastectomy with or without radiation therapy in the treatment of breast cancer. N Engl J Med 312:665–673, 1985.

8. Early Breast Cancer Trialists' Collaborative Group: Systemic treatment of early breast cancer by hormonal, cytotoxic, or immune therapy: 133 randomised trials involving 31,000 recurrences and 24,000 deaths among 75,000 women. Lancet 339:1–15, 71–85, 1992.

9. Rosen PP, Groshen S, Saigo PE, et al: A long-term follow-up study of survival in stage I (T1N0M0) and stage II (T1N1M0) breast carcinoma. J Clin Oncol 7:355–366, 1989.

10. Rosen PP, Groshen S, Saigo PE, et al: Pathological prognostic factors in stage I (T1N0M0) and stage II (T1N1M0) breast carcinoma: A study of 644 patients with median follow-up of 18 years. J Clin Oncol 7:1239–1251, 1989.

11. McGuire WL, Clark GM: Prognostic factors and treatment decisions in axillary-node-negative breast cancer. N Engl J Med 326:1756–1761, 1992.

12. McGuire WL: Estrogen receptor versus nuclear grade as prognostic factors in axillary node negative breast cancer. J Clin Oncol 6:1071–1072, 1988.

13. Clark GM, Mathieu M-C, Owens MA, et al: Prognostic signif-

icance of S-phase fraction in good-risk, node-negative breast cancer patients. J Clin Oncol 10:428–432, 1992.

14. Remvikos Y, Beuzeboc A, Zajdela N, et al: Correlation of pretreatment proliferative activity of breast cancer with the response to cytotoxic chemotherapy. J Natl Cancer Inst 81:1383–1387, 1989.

15. Nicholson S, Richard J, Sainsbury C, et al: Epidermal growth factor receptor (EGF): Results of a 6 year follow-up study in operable breast cancer with emphasis on the node negative subgroup. Br J Cancer 63:146–150, 1991.

16. Sahin AA, Ro J, Ro JY, et al: Ki-67 immunostaining in node negative stage I/II breast carcinoma. Significant correlation with prognosis. Cancer 68:549–557, 1991.

17. Wintzer HO, Zipfel I, Schulte-Monting J: Ki-67 immunostaining in human breast tumors and its relationship with prognosis. Cancer 67:421–428, 1991.

18. Predine J, Spyratos F, Prud'hommme JF, et al: Enzyme-linked immunosorbent assay of pS2 in breast cancers, benign tumors, and normal breast tissues: Correlation with prognosis and adjuvant hormone therapy. Cancer 69:2116–2123, 1992.

19. Chamness GC: Estrogen-inducible heat shock protein hsp27 predicts recurrence in node-negative breast cancer. Proc Am Assoc Cancer Res 30:252, 1989.

20. Daidone MG, Silvestrini R, D'Errico, et al: Laminin receptors, collagenase IV and prognosis in node-negative breast cancers. Int J Cancer 48:529–532, 1991.

21. Hennessy C, Henry JA, May FEB, et al: Expression of the antimetastatic gene nm23 in human breast cancer: An association with good prognosis. J Natl Cancer Inst 83:281–285, 1991

22. Thor AD, Moore DM, Edgerton SM, et al: Accumulation of p53 tumor supressor gene protein: An independant marker of prognosis in breast cancers. J Natl Cancer Inst 84:845–855, 1992.

23. Allred DC, Clark GM, Elledge R, et al: Association of p53 protein expression with tumor cell proliferation rate and clinical outcome in node-negative breast cancer. J Natl Cancer Inst 85:200–206, 1993.

24. Duffy MJ, O'Grady P, Devaney D, et al: Tissue-type plasminogen activator, a new prognostic marker in breast cancer. Cancer Res 49:6008–6014, 1989.

25. Tandon AK, Clark GM, Chamness GC, et al: Cathepsin-D and prognosis in breast cancer. N Engl J Med 322:297–302, 1990.

26. Ravdin PM: Evaluation of Cathepsin D as a prognostic factor in breast cancer. Breast Cancer Res Treat 24:219–226, 1993.

27. Ravdin PM, Tandon AK, Allred DC, et al: Cathepsin D by western blotting and immunochemistry: Failure to confirm correlations with prognosis in node-negative breast cancer. J Clin Oncol 12:467–474, 1994.

28. Paik S, Hazan ER, Fisher ER, et al: Pathological Findings from the National Surgical Adjuvant Breast and Bowel Project: Prognostic significance of erbB-2 protein overexpression in primary breast cancer. J Clin Oncol 8:103–112, 1990.

29. Toikkanen S, Helin H, Isola J, et al: Prognostic significance of HER-2 oncoprotein expression in breast cancer: A 30-year follow-up. J Clin Oncol 10:1044–1048, 1992.

30. Muss HB, Thor AD, Berry DA, et al: c-erbB-2 expression and response to adjuvant therapy in women with node-positive early breast cancer. N Engl J Med 330:1260–1266, 1994.

31. Folkman J: What is the evidence that tumors are angiogenesis dependent? (editorial). J Natl Cancer Inst 82:4–6, 1990.

32. Weidner N, Folkman J, Pozza F, et al: Tumor angiogenesis is an independant prognostic indicator in early-stage breast carcinoma. J Natl Cancer Inst 84:1875–1887, 1992.

33. Gasparini G, Weidner N, Bevilacqua, et al: Tumor microvessel density, p53 expression, tumor size, and peritumoral lymphatic vessel invasion are relevant prognostic markers in node-negative breast

carcinoma. J Clin Oncol 12:454–456, 1994.

34. Rosner D, Lane WW: Node-negative minimal invasive breast cancer patients are not candidates for routine systemic adjuvant therapy. Cancer 66:199–205, 1990.

35. Henderson IL, Harris JR, Kinne DW, et al: Cancer of the breast, in DeVita VT, Hellman S, Rosenberg SA (eds): Cancer: Principles and Practice of Oncology, 3rd ed, p 1206. Philadelphia, JB Lippincott, 1989.

36. Buzdar AU, Kau SW, Hortobagyi GN, et al: Clinical course of patients with breast cancer with 10 or more positive nodes who were treated with doxorubicin-containing adjuvant therapy. Cancer 69:448–452, 1992.

37. Meakin J, Allt WE, Beale FA, et al: Ovarian irradiation and prednisolone following surgery and radiotherapy for carcinoma of the breast. Can Med Assoc J 120:1221–1229, 1979.

38. Coombes R, Chilvers C, Paules T: Adjuvant aminoglutethimide therapy for postmenopausal patients with primary breast cancer, in Jones SE, Salmon SE (eds): Adjuvant Therapy of Cancer, 4th ed, pp 349–357. Orlando, Grune and Stratton, 1984.

39. Tally R, Segaloff A, Gregory E, et al: Adjuvant therapy of breast cancer with megestrol acetate. Breast Cancer Res Treat 3:323, 1983.

40. Ang PT, Buzdar AU, Smith TL, et al: Analysis of dose intensity in doxorubicin-containing adjuvant chemotherapy in stage II and III breast carcinoma. J Clin Oncol 7:1677–1684, 1989.

41. Misset JL, DeVassel F, Jasmis C, et al: Five-year results of the French adjuvant trial for breast cancer comparing CMF to a combination of Adriamycin, vincristine, cyclophosphamide, and fluorouracil, in Jones SE, Salmon SE (eds): Adjuvant Therapy of Cancer, 4th ed, pp 243–251. Orlando, Grune and Stratton, 1984.

42. Beuzeboc P, Mosseri V, Dorval E, et al: Adriamycin-based combination chemotherapy significantly improves overall survival in high risk premenopausal breast cancer patients. Adjuvant Therapy of Primary Breast Cancer 4th International Conference (abstract 55P). Sankt Gallen, Switzerland, February 26–29, 1992.

43. Coombs RC, Bliss JM, Marty M, et al: A randomized trial comparing adjuvant FEC with CMF in pre-menopausal patients with node-positive resectable breast cancer (abstract). Proc Am Soc Clin Oncol 10:31, 1991.

44. Carpenter JT, Velez-Garcia E, Aron BS, et al: Prospective randomized comparison of cyclophosphamide, doxorubicin, and fluorouracil vs cyclophosphamide, methotrexate and fluorouracil for breast cancer with positive axillary nodes (abstract). Proc Am Soc Clin Oncol 10:45, 1991.

45. Bonadonna G, Valagussa A, Zambetti M, et al: Milan adjuvant trials for stage I-II breast cancer, in Salmon SE (ed): Adjuvant Therapy of Cancer 5th ed, pp 211–221. New York, Grune and Stratton, 1987.

46. Abeloff MD, Gray R, Tormey DC, et al, for the Eastern Cooperative Oncology Group: A randomized comparison of CMFPT versus CMFPTH/VATHT and maintenance versus no maintenance tamoxifen in premenopausal, node-positive breast cancer patients, an ECOG study (abstract). Proc Am Soc Clin Oncol 10:43, 1991.

47. Perloff M, Norton L, Korzun N, et al: Advantage of an Adriamycin combination plus halotestin after initial cyclophosphamide, methotrexate, 5-FU, vincristine, and prednisone (CMFVP) for adjuvant therapy of node-positive stage II breast cancer. Proc Am Soc Clin Oncol 5:70, 1986.

48. Bonadonna G, Valagussa P, Zambetti M: Sequential Adriamycin-CMF in the adjuvant treatment of breast cancer with more than 3 positive axillary nodes. Proc Am Soc Clin Oncol 11:61, 1992.

49. Fisher B, Redmond C, Vickerham DL, et al: Doxorubicin-containing regimens for treatment of stage II breast cancer: National Surgical Adjuvant Breast and Bowel Project experience. J Clin Oncol 7:572–582, 1989.

50. O'Bryan R, Green S, O'Sullivan J, et al: A comparison of CMFVP for one year to short-term Adriamycin based chemotherapy for patients with receptor-negative node-positive operable breast cancer: An intergroup study (abstract). Proc Am Soc Clin Oncol 11:61, 1992.

51. Misset JL, Gil-Delgado M, Chollet PH, et al: Ten year results of the French trial comparing Adriamycin, vincristine, 5-fluorouracil and cyclophosphamide to standard CMF as adjuvant therapy for node positive breast cancer. Proc Am Soc Clin Oncol 11:54, 1992.

52. Buzdar AU, Hortobagyi GN, Smith TL, et al: Adjuvant therapy of breast cancer with or without additional treatment with alternate drugs. Cancer 62:2098–2104, 1988.

53. Ingle JN, Krook JE, Schaid DJ: Randomized trial in post-menopausal women with node-positive breast cancer: Observation versus adjuvant therapy with cyclophosphamide (C), 5-fluorouracil, prednisone (P) with or without tamoxifen (T): Results with seven year median follow-up. A collaborative trial of the North Central Cancer Treatment Group and Mayo Clinic. Sixth International Conference on the Adjuvant Therapy of Cancer (abstract 39). Tucson, Arizona, March 7–10, 1990.

54. Fisher B, Redmond C, Poisson S, et al: Increased benefit from addition of Adriamycin and cyclophosphamide (AC) to tamoxifen (Tam, T) for positive nodes, tamoxifen-responsive post-menopausal breast cancer patients: Results from NSABP B-16 (abstract). Proc Am Soc Clin Oncol 9:20, 1990.

55. Wolberg WH, Gray R, Falkson HC, et al: Adjuvant therapy of postmenopausal women with breast cancer: An ECOG phase III trial. Sixth International Conference on the Adjuvant Therapy of Cancer (abstract 50). Tucson, Arizona, March 7–10, 1990.

56. Bonadonna G, Valagussa P: Dose-response effect of adjuvant chemotherapy in breast cancer. N Engl J Med 304:10–15, 1981.

57. Hryniuk W, Bush H: The importance of dose intensity in chemotherapy of metastatic breast cancer. J Clin Oncol 2: 1281–1288, 1984.

58. Hryniuk W, Levine MN: Analysis of dose intensity for adjuvant chemotherapy trials in stage II breast cancer. J Clin Oncol 4:1162–1170, 1986.

59. Wood WC, Budman DR, Korzun AH, et al: Dose and dose intensity of adjuvant chemotherapy for stage II, node-positive breast carcinoma. N Engl J Med 330:1253–1259, 1994.

60. Dimitrov N, Anderson S, Fisher B, et al: Dose intensification and increased total dose of adjuvant chemotherapy for breast cancer: Findings from NSABP-22. Proc Am Soc Med Oncol 13:64, 1994.

61. Peters WP, Ross M, Vredenburgh JJ, et al: High-dose chemotherapy and autologous bone marrow support as consolidation after standard-dose adjuvant therapy for high-risk primary breast cancer. J Clin Oncol 11:1132–1143, 1993.

62. Lyding J, Damon L, Wolf J, et al: High dose cyclophosphamide, thiotepa and mitoxantrone with autologous bone marrow transplant for breast cancer. Proc Am Soc Clin Oncol 11:70, 1992.

63. Jaiyesimi IA, Buzdar AU, Sahin AA, et al: Carcinoma of the male breast. Ann Intern Med 117:771–777, 1992.

64. Holmes FA, Walters RS, Theriault RL: Phase II trial of taxol, an active drug in metastatic breast cancer. J Natl Cancer Inst 83:1797–1805, 1991.

65. Valero V, Walters RS, Theriault RL, et al: Phase II study of docetaxel (Taxotere) in anthracycline-refractory metastatic breast cancer. Proc Am Soc Clin Oncol 13:470, 1994.

66. Lluch A, Garcia-Conde J, Cassardo A, et al: Phase II trial with navelbine in advanced breast cancer, previously untreated. Proc Am Soc Clin Oncol 11:115, 1992.

67. Baselga J, Norton L, Shalaby R, et al: Anti HER-2 humanized monoclonal antibody (Mab) alone and in combination with chemotherapy against human breast carcinoma xenografts. Proc Am Soc Clin Oncol 13:63, 1994.

CHAPTER 20

Metastatic Breast Cancer

Mary K. Crow, MD,[1] Edward Soo, MD,[1] *and* Frankie A. Holmes, MD[2]

[1]Division of Medicine; [2]Department of Breast and Gynecologic Medical Oncology
The University of Texas M. D. Anderson Cancer Center, Houston, Texas

In 1995, it is projected that there will be 183,400 new cases of breast cancer and 46,240 deaths from the disease, despite an emphasis on early detection.[1] Fewer than 10% of patients will present with metastatic disease, but nearly 50% of newly diagnosed patients may eventually develop it. Unfortunately, advanced breast cancer is incurable. In a classic study of untreated patients, the median survival was 2.7 years from the onset of symptoms.[2] Most patients who relapse do so within 2 to 3 years after diagnosis of the primary tumor. In a minority of patients, the disease will recur 5 or more years after the initial diagnosis; 3% to 5% of patients remain in remission longer than 10 years.[2] Survival after relapse is directly related to the extent of disease, not the site of relapse, with the exception of disease in the central nervous system, which portends very short survival.[3]

MOLECULAR EVENTS IN BREAST CANCER METASTASIS

Recent data from work on cell lines and tumor specimens are beginning to elucidate a complex interaction between the tumor cell and its microenvironment. For a cancer cell to metastasize, a series of disparate events must occur. The cancer cell must penetrate various basement membranes, degrade the underlying mesenchymal tissues, gain access to blood and lymph vessels, and enter the stroma of the target organ.[4] Other important events include paracrine stimulation of growth factor receptors (possibly by the surrounding stromal cells), angiogenesis to support tumor growth, and the cancer cell's evasion of host immune surveillance.

Once the mechanisms of breast cancer metastasis are understood, they will become new targets for therapy. A number of experimental models of metastasis are under study.[5–7] Table 1 lists some important targets for phase I trials. Many human cancers, including breast cancer, can be regarded as stromal-dependent tumors[8]; disabling essential mechanisms that these cancers need for growth and support may represent an approach to their treatment.

DIAGNOSTIC WORKUP

History: Once metastatic disease is suspected, careful evaluation of the primary disease history, current symptoms, and existing comorbid disease is essential. The history of the primary disease should include a review of the initial presentation, stage of disease, hormone-receptor status pathology report, and treatment modalities employed. It may be helpful to review the primary histologic material to confirm the exact tumor type, estrogen and progesterone receptor status, and extent of nodal metastasis. Knowledge of the initial tumor type may yield clues about the sites of disease. For instance, infiltrating ductal carcinoma most commonly involves the lungs, pleura, and brain, whereas infiltrating lobular carcinoma most commonly involves the bone marrow, peritoneum, and retroperitoneal structures, such as the ureters.[9]

Other ancillary information, such as DNA ploidy, S-phase fraction, and the presence of oncogene products, such as c-*erbB*-2 (*HER-2/neu*) or *p53*, has been studied in primary breast cancer,[10] but the influence of these factors on metastatic disease progression is unclear. However, among patients who develop extraosseous metastatic disease, those with highly aneuploid tumors at initial presentation have significantly shorter survival than do patients with diploid tumors at initial presentation.[11]

The length of the disease-free interval and the menopausal status should be ascertained. Information on hot flashes, cyclic breast tenderness, premenstrual symp-

TABLE I

Selected Molecular Targets and Mechanisms in Breast Cancer

Target	Intervention
Epidermal growth factor receptor (EGFR)	Anti-EGFR monoclonal antibodies
c-*erbB*-2 (*HER2/neu*) overexpression	Anti-*neu* monoclonal antibodies
Insulin-like growth factor receptor (IGFR-I, II)	Anti-IGFR monoclonal antibodies
Matrix metalloproteases	Antisense or metalloprotease inhibitors
Angiogenesis	Fumagillin, alpha interferon

toms, serum follicle-stimulating hormone/luteinizing hormone (FSH/LH), and vaginal cytology is helpful in assessing the menstrual status of women who have undergone a hysterectomy.

Any current symptoms should be carefully evaluated to assess potential metastatic sites and tumor burden. Pain, weight loss, activity constraints, nutritional status, dental health, and psychological factors are also important in determining the optimal treatment. Any coexisting medical conditions should be noted because they may affect the choice of chemotherapeutic agents.

Physical Examination: A comprehensive physical examination is essential for establishing the initial baseline status. The usual sites of metastasis, including soft tissues, bones, lungs, and liver, should be assessed. Evaluation of the soft tissues includes a careful survey of all the lymph-node basins of the upper torso, with documentation of the size and location of enlarged nodes and assessment of the chest wall, operative site, and all breast tissue. These areas should be examined while the patient is in both seated and recumbent positions. Photographs or diagrams of these areas often add invaluable information for subsequent comparison. A complete neurologic examination can determine the need for specific diagnostic imaging. Ascites caused by peritoneal metastases is less common but not rare.

Laboratory Tests: A basic laboratory evaluation includes a complete blood count with differential, liver and renal function tests, and serum calcium determination. In addition, carcinoembryonic antigen (CEA) and CA 15-3 are potentially helpful in detecting or monitoring metastatic disease. CEA levels are is elevated in 40% to 50% of patients with metastases.[12,13] Benign, low elevations (3 to 10 ng/mL) can be found in patients with inflammatory disease of the gastrointestinal tract, in smokers with chronic bronchitis, and in patients with cystic breast disease.[14] The CA 15-3 test is a combination of two monoclonal antibodies bearing two reactive determinants directed against DF3 and MAM-6 antigens expressed on the mammary epithelial cells.[12,15] CA 15-3, which is much more sensitive than CEA, is elevated in 70% to 85% of patients with metastases. The false-positive rate of the CA 15-3 test is similar to that with CEA.[12,15] Unfortunately, the CA 15-3 test is not approved by the US Food and Drug Administration for evaluation of breast cancer.

Diagnostic Imaging: The chest radiograph is usually sufficient to assess the lungs unless there is a compressed bronchus or solitary lesion or the disease is primarily mediastinal. In addition to liver parenchymal involvement, metastases to periportal nodes with compression of

the biliary tree or hepatic/portal vessels may also occur; these metastases are best detected by computed tomographic scanning or ultrasonography. The liver-spleen scan is insufficiently detailed and should not be used. Hydroureter or hydronephrosis is the most common indication of retroperitoneal metastases, particularly in patients with signet-ring or lobular variants. Only 30% to 60% of patients with a true-positive bone scan have increased alkaline phosphatase levels.[16,17] Conversely, only 20% of patients with elevated alkaline phosphatase levels are disease free.[16]

If the bone scan shows areas of abnormal uptake, radiographs of the affected sites are necessary to confirm metastatic disease and to exclude benign etiologies. Impending fractures in the weight-bearing bones, such as the femur or humerus (if the patient is using crutches), or an unstable spine must be ruled out. Radiographic evaluation of the brain, leptomeninges, and spinal cord has a low yield unless the patient is symptomatic or has an abnormal neurologic finding.

Pathology: The histologic slides of the primary tumor should be reviewed and compared with biopsy results of lesions suspected of being metastases. Patients with solitary lesions, easily accessible lesions that may be confused with benign processes (such as chest-wall or lymph-node abnormalities), and suspicious lesions in patients with a disease-free interval longer than 5 years should undergo biopsy to confirm or rule out metastatic breast cancer. Estrogen and progesterone receptor status should be evaluated. Autopsy data from a 1993 study showed that second primary nonmammary malignancies, most commonly of the female genital and gastrointestinal systems, occurred in 11% of patients with breast cancer at a mean interval of nearly 7 years after diagnosis of primary breast cancer; half occurred in the first 4 years following diagnosis. In this series, the nonmammary primary tumor was the cause of death in 54% of patients, whereas breast cancer was the cause of death in 29%.[18]

TREATMENT

The selection of treatment is guided by the results of the previous evaluations, common sense, and the realization that metastatic breast cancer differs greatly in its clinical course from one patient to another. Reports of long-term follow-up in the era predating effective systemic therapy showed that a small fraction of patients survive for 10, 15, or even 20 years.[2] Metastatic disease often follows one of two patterns.[19,20] The first pattern is a relatively asymptomatic, indolent disease. Patients whose disease follows this pattern typically have primary disease that is estrogen receptor positive, a disease-free interval of longer than 2 years, and metastases to bone, soft-tissue, or non-life-threatening visceral sites. If such a patient has a small tumor burden and positive hormone receptors, hormonal therapies should be tried. Observation of incidental asymptomatic osteoblastic metastases until they become symptomatic is reasonable. The second pattern is a highly symptomatic, estrogen receptor-negative, aggressive, widely disseminated, life-threatening visceral disease. In patients with this type of metastatic disease, cytotoxic chemotherapy, with or without sequential radiation, is the treatment of choice.

The patient's age should not unduly influence the type of initial therapy. Although cytotoxic chemotherapy has not been studied extensively in elderly women, several studies have shown no difference in age-related response, time to treatment failure, survival, or major toxicity in women 70 years and older who received standard doses of conventional agents compared with younger women.[21]

Regardless of the regimen, only one systemic modality should be given at a time. The addition of hormones to chemotherapy is not generally recommended. Although the exact mechanism of action of most hormonal agents is not well understood, it is known that tamoxifen (Nolvadex), the most commonly used agent in hormonal therapy, arrests cells in the G_1 phase of the cell cycle. This is antagonistic to the action of most of the cytotoxic agents, the majority of which are most effective against cells actively progressing through the cell cycle.[22]

However, no adverse effect on response rate and survival has been reported with the use of combined hormonal and cytotoxic therapy in patients with metastatic disease[23]; in some postmenopausal women, the combination may increase the response rate by 10% to 20%.[24] Biopsy studies of metastatic lesions exposed to estrogenic recruitment before chemotherapy did show an increase in the fraction of cells in the S phase,[25] but estrogenic recruitment did not translate into improved response rates, time to disease progression, or median survival duration.[25,26] However, the risk of thromboembolic phenomena is increased when hormones and chemotherapy are combined, especially with regimens using cyclophosphamide (Cytoxan, Neosar), methotrexate, and fluorouracil (CMF) and prednisone.[27,28]

The choice of drugs for systemic therapy can be affected by any number of coexisting medical conditions. Diabetes may complicate the use of glucocorticoids, anabolic steroids, megestrol acetate, and neurotoxic drugs, such as vinblastine, cisplatin (Platinol), and paclitaxel (Taxol). Preexisting significant cardiovascular disease may also increase the potential cardiac toxicity of anthracyclines, mitoxantrone (Novantrone), mitomycin (Mutamycin), and high-dose cyclophosphamide. Cisplatin, the aminoglycosides, and ciprofloxacin (Cipro) can potentiate existing renal insufficiency; renal insufficiency may impair methotrexate clearance, and ureteral or urethral stenosis may enhance local cyclophosphamide toxicity. Doxorubicin (Adriamycin, Rubex), vincristine (Oncovin), vinblastine, and paclitaxel, which depend on hepatic clearance, may cause toxic reactions in patients with hyperbilirubinemia. Dementias of various causes seriously limit tolerance to any treatment.

At present, there is very little evidence that the biologic response modifiers have systemic efficacy in metastatic breast cancer. The one exception is intracavitary alpha interferon (IFN-α), which shows promise in the palliation of ascites or pleural effusions.[29]

Often overlooked in discussions with patients of the treatment of metastatic breast cancer is the important role of supportive services. Patients often require the services of social workers in obtaining compassionate-use drugs, financial assistance, hospital equipment, referral to counseling services, and disability payments. During their illness, patients may require consultation with experts in pain management and rehabilitative medicine. Women with minor children may require legal advice. Anticipation of the need for supportive services early in the course of a patient's illness and frank discussion of the nature of the disease often relieve anxiety and facilitate therapy.

Chemotherapy

Several clinical clues may predict the likelihood of response to treatment. Usually, better performance status, smaller tumor burden, and less prior exposure to chemotherapy all translate into a higher probability of response. In a previously untreated patient with a good performance status and small tumor burden, the response rate to chemotherapy ranges from 50% to 70%. If the patient has a poor performance status and an extensive tumor burden, the probability of response to chemotherapy is only 10% to 30%.[3,19] Age, menopausal status, hormone receptor status, and dominant disease site are not related to the probability of response to chemotherapy but are important to the response to hormonal therapy. With the exception of the central nervous system and the bones, the site of disease is less important than the volume of disease when estimating the probability of response.

Although current treatment modalities are palliative in most patients, some patients achieve durable complete or partial remission with standard-dose regimens after initial induction therapy. Restoring or maintaining response after initial treatment remains a therapeutic problem and an area of controversy. Some studies have suggested that although overall survival is unchanged, quality of life, time to disease progression, and tumor response are better in patients treated with maintenance chemotherapy after induction than in patients given intermittent chemotherapy for tumor progression.[30,31] In one study, reinduction with the same chemotherapeutic regimen for metastatic breast cancer showed an overall response rate of 18% and a time to treatment failure of 3 months, but 50% of the patients had life-threatening or severe toxic reactions. Response rates were high in patients initially in complete remission (44%) or partial remission (15%) but poor in patients with stable disease or no change.[32] Unfortunately, response rates decline rapidly with subsequent salvage attempts after induction therapy.

Several recent retrospective studies have shown overall response rates of 11% to 16% to either cytotoxic or hormonal salvage therapy after induction chemotherapy, but predicting who will benefit is still difficult.[33,34] These data are in agreement with the lack of enthusiasm among community medical oncologists for administering subsequent salvage regimens.[35] Clearly, the decision to pursue maintenance therapy after induction, subsequent salvage regimens, or observation and treatment for progression depends on tumor response, extent of palliation, and the patient's wishes.

Standard Regimens: Breast cancer is moderately sensitive to at least 25 agents; however, single-agent therapy is effective in only 20% to 30% of patients. Notably, the anthracyclines, alkylating agents, and taxanes produce response rates of 30% to 60% when given as single agents.[36-38] The most effective proven chemotherapeutic regimens are combinations of doxorubicin or its congeners, mitoxantrone, cyclophosphamide, methotrexate, and fluorouracil. Commonly used regimens are listed in Table 2.[39-41]

At the University of Texas M. D. Anderson Cancer Center, initial chemotherapy for metastatic breast cancer is usually a doxorubicin-based regimen, such as 5-fluorouracil, doxorubicin, and cyclophosphamide (FAC), with doxorubicin administered by a 48- to 72-hour infusion. The continuous infusion reduces nausea, vomiting, and cardiac damage.[42] Although doxorubicin is the most active single agent in the treatment of breast cancer, the difference in reported response rates between doxorubicin- and methotrexate-based regimens is only 10% to 15%, and differences in response duration and survival also have been small.[43-46]

The mean time to response to chemotherapy with these regimens varies with the site of disease. The mean time to response is 6 to 9 weeks in skin and nodes, 9 to 12 weeks in lungs, 15 to 18 weeks in liver, and 18 weeks in bone.[47] The median duration of response after the first remission is 9 to 12 months; this decreases to 3 to 6 months for subsequent remissions. The data from Coates et al[30] and Tannock et al[48] suggest that continuing therapy after response improves quality of life. Treatment is generally continued for an additional 3 to 6 months after the maximum response. Unfortunately, in many patients, the disease progresses by the time treatment is scheduled to be stopped. At this point, it is reasonable to consider a trial of a phase II regimen or other single agents that the patient has not received. Analysis of older clinical trials comparing survival advantage among patients treated with polychemotherapy vs single-drug chemotherapy in the phase II setting showed a very modest survival advantage (3.7 months) for patients receiving polychemotherapy.[49]

The heterogeneous behavior of metastatic breast cancer is such that some patients may still experience meaningful palliation with other standard drugs. Also, if the patient is more symptomatic from the increased tumor burden or the cumulative effect of prior treatments, toxicity is often increased. The median duration of survival is usually 24 to 30 months. Patients who have a complete remission tend to live longer than patients who have partial remissions or stable disease. However, patients whose disease is refractory to the initial chemotherapeutic regimen tend to do poorly, with a median survival of only 4 to 6 months regardless of the regimen used.[50,51]

Many phase II trials currently allow only one prior chemotherapeutic regimen for metastatic breast cancer. The expected benefits and toxicity of therapy should be clearly understood by the referring physician, the phase II investigator, and the patient.

Paclitaxel: Paclitaxel (Taxol) is the newest agent to show significant activity in untreated, heavily pretreated, and doxorubicin-refractory patients in phase I or II trials. Phase III trials comparing paclitaxel with standard regimens are ongoing. Paclitaxel is approved by the US Food and Drug Administration at a dose of 175 mg/m^2 by 3-hour infusion for treatment of breast cancer after failure of combination chemotherapy for metastatic disease or relapse within 6 months of adjuvant chemotherapy, provided that the previous chemotherapeutic regimen included an anthracycline.

The first reported phase II study of paclitaxel indicated an overall response rate of 56% (12% complete, 44% partial) in 25 evaluable patients, 14 of whom had previously received only adjuvant chemotherapy and 11 of whom had previously received chemotherapy for metastatic disease.[52] The median response duration was 9 months (range, 3 to 19 months), the median time to disease progression was 9 months (range, 1 to 20 months), and the median overall survival was 23 months (range, 5 to 29+ months). Only 8% of patients had progression of disease during therapy. This finding has been confirmed in phase II trials[38] of previously untreated metastatic disease. In most studies, 20% to 40% of patients had previously received adjuvant chemotherapy. Other studies have shown response rates with paclitaxel as a second-line or greater salvage regimen are 6% to 44%,[53,54] much higher than response rates with other cytotoxic drugs.

In vitro studies have demonstrated marginal cross-resistance between paclitaxel and doxorubicin.[55] Investigators at M. D. Anderson Cancer Center found that three of six doxorubicin-resistant patients responded to paclitaxel,[53] whereas investigators at Memorial Sloan-Kettering Cancer Center observed responses to paclitaxel in 38%, 32%, and 17% of patients who had received prior doxorubicin in one, two, and three regimens, respectively.[56] Gianni et al[57] found an overall response rate of 47% (three complete, four partial) in 15 patients with anthracycline-resistant metastatic breast cancer treated with 175 to 200 mg/m^2 paclitaxel given by 3-hour infusion every 21 days; the median response duration was only 7 months. Most recently, a phase I to II study using paclitaxel by 96-hour infusion in doxorubicin- or mitoxantrone-refractory patients defined the dose-limiting toxicity as mucositis and grade 4 granulocytopenia and the maximum tolerated dose as 140 mg/m^2, or as 105 mg/m^2 for patients with liver metastases and elevation of serum transaminase levels to more than 2.5 times the upper limit of normal.[58] The objective response rate was 48%, but an additional 15% of patients had clinically meaningful minor responses. The median progression-free survival was 27 weeks, and the overall survival was 43 weeks.[58]

The current optimal dose for paclitaxel in untreated, heavily pretreated, or doxorubicin-refractory metastatic breast cancer is under study. Paclitaxel schedules tested are 135, 175, or 250 mg/m^2 given by 24-hour continuous infusion or 135 or 175 mg/m^2 given over 3 hours every 21 days. The use of growth factors allows dose escalation, but neurotoxicity eventually becomes dose limiting.[59] Most phase II trials have used 24-hour infusion schedules with prophylactic steroids and H_1 and H_2 blockers to avoid the problem of hypersensitivity reactions (HSRs), seen in up to 18% of patients in phase I testing.[60] However, 3-hour infusions have recently been shown to be safe and less myelosuppressive and to have equivalent antitumor effect, at least in ovarian cancer.[61] A recent report of a phase I trial has also shown 1-hour infusion of paclitaxel to be safe.[62]

The recommended prophylactic regimen for HSRs in these studies is dexamethasone, 20 mg orally 12 and 6 hours prior to treatment, and diphenhydramine, 50 mg, with cimetidine, 300 mg intravenously 30 minutes prior to treatment; however, some studies have used dexamethasone, 20 mg intravenously, with cimetidine and diphenhydramine given 30 to 60 minutes before treatment. Starting doses of paclitaxel are usually decreased by 25% for patients who have been heavily pretreated, for example, patients who have received prior high-dose regimens, mitomycin, irradiation to more than 30% of marrow-containing bones, or two or more regimens and patients with poor tolerance to prior therapy manifested by frequent infections or delayed hematologic recovery. Paclitaxel doses must also be reduced significantly in patients with hepatic dysfunction manifested by elevated transaminases and bilirubin.[62a]

Paclitaxel has a unique pattern of toxicity. The side effects of paclitaxel given by 3- or 24-hour infusion can be divided into dose-dependent effects (for example, an early but brief granulocyte nadir, sensory and motor peripheral neuropathy, mucositis, and arthralgias/myalgias) and dose-independent effects (for example, total and sudden alopecia, HSRs, and rhythm disturbances).[63] Neuropathy may be cumulative but is reversible upon discontinuation of the drug. Mucositis is more pronounced with 96-hour infusion schedules, in which the dose is only 60% to 80% of the dose of 3- or 24-hour infusion schedules; however, prophylaxis for HSRs is not required.[58] Recently, optic-nerve disturbances causing photopsia, scotomata, and decreased visual acuity have been described in patients receiving more than 175 mg/m^2 by 3-hour infusion schedules; although most cases have been readily reversible with cessation of the infusion, some patients have sustained visual loss.[64,65] Radiation-recall dermatitis following paclitaxel infusion has also been described,[66] as has local irritation with extravasation.[67]

Given the high single-agent response rates of doxorubicin and paclitaxel, several groups of investigators have attempted to combine the two drugs[68] in phase I/II trials of previously untreated patients. However, there is emerging evidence from in vitro studies that concurrent doxorubicin and paclitaxel exposure, at least in cell lines, may be antagonistic. Paclitaxel might cause a G_2/M cell-cycle block, thereby leaving fewer cells in the S phase, the most doxorubicin-sensitive phase of the cell cycle.[69] When paclitaxel and doxorubicin are given by 24- or 72-hour infusion, either sequentially or concurrently, the re-

TABLE 2

Standard Chemotherapeutic Regimens in Metastatic Breast Cancer

Regimen	Drugs	Doses (mg/m^2)	Schedule
Initial chemotherapeutic regimens			
CMF—oral	Cyclophosphamide	100 mg PO total	Days 1 to 14 every 28 days
	Methotrexate	40 IV	Days 1 and 8 every 28 days
	Fluorouracil	600 IV	Days 1 and 8 every 28 days
CMF—IV	Cyclophosphamide	600 IV	Day 1 every 28 days
	Methotrexate	40 IV	Days 1 and 8 every 28 days
	Fluorouracil	600 IV	Days 1 and 8 every 28 days
FAC	Cyclophosphamide	500 IV	Day 1 every 21 days
	Doxorubicin	50 IV (or CI)	Day 1 every 21 days (48 to 72 hours)
	Fluorouracil	500 IV	Days 1 and 8 (or 4) every 21 days
VATH	Vinblastine	4.5 IV	Day 1 every 21 days
	Doxorubicin	45 IV	Day 1 every 21 days
	Thiotepa	12 IV	Day 1 every 21 days
	Halotestin	30 mg PO total	Daily
AC	Doxorubicin	60 IV	Day 1 every 21 days
	Cyclophosphamide	600 IV	Day 1 every 21 days
NFL-1	Mitoxantrone	12 IV	Day 1 every 21 days
	Fluorouracil	350 mg IV total	Days 1, 2, and 3 every 21 days
	Leucovorin	300 mg IV total	Each day before fluorouracil
NFL-2	Mitoxantrone	10 IV	Day 1 every 21 days
	Fluorouracil	1,000 IV over 24 h	Daily × 3 days every 21 days
	Leucovorin	350 IV over 15 min	Daily × 3 days every 21 days
Salvage regimens			
Paclitaxel	Paclitaxel	135 to 175/3 h IV	Every 21 days
		200 to 250/24 h IV	Every 21 days
		± G-CSF	
		140/96 h IV	Every 21 days
MV	Mitomycin	20 IV	Day 1 every 6 to 8 weeks
	Vinblastine	0.15 mg/kg IV	Day 1 every 3 to 4 weeks
2M	Mitoxantrone	6.5 IV	Day 1 every 21 days
	Methotrexate	30 IV	Day 1 every 21 days
(3M)	(Mitomycin)	(6.5 IV)	(Day 1 every 42 days)
Fluorouracil—CI	Fluorouracil	175 to 250 IV	By continuous infusion 2 to 3 weeks on, 1 to 2 weeks off; some do continuously
Doxorubicin	Doxorubicin	40 to 75 IV	Day 1 every 21 to 28 days
PE	Cisplatin	20 IV	Days 1 to 5 every 21 to 28 days
	Etoposide	60 IV	Days 1 to 5 every 21 to 28 days

CI = continuous infusion, G-CSF = granulocyte colony-stimulating factor (filgrastim)

sponse rates and duration are similar to those obtained when either drug is given alone. However, toxicities are schedule and sequence dependent. With concurrent 72-hour infusion of doxorubicin and paclitaxel, the gastrointestinal toxicity is primarily in the lower gastrointes-tinal tract and may include abdominal pain, diarrhea, and typhlitis.[70] When 24-hour infusion of paclitaxel is followed by 48-hour infusion of doxorubicin, stomatitis of the upper gastrointestinal tract is dose limiting,[68] whereas febrile neutropenia is dose limiting with the reverse sequence. Three-hour paclitaxel infusion followed by bolus infusion of doxorubicin has the same toxicity as the reverse sequence.[71] Pharmacokinetic data indicate that prior 24-hour infusion of paclitaxel reduces doxorubicin clearance, perhaps by altering the metabolism of doxorubicin in the liver.[72] Paclitaxel has been combined with cisplatin, carboplatin (Paraplatin), or cyclophosphamide in phase I studies,[73] and phase II trials of these combinations are ongoing. Because of the sequence-dependent toxicities that have been seen, combinations of paclitaxel with other drugs outside a clinical trial are not recommended.

Docetaxel: As initial therapy for metastatic disease, docetaxel (Taxotere) is at least as active as paclitaxel. In several phase II trials, docetaxel, at a dose of 100 mg/m² every 3 weeks, produced an overall response rate of 57% to 67% in patients previously untreated for metastatic disease,[74–76] with complete remissions in 15%, including patients with metastases to visceral sites, such as the liver. In one study of previously untreated patients,[74] the median duration of response was 44+ weeks; the median time to disease progression was 37+ weeks, and the median overall survival was 16+ months. Docetaxel is also active as salvage therapy; even in patients with anthracycline resistance, docetaxel produces an overall response rate of 60% (6% complete, 27% partial) and is highly active against liver metastases.[77–78] Overall response duration is reported as 38 weeks, and median time to disease progression is 23 weeks.[77] This makes docetaxel as active as or more active than conventional chemotherapy or paclitaxel for either initial or salvage chemotherapy for metastatic breast cancer. The activity of docetaxel in paclitaxel-refractory patients is unknown, and combinations of docetaxel with other drugs are currently being tested in phase I trials.[79]

However, docetaxel also has significant toxicities, some of which are unique. Grade 3 or 4 neutropenia and complete alopecia are common. Neurosensory toxicity appears to be less severe than it is with paclitaxel. Unique toxic effects result in skin changes, including erythema and desquamative dermatitis, onycholysis, and fluid retention. Fluid retention has been seen in responding patients with cumulative doses of docetaxel of 400 mg/m² and has necessitated cessation of therapy. Docetaxel has not been approved by the US Food and Drug Administration for the treatment of metastatic breast cancer outside clinical trials.

Vinorelbine: Vinorelbine (Navelbine), a semisynthetic vinca alkaloid, has been approved in France for non-small-cell lung cancer and breast cancer. In the United States, it has been approved for non-small-cell lung cancer but is still in phase II testing for breast cancer. From phase I testing, the recommended dose is 30 mg/m² intravenously per week. However, in most trials in the United States, investigators have not been able to administer the full dose. Often, the day-14 dose must be delayed because of neutropenia. A dose of 20 mg/m² appears to be more consistently tolerated. As a single agent in patients previously untreated for metastatic disease, vinorelbine produces overall response rates of 24% to 52%,[80–82] with average complete response and partial response rates of 7% and 34%, respectively. The median time to treatment failure is 6 months, the median duration of response is 9 months, and the median survival is 18 months[81] or not yet reached.[80]

Furthermore, vinorelbine is active in the salvage setting for patients who have received prior anthracyclines; the drug produces overall response rates of 16% to 36%.[83,84] Combinations of vinorelbine, 25 mg/m² intravenously on days 1 and 8, with doxorubicin, 50 mg/m² by short infusion on day 1 repeated every 21 days, produced an objective response in 74% of previously untreated patients (21% complete, 53% partial).[84] Responses were seen at all sites of disease, and no difference was noted in patients who had received anthracyclines in the adjuvant setting. The median duration of response was 12 months, and the median overall survival was 27.5 months. Neutropenia was seen, and in 10% of patients, treatment-related cardiotoxicity was noted.[85] Vinorelbine also has been combined with fluorouracil as initial therapy for metastatic disease; this combination produced an overall response rate of 70% in a small study.[86] Studies combining vinorelbine with paclitaxel are ongoing at M. D. Anderson and elsewhere.

Toxic reactions associated with vinorelbine include phlebitis at a peripheral-vein insertion site, myelosuppression, peripheral neuropathy, and myalgias. Transient increases in aspartate aminotransferase and alanine aminotransferase levels were reported in approximately 50% of patients but did not require discontinuation of therapy.[87] In up to 5% of patients, a unique respiratory toxic effect may occur; it includes both an acute reaction, which resembles bronchospasm and is readily reversible with bronchodilators, and a subacute reaction of cough and dyspnea, which occurs within 1 hour and is treated with steroids.[87]

Investigational Agents: Drug development has proceeded rapidly in the past few years in an attempt to find single agents with high activity and low toxicity that produce durable responses. Table 3 lists several of these agents.[88] Referral of patients to centers studying these agents should be encouraged when clinically appropriate.

TABLE 3

Investigational Agents for Metastatic Breast Cancer

Class	Agent
Alkylator	Temozolomide
	Adozelisin
Angiogenesis inhibitors	TNP-470
Antimetabolites	Edatrexate
	ICI D1694
	Gemcitabine
DNA intercalators	Losoxantone
	Piroxantrone
	Pyrazoloacridine
Retinoids (differentiating agents)	All-*trans*-retinoic acid (ATRA)
	N-(4-hydroxyphenyl) retinamide (4HPR)
Topoisomerase-1 inhibitors	Topotecan
	CPT-11
	9-amino camptothecin (9-AC)
Unknown mechanisms of action	Penclomidine

High-Dose Chemotherapy: "High-dose" chemotherapy refers to the administration of pulsed, large doses of cytotoxic drugs, which results in very high peak concentrations, whereas "dose intensity" refers to the amount of drug administered per unit of time, usually reported in mg/m²/wk.[89]

Autologous bone marrow or peripheral blood stem-cell infusion allows the dose intensity of the chemotherapeutic regimen to be escalated to the point of marrow aplasia. (This is addressed in detail in other chapters.) Until conclusive phase III trials are completed, high-dose chemotherapy with autotransplantation, although promising, is still considered investigational. Prospective trials comparing standard- and high-dose strategies are ongoing. High-dose chemotherapy may be a reasonable option for some patients. The overall response rate ranges from 6% to 94%, with a high fraction of complete responders (36%). Treatment-related mortality is 5% to 15%, but most patients (67%) have a relapse. Historic comparisons with patients treated with standard-dose chemotherapy have not shown an increase in median response duration and overall survival with the use of high-dose chemotherapy, although disease-free survival may be improved.[90-92]

One drawback to the current studies of high-dose chemotherapy is that the agents used to achieve marrow aplasia, for example, carmustine (BiCNU), etoposide (VePesid), or cisplatin, are not the most active agents in breast cancer. The optimal regimen would escalate active agents against breast cancer to a maximum tolerated dose determined by nonmyelosuppressive toxicities. Studies by Tannock et al[48] and Engelsman et al[93] and a retrospective analysis of previous trials by Hryniuk and Bush[94] support a relationship between dose intensity and response to initial chemotherapy in metastatic breast cancer for the combination of cyclophosphamide, fluorouracil, and either methotrexate or doxorubicin. The relationship between response and dose intensity for other active agents is either unproven or under study. Generally, the best results usually are seen in patients who have responded to induction therapies.

Serious toxic effects have been noted, however, especially with carmustine-containing regimens. Toxicity increases when comorbid conditions are present. These serious toxic effects include prolonged thrombocytopenia and immunosuppression, hepatic veno-occlusive disease, and interstitial pneumonitis. Mortality may decrease in the future with more experience and with the use of colony-stimulating factors, especially thrombopoietins, and autologous stem cells.

Complications: Because treatment of metastatic breast cancer is primarily palliative, it is important to anticipate and recognize the complications of chemotherapy. One of the most serious problems is neutropenia with fever or rigor; patients with this condition should be presumed to have sepsis until a complete evaluation proves otherwise. In anticipation of this complication, patients should be instructed to monitor their temperatures and to contact the physician promptly if the temperature rises to 38.3°C or higher, especially during the expected myelosuppressive period, which generally lasts from day 10 to day 18 after treatment is started (or earlier, from day 8 to day 10, for paclitaxel). If the patient has a temperature of 38.3°C or higher and has an absolute granulocyte count (the white blood cell count multiplied by the percentage of granulocytes) of less than 1,000/μL, or symptoms of toxemia or sepsis, intravenous broad-spectrum antibiotics effective against both gram-negative and gram-positive organisms should be started immediately after cultures are obtained. Gram-positive coverage is crucial if the patient has an indwelling catheter. At M. D. Anderson, we generally use a combination of anti-pseudomonal penicillin or third-generation cephalosporin with vancomycin or clindamycin. Antibiotic use should be tailored to an institution's prevailing organisms and susceptibility patterns.

Many oncologists use hematopoietic growth factors

empirically to increase or maintain dose intensity by reducing the incidence of febrile neutropenic events and infections, shortening hospitalizations, and obviating the need for antibiotics; however, there is no evidence that this practice produces a survival benefit.[95] In addition, the benefit of receiving hematopoietic growth factors with empiric antibiotic therapy during febrile neutropenia is unknown.[96] However, in the presence of a documented infection, a granulocyte count of 1,000/μL or lower, or an expected period of granulocytopenia exceeding 5 to 7 days, the use of growth factors is probably warranted.[97]

Stomatitis may be prevented or reduced by attending to any dental problems seen during the prechemotherapy dental evaluation and instructing the patient in appropriate oral hygiene. Herpes infection must be entertained as a diagnosis if the patient develops oral lesions that are particularly painful, punched out in appearance, or located on the hard palate. Doxorubicin, fluorouracil, and paclitaxel given by infusion may increase the incidence of mucositis and diarrhea and can exacerbate hemorrhoids. Attention to oral and rectal hygiene, as well as the use of topical oral analgesia, antimotility agents, and sitz baths, can prevent or reduce the severity of these complications. If severe odynophagia occurs, a barium swallow is indicated to assess for *Candida* esophagitis. An appropriate antiemetic or combination of antiemetics before, during, and after chemotherapy is important to prevent and control nausea and vomiting. Thrombosis or infection in chronic indwelling catheters can be prevented by appropriately timed heparin injections and dressing changes. Recently, Fraschini et al have shown that the use of the thrombolytic agent urokinase, instead of heparin, in implanted venous access devices may reduce the incidence of both infection and thrombosis.[98]

Hormonal Therapy

Principles: When systemic therapy is indicated, endocrine therapy is an appropriate first step in patients with the following clinical characteristics: indolent disease course; positive estrogen-receptor (ER) or progesterone-receptor (PR) status; disease-free interval longer than 2 to 5 years; postmenopausal status; or disease limited to the soft tissues, such as the nodes, chest wall, or skin. Other indications are cachexia, failure to thrive, and anorexia. Currently, hormonal castration obviates surgery as a first choice; there is no indication for adrenalectomy or hypophysectomy. There are no conclusive data to support combined hormonal treatments. In trials of combinations, some minimal increases in response rate were seen, but there was no significant improvement in survival, and additional toxicity was observed.[99-101]

There are three clinical approaches to estrogen deprivation of breast tumors. One approach is to block estrogen by use of antiestrogens (such as tamoxifen) or androgens (such as halotestin); the probability of response depends on the status of hormone receptors in the tumor. The second approach is to inhibit gonadotropin-induced estrogen production by use of gonadotropin agonist-antagonists (luteinizing hormone-releasing hormone [LHRH] inhibitory agents), which are less effective in postmenopausal women.[102] The third approach is to decrease estrogen biosynthesis by inhibiting the aromatase enzyme, which catalyzes the final step in estrogen production in humans. This does not completely block ovarian estrogen production in premenopausal women, and there is concern that use of a single agent may cause a reflex increase in gonadotropin levels and result in an ovarian hyperstimulation syndrome. Thus, aromatase inhibitors (for example, aminoglutethimide) should be used primarily in postmenopausal women[103]; they are not effective in premenopausal women.[104]

Hormone Receptors and Response: The probability of response to hormone therapy is directly related to the status of hormone receptors. If the tumor is negative for both ER and PR, the probability of response is less than 10%. If ER is negative and PR is positive or vice versa, the response rate is 30% to 60%. Finally, if both ER and PR are positive, the response rate ranges from 75% to 80%.[105] The quantitative ER level also correlates positively with the response rate, as seen in Table 4.[106] Recently, quantitative PR levels have been shown to correlate significantly and independently with increased response to tamoxifen, longer time to treatment failure, and longer overall survival in patients with ER-positive tumors.[107]

Approximately 30% of women whose ER status is unknown will respond to the first hormonal manipulation. Of patients with a prior history of hormonal re-

TABLE 4

Correlation of Estrogen Receptor Levels With Response Rates

Estrogen receptor level (fmol/mg protein)	Response rate (%)
0–9	3/33 (9%)
10–20	3/10 (30%)
21–49	7/11 (63%)
> 50	24/31 (77%)

Adapted, with permission, from Allegra JC, Lippman ME, Thompson EB, et al: Eur J Cancer 16:323–331, 1980

sponse, 33% to 50% will respond to another hormonal regimen. Patients with low-volume disease and better performance status generally have higher response rates. The duration of first response is usually 9 to 12 months, similar to that with chemotherapy. The side-effect profile aids in the determination of which hormonal therapy to use, because the efficacy of all agents is nearly equal.[19,108,109] Additionally, for patients whose tumors are unusually sensitive to hormonal manipulation, retreatment with a previously effective agent may again be effective if a long interval has elapsed since it was discontinued.

Side Effects: Endocrine therapy is usually milder and more tolerable than cytotoxic chemotherapy. However, several unique complications of endocrine therapy should be anticipated. One such complication, flare, is defined clinically by an abrupt, diffuse onset of musculoskeletal pain, increased size of skin lesions, or erythema surrounding the skin lesion within the first month of endocrine therapy. There is no published evidence that tumor growth rates increase during this period. The most serious manifestation of flare is hypercalcemia, which can be seen with all hormonal therapies except aminoglutethimide and castration. Hypercalcemia usually occurs in patients with bone metastases and manifests within the first 2 weeks after treatment. The underlying mechanism is the predominating early agonist effect of hormonal agents. Low doses of prednisone (10 to 30 mg/d) may abrogate the initial flare of bone pain. The patient should be instructed about the possibility of flare and should undergo serum calcium level monitoring on a weekly basis for the first 2 weeks. If hypercalcemia develops, the calcium level should be controlled and treatment continued, provided the serum calcium level is lower than 14 mg/dL.

All hormonal regimens except the aromatase inhibitors may cause weight gain. This side effect is most common with progestins, which can lead to both a true increase in weight, from their anabolic effect, and fluid retention, secondary to their glucocorticoid effect. Progestins are the drugs most likely to cause thromboembolism; tamoxifen is the next most likely drug to cause this complication. Both drugs have been reported to prolong the prothrombin time in patients who are also receiving warfarin.[110,111]

Active Agents and Complications: Table 5 summarizes the current recommended hormonal treatment sequences for both premenopausal and postmenopausal women.[108] Whether tamoxifen or progestins are the preferred initial therapy in postmenopausal women, is still a subject of debate,[112] but the side-effect profile often

TABLE 5

Recommended Hormonal Treatment Sequences for Metastatic Breast Cancer

Therapy	Premenopausal	Postmenopausal
First line	Tamoxifen or an LHRH antagonist	Tamoxifen or a progestin
Second line	LHRH antagonist or a progestin	Progestin or tamoxifen
Third line	Androgen	Aromatase inhibitor, eg, aminoglutethimide or anastrozole
Fourth line	Diethylstilbestrol or oophorectomy [a]	Androgen

LHRH = leuteinizing hormone-releasing hormone

[a] Oophorectomy may be considered in patients who are premenopausal or within 1 year of their last menstrual period.

Adapted, with permission, from Buzdar AU: Semin Surg Oncol 6:77–82, 1990.

dictates the choice. Several studies have shown increased response rates, improved median time to treatment failure, and improved survival with high-dose medroxyprogesterone acetate as the initial therapy, but toxicity in terms of thromboembolic events, weight gain, increased systolic blood pressure, and fatigue is increased with the use of this drug.[113,114] The aromatase inhibitor 4-OHA (4-hydroxyandrostenedione, Lentaron) is effective and widely used in the United Kingdom. It is administered intramuscularly every 2 weeks.[115] This drug is not approved for use in the United States.

Tamoxifen: Tamoxifen is one of the least toxic hormones used in the treatment of breast cancer. Its most frequent side effect is hot flashes. Mild nausea may occur but usually disappears after a few weeks of therapy. These side effects are rarely severe enough to discontinue the regimen. Transient thrombocytopenia and, rarely, leukopenia have been seen during the first week of treatment, but they usually require no monitoring. A minority of patients experience depression and weight gain.[116,117] A dose of 20 mg at bedtime is often better tolerated than 10 mg twice daily.[118]

Concern over the safety of tamoxifen in the adjuvant setting for primary breast cancer has emerged and may affect its use in the patient with low-volume, asymptomatic metastatic disease who may have a long anticipated survival. Recent reports have found that women receiving adjuvant tamoxifen for primary breast cancer for 2 years or greater have a 2- to 6-fold increase in endometrial cancer than women in the general population.[119,120] While data on the incidence of endometrial cancers developing in women taking tamoxifen for metastatic breast cancer is lacking, women with an intact uterus should undergo annual pelvic examinations and endometrial ultrasonography or biopsy, or both, should be performed when there is any abnormal finding or history of bleeding.

Megestrol Acetate: The most commonly used progestin is megestrol acetate (Megace). Like tamoxifen, it may cause mild nausea, flare, and hot flashes, but it is also associated with more thromboembolic effects, weight gain, glucose intolerance, and increase in blood pressure. In patients who have an intact uterus, vaginal bleeding will occur when progestins are discontinued, and patients should be so advised. A minority of patients will experience an Addisonian syndrome after withdrawal of progestins because of the glucocorticoid effects of these agents.

Aminoglutethimide: The major side effect of aminoglutethimide (Cytadren), which is closely related to the rarely used sedative-hypnotic glutethimide, is sedation. Initially, up to one third of treated patients may experience lethargy, but this may be ameliorated by initiating treatment at a lower dose, 250 mg twice daily, with full replacement doses of hydrocortisone. One recommended regimen is hydrocortisone, 10 mg in both the morning and afternoon with 20 mg at bedtime; alternatively, cortisone acetate, 25 mg in the morning and 12.5 mg in the evening, may be associated with fewer Cushingoid symptoms. Fludrocortisone acetate (Flurinef), 0.1 mg every other day or three times a week, may also be required for mineralocorticoid replacement. After 1 to 2 weeks, the therapeutic dose, 250 mg every 6 hours, may be started. In addition, during the initial 2 to 3 weeks of therapy, nearly 25% of patients develop a maculopapular, erythematous, pruritic rash that usually disappears without additional treatment. Some patients require a transient increase in steroid dosages.[104,109] A total of 5% to 10% of patients develop a "flu-like" syndrome of myalgia and fever that requires discontinuation of the drug. Recent data suggest that a lower dose of aminoglutethimide (250 mg twice daily) may be as effective as the standard dose of 1,000 mg daily. 4-OHA is better tolerated than aminoglutethimide, with reported side effects including pain at the injection site, hot flashes, lethargy, rash, transient leukopenia, facial swelling, and, rarely, anaphylaxis.[121]

Metastases at Specific Sites

Isolated Hepatic Metastases: In a review of 1,171 patients who received chemotherapy for metastatic breast cancer at M. D. Anderson, 233 (20%) had liver metastases, either isolated or with other sites of metastatic disease.[122] Standard treatment of liver metastases is chemotherapy, although hormonal therapies may provide a transient benefit in asymptomatic patients with low-volume, ER-positive disease. Resection of liver metastases cannot be recommended, except in selected cases.[123] Hepatic artery infusion of chemotherapeutic agents may expose the tumor to a higher drug concentration. The overall response rate to intra-arterial infusion therapy is 50%.[124,125] No phase III trials have been performed to compare this approach with standard intravenous therapy. Reported phase II trials for breast cancer have used intra-arterial infusion of fluorouracil, fluorouracil plus mitomycin, floxuridine (FUDR), vinblastine, cisplatin plus vinblastine, or FAC.[126] The potential side effects are chemical cholecystitis, gastric ulceration, pancreatitis, sclerosing cholangitis (more common with chronic use of fluorouracil or floxuridine), and occlusion of the femoral artery. A high response rate can be seen in patients with liver-predominant disease, but the impact of intra-arterial infusion therapy on overall survival remains unknown.

Bone Metastases: Breast cancer metastases to bone are lytic (48%), blastic (13%), or mixed (38%) or a diffuse osteoporosis without bone destruction (1%); they are the initial metastases in 29% to 46% of patients with breast cancer and may develop in up to 70% of patients during the course of the disease.[127] Although patients with bone-predominant or bone-only metastases often have prolonged survival, this is usually offset by substantial clinical morbidity. Clinically, bone metastases manifest as pain, pathologic fracture, limited mobility, hypercalcemia, nerve-root or spinal-cord compression, and compromised hematopoiesis. Because patients with bone metastases often have metastases to other sites as well, the first approach is to employ the most effective systemic therapy. Localized complications are managed by orthopedic surgery or neurosurgery with or without external-beam radiation; the optimal dose and fractionation schedule are controversial.[128] The response to chemotherapy or external-beam radiation often parallels the systemic response and is notoriously difficult to measure by plain films or nuclear bone scans.[129] Treatment of bone metastases can be undertaken either as an adjunct to anticancer therapy or as palliation of bone pain when the patient's tumor is refractory to further therapy.

Understanding the pathogenesis of malignant bone disease has allowed for the development of therapies specifically targeted to the skeleton. Bone-seeking radio-isotopes have been developed in an attempt to deliver medium- to high-energy beta radiation directly to tumor-involved sites in the skeleton while sparing normal tissues. One of the most promising agents to date has been strontium 89 (^{89}Sr).[130] This radioisotope is chemically similar to calcium, is preferentially deposited in skeletal tissue, and may be absorbed 10-fold more by bone metastases than by bone marrow. It is most efficacious in *blastic* bony metastases. Its biologic half-life is longer than 50 days at sites of bone metastases, compared with 14 days in normal bone; its physical half-life allows for a long shelf-life in the pharmacy. Most studies have used relief of bone pain as the principal endpoint; its effect on overall survival, fracture rate, and other markers of tumor progression is unknown. A total of 50% to 89% of patients with breast cancer experience moderate or greater pain relief. Side effects are limited to a transient flare in bone pain 1 to 2 days after injection in 15% of patients (usually predictive of a clinical response) and mild, reversible thrombocytopenia and leukopenia 5 to 6 weeks after treatment.

Bisphosphonates are synthetic analogs of the endogenous substance pyrophosphate and are capable of regulating bone turnover by inhibiting osteoclast activity by mechanisms that are not well understood. They are used clinically to treat Paget's disease of bone, osteoporosis, and hypercalcemia, and they have been evaluated for the treatment of bone metastases in breast and prostate cancer and multiple myeloma.[131] Three bisphosphonates are currently available: etidronate (Didronel), pamidronate (Aredia), and clodronate. (Clodronate and the oral formulation of pamidronate have not been approved in the United States.)

Several double-blind, placebo-controlled studies have suggested that prophylactic oral clodronate or pamidronate treatment of patients with metastatic breast cancer reduces osseous complications, such as hypercalcemic events, vertebral fractures, and bone pain, and promotes healing of osteolytic lesions.[132–135] In two studies, a survival benefit was seen.[136] These data, which suggest that the bisphosphonates also inhibit tumor growth in bone, are the basis for planned studies in the adjuvant setting. Side effects, mainly nausea and vomiting, led to drug discontinuance for some patients. Studies of less toxic oral bisphosphonates are ongoing. Pamidronate can be given safely intravenously in high doses (90 mg intravenously) in an outpatient setting on a monthly basis without significant side effects; it relieves bone pain and promotes healing of lytic lesions in 25% of patients.[137]

Stage IV—No Evidence of Disease: In 1% to 10% of patients who have metastatic breast cancer, the metastasis is an isolated lesion in a location from which it can be removed by either irradiation or surgery; the disease is then classified as stage IV with no evidence of disease (NED). From 50% to 80% of patients with stage IV-NED disease develop systemic disease within 2 years despite curative local therapies. The 5-year survival rate ranges from 4% to 36%.[138–140] The most common situation involves patients with an isolated chest-wall recurrence; 50% have distant metastases upon further investigation and 25% develop other metastases within several months. The remaining 25% have a single, isolated lesion. Half of chest-wall nodules are solitary and near the mastectomy incision. If they are not controlled, these nodules have a significant impact on the quality of life. The dismal survival rates after a chest-wall recurrence are quite different from those after a recurrence in a breast treated by conservative surgery and irradiation; 50% to 60% of these patients can be salvaged with surgery alone.[141] There is some disagreement in the literature about whether local or systemic therapy is more appropriate. It is reasonable to provide the optimum local regimen with surgery and irradiation whenever possible. Although the use of systemic therapy is controversial, the literature supports the use of CMF or FAC for 6 to 8 cycles, tamoxifen, or both in sequence or combined.[142,143]

Brain Metastases: Metastases to the brain are usually a late finding. The overall incidence of brain metastases in autopsy studies is 30%; only 10% of patients with brain metastases were symptomatic during life.[144] Headache may occur in approximately 50% of affected patients. Computed tomography or magnetic resonance imaging with contrast is the diagnostic test of choice. The median survival after diagnosis is 4 months, with a wide range.[145] A patient with an isolated, resectable brain metastasis may improve after surgery followed by radiation therapy.[146] However, whole-brain irradiation is the treatment of choice in patients with multiple brain lesions or widespread or uncontrolled metastatic disease. Because seizure occurs in only 20% to 30% of patients with brain metastases, only these patients require anticonvulsants.[147] Of note, there is an association between the development of erythema multiforme or the Stevens-Johnson syndrome in patients receiving phenytoin and corticosteroids during whole-brain irradiation.[148]

Leptomeningeal Disease: Metastases to the leptomeninges occur in approximately 1% to 5% of patients with metastatic breast cancer. They usually present as progressive neurologic dysfunction involving multiple central nervous system sites. Untreated, they usually are fatal in 4 to 6 weeks. Clinically, symptoms and signs are grouped by the site of origin: cerebrum, cranial nerve, or spinal cord. Treatment consists of whole-brain irradiation and intrathecal chemotherapy with methotrexate or thiotepa (Thioplex). Systemic chemotherapy alone is ineffective, although there are reports of high levels of the active metabolite of thiotepa achieving potentially therapeutic cerebrospinal fluid levels after intravenous administration.[149] Neurotoxic effects from radiation and chemotherapy are additive. Median survival from the time of diagnosis is 6 months in responders but only 6 weeks in nonresponders.[150-151]

Epidural Metastases: In several large series, breast cancer was the most common malignancy to cause epidural compression of the spinal cord and cauda equina. Approximately 60% to 70% of these patients will have multiple lesions in the vertebral column; the thoracic spine is the most frequently affected site, followed by the lumbosacral spine and the cervical spine.[152-155] In patients with bony metastases, complaints of back pain, weakness, sensory loss, or sphincter dysfunction should arouse suspicion of spinal cord compression. Early diagnosis and treatment are imperative in preventing any further neurologic damage. Magnetic resonance imaging with gadolinium is the diagnostic method of choice; computed tomographic scanning with contrast is also informative. Myelography is painful and potentially dangerous. Treatment usually consists of high-dose steroids and radiation.[153-155] However, surgery can be considered in a patient who develops compression at a previously irradiated site. Surgery should also be considered a reasonable choice when the diagnosis is in question or in patients with neurologic deterioration despite radiation therapy.[156,157] Once spinal-cord compression develops, treatment may not restore any function that was lost, but it can prevent any further deterioration.

Evaluation of Treatment Response

The assessment of response should not be based on a single test but, rather, on the examination of the patient as a whole. Patients should be examined at regular intervals to ensure that therapy continues to be beneficial. The examination begins with a history and physical examination, with attention given to known sites of metastases and the clinical symptoms associated with these metastases. A history of improvement in clinical symptoms may provide some clinical evidence of response. Examples of such improvement include a reduction in the levels and locations of pain in patients with bony metastases; a decrease in pulmonary symptoms in patients with intrathoracic involvement; and a reduction in symptoms of anorexia, weight loss, malaise, and right upper-quadrant pain in patients with known liver metastases.

All lesions accessible to physical examination should be measured and compared with baseline and prior measurements. Any neurologic finding, nonspecific headache, nausea, or vomiting should be evaluated by further diagnostic studies.

The biologic markers CEA and CA 15-3 generally parallel the clinical course. However, they may also rise paradoxically after a new treatment is initiated.[158,159] If the patient has liver metastases, liver function studies usually improve with effective therapy. However, some chemotherapeutic agents, such as methotrexate, doxorubicin, and the androgen hormones, may produce elevations in transaminase levels. Although alkaline phosphatase is a marker of bone and liver disease, its levels also may rise with healing of bone lesions. Serum calcium levels rise during the flare response, which may begin within the first 2 weeks after treatment. A later rise in this parameter may indicate progressive disease.

The computed tomographic scan is effective in monitoring liver and abdominal metastases. Although thoracic computed tomographic scanning is more sensitive than chest x-rays in defining the sizes of intrathoracic metastases, chest x-rays are usually sufficient to evaluate responses. Bone response can be difficult to assess if the disease is primarily blastic. Improvement of lytic lesions appears on the radiograph as no change, a rim of calcification, or complete reossification. If the lytic or blastic lesion responds to treatment, the nuclear bone scan will initially show increasing intensity in the previously demonstrated lesions but no new lesions. After the healing has stopped and the bones are metabolically quiet, the intensity usually decreases. Thus, the nuclear bone scan is useful in detecting the sites of bony metastases, especially when patients develop new symptoms and plain radiographs are normal. However, reliance on the nuclear bone scan alone to determine response may be misleading.[129] In some patients, metastatic disease involves the bone marrow more than the cortical bone. Magnetic resonance imaging is the only modality that will effectively image bone and bone marrow (generally the vertebral bodies).

CONCLUSIONS

Metastatic breast cancer remains a challenging disease to manage in the 1990s. Most patients are best managed with the judicious use of local and systemic therapies to achieve maximum palliation with minimal toxicity. However, decades of research on basic tumor biology, mechanisms of resistance, drug development, radiopharmaceuticals, and hematopoietic growth factors have yielded many promising approaches for combating this common and disabling disease. Most of these approaches are being tested clinically, and many are available through clinical trials for interested patients.

Acknowledgments: The authors appreciate the secretarial assistance of Judy Dillon.

REFERENCES

1. Wingo PA, Tong T, Bolden S: Cancer statistics, 1995. CA Cancer J Clin 45:8–30, 1995.

2. Bloom HJG: Natural history of untreated breast cancer (1805-1933). Br Med J 1:213–221, 1962.

3. Swenerton KD, Legha SS, Smith T, et al: Prognostic factors in metastatic breast cancer treated with combination chemotherapy. Cancer Res 39:1552–1562, 1979.

4. Liotta LA: Cancer invasion and metastasis. JAMA 263:1123–1126, 1990.

5. Bae S-N, Arand G, Azzam H, et al: Molecular and cellular analysis of basement membrane invasion by human breast cancer cells in Matrigel-based in vitro assays. Breast Cancer Res Treat 24:241–255, 1993.

6. Brunner N, Boysen B, Romer J, et al: The nude mouse as an in vivo model for human breast cancer invasion and metastasis. Breast Cancer Res Treat 24:257–264, 1993.

7. Porter-Jordan K, Lippman ME: Overview of the biologic markers of breast cancer. Hematol Oncol Clin North Am 8:73–100, 1994.

8. Van den Hooff A: The role of stromal cells in tumor metastasis: A new link. Cancer Cells 3:186-187, 1991.

9. Jain S, Fisher C, Smith P, et al: Patterns of metastatic breast cancer in relation to histological type. Eur J Cancer 29A(suppl):2155–2157, 1993.

10. McGuire WL, Clark GM: Prognostic factors and treatment decision in axillary-node-negative breast cancer. N Engl J Med 326:1756–1761, 1992.

11. De Lena M, Romero A, Rabinovich M, et al: Metastatic pattern and DNA ploidy in stage IV breast cancer at initial diagnosis: Relation to response and survival. Am J Clin Oncol 16:245–249, 1993.

12. Hayes DF, Zurawski VRJ, Kufe DW: Comparison of circulating CA 15-3 and carcinoembryonic antigen levels in patients with breast cancer. J Clin Oncol 4:1542–1550, 1986.

13. Tormey D, Waalkes T: Clinical correlation between CEA and breast cancer. Cancer 42:1507-1511, 1978.

14. Lee YN: Carcinoembryonic antigen as a monitor of recurrent breast cancer. J Surg Oncol 20:109–114, 1982.

15. Tondini C, Hayes DF, Gelman R, et al: Comparison of CA 15-3 and carcinoembryonic antigen in monitoring the clinical course of patients with metastatic breast cancer. Cancer Res 48:4107–4112, 1988.

16. White DR, Maloney JJ III, Muss HB, et al: Serum alkaline phosphatase determination: Value in the staging for advanced breast cancer. JAMA 242:1147–1149, 1979.

17. Khansur T, Haick A, Patel B, et al: Evaluation of bone scan as a screening workup in primary and local regional recurrence of breast cancer. Am J Clin Oncol 10:167–170, 1987.

18. Mamounas EP, Perez-Mesa C, Penetrante RB, et al: Patterns of occurrence of second primary nonmammary malignancies in breast cancer patients: Results from 1382 consecutive autopsies. Surg Oncol 2:175–185, 1993.

19. Henderson IC, Canellos GP: Cancer of the breast: The past decade. N Engl J Med 302:17–30, 1980.

20. Tormey DC, Gelman R, Band PR, et al: Comparison of induction chemotherapies for metastatic breast cancer. Cancer 50:1235–1244, 1982.

21. Muss HB: The role of chemotherapy and adjuvant therapy in management of breast cancer in older women. Cancer 74:2165–2171, 1994.

22. Hug V, Hortobagyi GN, Drewinko B, et al: Tamoxifen citrate counteracts the antitumor effects of cytotoxic drugs in vitro. J Clin Oncol 3:1672–1677, 1985.

23. Australian and New Zealand Breast Cancer Trial Group: A randomized trial in postmenopausal patients with advanced breast cancer comparing endocrine and cytotoxic therapy given sequentially or in combination. J Clin Oncol 4:186–193, 1986.

24. Mouridsen HT, Rose CJ, Engelsman E, et al: Combined cytotoxic and endocrine therapy in postmenopausal patients with advanced breast cancer: A randomized study of CMF vs CMF plus tamoxifen. Eur J Clin Oncol 21:219–299, 1985.

25. Fabian CJ, Kimler BF, McKittrick R, et al: Recruitment with high physiological doses of estradiol preceding chemotherapy: Flow cytometric and therapeutic results in women with locally advanced breast cancer—A Southwest Oncology Group study. Cancer Res 54:5357–5362, 1994.

26. Paridaens R, Heuson JC, Veyret JC, et al: Assessment of estrogenic recruitment before chemotherapy in advanced breast cancer: A double-blind randomized study. J Clin Oncol 11:1723–1728, 1993.

27. Levin MN, Gent M, Hirsh J, et al: The thrombogenic effect of anticancer drug therapy in women with stage II breast cancer. N Engl J Med 318:404–407, 1988.

28. Goodnough LT, Saito H, Manni A, et al: Increased incidence of thromboembolism in stage IV breast cancer patients treated with a five-drug chemotherapy regimen. Cancer 54:1264–1268, 1984.

29. Markowitz A: Beneficial effects of intracavitary interferon-alpha 2B: A phase I study of patients wivth ascites or pleural effusion (abstract 841). Proc Am Soc Clin Oncol 11:258, 1992.

30. Coates A, Gebski V, Stat M, et al: Improving the quality of life during chemotherapy for advanced breast cancer. N Engl J Med 317:1490–1495, 1987.

31. Muss HB, Case LD, Richards II F, et al: Interrupted versus continuous chemotherapy in patients with metastatic breast cancer. N Engl J Med 325:1342–1348, 1991.

32. Falkson G, Gelman R, Glick J, et al: Reinduction with the same cytostatic treatment in patients with metastatic breast cancer: An Eastern Cooperative Oncology Group study. J Clin Oncol 12:45–49, 1994.

33. Porkka K, Blomqvist C, Rissanen P, et al: Salvage therapies in women who fail to respond to first-line treatment with fluorouracil, epirubicin, and cyclophosphamide for advanced breast cancer. J Clin Oncol 12:1639–1647, 1994.

34. Gregory WM, Smith P, Richards MA, et al: Chemotherapy of advanced breast cancer: Outcome and prognostic factors. Br J Cancer 68:988–995, 1993.

35. Benner SE, Fetting JH, Brenner MH: A stopping rule for standard chemotherapy for metastatic breast cancer: Lessons from a survey of Maryland medical oncologists. Cancer Invest 12:451–455, 1994.

36. Hoogstraten B, Fabian C: A reappraisal of single drugs for advanced breast cancer. Cancer Clin Trials 2:101–198, 1979.

37. Taylor SG IV, Gelber R: Experience of the Eastern Cooperative Oncology Working Group with doxorubicin as a single agent in patients with previously untreated breast cancer. Cancer Treat Rep 66:1594–1595, 1982.

38. Arbuck SG, Dorr A, Friedman MA: Paclitaxel (Taxol) in breast cancer. Hematol Oncol Clin North Am 8:121–140, 1994.

39. Greenberg EF: The treatment of metastatic breast cancer. CA

Cancer J Clin 41:242–256, 1991.

40. Cameron DA, Gabra H, Leonard RCF: Continuous 5-fluoro-uracil in the treatment of breast cancer. Br J Cancer 70:120–124, 1994.

41. Fisher B, Osborne CK, Margolee R, et al: Neoplasms of the breast, in Holland JI, Frei E III, Bast RC, et al (eds): Cancer Medicine, pp 1706–1774. Philadelphia, Lea & Febiger, 1993.

42. Hortobagyi GN, Frye D, Buzdar AU, et al: Decreased cardiac toxicity of doxorubicin administered by continuous intravenous infusion in combination chemotherapy for metastatic breast carcinoma. Cancer 63:37–45, 1989.

43. Smalley RV, Lefante J, Bartolucci A, et al: A comparison of cyclophosphamide, Adriamycin, and 5-fluorouracil (CAF) and cyclophosphamide, methotrexate, 5-fluorouracil, vincristine, and prednisone (CMFVP) in patients with advanced breast cancer: A Southwestern Cancer Study Group project. Breast Cancer Res Treat 3:209–220, 1983.

44. Bull JM, Tormey DC, Li SH, et al: A randomized comparative trial of Adriamycin versus methotrexate in combination drug therapy. Cancer 41:1649–1657, 1978.

45. Tormey DC, Weinberg VE, Leone LA, et al: A comparison of intermittent vs. continuous and of Adriamycin vs. methotrexate 5-drug chemotherapy for advanced breast cancer: A Cancer and Leukemia Group B study. Am J Clin Oncol 7:231–239, 1984.

46. Muss HB, White DR, Richards F III, et al: Adriamycin versus methotrexate in 5-drug combination chemotherapy for advanced breast cancer. Cancer 42:2141–2148, 1978.

47. Mattson W, Areidi A, von Eyben F, et al: Phase II study of combined vincristine, Adriamycin, cyclophosphamide, and methotrexate with citrovorum factor in metastatic breast cancer. Cancer Treat Rep 61:1527–1531, 1977.

48. Tannock IF, Boyd NF, DeBoer G, et al: A randomized trial of two dose levels of cyclophosphamide, methotrexate, and fluorouracil chemotherapy for patients with metastatic breast cancer. J Clin Oncol 6:1377–1387, 1988.

49. Ahmann DL, Schaid DJ, Bisel HF, et al: The effect on survival of initial chemotherapy in advanced breast cancer: Polychemotherapy versus single drug. J Clin Oncol 12:1928–1932, 1987.

50. Legha SS, Buzdar AU, Smith TL, et al: Complete remission in metastatic breast cancer treated with combination drug therapy. Ann Intern Med 91:847–852, 1979.

51. Fischer J, Rose CJ, Rubens RD: Duration of complete response to chemotherapy in advanced breast cancer. Eur J Cancer Clin Oncol 18:747–753, 1982.

52. Holmes FA, Walters RS, Theriault RL, et al: Phase II trial of Taxol, an active drug in the treatment of metastatic breast cancer. J Natl Cancer Inst 83:1797–1805, 1991.

53. Holmes FA, Valero V, Theriault RL, et al: Phase II trial of Taxol in metastatic breast cancer refractory to multiple prior treatments. Proc Am Soc Clin Oncol 12:91, 1993.

54. Seidman AD, Barrett S, Hudis C, et al: Three hour Taxol infusion as initial (I) and as salvage (S) chemotherapy of metastatic breast cancer (MBC). Proc Am Soc Clin Oncol 13:66, 1994.

55. Waud WR, Gilber KS, Steadman D, et al: Cross-resistance of drug-resistant murine P388 leukemias to taxol in vivo. Cancer Chemother Pharmacol 31:255–257, 1992.

56. Seidman AD, Crown JPA, Reichman BS, et al: Lack of clinical cross-resistance of Taxol with anthracyclines (A) in the treatment of metastatic breast cancer (MBC). Proc Am Soc Clin Oncol 12:63, 1993.

57. Gianni L, Capri G, Munzone E, et al: Paclitaxel (Taxol) efficacy in patients with advanced breast cancer resistant to anthracyclines. Semin Oncol 21(suppl 5):29–33, 1994.

58. Wilson WH, Berg SL, Bryant G, et al: Paclitaxel in doxorubicin-refractory or mitoxantrone-refractory breast cancer: A phase I/II trial

of 96-hour infusion. J Clin Oncol 12:1621–1629, 1994.

59. Seidman AD, Norton L, Reichman BS, et al: Preliminary experience with paclitaxel (Taxol) plus recombinant human granulocyte colony-stimulating factor in the treatment of breast cancer. Semin Oncol 20(suppl 3):40–45, 1993.

60. National Cancer Institute Clinical Brochure: Taxol (NSC 125973). Division of Cancer Treatment. Bethesda, Maryland, NCI, 1991.

61. Eisenhauer EA, Wim W, ten Bokkel Huinink WW, et al: European-Canadian randomized trial of paclitaxel in relapsed ovarian cancer: High-dose versus low-dose and long versus short infusion. J Clin Oncol 12:2654–2666, 1994.

62. Hainsworth JD, Greco FA: Paclitaxel administered by 1-hour infusion: Preliminary results of a phase I/II trial comparing two schedules. Cancer 74:1377–1382, 1994.

62a. Venook AP, Egorin M, Brown TD, et al: Paclitaxel (Taxol) in patients with liver dysfunction (CALGB 9264). Proc Am Soc Clin Oncol 13:139, 1994.

63. Rowinsky, EK, Eisenhauer EA, Chaudhry V, et al: Clinical toxicities encountered with paclitaxel (Taxol). Semin Oncol 20(suppl 3):1–15, 1993.

64. Seidman AD, Barrett S, Canezo S: Photopsia during 3-hour paclitaxel administration at doses greater than 250 mg/m2 (letter). J Clin Oncol 12:1741–1742, 1994.

65. Capri G, Munzone E, Tarenzi E, et al: Optic nerve disturbances: A new form of paclitaxel neurotoxicity (letter). J Natl Cancer Inst 86:1099–1101, 1994.

66. Raghavan VT, Bloomer WD, Merkel DE: Taxol and radiation recall dermatitis (letter). Lancet 341:1354, 1993.

67. Ajani JA, Dodd LG, Daughtery K, et al: Taxol-induced soft-tissue injury secondary to extravasation: Characterization by histopathology and clinical course. J Natl Cancer Inst 86:51–53, 1994.

68. O'Shaughnessy JA, Fisherman JS, Cowan KH: Combination paclitaxel (Taxol) and doxorubicin therapy for metastatic breast cancer. Semin Oncol 21(suppl 8):19–23, 1994.

69. Hahn SM, Liebmann JE, Cook J, et al: Taxol in combination with doxorubicin or etoposide: Possible antagonism in vitro. Cancer 72:2705–2711, 1993.

70. Pestalozzi BC, Sotos GA, Choyke PL, et al: Typhlitis resulting from treatment with Taxol and doxorubicin in patients with metastatic breast cancer. Cancer 71:1797–1800, 1993.

71. Gianni L, Straneo M, Capri G, et al: Optimal dose and sequence finding study of paclitaxel (P) by 3 H infusion combined with bolus doxorubicin (D) in untreated metastatic breast cancer patients (pts). Proc Am Soc Clin Oncol 13:74, 1994.

72. Holmes FA, Newman RA, Madden T, et al: Schedule dependent pharmacokinetics (PK) in a phase I trial of Taxol (T) and doxorubicin (D) as initial chemotherapy for metastatic breast cancer. Ann Oncol 5(suppl 5):197, 1994.

73. Verweij J, Clavel M, Chevalier B: Paclitaxel (Taxol) and docetaxel (Taxotere): Not simply two of a kind. Ann Oncol 5:495–505, 1994.

74. Chevallier B, Fumoleau P, Kerbrat P, et al: Docetaxel is a major cytotoxic drug for the treatment of advanced breast cancer: A phase II trial of the clinical screening cooperative groups of the European Organization for Research and Treatment of Cancer. J Clin Oncol 13:314–322, 1995.

75. Trudeau ME, Eisenhauer EA, Lofters W, et al: Phase II study of Taxotere as first line chemotherapy for metastatic breast cancer (MBC): A National Cancer Institute of Canada Clinical Trials Group (NCIC CTG) study. Proc Am Soc Clin Oncol 12:64, 1993.

76. Seidman AD, Hudis C, Crown JPA, et al: Phase II evaluation of Taxotere (RP56976, NCS628503) as initial chemotherapy for

metastatic breast cancer. Proc Am Soc Clin Oncol 12:63, 1993.

77. ten Bokkel Huinink WW, Prove AM, Piccart M, et al: A phase II trial with docetaxel (Taxotere) in second line treatment with chemotherapy for advanced breast cancer. Ann Oncol 5:527–532, 1994.

78. Valero V, Walters RS, Theriault RL, et al: Phase II study of Taxotere in refractory metastatic breast cancer (RMBC). Eur J Cancer 29A(suppl 6):S83, 1993.

79. Verweij J, Planting AST, van der Burg MEL, et al: A phase I study of docetaxel and cisplatin in patients with solid tumors. Proc Am Soc Clin Oncol 13:148, 1994.

80. Romero A, Rabinovich MG, Vallejo CT, et al: Vinorelbine as first-line chemotherapy for metastatic breast carcinoma. J Clin Oncol 12:336–341, 1994.

81. Fumoleau P, Delgado FM, Delozier T, et al: Phase II trial of weekly intravenous vinorelbine in first-line advanced breast cancer chemotherapy. J Clin Oncol 11:1245–1252, 1993.

82. Weber, B, Boegel C, Jones S, et al: A US multicentre phase II trial of Navelbine in advanced breast cancer. Proc Am Soc Clin Oncol 12:61, 1993.

83. Degardin M, Bonneterre J, Hecquet B, et al: Vinorelbine (Navelbine) as a salvage treatment for advanced breast cancer. Ann Oncol 5:423–426, 1994.

84. Marty M, Leandri S, Extra JM, et al: A phase II study of vinorelbine (NVB) in patients (PTS) with advanced breast cancer. Proc Am Assoc Cancer Res 30:256, 1989.

85. Spielmann M, Dorval T, Turpin F, et al: Phase II trial of vinorelbine/doxorubicin as first-line therapy of advanced breast cancer. J Clin Oncol 12:1764–1770, 1994.

86. Dieras V, Extra JM, Morvan F, et al: Phase II study of Navelbine and fluorouracil in metastatic breast cancer patients using a group sequential design. Breast Cancer Res Treat 16:161, 1990.

87. Hohneker JA: A summary of vinorelbine (Navelbine) safety data from North American clinical trials. Semin Oncol 21(suppl 10):42–47, 1994.

88. Abrams JS, Moore TD, Friedman M: New chemotherapeutic agents for breast cancer. Cancer 74:1164–1176, 1994.

89. Livingston RB: Dose intensity and high dose therapy: Two different concepts. Cancer 74(suppl 3):1177–1183, 1994.

90. Eddy DM: High-dose chemotherapy with autologous bone marrow transplantation for the treatment of metastatic breast cancer. J Clin Oncol 10:657–670, 1992.

91. Meropol NJ, Overmoyer BA, Stadtmauer EA: High-dose chemotherapy with autologous stemm cell support for breast cancer. Oncology 6:53–63, 1992.

92. Peters WP, Ross M. Vredenburgh JJ, et al: High-dose chemotherapy and autologous bone marrow support as consolidation after standard-dose adjuvant therapy for high-risk primary breast cancer. J Clin Oncol 11:1132–1143, 1993.

93. Engelsman E, Klijn JC, Rubens RD, et al: 'Classical' CMF versus a 3-weekly intravenous CMF schedule in postmenopausal patients with advanced breast cancer. Eur J Cancer 27:966–970, 1991.

94. Hryniuk W, Bush H: The importance of dose intensity in the chemotherapy of metastatic breast cancer. J Clin Oncol 2:1281–1288, 1984.

95. Canellos GP, Demetri GD: Myelosuppression and 'conventional' chemotherapy: What price, what benefit? (editorial). J Clin Oncol 11:1–2, 1993.

96. Lieschk GJ, Burgess AW: Granulocyte colony-stimulating factor and granulocyte-macrophage colony-stimulating factor (second of 2 parts). N Engl J Med 327:99–106, 1992.

97. American Society of Clinical Oncology Recommendations for the Use of Hematopoietic Colony-Stimulating Factors: Evidence-based, clinical practice guidelines. J Clin Oncol 12:2471–2508, 1994.

98. Fraschini G, Poneso P, Wang Z, et al: Urokinase prophylaxis of central venous ports reduces thrombotic and infectious complications. Eur J Cancer 27(suppl 2):S289, 1991.

99. Ingle JN, Green SF, Ahmann DL, et al: Randomized trial of tamoxifen alone or combined with aminoglutethimide and hydrocortisone in women with metastatic breast cancer. J Clin Oncol 6:958–964, 1986.

100. Smith IE, Harris AL, Stuart-Harris RC, et al: Combination treatment with tamoxifen and aminoglutethimide in advanced breast cancer. Br Med J 286:1615–1616, 1983.

101. Powles TJ, Ashley S, Ford HT, et al: Treatment of disseminated breast cancer with tamoxifen, aminoglutethimide, hydrocortisone, and danazol, used in combination or sequentially. Lancet I:1369–1372, 1984.

102. Saphner T, Troxel AB, Tormey DC, et al: Phase II study of goserelin for patients with postmenopausal metastatic breast cancer. J Clin Oncol 11:1529–1535, 1993.

103. Goss PE, Gwyn KMEH: Current perspectives on aromatase inhibitors in breast cancer. J Clin Oncol 12:2460–2470, 1994.

104. Stuart-Harris RC, Smith IE: Aminoglutethimide in the treatment of advanced breast cancer. Cancer Treat Rev 11:189–204, 1984.

105. McGuire WL, DeLa Garza M, Chamness GC: Evaluation of estrogen receptor assays in human breast cancer tissues. Cancer Res 37:637–639, 1977.

106. Allegra JC, Lippman ME, Thompson EB, et al: Estrogen receptor status: An important variable in predicting response to endocrine therapy in metastatic breast cancer. Eur J Cancer 16:323–331, 1980.

107. Ravdin PM, Green SF, Dorr TM, et al: Prognostic significance of progesterone receptor levels in estrogen receptor-positive patients with metastatic breast cancer treated with tamoxifen: Results of a prospective Southwest Oncology Group study. J Clin Oncol 10:1284–1291, 1992.

108. Buzdar AU: Current status of endocrine treatment of carcinoma of the breast. Semin Surg Oncol 6:77–82, 1990.

109. Muss HB: Endocrine therapy for advanced breast cancer: A review. Breast Cancer Res Treat 21:15–26, 1992.

110. Lundgren S, Kvinnsland S, Utaakes E, et al: Effect of oral high-dose progestins on the disposition of antipyrine, digitoxin, and warfarin in patients with advanced breast cancer. Cancer Chemother Pharmacol 18:270–275, 1986.

111. Tenni P, Lalich DL, Byrne MJ: Life-threatening interaction between tamoxifen and warfarin. Br Med J 298:93, 1989.

112. Gill PG, Gebski V, Snyder R, et al: Randomized comparison of the effects of tamoxifen, megestrol acetate, or tamoxifen plus megestrol acetate on treatment response and survival in patients with metastatic breast cancer. Ann Oncol 4:741–744, 1993.

113. Muss HB, Case LD, Atkins JN, et al: Tamoxifen versus high-dose oral medroxyprogesterone acetate as initial endocrine therapy for patients with metastatic breast cancer: A Piedmont Oncology Association study. J Clin Oncol 12:1630–1638, 1994.

114. Castiglione-Gertsch M, Pampallona S, Varini M, et al: Primary endocrine therapy for advanced breast cancer: To start with tamoxifen or with medroxyprogesterone acetate? Ann Oncol 4:735–740, 1993.

115. Dowsett M, Coombes RC: Second-generation aromatase inhibitor: 4-hydroxy-androstenedione. Breast Cancer Res Treat 30:81–87, 1994.

116. Mouridson H, Palshof T, Patterson J, et al: Tamoxifen in advanced breast cancer. Cancer Treat Rev 5:131–141, 1978.

117. Heel C, Brogden RN, Speight TM, et al: Tamoxifen: A review of its pharmacological properties and therapeutic use in the treatment

of breast cancer. Int J Curr Ther Appl Pharmacol Rev 16:1–24, 1978.

118. Buzdar AU, Hortobagyi GN, Frye D, et al: Bioequivalence of 20-mg once daily tamoxifen relative to 10-mg twice daily tamoxifen regimens for breast cancer. J Clin Oncol 12:50–54, 1994.

119. Fisher B, Costantino JP, Redmon CK, et al: Endometrial cancer in tamoxifen-treated breast cancer patients: Findings from the National Surgical Adjuvant Breast and Bowel Project (NSABP) B-14. J Natl Cancer Inst 86:527–537, 1994.

120. van Leeuwen FE, Benraadt J, Coebergh JWW, et al: Risk of endometrial cancer after tamoxifen treatment of breast cancer. Lancet 343:448–452, 1994.

121. Coombes RC, Goss PE, Dowsett M, et al: 4-Hydroxy androstenedione treatment for postmenopausal patients with advanced breast cancer. Steroids 50:245–252, 1987.

122. Zinser JW, Hortobagyi GN, Buzdar AU, et al: Clinical course of breast cancer patients with liver metastases. J Clin Oncol 5:773–782, 1987.

123. Nims TA: Resection of the liver for metastatic cancer. Surg Gynecol Obstet 158:46–48, 1984.

124. Fraschini G, Fleishman G, Charnsangavej C, et al: Continuous 5-day infusion of vinblastine for percutaneous hepatic arterial chemotherapy for metastatic breast cancer. Cancer Treat Rep 71:1001–1005, 1987.

125. Fraschini G, Fleishman G, Yap HY, et al: Percutaneous hepatic arterial infusion of cisplatin for metastatic breast cancer. Cancer Treat Rep 71:313–315, 1987.

126. Fraschini G, Esparza L, Theriault RL, et al: Frontline arterial infusion chemotherapy in breast cancer patients with liver metastases. Proc Am Assoc Cancer Res 33:261, 1992.

127. Scheid V, Buzdar AU, Smith TL, et al: Clinical course of breast cancer patients with osseous metastasis treated with combination chemotherapy. Cancer 58:2589–2593, 1986.

128. Price P, Hoskin PJ, Easton D, et al: Prospective randomized trial of single and multifraction radiotherapy schedules in the treatment of painful bony metastases. Radiother Oncol 6:247–255, 1986.

129. Hortobagyi GN, Libshitz HI, Seabold JE: Osseous metastases of breast cancer: Clinical, biochemical, radiographic, and scintigraphic evaluation of response to therapy. Cancer 53:577–582, 1984.

130. Robinson RG, Preston DF, Baxter KG, et al: Clinical experience with strontium-89 in prostatic and breast cancer patients. Semin Oncol 20(suppl 2):44–48, 1993.

131. Averbuch SD: New bisphosphonates in the treatment of bone metastases. Cancer 72:3443–3452, 1993.

132. van Breukelen FJM, Bijvoet OLM, van Oosterom AT, et al: Inhibition of osteolytic bone lesions by (3-amino-1-hydroxypropylidene)-1,1-bisphosphonate. Lancet I:803–805, 1979.

133. van Holten-Verzantvoort ATH, Bijvoet OLM, Cleton FJ, et al: Reduced morbidity from skeletal metastasis in breast cancer patients during long-term bisphosphonate treatment. Lancet 2:983–985, 1987.

134. Paterson AHG, Powles TJ, Kanis JA, et al: Double-blind controlled trial of oral clodronate in patients with bone metastases from breast cancer. J Clin Oncol 11:59–65, 1993.

135. Elomaa I, Blomqvist C, Grohn P, et al: Long-term controlled trial with diphosphatate in patients with osteolytic bone metastases. Lancet I:146–149, 1983.

136. Elomaa I, Blomqvist C, Porkka L, et al: Treatment of skeletal disease in breast cancer: A controlled clodronate trial. Bone 8(suppl 1):553–555, 1987.

137. Glover D, Lipton A, Keller A, et al: Intravenous pamidronate disodium treatment of bone metastases in patients with breast cancer. Cancer 74:2949–2955, 1994.

138. Beck TM, Hart NE, Woodard DA, et al: Local or regionally recurrent carcinoma of the breast: Results of therapy in 121 patients.

J Clin Oncol 1:400–405, 1983.

139. Gilliland MD, Barton RM, Copeland III EM: The implications of local recurrence of breast cancer as the first site of therapeutic failure. Ann Surg 197:284–287, 1983.

140. Toonkel LM, Fix I, Jacobsen LH, et al: The significance of local recurrence of carcinoma of the breast. Int J Radiat Oncol Biol Phys 9:33–39, 1983.

141. Abner AL, Recht A, Eberlein T, et al: Prognosis following salvage mastectomy for recurrence in the breast after conservative surgery and radiation therapy for early-stage breast cancer. J Clin Oncol 11:44–48, 1993.

142. Buzdar AU, Blumenschein GR, Montague ED, et al: Combined modality approach in breast cancer with isolated multiple metastases. Am J Clin Oncol 6:45–50, 1984.

143. Holmes FA, Buzdar AU, Kau SW, et al: Combined-modality approach for patients with isolated recurrences of breast cancer (IV-NED): The M. D. Anderson experience. Breast Dis 7:7–20, 1994.

144. Posner JB: Neurological complications of systemic cancer. Med Clin North Am 63:783–800, 1979.

145. DiStefano A, Yap HY, Hortobagyi GN, et al: The natural history of breast cancer patients with brain metastasis. Cancer 44:1913–1918, 1979.

146. Patchell RA, Tibbs PA, Walsh JW, et al: A randomized trial of surgery in the treatment of single metastasis to the brain. N Engl J Med 322:494–500, 1990.

147. Cohen N, Strauss G, Lew R, et al: Should prophylactic anticonvulsants be administered to patients with newly diagnosed cerebral metastases? A retrospective analysis. J Clin Oncol 6:1621–1624, 1988.

148. Delattre J-Y, Safai B, Posner JB: Erythema multiforme and Stevens-Johnson syndrome in patients receiving cranial irradiation and phenytoin. Neurology 38:194–198, 1988.

149. Heideman RI, Cole DE, Balis F, et al: Phase I and pharmacokinetic evaluation of Thiotepa in the cerebrospinal fluid and plasma of pediatric patients: Evidence for dose-dependent plasma clearance of Thiotepa. Cancer Res 49:736–741, 1989.

150. Chamberlain MC: Current concepts in leptomeningeal metastasis. Curr Opin Oncol 4:533–539, 1992.

151. Wasserstrom WR, Glass JP, Posner JB: Diagnosis and treatment of leptomeningeal metastasis from solid tumors: Experience with 90 patients. Cancer 49:759–772, 1982.

152. Stillman MJ, Foley KM: Breast cancer and epidural spinal cord compression: Diagnosis and therapy, in Harris JR, Hellman S, Henderson IC, et al (eds): Breast Diseases, 2nd ed, pp 688–700. Philadelphia, JB Lippincott, 1991.

153. Byrne TN: Spinal cord compression from epidural metastases. N Engl J Med 327:614–619, 1992.

154. Ratanatharathron V, Powers WE: Epidural spinal compression from metastatic tumors: Diagnosis and guidelines for management. Cancer Treat Rev 18:55–71, 1991.

155. Harrison KM, Muss HB, Ball MR, et al: Spinal cord compression in breast cancer. Cancer 55:2839–2844, 1985.

156. Cybulski GR: Methods of surgical stabilization for metastatic disease of the spine. Neurosurgery 25:240–252, 1989.

157. Sundaresan N, DiGiancinto GV, Hughes JEO: Surgical treatment of spinal metastases. Clin Neurosurg 33:503, 1986.

158. Loprinzi CL, Tormey DC, Rasmussen P, et al: Prospective evaluation of carcinoembryonic antigen levels and alternating chemotherapeutic regimen in metastatic breast cancer. J Clin Oncol 4:46–56, 1986.

159. Hayes DF, Kiang DT, Kortan A, et al: CA15-3 and CEA spikes during chemotherapy for metastatic breast cancer. Proc Am Soc Clin Oncol 7:38, 1988.

CHAPTER 21

Special Issues in Breast Cancer Management

Vance Wright-Browne, MBBS, *and* Richard L. Theriault, DO

Division of Medicine, The University of Texas M. D. Anderson Cancer Center, Houston, Texas

This chapter will examine several controversial or uncommon topics in breast cancer: use of dose-intensive therapy, estrogen replacement therapy, male breast cancer, and breast cancer in pregnancy. The section on dose-intensive therapy will trace the development and clinical rationale for the use of this therapy. For additional information, the reader is referred to the section on autologous bone marrow transplantation. Estrogen replacement therapy in patients previously treated for breast cancer is an area of active investigation and controversy. Available information is reviewed, and ongoing studies are discussed. Male breast cancer and breast cancer in pregnancy are uncommon conditions. The relevant literature is summarized and presented.

DOSE-INTENSIVE THERAPY FOR BREAST CANCER

Dose-intensive therapy for breast cancer is an area of intense clinical investigation; several major trials are underway to evaluate the effect of this therapy in various patient groups. This section summarizes the current concepts of dose intensity, outlines the areas of controversy, and discusses studies to date of the efficacy and appropriate clinical applications of this technique.

Background

Evaluation of the effect of dose intensity on the outcome of breast cancer chemotherapy began in the 1980s. There were several precipitating factors: (1) the emerging success of dose-intensive therapy with autologous bone marrow transplantation for leukemias and lymphomas[1-4]; (2) evidence of the efficacy of dose-intensive therapy with or without bone marrow support for solid tumors, including breast cancer[5-14]; and (3) the publication of retrospective reviews that suggested a reduced relapse rate in patients receiving higher doses of chemotherapeutic agents.[15-17]

In laboratory animals with cancer, drug dose is proportional to cure.[18] However, tumor types and dose schedule do modify the magnitude of this effect.[19] A clinical correlation between dose and response has long been recognized as well.[20-22] The lack of complete response is often tied to drug resistance,[18] which can be overcome by increasing the dose. The availability of agents that enhance hematopoietic recovery, including the cytokines and autologous hematopoietic elements from the bone marrow or the peripheral blood, has allowed the escalation of doses of chemotherapeutic agents.[23] Peters et al demonstrated the possibility of administering cyclophosphamide (Cytoxan, Neosar), cisplatin (Platinol), and carmustine (BiCNU) at escalated doses.[24]

The alkylating agents exhibit a number of features that prompted their investigation of dose-intensive therapy. Most alkylating agents at conventional doses share a common dose-limiting toxic effect, myelosuppression. Marrow autografting permits dose escalation to the level at which dose-limiting nonhematologic toxic effects occur. The nonhematologic toxic effects vary with each agent (Table 1), allowing combination therapy without additive toxicity.[18] With bone marrow support, the dose of an alkylating agent can be escalated to 5 to 20 times the standard dose before nonmyelosuppressive dose-limiting toxic effects occur.[23]

Schabel was the first to demonstrate that the presence of resistance to an alkylating agent did not imply cross-resistance to other alkylating agents.[25] Schabel et al also demonstrated that the toxic effects of the alkylating agents were not additive and that the therapeutic effects of these agents were synergistic.[26] Resistance to alkylating agents is of a low level, is difficult to produce by selection pressure,[18] and can be overcome by increasing the dose 5 to 10 times.[25]

The steep dose-response curve of alkylating agents has been previously described (Figure 1).[19] However, the dose-response curve for solid tumors is less steep than that for the more sensitive hematologic malignancies.[27]

The first evidence that chemotherapy could potentially cure breast cancer came from adjuvant chemotherapy trials, in which the death rate was 20% to 30% lower in premenopausal women who received chemotherapy than in those who did not.[28] This difference was presumably due to the eradication of micrometastatic disease by chemotherapy. Gelber and Goldhirsch reviewed the validity of this type of overview analysis and concluded that in the case of early breast cancer, the conclusions drawn were likely to be valid.[29]

TABLE I

Dose-Limiting Toxicity Associated With Alkylating Agent Use

Drug	Dose-limiting toxicity associated with standard dose therapy	Dose-limiting toxicity associated with therapy utilizing bone marrow support
Cyclophosphamide	Myelosuppression	Hemorrhagic myocarditis
Cisplatin	Myelosuppression	Nephrotoxicity, neurotoxicity
Carmustine	Myelosuppression	Pulmonary fibrosis, toxic hepatitis
Melphalan	Myelosuppression	Mucositis
Busulfan	Myelosuppression	Anorexia, veno-occlusive disease, autoimmune disease
Thiotepa	Myelosuppression	Mucositis, CNS syndromes

CNS = central nervous system
Adapted, with permission, from Peters WP: Dose intensification using combination alkylating agents and autologous bone marrow support in the treatment of primary and metastatic breast cancer, in Effect of Therapy on Biology and Kinetics of the Residual Tumor, Part B. Clinical Aspects, pp 185–194. New York, Wiley Liss, 1990.

FIGURE I

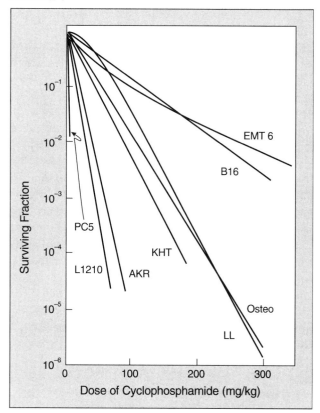

Single-dose cyclophosphamide survival curves in various in vivo experimental tumors. A variety of techniques were performed to assay the surviving fraction of tumor cells, and these assays were performed 24 hours after injection of the drug. Qualitatively similar curves were obtained with carmustine, lomustine, and vincristine. The tumors include AKR lymphoma, L1210 leukemia, KHT sarcoma, EMT6 carcinoma, osteosarcoma, PC5 astrocytoma, B16 melanoma, and LL lung carcinoma. Reprinted, with permission, from Frei E III and Canellos GP.[19]

Data on metastatic breast cancer suggest that the achievement of complete response (CR) may be important because only patients who entered CR had prolonged survival.[30–32] The duration of CR in standard chemotherapy trials has been shown to be inversely related to the bulk of metastatic tumor.[30] It was suspected that dose-intensive therapy might increase the number of patients entering CR or prolong this CR further,[33] suggesting that chemotherapy might be curative in a fraction of patients with metastatic disease.

However, this inference may not be correct. Macrometastatic disease may be less sensitive to chemotherapy than is micrometastatic disease for a number of reasons. Patients with established metastases have a large tumor burden with an increased likelihood of resistant cells. Metastatic tumors are associated with hypovascularity, poor perfusion of tumor by chemotherapy, hypoxia, low growth fraction, and increased mutation rates and, therefore, a greater propensity for drug resistance.[18]

Methods of Calculating Dose Intensity

Cumulative Dose: In a retrospective analysis of the data in the first two Milan trials, Bonadonna et al calculated dose intensity as a function of cumulative total dose (total dose actually administered expressed as a percentage of optimal dose).[17] Their results demonstrated that patients administered the highest dose of chemotherapy (85% or more of the optimal dose) had a significantly better disease-free survival rate than did control patients in the first trial or patients administered less than 65% of the optimal dose in either trial. These differences persisted after 10 years of follow-up.[34] Similar retrospective analyses have had mixed results.[20]

Confounding biases in the analysis of these data may include patient age and performance status. Patients with a good performance status might be expected to tolerate higher doses of therapy. In addition, there is a highly significant correlation between performance status and response rate, response duration, and survival.[35] Furthermore, patients whose disease progressed during therapy were included in the lower dose group, worsening the outcome statistics for that group.

Dose Rate: In a second type of retrospective analysis, Hryniuk examined dose rate rather than cumulative doses of planned chemotherapy.[36] He defined dose intensity as the amount of drug given per unit of time, expressed as $mg/m^2/wk$, regardless of schedule. Limitations of this model include the assumption that scheduling does not directly determine tumor cell kill. Additionally, the model may be applicable only after a threshold dose intensity has been reached.[36–38]

Using this model, Hryniuk demonstrated an association between dose intensity and response duration in patients with metastatic breast cancer[15] and in those receiving adjuvant therapy.[39,40] In a retrospective analysis, Hryniuk and Levine assigned a dose-intensity score to chemotherapy administered in an adjuvant setting in a series of published trials.[39] The standard was the Cooper et al regimen of cyclophosphamide, methotrexate, and fluorouracil (CMF) plus vincristine (Oncovin) and prednisone (CMFVP).[41] A high and positive correlation coefficient, statistically significant for all patient subsets, was found when 3-year disease-free survival was correlated with dose intensity in a linear regression analysis (Figure 2).

Peak Drug Dose: In the bone marrow transplant setting, peak drug dose is often the calculation used to represent dose intensity. This method emphasizes peak drug dose, as compared with the method of Hryniuk, which calculates cumulative drug dose over a defined period.[20]

Early Studies of Dose Intensity

Dose intensive chemotherapy, with or without autologous bone marrow transplantation (ABMT), was initially examined in patients with treatment-refractory or recurrent cancer. Trials usually involved small numbers of heavily pretreated patients with a variety of malignancies and were rarely randomized. Of several drugs examined in the single-agent setting using autologous marrow support, active drugs included melphalan,[6,10,11] cyclophosphamide,[7,24] thiotepa (Thioplex),[24] fluorouracil,[42] and carmustine.[24]

O'Bryan et al[43] performed a dose-escalation trial of doxorubicin (Adriamycin, Rubex) for refractory malignancies using doses ranging from 25 to 75 mg/m^2 every 3 to 4 weeks. Only patients with breast cancer who had

FIGURE 2

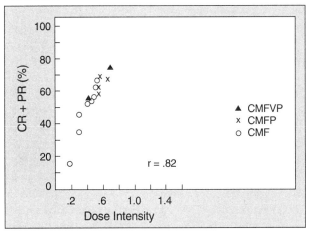

Response rate vs average relative dose intensity of CMF. Calculations are from doses actually delivered after reductions for toxicity. Dose intensities are relative to the regimen of Cooper and Holland. Reprinted, with permission, from Hryniuk W and Bush H.[15]

received multiple prior chemotherapeutic regimens showed a dose-response effect. Of 34 patients, eight (24%) with heavy prior exposure to chemotherapy responded to 50 mg/m^2. There were two responses to 25 mg/m^2.

Forastiere et al[44] treated patients who had metastatic breast cancer with 60 mg/m^2 or 120 mg/m^2 of cisplatin every 3 weeks and noted four short-lived partial responses, primarily in soft tissue and the lung, at the higher dose. There were no responders at the lower dose. One of five patients who were crossed over to the higher dose arm responded. Kolaric and Roth[45] found 13 complete responders in 35 patients with metastatic breast cancer using high-dose cisplatin given by continuous infusion. Although rapid and frequent responses were obtained in patients with treatment-resistant breast cancer, dose escalation was limited by unexpected dose-related toxic effects.[46]

Antman has reviewed the single-agent data in patients with failed or refractory breast cancer. She found that all complete responses were obtained with alkylating agents (melphalan [Alkeran] or thiotepa) and that these alkylating agents initiated a response rate of 39% compared with 16% for nonalkylating agents.[47]

Only one nonrandomized study has prospectively compared patients treated with high-dose therapy with patients treated with standard doses of chemotherapy.[48] Vincent et al compared the survival of patients treated with 140 to 200 mg/m^2 of melphalan with that of patients administered conventional therapy. Patients had already had responses to induction therapy. Based on performance status, partial or complete response to chemotherapy, and minimal disease burden, 15 patients were selected to receive high-dose melphalan with autologous bone marrow rescue. There were three treatment-related deaths in the high-dose group. Of the 12 assessable patients, 11 had relapses. The median survival was 7 months. The overall survival rate of the two groups was the same.[48]

Dose-intensive combination chemotherapy without autologous marrow infusion has also been studied. Six trials examined the CMF regimen in a prospective randomized fashion in patients with metastatic breast cancer.[49–54] Although five trials have shown an increased response rate with higher-dose CMF,[49–53] only two have demonstrated an increase in survival,[49,52] and in only one did the survival advantage achieve statistical significance.[49] Tannock et al[49] demonstrated a positive dose-response effect using a relative dose intensity of 2 for the high- and low-dose CMF regimens compared. A significant difference in response rate (11% vs 30%) and survival (13 vs 16 months) was found.[49] When adjustments were made for inequalities noted between the two groups for the time from first relapse to randomization, the significance of the dose response effect was diminished.

Other important trials examining dose intensity include the Ludwig trial group study of CMF with (n = 250) or without (n = 241) prednisone. Patients who received prednisone required fewer dose reductions for hematologic toxicity, receiving an average of 83% of the full CMF doses compared with 72% of full doses in patients treated with CMF alone ($P < .001$). However, at a median follow-up of 48 months, there was no significant difference in disease-free or overall survival between the two groups.[55]

The Cancer and Leukemia Study Group B (CALGB) randomized patients to receive one of two different dose schedules of CMFVP. The dose intensities actually delivered, as calculated by the system of Hryniuk and Levine,[39] were 84% and 76%. However, this significant difference in dose intensity did not result in a significant difference in disease-free or overall survival after a median follow-up of 45 months.[56]

In a follow-up study, the CALGB enrolled more than 800 patients in a three-arm comparison of cyclophosphamide, doxorubicin, and fluorouracil (CAF) at high doses for 4 months, intermediate doses for 6 months, or low doses for 4 months.[57] The high-dose regimen comprised 600 mg/m² of cyclophosphamide on day 1, 60 mg/m² of doxorubicin on day 2, and 600 mg/m² of fluorouracil on days 1 and 8. The moderate- and low-dose regimens used two thirds and one half, respectively, of the doses in the high-dose regimen. At a median follow-up of 3.4 years, results for 1,529 women were published. The women treated with high or moderate dose intensity had a significantly higher disease-free survival rate (74% and 70%, respectively, at 3 years) and overall survival rate than did women treated with the low-dose regimen (63% disease-free survival rate at 3 years).

Some of these of these large trials[49,57] suggest a positive correlation between dose intensity and disease response. However, the effect appears to be modest and is associated with a significant increase in toxicity.

High-dose epirubicin has also been studied in a randomized fashion as a single-agent[58] and as part of a combination regimen for breast cancer.[59] There was no difference in response rates between standard and high doses in the combination regimen[59]; a higher response rate was seen with high-dose single-agent epirubicin,[58] but this did not affect overall survival or the progression-free interval.

Hortobagyi et al used the M. D. Anderson Cancer Center regimen of fluorouracil, doxorubicin, and cyclophosphamide (FAC) in a randomized trial treating patients with a dose intensity of 1 or 3. Patients were placed in a protective environment and given supportive care and cytokines. Overall response rates were identical (78%), as were CR rates. No difference was seen in median survival (20 months for both groups).[60] The toxicity of the high-dose regimen was considerably higher. It was concluded that the extramedullary toxicity of FAC was severe enough to preclude further dose escalation, which might have produced a therapeutic difference.[61] Hortobagyi et al have also reviewed the M.D. Anderson Cancer Center experience with dose intensity.[61] It is notable that in all trials at M. D. Anderson between July 1973 and June 1976, patients who received higher doses of chemotherapy had a higher response rate and a longer survival duration. The correlation of response rate with drug dose was highly statistically significant, whereas the correlation with survival showed a trend that did not reach statistical significance.[61] Similar correlations were also seen in the institution's adjuvant therapy trials.[62]

High-Dose Chemotherapy With or Without Hematopoietic Support

Early trials of high-dose chemotherapy with hematopoietic support in patients with metastatic breast cancer were often small, were seldom randomized, and produced mixed results. Important positive observations for high-dose chemotherapy with hematopoietic support included the following: a higher overall response rate (70% to 80%) than that of standard-dose therapy (50% to 60%) and a higher complete response rate (30% to 40%) than that of standard therapy (10%). Failure to respond to prior chemotherapy appeared to reduce the rate of CR to high-dose therapy substantially. Conversely, patients who responded to standard chemotherapy had a very high rate of CR to high-dose chemotherapy (70% to 80%).

Metastatic Disease: High-dose chemotherapy for metastatic breast cancer has been used in pretreated patients, as initial therapy in patients with or without a history of adjuvant therapy, and as consolidation of an initial response to conventional-dose therapy.[20]

Pretreated patients were the first to be examined. In this group, high-dose chemotherapy with ABMT has not substantially improved disease-free survival in patients with advanced treatment-refractory disease. The duration of response of 2 to 5 months without maintenance therapy approximates that achieved with a second-line regimen of standard-dose therapy.[63] Patients with advanced refractory disease, which easily justifies the use of aggressive high-dose therapy, thus appear to be the ones least likely to benefit from the treatment.

In 1988, Peters et al[64] published results of a study that examined the effect of high-dose combination alkylating agents with bone marrow support as initial treatment of metastatic breast cancer. They evaluated 22 premenopausal, estrogen-receptor (ER)-negative patients; 12 (55%) of 22 obtained a CR. The median duration of response in complete responders was 9 months. Five patients died of therapy-related complications. The median disease-free survival and overall survival were not improved (7.0 months and 10.1 months, respectively). However, 3 of the 22 patients remain in continuous unsustained remission at 3.3 to 6.4 years.[65]

Spitzer et al[66] evaluated high-dose cyclophosphamide, etoposide (VePesid), and cisplatin (CVP) for hormonally unresponsive metastatic breast cancer. Following induction therapy with doxorubicin and cyclophosphamide, patients received two courses of CVP. There was a 65% CR rate and a 27% partial response rate.[66]

Table 2 outlines some of the trials of high-dose chemotherapy with ABMT for metastatic disease (20 patients or more) for which survival data are available.[65-77] Important points include the lower response rate seen in patients with treatment-refractory disease compared with that in patients in whom ABMT was used as the first-line therapy for metastatic disease. Although there is no difference in overall survival when these results are

compared with those for standard chemotherapy, the presence of long-term survivors (10% to 15%) in the study population is noteworthy. The ability to achieve similar results with dose-intensive therapy without hematopoietic support is controversial. Some studies appear to achieve comparable results without the use of ABMT. The Eastern Cooperative Oncology Group evaluated 80 premenopausal women who had positive or unknown ER status and who were treated with CAF plus oophorectomy and 50 women with ER-negative disease who were treated with CAF alone. The response rate was 80% in the ER-positive/unknown group (with a CR of 37%) and was 70% in the ER-negative group.[78] Bezwoda et al[79] conducted a small randomized study of high-dose cyclophosphamide, 60 mg/kg, etoposide, 2.5 g/m^2, and mitoxantrone (Novantrone), 12 mg/m^2, compared with standard doses of a similar regimen (cyclophosphamide, 600mg/m^2, mitoxantrone, 12mg/m^2, vincristine, 1.4 mg/m^2) in 33 patients. Of the 16 patients in the high-dose arm, the response rate was 100% (50% CR) vs a response rate of 50% among the 17 patients in the standard-dose arm. No ABMT was used. Follow-up data was not given.

The Dana-Farber Cancer Institute recently published an update of its experience with ABMT for metastatic breast cancer.[80] A progression-free rate of 19% was found in patients with metastatic disease at a median follow-up of 40 months. Other large centers have also reviewed their data, with similar findings.[71,81]

Antman and Gale[63] evaluated 27 trials in 172 patients who received single or multiagent chemotherapy with ABMT, with or without radiation. The overall response rate was 58%. The response rate was highest in trials involving multiple alkylating agents (76%) or previously untreated patients (81%).[63] Patients with chemotherapy-sensitive disease, good performance status, and few sites of metastatic disease appear to derive the most benefit from high-dose therapy with ABMT.[82] Dunphy et al[83] examined the factors that predict long-term survival of metastatic breast cancer patients treated with high-dose chemotherapy and bone marrow support. These factors include the absence of relapse in the liver or soft tissue, few metastatic sites, and a disease-free interval longer than 1 year from initial diagnosis to detection of stage IV disease.

Given the disappointing results of high-dose therapy with ABMT in its overall application to patients with metastatic breast cancer, attention has turned to the use of this treatment to intensify a substantial response to induction chemotherapy. This strategy has been evaluated by a number of authors[74-77] (Table 2). Common features of these studies include use of this therapy as initial treat-

TABLE 2

Clinical Trials of High-Dose Chemotherapy With ABMT in 20 or More Patients

Author	Evaluated patients	Response rate (%)[a]	Complete response (%)	Regimen	Median disease-free survival (mo)	Median survival (mo)	Comments
Bouleuc[67]	91	59	18.8	Ifosfamide/epirubicin	18	36	
Spitzer[66]	25	95	65	NA	13.5	20	ER-negative/hormone unresponsive
Israel[68]	30	93	40	Cyclophosphamide/ fluorouracil	NA	NA	No prior chemotherapy[b;] 43-month survival 52%
Peters[65]	22	73	54	Cyclophosphamide/ cisplatin with carmustine or mitoxantrone	NA	10.1	No prior chemotherapy[b]
Nabholtz[69]	20	57.9		Cyclophosphamide/ mitoxantrone/ vinblastine	NA	9	Refractory
	19	100	58		NA	NA	Initial therapy[b]
Antman[70]	29	NA	44.8	Cyclophosphamide/ thiotepa/carboplatin	NA	NA	One toxic death
Grad[71]	23	NA	NA	Cyclophosphamide/ thiotepa/carmustine	9		Stem cells
	79			Cyclophosphamide/ thiotepa			
Vredrenburgh[72]	30	50	7	Ifosfamide/carboplatin	NA	NA	Three toxic deaths
de Vries[73]	30	NA	NA	Melphalan/mitoxantrone	27	NA	One toxic death; NED [d] prior to ABMT
Dunphy[c 74]	58		55	Cyclophosphamide/ cisplatin/epirubicin	13	NA	Two courses. 9% mortality
Jones[c 75]	45		58	Cyclophosphmide/ cisplatin/carmustine	NA	NA	18% mortality
Kennedy[c 76]	30		37	Cyclophosphamide/ thiotepa	13	NA	0% mortality Purged marrow
Williams[c 77]	27		48	Cyclophosphamide/ thiotepa	10	NA	15% mortality

[a] Complete response plus partial response   [b] No prior therapy for metastatic disease   [c] Intensification studies   [d] No evidence of disease
ABMT = autologous bone marrow transplantation, ER = estrogen receptor, NA = not available

ment of metastatic disease and selection of only patients with a favorable response to induction therapy and, consequently, a very high rate of CR. deVries et al[73] have extended this strategy; using myeloablative therapy in 30 patients who had metastatic disease, they achieved CR prior to high-dose therapy. The median disease-free survival was 27 months.

The results of high-dose chemotherapy with ABMT in patients with metastatic cancer have provided a number of lessons for further application of this technique.

(1) Success of bone marrow transplantation in the treatment of leukemia/lymphoma has been dependent on pretransplant reduction in tumor burden by remission-induction chemotherapy.[3,4] In breast cancer, the approach

to this problem has been to induce maximum tumor regression, hopefully a CR, prior to intensification therapy.

(2) The most powerful predictor of long-term disease-free survival following bone marrow transplantation for non-Hodgkin's lymphoma has been response to chemotherapy before transplantation.[4] Breast cancer trials have mirrored this,[63] and many trials are using ABMT only in patients who respond to induction chemotherapy.

(2) The rate of CR appears to be increased by the following: the use of three or more agents; the use of agents that are individually effective in the treatment of breast cancer; the use of agents with steep dose-response curves that are maintained through multiple logs of tumor stem-cell death. The optimal agent for a curative regimen should maintain fractional tumor kill through multiple logs, ie, a straight line on semilog plots[40]; the use of minimally cross-resistant or non-cross-resistant agents; the use of agents with experimentally or clinically demonstrated synergism; the use of agents whose tolerable doses in the setting are at least 5-fold the standard maximum safe doses; and the use of agents with nonmyelosuppressive dose-limiting toxic effects that are sufficiently different from the agents may be used in combination in the ABMT setting without significant compromise of the doses.

Adjuvant Therapy: The superior response to high-dose chemotherapy with ABMT in patients with a small tumor burden in the metastatic setting prompted the study of this technique in patients with locoregional disease who were at high risk for relapse. The prognosis for patients with stage II breast cancer with 10 or more involved axillary lymph nodes is extremely poor. The median time to relapse despite adjuvant chemotherapy is 1 year. The median survival is 3.4 years, and long-term disease-free survival occurs in only 20% of patients.[34] Buzdar et al[84] examined the outcome of patients with 10 or more positive nodes who had received doxorubicin-containing adjuvant chemotherapy; the estimated disease-free survival rate at 5 years was 41%.

Given these poor outcomes, trials have examined dose-intensive therapy with and without hematopoietic support in this patient group. Hudis et al[85] treated 60 patients with high-risk node-positive primary breast cancer (more than four ipsilateral axillary nodes) with doxorubicin for four courses followed by high-dose cyclophosphamide for three courses, without bone marrow support. All planned treatment was completed in 97% of patients. At 15-month follow-up, the actuarial relapse-free survival rate was 84% (standard error 5%). A Johns Hopkins pilot study[86] of 53 women with 10 or more

positive nodes treated with CAF, methotrexate, and leucovorin rescue but no hematopoietic support had an actuarial disease-free survival rate of 61%.

Blumenschein et al[87] recently demonstrated response rates comparable to Peters's response rate with high-dose alkylating therapy and ABMT[88] using standard-dose chemotherapy and regional radiotherapy. They achieved a disease-free survival rate of 80% at 4 years. Cocconi et al[89] published a randomized trial of conventional vs intensive sequential chemotherapy as adjuvant treatment of stage II breast cancer with ten or more involved axillary nodes. Group 1 received six cycles of standard CMF; group 2 received intensive sequential chemotherapy including three cycles of cisplatin-etoposide, three cycles of CMF, and three cycles of fluorouracil, leucovorin, and doxorubicin. A total of 108 patients were entered in the study. No ABMT was used. Two-year actuarial disease-free survival rates were 53% and 58%, respectively, a difference that was not statistically significant.

In a study by de Graaf et al[90] of 24 patients with more than five involved axillary nodes, patients were treated with induction chemotherapy followed by myeloablative therapy with marrow support, regional radiotherapy for extranodal disease, and tamoxifen. The 5-year disease-free survival rate is predicted to be 84%. Two patients died of treatment-related toxicity. Peters et al[88] treated 102 women with high-risk disease involving 10 or more axillary lymph nodes. Patients were treated with four cycles of standard-dose cyclophosphamide, doxorubicin, and fluorouracil, followed by high-dose cyclophosphamide, cisplatin, and carmustine with autologous bone marrow support. Of 85 evaluable patients, at a median follow-up of 2.5 years the actuarial event-free survival rate was 72%. The therapy-related death rate was 12%, and pulmonary toxic effects occurred in 31% of patients. Table 3 lists the trials of high-dose adjuvant therapy with ABMT published to date. Ongoing trials include CALGB 8451, CALGB 9082, and MDACC DM 89-102.

Inflammatory Breast Cancer: Gisselbrecht et al[93] treated eight patients with inflammatory breast cancer using a regimen of cyclophosphamide and total-body irradiation with ABMT following induction chemotherapy. All patients responded, and none had a relapse at the time of the report, although all follow-up was shorter than 1 year.

Israel et al[94] treated 25 consecutive cases of inflammatory breast cancer with high-dose cyclophosphamide and fluorouracil given in 5-day courses every 3 weeks for 2 years. The median disease-free survival was 46 months, and expected median survival was longer than 6 years.

Extra et al[95] randomized patients with inflammatory breast cancer to receive intensive chemotherapy with or

TABLE 3

High-Dose Chemotherapy With ABMT as Adjuvant Intensification for Patients With More Than Four Positive Nodes

Author	Evaluated patients	Number of positive axillary nodes	Regimen	Disease-free survival	Toxic deaths	Hematopoietic support
Abeloff[86]	53	≥ 10	Cyclophosphamide/ doxorubicin/methotrexate vincristine/fluourouracil	80% (3 yr)	None	No
de Graaf[90]	24	> 5	Methotrexate/fluorouracil doxorubicin/vincristine	84% (5 yr)	2	Yes
Peters[88]	85	> 10	Cyclophosphamide/ cisplatin/busulfan	72% (2.5 yr)	10	Yes
Hudis[85]	60	> 4	Doxorubicin, cyclophos-phamide	84% (15 mo)	None	No
Somlo[92]	79	≥ 10[a]	Doxorubicin/etoposide/ cyclophosphamide or cisplatin/etoposide/cyclo-phosphamide	NA	1	Yes
Overmoyer[91]	29	≥ 10[a]	Busulfan/cyclophospha-mide:cisplatin/cyclophospha-mide/carmustine:cyclophos-phamide/carboplatin/carmustine	85% (3 yr)	1	Yes

NA = not available
[a] Included patients with locally advanced and/or inflammatory disease

without ABMT. A total of 67 patients were treated with high-dose cyclophosphamide (122 mg/m^2) and epirubicin (75 mg/m^2) for six cycles. This regimen was followed by mastectomy, local irradiation, and CMF/FAC/FMV(methotrexate, vinblastine, fluorouracil) in 54 patients or ABMT intensification in 13 patients. The chemotherapy used for dose intensification was not stated. At the time of mastectomy, pathologic response of the tumor was complete in 7 patients (10%) and major in 25 (37%). The actuarial 4-year progression-free survival rate was 54%; the outcome seemed to be influenced mainly by pathologic response and not by the use of ABMT. High-dose therapy combined with surgery and local irradiation to the chest wall is also used for treatment of locally advanced unresectable disease, including stage IIIB and inflammatory breast cancer.

Ayash et al [96] treated 16 patients, rendering them all disease-free, with induction therapy with doxorubicin, local therapy, followed by high-dose cyclophosphamide, thiotepa, and carboplatin (Paraplatin) with ABMT.

Other Important Issues: The mortality rate with conventional-dose chemotherapy is 2% to 4%, whereas with high-dose chemotherapy the rate ranges from 3% to 24%.[47] Concerns have been raised about treating patients

who are responding well to standard chemotherapy with potentially deadly myeloablative intensification regimens and about treating high-risk patients who are free of disease with therapy that has such high potential morbidity and mortality.

Breast Cancer Micrometastases: The presence of breast cancer stem cells in the autograft and the role, if any, of transplanted cancer cells in the relapse rate are areas of investigation. The role of either overt or occult bone marrow involvement in ABMT is unknown. More than 40% of patients with metastatic breast cancer and 55% of patients with bony metastases (documented by positive bone scan or plain radiographs) have morphologically involved bone marrow.[97] Patients also may have morphologically undetected bone marrow involvement.

Redding et al[98] demonstrated that 31 (28%) of 110 patients with "negative" bone marrow had positive findings by immunocytochemical techniques. However, the viability of these positive cells has been called into question, prompting evaluation of more specific monoclonal techniques.[99] Cote et al[100] followed 49 stage I and II patients, 18 of whom had bone marrow micrometastases identified by monoclonal antibody staining techniques. At a median follow-up of 30 months, 12 patients had had recurrences. A 2-year projection indicated that the presence of bone marrow micrometastases was positively correlated with the risk of relapse. The fact that at least some of these micrometastases are viable has also been shown by Mann et al,[101] who, using long-term marrow cultures, detected metastatic breast carcinoma in the morphologically normal marrow of a patient awaiting autotransplantation. The effect of such contamination on patient survival and the rate of relapse remains controversial.

Purging has been studied as a method of potentially reducing bone marrow contamination by breast cancer micrometastases. Monoclonal breast cancer cell antibodies conjugated to toxins,[102] soybean agglutinin-bound magnetic beads that bind selectively to breast cancer cells,[103] and 4-hydroxy-peroxycyclophosphamide (4-HC)[104] are some of the modalities that have been studied. Shpall et al[105] recently demonstrated that patients who have morphologically detectable tumor in bone marrow have a shorter survival than patients without morphologically detectable tumor in bone marrow, and that purging before ABMT prolongs the disease-free interval.

Peripheral Stem Cells: Rapid reengraftment has been demonstrated with peripheral stem cells, and they are now frequently used as the sole hematopoietic support following myeloablative therapy. There are data[106] showing identical engraftment patterns to unselected stem-cells with CD34-positive peripheral stem-cells derived by positive selection. This selection was thought to decrease contaminating tumor cells by approximately 3 logs. The clinical significance of this 3-log reduction in contaminating tumor cells is unknown.

The Role of Cytokines: In randomized trials, the hematopoietic growth factors granulocyte-colony-stimulating factor (G-CSF, filgrastim [Neupogen]) and granulocyte-macrophage colony-stimulating factor (GM-CSF, sargramostim [Leukine]) have been found to decrease the time to reengraftment[107–109] and, in the case of the former, to decrease the duration of neutropenia and associated morbidity.[110] The availability of hematopoietic growth factors allows the use of high-dose cyclophosphamide, thus maximizing its dose-response relationship[24] while reducing the time to reengraftment.[111] G-CSF has also been shown to accelerate the time to reengraftment after a high-dose chemotherapy regimen that utilized marrow purged with 4-HC.[112]

Conclusions

The role of high-dose chemotherapy in breast cancer remains under active investigation. Clearly, its role will not be as broad as was initially hoped. Rather, high-dose chemotherapy may be most appropriate for certain subgroups of patients whose characteristics are still being defined. Current reviews explore the topic further.[113–115]

ESTROGEN REPLACEMENT THERAPY IN BREAST CANCER

The use of estrogen replacement therapy (ERT) in postmenopausal women has increased dramatically over the past 10 years. Estrogen replacement in postmenopausal women has been demonstrated to maintain bone mineral density,[116] to reduce the rate of hip fracture by 30% to 60%,[116–118] and to decrease the incidence of coronary artery disease in postmenopausal women.[119–121] The long-term use of ERT has been shown to benefit women studied in a case-control fashion,[122] leaving little doubt about the beneficial effect of estrogens on postmenopausal morbidities.

At the same time, the incidence of breast cancer has increased, with an estimated 182,000 cases expected to be diagnosed in 1995,[123] making it one of the most common malignancies. The proven benefit of adjuvant therapy to disease-free and overall survivals in women with resectable disease has sharply increased the proportion of patients with breast cancer who are exposed to chemotherapy and its associated morbidities.[28] Prominent among these is amenorrhea due to primary ovarian failure.[124]

The incidence of postchemotherapy amenorrhea is age and drug dependent. Among those who experience amenorrhea, ovarian failure is permanent in 57% of women age 40 years or younger and in 96% of women older than age 40.[125] The cyclophosphamide/methotrexate/fluorouracil regimen produces amenorrhea in 53% of women younger than age 35 years, in 84% of patients 35 to 44 years, and in 94% of women age 45 or older.[126] There is an inverse relation between age and the duration of treatment required to produce ovarian suppression with CMF.[127] With doxorubicin-containing regimens, which are used at M. D. Anderson Cancer Center, amenorrhea occurs in 80% of premenopausal women. In a review of the M. D. Anderson experience, the incidence of amenorrhea was 0% in patients younger than 30 years, 33% in patients 30 to 39 years, 96% in women 40 to 49 years, and 100% in patients older than 50 years. This was reversible in 50% of women younger than 40 but was permanent in the majority of patients older than 40.[128]

Atrophic vaginitis, dyspareunia, hot flashes, and sleep disturbance are the most immediate effects of estrogen deficiency. However, the long-term effects of premature coronary artery disease, osteoporosis, and increased rate of hip fracture have greater potential morbidity.

Several nonhormonal treatment alternatives are available for menopausal symptoms (Table 4). However, they are ineffective in the majority of patients, and many have unpleasant side effects. They also lack the long-term benefits of ERT.

Vassilopoulou-Sellin and Zolinski[129] evaluated the attitudes of breast cancer survivors toward ERT and found that most (78%) had concerns about the risk of cancer recurrence; however, almost half (44%) were willing to consider ERT under medical supervision.

The issue of ERT has thus become one of immense importance, with a profound ability to influence the quality of life of breast cancer survivors.

The standard of care is to discourage the use of ERT in survivors of breast cancer . The American College of Obstetricians and Gynecologists, while supporting the use of ERT in postmenopausal women, considers breast cancer a contraindication.[130] Evaluation of the role of ERT for survivors of breast cancer has focused on indirect data on the action of estrogens in breast carcinogenesis and the effect of ERT on the outcome of patients who develop breast cancer while receiving ERT.

Effects of Estrogens on Breast Cancer

Estrogens have two effects with respect to breast cancer. First, estrogen is probably a promoter in the two-step model of breast carcinogenesis. Estradiol is the most powerful promoter of breast carcinogenesis in animal models. Nonestradiol estrogens are either weak promoters or function as antipromoters and protect against carcinogenesis.[131] Second, estrogen functions as a growth factor for the tumor. Estradiol is the most potent growth factor of the estrogens. Any estrogen that binds to the estrogen receptor in ER-positive tumors and inhibits estradiol will inhibit tumor growth.[132]

In vitro studies show that low-dose estrogen stimulates and high-dose estrogen inhibits breast cancer cell growth.[133] Estrogen has been successfully used to treat metastatic breast cancer, demonstrating a therapeutic antitumor effect.[134,135] The doses of estrogens used for breast cancer treatment are pharmacologic and not physiologic, and this may account for the inhibitory effect seen in the clinical setting.[136] Stoll[135] treated 105 patients with postmenopausal breast cancer with an oral contraceptive containing estrogen [17-alpha-ethinylestradiol (0.15 mg)] and a progestin [17-alpha-ethinylestrenol (5 mg)] and found that a significant proportion of patients with measurable soft-tissue disease had partial responses.[135]

The association between the use of ERT and the development of primary breast cancer is controversial. Several studies have found a slight but statistically signif-

TABLE 4

Physiologic Consequences of Estrogen Deprivation and Nonhormonal Treatment Alternatives

Estrogen deficiency consequence	Treatment alternatives
Vasomotor instability	Bellergal, clonidine, progesterone, herbal
Genitourinary atrophy	Topical estrogen creams
Dyspareunia	Vaginal lubricants
Osteoporosis	Calcium, bisphosphonates calcitonin, ? fluoride
Cardiovascular disease, dyslipidemia-related	Bile acid-binding resins, fibric acid derivatives, HMC-CoA reductase inhibitors, nicotinic acid, antioxidants

Adapted, with permission, from Vassilopoulou-Sellin R: Estrogen-replacement therapy in women at increased risk for breast cancer. Breast Cancer Res Treat 28:167–177, 1993.

icant increased risk of breast cancer associated with the use of oral estrogens.[137–140] Bergkvist et al[141] studied the issue in postmenopausal women, focusing on 653 women who responded to a questionnaire and extrapolating these data to draw conclusions about 23,244 women who had received estrogens from 1977 to 1980. The relative risk of breast cancer reached 1.7 after 9 years of ERT. The increased risk was associated only with the use of estradiol; no increase was found with the use of conjugated estrogens. Study weaknesses included the study design (case-cohort) and reliance on the responses of 653 women to draw inferences about a much larger group.

In contrast, Hunt et al[142] found a reduction in the overall incidence of breast cancer in their long-term surveillance of 4,544 ERT users, who had a relative risk of breast cancer of .55 compared with national rates. These studies suggest that ERT using conjugated estrogens does not promote carcinogenesis in postmenopausal women with no prior history of breast cancer. Similarly, Dupont et al,[143] in a recent meta-analysis, concluded that the use of low-dose (0.625 mg/d) conjugated estrogens for several years does not appreciably increase the risk of breast cancer, and Henrich concurred.[144]

If estrogens stimulate breast cancer growth, postmenopausal women diagnosed with breast cancer should have a better prognosis than women who are diagnosed prior to menopause. In fact, however, the prognosis of postmenopausal women is worse when compared with that of premenopausal women.[145]

If the tumor-promoter effect of estrogen that is demonstrable in the laboratory has clinical significance, women who develop breast cancer while receiving ERT would be expected to have a poor prognosis. However, the opposite is the case, and several studies have demonstrated a significantly better prognosis for women using hormonal therapy who develop breast cancer than their counterparts who were not receiving ERT.[146,147]

Gambrell[146] evaluated the effect of ERT on breast cancer survival in 256 postmenopausal women. In this prospective trial, the mortality rate was 46% among patients not using the hormone and 22% among regular hormone users ($P < .002$). More of the hormone users had negative lymph nodes (57%) than did nonusers (42%); the death rate within the node-negative group was 8% for hormone users and 22% for nonusers.

In addition, Henderson et al[147] observed a 19% reduction in the breast cancer mortality rate among 4,988 ERT users compared with 3,865 nonusers who subsequently developed breast cancer. Furthermore, in a study of patients with breast cancer who had received ERT, Bergkvist et al[148] found a reduction in mortality of 40% but only in patients 50 years or older. The effect was most pronounced in women who were still receiving or had recently discontinued (within 1 year) ERT. The relative survival rate was higher by about 10% in patients who had received ERT than in patients who had never received ERT. These survival curves are shown in Figure 3.

Nevertheless, there remains a concern that select subgroups of the population will be adversely affected by the use of ERT. Some studies have suggested that long-term ERT (10 years or longer) does increase the risk of breast cancer.[149]

Mammographic Changes Associated With ERT

Yearly mammograms are recommended for screening in all women who have a history of breast cancer and in women older than 50 years. A concern is that ERT may produce changes in breast density that would decrease the sensitivity of mammography. In a matched cohort study of 405 women who underwent screening mammography, Bland et al[150] demonstrated no increase in breast density among ERT users. However, patients treated with ERT had an increased frequency of a more glandular parenchymal pattern, which may increase the interpretation error rate. In a retrospective study of 50 postmenopausal women receiving ERT, Stomper et al found that 25% of the women developed increased parenchymal density.[151] They suggested that this might decrease the sensitivity of mammography for early detection of breast cancer.

FIGURE 3

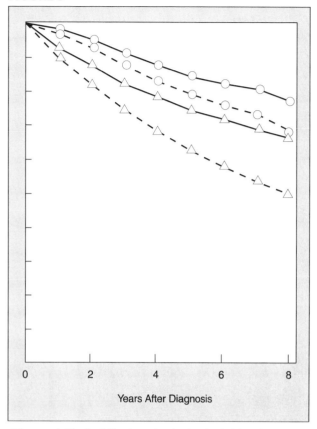

Observed (dashed line) and relative (solid line) survival in 261 patients with breast cancer with previous estrogen therapy (circles) and 6,617 such patients without previous estrogen therapy (triangles). Uppsala Health Care Region, Sweden, 1977–1986. Modified from Bergkvist L et al: Prognosis after breast cancer diagnosis in women exposed to estrogen and estrogen-progestogen replacement therapy. Am J Epidemiol 130:221–228, 1989. Reprinted, with permission, from DiSaia PJ.[180]

Berkowitz et al compared the mammograms of individual women obtained with and without ERT.[152] Increased parenchymal density on mammograms obtained during ERT was shown in only 17% of these women.

The Role of Tamoxifen

Tamoxifen (Nolvadex) is a weak estrogen that is widely used in the treatment of metastatic disease and in the adjuvant setting. An overview of breast cancer treatments has suggested that tamoxifen might benefit all women with invasive tumors.[153] Tamoxifen reduces the incidence of cancer in the contralateral breast of women with a history of breast cancer.[153] Among eight prospec-

TABLE 5

Estrogen Replacement Therapy in Women With Background of Breast Cancer: Preliminary Data of Prospective Study [a]

	Randomized study		Off study group, (+) ERT
	(+) ERT	(−) ERT	
Number of patients	12	12	16
Median age in yr (range)	46 (40-60)	45 45 (36-54)	47 47 (29-68)
Tumor, F/U [b]			
ER (−), < 10 y	6	7	7[c]
ER (?), > 10 y	6	5	5[c]
Motive			
Dyspareunia	8	4	4
Flashes	5	6	6
Depression	4	1	3
Heart risk	1	—	1
Osteoporosis	—	1	3
Lipids [c]			
Cholesterol (mg/100 mL)	232 ± 10	219 ± 10	226 ± 8
HDL	61 ± 4	60 ± 6	56 ± 5
LDL	146 ± 9	130 ± 9	140 ± 11
Triglycerides	143 ± 22	169 ± 26	184 ± 33
Hormones [c]			
FSH (mIU/mL)	82 ± 8	107 ± 10	78 ± 11
Bone mineral density[e,f]			
Vertebral spine	95 ± 4	90 ± 8	94 ± 4
(R) fem neck	97 ± 5	91 ± 4	88 ± 4
(L) fem neck	95 ± 5	88 ± 3	90 ± 3

ER = estrogen receptor, ERT = estrogen-replacement therapy, FSH = follicle-stimulating hormone, HDL = high-density lipoprotein, LDL = low-density lipoprotein

[a] As of 12/15/92

[b] Tumor = tumor ER status; F/U = duration of follow-up since cancer diagnosis.

[c] In off study patients, the interval since diagnosis is quite variable: the remaining four patients had ER (+) tumors

[d] Values = mean ± SEM

[e] Bone mineral density in g/cm² is expressed as percentage relative to sex- and age-matched normal controls

Adapted, with permission, from Vassilopoulou-Sellin R, Theriault RL: Randomized prospective trial of estrogen replacement therapy in women with a history of breast cancer. Monogr Natl Cancer Inst 16:153–159, 1994.

tive, randomized trials of tamoxifen vs no adjuvant therapy, the reduction in relative risk of contralateral breast cancer was 35% for women receiving tamoxifen.[154] Because of its estrogenic properties, tamoxifen also maintains bone mass and reduces death from heart attack by nearly 20% in postmenopausal women.[155–158]

Tamoxifen's mechanism of action was initially thought to be mediated through its antiestrogenic effects on the estrogen receptor. However, its effectiveness in pre-menopausal women with high levels of estrogen, which should competitively inhibit the effect of tamoxifen, has raised questions about this mechanism.

Tamoxifen has also been shown to inhibit the mitogenic effect of growth factors on breast cancer cells in the total absence of estrogens.[159] This suggests a non-estrogen-dependent effect of tamoxifen on the proliferation of breast cancer. Further research has demonstrated several other effects of tamoxifen on breast cancer cells, including increasing the secretion of inhibitory growth factors and decreasing the secretion of stimulatory growth factors.[160] Other suggested mechanisms of action have been outlined. These include inhibition of protein kinase c,[161] binding to calmodulin, a protein that plays a role in DNA synthesis,[162] and stimulation of natural killer cell activity.[163] Dose-dependent effects on the clonogenicity of breast tumor cells have been demonstrated.[164]

A concern over the concurrent administration of estrogen and tamoxifen is that estrogen might antagonize the effect of tamoxifen on tumor cells. However, the response of premenopausal women to tamoxifen, despite their high levels of circulating estradiol,[165–168] suggests that this is not the case. In the National Surgical Adjuvant Breast and Bowel Project B-14,[169] women with node-negative estrogen receptor-positive breast cancer were randomly assigned to receive either tamoxifen or placebo for 5 years after surgery. Premenopausal women derived a greater disease-free survival benefit from tamoxifen than did postmenopausal women. This indicates that the effect of endogenous estrogens was not deleterious to the anticancer effect of tamoxifen. Furthermore, in the British Breast Cancer Prevention Trial,[170] which uses tamoxifen as the preventive agent, postmenopausal women who experience severe hot flashes are given ERT, apparently with no ill effects. It has also been suggested that the benefits to heart and bone may be accentuated by combined tamoxifen and ERT.[154]

ERT and Breast Cancer Relapse

The most important question to be answered with the use of ERT in women who have been previously treated for breast cancer is, will ERT increase the rate of relapse? No controlled randomized trials have been published to date, but several small series have been reported. Stoll[171] reported on postmenopausal women who received 0.625 mg of conjugated equine estrogens and 0.15 mg of norgestrel per day. Patients were followed for 2 years, and no relapses occurred.

Wile et al[172] conducted a case-control study of 25 breast cancer survivors who received various types of ERT. The average interval between the diagnosis of malignancy and the start of ERT was 2 years; ERT was initiated in 17 patients less than 2 years after the primary diagnosis. Each patient was matched with two non-ERT users for age, stage of disease, and duration of observation. There were one cancer-related death in the treatment group and two in the control group. At further follow-up (mean, 35 months), three women receiving ERT had had relapses, and no non-ERT users had had a relapse.[132] The three relapses all occurred in the group in which ERT was initiated less than 2 years after the initial diagnosis of malignancy. In the overall group, two patients with positive lymph nodes were disease-free at 35 and 50 months.

Eden et al[173] conducted a case-control study of 901 survivors of breast cancer, 90 of whom received combined continuous estrogen and moderate-dose progesterone for relief of menopausal symptoms. Patients were matched for age at disease-free interval prior to the start of ERT. Significantly fewer tumor recurrences were seen in the ERT group. DiSaia et al[174] reported on their experience with 77 survivors of breast cancer who received ERT and were followed for up to 15 years (median follow-up, 59 months). The majority of patients (43 of 70) had stage I disease. Ninety-two percent had no evidence of recurrent disease at the time of the report.

Future Studies

Vassilopoulou-Sellin and Theriault[175] have instituted a prospective randomized study of ERT in postmenopausal survivors of breast cancer. The aims of the study include the development of specific benefit vs risk criteria that can be used in a clinical setting. Patients are eligible if they have survived stage I or II ER-negative breast cancer with no evidence of disease for at least 2 years or if they had unknown receptor status and no evidence of disease for at least 10 years. Patients with ER-positive disease and patients with carcinoma in situ are excluded, as are patients taking tamoxifen. Daily conjugated estrogens are being administered at a dose of 0.625 mg/d on days 1 through 25. Progesterone is not administered. Parameters of benefit and risk will be measured to detect a 10% change in disease-free survival for up to 5 years. The most recent published data on the trial are shown in Table 5.

Conclusions

While the beneficial effects of ERT in postmenopausal women are definite and substantial, it must be remembered that both ERT[176–178] and tamoxifen[179] increase the risk of endometrial cancer, the former by four to eight times compared with that of the general population. This risk remains elevated even after the use of estrogens has been discontinued.[178]

Several reviews have summarized the current controversy on the assessment of the risk-benefit ratio of ERT in survivors of breast cancer.[154,180,181] Opinions range from advocating the use of ERT in all patients with breast cancer who desire it to avoiding estrogens altogether in survivors of breast cancer and using nonhormonal therapies, progestogens, and tamoxifen to treat the symptoms of menopause.[182] This divergence of opinion highlights the need for scientific study in this area.

MALE BREAST CANCER

About 1% of all breast cancer cases occur in men. Age-standardized rates of breast cancer in men are 1.5 to 3.0 per million. It is estimated that 1,400 men will develop the disease in the United States in 1995 and that approximately 300 men will die of the disease this year.[123] About 1.35% to 1.5% of all cancers in men are breast cancer.[183]

Epidemiology and Etiology

The highest rates of male breast cancer are reported in Brazil and the lowest in Japan and Costa Rica.[183] The male to female ratio is higher among blacks than among whites in the United States[184] and Africa.[185] A higher incidence of male breast cancer is found in Jewish men compared with non-Jewish men, both in Israel[186,187] and in the United States.[186]

Exposures to electromagnetic fields,[188] heat,[189,190] and sex steroids[183,191] have been suggested to increase the risk of breast cancer in men. In a case-control study by Rosenbaum et al,[189] 71 men with breast cancer were compared with 256 healthy male controls. The authors found an elevated risk associated with heat exposure but not with electromagnetic fields. Demers et al[188] found an elevated risk (relative risk, 1.8; 95% confidence intervals 1.0 to 3.7) associated with exposure to electromagnetic fields in a case-control study of 227 men with breast cancer. Well-described associations with male breast cancer include prior breast or testicular pathology and liver disease[186,191,192] However, Thomas et al[193] found no association between liver disease and male breast cancer in their study. A family history of breast cancer,[183,190] particularly in males,[183,192] and a family history of prostate cancer[194] have also been shown to confer an increased risk of male breast cancer. The breast cancer risk of men with Klinefelter's syndrome is also increased[192,195] and is estimated to be 20 times that of the general male population,[183] thus approaching an incidence of 3%.[195] Interestingly, a family history of male breast cancer appears to confer an increased risk on female relatives similar to that of female breast cancer.[196] However, familial male breast cancer has been recently demonstrated not to be linked to the BRCA1 locus on chromosome 17q.[197] BRCA2 appears to be associated with male breast cancer, and was localised to chromosome 13q.[198] Figure 4 summarizes the etiologic factors associated with male breast cancer.

Pathology

The majority of breast cancers in men are epithelial. About 80% to 90% are carcinomas, most often infiltrating ductal histology.[199] Ductal carcinoma in situ comprises 3% to 7% of cases.[200] Mucinous, medullary, tubular, and inflammatory breast carcinomas have all been seen in men.[199] Paget's disease,[201] cystosarcoma phyllodes,[202,203] and small cell carcinoma of the breast[204] have also all been described in men. Heller et al[205] reviewed the pathologic findings in a series of male breast cancers and compared them with female breast cancers. The distribution of histologic subtypes and the pattern of distant metastases were the same in men and women. Hultborn et al[206] had similar findings. It was once thought that lobular carcinoma could not occur in the male breast because of the absence of the terminal lobular unit; however, 16 cases of lobular carcinoma in men have now been described in the literature and have been recently reviewed.[207]

Ninety-two cases of ductal carcinoma in situ in men have been described in the literature and have been recently reviewed.[200] All patients presented with a mass or nipple discharge. Of the 33 patients in whom axillary lymph-node dissection was performed, none had positive nodes. It has been suggested that axillary dissection should not be performed in this subset of men unless the primary tumor is 2.5 cm or larger.[208] A similar recommendation has been made for women.[209]

Clinical Features

The most common presenting feature in men with breast cancer is a painless lump in the subareolar region or upper outer quadrant, occurring in 60% to 90% of cases.[194,210–218] Nipple discharge (bloody or nonbloody) is the second most frequent presenting feature. Mastalgia, nipple pruritus and eczematoid changes (as seen in Paget's disease), and symptoms from distant metastases are sometimes presenting symptoms. Several series have described a delay of several months in presentation to a physician.

Median age at diagnosis is 68 years,[183] though older series have quoted a younger median age.[210] Breast cancer associated with Klinefelter's syndrome is seen in a younger age group.[183] Cases have been described in a 5-year-old boy and a 92-year-old man.[183]

FIGURE 4

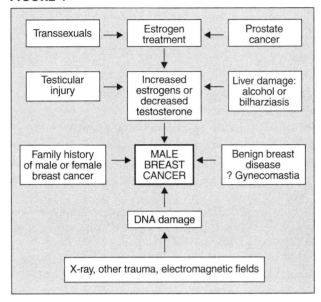

Schematic diagram of the possible relationship between male breast cancer and various risk factors. Reprinted, with permission, from Sasco AJ et al.[183]

A slight preponderance of left-sided tumors, similar to that observed in women, has been noted.[183] Bilateral tumors are present in 1% to 1.5% of male patients.[210,215,217] In a series of 444 men with breast cancer, 54% were node-positive. Several retrospective analyses of the clinical features and outcomes of series of patients have been published.[194,210–224]

Diagnosis

The differential diagnosis for a man with a breast lump includes gynecomastia,[210] mastitis,[215] and fibroadenoma.[203] In contrast to the unilateral, painless, indurated lump commonly seen with breast cancer, gynecomastia is often bilateral, freely mobile, subareolar, and moderately tender. Mammography can be useful in differentiating gynecomastia from male breast cancer.[225] The incidence of preceding gynecomastia in men with breast cancer is influenced by recall bias but has been quoted as 1% to 12%.[183] The radiographic features of malignancy and other breast diseases in men have been reviewed.[225–227] Jackson and Gilmor[227] reviewed sonograms and mammograms obtained over a 3-year period for 41 men who had breast enlargement. The appearances of benign and malignant disease overlapped with both modalities, and the authors recommended that both be used in the evaluation of breast pathology in males. On the other hand, Dershaw[228] reviewed 94 mammograms done for the evaluation of male breast disease and found that gyneco-

TABLE 6

Survival Data From Published Series of More Than 100 Male Breast Cancer Patients

Author	No. of patients	Overall survival		Disease-free survival			
				Node negative		Node positive	
		5-year	10-year	5-year	10-year	5-year	10-year
Gough[214]	124	57	31	68	NA	55	NA
Borgen[215]	104	85	NA	87	NA	30	NA
Ramantanis[218]	138	NA	NA	57	NA	31	NA
Cutuli[194]	444	65	36	NA	52	NA	28
Salvadori[222]	170	54.3	26.9				
Ciatto[223]	150	65	39	62	46	40	20
van Geel[219]	104	54	26.3				
Ribeiro[224]	301	52	38				

mastia was easily differentiated from malignancy in all but one case. However, there were only three carcinomas in his series. Borgen et al[215] found an 8% false-negative rate in the 50 patients in their series who had a mammogram; 58% had a mass, and 35% had other mammographic findings.

Men with dominant masses or inflammatory changes in the breast, or both, should undergo aspiration or surgical biopsy.[229] Fine-needle aspiration is the appropriate initial step to obtain a pathologic diagnosis.[230–231] If this is inconclusive, it is mandatory to proceed to a surgical biopsy.

Staging

Breast tumors in men are staged using the standard T (tumor size), N (nodal status), M (distant metastases) system. Male patients with breast cancer have a high incidence of T4 tumors, 69% in the series by Lartigau et al.[213] There is also high incidence of regional nodal metastases, 54% in the series of Cutuli et al[194]; in the same series, 40 of 444 patients presented with distant metastases. Heller et al[205] noted fewer men with T2N0 disease and more with T1N1 disease than in a similar group of women. T1N1 disease has a poorer prognosis than T2N0 disease, and this may contribute to the relatively poorer prognosis in men with stage II disease compared to women with a similar stage of disease.

Prognosis

Hormonal Status: Men with breast cancer have a high frequency of hormone receptor positivity: 75% to 85%.[215,232–234] Estrogen receptor (ER) positivity ranges from 80% to 83% and is slightly more frequent than progesterone receptor positivity which ranges from 70% to 76%.[210,215,232] It is not clear whether progesterone receptor positivity increases response to hormonal therapy.[235] A 76% incidence of epidermal growth factor positivity has also been described.[236] The clinical significance of this is unknown.

The high incidence of hormone receptor positivity led to the use of hormonal therapy in male patients with metastatic breast cancer, with a response rate of 80% in receptor-positive patients.[232]

Prognostic Factors: Axillary nodal involvement at the time of diagnosis remains the strongest predictor of prognosis.[197,216,237,238] In a recent series by Lartigau et al,[213] the 10-year survival rate was 55% for node-negative men vs 22% for node-positive men. Digenis et al[232] studied a series of 41 men with breast cancer and observed the following 5- and 10-year survival rates after all treatments: stage I, 100% and 100%; II, 65% and 52%; III, 55% and 22%; and IV, 0% and 0%. These data are similar to historical survival data for women with breast cancer[237] and conflict with earlier studies that suggested a poorer prognosis in men.[238,239] Table 6 shows the 5 and 10 year survival rates with a breakdown by nodal status, of all series with more than 100 patients.[194,214,215,218,219,222–224] Tumor size,[213,240] pathologic stage,[214] hormonal status,[241] duration of symptoms,[215] and tumor grade[214,242] are also important prognostic factors. Well-differentiated tubular carcinoma has a less favorable prognosis than do mucinous, cystic, papillary, or medullary types.[242] A recent report demonstrated a prognostic significance of the degree of proliferative activity in the tumor but no prognostic value of receptor status.[243]

The prognostic importance of other features such as flow cytometry, S phase, thymidine labeling index, and ploidy remain under active investigation.[244]

Treatment of Local-Regional Disease

Control of local disease is the first principle of breast cancer therapy, regardless of gender. Modified radical mastectomy or simple mastectomy with irradiation are the treatments of choice in men. There is no survival advantage from radical mastectomy.[232] Radical mastectomy is done only if the tumor involves the pectoral muscles. Men whose general condition precludes major surgery can be treated with lumpectomy or tumor excision followed by irradiation of the chest wall and regional nodes.[211] Adjuvant radiotherapy decreases local recurrence but does not change survival.[199]

Adjuvant Chemotherapy: Adjuvant chemotherapy in men with breast cancer was first investigated using combination regimens. Bagley et al[245] treated 24 stage II node-positive men with cyclophosphamide, methotrexate, and fluorouracil (CMF) within 4 weeks of mastectomy. Median follow-up was 46 months. Median overall survival was 98 months, and the projected 5-year survival rate exceeded 80%.

Ben-Baruch et al[246] presented a cohort of 31 men treated with 12 cycles of CMF following local therapy. Cancer survival was significantly improved in the treated group compared with historical controls taken from the Surveillance, Epidemiology, and End Results data. Historical controls had stage II node-positive male breast cancer and were individually matched to the treatment group within 5 years of age and 5 years of diagnosis. Patel et al[247] treated 11 node-positive men with stage II or III disease with fluorouracil, doxorubicin, and cyclophosphamide (FAC). With a median follow-up of 52 months, four patients had recurrent disease. The 5-year survival rate was greater than 85%. This compares very favorably with the 30% 5-year survival rate demonstrated in a retrospective series of male patients treated with local therapy only.[240]

Adjuvant Hormonal Therapy: The success of hormonal therapy in treating metastatic disease[248] plus data suggesting an increase in disease-free survival when tamoxifen was used as an adjuvant agent in women[249] prompted Ribeiro and Swindell[250] to study the use of adjuvant tamoxifen for male breast cancer. Thirty-nine stage II (all axillary node-positive) or operable stage III patients treated with adjuvant tamoxifen had a 5-year

survival rate of 61%, compared with 44% for historical controls. The disease-free survival rates for tamoxifen-treated and control patients were 56% and 28%, respectively.

Treatment of Metastatic Disease

Men who present with distant metastases from breast cancer have a median survival of 26.5 months.[232] The high incidence of receptor positivity resulted in early interest in hormonal manipulation for metastatic breast cancer in men.

Hormonal Manipulation: An overall response rate of 55% to 80% has been seen in men with metastatic breast disease who were treated with hormonal ablation.[229] Response to orchiectomy, the earliest form of hormonal ablation, is not age related. However, orchiectomy is poorly tolerated psychologically.[251] Adrenalectomy and hypophysectomy are virtually never used because of irreversible side effects and the availability of less morbid alternatives.[240]

A number of publications have described the clinical response of male breast cancer to total androgen blockade.[252–256] Doberauer et al[256] observed a partial response in one of five men treated with the luteinizing hormone-releasing hormone analog buserelin; this 12-month remission was reinduced at relapse for an additional 24 months by the addition of the antiandrogen flutamide. Lopez et al[253] treated 11 men with recurrent or progressive cancer of the breast with buserelin and cyproterone acetate. Objective responses were observed in seven patients and lasted 9 to 24 months; three additional patients had stable disease for 5 months. Cyproterone acetate used as a single agent has been compared with a combination of buserelin and cyproterone acetate. Though there was a trend favoring the combination, no statistically significant difference was demonstrated.[255] Clinical worsening of disease during the first week of treatment with cyproterone acetate and luteinizing hormone releasing hormone analogs was not seen. Side effects of androgen blockade include decrease or loss of libido, impotence, and hot flashes.[252,253,256]

While it is clear that these regimens utilizing total androgen blockade are effective, they have not been compared with standard hormonal therapy to determine which therapy has the greater efficacy.

The overall response rate with tamoxifen is between 32% and 75% and rises to between 44% and 81% if the tumors are ER positive.[241,257] The high rate of hormone receptor positivity in men has resulted in a large body of literature on the use of tamoxifen.[241,257–60] It is the drug of choice in hormone receptor-positive men with recurrent or metastatic breast cancer. However, the rate of discontinuing tamoxifen because of side effects is much higher in men (20%) than in women (4.1%). Prominent side effects in men include a decrease in libido (29%), hot flashes (20%), and weight gain (25%).[261] Responses to tamoxifen have been seen after both response and failure-to-respond to orchiectomy, suggesting that tamoxifen and orchiectomy may be non-cross-resistant.[262]

Other hormonal agents that have been used include progestins such as megestrol acetate,[263] medroxyprogesterone acetate,[264] aminoglutethimide,[241] and estrogens.[265] Pannuti et al[264] reported a partial response in five of six patients, with a median response duration of 7 months, with high-dose medroxyprogesterone acetate. Patients with ER-positive tumors that fail to respond to initial endocrine manipulation may still respond to other forms of hormonal therapy.[229]

Hormone-induced tumor flares have been seen in men started on new hormonal therapy as treatment for metastatic disease.[266] It has been suggested that these flares may be a sign of hormonal dependency. Therapy should not be abandoned; rather, the patient should be treated for pain until the episode has resolved.

Kinne and Hakes[251] recently summarized the literature on hormone manipulation in male breast cancer. They found an overall response rate of 51%, reaching 71% if the tumor is ER positive.

Chemotherapy: Chemotherapy can improve the prognosis of men with advanced breast cancer.[251] Overall chemotherapy response rates are around 35% to 45%.[267,268] Yap et al[268] reviewed the M. D. Anderson chemotherapy experience for metastatic disease in 1980. Of 18 men, 11 demonstrated a response (complete or partial) to chemotherapy. Median survival for this group was 23 months, compared with 14.5 months for men who failed to demonstrate any chemotherapeutic response ($P < .05$). They found a similar response rate of male breast cancer to chemotherapy as seen in female breast cancer. Lopez et al[267] also found a response rate comparable to that seen in female breast cancer. They also found that doxorubicin-containing regimens seemed superior to regimens without doxorubicin, such as CMF. Single-agent chemotherapy (vinblastine or triethylenethiophosphoramide) has proved to be less effective than combination therapy.[267] Responses to chemotherapy tend to be faster but less durable than those with hormonal manipulation.[224,267] For these reasons, chemotherapy is often reserved for men who have clearly failed to respond to hormonal manipulation. Responses to both chemotherapy and hormonal manipulation have been observed in all organs, including lung, liver, and bone.

BREAST CANCER AND PREGNANCY

The simultaneous occurrence of breast cancer and pregnancy is rare. The reported incidence of pregnancy is 1 in 3,000 to 5,000 breast cancer cases,[269] though some authors quote a rate as high as 1% to 3% of all breast cancers.[270–273] The incidence in Japan is quoted as 0.76%.[274] Pregnant patients represent 10% to 15% of breast cancer patients younger than 40 years.[275] There is evidence that the incidence of breast cancer in premenopausal women is rising, and as more women delay childbearing, the simultaneous presentation of breast cancer and pregnancy may increase. The incidence of breast cancer during pregnancy is no higher than the incidence in any premenopausal woman.[277]

Diagnosis

Women with pregnancy-associated breast cancer have clearly been shown to present at a later stage than do nonpregnant women. Zemlickis et al[273] demonstrated a relative risk of 2.5 (confidence interval, 1.1 to 5.3) of presenting with stage IV disease and a decreased chance of diagnosis during stage I , for pregnant patients compared with age-matched nonpregnant controls. A number of series have demonstrated a diagnostic delay in pregnant women with a breast abnormality ranging from 2 to 15 months longer than in nonpregnant women.[271,276,277] The reasons for this include physiologic hypertrophy of the breast and engorgement, which may mask a lump, and the fact that most gestational abnormalities of the breast are benign.[276] Lumps are often followed clinically for many months in pregnant women. Coincident pathology, such as mastitis, has been reported in up to 30% of breast cancers diagnosed during pregnancy.[278] Other issues apart from delayed diagnosis may play a role in the more advanced stage at presentation. For example, the effect of the high levels of circulating prolactin found during pregnancy on the growth of breast cancer is unknown.[279] The impact of the altered immunocompetence and decreased activity of mitogens found during pregnancy is also unknown.[280,281]

Mammography is rarely performed in pregnant women because of the perceived risk of harm to the fetus.[276,282] In addition, it has been stated that increased breast density during pregnancy makes mammography interpretation difficult.[276] However, in a retrospective review of 23 women diagnosed with breast cancer during or within 1 year following pregnancy, who had a mammogram performed prior to biopsy, mammographic evidence of breast cancer was present in 18 (78%) of 23 cases.[282] Breast sonography has less risk, and in the six patients examined by Liberman et al[282] with this technique, all had a solid mass detected. Similarly, the accuracy of sonography was 93% (39 of 42) in a series by Ishada et al.[274] Sonography appears to be safe and sensitive in the evaluation of a breast abnormality.

Pathology

There is no difference in tumor type between pregnant and nonpregnant women,[274] and the incidence of inflammatory carcinoma in pregnant women is 1.5% to 4%, identical to that of nonpregnant women.[283] However, the number of pregnant patients with vascular and lymphatic invasion is higher,[274] as are the mean tumor size and number of lymph-node metastases. The presence of estrogen receptors (ERs) and progesterone receptors(PRs) has shown a trend toward a lower incidence in pregnant patients, perhaps because of patient age.[271,283,284] The exception has been a single case-control study[274] which suggested an independent trend toward higher levels of ER-positivity in pregnant patients. ER-negative tumors, regardless of pregnancy status, have a biologically aggressive course and carry a poor prognosis,[285] and it is thought that this may contribute to a worse outcome in pregnant patients. Assay of ER status during pregnancy may result in excessive false-negatives because of high levels of circulating estrogens saturating all available ER sites.[276] Though the diagnosis of malignancy may be made by fine-needle aspiration, a surgical biopsy is required to document the presence or absence of tumor invasion.[286]

Staging

The most accurate means of assessing the pregnant patient are a detailed history and physical examination with particular attention to tumor size, nodal involvement, and assessment for metastatic disease including the musculoskeletal and central nervous systems. Mammography and extensive nuclear scanning should be done only if the information is vital to treatment planning.[286] Any such procedure should be done with appropriate precautions to protect the fetus. A chest radiograph can be safely obtained with proper shielding.[286] Aggressive hydration to aid in excretion of the isotope should precede all bone scans.[276] Laboratory studies should include a complete blood count, biochemical profile, and analysis for tumor markers.

Prognosis

It has been shown that outcome in patients with concurrent breast cancer and pregnancy is the same as for their nonpregnant counterparts when adjustment is made

TABLE 7

First Trimester Chemotherapy Exposure and Fetal Malformations

Agent	Number of exposed patients	Number of malformed fetuses
Aminopterin	52	10
Methotrexate	3	3
Vinca alkaloids	14	1
Alkylating agents	44	6

Adapted from Doll DC, Ringenberg QS, Yarbro JW, et al: Antineoplastic agents and pregnancy. Semin Oncol 16:337–346, 1989.

for age and stage of disease.[287,288] Pregnant patients do present with more advanced disease. Various studies show that 56% to 89% of patients who present with breast cancer during pregnancy are lymph-node positive.[289] Most series report identical actuarial and disease-free survival rates in gestational and nongestational breast cancer once patients are matched for age and stage.[273,283,287,289,290] Von Schoultz et al[290] recently published a study on 173 women who were diagnosed with pregnancy in the 5 years preceding or following the diagnosis of breast cancer. These women were compared with 1,740 women with breast cancer who were not pregnant during that period. Though women with a pregnancy before diagnosis of breast cancer had slightly larger tumors than did the control group, they did not differ with respect to nodal status or ER status. Their prognosis was the same when compared with that of the control group. However, some studies suggest that pregnant patients do have a worse prognosis.[291,292] Guinee et al[292] recently completed a large multicenter review of 407 women aged 20 to 29 years. For women whose breast cancers were diagnosed during pregnancy, the risk of dying from breast cancer was significantly greater than that of women with breast cancer who had never been pregnant (relative risk, 3.26; 95% confidence interval, 1.81 to 5.87; $P = .0004$). The risk remained significant ($P = .023$) when adjustment was made for the number of axillary nodes and tumor size. Age at the time of pregnancy is an inconsistent prognostic factor. Clark and Reid found that survival was worse in those older than age 40,[283] while Ribeiro et al found no association with age.[287]

Treatment

There is no justification for delaying in treatment in pregnant women with breast cancer. Termination of the pregnancy is not routinely indicated.[270,287,293]

Local treatment remains a modified radical mastectomy. Maternal morbidity from surgery and general anesthesia is low.[294] Fetal risk is low unless complications (shock, hypotension) occur.[294] Milk production should be suppressed by bromocriptine to reduce the size and vascularity of the breasts preoperatively and to lessen the risk of infection and milk fistulae.[276]

Chemotherapy and Hormonal Therapy: Chemotherapy has the highest likelihood of affecting the baby during embryogenesis.[295] Nevertheless, adjuvant chemotherapy in appropriate patients should not be withheld because of fear of potential fetal morbidity. Doll et al reviewed the reported adverse effects of in utero chemotherapy exposure and found a rate of fetal malformation of 19% in the first trimester.[296] Chemotherapy should therefore be delayed until the first trimester is past. The risk of fetal malformation secondary to chemotherapy administered during the second and third trimesters has been estimated at 2%.[296] Alkylating agents, aminopterin and methotrexate have all shown evidence of associated fetal malformations (Table 7). Turchi and Villaris[297] reported on 28 pregnancies following treatment with anthracyclines; 24 normal infants were born, 4 infants were reported to have reversible defects.

The effect of cytotoxic therapy on the maintenance of the integrity of the placental barrier is largely unstudied. It has been suggested that the anthracyclines and other agents may be prevented from entering the fetal circulation by the high levels of MDR1 protein localized in the placental membrane.[298]

Ovarian ablation, by surgery or radiation, has no place in the treatment of pregnant women.[283] Postpartum breast feeding should be avoided because cyclophosphamide is secreted in breast milk.

Radiation Exposure: The effects of radiation on the fetus depend on the gestational age at the time of exposure.[276] It is estimated that a 12-week shielded fetus will receive a dose secondary to internal scatter radiation of up to 30 cGy with a standard 5,000 cGy course of radiotherapy.[299] Radiation should be avoided if at all possible during the first trimester, as the period of organogenesis is the most sensitive to radiation. In the second and third trimesters, the risk is primarily that of microcephaly and of childhood cancer developing in later years. Lower nonmorbid doses from scatter radiation have been quoted in other studies.[300]

Subsequent Pregnancy

Posttreatment fertility in breast cancer patients has been looked at in several studies. Richards et al's study[301] of cyclophosphamide, methotrexate, and fluorouracil

showed a 37% incidence of premature menopause in women 40 years or younger. Doxorubicin-containing regimens at M. D. Anderson produce amenorrhea in 96% of women 40 to 49 years old, but no woman younger than 30 years has developed amenorrhea. Half of women younger than 40 who become amenorrheic resume menstruating following cessation of chemotherapy.[128]

Following treatment of breast cancer, there is a concern about the safety of subsequent pregnancy. The fear is that sustained increases in the levels of estrogen and progesterone during pregnancy will stimulate the growth of occult metastatic disease. In the past, patients were advised to avoid pregnancy for at least 2 years after breast cancer treatment so that the endocrine stimulus would not activate occult systemic disease. However, Mignot et al[302] have reported that survival rates were no different in women who conceived within 6 months after breast cancer treatments were completed compared with a control group.

Peters and Meakin[303] have demonstrated that stage for stage, patients who become pregnant after breast cancer do better than their nonpregnant counterparts. The selection bias that patients who are able to become pregnant after chemotherapy were probably the group with a superior performance status and less disease is evident. Despite this, it is clear that these women do not do any worse than their nonpregnant counterparts, suggesting no role of pregnancy in disease recurrence. In Sutton et al's series,[304] there were 33 pregnancies in 25 (11%) of 227 breast cancer patients younger than 35. Of these pregnancies, 10 were terminated, 2 ended with spontaneous abortion, and 19 had resulted in live births, with no fetal malformations. Two patients were still pregnant at the time of the report. Donegan found a comparable rate of 7%.[305]

Conclusions

In conclusion, breast cancer associated with pregnancy poses several treatment challenges. Local therapy should never be delayed. Careful management and avoidance of chemotherapy and radiation exposure during the first trimester should help to produce a positive outcome for both mother and fetus.

REFERENCES

1. Thomas ED, Clift RA, Buckner CD: Marrow transplantation for patients with acute non-lymphoblastic leukemia who achieve a first remission. Cancer Treat Rep 66:1463–1466, 1982.

2. Appelbaum FR, Thomas ED: Review of the use of marrow transplantation in the treatment of non-Hodgkin's lymphoma. J Clin Oncol 1:440–447, 1983.

3. Philip T, Armitage JO, Spitzer G, et al: High-dose therapy and

autologous bone marrow transplantation after failure of conventional chemotherapy in adults with intermediate or high grade non-Hodgkin's lymphoma. N Engl J Med 316:1493–1498, 1987.

4. Takvorian T, Canellos GP, Ritz J, et al: Prolonged disease free survival after autologous bone marrow transplantation in patients with non-Hodgkin's lymphomas with poor prognosis. N Engl J Med 316:1499–1515, 1987.

5. Levin L, Hryniuk W: The application of dose-intensity to problems in chemotherapy of ovarian and endometrial cancer. Semin Oncol 14(4 suppl 4):12–19, 1987.

6. Maraninchi D, Gastaut JA, Herre P, et al: High dose melphalan and autologous marrow transplant in adult solid tumors. Clinical responses and preliminary evaluation of different strategies. Monograph Ser Eur Organ Res Treat Cancer 14:145–150, 1984.

7. Mulder NH, Meinesz AF, Sleijfer DT, et al: High dose etoposide with or without cyclophosphamide and autologous bone marrow transplantation in solid tumors. Monograph Ser Eur Organ Res Treat Cancer 14:125–130, 1984.

8. Douer D, Champlin RE, Ho WG, et al: High-dose combined modality therapy and autologous bone marrow transplantation in resistant cancer. Am J Med 71:973–976, 1981.

9. Wolff SN, Fer MF, McKay CM, et al: High dose VP-16-213 and autologous bone marrow transplant for refractory malignancies: A phase I study. J Clin Oncol 1:701–705, 1983.

10. Lazarus HM, Herzig RH, Graham Pole J: Intensive melphalan chemotherapy and cryopreserved autologous bone marrow transplantation for the treatment of refractory cancer. J Clin Oncol 1:359–367, 1983.

11. Corringham R, Gilmore M, Prentice HG, et al: High dose melphalan with autologous bone marrow transplant. treatment of poor prognosis tumors. Cancer 52:1783–1787, 1983.

12. Tobias JS, Weiner RS, Griffiths CT, et al: Cryopreserved autologous marrow infusion following high-dose cancer chemotherapy. Eur J Cancer 13:269–277, 1977.

13. Ariel IM: Treatment of disseminated cancer by intravenous hydroxyurea and autogenous bone marrow transplants: Experience with 35 patients. J Surg Oncol 7:331–335, 1975.

14. Bone marrow autotransplantation in man. Report of an international group. Lancet 2:960–962, 1986.

15. Hryniuk W, Bush H: The importance of dose intensity in chemotherapy of metastatic breast cancer. J Clin Oncol 2:1281–1288, 1984.

16. Hryniuk W: The influence of dose intensity in the outcome of chemotherapy, in Hellman S, DeVita V, Rosenberg S (eds): Advances in Oncology, pp 121–124. Philadelphia, JB Lippincott, 1988.

17. Bonadonna G, Valagussa P, Rossi A, et al: Dose-response effect of adjuvant chemotherapy in breast cancer. N Engl J Med 304:10–15, 1981.

18. Frei E III, Antman K, Teicher B, et al: Bone marrow autotransplantation for solid tumors—prospects. J Clin Oncol 7:515–526, 1989.

19. Frei E III, Canellos GP Dose: A critical factor in cancer chemotherapy. Am J Med 69:585–594, 1980.

20. Henderson IC, Hayes DF, Gelman R: Dose response in the treatment of breast cancer: A critical review. J Clin Oncol 6:1501–1515, 1988.

21. vonHoff DD, et al: Use of in-vitro dose-response effects to select antineoplastics for high-dose or regional administration regimens. J Clin Oncol 4:1827–1834, 1986.

22. Schabel FM, et al: Increasing the therapeutic response rates to anticancer drugs by applying the basic principles of pharmacology. Cancer 54:1160–1167, 1984.

23. Herzig G: Autologous marrow transplant in cancer therapy. Hematology 9:1–24, 1981.

24. Peters WP, Eder J, Hannes WD, et al: High dose combination alkylating agents and autologous bone marrow support: A phase I trial. J Clin Oncol 4:646–654, 1986.

25. Schabel FN: Patterns of resistance and therapeutic synergism among alkylating agents. Antibiot Chemother 23:200–215, 1978.

26. Schabel FN, Griswold DP Jr, Corbett TH, et al: Testing therapeutic hypotheses in mice and man: Observations on the therapeutic activity against advanced solid tumors in mice treated with anticancer drugs that have demonstrated or potential clinical utility for treatment of advanced solid tumors in man, in DeVita VT, Busch H (eds): Methods in Cancer Research, pp 3–5. New York Academic Press, 1979.

27. Peters WP: Dose intensification using combination alkylating agents and autologous bone marrow support in the treatment of primary and metastatic breast cancer: A review of the Duke Bone Marrow Transplantation Program experience, in Effects of Therapy on Biology and Kinetics of the Residual Tumor, Part B: Clinical Aspects, pp 185–194. New York, Wiley-Liss, 1990.

28. Early Breast Cancer Trialists' Collaborative Group: Systemic treatment of early breast cancer by hormonal, cytotoxic or immune therapy. Lancet 339:1–15, 71–85, 1992.

29. Gelber RD, Goldhirsch A: The concept of an overview of clinical trials with special emphasis on early breast cancer. J Clin Oncol 4:1696–1703, 1986.

30. Legha SS, Buzdar AU, Smith TL, et al: Complete remissions in metastatic breast cancer treated with combination drug therapy. Ann Intern Med 91:847–852, 1979.

31. Decker DA, Ahmann DL, Bisel HF, et al: Complete responders to chemotherapy in metastatic breast cancer: Characterization and analysis. JAMA 242:2075–2079, 1979.

32. Swenerton KD, Legha SS, Smith T, et al: Prognostic factors in metastatic breast cancer treated with combination chemotherapy. Cancer Res 39:1552–1562, 1979.

33. Ahmann DL, Bisel HF, Hahn RG, et al: An analysis of a multiple drug program in the treatment of patients with advanced breast cancer utilising 5 fluorouracil, cyclophosphamide, and prednisone with and without vincristine. Cancer 36:1925–1935, 1975.

34. Bonadonna G, Valagussa P, Rossi A, et al: Ten year experience with CMF-based adjuvant chemotherapy in resectable breast cancer. Breast Cancer Res Treat 5:95–115, 1985.

35. Ogawa M, Mukaiyama T: Treatment strategy to obtain cure for recurrent advanced breast cancer. Gian to Kagaku Ryoho 21(suppl 2):259–263, 1994.

36. Hryniuk W: The impact of dose intensity on the design of clinical trials. Semin Oncol 14:65–74, 1987.

37. Hryniuk WH, Figueredo A, Goodyear H: Applications of dose intensity to problems in chemotherapy in breast and colorectal cancer. Semin Oncol 14(suppl 4):3–11, 1987.

38. Dembo AJ: Time dose factors in chemotherapy: Expanding the concept of dose intensity. J Clin Oncol 5:94–96, 1987.

39. Hryniuk W, Levine MN: Analysis of dose intensity for adjuvant chemotherapy trials in stage II breast cancer J Clin Oncol 4:1162–1170, 1986.

40. Hryniuk WN, Bonadonna G, Valagussa P: The effect of dose intensity in adjuvant chemotherapy, in Grune SE (ed): Adjuvant Therapy of Cancer, vol 5, pp 13–24. Philadelphia, Grune & Stratton, 1987.

41. Cooper RG, Holland JF, Glidewell O: Adjuvant chemotherapy of breast cancer. Cancer 44:793–798, 1979.

42. Marini G, Simoncini E, Zamboni A, et al: 5-fluorouracil and high-dose folinic acid as salvage treatment of advanced breast cancer: An update. Oncology 44:336–340, 1987.

43. O'Bryan RM, Baker LH, Gottlieb JE, et al: Dose response

evaluation of Adriamycin in human neoplasia. Cancer 39:1940–1948, 1977.

44. Forastiere AA, Hakes TB, Wittes JT, et al: Cisplatin in the treatment of metastatic breast carcinoma. A prospective randomized trial of two dosage schedules. Am J Clin Oncol 5:243–247, 1982.

45. Kolaric K, Roth A: Phase II clinical trial of cis-dichlorodiammine platinum (cis-DDP) for antitumorigenic activity in previously untreated patients with metastatic breast cancer. Cancer Chemother Pharmacol 11:108–112, 1993.

46. Peters WP, Eder HP, Henner WD, et al: Novel toxicities associated with high dose combination alkylating agents and autologous bone marrow support, in Dicke KA, Spitzer G, Zander AR (eds): Autologous Bone Marrow Transplantation, pp 231–235. Houston, The University of Texas M. D. Anderson Hospital and Tumor Institute at Houston, 1985.

47. Antman K: Dose-intensive therapy in breast cancer, in Armitage JO, Antman KA (eds): High Dose Cancer Chemotherapy: Pharmacology, Hematopoietins, Stem cells. Baltimore, Williams and Wilkins 1992.

48. Vincent MD, Powles TJ, Coombes RC, et al: Late intensification with high-dose melphalan and autologous bone marrow support in breast cancer patients responding to conventional chemotherapy. Cancer Chemother Pharmacol 21:255–260, 1988.

49. Tannock IF, Boyd NF, DeBoer G, et al: A randomized trial of two dose levels of cyclophosphamide, methotrexate and fluorouracil chemotherapy for patients with metastatic breast cancer. J Clin Oncol 6:1377–1387, 1988.

50. Engelsman E, Rubens R, Klija J, et al: Comparison of "classical CMF" with three-weekly intravenous CMF schedule in postmenopausal patients with advanced breast cancer: An EORTC study (trial 10808) (abstract). Proc Eur Organ Res Treat Cancer 1:7, 1987.

51. Beretta G, Tabiadon D, Tedeschi L, et al: Front-line treatment with CMF—Variations for advanced breast carcinoma. A randomized study (abstract 302). Proc Am Soc Clin Oncol 5:77, 1986.

52. Carmo-Pereira J, Costa FO, Henriques V, et al: A randomized trial of cyclophosphamide, methotrexate, 5-fluorouracil and prednisone in advanced breast cancer. Cancer Chemother Pharmacol 17:87–90, 1986.

53. Hoogstraten B, George S, Samal B: Combination chemotherapy and Adriamycin in patients with advanced breast cancer. Cancer 38:13–20, 1976.

54. Smalley RV, Murphy S, Huguley CM: Combination versus sequential five-drug chemotherapy in metastatic adenocarcinoma of the breast. Cancer Res 36:3911–3916, 1976.

55. Ludwig Breast Cancer Study Group: A randomized trial of adjuvant combination chemotherapy with or without prednisone in premenopausal breast cancer patients with metastases in one to three axillary nodes. Cancer Res 45:4454–4459, 1985.

56. Korzun A, Norton L, Perloff M, et al: Clinical equivalence despite dosage differences of two schedules of cyclophosphamide, methotrexate, 5-fluorouracil, vincristine, and prednisone (CMFVP) for adjuvant therapy of node-positive stage II breast cancer (abstract). Proc Am Soc Clin Oncol 7:A12, 1988.

57. Wood WC, Budman DR, Korzun AH, et al: Dose and dose intensity of adjuvant chemotherapy for stage II, node positive breast carcinoma. N Engl J Med 330:1253–1259, 1993.

58. Habeshaw T, Paul R, Jones R, et al: Epirubicin at two dose levels with prednisolone as treatment for advanced breast cancer: The results of a randomized trial. J Clin Oncol 9:295–304, 1991.

59. French Epirubicin Study Group: A prospective randomized trial comparing epirubicin monochemotherapy to two fluorouracil, cyclophosphamide, and epirubicin regimens differing in epirubicin dose in advanced breast cancer patients. J Clin Oncol 9:305–312, 1991.

60. Hortobagyi GN, Bodey SP, Buzdar AU, et al: Evaluation of high-dose versus standard FAC chemotherapy for advanced breast cancer in protected environment units: A prospective randomized study. J Clin Oncol 5:354–364, 1987.

61. Hortobagyi GN, Dunphy F, Buzdar AU, et al: Dose intensity studies in breast cancer—Autologous bone marrow transplantation, in Effects of Therapy on Biology and Kinetics of the Residual Tumor, Part B: Clinical Aspects, pp 195–209. New York, Wiley-Liss, 1990.

62. Buzdar AU, et al: Significance of drug dose, timing and radiotherapy in adjuvant therapy of breast cancer, in Mathe G (ed): Recent Results in Cancer Research, pp 141–147. New York, Springer-Verlag, 1984.

63. Antman K, Gale RP: Advanced breast cancer: High dose chemotherapy and bone marrow autotransplants. Ann Intern Med 108:570–574, 1988.

64. Peters WP, Shpall EJ, Jones RB, et al: High dose combination alkylating agents with bone marrow support as initial treatment for metastatic breast cancer. J Clin Oncol 6:1368–1376, 1988.

65. Peters WP, Shpall EJ, Jones RB, et al: High-dose combination cyclophosphamide (CPA), cisplatin (cDDP), and carmustine (BCNU) with bone marrow support as initial treatment for metastatic breast cancer. Three to six year follow-up. Proc Am Soc Clin Oncol 9:31, 1990.

66. Spitzer G, Dunphy F, Buzdar AU, et al: High dose cytoxan/ VP16/ platinum (CVP) intensification for hormonally unresponsive (HU) metastatic breast cancer (abstract 50). Proc Am Soc Clin Oncol 7:14, 1988.

67. Bouleuc C, Rousseau F, Extra JM, et al: Intensive induction chemotherapy with cyclophosphamide and epirubicin in patients with metastatic breast cancer. Ann Oncol 3(suppl 5):114, 1992.

68. Israel L, Breau JL, Aguilere J: High-dose cyclophosphamide and high-dose 5-fluorouracil. A new first line regimen for advanced breast cancer. Cancer 53:1655–1659, 1984.

69. Nabholtz JM, Gulck S, Fargeot P, et al: High-dose chemotherapy with mitoxantrone, cyclophosphamide, vinblastine or carboplatin with bone marrow support in metastatic breast cancer: Role of autologous peripheral blood stem cell transplantation and cytokines (abstract). Int Ass Br Ca Res A87, 1993.

70. Antman K, Ayash L, Elias A, et al: A phase II study of high-dose cyclophosphamide, thiotepa and carboplatin with autologous marrow support in women with measurable advanced breast cancer responding to standard dose therapy. J Clin Oncol 10:102–110, 1992.

71. Grad G, Lane N, Zimmerman T, et al: High dose chemotherapy and autologous stem cell support in metastatic breast cancer: The University of Chicago experience (abstract). Proc Am Soc Clin Oncol 13:A94, 1994.

72. Vredenburgh J, Ross M, Hussein A, et al: A phase I trial of ifosfamide (I), carboplatin (C) and melphalan (M) with hematopoietic support for advanced metastatic breast cancer (abstract). Proc Am Soc Clin Oncol 13:A185, 1994.

73. deVries EG, Rodenhuis S, Schouten HC, et al: Phase II study of intensive chemotherapy with autologous bone marrow transplantation in patients in complete remission of disseminated breast cancer (abstract). Proc Am Soc Clin Oncol 13:A151, 1994.

74. Dunphy FR, Spitzer G, Buzdar AU, et al: Treatment of estrogen receptor-negative or hormonally refractory breast cancer with double high-dose chemotherapy intensification and bone marrow support. J Clin Oncol 8:1207–1216, 1990.

75. Jones RB, Shpall EJ, Ross M, et al: AFM induction chemotherapy followed by intensive alkylating agent consolidation with autologous bone marrow support (ABMS) for advanced breast cancer. Current results (abstract). Proc Am Soc Clin Oncol 9:30, 1990.

76. Kennedy M, Beveridge R, Rowley R, et al: High-dose chemotherapy with reinfusion of purged autologous bone marrow following dose intense induction as initial therapy for metastatic breast cancer. J Natl Cancer Inst 83:920–926, 1991.

77. Williams SF, Mick R, Desser R, et al: High-dose consolidation therapy with autologous stem cell rescue in stage IV breast cancer. J Clin Oncol 7:1824–1830, 1989.

78. Falkson G, Gelman RS, Tormay DC, et al: Treatment of metastatic breast cancer in premenopausal women using CAF with or without oophorectomy. An Eastern Cooperative Oncology Group study. J Clin Oncol 5:881–889, 1987.

79. Bezwoda WR, Seymour L, Vorobiof DA: High-dose cyclophosphamide, mitoxantrone and VP-16 (HC-CNV) as first-line treatment for metastatic breast cancer. Proc Am Soc Clin Oncol 11:A81, 1992.

80. Ayash LJ, Elias A, Wheeler C, et al: High-dose chemotherapy with autologous stem cell support for breast cancer: A review of the Dana-Farber Cancer Institute/Beth Israel Hospital experience. J Hematother 2:507–511, 1993.

81. Samlo G, Doroshow JH, Forman SJ, et al: High dose doxorubicin, etoposide and cyclophosphamide with stem cell reinfusion in patients with metastatic or high-risk primary breast cancer. City of Hope Bone Marrow Oncology Team. Cancer 73:1678–1685, 1994.

82. Myers SE, Williams SF: Role of high-dose chemotherapy and autologous stem cell support in treatment of breast cancer. Hematol Oncol Clin North Am 7:631–645, 1993 .

83. Dunphy FR, Spitzer G, Fornoff JE, et al: Factors predicting long-term survival for metastatic breast cancer patients with high-dose chemotherapy and bone marrow support. Cancer 73:2157–2167, 1994.

84. Buzdar AU, Kau SW, Hortobagyi GN, et al: Clinical course of patients with breast cancer with ten or more positive nodes who were treated with doxorubicin-containing adjuvant therapy. Cancer 69:448–452, 1992.

85. Hudis C, Lebwohl D, Crown J, et al: Dose intensive sequential crossover adjuvant chemotherapy for women with high-risk node-positive primary breast cancer, in Solomon SE (ed): Adjuvant Therapy of Cancer, pp 214–219. Philadelphia, JB Lippincott.

86. Abeloff MD, Beveridge RA, Donehower RC, et al: Sixteen week dose intense chemotherapy in adjuvant treatment of breast cancer. J Natl Cancer Inst 82:570–574, 1990.

87. Blumenschein G, Jampolis S, DiStefano A: CAVe/XRT/McCFUD as an alternative to high-dose chemotherapy (HDC) and autologous bone marrow support (ABMS) for patients (pts) with advanced primary breast cancer (abstract). Proc Am Assoc Cancer Res 35:A1149, 1994.

88. Peters WP, Ross M, Vredenburg JJ, et al: High-dose chemotherapy and autologous bone marrow support as consolidation after standard-dose adjuvant therapy for high-risk primary breast cancer. J Clin Oncol 11:1132–1143, 1993.

89. Cocconi G, Algeri R, Contu A, et al: Randomized trial of conventional versus a more intensive sequential chmeotherapy as adjuvant treatment for Stage II breast carcinoma with greater than or equal to 10 involved axillary nodes (meeting abstract). Proc Am Soc Clin Oncol 13:A49, 1994.

90. de Graaf H, Willemse PH, de Vries EG, et al: Intensive chemotherapy with autologous bone marrow transfusion as primary treatment in women with breast cancer and more than five involved axillary lymph nodes. Eur J Cancer 30A:150–153, 1994.

91. Overmoyer B, Dannley R, Goormastic M et al: Consolidation for high risk breast cancer with high-dose chemotherapy and autologous bone marrow rescue (abstract). Proc Am Soc Clin Oncol 13:A174, 1994.

92. Somlo G, Doroshow JH, Forman S, et al: High dose chemotherapy (HDCT) with stem cell rescue (SCR) for high risk breast cancer (HRBC) (meeting abstract). Proc Am Soc Clin Oncol 13:A217, 1994.

93. Gisselbrecht E, Lepage M, Espie JM, et al: Cyclophosphamide, total body irradiation with autologous bone marrow infusion as consolidation for inflammatory and metastatic breast cancer (abstract 255). Proc Am Soc Clin Oncol 6:65, 1987.

94. Israel L, Breau JL, Morere JF: Two years of high dose cyclophosphamide and 5-fluorouracil followed by surgery after 3 months for acute inflammatory breast carcinomas. A phase II study of 25 cases with a median follow-up of 35 months. Cancer 57:24–28, 1986.

95. Extra JM, Bourstyn E, Espie M, et al: Intensive induction chemotherapy followed by mastectomy in inflammatory breast carcinoma (abstract 233). Proc Am Soc Clin Oncol 12, 1993.

96. Ayash L, Lynch J, Cruz J et al: High-dose multimodality therapy for locally unresectable or inflammatory (stage IIIB) breast cancer (meeting abstract). Proc Am Soc Clin Oncol 12:A158, 1993.

97. Ingle JN, Tormey DC, Tan KH: The bone marrow examination in breast cancer. Diagnostic considerations and clinical usefulness. Cancer 41:1670–1674, 1978.

98. Redding WH, Monaghan P, Coombes RC, et al: Detection of micrometastases in patients with primary breast cancer. Lancet 2:1271–1274, 1983.

99. Giai M, Natoli C, Sismondi P, et al: Bone marrow micrometastases detected by a monoclonal antibody in patients with breast cancer. Anticancer Res 10:119–122, 1990.

100. Cote RJ, Posen PP, Lesser ML, et al: Prediction of early relapse in patients with operable breast cancer by detection of occult bone marrow micrometastases. J Clin Oncol 9:1749–1756, 1991.

101. Joshi SS, Kessinger A, Mann SL et al: Detection of malignant cells in histologically normal bone marrow using culture techniques. Bone Marrow Transplant 1(3):303–310, 1987.

102. Combes C, Powles T, Buckman R, et al: In vitro and in vivo effect of a monoclonal antibody-toxin conjugate for use in autologous bone marrow transplantation for patients with breast cancer. Cancer Res/Rev 46:4217–4220, 1986.

103. Morecki S, Margel S, Pavlotsky, et al: Purging of breast cancer cells in preparation for autologous bone marrow transplantation. Bone Marrow Transplant 1:357–363, 1987.

104. Kaizer H, Stuart RK, Brookmeyer R, et al: Autologous bone marrow transplantation in acute leukemia: A phase I study of in vitro treatment of marrow with 4-hydroxyperoxycyclophosphamide to purge tumor cells. Blood 65:1504–1510, 1985.

105. Sphall EJ, Franklin WA, Jones RB, et al: Transplantation of CD34 positive (+) marrow and /or peripheral blood progenitor cells (PBPCS) into breast cancer patients following high dose chemotherapy. Proc Am Soc Hem Ann Meet A1571:396a, 1994.

106. Brugger W, Henschler R, Heimfeld S: Positively selected autologous blood CD34+ cells and unseparated peripheral blood progenitor cells mediate identical hematopoietic engraftment after high dose VP16, ifosfamide, carboplatin and epirubicin. Blood 84:1421–1426, 1994.

107. Nemunaitis J, Rabinowe SN, Singer JW, et al: Recombinant granulocyte-macrophage colony-stimulating factor after autologous bone marrow transplantation for lymphoid cancer. N Engl J Med 324:1773–1778, 1991.

108. Sheridan WP, Morstyn G, Wolf M, et al: Granulocyte colony-stimulating factor and neutrophil recovery after high-dose chemotherapy and autologous bone marrow transplantation. Lancet 14:891–895, 1989.

109. Peters WP: Use of cytokines during prolonged neutropenia associated with autologous bone marrow transplantation. Rev Infect

Dis 13:993–996, 1991.

110. Taylor KM, Jagannath S, Spitzer G, et al: Recombinant human granulocyte colony-stimulating factor hastens granulocyte recovery after high-dose chemotherapy and autologous bone marrow transplantation in Hodgkin's disease. J Clin Oncol 7:1791–1799, 1989.

111. Laughlin MJ, Kirkpatrick G, Sabiston N, et al: Hematopoietic recovery following high-dose combined alkylating agent chemotherapy and autologous bone marrow transplant in patients: clinical trials of CSF factors G-CSF, GM-CSF, IL1, IL2, M-CSF. Ann Hematol 67:267–276, 1993.

112. Passos-Coelho J, Davidsn NE, Noga S: G-CSF accelerates hematopoietic recovery after high dose chemotherapy and 4-hydroxyperoxycyclophosphamide purged autologous bone marrow transplantation in patients with metastatic breast cancer (meeting abstract 1614). Proc Am Soc Clin Oncol 12, 1993.

113. Vaughan WP: Autologous bone marrow transplantation in the treatment of breast cancer: Clinical and technologic strategies. Semin Oncol 20(5 suppl 6):55–58, 1993.

114. Tajima T, Tokuda Y, Okumura T, et al: Chemotherapy with autologous stem cell support for breast cancer. Japan J Cancer Chemother 21(suppl 2):255–258, 1994.

115. Eddy DM: High-dose chemotherapy with autologous bone marrow transplantation for the treatment of metastatic breast cancer. J Clin Oncol 10:652–670, 1992.

116. Kiel DP, Felson DT, Anderson JJ, et al: Hip fracture and the use of estrogens in postmenopausal women. N Engl J Med 317:1169–1174, 1987.

117. Grady D, Rubin SM, Petitti DB, et al: Hormone therapy to prevent disease and prolong life in postmenopausal women. Ann Intern Med 15:1016–1037, 1992.

118. Weiss NS, Ure CL, Balard JH, et al: Decreased risk of fractures of the hip and lower forearm with postmenopausal use of estrogens. N Engl J Med 303:1195–1198, 1980.

119. Stampfer MJ, Colditz GA, Willett WC, et al: Postmenopausal estrogen therapy and cardiovascular disease: 10 year follow-up from the Nurses' Health Study. N Engl J Med 325:756–762, 1991.

120. Barrett-Connor E, Bush TL: Estrogen and coronary heart disease in women. JAMA 265:1861–1867, 1991.

121. Lobo RA: Cardiovascular implications of estrogen replacement therapy. Obstet Gynecol 75(suppl 4):18–25s, 1990.

122. Lafferty FW, Fiske ME: Postmenopausal estrogen replacement: A long-term cohort study. Am J Med 97:66–76;1994.

123. Boring CC, Squires TS, Tong T, et al: Cancer statistics 1995: CA Cancer J Clin 45(1):12–13, 1995.

124. Samaan NA, DeAsis DN, Buzdar AU, et al: Pituitary ovarian function in breast cancer patients on adjuvant chemoimmunotherapy. Cancer 41:2084–2087, 1987.

125. Bonadonna G, Valagussa P, Rossi A, et al: CMF adjuvant chemotherapy in operable breast cancer, in Jones SE, Salmon SS (eds): Adjuvant Therapy of Cancer II, pp 227–235. New York, Grune and Stratton, 1979.

126. Mehta RR, Beattie CN, Das Gupta T: Endocrine profile in breast cancer patients receiving chemotherapy. Breast Cancer Res Treat 20:125–132, 1991.

127. Dristan AM, Schwartz MK, Fracchia AA, et al: Endocrine consequences of CMF adjuvant therapy on premenopausal and postmenopausal breast cancer patients. Cancer 51:803–807, 1983.

128. Hortobagyi GN, Buzdar AU, Mareus CE, et al: Immediate and long-term toxicity of adjuvant chemotherapy regimens containing doxorubicin in trials of the M. D. Anderson Hospital and Tumor Institute. NCI Monogr 1:105–109, 1986.

129. Vassilopoulou-Sellin R, Zolinski C: Estrogen replacement therapy in women with breast cancer: A survey of patient attitudes. Am J Med Sci 304:145–149, 1992.

130. American College of Obstetrics and Gynecology: Hormone replacement therapy, p 166. Washington DC, American College of Obstetrics and Gynecology, 1992.

131. Spratt JS, Donegan WL, Greenberg RA: Epidemiology and etiology, in Donegan WL, Spratt JS (eds): Cancer of the Breast, 3rd ed, pp 56–58. Philadelphia, WB Saunders, 1988.

132. Wile AG, Opfell RW, Margileth DA: Hormone replacement therapy in previously treated breast cancer patients. Am J Surg 165:372–375, 1993.

133. Lippman M, Bolan G, Huff K: The effects of oestrogens and antiestrogens on hormone-responsive human breast cancer in long-term tissue culture. Cancer Res 36:4595–4601, 1976.

134. Sheth SP, Allegra JC: Endocrine therapy of breast cancer, in Bland KI, Copeland EM III (eds): The Breast, pp 939–940. Philadelphia, WB Saunders, 1991.

135. Stoll BA: Effect of Lyndiol, an oral contraceptive, on breast cancer. Br Med J 3:150–153, 1967.

136. Eden JA: Oestrogen and the breast 2: The management of the menopausal woman with breast cancer. Med J Aust 157:247–250, 1992.

137. Hoover R, Gray LA Sr, Cole P, et al: Menopausal estrogens and breast cancer. N Engl J Med 295:401–405, 1976.

138. Byrd BF Jr, Burch JC, Vaughn WK: The impact of long term estrogen support after hysterectomy. Ann Surg 185:574–580, 1977.

139. Sartwell PE, Arthes FG, Tonascia JA: Exogenous hormones, reproductive history and breast cancer. J Natl Cancer Inst 59:1589–1592, 1977.

140. Ross RK, Paganini-Hill A, Gerkins VA, et al: A case-control study of menopausal estrogen therapy and breast cancer. JAMA 243:1635–1639, 1980.

141. Bergkvist L, Adami HO, Persson I, et al: The risk of breast cancer after estrogen and estrogen/progestin replacement. New Engl J Med 321:293–297, 1989.

142. Hunt K, Vessley M, McPherson K, et al: Long-term surveillance of mortality and cancer incidence in women receiving hormone replacement therapy. Br J Obstet Gynaecol 94:620–635, 1987.

143. Dupont WD, Page DL: Menopausal estrogen replacement therapy and breast cancer. Arch Intern Med 151:67–72, 1991.

144. Henrich JB: The postmenopausal estrogen/breast cancer controversy. JAMA 268:1900–1902, 1992.

145. Adami HO, Malker B, Holmberg L, et al: The relation between survival and age at diagnosis in breast cancer. N Engl J Med 315:559–563, 1986.

146. Gambrell DR: Proposal to decrease the risk and improve the prognosis in breast cancer. Am J Obstet Gynecol 150:119–128, 1984.

147. Henderson BE, Paganini-Hill A, Ross RK: Decreased mortality in users of estrogen-replacement therapy. Arch Intern Med 151:75–78, 1991.

148. Bergkvist L, Adami HO, Persson I, et al: Prognosis after breast cancer diagnosis in women exposed to estrogen and estrogen-progestogen replacement therapy. Am J Epidemiol 130:221–228, 1989.

149. Armstrong BK: Oestrogen therapy after the menopause: Boon or bane?. Med J Aust 148:213–214, 1988.

150. Bland KI, Buchanan JB, Weisberg BF, et al: The effect of exogenous estrogen replacement therapy of the breast: Breast cancer risk and mammographic parenchymal patterns. Cancer 45:3027–3033, 1980.

151. Stomper PC, van Voorhis BJ, Ravnikar VA, et al: Mammographic changes associated with postmenopausal hormone replacement therapy: a longitudinal study. Radiology 174:487–490, 1990.

152. Berkowitz JE, Gatewood M, Goldblum LE, et al: Hormonal replacement therapy: Mammographic manifestations. Radiology

174:199–201, 1990.

153. Nayfield SG, Karp JE, Ford LG, et al: Potential role of tamoxifen in prevention of breast cancer. J Natl Cancer Inst 83:1450–1458, 1991.

154. Cobleigh MA, Beris RF, Bush T, et al: Estrogen replacement therapy in breast cancer survivors: A time for change. JAMA 272:540–545, 1994.

155. Love RR, Mazess RB, Barden HS, et al: Effects of tamoxifen on bone marrow density in postmenopausal women with breast cancer. N Engl J Med 326:852–856, 1992.

156. Love RR, Mazess RB, Tormay DC, et al: Bone mineral density in women with breast cancer treated with adjuvant tamoxifen for at least two years. Breast Cancer Res Treat 12:297–301, 1988.

157. Turkan S, Siris E, Seldin D, et al: Effects of tamoxifen on spinal bone density in women with breast cancer. J Natl Cancer Inst 81:1086–1088, 1989.

158. McDonald CC, Stewart HJ: Fatal myocardial infarction in the Scottish Adjuvant Tamoxifen Trial: The Scottish Breast Cancer Committee. Br Med J 303:435–437, 1991.

159. Vignon F, Bouton MN, Rochefort H: Antiestrogens inhibit the mitogenic effect of growth factors on breast cancer cells in the total absence of estrogens. Biochem Biophys Res Commun 146:1502–1508, 1987.

160. Sunderland MC, Osborne CK: Tamoxifen in premenopausal women with metastatic breast cancer: A review. J Clin Oncol 9:1283–1295, 1991.

161. O'Brien CA, Liskamp RM, Solomon DH, et al: Inhibition of protein kinase c by tamoxifen. Cancer Res 45:2462–2465, 1985.

162. Lam H-YP: Tamoxifen is a calmodulin antagonist in the activation of cAMP phosphodiesterase. Biochem Biophys Res Commun 118:27–32, 1984.

163. Mandeville R, Ghali SS, Chasseau JP: In vitro stimulation of human NK activity by an estrogen antagonist (tamoxifen). Eur J Cancer Clin Oncol 20:983–985, 1984.

164. Hug V, Hortobagyi GN, Drewinke B, et al: Tamoxifen-citrate counteracts the anti-tumor effects of cytotoxic drugs in vitro. J Clin Oncol 3:1672–1677, 1985.

165. Jordan VC, Fritz NF, Tormey DC: Endocrine effects of adjuvant chemotherapy and long term tamoxifen administration on node-positive patients with breast cancer. Cancer Res 47:624–630, 1987.

166. Sherman BM, Chapler FK, Crickard K: Endocrine consequences of continous antiestrogen therapy with tamoxifen in premenopausal women. J Clin Invest 64:398–404, 1979.

167. Margreiter R, Wiegele J: Tamoxifen for premenopausal patients with breast cancer. Cancer Res Treat 4:45–49, 1984.

168. Planting AS, Alexieva-Figusch J, Blonkivd-Wijst J, et al: Tamoxifen therapy in premenopausal womwn with metastatic breast cancer. Cancer Treat Rep 69:363–368, 1985.

169. Fisher B, Costantino J, Redmond C, et al: A randomized clinical trial evaluating tamoxifen in the treatment of patients with node negative breast cancer who have estrogen receptor negative or positive tumors. N Engl J Med 320:479–484, 1989.

170. Powles TJ: Tamoxifen and oestrogen replacement (letter). Lancet 336:48, 1990.

171. Stoll BA: Hormone replacement therapy in women treated for breast cancer. Eur J Cancer Clin Oncol 25:1909, 1989.

172. Wile AG, Opfell DA, Margileth DA, et al: Hormone replacement therapy does not affect breast cancer outcome (abstract). Proc Am Soc Clin Oncol 10:58, 1991.

173. Eden JA, Bush T, Nand S, et al: The Royal Hospital for Women Breast Cancer Study: A case-controlled study of combined continuous hormone replacement therapy amongst women with a personal history

of breast cancer. Med J Aust (in press).

174. Disaia PJ, Odicino F, Grosen EA, et al: Hormone replacement therapy in breast cancer. Lancet 342:1242, 1993.

175. Vassilopoulou-Sellin R, Theriault RL: Randomized prospective trial of estrogen-replacement therapy in women with a history of breast cancer. J Natl Cancer Inst Monogr 16:153–159, 1994.

176. Smith DC, Prentice R, Donovan JJ, et al: Association of exogenous estrogen and endometrial carcinoma. N Engl J Med 293:1164–1167, 1975.

177. Ziel HK, Finkler WD: Increased risk of endometrial carcinoma among users of conjugated estrogens. N Engl J Med 293:167–1170, 1975.

178. Mack TM, Pike HC, Henderson BE, et al: Estrogens and endometrial cancer in a retirement community. N Engl J Med 294:1262–1267, 1976.

179. Fornander T, Rutqvist LE, Cedermark B, et al: Adjuvant tamoxifen in early breast cancer: occurrence of new primary cancers. Lancet 1:117–120, 1989.

180. Disaia PJ: Hormone replacement therapy in patients with breast cancer. A reappraisal. Cancer 71:1490–1500, 1993.

181. Spicer D, Pike MC, Henderson BE: The question of estrogen replacement therapy in patients with a prior diagnosis of breast cancer. Oncology 4:49–55, 1990.

182. Tamoxifen and standard estrogen replacement in breast cancer patients: Four clinical views. Oncology 5:137–139, 1991.

183. Sasco AJ, Lowenfels AB, Pasker-de-Jong P: Epidemiology of male breast cancer. A meta-analysis of published case-control studies and discussion of selected aetiological factors. Int J Cancer 53:538–549, 1993.

184. Simon MS, McKnight E, Schwartz A, et al: Racial differences in cancer of the male breast. Fifteen year experience in the Detroit metropolitan area. Breast Cancer Res Treat 21:55–62, 1992.

185. Ajayi DOS, Osegbe DN, Ademiluyi SA: Carcinoma of the male breast in West Africans and a review of world literature. Cancer 50:1664–1667, 1982.

186. Mabuchi K, Bross DS, Kessler II: Risk factors for male breast cancer. J Nat Cancer Inst 74:371–375, 1985.

187. Steinitz Z, Katz L, Ben-Hur M: Male breast cancer in Israel: Selected epidemiological aspects. Isr J Med Sci 17:816–821, 1981.

188. Demers PA, Thomas DB, Rosenblatt KA, et al: Occupational exposure to electromagnetic fields and breast cancer in men. Am J Epidemiol 15(134):340–347, 1991.

189. Rosenbaum PF, Vena JE, Zielezny MA, et al: Occupational exposure associated with male breast cancer. Am J Epidemiol 139:30–36, 1994.

190. L'Enfant-Pejovic MH, Mlika-Cabanne N, Bourchardy C, et al: Risk factors for male breast cancer: A Franco-Swiss case-control study. Int J Cancer 15:45(4):661–665, 1990.

191. Thomas DB: Breast cancer in men. Epidemiol Rev 15:220–231, 1993.

192. Casagrande JT, Hanisch R, Pike MC, et al: A case-control study of male breast cancer. Cancer Res 48:1326–1330, 1988.

193. Thomas DB, Jiminez LM, McTiernan A, et al: Breast cancer in men: Risk factors with hormonal implications. Am J Epidemiol 135:734–738, 1992.

194. Cutuli BF, Florentz P, Lacroze M, et al: Male breast cancer: Analysis of 444 cases by the French Federation of Cancer Centers, in Pisa Symposia in Oncology. Breast Cancer: From Biology to Therapy (abstract), October 19–21, 1992, Pisa, Italy, p 65, 1992.

195. Evans DB, Crichlow RW: Carcinoma of the male breast and Klinefelter's syndrome: Is there an association? Cancer J Clin 37:246–251, 1987.

196. Anderson DE, Badzioch MD: Breast cancer risks in relatives

of male breast cancer patients. J Natl Cancer Inst 84(14):1114–1117, 1992.

197. Stratton MR, Ford D, Neuhasen S, et al: Familial male breast cancer is not linked to the BRCA1 locus on chromosome 17q. Nat Genet 7:103–107, 1994.

198. Collins N, McManus M: Consistent loss of the wild type allele in breast cancers from a family linked to the BRCA2 gene on chromosome 13q12-13. Oncogene 10(8):1673–1675, 1995.

199. Erlichman C, Murphy KC, Elkahim T: Male breast cancer: A 13 year review of 89 patients. J Clin Oncol 2:903–909, 1984.

200. Camus MG, Joshi MG, Mackarem G, et al: Ductal carcinoma in situ of the male breast. Cancer 74:1289–1293, 1994.

201. Gupta S Khanna NN, Khanna S: Paget's disease of the male breast: A clinicopathologic study and collective review. J Surg Oncol 22:151–156, 1983.

202. Pantoja E, Llobet RE, Lopez E: Gigantic cystosarcoma phylloides in a man with gynecomastia. Arch Surg 111:611, 1976.

203. Ansah-Boateng Y, Tavasoli FA: Fibroadenoma and cystosarcoma phylloides of the male breast. Mod Pathol 5:114–116, 1992.

204. Giffler RF, Kay S: Small-cell carcinoma of the male mammary gland. A tumor resembling infiltrating lobular carcinoma. Am J Clin Pathol 66:715–722, 1976.

205. Heller KS, Rosen PP, Schottenfeld D, et al: Male breast cancer: A clinicopathologic study of 97 cases. Ann Surg 188:60–65, 1978.

206. Hultborn R, Friberg S, Hultborn KA: Male breast carcinoma. I. A study of the total material reported to the Swedish Cancer Registry 1958–1967, with respect to clinical and histopathologic parameters. Acta Oncol 26:241–256, 1987.

207. Michaels BM, Nunn CR, Roses DF: Lobular carcinoma of the male breast. Surgery 115:402–405, 1994.

208. Lagios MD, Westdahl PR, Margolin FR, et al: Duct carcinoma in situ: Relationship of extent of noninvasive disease to the frequency of occult invasion, multicentricity, lymph node metastases, and short-term treatment failures. Cancer 50:1309–1314, 1982.

209. Silverstein MJ, Rosser RJ, Gierson ED, et al: Axillary lymph node dissection for intraductal breast carcinoma: Is it indicated? Cancer 59:1819–1824, 1987.

210. Crichlow RW: Carcinoma of the male breast. Surg Gynecol Obstet 134:1011–1019, 1972.

211. Robinson R, Montague ED: Treatment results in males with breast cancer. Cancer 49:403–406, 1982.

212. Scheike O: Male breast cancer 5. Clinical manifestations in 25 cases in Denmark. Br J Cancer 28:552–561, 1973.

213. Lartigau E, el-Jabbour JN, Dubray B, et al: Male breast carcinoma: A single centre report of clinical parameters. Clin Oncol (R Coll Radiol) 6:162–166, 1994.

214. Gough DB, Donohue JH, Evans MM, et al: A 50-year experience of male breast cancer: Is outcome changing? Surg Oncol 2:325–333, 1993.

215. Borgen PI, Wong GY, Vlamis V, et al: Current management of male breast cancer. A review of 104 cases. Ann Surg 215:451–457, 1992.

216. Mani S, Ahmad YH, Papac RJ: Male breast cancer: Risk factors and clinical features (abstract 157). Proc Am Soc Clin Oncol 11:1992.

217. Allain YM, Mermod B, Malkani K: Breast Cancer in men. Twenty three cases and general review. J Eur Radiother 9:115–120, 1988.

218. Ramantanis G, Bebeas S, Garas JG: Breast cancer in the male: A report of 138 cases. World J Surg 4:621–624.

219. van Geel AN, van Slooten EA, Mavrunac M, et al: A retrospective study of male breast cancer in Holland. Br J Surg 72:724–727, 1985.

220. Spence RA, Mckenzie G, Anderson JR, et al: Long-term survival following cancer of the male breast in Northern Ireland. A report of 81 cases. Cancer 55:648–652, 1985.

221. Hultborn R, Friberg S, Hultborn KA, et al: Male breast carcinoma II. A study of the total material reported to the Swedish Cancer Registry 1958–1967, with respect to treatment, prognostic factors and survival. Acta Oncol 26:327–341, 1987.

222. Salvadori B, Saccozzi R, Manzari A, et al: Prognosis of breast cancer in males: An analysis of 170 cases. Eur J Cancer 30A:930–935, 1994.

223. Ciatto S, Zossa A, Bonardi R, et al: Male breast carcinoma: Review of a multicenter series of 150 cases. Coordinating Center and Writing Committee of FONCAM (National Task Force for Breast cancer), Italy. Tumori 76:555–558, 1990.

224. Ribeiro G: Male breast carcinoma—A review of 301 cases from the Christie Hospital and Holt Radium Institute, Manchester. Br J Cancer 51:115–119, 1985.

225. Kalisher L, Peyster R: Xerographic manifestations of male breast disease. Am J Roentgenol Radium Ther Nucl Med 125:656–661, 1975.

226. Michels LG, Gold RH, Arndt RD: Radiography of gynecomastia and other disorders of the male breast. Radiology 122:117–122, 1977.

227. Jackson VP, Gilmor RL: Male breast carcinoma and gynecomastia: comparison of mammography with sonography. Radiology 149:533–536, 1983.

228. Dershaw DD: Male mammography. Am J Roentgenol 146:127–131, 1986.

229. Jaiyesimi IA, Buzdar AU, Sahin AA, et al: Carcinoma of the male breast. Ann Intern Med 117:771–777, 1992.

230. Gupta RK, Naran S, Simpson J: The role of fine needle aspiration cytology (FNAC) in the diagnosis of breast masses in males. Eur J Surg Oncol 14:317–320, 1988.

231. Bhagat P, Kline TS: The male breast and malignant neoplasms. Diagnosis by aspiration biopsy cytology. Cancer 65:2338–2341.

232. Digenis AG, Ross CB, Morrison JG, et al: Carcinoma of the male breast: A review of 41 cases. South Med J 83:1162–1167, 1990.

233. Gupta N, Cohen JL, Rosenbaum C, et al: Estrogen receptors in male breast cancer. 46:1781–1784, 1980.

234. Pegoraro RJ, Nirmul D, Joubert SM: Cytoplasmic and nuclear estrogen and progesterone receptors in male breast cancer. Cancer Res 42:4812–4814, 1982.

235. Everson RB, Lippman ME, Thompson EB, et al: Clinical correlations of steroid receptors and male breast cancer. Cancer Res 40:991–997, 1980.

236. Fox SB, Rogers S, Day CA, et al: Oestrogen receptor and epidermal growth factor receptor expression in male breast carcinoma. J Pathol 166:13–18, 1992.

237. Henderson IC, Canellos GP: Cancer of the breast: The past decade. N Engl J Med 202:278–290, 1980.

238. Norris HJ, Taylor HB: Carcinoma of the male breast. Cancer 23:1422–1435, 1969.

239. Crichlow RW: Breast cancer in men. Semin Oncol 1:145–152, 1974.

240. Yap H, Tashima C, Blumenschein G, et al: Male breast cancer: A natural history study. Cancer 44:748–754, 1979.

241. Lopez M, Di Lauro L, Lazzaro, et al: Hormonal treatment of disseminated male breast cancer. Oncology 42:345–349, 1985.

242. Visfeldt J, Scheike: Male breast cancer. Histologic typing and grading of 187 Danish cases. Cancer 32:985–990, 1973.

243. Pich A, Margaria E, Chiusa L: Proliferative activity is a significant prognostic factor in male breast carcinoma. Am J Pathol 145:481–489, 1994.

244. Olsson H, Alm P, Baldetorp B, et al: A comparison of DNA content and hormone receptor concentration in malignant breast tumors in males and females (abstract). Proc Am Soc Clin Oncol 10:A141, 1991.

245. Bagley C, Wesley M, Young R, et al: Adjuvant chemotherapy in males with cancer of the breast. Am J Clin Oncol 10:55–60, 1987.

246. Ben-Baruch N, Giusti R, Steinberg SM, et al: Adjuvant chemotherapy in stage II node-positive male breast cancer (abstract 164). Proc Am Soc Clin Oncol 11, 1992.

247. Patel H, Buzdar AU, Hotrobagyi G: Role of adjuvant chemotherapy in male breast cancer. Cancer 64:1583–1585, 1989.

248. Kantarjian H, Yap H-Y, Hortobagyi GN, et al: Hormonal therapy for metastatic breast cancer. Arch Intern Med 143:237-240, 1983.

249. Fisher B, Costantino J, Redmond C, et al: A randomized clinical trial evaluating tamoxifen in the treatment of patients with node negative breast cancer who have estrogen receptor positive or negative tumors. N Engl J Med 320:479–484, 1989.

250. Ribeiro G, Swindell R: Adjuvant tamoxifen for male breast cancer. Br J Cancer 65:252–254, 1992.

251. Kinne DW, Hakes TB: Male breast cancer, in Harris J (ed): Breast Diseases, pp 782–790. Philadelphia, JB Lippincott, 1991.

252. Lopez M, Di Lauro L, Vici P, et al: Cyproterone acetate (CPA) +/- buserelin (BUS) in the treatment of metastatic male breast carcinoma. Ann Oncol 3(suppl 5):88, 1992.

253. Lopez M, Natali M, Di Lauro L, et al: Combined treatment with buserelin and cyproterone acetate in metastatic male breast cancer. Cancer 72:502–505, 1993.

254. Tsai DC, Kim CR, Lee DJ: Treatment of carcinoma of the male breast (abstract 212). Proc Am Soc Clin Oncol 12, 1993.

255. Di Lauro L, Vici P, Carpano S, et al: Cyproterone acetate (CPA) alone or with LHRH analogs in metastatic male breast carcinoma (MBC) (abstract 177). Proc Am Soc Clin Oncol 13, 1994.

256. Doberauer C, Nerderle N, Schmidt CG: Advanced male breast cancer treatment with the LHRH analogue buserelin alone or in combination with the antiandrogen flutamide. Cancer 62:474–478, 1988.

257. Aisner J, Ross DD, Wiernih PH: Tamoxifen in advanced male breast cancer. Arch Intern Med 139:480–481, 1979.

258. Hortobagyi GN, DiStefano A, Legha SS, et al: Hormonal therapy with tamoxifen in male breast cancer. Cancer Treat Rep 63:539–541, 1979.

259. Patterson JS, Battersby LA, Bach BK: Use of tamoxifen in advanced male breast carcinoma. Cancer Treat Rep 64:801–804, 1980.

260. Bezwoda WR, Hesdorffer C, Dansey R, et al: Breast cancer in men: Clinical features, hormone receptor status, and response to therapy. Cancer 60:1337–1340, 1987.

261. Anelli TF, Anelli A, Tran N, et al: Tamoxifen administration is associated with a high rate of treatment-limiting symptoms in male breast cancer patients. Cancer 74:73–77, 1994.

262. Tirelli U, Tumolo S, Talamini R, et al: Tamoxifen before and after orchiectomy in advanced male breast cancer. Cancer Treat Rep 66:1882, 1982.

263. Mitsuyasu R, Bonomi P, Anderson K, et al: Response to megesterol in male breast cancer. Arch Int Med 141:809–810, 1981.

264. Pannuti F, Martoni A, Busitti L, et al: High dose medroxyprogesterone acetate in advanced male breast cancer. Cancer Treat Rep 66:1763–1765, 1982.

265. Ribeiro GG: The results of diethylstilboestrol therapy for recurrent and metastatic carcinoma of the male breast. Br J Cancer 33:465–467, 1976.

266. Thomas C Jr, Bonomi P: Hormone-induced hypercalcemic tumor flares in a male with breast cancer (abstract 1010). Proc Assoc Cancer Res 30, 1989.

267. Lopez M, Dilauro L, Papaldo P, et al: Chemotherapy in metastatic male breast cancer. Oncology 42:205–209, 1985.

268. Yap HY, Tashima CK, Blumenschein GR, et al: Chemotherapy for advanced male breast cancer. JAMA 243:1739–1741, 1980.

269. Ribeiro O, Palmer M: Breast carcinoma associated with pregnancy: A clinician's dilemma. Br Med J 2:1524–1527, 1977.

270. Hoover HC Jr: Breast cancer during pregnancy and lactation. Surg Clin North Am 70:1151–1163, 1990.

271. Nugent P, O'Connell TX: Breast cancer and pregnancy. Arch Surg 120:1221–1224, 1985.

272. Allen HH, Nisker JA: Cancer in pregnancy. Therapeutic guidelines, in Allen HH, Nisker JA (eds): Cancer in pregnancy: An overview, pp 3–8. New York, Futura Publications, 1988.

273. Zemlickis D, Lishner M, Degendorfer P, et al: Maternal and fetal outcome after breast cancer in pregnancy. Am J Obstet Gynecol 166:781–787, 1992.

274. Ishida T, Yokoe T, Kasumi F, et al: Clinicopathologic characteristics and prognosis of breast cancer patients associated with pregnancy and lactation: Analysis of case-control study in Japan. Jpn J Cancer Res 83:1143–1149, 1992.

275. Gloeckler Ries LA, Hankey BF, Edwards BK (eds): Cancer Statistics Review: 1973–1987, section II.1–II.49. Bethesda, MD, National Cancer Institute, U.S. Department of Health and Human Services,

276. Saunders CM, Baum M: Breast cancer and pregnancy: A review. J R Soc Med 86:162–165, 1993.

277. Max MH, Klamer TW: Pregnancy and breast cancer. South Med J 76:1088–1090, 1983.

278. Byrd BF, Bayer DS, Robertson JC, et al: Treatment of breast tumors associated with pregnancy and lactation. Ann Surg 155:940–947, 1962.

279. Bonneterre J, Peyrat JP, Beuscart R, et al: Biological and clinical aspects of prolactin receptors (PRL-R) in human breast cancer. J Steroid Biochem Mol Biol 37:977–981, 1990.

280. Strelkauskas AJ, Wilson BS, Dray S, et al: Inversion of levels of T and B cells in early pregnancy. Nature 258:331–332, 1975.

281. Purtilo DT, Hallgren HM, Yunis EJ: Depressed maternal lymphocyte response to phytohemagglutinin in human pregnancy. Lancet 1:769-771, 1972.

282. Liberman L, Giess CS, Dershaw DD, et al: Imaging of pregnancy-associated breast cancer. Radiology 191:245–248, 1994.

283. Clark RM, Reid J: Carcinoma of the breast in pregnancy and lactation. Int J Radiat Oncol Biol Phys 4:693–698, 1978.

284. Wallack MK, Wolf JA, Bedwanek J, et al: Gestational carcinoma of the female breast. Curr Probl Cancer 7:1–58, 1983.

285. Zinns JS: The association of pregnancy and breast cancer. J Reprod Med 22:297–301, 1979.

286. Theriault RL, Stallings CB, Buzdar AU: Pregnancy and breast cancer: Clinical and legal issues. Am J Clin Oncol 15:535–539, 1992.

287. Ribeiro G, Jones DA, Jones M: Carcinoma of the breast associated with pregnancy. Br J Surg 73:607–609, 1986.

288. Schlanger H, Ben Yose FR, Baras M, et al: The effect of pregnancy at diagnosis in the prognosis in breast cancer. European Association for Cancer Research 10th Biennial Meeting, September 1989.

289. Peters MV: The effect of pregnancy in breast cancer, in Forrest APM, Kunkler PB (eds): Prognostic Factors in Breast Cancer, pp 65–89. Baltimore, Williams and Wilkins, 1968.

290. von Schoultz E, Hemming J, Wilking N, et al: Influence of prior and subsequent pregancy on breast cancer prognosis. J Clin Oncol 13:430–434, 1995.

291. Mauer WP: Carcinoma of the breast in pregnancy and lactation. Breast 4:12–15, 1979.

292. Guinee VF, Olson H, Moller T, et al: Effect of pregnancy on prognosis for young women with breast cancer. Lancet 343:1587–1589, 1994.

293. Kitchen PR, McLennan R: Breast cancer and pregnancy. Med J Aust 147:337–339, 1987.

294. Pedersen H, Finster M: Anesthetic risk in the pregnant surgical patient. Anesthesiology 51:439–451, 1979.

295. Sutcliffe SB: Treatment of neoplastic disease during pregnancy: Maternal and fetal effects. Clin Invest Med 8:333–338, 1985.

296. Doll D, Ringenberg Q, Yarbro J: Management of cancer during pregnancy. Arch Intern Med 148:2058–2064, 1988.

297. Turchi J, Villaris C: Anthracyclines in the treatment of malignancy in pregnancy. Cancer 61:435–440, 1988.

298. Sugawara I, Kataoka I, Morishita Y, et al: Tissue distribution of P-glycoprotein encoded by a multidrug-resistant gene as revealed by a monoclonal antibody, MRK 16. Cancer Res 48:1926–1929, 1988.

299. van der Vange N, van Dongen JA: Breast cancer and pregnancy. Eur J Surg Oncol 17:1–8, 1991.

300. National Council on Radiation Protection and Measurements: Medical radiation exposure of pregnant and potentially pregnant women (CRP report #54), p 32. National Council on Radiation Protection and Measurement, 1979.

301. Richards MA, O'Reilly SM, Howell A, et al: Adjuvant cyclophosphamide, methotrexate and fluorouracil in patients with axillary node positive breast cancer: An update of the Guy's and Manchester trial. J Clin Oncol 8:2032–2039, 1990.

302. Mignot L, Morvan F, Berdah J, et al: Pregnancy after breast cancer: Results of a case study. Presse Med 15:1961–1964, 1986.

303. Peters M, Meakin J: The influence of pregnancy in carcinoma of the breast. Prog Clin Cancer 1:471–506, 1965.

304. Sutton R, Buzdar A, Hortobagyi G: Pregnancy and offspring after adjuvant chemotherapy in breast cancer patients. Cancer 65:847–850, 1990.

305. Donegan WL: Mammary carcinoma and pregnancy, in Donegan WL, Spratt JS (eds): Cancer of the Breast, pp 679–688. Philadelphia, WB Saunders, 1985.

SECTION 6

GYNECOLOGIC MALIGNANCIES

CHAPTER **22**   **Ovarian Cancer**

CHAPTER **23**   **Gestational Trophoblastic Tumors**

CHAPTER **24**   **Carcinoma of the Uterine Cervix**

CHAPTER **25**   **Tumors of the Uterine Corpus**

Ovarian Cancer

Eleni Diamandidou, MD, John J. Kavanagh, MD, Creighton L. Edwards, MD, *and* Andrzej P. Kudelka, MD

Division of Medicine and Department of Gynecologic Oncology
The University of Texas M. D. Anderson Cancer Center, Houston, Texas

Ovarian cancer is the sixth most common cancer, with 26,600 new cases expected in 1995. It is the fourth most common cause of cancer-related deaths in American women of all ages and the most frequent cause of death from gynecologic malignancies in the United States. It accounts for 14,500 deaths annually. The median age at diagnosis is about 62 years, and incidence rises rapidly after age 60.[1]

In the United States, the lifetime risk of developing ovarian cancer is 1 in 70.[2] Internationally, the lifetime risk of developing ovarian cancer is highest in Sweden (1.73%), followed by the United States (1.53%), the United Kingdom (1.25%), South Europe (1.11%), South America (0.87%), India (0.75%), and Japan, with the lowest incidence (0.47%).[2]

ETIOLOGY

The etiology of ovarian cancer is unknown. Numerous studies have sought any possible link between environmental, dietary, reproductive, endocrine, viral, and hereditary factors and the risk of developing ovarian cancer.

The strongest risk factor for ovarian cancer identified to date is a familial pattern of ovarian cancer, which is reported in about 7% of women with the disease.[3] There are two types of familial patterns: hereditary syndromes and familial history.

Hereditary ovarian cancer syndromes refer to (a) site-specific ovarian cancer syndromes; (b) ovarian and breast cancer (breast/ovarian cancer syndrome); and (c) non-polyposis colorectal cancer, endometrial cancer, and ovarian cancer (Lynch II syndrome) within two or more generations of a kindred.[4] The hereditary ovarian cancer syndrome accounts for less than 1% of ovarian cancers and less than 3% of cancers among women with familial evidence of ovarian cancer.[5] In some families, an autosomal dominant mode of inheritance has been shown and may increase one's lifetime risk of developing ovarian cancer up to 50%.[4–9]

The family history pattern of ovarian cancer, which is much more common than the hereditary syndrome, applies to families with isolated cases of ovarian cancer. Often, this is only one relative, with no evidence of hereditary disease. Of women with ovarian cancer, 7% report a family history of the disease.[3,5] The lifetime risk of ovarian cancer ranges from 1.2% to 3.7% in a 50-year-old woman with a family history of ovarian cancer in a first-degree relative and up to 5.5% in a woman with two or three first-degree relatives with ovarian cancer (Table 1).[5,10,11]

Two other reported risk factors for ovarian cancer have been consistently shown to reduce the risk for this cancer: the use of oral contraceptives[10,11] and increasing number of pregnancies (Table 1).[10] Though there is no definite explanation for the correlation between risk and either of these factors,[10,11] two theories have been offered: the excess gonadotropin secretion theory by Cramer and Welch[12] and the incessant ovulation theory by Fathala.[13]

Other risk factors have also been studied: asbestos-talc powder absorption through the vagina or cervix, increased dietary galactose consumption and low serum levels of galactose-1-phosphatase uridyltransferase, in-

TABLE I

Risk Factors for Ovarian Cancer

Risk factor	Relative risk	Lifetime risk for ovarian cancer (%)[a]
No risk factors	1.0	1.2
Familial ovarian cancer syndrome	Unknown	≤ 50
One first- or second-degree relative with ovarian cancer	3.1[b]	3.7
Two or three relatives with ovarian cancer	4.6[b]	5.5
Oral contraceptive pill use	0.65[c]	0.8
Pregnancy	0.5[d]	0.6

[a] Risk for cancer in a 50-year-old woman. Calculated from relative risk estimates and ovarian cancer incidence data from the SEER (Surveillance, Epidemiology, and End-Result) program.[10,11] Calculations assume that a family history of ovarian cancer is relatively uncommon.
[b] Based on data in reference 5.
[c] Based on data in references 10 and 11.
[d] Based on data in reference 10.
Adapted from Carlson KJ: Screening for ovarian cancer. Ann Intern Med, 121:124–132, 1994.

creased fat consumption, menstrual history, age at first pregnancy, infertility, and hormonal replacement treatment.[14-16] None, however, has shown a consistent and significant effect on ovarian cancer risk.[16,17] No association has been found between ovarian cancer and the use of coffee, alcohol, or tobacco.[18]

SCREENING

The main purpose of a screening test is to increase survival by allowing diagnosis of disease at a more localized and curable stage (Table 2).[19-24] However, there is no evidence to date that treatment of ovarian cancer detected in its early stages by currently available screening methods lowers the cause-specific mortality.[25]

Available Screening Techniques

Physical Examination: Pelvic examination is of limited value in screening asymptomatic women for ovarian cancer. Its sensitivity and specificity in detection of adnexal masses have not been well established. Sensitivity increases with the size of the mass. In about two thirds of patients, disease is disseminated by the time it is palpable. Yet, pelvic examination is still too insensitive to serve as the sole screening test.[26] However, some studies suggest that a pelvic examination by a highly skilled examiner may reveal early-stage ovarian cancer.

Abdominal/Transvaginal Ultrasound: In diagnosing ovarian cancer, the morphology and size of the mass are the most important factors. Uniform hypoechogenic or entirely cystic patterns are usually of no concern, as opposed to complex or solid patterns.[27,28] Also important to consider is that cyclic changes in ovary size during the menstrual cycle can give an abnormal transvaginal ultrasound (TVUS); therefore, an abnormal TVUS always needs to be repeated. Screening studies have shown specificities as high as 97.6% with TVUS and between 76% and 97% with abdominal ultrasound (US) and sensitivities between 80% and 100% for either method. Although TVUS and, to a lesser degree, abdominal US can detect diseases at early stages, more extended studies of larger populations are needed to confirm the exact sensitivity and specificity.[29]

CA125: CA125 is an antigenic determinant on a glycoprotein shed into the bloodstream by malignant cells derived from coelomic epithelium.[30] Serum levels of CA125 are increased in about 80% of patients with epithelial ovarian cancers, more frequently in patients with nonmucinous histologic types. Levels of CA125 are also increased in patients with endometrial and pancreatic cancer. They may be increased in patients with some benign conditions, including endometriosis and uterine leiomyoma; in patients with pelvic inflammatory disease (PID), in early pregnancy, and with benign ovarian cysts; and in patients with cirrhosis and pericarditis.[30]

The serum level of CA125 fluctuates during the menstrual cycle.[31] Consequently, screening with CA125 in premenopausal women has been little studied. At a reference level of 35 μ/mL, the sensitivity of CA125 as a marker of clinically diagnosed ovarian cancer ranges from 61% to 96%: 25% to 75% for stage I and 67% to 100% for stage II.[29] The reported specificity is 98.6% to 99.2%.[29] In about one third of women who ultimately develop cancer, CA125 levels rise above 35 μ/mL 18 months before the disease is clinically detected.[32]

Combined Ultrasound and CA125: The positive predictive value of an abnormal US test is less than 1% for women at average risk and 2% for women with a history of ovarian cancer in one relative. For CA125, the positive predictive value is 3% for women at average risk and 10% for women with one or more relatives with ovarian cancer (Table 3).[2,33] In a large British study whose primary screen was CA125 followed by US, CA125 levels achieved a positive predictive value of 27%.[29] However, even though the combined specificity of US and CA125 is high, only one of every two early-stage ovarian cancers can be so detected.

A recent study showed that combined screening with CA125 and the tumor-associated antigens M-CSF and OVX1 increases the sensitivity of the screening in patients with stage I ovarian cancer: At least one of the serum markers was elevated in 98% of patients with

TABLE 2

Stage at Clinical Presentation and Mortality from Ovarian Cancer

Stage	Definition	Patients in stage at clinical detection (%)[a]	Five-year survival (%)[b]
I	Confined to ovaries	25	73
II	Extension within pelvis	8	45
III	Intraperitoneal metastases outside pelvis or positive retroperitoneal nodes	52	21
IV	Distant metastases	15	17

[a] Derived from references 19 and 21–24. [b] Derived from references 19 and 20.   Adapted from Carlson KJ: Screening for ovarian cancer. Ann Intern Med, 121:124–132, 1994.

TABLE 3

Predictive Value of Annual Screening with Ultrasound or CA125 in Women 50 Years of Age and Older [a]

| Screening method | Predictive value of positive test (%) | |
	Women at average risk	Women with one relative with ovarian cancer
Ultrasound [b]	0.7	2
CA125 [c]	3	10

[a] Prevalence at annual screening = 0.0005.   [b] Sensitivity, 85%; specificity, 93.8%   [c] Sensitivity, 78%; specificity, 98.9%.
Adapted from Carlson KJ: Screening for ovarian cancer. Ann Intern Med, 121:124–132, 1994.

stage I ovarian cancer, yet the true specificity in the study was moderate. Elevations of one or more serum tumor markers should be further evaluated by TVUS to increase the specificity in apparently healthy women.[34] Having recognized the need to determine whether the available screening can decrease the mortality of ovarian cancer by early detection, the US National Cancer Institute (NCI) has instituted a trial of screening for ovarian cancer in women aged 60 to 74 years using CA125, TVUS, and pelvic examination.[35] To date, 17,000 women have been accrued to this study. Results of this trial are eagerly awaited.[36]

The benefits of screening a woman who has one or no first-degree relatives with ovarian cancer are unproven. There is currently no evidence to support routine screening in these women. However, participation in clinical trials is an appropriate option. There are inconclusive data that screening benefits women with two or more first-degree relatives who have ovarian cancer; however, women with two or more affected family members have a 3% chance of having a hereditary ovarian cancer syndrome. Though there are no data showing that screening these high-risk women reduces their mortality, rectovaginal and pelvic examination at least annually is recommended. The Consensus Panel further recommends measurement of CA 125 levels, TVUS, and consideration of prophylactic bilateral oopherectomy at age 35 or completion of childbearing. These recommendations are of uproven value and controversial.[36]

Biology, Immunology, Tumor Markers, and Pathogenesis

Steroid Hormones: Many ovarian cancers have histologic characteristics of classic endocrine-responsive tissues. This alone suggests a role for hormones in the etiology and progression of such cancers.[37] Many studies show the presence of estrogen receptors in a high percentage of ovarian tumor specimens; estrogen has been shown to stimulate the growth of ovarian cancer cell lines. Progesterone and androgen receptors have also been reported in ovarian cancer specimens.[37] As for gonadotropin, there are conflicting reports as to the presence of its receptors in ovarian cancer.[37] Finally, experimental data indicate a role for peptide hormones in the regulation of growth or function of normal or neoplastic ovarian surface epithelial cells.

Growth Factors and Cytokines: Because it localizes to the peritoneal cavity, ovarian cancer is amenable to immune analysis and experimental immunotherapy. It has even been suggested that the intraperitoneal growth of ovarian cancer may be related to the local deficiency of antitumor immune effector mechanisms.[38,39]

Several cytokines and growth factors have been studied in this respect. For instance, levels of interleukin-10 (IL-10) and interleukin-6 (IL-6) are particularly elevated in ovarian cancer ascites.[40,41] Also, preliminary studies have shown that on one hand, endogenously produced IL-6 can protect tumor cells from natural killer cell-mediated killing[41] and that on the other hand, high levels of IL-10 may play a role in immune responsiveness and the promotion of tumor growth.[40,42-44]

Epidermal growth factor (EGF) receptors have been detected in a high percentage of ovarian cancer specimens, and overexpression of the receptor has been correlated with poor prognosis.[37] The effects of tumor growth factor (TGF)-beta, which is closely related to epidermal growth factor (EGF), are mediated through the EGF receptor, and TGF-beta has been shown to inhibit the growth of normal surface epithelium and some ovarian cancer cell lines.[37] Furthermore, fibroblast growth factor (FGF) was shown in one study to be mitogenic in one of four ovarian cancer cell lines.[37] Receptors for two other factors, c-Erb-2 and c-Fms, have been identified, and increased levels of their oncogenes have been correlated with poor prognosis.[45,46]

Oncogenes: Recent efforts have focused on the role of oncogenes in ovarian cancer. *HER-2/neu* is the most studied. Normal ovarian epithelium expresses low to moderate levels of *HER-2/neu*[47]; however, as studies have shown, overexpression of this oncogene may impart a biologic advantage to tumor cells by enhancing their resistance to cytotoxicity.[48] *HER-2/neu* is overexpressed in about 30% of ovarian malignancies and appears to indicate poor clinical prognosis and poor survival. *HER-2/neu* thus has the potential to be clinically useful as both a prognostic marker and a potential therapeutic target for ovarian cancer.[47,49,50]

Antioncogenes have also been studied, notably the tumor suppressor gene *p53*. The loss of normal *p53* function, due to mutation and overexpression or to deletion of the normal *p53* gene, is often associated with a malignant phenotype. The *p53* gene is located on chromosome 17p and has been seen to be overexpressed and mutated in about 30% to 50% of ovarian cancers.[51–53] Another antioncogene, *MDR-1*, is specifically stimulated by mutant *p53* and repressed by wild-type *p53*, implying an increased drug resistance and a growth advantage in cells that express a mutated *p53* gene.[54]

Tumor necrosis factor (TNF)-alpha, levels of which are also increased in ascites, has been shown to upregulate *p53* mRNA expression and to induce apoptosis in an ovarian cancer cell line.[55] TNF-alpha also was recently found to follow a distinct pathway in inducing apoptosis.[56] Upregulation by TNF-alpha of the mutated oncogene *p53* could induce the proliferation of ovarian cancer cells, whereas its upregulation of wild-type *p53* would induce apoptosis.[57,58]

The prognostic value of the preoperative CA125 level in epithelial ovarian cancer is debatable.[59,60] Most aggressive tumors are not necessarily those with the highest CA125 levels. Although the highest CA125 levels are seen in the most poorly differentiated tumors, there is no big difference in the percentages of patients with low-grade and high-grade tumors who have elevated CA125 level.[61,62] This suggests that the absolute level of CA125 does not relate to the volume of ovarian tumor; furthermore, the expression of CA125 in tissue shows no association with tumor grade, DNA ploidy, or S-phase fraction.[63]

DNA Ploidy Analysis: DNA ploidy, which is the expression of a cell's nuclear DNA content, is an independent prognostic factor.[64] Aneuploidy increases with age, stage, histology other than serous and mucinous, and degree of atypia and in the presence of *Pseudomyxoma peritonei*. In patients with invasive cancer, most tumors are aneuploid; most borderline tumors are diploid. To establish an individual tumor's ploidy, at least two biopsies from the solid tumor are required. S-phase fraction is currently not a reliable prognostic factor.[37]

Other Prognostic Factors: Prognostic factors are tumor-related characteristics that determine the biologic behavior and risk of death from the disease and whose predictive value may change during the course of treatment and thereafter. The main prognostic factors in early ovarian cancer (stage I to IIA) are International Federation of Obstetricians and Gynecologists (FIGO) stage, histologic grade, histologic type, and age.[65,66] Ovarian

cancer is discovered early in fewer than 30% of patients; in such cases, the 5-year survival is good, ranging from 51% to 98%.[65,67,68] Unfortunately, however, the histologic grading of ovarian tumors is based on subjective criteria and varies widely between and among observers.[69–71] To improve on this shortcoming, DNA flow-cytometric analysis has been introduced in recent years as a tool for assessing prognosis.

All studies agree that most borderline malignant tumors are diploid and that the few patients with aneuploid tumors have a worse prognosis.[72–74] Among stage I (early ovarian cancer) patients, diploid tumors are associated with an extremely good survival, independent of adjuvant treatment. The 5-year disease-free survival for patients with diploid tumors is 90% vs 64% for those with aneuploid tumors.[75,76]

Factors associated with a poor prognosis in advanced ovarian cancer (stage III or IV) fall into two subgroups (as determined by multivariate analysis in clinical trials):

(1) Variables prior to systemic treatment predictive of survival: residual tumor > 1 cm diameter, FIGO stage IV, poorer performance status, older age, undifferentiated tumor, presence of ascites, 20 or more sites of disease, clear cell or mucinous histology, aneuploid and polyploid tumors, clonogenic growth in vitro, treatment center.[77–79]

(2) Variables at the time of relapse predictive of time to progression: less than 180 days from last chemotherapy, poorer performance status, mucinous histology, larger number of sites of disease, best previous response to chemotherapy vs progression, serum CA125 levels.[80] Low-risk patients with invasive advanced carcinomas are younger than 40; have tumors that are euploid, stage III, serous and/or endometrioid type, and grade 1; and have no residual tumors. The high-risk patients are older than 70; have tumors that are aneuploid, stage IV, clear cell and/or unclassified type, and grade III; and have bulky disease.[37]

Postoperative residual tumor volume may simply reflect the natural biology and history of the disease. Tumors that are more advanced are more difficult to resect and therefore associated with larger residual disease. Therefore, how advanced the tumor was before debulking may be more important than how much disease was left behind.[79] Other features, such as the type of chemotherapy, the intrinsic chemosensitivity of the tumor, and the presence of other biologic variables, may be as important as or even more important than the extent of the surgery.[81–86] Indeed, Heintz et al found that factors influencing the ability to perform optimal cytoreductive surgery were the same as those influencing disease-free and overall survival.[82]

The literature on second-look surgery in ovarian cancer covers its diagnostic, prognostic, and therapeutic aspects. The earlier assumption that a negative second-look surgery is associated with excellent survival is clearly not true,[87,88] since it is now quite clear that at least 30% to 50% of patients with no pathologic evidence of disease will experience a relapse.[88–91] Furthermore, patients with grade 3 tumors or grossly visible disease at completion of initial surgery also are at high risk. The question then remains whether additional treatment will affect outcome in these high-risk patients (survival difference).[89–91]

Some investigators have attempted to quantify the impact of pretreatment prognostic factors on survival and to construct from these factors a prognostic index (PI). Five pretreatment characteristics so far used in calculating the PI are performance status, FIGO stage, residual tumor size, tumor grade, and presence of ascites.[85,92,93] Future prognostic factors under study and which have produced promising results include *p53* immunostaining of epithelial ovarian cancers. It has been shown that those individuals whose tumors express excessive amounts of mutated *p53* experience shorter overall survival. However, those same studies failed to show that *p53* expression is an independent prognostic factor.[94]

PATHOLOGY AND STAGING

The ovarian stroma and epithelium are of the same mesodermal origin.[95] The epithelium lining the ovary and the peritoneum is similar to the coelomic epithelium that gives rise to the fallopian tube, uterus, cervix, and müllerian duct and from which approximately 75% of all primary ovarian neoplasms arise.

"Epithelial" ovarian tumors contain varying amounts and activities of the gonadal mesenchyma and are all potentially hormone producing. They are classified according to cell type and behavior as benign, borderline malignant or of low malignant potential, or malignant.

Criteria for the diagnosis of borderline malignant tumors are as follows: (1) epithelial proliferation with papillary formation and pseudostratification; (2) nuclear atypia and increased mitotic activity; and (3) absence of true stromal invasion (20% to 25% of borderline malignant tumors have truly spread beyond the ovary, although rare examples of microinvasion have been reported; the prognosis of these tumors is determined by the nature of metastatic implants).

The major cell types of epithelial tumors are serous, mucinous, endometrioid, clear cell, transitional, and undifferentiated. The importance of distinguishing among different epithelial subtypes lies in their different biologic behaviors, likelihood of spread, and consequent variation in prognosis and treatment. For the invasive epithelial carcinomas, however, the current consensus is that histologic type has limited prognostic significance independent of clinical stage, extent of residual disease, and histologic grade.

Serous Tumors: Serous tumors represent 50% of epithelial ovarian tumors. Of these, 10% are borderline malignant serous tumors and 50% occur before the age of 40. The 5-year survival is 80% to 90%. Malignant calcified psammoma bodies are found in 80% of serous carcinomas.

Mucinous Tumors: Mucinous tumors make up 8% to 10% of epithelial ovarian tumors. These tumors may reach enormous size, filling the entire abdominal cavity. The tumors are bilateral in 8% to 10% of cases, and the mucinous lesions are intraovarian in 95% to 98% of cases. *Pseudomyxoma peritonei* is most commonly secondary to an ovarian mucinous carcinoma.

Endometrioid Tumors: Overall, 6% to 8% of epithelial ovarian tumors resemble endometrial adenocarcinoma, and both types occur simultaneously as synchronous primary tumors in 30% of cases. Identification of multifocal disease is important because patients with disease metastatic from the uterus to the ovaries have a 5-year survival rate of 30% to 40%. Those with synchronous multifocal disease have a 5-year survival rate of 75% to 80%. Concurrent endometriosis is present in 10% of cases. The malignant potential of endometriosis is very low, although a transition from benign to malignant epithelium may be seen.

Adenocarcinoma with benign-appearing squamous metaplasia has an excellent prognosis. Conversely, mixed adenosquamous carcinoma (malignant glandular and squamous epithelial) has a very poor one.

Clear-Cell Carcinomas: Clear-cell carcinomas occur in 5% of cases and may also be associated with endometriosis or endometrial cancer. Often the clear-cell type coexists with other cell types. It is sometimes associated with hypercalcemia or hyperpyrexia and metastatic disease. These tumors have a worse prognosis than others.

Small-Cell Carcinomas: Small-cell carcinomas are rare, occasionally associated with neuroendocrine features, and usually have a poor prognosis.

Brenner Tumors: Brenner tumors can be malignant, borderline, or benign; they are very rare.

Transitional-Cell Tumors: Some primary ovarian carcinomas resemble transitional-cell carcinoma of the urinary bladder without a recognizable Brenner tumor. Ovarian carcinomas that are more than 50% transitional-cell tumors are more sensitive to chemotherapy and have a more favorable prognosis.[96]

Undifferentiated Carcinomas: Undifferentiated carcinomas make up 17% of epithelial ovarian tumors, and the prognosis for patients with these tumors is poor.

Peritoneal Mesotheliomas: Peritoneal mesotheliomas are characterized by carcinomatosis with peritoneal epithelium as the primary source. The ovaries are not involved with tumor, or only their surfaces are involved. Women with such tumors may have a remote history of oophorectomy.

Histologic Grading

Two histologic grading systems are in common use. *The pattern system* considers the general microscopic appearance of a lesion. Lesions range from grade 1 (well differentiated) to grade 2 (moderately differentiated and predominantly glandular) to grade 3 (poorly differentiated and predominantly solid). *Broder's grading system* classifies lesions from grade 1 to 4, depending on the lesions' cytologic and nuclear characteristics. This system assumes grade 4 to be an undifferentiated lesion. Pathologists usually use a combination of both systems.

The value of grade as an independent prognostic variable has not been fully clarified. A number of reports state that tumor grade may be of value in early-stage ovarian cancer but that its value falls off in patients with advanced-stage disease.

Objective signs of ovarian carcinoma are nonspecific and include a pelvic mass, ascites, pleural effusion, and occasionally supraclavicular lymphadenopathy. Patients with ovarian cancer may occasionally present with various types of paraneoplastic conditions, such as humorally mediated hypercalcemia (clear-cell, small-cell), cerebellar degeneration (associated with antibodies to Purkinje's cells), the sudden appearance of seborrheic keratosis (a sign of Leser-Trelat syndrome), or chronic intravascular coagulation (Trousseau's syndrome). Preoperative evaluation should include a barium enema, an abdominal/pelvic computed tomography (CT) scan, blood chemistries, chest x-ray, and CA125 measurement. If symptoms of obstruction are present, an upper gastrointestinal (GI) series may be indicated. Mammograms may be helpful in ruling out metastatic breast cancer. Ascitic or pleural fluid should be tapped and examined.

A full staging laparotomy should be performed, the essential steps of which are listed in Table 4. Meticulous surgical staging for early-stage ovarian cancer is very important and should include the following: peritoneal washing; palpation of all peritoneal surfaces, including the diaphragm; bilateral salpingo-oophorectomy and to-

TABLE 4

Surgical Staging of Ovarian Cancer

Midline vertical incision

Evacuation and cytologic analysis of ascites

If ascites absent, cytologic washing of pelvis and paracolonic gutters

Inspection and palpation of the subdiaphragmatic areas, intraperitoneal contents, and retroperitoneal areas, including pancreas

Frozen section of ovarian mass (unilateral or bilateral)

If carcinoma on frozen section, hysterectomy and bilateral salpingo-oophorectomy

Omentectomy with optimal bulk reduction of remaining tumor masses

Relief of intestinal obstruction by resection or colostomy

If disease limited to ovaries, multiple biopsies including the paracolonic gutters, cul-de-sac, lateral pelvic walls, vesicouterine reflection, subdiaphragmatic sites, and intra-abdominal areas

Ipsilateral and para-aortic lymph-node sampling if conservative therapy planned

tal abdominal hysterectomy (although a unilateral salpingo-oophorectomy without hysterectomy may be considered for those patients with low-risk early-stage disease who wish to maintain fertility); biopsy of suspicious nodules; infracolic omentectomy; multiple peritoneal biopsies including paracolic gutters, pouch of Douglas, and diaphragm; and ipsilateral pelvic lymph nodes.[97]

Repeat surgery for staging may be indicated in patients who have been inadequately staged and in whom this will provide further information that will affect treatment. After surgery is completed, the patient's histologic grade, stage, and residual disease should be characterized.

FIGO staging criteria, whose prognostic value is well established, are used to stage these tumors (Table 5). According to FIGO, stage I has a 5-year survival rate of 80% to 90%; stage II has a 5-year survival rate of 40% to 60%; stage III has a 5-year survival rate of 10% to 15%; and stage IV has a 5-year survival rate of less than 5%. Differences in survival among patients with the same FIGO stage of disease may indicate incomplete staging. This may limit stage as a prognostic factor. Frequently unrecognized sites of disease include the pelvic lymph nodes, cul-de-sac peritoneum, para-aortic nodes, omentum, and diaphragm.

TABLE 5

FIGO Staging for Ovarian Carcinoma (1988)

Stage I	Growth limited to the ovaries	
Stage IA	Growth limited to one ovary; no ascites; no tumor on the external surface; capsule intact	
Stage IB	Growth limited to both ovaries; no ascites; no tumor growth on the external surfaces; capsules intact	
Stage IC	Stage IA or IB tumor, but with tumor on surface of one or both ovaries or with ruptured capsule; or ascites present containing malignant cells or positive peritoneal washings	
Stage II	Growth involving one or both ovaries; pelvic extension	
Stage IIA	Extension and/or metastases to the uterus and/or tubes	
Stage IIB	Extension to other pelvic tissues	
Stage IIC	Either stage IIA or IIB tumor, but with tumor on surface of one or both ovaries or ruptured capsules, or ascites containing malignant cells or positive peritoneal washings	
Stage III	Tumor involving one or both ovaries with peritoneal implants outside the pelvis and/or positive retroperitoneal or inguinal nodes; superficial liver metastases; tumor limited to true pelvis but with histologically proven malignant extension to small bowel or omentum	
Stage IIIA	Tumor grossly limited to the true pelvis with negative nodes but with histologically confirmed microscopic seeding of abdominal peritoneal surfaces	
Stage IIIB	Tumor involving one or both ovaries with histologically confirmed implants of abdominal peritoneal surfaces, none extending 2 cm in diameter; nodes are negative	
Stage IIIC	Abdominal implants greater than 2 cm in diameter and/or positive retroperitoneal or inguinal nodes	
Stage IV	Growth involving one or both ovaries with distant metastases; if pleural effusion is present there must be positive cytology to allot a case to stage IV; parenchymal liver metastases indicates stage IV	

Surgery

The rationale for cytoreductive surgery is based on kinetic as well as retrospective studies, which have shown that patients with small-volume residual disease following initial surgery respond better to subsequent chemotherapy and survive longer. Cytoreductive surgery in properly selected patients probably helps palliate intestinal obstruction and abdominal discomfort. However, there are no prospective, randomized studies to prove the survival benefit of cytoreductive surgery.[98] In fact, several retrospective studies recently have questioned the value of initial cytoreductive surgery in the long-term prognosis of patients with advanced disease.[87]

One recent meta-analysis[88] of patients with advanced disease treated with platinum-based chemotherapy shows that patients who had maximum cytoreductive surgery had only a small increase in mean survival time. Two large retrospective trials,[89,90] one that included patients with stage III disease and one that included patients with stage IV disease, failed to show that initial cytoreductive surgery prolonged survival. Some studies have advocated extensive debulking procedures, including bowel resection and peritoneal stripping.[99,100] However, in a study of 302 patients with advanced epithelial ovarian cancer, Potter found that patients who had extensive debulking surgery showed no improved survival over those who did not.[101]

Together, these studies suggest that survival in patients with advanced bulky ovarian carcinoma is influenced by many factors other than the surgeon's technical ability to cytoreduce tumor bulk. Instead, tumor biology probably plays an important but undefined role in the natural history of the disease.

Nevertheless, in the absence of a prospective randomized trial, the standard practice remains cytoreductive surgery when it can be accomplished with acceptable morbidity. The importance of secondary cytoreduction following chemotherapy, however, remains controversial, since there is no evidence to suggest that second-look laparotomy prolongs survival.[91,102]

Secondary Cytoreduction

The information obtained at a second look is primarily prognostic. However, information from a negative second look is of limited clinical benefit: in 30% to 50% of patients who obtain a surgically confirmed complete response (CR), disease will recur.[88–91] Nevertheless, as one randomized study reports, patients with recurrent or progressive ovarian cancer who had optimal (less than 2 cm) secondary cytoreduction survived longer (mean, 27.1 months) than those who had unsuccessful surgery (mean, 9 months).[103]

In a large European study, patients who had undergone primary surgery and had residual tumors larger than 1 cm received three cycles of cisplatin chemotherapy. Then the patients with responding disease were randomly assigned to have either interval debulking surgery (IDS) and chemotherapy or no surgery followed by further chemotherapy. In both groups, 84% of patients received at least six cycles of chemotherapy. Median survival for the IDS patients was 26 months vs 19 months for the chemotherapy patients.[104] This finding suggests that further studies are needed to determine the role of secondary debulking surgery. Berek et al[105] have even gone so far as to suggest that the focus should be on whether any intervention during or after secondary surgery can improve survival, since salvage therapies may have an even greater negative impact on quality of life than second-look surgery.

TREATMENT

Chemotherapy

The standard present practice of following cytoreductive surgery with platinum-based chemotherapy fails to cure the vast majority of patients with advanced disease. Chemotherapy's role at present is largely palliative. However, at a recent consensus meeting on the treatment of advanced ovarian cancer, there was agreement that after appropriate cytoreductive surgery, platinum-based chemotherapy yields superior response rates, progression-free survival, and superior survival rates.[106] The meeting participants also concluded that carboplatin (Paraplatin) is an acceptable option in patients with suboptimal disease (stage III or IV) but should not replace cisplatin in patients with potentially curable small-volume disease. Investigators at a recent symposium came to the same conclusion.[107]

The above statements raise one of the most common concerns in treating ovarian cancer: the issue of carboplatin vs cisplatin. A recent meta-analysis[108] that incorporated data from two trials, including survival data from over 2,000 patients, compared carboplatin and cisplatin treatment groups; it failed to demonstrate any significant differences in overall survival between the two groups. A similar conclusion came from two large North American

trials: a trial by the Southwest Oncology Group[109] (342 patients with stage III or IV disease randomized to receive cisplatin, 100 mg/m^2, plus cyclophosphamide, 600 mg/m^2, or carboplatin, 300 mg/m^2, plus cyclophosphamide, 600 mg/m^2) and a trial by the National Cancer Institute of Canada[110] (447 patients randomized to cisplatin 75 mg/m^2, plus cyclophosphamide vs carboplatin/cyclophosphamide). All three of these trials failed to demonstrate a significant difference in overall survival, though the carboplatin regimen was found to have a better therapeutic index and to produce a better quality of life.[109,110] In contrast, a recent French trial[111] involving 144 patients with stage III or IV disease who received either cisplatin or carboplatin demonstrated very different results, as seen in Table 6.[109–115] The doses of cyclophosphamide (500 mg/m^2) and doxorubicin (40 mg/m^2) were the same in both groups. The pathologic complete remission and overall response rates were significantly higher in the cisplatin arm than in the carboplatin arm (33% vs 15% and 73% vs 47%, respectively). The median survival time was 27.9 months for the cisplatin arm and 20.6 months for the carboplatin arm. The actual delivered dose intensity of the drugs in the two arms was not reported.[111]

Another issue is the addition of doxorubicin to cisplatin or cyclophosphamide regimens. The recent consensus[87] is that either cyclophosphamide (750 mg/m^2) plus cisplatin (75 mg/m^2) every 3 weeks or cyclophosphamide (500 mg/m^2) plus doxorubicin (50 mg/m^2) plus cisplatin (50 mg/m^2) every 3 weeks (CAP) is acceptable standard therapy. However, four prospective randomized trials[116–119] comparing cisplatin and cyclophosphamide with the CAP regimen failed to show statistically significant differences in overall survival.

The largest of the above trials was that of the Italian Cooperative Gynecologic Oncology Group (GICOG), which randomized 529 patients to receive CAP, cisplatin/cyclophosphamide, or single-agent cisplatin.[116] No statistical difference was seen in overall survival (minimum follow-up, 5 years) among the three groups. Meta-analysis of the above four trials[120] revealed a 6-year survival advantage of 7% in patients receiving the doxorubicin-containing regimen, but it remains unclear whether the benefit was a result of doxorubicin or the greater dose intensity reached by adding it.

A third and still controversial issue is the number of cycles of chemotherapy to be given. Most studies report 5 to 10 courses of treatment, and it is generally agreed that most responses occur within four courses of chemotherapy. Two prospective randomized trials failed to demonstrate any significant benefit for more prolonged treatment.[121,122] The current recommendation is to give at least

TABLE 6

Carboplatin vs Cisplatin in Combination Chemotherapy for Advanced Ovarian Cancer

Group	Number of patients	Carb/cis dose (mg/m²)	Carb/cis PDI (mg/m²/wk)	Combine with drug	SOD %	Carb/cis PCR (%)	Carb/cis median PFS (mo)	Carb/cis median survival (mo)
NCIC [110]	417	300/75	75/18.75	CTX	59 [a]	11/15	13.4/12.9	25.8/23.8
EORTC [112]	342	350/100	70/20	DOX CTX HMM	63 [b]	23/27	13.1/16.8	22.7/24.6
SWOG [109]	291	300/100	75/25	CTX	100 [a]	8/7	NA	19.8/17.4
GONO [113]	164	200/50	50/12.5	DOX CTX	66 [a]	14/20	15.5/13.2	23.1/22.6
ARTAC [111]	144	300/75	75/18.75	DOX CTX	NA	10/25	NA	20.6/27.9
NCCTG/ Mayo [114]	103	150/60	37.5/15	CTX	35 [a]	NA	12.0/17.0	20.0/27.0
UK [115]	56	300/100	75/25	CTX	77 [a]	NA	24.0/13.0	24.0/19.0

carb = carboplatin, cis = cisplatin, CTX = cyclophosphamide, DOX = doxorubicin, HMM = hexamethylmelamine (altretamine), NA = not available, PCR = pathologic complete response, PDI = planned dose intensity 20 mg/m²/d × 5, PFS = progression-free survival, SOD = suboptimally debulked

[a] Lesions > 2 cm   [b] Lesions > 1 cm

six courses of treatment. There is no evidence so far to show that additional treatment produces any benefit.

Dose Intensity

The importance of dose intensity (DI) (mg/m²/time period) in relation to clinical outcome in ovarian cancer has been analyzed by several investigators. In particular, three large prospective randomized trials have failed to consistently demonstrate a clinically significant improvement with high-dose chemotherapy.[123–125] The Hong Kong trial included stage III to IV patients who showed improved survival with high-dose regimens, but the patient population was small and staging criteria were not uniform.[125] The large Scottish trial[124] also showed a difference in survival but included in its population optimally debulked patients with stage IC to IV disease. However, a separate analysis by the Scottish investigators of patients with advanced ovarian cancer still showed a difference favoring the high-dose arm with respect to progression-free and overall survival. Patients on the high-dose arm received the same number of treatment cycles as those in the low-dose arm, and as a result the total dose of cisplatin was 67% higher.

The Gynecologic Oncology Group (GOG) trial of patients with suboptimal stage III or IV disease failed to demonstrate any survival advantage for the high-dose chemotherapy arm.[123] However, it is important to note that the final assessment of clinical response was based on a relatively small subset of patients with measurable disease (34%), and that in this study the high-intensity arm consisted of only four courses of chemotherapy (Table 7).[116,122–125] It is possible that a greater increase in dose intensity was required to produce clinically meaningful improvement in patients with advanced disease. A central problem, however, with evaluation of dose intensity in ovarian cancer is that multiple chemotherapy-related toxicities preclude marked increases in dose intensity for prolonged periods.

Paclitaxel

Single-Agent Therapy: Three phase II trials with paclitaxel (Taxol) as a single agent without cytokine support have been completed (Table 8).[126–134] A total of 110 patients with advanced ovarian cancer were involved.[126–128,131,135–137] The paclitaxel dose ranged from 100 mg/m² to 250 mg/m² infused over 24 hours every 3 weeks. Overall, in 20% to 37% of patients tumor regressed partially, and in seven patients regression was complete. Responses were 40% to 50% in platinum-sensitive tumors and 24% to 30% in platinum-resistant tumors. At least two patients with platinum-resistant disease achieved a CR. The median duration of response was 6 months. The overall median survival was 11 months (17 months in patients with platinum-sensitive tumors and 9 months in those with platinum-resistant tumors).[131] The major toxic effect was granulocytopenia.

TABLE 7

Randomized Trials of Cisplatin/Cyclophosphamide Dose Intensity

Group	Disease stage	Number of patients	Drug regimens	Dose intensity	Cumulative dose	Assigned increase in dose intensity in the intensified arm	Results
Hong Kong [125]	Stage III/IV	60	Cisplatin 100 mg/m^2 + CTX 1,000 mg/m^2 vs cisplatin 50 mg/m^2 + CTX 1,000 mg/m^2 × 6 cycles	+	+	× 2	3-year survival rates: higher dose = 60%, lower dose = 30%
GOG [123]	Untreated, suboptimal stage III/IV	458	Cisplatin 100 mg/m^2 + CTX 1,000 mg/m^2 × 4 vs cisplatin 50 mg/m^2 + CTX 500 mg/m^2 × 8	+	−	× 2	Median survival duration: higher dose = 21.9 mo, lower dose = 18.9 mo
Scottish [124]	Stage I-IV	165	Cisplatin 100 mg/m^2 + CTX 750 mg/m^2 vs cisplatin 50 mg/m^2 + CTX 750 mg/m^2 × 6 cycles	+	−	× 2	Median survival duration: higher dose = 28.5 mo, lower dose = 17.2 mo
Italian [116]	Stage III/IV	296	Cisplatin 75 mg/m^2 every 3 wk × 6 vs cisplatin 50 mg/m^2 every wk × 9 cycles	+	−	× 2	Median survival duration: higher dose = 36 mo, lower dose = 33 mo
Danish [122]	Stage II-IV	78	AUC escalation from: 3-8 mg/ml/min	+	+	AUC × 4 vs AUC × 8	Higher PCR; survival too early for analysis

CTX = cyclophosphamide, PCR = pathologic complete response

Patients With Multiple Prior Regimens: The NCI-designated Comprehensive Cancer Centers provide paclitaxel (135 mg/m^2) in a 24-hour infusion to patients with ovarian cancer who have failed at least three prior treatments.[129] In a study of response rates, Trimble et al found that 22% of patients had objective responses to this regimen (4% CR, 18% PR) and that the median survival was 9 months.

Dose Intensification With Cytokines: The effect of dose intensification of paclitaxel on outcome is suggestive in ovarian cancer[127]; efforts have been made to better define dose intensification with paclitaxel in this disease.[132–134,138] Paclitaxel was given as a single agent at 250 mg/m^2 over 24 hours to patients with platinum-resistant ovarian carcinoma. Granulocyte colony-stimulating factor (G-CSF, filgrastim [Neupogen]) also was administered starting 24 hours after completion of paclitaxel infusion. Objective tumor response was seen in 48% of patients. The duration of response was 6 months and the

median survival was 12 months.

Dose and Schedule Study: A joint European-Canadian trial coordinated by the NCI of Canada prospectively randomized patients to two dose levels of paclitaxel (135 mg/m^2 or 175 mg/m^2) and two different infusion schedules (3 or 24 hours).[130] Responses were more frequent at larger doses (20% vs 15%) and with longer infusion (19% vs 16%). Though neither of these differences in response was statistically significant, paclitaxel at 175 mg/m^2 given over 3 hours was recommended in that study.

Combinations in Primary Treatment: In 1993, the GOG presented in abstract form the preliminary results of a trial using paclitaxel in combination with other agents as front-line chemotherapy in suboptimally debulked stage III/IV disease.[139] At the 1995 meeting of the American Society of Clinical Oncology, the same group[140] presented the 5-year follow-up data from this trial comparing paclitaxel plus cisplatin with cisplatin plus cyclophosphamide as first-line therapy in advanced-stage III/

TABLE 8

Studies of Paclitaxel in Advanced and Refractory Ovarian Cancer

Institution	Number of patients	Dose (mg/m²)	Overall response	CR % (number)	Median survival (mo)
Single agent					
JHOC [126]	40	135 (110-170)	30%	2.5 (1)	8.2
GOG [127]	41	170 (decreasing)	37%	12 (5)	15.9
Einstein [128]	30	180–250	20%	3 (1)	6.5
NCI-TRC [129]	619	135	22%	3	9
European/	195	135	15%	1 (2)	11
Canadian [130]	187	175	20%	2 (4)	11.5
High dose (with G-CSF)					
NCI [131,132]	44	250	48%	14	11.5
M. D. Anderson [133,134]	48	250	48%	4	12

CR = complete response, G-CSF = granulocyte colony-stimulating factor, GOG = Gynecologic Oncology Group, JHOC = Johns Hopkins Oncology Center, NCI = National Cancer Institute, TRC = Treatment Referral Center   Adapted from Holmes et al: Current status of clinical trials with paclitaxel and docetaxel, in Georg GI, Cuen TC, Ojiwa I, et al (eds): ACS Symposium-in-Print. Taxane Anticancer Agent: Basic Science and Current Status, 3:31–57, 1994.

IV ovarian cancer. Patients were randomized to receive either 750 mg/m² cyclophosphamide and 75 mg/m² cisplatin or 135 mg/m² of paclitaxel and 75 mg/m² of cisplatin. The reported toxicity was lower for the paclitaxel/cisplatin arm. Clinical response was 64% in the cisplatin/cyclophosphamide (CP) group and 77% in the paclitaxel/cisplatin (TP) group. The median progression-free survival was 12.9 months for the CP group and 18 months for the TP group. The median overall survival was 24.4 months for the CP group and 37.5 for the TP group. Only approximately one third of the patients in the cyclophosphamide study arm were treated with paclitaxel on relapse. The overall survival of this subgroup has not been reported. Of further interest is the observation that the cisplatin dose was higher in the paclitaxel arm.[141] The European Organization for Research and Treatment of Cancer (EORTC) and NCI of Canada Clinical Trials Group plan to confirm and possibly extend these findings in both optimal and suboptimal patients, including those with early disease who are at high risk of relapse.

Intraperitoneal Chemotherapy: The rationale for intraperitoneal (IP) chemotherapy is based primarily on patterns of spread of epithelial ovarian cancer. It has been shown that IP platinum produces objective responses in patients with small-volume residual ovarian cancer. In a phase III Southwest Oncology Group (SWOG)-GOG-ECOG study, the results of which were presented at the 1995 ASCO meeting, patients with optimal (less than 2 cm) residual stage III disease were randomized to receive either six courses of IP platinum (100 mg/m²) and IV cyclophosphamide (600 mg/m²) or IV platinum (100 mg/m²) and IV cyclophosphamide (600 mg/m²). Median follow-up was 47 months in the IP arm and 44 months in the IV arm. Survival in the IP arm was 49 months, and in the IV arm, 41 months.[142] The IP platinum approach is also under study in patients who have achieved a surgically confirmed CR to determine whether disease recurrences can be prevented or delayed.[143] Intraperitoneal administration of paclitaxel appears promising, but first, a prospective randomized trial of IP vs IV paclitaxel is required to determine the relative efficacy of the different routes of administration.[144]

It is very important to point out that IP chemotherapy should be used in patients with small-volume disease or no residual disease in light of poor penetration of IP tumor nodules by most antineoplastic agents. Moreover, IP therapy in patients with ovarian cancer may be limited by the frequent presence of extraperitoneal disease.

Other Chemotherapeutic Agents

Docetaxel (Taxotere) is a semisynthetic compound structurally related to paclitaxel. The toxicity of docetaxel is in many ways similar to that of paclitaxel. However, prolonged treatment with docetaxel increases skin toxicity and produces significant edema. When used as a single agent in advanced (stage IV) platinum-refractory ovarian cancer, the rate of response to docetaxel is 25% to 32%.[145]

Etoposide (VePesid) has produced reported response rates of up to 30%, but more typically 10% to 20%. In patients with platinum-refractory disease who were given 100 mg doses of etoposide orally for 14 days every 21 days, the response rate was about 26%.[146] Immediately after failing paclitaxel therapy, patients show a minimal response rate to etoposide.[147]

Altretamine (Hexalen): In patients with platinum-resistant measurable disease who were administered 600-mg/m^2/d doses of altretamine for 5 days every 4 weeks, no objective responses were noted.[148]

Gemcitabine is a primary antimetabolite that closely resembles cytarabine. In patients with platinum-refractory disease who received 800-mg/m^2 doses weekly for 3 weeks, 19% had a partial response.[149] We plan to study this drug at higher doses.

Topoisomerase I Inhibitors: Topotecan, a semisynthetic camptothecin derivative,[150–152] has shown activity in both preclinical and phase I studies. For example, 30 women with ovarian cancer refractory to cisplatin or carboplatin and no prior taxane therapy were treated with a starting dose of 1.5 mg/m^2/d for 5 days every 21 days. The result was a 14% partial response rate with a median duration response of 9 months and a median survival of all treated patients of 10 months.[153]

CPT-11: This drug produced an 18% to 28% objective response rate and a 23% response rate in patients who received prior platinum therapy.[154–157]

Ifosfamide (Ifex): The response rate of platinum-refractory ovarian cancer to ifosfamide is 13%.[158]

Hormones: There has been relatively little prospective evaluation of hormonal therapy in ovarian cancer. Nevertheless, there are several reports of responses to various hormonal treatments (eg, progestational agents, antiandrogens, gonadotropin agonists, and tamoxifen [Nolvadex]) ranging from 10% to 20% and an additional 10% to 20% stabilization of disease in patients treated with prior chemotherapy and platinum-resistant tumors.[159–161]

RADIATION THERAPY

Radiation therapy has been used to treat ovarian carcinoma in two situations: (1) as adjuvant therapy for stages I to III disease without residual tumor after surgery and (2) as consolidation after chemotherapy in advanced disease with minimal residual tumor at second-look laparotomy.[162] Whole abdominal radiation (WAR) and IP isotopes have been used in the adjuvant setting. Review of the randomized and nonrandomized data for WAR suggest that it can help prolong disease-free survival in early-stage ovarian cancer.[163] Unfortunately, no prospective randomized trial has compared WAR with a cisplatin-containing regimen.

However, three papers concerning the use of intraperitoneal ^{32}P have been published. After conducting a study that included patients with FIGO stage I or II disease, Soper et al[164] concluded that ^{32}P is not effective in the adjuvant setting. Spanos et al[165] gave no information about survival. Vergote et al studied patients with stage I ovarian cancer who were randomly assigned to receive either six courses of cisplatin or intraperitoneal ^{32}P.[166] There was no difference in response between the two groups, but complications (ie, bowel obstruction) were more frequent in the ^{32}P-treated group.

To date, there is no proof that adjuvant radiation therapy is superior to other treatment modalities. However, it is clear from two studies of consolidation radiation therapy that the related complications are significant. Hoskins et al evaluated patients with stage III or IV disease and found a 10-year overall survival of 4%.[167] Whelan et al evaluated 105 patients and found no survival advantage and an increased risk (8.6%) of complications (bowel obstruction).[168] Overall, the complication rate of radiation therapy as consolidation treatment is considerable and the effect on survival unremarkable.

DRUG RESISTANCE

Ovarian cancer is a good model in which to investigate chemotherapeutic resistance because both intrinsic and acquired resistance are apparent. Approximately 50% of ovarian carcinomas are intrinsically resistant to conventional chemotherapy. The natural history of the disease after relapse is characterized by the eventual development of broad cross-resistance to various treatments. Patients with relapses within 6 months of a complete response have only a 10% to 20% chance of responding to platinum retreatment, whereas those with treatment-free intervals of 21 months or longer have a 90% response rate.[169] In general, drug resistance may result from alterations in host-drug metabolism, from the spread of tumor cells to sites poorly accessible to chemotherapy, and/or from biochemical changes at the cellular or subcellular level.

To date, there is no modulator of drug resistance that benefits refractory ovarian cancer patients. However, general mechanisms of resistance that may be able to be manipulated are currently under investigation. They include efflux by multidrug resistance (MDR) pumps and other transport proteins, intracellular drug inactivation either by enzymatic detoxification (by glutathione transferases) or by binding to thiol-rich proteins (eg, metallothionein) or glutathione, repair of cytotoxic DNA adducts, alterations in tubulin structure, and enhancement of signal transduction pathways that include growth factors.[37]

ABMT and PBSC Support

High-Dose Chemotherapy Approaches That Require Cytokines: Two such approaches are autologous bone marrow transplant (ABMT) and peripheral blood stem cell (PBSC) support. Patients with drug-sensitive, small-volume disease are good candidates for high-dose chemotherapy approaches that require cytokines. To date, however, there is no conclusive evidence that high-dose therapy with ABMT benefits any subset of patients with epithelial ovarian cancer.

The major obstacle is that giving such high-dose chemotherapy in a single course produces a dose-dependent antitumor effect; this, in turn, can induce a high but not durable response rate in patients with advanced disease.[170,171] A single intensification course is inadequate because of the low-growth fraction of tumor cells, which comprises a significant number of clonogenic tumor cells, and is unaffected by most chemotherapeutic agents. Since dose intensity is important in achieving responses in ovarian cancer, a viable alternative to ABMT is to administer repeated courses of dose-intensified therapy with PBSC support.[172-174]

The first phase I and II trials with ABMT included patients with refractory ovarian carcinoma.[175,176] Most of the regimens included high doses of alkylating agents; some used carboplatin and/or mitoxantrone (Novantrone).[177-180] However, patients with responsive residual disease are more likely to respond to high-dose chemotherapy since they are not too heavily pretreated and their likelihood of drug resistance is less. With this in mind, French investigators evaluated high-dose melphalan (Alkeran) treatment with ABMT as salvage or consolidation treatment in 35 patients. After a median follow-up of 23 months, 19 patients were alive, and projected survival at 54 months was 47%.[181]

In another French study, Dauplat et al evaluated 14 patients who received similar treatment.[182] All patients were treated with high-dose melphalan and autologous bone marrow support after a second-look operation. The median follow-up after the second-look operation was 43 months. Five patients (35.7%) remain disease free at 30 to 60 months. The actuarial 3-year survival rate was 64%.[182]

Later, Legros et al evaluated patents who had received high-dose melphalan chemotherapy following induction therapy. They reported a median survival of 47 months with 69% alive at 3 years and 33% at 5 years.[183] Further

clinical trials now underway are examining the efficacy and feasibility of high-dose chemotherapy with PBSC as front-line therapy.[175]

Biological Therapy

Interferon is the most studied biological used against ovarian carcinoma. When administered intraperitoneally, it has produced response rates of 30% to 50% in patients with minimal residual disease. Other studies are underway with different combinations of biological agents, including retinoids, interleukins, and interferons, but results are preliminary.[184-186]

Immunotherapy

Ovarian cancer has a number of clinical features that make it well suited for monoclonal antibody (MoAb)-directed therapy. Because it remains primarily within the peritoneal cavity, ovarian cancer is a possible target for the IP use of MoAbs.[187] In the past, radioactive MoAbs have been used to deliver therapeutic doses of radiation to malignant tumors. The most studied of these are rhenium-186 and yttrium-90.[188] Radioactive MoAbs have already been used to palliate ascites, and delivery of meaningful radiation doses for this purpose is now possible with 40 mCi of yttrium-90.[189] Relief of ascites was reported in two studies using AB263I131 or H MFGY90.[190,191]

MoAb-directed therapy also might be possible through the use of immunotoxins. Indeed, the therapeutic activity of immunotoxins has already been demonstrated in studies of human ovarian cancers in mice.[192] The most frequently used immunotoxins are plant toxins (ricin and abrin) and bacterial toxins (*Pseudomonas* and diphtheria). However, clinical trials of immunotoxins have been hampered by several features of these agents. In particular, immunotoxins are only cytotoxic to cells that express the appropriate antigen and that internalize the MoAb toxin.

One other promising approach to immunotherapy of ovarian cancers involves tumor-infiltrating lymphocytes. Such cells have been expanded from malignant lesions and reinfused intraperitoneally with low-dose interleukin-2 (aldesleukin [Proleukin]) to reduce ascites.[193]

Gene Therapy

A recent and powerful approach to treating ovarian cancers is gene therapy, especially that involving the *MDR* gene. The rationale behind *MDR* gene transduction into hematopoietic stem cells is to protect against the toxic effects of high-intensity chemotherapy and to overcome tumor drug resistance.

At M. D. Anderson, we introduce *MDR* gene into marrow cells to protect them from paclitaxel. Once the marrow is returned to the patient, continued intensive therapy can then be given cyclically. With each therapy cycle, the marrow should become increasingly enriched with chemotherapy-resistant stem cells, because cells not transduced with *MDR* gene should die, while those containing chemotherapy resistance factors continue to grow. This, in turn, should permit more intensive therapy with paclitaxel.[194] A study of *MDR* gene therapy is underway at M. D. Anderson Cancer Center. Ten patients have already been enrolled.

REFERENCES

1. National Center for Health Statistics: Vital statistics of the United States, 1991. Washington, DC, Public Health Service, 1994.

2. World Health Organization: World Health Statistics Annuals: 1987–1992. Geneva, Switzerland, World Health Organization, 1987–1992.

3. Schildkraut JM, Thompson WD: Familial ovarian cancer: A population-based case control study. Am J Epidemiol 128:456–466, 1988.

4. Lynch HT, Conway T, Lynch J: Hereditary ovarian cancer: Pedigree studies, part II. Cancer Genet Cytogenet 52:161–183, 1991.

5. Kerlikowske K, Brown JS, Grady DG: Should women with familial ovarian cancer undergo prophylactic oophorectomy? Obstet Gynecol 80:700–707, 1992.

6. Lynch HT, Kullander S: Cancer Genetics, in Women, p 95, Boca Raton, FL, CRC Press, 1987.

7. Lynch HT, Watson P, Bewtra C, et al: Hereditary ovarian cancer: Heterogeneity in age at diagnosis. Cancer 67:1460–1466, 1991.

8. Amos CI, Shaw GL, Tucker MA, et al: Age at onset for familial epithelial ovarian cancer. JAMA 268:1896–1899, 1992.

9. Lynch HT, Fitzsimmons M, Conway TA, et al: Hereditary carcinoma of the ovary and associated cancers: A study of two families. Gynecol Oncol 36:48–55, 1990.

10. Whittemore AS, Harris R, Huyre J: Characteristics relating to ovarian cancer risk: Collaborative analysis of twelve US case-control studies. II. Invasive epithelial ovarian cancers in white women. Am J Epidemiol 136:1184–1203, 1992.

11. Haukinson SE, Colditz GA, Hunter DJ, et al: A quantitative assessment of oral contraceptive use and risk of ovarian cancer. Obstet Gynecol 80:708–714, 1992.

12. Gardner WU: Hormonal imbalances in tumorigenesis. Cancer Res 8:397, 1948.

13. Fathala MR: Incessant ovulation: A factor in ovarian neoplasia. Lancet 2:163, 1971.

14. Cramer DW, Welch WR, Scully RE, et al: Ovarian cancer and talc: A case control study. Cancer 50:372, 1982.

15. Whittemore AS, Wu ML, Paffenbarger RS, et al: Personal and environmental characteristics related to epithelial ovarian cancer: II. Exposure to talcum powder, tobacco, alcohol and coffee. Am J Epidemiol 128:1228, 1988.

16. Cramer DW, Willet WC, Bell DA, et al: Galactose consumption and metabolism in relation to the risk of ovarian cancer. Lancet 2:66, 1989.

17. Piver MS, Mattlin C: A case-control study of milk-drinking and ovary cancer risk. Am J Epidemiol 132:871–876, 1990.

18. Cramer DW, Welch WR, Hutchison GB, et al: Dietary animal fat in relation to ovarian cancer risk. Obstet Gynecol 63:833, 1984.

19. Annual report on the results of treatment in gynecological cancer: Twenty-first volume: Statements of results obtained in patients treated in 1982 to 1986, inclusive 3 and 5-year survival up to 1990. Int J Gynaecol Obstet 36(suppl):238–277, 1991.

20. Goswamy RK, Campbell S, Whitehead MI: Screening for ovarian cancer. Clin Obstet Gynecol 10:621–643, 1983.

21. Sassone AM, Timor-Tritsch IE, Artner A, et al: Transvaginal sonographic characterization of ovarian disease: Evaluation of a new scoring system to predict ovarian malignancy. Obstet Gynecol 78:70–76, 1991.

22. Bourne T, Campbell S, Steer C, et al: Transvaginal colour flow imaging: A possible new screening technique for ovarian cancer. Br Med J 299:1367–1370, 1989.

23. Kurjak A, Zalud I, Alfirevic Z: Evaluation of adnexal masses with transvaginal color ultrasound. J Ultrasound Med 10:295–297, 1991.

24. Schilthuis MS, Aalders JG, Bouma J, et al: Serum CA125 levels in epithelial ovarian cancer: Relation in findings at second look operations and their role in the detection of tumor recurrence. Br J Obstet Gynaecol 94:202–207, 1987.

25. Bourne T, Reynolds D, Campbell S: Ovarian cancer screening. Eur J Cancer 27:655–659, 1991.

26. Griffiths CT, Parker L: Cancer of the ovary, in Knapp RC, Berkowitz RS (eds): Gynecologic Oncology, pp 313–375. New York, MacMillan, 1986.

27. van Nagell JJ, Higgins R, Donaldson E, et al: Transvaginal sonography as a screening method for ovarian cancer: A report of the first 1000 screened. Cancer 65:573–577, 1990.

28. Grauberg S, Wikland M, Jansson I: Microscopic characterization of ovarian tumors and the relation to the histological diagnosis: Criteria to be used for ultrasound evaluation. Gynecol Oncol 35:139–144, 1989.

29. Carlson KJ, Skates SJ, Singer DE: Screening for ovarian cancer. Ann Intern Med 121:124–132, 1994.

30. Jacobs F, Bast RC Jr: The CA-125 tumor associated antigen: A review of the literature. Hum Reprod 4:1–12, 1989.

31. Pittaway DE, Fayez JA: Serum CA-125 antigen levels increase during menses. Am J Obstet Gynecol 156:75–76, 1987.

32. Zurawski VR Jr, Orgaseter H, Andersen A, et al: Elevated serum CA125 levels prior to diagnosis of ovarian neoplasia: Relevance for early detection of ovarian cancer. Int J Cancer 42:677–680, 1988.

33. Howe HL: Age-specific hysterectomy and oophorectomy prevalence rates and the risks for cancer of the reproductive systems. Am J Public Health 74:560–563, 1984.

34. Wollas RP, Yu Feng J, Jacobs KNJ, et al: Elevation of multiple serum markers in patients with stage I ovarian cancer. J Natl Cancer Inst 85:1748–1751, 1993.

35. Kramer BS, Gonagan J, Prorok PC, et al: A National Cancer Institute sponsored screening trial for prostatic, lung, colorectal, and ovarian cancers (PLCO). Cancer 71:589–593, 1993.

36. National Institutes of Health Consensus Statement: Ovarian cancer screening, treatment, and follow-up. NIH, 12(3), April 5–7, 1994.

37. Berek JS, Martinez-Maza O, Hamilton T, et al: Molecular and biological factors in the pathogenesis of ovarian cancer. Semin Oncol 4(suppl):S3–16, 1993.

38. Elsasser-Beile V, von Kleist S, Sauther W, et al: Impaired cytokine production in whole blood cell cultures of patients with gynecological carcinomas in different clinical stages. Br J Cancer 68:32–36, 1993.

39. Garzetti GG, Gignitti M, Giavattini A, et al: Natural killer cell activity and progression free survival in ovarian cancer. Gynecol Obstet Invest 35:118–120, 1993.

40. Gotlieb WH, Abrams JS, Watson JM, et al: Presence of IL-10

in the ascites of patients with ovarian and other intra-abdominal cancers. Cytokine 4:385–390, 1992.

41. Ray A, Tatter SB, Santhanam V, et al: Regulation of expression of IL-6: Molecular and clinical studies. Ann NY Acad Sci 557:353–361, 1989.

42. Fiorentino DF, Zlotuik A, Mosmann TR, et al: IL-10 inhibits cytokine production by activated macrophages. J Immunol 147:3815–3822, 1991.

43. Bogdan C, Vodovotz Y, Nathan C: Macrophage deactivation by IL-10. J Exp Med 174:1549–1555, 1991.

44. de Waal Malefyt R, Abrams J, et al: IL-10 inhibits cytokine synthesis by human monocytes. J Exp Med 174:1209–1226, 1991.

45. Berchuck A, Bast RC Jr, Kohler M: Oncogenes in ovarian cancer. Hematol Oncol Clin North Am 6:813–827, 1992.

46. Kommoss F, Bauknecht T, Birmelin G, et al: Oncogene and growth factor expression in ovarian cancer. Acta Obstet Gynecol Scand 155(suppl):19–24, 1992.

47. Berchuck A, Marks JR, Bast RC Jr: Expression of the epidermal growth factor receptor, HER-2/neu, and P53 in ovarian cancer, in Sharp F, Mason WP, Creasman W (eds): Ovarian Cancer 2: Biology, Diagnosis, and Management, pp 53–59, 1992.

48. Lichtenstein A, Berenson J, Gera JF, et al: Resistance of human ovarian cancer cells to tumor necrosis factor and lymphokine-activated killer cells: Correlation with expression of HER-2/neu oncogenes. Cancer Res 50:7364–7370, 1990.

49. Slamon DJ, Goddphin W, Jones LA, et al: Studies of HER-2/neu proto-oncogene in human breast and ovarian cancer. Science 244:707–712, 1989.

50. Berchuck A, Kamel A, Whitaker R, et al: Overexpression of HER-2/neu is associated with poor survival in advanced epithelial ovarian cancer. Cancer Res 50:4087–4091, 1990.

51. Marks JR, Davidoff AM, Kerus BJ, et al: Overexpression and mutation of P53 in epithelial ovarian cancer. Cancer Res 51:2979–2984, 1991.

52. Okamoto A, Sameshima Y, Yokoyama S, et al: Frequent allelic losses and mutations of the P53 gene in human ovarian cancer. Cancer Res 51:5171–5174, 1991.

53. Mazars R, Pujol P, Mandelonde T, et al: P53 mutations in ovarian cancer: A late event? Oncogene 5:1685–1690, 1991.

54. Chin KV, Veda K, Pastan I, et al: Modulation of activity of the promoter of the human MDR I gene by ras and P53. Science 255:459–462, 1992.

55. Gotlieb WH, Watson JM, Rezai AR, et al: Cytokine-induced modulation of tumor suppressor gene expression in ovarian cancer cells: Up-regulation of P53 gene expression and induction of apoptosis by tumor necrosis factor-alpha. Am J Obstet Gynecol 4:1121–1128, 1994.

56. Wong GHW, Goeddel DV: Fas antigen and P55 TNF receptor signal apoptosis through distinct pathways. J Immunol 52:1751–1755, 1994.

57. Wu S, Boyer CM, Whitaker RS, et al: Tumor necrosis factor alpha as an autocrine and paracrine growth factor for ovarian cancer: Monokine induction of tumor cell proliferation and tumor necrosis factor alpha expression. Cancer Res 53:1939–1944, 1993.

58. Naylor MS, Stamp GW, Foulkes WD, Eccles D, et al: Tumor necrosis factor and its receptors in human ovarian cancer: Potential role in disease progression. J Clin Invest 91:2194–2206, 1993.

59. Cruickshank DJ, Fullerton WT, Klapper A: The clinical significance of preoperative serum CA125 ovarian cancer. Br J Obstet Gynecol 94:692–695, 1987.

60. Mobus V, Kreinberg R, Crowbuch G, et al: Evaluation of CA125 as prognostic and predictive factor in ovarian cancer. J Tumour Marker Oncol 3:251–258, 1988.

61. Tholander B, Taube A, Lindgren A, et al: Pretreatment serum

levels of CA125, CEA, tissue polypeptide antigen, and placental alkaline phosphatase in patients with ovarian carcinoma: Influence of histological type, grade of differentiation, and clinical stage of disease. Gynecol Oncol 39:26–33, 1990.

62. Zanaboni F, Vergadoro F, Presti M, et al: Tumour antigen CA 125 as a tumor marker of ovarian epithelial carcinoma. Gynecol Oncol 28:61–67, 1987.

63. Tholander B, Lindgren A, Taube A, et al: Immunohistochemical detection of CA 125 and CEA in ovarian tumors in relation to corresponding preoperative S levels. Int J Gynecol 2:263–270, 1992.

64. Karen J: DNA ploidy in epithelial ovarian malignancies: Prognostic value and therapeutic implications. Norwegian Cancer Society, 1993. Thesis.

65. Sigurdsson K, Alm P, Gullberg B: Prognostic factors in malignant epithelial ovarian tumors. Gynecol Oncol 15:370–380, 1983.

66. Dembo AJ, Davy M, Stenwig AE, Berle EJ, et al: Prognostic factors in patients with stage I epithelial ovarian cancer. Obstet Gynecol 75:263–273, 1990.

67. Petterson F, Coppleson M, Creasman W, Ludwig H, et al: Annual report on the result of treatment in gynecological cancer, pp 110–151. Stockholm, International Federation of Gynecology and Obstetrics, 1988.

68. Young RC, Walton LA, Ellenberg SS, et al: Adjuvant therapy in stage I and stage II epithelial ovarian cancer. N Engl J Med 322:1021–1027, 1990.

69. Hernandez E, Bhagavan BS, Parmley TH, Rosenbein NB: Interobserver variability in the interpretation of epithelial ovarian cancer. Gynecol Oncol 17:117–123, 1984.

70. Baak JPA, Langley FA, Talerman A, et al: Interpathologist and intrapathologist disagreement in ovarian tumor grading and typing. Anal Quant Cytol Histol 8:354–357, 1986.

71. Cramer SF, Roth LM, Ulbright TM, et al: Evaluation of the reproducibility of the WHO classification of common ovarian cancers. Arch Pathol Lab Med 111:819–829, 1987.

72. Klemi PJ, Jaensuu H, Kilholma P, et al: Clinical significance of abnormal nuclear DNA content in serous ovarian tumors. Cancer 62:2005–2010, 1988.

73. Erhardt K, Auser G, Bjorkualm E, et al: Prognostic significance of nuclear DNA content in serous ovarian tumors. Cancer Res 44:2198–2202, 1984.

74. Dietel M, Arps H, Rohlff A, et al: Nuclear DNA content of borderline tumors of the ovary: Correlation with histology and significance for prognosis. Virchows Arch Pathol Anat Histopathol 409:829–836, 1986.

75. Tazelaar HA, Bostwick DG, Balloy SC, et al: Conservative treatment of borderline ovarian tumors. Obstet Gynecol 66:417–422, 1985.

76. Chambers JT, Merino MJ, Kohory EI, et al: Borderline ovarian tumors. Am J Obstet Gynecol 59:1088–1094, 1988.

77. Alberts DS, Dahlberg S, Green SJ, et al: Analysis of patient age as an independent prognostic factor for survival in a phase III study of cisplatin-cyclophosphamide vs carboplatin-cyclophosphamide in stage III (suboptimal) and IV ovarian cancer: A SWOG study. Cancer 71:2(suppl):618–627, 1993.

78. deSouza PL, Friedlander ML: Prognostic factors in ovarian cancer. Hematol Oncol Clin North Am 6:4:761–781, 1992.

79. Omura GA, Brady MF, Homesley HD, et al: Long-term follow up and prognostic factor analysis in advanced ovarian carcinoma: The GOG experience. J Clin Oncol 9:1138–1150, 1991.

80. Hoskins PJ, O'Reilly SE, Swenerton KD: The "failure free interval" defines the likelihood to resistance to carboplatin in patients with advanced epithelial ovarian cancer previously treated with cisplatin: Relevance to therapy and new drug testing. Int J Gynecol Cancer

1:205–208, 1991.

81. Levin L, Lund B, Heintz AP: Advanced ovarian cancer: An overview of multivariate analysis of prognostic variables with special reference to the role of cytoreductive surgery Ann Oncol 4 (suppl 4):S23–29, 1993.

82. Heintz APM: Surgery in advanced ovarian carcinoma: Is there proof to show the benefit? Eur J Surg Oncol 14:91–99, 1988.

83. Gershenson DM, Copeland LJ, Wharton JT, et al: Prognosis of surgically determined complete responders in advanced ovarian cancer. Cancer 55:1129–1135, 1985.

84. Bertelsen E, Hansen MK, Pedersen PH, et al: The prognostic and therapeutic value of second look laparotomy in advanced ovarian cancer. Br J Obstet Gynaecol 95:1231–1236, 1988.

85. van Houwelingen JC, Ten Bokkel Huinink WW, van der Burg MEL, et al: Predictability of the survival of patients with advanced ovarian cancer. J Clin Oncol 7:769–773, 1989.

86. Hartmann LC, Podratz KC, Keeney GL, et al: Prognostic significance of P53 immunostaining in epithelial ovarian carcinoma. J Clin Oncol 12:64–69, 1994.

87. Ozols RF: Ovarian cancer: Part II. Treatment. Curr Probl Cancer 16:63–126, 1992.

88. Hunter RW, Alexander NDE, Stouter WA, et al: Metaanalysis of surgery in advanced ovarian carcinoma: Is maximum cytoreductive surgery an independent determinant of prognosis? Am J Obstet Gynecol 166:504–511, 1992.

89. Hoskins WJ, Bundy BN, Thigpen JT, et al: The influence of cytoreductive surgery on recurrence-free interval and survival in small volume stage III epithelial ovarian cancer: A Gynecologic Oncology Group study. Gynecol Oncol 47:159–166, 1992.

90. Goodman HM, Harlow BL, Sheets EE, et al: The role of cytoreductive surgery in the management of stage IV epithelial ovarian carcinoma. Gynecol Oncol 46:367–371, 1992.

91. Potter ME, Hatch KD, Soong SJ, et al: Second look laparotomy and salvage therapy: A research modality only? Gynecol Oncol 44:3–9, 1992.

92. Lund B, Williamson P, van Houwelingen HC, et al: Comparison of the predictive power of different prognostic indices for survival in patients with advanced ovarian cancer. Cancer Res 50:4626–4629, 1990.

93. Morgan MA, Noumoff JS, King S, et al: A formula for predicting the risk of a positive second look laparotomy in epithelial ovarian cancer: Implications for a randomized trial. Obstet Gynecol 80:944–948, 1992.

94. Hartmann L, Podratz K, Keeney G, et al: Prognostic significance of p53 immunostaining in epithelial ovarian cancer. J Clin Oncol 12:64–69, 1994.

95. Berek JS, Hacker NF: General principles in oncology, in Berek JS, Hacker NF, (eds): Practical Gynecologic Oncology 2nd Ed, pp 117–174. Baltimore, Williams & Wilkine, 1994.

96. Silva EG, Robey-Cafferty SS, Smith TL, et al: Ovarian carcinomas with transitional cell carcinoma pattern. Am J Clin Pathol 93:457, 1990.

97. Allan DG, Baak J, Belpomme D, et al: Advanced epithelial ovarian cancer: 1993 consensus statements. Ann Oncol 4 (suppl 4):83–89, 1993.

98. Ozols, RF: Semin Oncol 21(2):suppl 2:1–9, 1994.

99. Haker F, Berek S, Lagasse D, et al: Primary cytoreductive surgery for epithelial ovarian cancer. Obstet Gynecol 61:413–420, 1983.

100. Delgado G, Oram H, Petrilii S: Stage III epithelial ovarian cancer: The role of maximal surgical reduction. Gynecol Oncol 18:293–298, 1984.

101. Potter M, Partridge E, Hatch K, et al: Primary surgical therapy of ovarian cancer: How much and when? Gynecol Oncol 40:195–200, 1991.

102. Friedman JB, Weiss NS: Second thoughts about second look laparotomy in advanced ovarian cancer. N Engl J Med 322:1079–1082, 1990.

103. Segna RA, Dottino PR, Mandeli JP, et al: Secondary cytoreduction for ovarian cancer following cisplatin therapy. J Clin Oncol 11:434–439, 1993.

104. van der Burg MEL, van Lent M, Kobiersca A, et al: The effect of debulking surgery after induction chemotherapy on the prognosis in advanced epithelial ovarian cancer. N Engl J Med 332:629–634, 1995.

105. Berek JS: Second look vs second nature. Gynecol Oncol 44:1–2, 1992.

106. Allen DG, Baak J, Belpomme D, et al: Consensus group on advanced epithelial ovarian Cancer: 1993 consensus statement. Ann Oncol 4(suppl):83–89, 1993.

107. Vermorgen JB, ten Bokkel Huinink WW, Eisenhauer A, et al: Carboplatin vs cisplatin. Ann Oncol 4(suppl 4):41–48, 1993.

108. Advanced Ovarian Cancer Trialist Group: Chemotherapy in advanced ovarian cancer: An overview of randomized clinical trials. Br Med J 303: 884–893, 1991.

109. Alberts DS, Green S, Hanningan EV, et al: Improved therapeutic index of carboplatin plus cyclophosphamide vs cisplatin plus cyclophosphamide: Final report by the Southwest Oncology Group of a phase III randomized trial in stages III and IV ovarian cancer. J Clin Oncol 10:706–717, 1992.

110. Swenerton K, Jeffrey J, Stuart G, et al: Cisplatin-cyclophosphamide vs carboplatin-cyclophosphamide in advanced ovarian cancer: A randomized phase III study of National Cancer Institute of Canada Clinical Trial Group. J Clin Oncol 10:718–726, 1992.

111. Belpomme D, Bugat R, Rives M, et al: Carboplatin vs cisplatin in association with cyclophosphamide and doxorubicin as first line therapy in stage III-IV ovarian carcinoma: Results of an ARTAC phase III trial (abstract). Proc Am Soc Clin Oncol 11:227, 1992.

112. ten Bokkel-Huinink WW, van der Burg MCL, Van Oosterom AT, et al: Carboplatin combination therapy for ovarian cancer. Cancer Treat Rep 15:9–15, 1988.

113. Conte PF, Bruzzone M, Caruino F, et al: Carboplatin, doxorubicin, and cyclophosphamide vs cisplatin, doxorubicin, and cyclophosphamide: A randomized trial in stage III-IV epithelial ovarian carcinoma. J Clin Oncol 9:658–663, 1991.

114. Edmondson JH, McCormack GM, Wieand HS, et al: Cyclophosphamide cisplatin vs cyclophosphamide-carboplatin in stage III-IV ovarian carcinoma: A comparison of equally myelosuppressive regimens. J Natl Cancer Inst 81:1500–1504, 1989.

115. Gurney H, Crowther D, Anderson H, et al: Five-year follow-up and dose delivery analysis of cisplatin, iproplatin, or carboplatin in combination with cyclophosphamide in advanced ovarian carcinoma. Ann Oncol 1:427–433, 1990.

116. GICOG: Randomized comparison of cisplatin with cyclophosphamide/cisplatin and with cyclophosphamide/doxorubicin/cisplatin in advanced ovarian cancer. Lancet 2:353–359, 1989.

117. Omura GA, Bundy BN, Berek JS, et al: Randomized trial of cyclophosphamide plus cisplatin with or without doxorubicin in ovarian carcinoma: A GOG study. J Clin Oncol 7:457–465, 1989.

118. Bertelsen K, Jakobsen A, Andersen JE, et al: A randomized study of cyclophosphamide and cisplatinum with or without doxorubicin in advanced ovarian carcinoma. Gynecol Oncol 28:161–169, 1987.

119. Conte PF, Bruzzon M, Chiara S, et al: A randomized trial comparing cisplatin plus cyclophosphamide vs cisplatin, doxorubicin, and cyclophosphamide in advanced ovarian cancer. J Clin Oncol 4:965–971, 1986.

120. Ovarian Cancer Meta-Analysis Project: Cyclophosphamide +

cisplatin vs cyclophosphamide, doxorubicin, and cisplatin chemotherapy of ovarian carcinoma: A meta-analysis. J Clin Oncol 9:166–167, 1991.

121. Hakes TB, Cholas E, Hoskins WJ, et al: Randomized prospective trial of 5 vs 10 cycles of cyclophosphamide, doxorubicin, and cisplatin in advanced ovarian carcinoma. Gynecol Oncol 45:284–289, 1992.

122. Bertelsen IF, Jakobsen A, Hansen MK, et al: A randomized trial of six vs twelve cycles of cyclophosphamide, Adriamycin, in advanced ovarian cancer (abstract). Proc Am Soc Clin Oncol 8:15, 1989.

123. McGuire WP, Hoskins WJ, Brady MF, et al: A phase III trial of dose intense (DI) vs standard dose (DS) cisplatin and Cytoxan, in advanced ovarian cancer (abstract). Proc Am Soc Clin Oncol 11:718, 1992.

124. Kaye SB, Lewis CR, Paul J, et al: Randomized study of two doses of cisplatin with cyclophosphamide in epithelial ovarian cancer. Lancet 340:329–333, 1992.

125. Ngam HY, Choo YC, Cheung M, et al: A randomized trial of high dose vs low dose cisplatin combined with cyclophosphamide in the treatment of advanced ovarian cancer. Chemotherapy 35:221–227, 1989.

126. McGuire WP, Ravinsky EK, Rosenstein NB, et al: Taxol: A unique antineoplastic agent with significant activity in advanced ovarian epithelial neoplasms. Ann Intern Med 11:273–279, 1989.

127. Thigpen T, Blessing J, Ball H, et al: Phase II trial of Taxol as second-line therapy for ovarian carcinoma. Proc Am Soc Clin Oncol 9:604, 1990.

128. Einzig AI, Wiernik P, Sasloff J, et al: Phase II study and long-term follow-up of patients treated with Taxol for advanced ovarian adenocarcinoma. J Clin Oncol 10:1748–1753, 1992.

129. Trimble E, Adams J, Vena D, et al: Paclitaxel for platinum-refractory ovarian cancer: Results from the first 1,000 patients registered to National Cancer Institute Treatment Referral Center 9103. J Clin Oncol 11:2405–2410, 1993.

130. Eisenhauer E, ten Bokkel-Huinink W, Swenerton K, et al: Toxicity of Taxol: A European-Canadian trial of high- vs low-dose and short vs long infusion in ovarian cancer coordinated by the NCI Canada Clinical Trial group (NCIC CTG) (meeting abstract). Second National Cancer Institute Workshop on Taxol and Taxus. September 23-24, 1992, Alexandria, VA, National Cancer Institute.

131. McGuire WP: Paclitaxel in the treatment of ovarian cancer, in American Society of Clinical Oncology Educational Book, pp 204–213. 3014 Annual Meeting, Dallas Texas, 1994.

132. Sarosy G, Kohn E, Stowe A, et al: Phase I study of Taxol and granulocyte colony-stimulating factor in patients with refractory ovarian cancer. J Clin Oncol 10:1165–1170, 1992.

133. Kavanagh J, Kudelka A, Edwards C, et al: A randomized crossover trial of parenteral hydroxyurea vs high-dose Taxol in cisplatin/carboplatin-resistant epithelial ovarian cancer. Proc Am Soc Clin Oncol 13:259, 1993.

134. Kavanagh J, Kudelka A: Unpublished results updated survival data, October 1994.

135. Colombo N, Pitteli MR, Parma G, et al: Cisplatin dose intensity in advanced ovarian cancer: A randomized study of conventional dose vs dose-intense cisplatin monochemotherapy (abstract 806). Proc Am Soc Clin Oncol 12:255, 1993.

136. Calvert AH, Newell DR, Gumbrell LA, et al: Carboplatin dosage: Prospective evaluation of a simple formula based on renal function. J Clin Oncol 7:1748–1756, 1989.

137. McGuire WP, Hoskins WJ, Brady MF, et al: A phase III trial comparing cisplatin-Cytoxan and cisplatin-Taxol in advanced ovarian cancer. Proc Am Soc Clin Oncol 12:255, 1993.

138. Sarosy G, Kohn E, Link C, et al: Taxol dose intensification

(DI) in patients with recurrent ovarian cancer. Proc Am Soc Clin Oncol 11:716, 1992.

139. McGuire WP, Hoskins WJ, Brady MF, et al: A phase III trial comparing cisplatin/Cytoxin and cisplatin/Taxol in advanced ovarian cancer. Proc Am Soc Clin Oncol 12:55, 1993.

140. McGuire WP, Hoskins WJ, Brady MF, et al: Taxol and cisplatin (TP) improves outcome in advanced ovarian cancer (AOC) as compared to cytoxan and cisplatin (CP) (abstract 771). Proc Am Soc Clin Oncol 14:275, 1995.

141. McGuire W: International Gynecologic Cancer Society meeting, Philadelphia, September 1995.

142. Alberts DS, Liu PY, Hannigan EV, et al: Phase III study of intraperitoneal (IP) cisplatin (CDDP)/intravenous (IV) cyclosphosphamide (CPA) vs IV CDAP/IV CPA in patients with optimal disease stage III ovarian cancer: A SWOG-GOG-ECOG intergroup study (abstract 760). Proc Am Soc Clin Oncol 14:273, 1995.

143. Markman M, Richman B, Hakes T, et al: Response to second-line cisplatin-based intraperitoneal therapy in ovarian cancer: Influence of prior response to intravenous cisplatin. J Clin Oncol 9:1801–1805, 1991.

144. Markman M, Rowinsky E, Hakes T, et al: Phase I trial of intraperitoneal Taxol: A Gynecologic Oncology Group study. J Clin Oncol 10:1485–1491, 1992.

145. Hansen HH, Eisenhauer EA, Hansen M, et al: New cytostatic drugs in ovarian cancer. Ann Oncol 4(suppl 4):63–70, 1993.

146. Hoskins PJ, Swenerton KD: Oral etoposide is active against platinum resistant ovarian cancer. J Clin Oncol 12:60–63, 1994.

147. Kavanagh JJ, Tresukosol D, Gonzales DeLeon C, et al: Phase II study of prolonged oral etoposide in refractory ovarian cancer. Int J Gynecol Cancer 5:351–354, 1995.

148. Hauge MD, Long HJ, Hartmann LC, et al: Phase II trial of intravenous hexamethylmelamine in patients with advanced ovarian cancer. Invest New Drugs 10:299–301, 1992.

149. Lund B, Hausey OP, Theilade K, et al: Phase II study of gemcitabine 2,2'-difluorodeoxycytidine in previously treated ovarian cancer patients. J Natl Cancer Inst 86(20):1530–1533, 1994.

150. Chabner BA: Camptothecins. J Clin Oncol 10:3–4, 1992.

151. Burris HA, Rothenberg ML, Kuhn JG, et al: Clinical trials with the topoisomerase I inhibitors. Semin Oncol 19:663–669, 1992.

152. Slichenmyer WJ, Rowinsky EK, Donehower RC, et al: The current status of camptothecin analogues as antitumor agents. J Natl Cancer Inst 85:271–291, 1993.

153. Kudelka AP, Edwards CL, Freedman RS, et al: An open phase II study to evaluate the efficacy and toxicity of topotecan administered intravenously as 5 daily infusions every 21 days to women with advanced epithelial ovarian carcinoma (abstract). Proc Am Soc Clin Oncol 12:259, 1993.

154. Mori H, Itoh N, Kondoh H, et al: Treatment of recurrent gynecologic malignancies with a new camptothecin derivative. Eur J Cancer 28:613, 1993.

155. Takeuchi S, Takamizawa H, Takeda Y, et al: Clinical study of CPT-11, a camptothecin derivative, on gynecological malignancy (abstract). Proc Am Soc Clin Oncol 10:189, 1991.

156. Noda K, et al: Late phase II study of CPT-11: New camptothecin derivative, in cervical and ovarian carcinoma, p 271. Proceedings of the 13th World Congress of Gynecology and Obstetrics (FIGO) (abstract). 1991.

157. Takeuchi S, Dobashi K, Fujimoto S, et al: A late phase II study of CPT-11 on uterine cervical cancer and ovarian cancer. Jpn J Cancer Chemother 8:1681–1689, 1991.

158. Hakes T, Markway M, Reichman B, et al: Ifosfamide therapy of ovarian cancer previously treated with cisplatin and Cytoxan (abstract). Proc Am Soc Clin Oncol 10:185, 1991.

159. Kavanagh JJ, Roberts W, Townsend P, et al: Leuprolide

acetate in the treatment of refractory or persistent epithelial ovarian cancer. J Clin Oncol 7:115–118, 1989.

160. Ahlgren JD, Ellison NM, Gottlieb RJ, et al: Hormonal palliation of chemoresistant ovarian cancer: Three consecutive phase II trials of the Mid-Atlantic Oncology Program. J Clin Oncol 11:1957–1968, 1993.

161. Sevelda P, et al: Goserelin alpha GnRH analogue as third-line therapy of refractory ovarian cancer. Int J Gynecol Cancer 2:160–162, 1992.

162. Bertlesen K, Jacobsen A: Radiotherapy for gynecologic cancers. Curr Opin Oncol 5:885–894, 1993.

163. Smith JP, Rutledge FN, Delclos L, et al: Postoperative treatment of early cancer of the ovary: A random trial between postoperative irradiation and chemotherapy. J Natl Cancer Inst 42:149–153, 1975.

164. Soper JT, Berchuck A, Dopdge R, et al: Adjuvant therapy with intraperitoneal chronic phosphate (P-32) in women with early ovarian carcinoma after comprehensive surgical staging. Obstet Gynecol 79:993–997, 1992.

165. Spanos WJ, Day T, Abner A, et al: Complications in the use of intra-abdominal P-32 for ovarian carcinoma. Gynecol Oncol 45:243–247, 1992.

166. Vergotte IB, DeVos LN, Abeler VM, et al: Randomized trial comparing cisplatin with radioactive phosphorus or whole-abdomen irradiation as adjuvant treatment of ovarian cancer. Cancer 63:741–749, 1992.

167. Hoskins PJ, O'Reilly SE, Swenerton KD, et al: 10 year outcome of patients with advanced epithelial ovarian carcinoma treated with cisplatin-based multimodality therapy. J Clin Oncol 10:1561–1568, 1992.

168. Whelan TJ, Dembo AJ, Bush RS, et al: Complications of whole abdominal and pelvic radiotherapy following chemotherapy for advanced ovarian cancer. Int J Radiat Oncol Biol Phys 22:853–858, 1992.

169. Blackledge G, Lawton R, Redman C, et al: Response of patients in phase II studies of chemotherapy in ovarian cancer: Implications for patient treatment and the design of phase II trials. Br J Cancer 59:650–653, 1989.

170. Cure H, Legros M, Fleury J, et al: High-dose chemotherapy and autologous bone marrow transplantation in advanced epithelial ovarian cancer. Bone Marrow Transplant 10(suppl 2):50, 1992.

171. Menichella G, Pierelli L, Foddai ML, et al : Autologous blood stem cell harvesting and transplantation in patients with advanced ovarian cancer. Br J Haematol 79:444–450, 1991.

172. Herrmann F, Brugger W, Kanz L, et al : In vivo biology and therapeutic potential of hematopoietic growth factors and circulating progenitor cells. Semin Oncol 19:422–431, 1992.

173. Korbling M, Juttner C, Henon P, et al: Autologous blood stem cell vs bone marrow transplant. Bone Marrow Transplant 10(suppl 10):144–148, 1992.

174. Shea TC, Mason JR, Storniolo AM, et al: Sequential cycles of high dose carboplatin administered with recombinant human granulocyte-macrophage colony-stimulating factor and repeated infusions of autologous peripheral blood progenitor cells: A novel and effective method for delivering multiple courses of dose-intensive therapy. J Clin Oncol 10:464–473, 1992.

175. Sypall EJ, Stemmer SM, Bearman SI, et al: High dose chemotherapy with ABMT support for the treatment of epithelial ovarian carcinoma, in Markman M, Hoskins WJ, (eds): Cancer of the Ovary, pp 327–338. Raven Press, New York, 1993.

176. Schilder RJ: High dose chemotherapy with autologous haematopoietic cell support in gynecologic malignancies. Principles Practice Gynecol Oncol Updates 1(3):1–14, 1993.

177. Shea TC, Flaherty M, Elias A, et al: A phase I clinical and pharmacokinetic study of carboplatin and ABMT. J Clin Oncol 7:651–661, 1989.

178. Shpall EJ, Pearson-Clarke D, Soper JT, et al: High dose alkylating agent chemotherapy with ABMT in patients with stage III/IV epithelial ovarian cancer. Gynecol Oncol 38:386–391, 1990.

179. McKenzie RS, Alberts DA, Bishop MR, et al: Phase I trial of high-dose cyclophosphamide (CY), mitoxantrone (Mx), and carboplatin (CB) with ABMT in female malignancies: Pharmacologic levels of mitoxantrone and high response rate in refractory ovarian carcinoma (abstract). Proc Am Soc Clin Oncol 10:186, 1991.

180. Viens P, Maraniuch D: High dose chemotherapy and ABMT for common epithelial ovarian cancer, in Armitage JO, Autman KH, (eds): High Dose Cancer Therapy: Pharmacology Hematopoietins Stem Cells, pp 729–734. Baltimore, MD, Williams and Wilkins, 1992.

181. Viens P, Maraniuch D, Legros M, et al: High dose melphalan and autologous marrow rescue in advanced epithelial ovarian carcinomas: A retrospective analysis of 35 patients treated in France. Bone Marrow Transplant 5:227–233, 1990.

182. Dauplat J, Legros M, Condat P, et al: High-dose melphalan and autologous bone marrow support for treatment of ovarian cancer with positive second-look operation. Gynecol Oncol 34:294–298, 1989.

183. Legros M, Fleury J, Cure H, et al: High dose chemotherapy and ABMT in 31 advanced ovarian cancers: Long-term results (abstract). Proc Am Soc Clin Oncol 11:222, 1992.

184. Berek J, Hacker NF, Lechtenstein A, et al: Intraperitoneal recombinant α–interferon for "salvage" immunotherapy in stage III epithelial ovarian cancer: A Gynecologic Oncology Group study. Cancer Res 45:4447–4453, 1985.

185. Willemse PHB, Devries EGE, Mulder NH, et al: Intraperitoneal human recombinant interferon alpha-2 in minimal residual ovarian cancer. Eur J Cancer 26:353, 1990.

186. Pujade-Lauraine E, Guastella JP, Colombo N: Intraperitoneal recombinant human interferon gamma (IFN-G) in residual ovarian cancer: Efficacy is independent of previous response to chemotherapy. Proc Am Soc Clin Oncol 2:225, 1992.

187. Rubin SC: Monoclonal antibodies in the management of ovarian cancer. Cancer 71(4 suppl):1602–1612, 1993.

188. Wessels BW, Rogus RD: Radionuclide selection and model absorbed dose calculations for radiolabeled tumor-associated antibodies. Med Phys 11:638–645, 1984.

189. Kavanagh JJ, Kudelka AP, Freedman R, et al: The amelioration of toxicity of intraperitoneal monoclonal Ab 90Y-B72.3 with EDTA: A phase I study in refractory ovarian cancer (abstract 1332). Proc Am Assoc Cancer Res 34:223, 1993.

190. Buckman R, DeAugelis C, Shan P, et al: Intraperitoneal therapy of malignant ascites associated with carcinoma of ovary and breast using radioiodined monoclonal Ab 2G3. Gynecol Oncol 47:102–109, 1992.

191. Stewart JS, Hird V, Snook D, et al: Intraperitoneal yttrium-90 labeled monoclonal antibody in ovarian cancer. J Clin Oncol 8:1941–1950, 1990.

192. Fitzgerald DJ, Bjorn MJ, Ferris J: Antitumor activity of an immunotoxin in a nude mouse model of human ovarian cancer. Cancer Res 47:1407–1410, 1987.

193. Freedman RS, Edwards CL, Kavanagh JJ, et al: Intraperitoneal adoptive immunotherapy of epithelial ovarian cancer with recombinant interleukin-2 expanded tumor infiltrating lymphocytes plus low-dose rIL-2. Proc Am Soc Clin Oncol 12:263, 1993.

194. Hanania E, Deisseroth A: Serial transplantation shows that early hematopoietic precursor cells are transduced by MDR-1 retroviral vector in a mouse gene therapy model: Cancer Gene Therapy 1:21–25, 1994.

CHAPTER 23

Gestational Trophoblastic Tumors

Ray D. Page, DO, PhD, Andrzej P. Kudelka, MD,
Ralph S. Freedman, MD, PhD, *and* John J. Kavanagh, MD
Section of Gynecologic Medical Oncology and Gynecologic Oncology
The University of Texas M. D. Anderson Cancer Center, Houston, Texas

Gestational trophoblastic tumors (GTTs) encompass a spectrum of neoplastic disorders that arise from placental trophoblastic tissue after abnormal fertilization. GTTs are classified histologically into four distinct groups: hydatidiform mole (complete and partial), chorioadenoma destruens (invasive mole), choriocarcinoma, and placental site tumor.[1,2] Most commonly, GTT results in a hydatidiform "molar" pregnancy characterized by the lack of a fetus, trophoblastic hyperplasia, edematous chorionic villi, and a loss of normal villous blood vessels.[3,4]

Most molar pregnancies spontaneously resolve after uterine evacuation with no further sequelae. However, at any time during or after gestation, malignant transformation may occur in approximately 10% to 20% of molar pregnancies. Nearly two thirds of these cases have an invasive mole confined to the uterus (chorioadenoma destruens), and in one third, choriocarcinoma characterized by distant metastatic spread develops.[5,6] Placental site tumors are rare neoplasms derived from intermediate trophoblast cells of the placenta, which are identified by cellular secretion of placental lactogen and small amounts of beta-human chorionic gonadotropin (hCG).[7]

In the United States, GTTs are uncommon and account for less than 1% of gynecologic malignancies; however, knowledge of the natural history and management of GTTs is important because of this tumor's potential for cure with appropriate therapy. More than 40 years ago, women with choriocarcinoma had a 95% mortality rate. Today, with the advent of effective chemotherapy and the development of a reliable tumor marker (beta-hCG), a cure rate of 90% to 95% is observed for choriocarcinoma.

Current studies continue to characterize GTT, and in recent years, much has been elucidated about the pathology, molecular biology, diagnosis, and treatment of this malignancy.

EPIDEMIOLOGY AND ETIOLOGY

In the United States, a hydatidiform mole develops in approximately 1 in 1,000 to 2,000 pregnancies.[8,9] Molar pregnancies are reported in approximately 3,000 patients per year, and malignant transformation occurs in 6% to 19% of these cases.[5,10] Complete molar pregnancies occur in 1 in 40 molar pregnancies, 1 in 15,000 abortions, and 1 in 150,000 normal pregnancies.[11] Overall, approximately 80% of cases of GTTs, are hydatidiform moles, 15% are chorioadenoma destruens, and 5% are choriocarcinomas. Choriocarcinoma is associated with an antecedent mole in 50% of cases, a history of abortion in 25%, term delivery in 20%, and ectopic pregnancy in 5%.

True estimates of the incidence of molar pregnancies are difficult to obtain because of considerable worldwide variation in the presentation and management of both normal and abnormal pregnancies. Early evaluations suggest a 5- to 15-fold greater incidence in the Far East and Southeast Asian countries than in the United States, with as many as 1 in 120 pregnancies in Taiwan being molar.[12] More recent studies show that in most parts of the world, the incidence of hydatidiform mole is approximately 1 in 1,000, whereas Japan and Vietnam report an incidence as high as 1 in 500.[13]

Ethnic and racial differences also may contribute to the variable incidence of GTTs. In one study, African-American women in the United States were estimated to have a higher GTT incidence than white women,[14] but the findings of another study did not support this estimation.[15] Native Alaskans were found to have an incidence rate three- or fourfold that of white women.[16] A Hawaiian study demonstrated a lower GTT rate in white and native Hawaiians than in Filipino and Japanese populations.[17] In the United Arab Emirates, women born in the Persian Gulf region had a higher GTT incidence than that of women of Arab and Asian origin.[18] Other investigators, however, have found racial differences to play a minor role in GTT. The observation that Malaysian, Indian, and Chinese populations within Kuala Lumpur have similar incidences of molar disease implies a lesser role for cultural or racial differences in the etiology of GTT.[19]

Although the etiology of GTT is not well understood, the occurrence of this tumor has been associated with several factors: extremes of reproductive age (younger than 20 and older than 40 years), prior molar pregnancy, lower socioeconomic class, and particular ABO blood groups. Women older than age 40 have as much as a fivefold increased risk of molar pregnancy.[15,20] In Singapore, the incidence of molar pregnancy in women older than 45 years was found to be 1 in 72 pregnancies.[21] In general, for women younger than age 20, a relative risk of 1.5- to 2-fold has been reported.[15,20,22] Younger patients have an improved prognosis, with a long-term disease-free survival rate of 85.4%, compared with 77.8% for women older than age 40. Paternal age does not confer an increased risk of molar pregnancy.[17]

A history of a previous hydatidiform mole is an established risk factor for GTT. Women with a previous molar pregnancy have up to a 10 times greater risk of developing a second molar pregnancy.[20] Furthermore, women who have had a prior molar pregnancy have at least a 1,000-fold increased risk of choriocarcinoma, compared with women who have had a normal pregnancy. The New England Trophoblastic Disease Center demonstrated the increased risk of subsequent molar pregnancy to be 1%. Thus, a normal future reproductive outcome generally can be anticipated after such a pregnancy.[23] Nevertheless, these women should be closely monitored with a first-trimester ultrasound, pathology review of the placenta, and beta-hCG measurements 6 weeks postpartum.

Lower socioeconomic status has been associated with a greater frequency of GTT. In the Philippines, women of lower socioeconomic standing have a rate of molar disease 10 times higher than that of affluent populations.[24] Likewise, Bertini reported a higher incidence of GTT among Israeli women of poorer Middle Eastern and African heritage than that in women of European descent.[25] Moreover, as the standard of living improved for Israeli women of Middle Eastern origin, the incidence of GTT declined. In the Western Hemisphere, the rate of molar pregnancy is 10 times higher in Mexicans than in other North Americans.

The relationship of GTT incidence to different geographic regions, cultures, and socioeconomic statuses suggests that diet and nutrition may contribute to the etiology of this disease. The results of most studies addressing deficiencies in animal protein, animal fat, and beta-carotene have been equivocal.

Parazinni and colleagues reported that low beta-carotene consumption was associated with GTT.[26] Further studies are needed to delineate the dietary contributions to this disease. Cigarette smoking has no strong association with GTT.[27]

The ABO blood groups of parents appear to be related to the development of choriocarcinoma. There is a particular risk for women in blood group A who are married to men in blood group O.[28] Thus far, human lymphocyte antigen (HLA) studies have been inconclusive in clarifying the significant association of the ABO blood group with GTT.

PATHOGENESIS AND CELL BIOLOGY

Normal fertilization results from the union of a single sperm and egg, which is followed by rapid cell division and the creation of an embryo. Early embryonic differentiation gives rise to trophoblasts, specialized epithelial cells responsible for connecting the embryo to the uterus and for developing the placenta and villi. This is a remarkable event involving activated transcription factors, cytokines, hormone secretion, cell-adhesion molecules, and immunologic activity.[29] The ability of normal trophoblasts to invade the endometrium is strikingly similar to the invasive behavior of cancer. However, in GTT, uncontrolled growth and invasion of trophoblasts occurs and is a result of chromosomal abnormalities and altered cell biology.

GTTs arise from the abnormal union of sperm and egg. This often occurs when a normal sperm fertilizes an ovum in which the female genetic material is extruded, followed by the duplication of paternal chromosomes and nondivision at the first blastomere mitosis, or alternatively, the sperm is diploid due to the absence of the second meiotic division, resulting in a totally chromosomal paternal zygote. This event results in abnormalities of the trophoblast[30] and probably in early embryo death.[31] This aberrant fertilization creates specific genetic abnormalities and results in distinct pathologic characteristics. Based on these morphologic and cytogenetic features, Szulman and Surti divided hydatidiform moles into two unique syndromes: complete (classic) and partial (Table 1).[3,4]

In addition, the roles of proto-oncogenes, tumor-suppressor genes, cytokines, and growth factors also are contributing to our understanding of GTT and tumor progression.

Pathology

Hydatidiform moles, invasive moles, and choriocarcinomas have distinct morphologic features. Moles are described as partial or complete (classic) based on their morphologic, karyotypic, and clinical features.[3,4] Complete moles are distinguished by the complete absence of normal villi and by chromosomal material that is virtually always of paternal origin. Partial moles are characterized grossly by an admixture of normal and hydropic villi, a triploid karyotype, and the presence of both maternal and paternal chromosomal material.

Complete moles usually are detected during the second trimester and are identified by total hydatidiform enlargement of the villi, which are enveloped by hyper-

TABLE I

Characteristics of Complete and Partial Moles

Feature	Complete	Partial
Villous edema	Diffuse	Focal
Trophoblastic hyperplasia	Diffuse	Focal
Embryonic tissue	None	Present
Persistent HCG	20%	0.5%
Karyotype	46XX (90%)	69XXY (90%)
Genetic parentage	Paternal	Biparental

plastic and atypical trophoblasts.[32] There is a notable absence of any embryonic or amniotic remnant. More than 90% of classic moles demonstrate a 46XX karyotype, which has been demonstrated to be of paternal origin by fluorescent banding polymorphic analysis.[33] Approximately 20% of complete moles give rise to persistent trophoblastic disease.[34]

Partial moles, in contrast, are more commonly accompanied by an identifiable embryo or amniotic membranes. These moles are described as partial because the hydatidiform changes in the villi tend to be focal. The hydropic villi usually are irregularly scalloped and have stromal hyperplastic inclusions.[4] The villous capillaries appear to be functional, because they possess the same proportion of nucleated fetal erythrocytes as are found in the embryo. In partial moles, hydatidiform change occurs at a slower rate, and the proportion of relatively normal villi appears to correlate with the fetal survival rate. Maturation of mesenchymal elements is only minimally delayed, and there is a paucity of fibroblast karyorrhexis. Partial moles are usually aneuploid and most often exhibit an XXY karyotype, which is thought to be secondary to dispermic fertilization of the ovum with retention of the maternal genome. Approximately 2% of partial moles undergo malignant degeneration. Because of this sporadic malignant potential, follow-up and treatment of patients with partial moles are the same as for patients with complete moles.

Locally invasive moles have the same histologic features as complete moles and, in addition, are characterized by myometrial invasion without involvement of intervening endometrial stroma.[35] Invasive moles are typically diagnosed approximately 6 months after molar evacuation. They tend to invade locally, causing hemorrhage and necrosis. Rarely, uterine perforation results. Hematogenous metastasis may occur, often to the lungs.

Occasionally, metastatic deposits display hydropic villi, rather than the sheets of anaplastic cells that typify metastatic choriocarcinoma.

Choriocarcinomas have a unique histology that is distinct from that of the moles.[11] The tumor is grossly red and granular and exhibits extensive necrosis and hemorrhage. Microscopically, the neoplasm is composed of a disordered array of syncytiotrophoblastic and cytotrophoblastic elements, frequent mitoses, and multinucleated giant cells. Vascular invasion occurs early, with resultant metastases to the lungs, vagina, brain, kidneys, liver, and gastrointestinal tract.

Placental site tumors are rare. They are derived from intermediate trophoblast cells of the placenta, which are identified by the secretion of placental lactogen and small amounts of beta-hCG.[36] Occasionally, after a complete hydatidiform mole is removed, an unusual complication develops, characterized by a proliferation of intermediate trophoblast-forming nodules in the endometrium and myometrium.[37] There are usually numerous nodules, which appear microscopically as cells with oval nuclei, and an abundant eosinophilic cytoplasm. No chorionic villi are seen. These tumors usually present as nodules confined to the endometrium and myometrium, produce a mild elevation in the hCG titer, do not respond well to chemotherapy, and may progress. In such instances, the lesions should be located and surgically removed to avoid unnecessary and ineffective chemotherapy.

Cytogenetics

Pathologic characteristics alone generally do not allow adequate discrimination of molar pregnancies. With the advent of cytogenetic techniques, such as chromosomal banding and restriction fragment-length polymorphism analysis of DNA, unique chromosomal patterns of molar pregnancies were discovered,[33,38] allowing a recognizable distinction between complete and partial moles.[3,39]

Using chromosomal banding, Kajii and Ohama first reported that complete moles contained only paternal chromosomes.[33] Yamashita and colleagues confirmed this finding by showing that when paternal heterozygotes for the HLA locus give rise to a mole, the HLA expression of the molar tissue is homozygous.[40] Approximately 85% to 92% of complete moles have a 46XX karyotype,[33,41] which results from fertilization of an egg by a haploid sperm (23X) that undergoes duplication to create a diploid set of chromosomes. Why the loss of maternal DNA takes place is uncertain; it may involve extrusion of maternal chromosomes or fertilization of an empty egg. Regardless of the mechanism, the finding of maternal mitochondrial DNA suggests that moles result from an abnormal fertilization event.[42]

Approximately 4% to 15% of complete moles have a 46XY karyotype,[43,44] which results from dispermy, in which two spermatozoa (23X and 23Y) fertilize an empty ovum. There is no strong evidence that dispermic or Y chromosome-containing moles have greater malignant potential than the monospermic 46XX karyotype.[45] Fisher and colleagues also found that nearly 5% of complete moles are heterozygous 46XX.[44] A 46YY mole has not been reported because the X chromosome is probably required for survival.

The typical partial mole has a triploid karyotype (69 chromosomes), and both paternal and maternal chromosomes are present.[3] The most common sex chromosome arrangement is XXY. The triploid genotype can result in two phenotypes. If the extra haploid chromosome is of paternal origin, a partial mole arises; if it is of maternal origin, a fetus develops.[46]

Growth Factors and Oncogenes

The excess of paternal chromosomes in moles probably contributes to the induction of trophoblastic hyperplasia. The genomic imbalance may cause changes in the gene expression of growth factors located on the paternal allele.[47] An insulin-like growth factor (IGF2) specifically located on the paternal allele may be inappropriately expressed in molar pregnancies, thus stimulating uncontrolled growth.

Both normal placentas and molar pregnancies contain paternal antigens; therefore, upon implantation, an immunologic response is initiated with infiltration of lymphocytes and macrophages and secretion of cytokines.[29] The growth of choriocarcinoma may be related to the abundant expression of epidermal growth factor (EGF) receptor. Macrophage-derived cytokines—interleukin (IL-1-alpha, IL-1-beta), and tumor necrosis factor—can suppress cell growth and increase EGF receptor expression in choriocarcinoma cell lines, thus acting as paracrine mediators of cell growth.[48]

The contribution of several oncogenes to the malignant transformation of GTT also has been examined. Growth regulation in the trophoblast recently has been found to be associated with expression of the transcription factor Mash-2.[49] Cheung et al have demonstrated increased expression of c-fms RNA in complete moles compared with that in normal placentas.[50] In choriocarcinoma, increased expression of c-myc and ras RNA has been observed.[51] At present, the significance of these findings is uncertain. Because trophoblasts are, by nature, rapidly dividing and invasive, increased expression of these oncogenes may be essential for normal cell function. Further studies are needed to elucidate these findings. Recently, expression of the c-erb B-2 oncogene product in persistent GTT was examined and found to have no significant contribution.[52] Thus far, no gene mutations or rearrangements in GTT have been reported.

Progression of some tumors has been associated with the inactivation of tumor suppressor genes. The inactivation of p53 by mutation of the p53 gene has been observed in nearly 50% of patients with ovarian cancer.[53] Expression of p53 in hydatidiform moles has recently been studied.[54] Expression of p53 in moles was observed to be increased over that in normal trophoblasts. No p53 mutations were found. Persaud and colleagues further noted an overaccumulation of p53 protein in 50% of choriocarcinomas and 78% of hydatidiform moles but none in partial mole and normal placenta.[55] Increased p53 expression may thus be an attempt to abrogate excessive trophoblastic proliferation in hydatidiform moles.

CLINICAL PRESENTATION

Several clinical features typify hydatidiform moles and metastatic trophoblastic disease.

Complete Mole

The classic signs of a molar pregnancy include the absence of fetal heart sounds, physical evidence of a uterus that is larger than expected for gestational age, and vaginal bleeding. Although an intact fetus may coexist with a partial mole, this occurs in fewer than 1 in 100,000 pregnancies.

The most common presenting symptom of molar pregnancy is vaginal bleeding, reported in up to 97% of patients.[56] Intrauterine clots may undergo oxidation and liquefaction, producing pathognomonic prune juice-like fluid. Rarely, spontaneous expulsion of grape-like villi will provide the diagnosis of hydatidiform mole. Prolonged or recurrent bleeding may result in iron-deficiency anemia. Symptoms of anemia occur in approximately 50% of patients at the time of diagnosis.

Abdominal pain may result from excessive uterine enlargement or prominent theca luteal cysts. An abdominopelvic examination may reveal a uterus larger than expected for the gestational date and with an irregular contour. Ovarian masses resulting from theca-luteal cysts may be palpable. Theca-luteal cysts, caused by hCG-induced hyperstimulation of both ovaries in about 50% of patients, may result in pelvic pressure or fullness. Usually, these cysts regress spontaneously after uterine evacuation; however, their rupture or tension can cause acute abdominal symptoms occasionally requiring surgery.

Early toxemia (hypertension, proteinuria, and edema) presenting during the first or second trimester is not uncommon in molar pregnancy. Toxemia, which was observed in 27% of patients at the New England Trophoblastic Disease Center,[23] is thought to be precipitated by the release of large amounts of vasoactive substances from necrotic trophoblastic tissue. Very rarely, eclamptic convulsions may occur in this setting.

Hyperemesis gravidarum—protracted nausea and vomiting during pregnancy—is observed in approximately 10% of women with GTT. The mechanism is not well understood.

Hyperthyroidism is seen in approximately 7% of molar pregnancies. An elevation of triiodothyronine (T3) and thyroxine (T4) levels is observed more commonly than are the clinical manifestations of tachycardia, sweating, weight loss, and tremor. These hormonal elevations are presumed to be secondary to the structural similarity of hCG to thyroid-stimulating hormone (TSH); thus, markedly elevated hCG levels intrinsically stimulate thyroid activity.[57] However, the findings surrounding the correlation of thyroid function to hCG level are conflicting and suggest that other substances elaborated from GTT are responsible for the hyperthyroidism.[58] Rarely, patients may develop thyroid storm, which may be precipitated by surgical stress during molar evacuation. In such cases, the administration of beta-adrenergic blockers is prudent.

Because placental tissues are rich in thromboplastin-like substances, the extrinsic coagulation pathway is occasionally activated, resulting in the consumption of platelets and clotting factors. In rare instances, frank disseminated intravascular coagulation and microangiopathic hemolytic anemia may develop; these life-threatening emergencies usually resolve with molar evacuation.

Partial Mole

Patients with partial mole do not have the same clinical features as those with complete mole; fewer than 10% of patients with the former have uterine enlargement. Goldstein and Berkowitz reviewed the cases of 81 patients with partial mole and found that none had prominent theca-luteal cysts, hyperthyroidism, or respiratory insufficiency and only 1 had toxemia.[59] The diagnosis of partial mole was usually made after histologic review of curettage specimens.

Metastatic Trophoblastic Disease

Metastatic GTT is reported in 6% to 19% of patients after molar evacuation.[5,10] Metastases sometimes have an identical histology to that of molar disease, but the vast majority are choriocarcinomas. Metastatic spread is hematogenous. Because of its extensive vascular network, metastatic GTT often produces local, spontaneous bleeding. Berkowitz et al at the New England Trophoblastic Disease Center (NETDC) reported that the common metastatic sites of GTT are the lungs (80%); vagina (30%); pelvis (20%); liver (10%); brain (10%); and bowel, kidneys, and spleen (5% each).[23]

Pulmonary metastases are quite common (80% of patients with metastatic disease)[56] and occur when trophoblastic tissue enters the circulation via uterine venous sinuses. Most often this happens spontaneously, but it also may occur after molar evacuation. Because choriocarcinoma is a vascular tumor, hemoptysis is a frequent symptom of lung involvement. Other symptoms include chest pain, dyspnea, and cough. Pulmonary hypertension also may develop. In some cases, an asymptomatic lesion on a chest x-ray or computed tomographic (CT) scan may be the only sign of pulmonary involvement.[60] The radiologic features may be protean or subtle and include alveolar, nodular, and miliary patterns.[61] Pleural effusions may also be present. Pulmonary metastases can be extensive and can cause respiratory failure and death.

Right upper-quadrant pain has been observed when hepatic metastases stretch Glisson's capsule. Gastrointestinal lesions may result in severe hemorrhage or in perforation with peritonitis, both of which require emergency intervention. Vaginal examination may reveal bluish metastatic deposits; these and other metastatic sites should not undergo biopsy because severe uncontrolled bleeding may occur.

Central nervous system (CNS) involvement from metastatic GTT suggests widespread disease and has a poor prognosis. CNS metastases are clinically evident in 7% to 28% of patients with metastatic choriocarcinoma.[22,30,56,62] Bakri and colleagues reported a 17% incidence of patients with GTT metastatic to the brain.[63] These patients had presenting neurologic symptoms of headache, hemiparesis, vomiting, dizziness, coma, grand mal seizure, visual disturbances, aphasia, and slurred speech. Some patients had multiple neurologic complaints, and a few were asymptomatic. All patients had concurrent pulmonary metastases. Cerebral metastases tend to respond favorably to both radiotherapy and chemotherapy.

DIAGNOSTIC STUDIES

Although the clinical presentation may suggest a diagnosis of GTT, certain laboratory studies, particularly a determination of the patient's beta-hCG level, and radiographic studies are needed to confirm this diagnosis.

Laboratory Studies

The blood count will usually reveal anemia of mixed morphologic characteristics. If disseminated intravascular coagulation is present, thrombocytopenia, prolonged clotting times, and consumption of coagulation factors may be observed. Uncommonly, blood chemistry studies may reveal hepatic or renal abnormalities.

Thyroid function studies should be performed in all patients with a clinical history or physical examination suggestive of hyperthyroidism. Abnormal thyroid function, manifested as an elevated T4 level, is not uncommon in GTT. Metastatic deposits in the kidneys or gastro-intestinal tract may reveal themselves by hematuria or hematochezia.

Tumor Markers: A well-characterized glycoprotein hormone secreted by the syncytiotrophoblast, hCG is essential to maintaining normal function of the corpus luteum during pregnancy.[64] This hormone has an alpha-subunit identical to the alpha-subunit of the pituitary hormones and a beta-subunit (beta-hCG) that confers the hormone's unique biologic activity. The presence of hCG appears approximately 8 days after ovulation, and its concentration doubles every 2 to 4 days, until it peaks at 10 to 12 weeks of gestation; thereafter, beta-hCG levels decline steadily. Because all trophoblastic tumors secrete beta-hCG, this hormone serves as an excellent marker for tumor activity in the nonpregnant patient.[65–67] The beta-hCG level will always be elevated in a molar pregnancy and, therefore, should be measured in all suspected cases.

CA-125 may also have a role as a marker for GTT. In patients with complete hydatidiform mole, the CA-125 level was elevated; more significant was the association of the degree of CA-125 elevation with the development of persistent GTT.[68]

Serial beta-hCG levels should be monitored during therapy to ensure adequate treatment. The level of beta-hCG is roughly proportional to the tumor burden and inversely proportional to therapeutic outcome. The approximately 10% to 20% of patients with hydatidiform mole who are not cured by local therapy or do not achieve a spontaneous remission can be identified by a rising or plateauing beta-hCG titer on serial determinations after the evacuation of a mole. These patients are considered to have persistent trophoblastic disease and require additional therapy.

Special Test: The ratio of beta-hCG in serum to beta-hCG in the cerebral spinal fluid (CSF) may contribute to the detection of brain metastases in GTT. A serum:CSF beta-hCG ratio of less than 60:1 is considered a positive predictor for brain metastases. Athanassiou et al com-

pared brain CT scans with serum:CSF beta-hCG ratios for the detection of intracranial metastatic disease.[69] Of 19 patients who underwent CT and measurement of serum:CSF beta-hCG ratios, 11 patients had positive brain CT scans and positive serum:CSF beta-hCG ratios, 7 had disease demonstrated by CT scan alone, and 1 patient had a positive ratio but a negative CT scan. No patient with both a negative CT scan and a negative ratio was found to have metastases on an isotope scan. Bagshawe and Harland reported similar results, with 29 of 33 patients who had CT-documented GTT brain involvement also having a positive serum:CSF beta-hCG ratio.[70]

Radiologic Studies

Because 70% to 80% of patients with metastatic GTT have lung involvement, a chest x-ray should always be performed.[56,71] Although this x-ray usually demonstrates nodular metastases, the patterns of metastatic disease can range from atelectatic areas to subtle pleural abnormalities. A CT scan often is helpful in evaluating these nonspecific areas.

Because it has been demonstrated that 97% to 100% of patients with CNS disease from choriocarcinoma have concomitant pulmonary metastases, a CNS workup in asymptomatic patients with normal chest x-rays is not routinely warranted.[69] If the chest x-ray is abnormal, or if beta-hCG levels plateau or rise during treatment, a more thorough evaluation for metastatic disease is indicated. CT scans of the brain, abdomen, and pelvis should be performed to evaluate other likely sites of metastatic spread.

Historically, angiography and amniography were important procedures used in the diagnosis of intrauterine molar disease, but today, ultrasonography is the preferred diagnostic modality. Ultrasonography is a reliable, safe, economical, and relatively simple method for confirming the diagnosis of GTT. It is also useful in identifying embryonic remnants. More recently, transvaginal color-flow Doppler ultrasonography has become increasingly useful in the diagnosis and assessment of GTT.[72]

Magnetic resonance imaging (MRI) may be useful in equivocal cases, particularly for evaluating the cerebellum and brain stem. MRI may replace CT because of the former's superior imaging characteristics of vascular metastases and improved definition of the brain stem and cerebellum, which are sites of occult metastases. The presence of intrauterine or ovarian disease also may be detected by MRI of the pelvis.

STAGING

Staging systems attempt to define prognostic groups that can direct a rational therapeutic strategy. Such crite-

TABLE 2

WHO Prognostic Scoring for Gestational Trophoblastic Disease

Prognostic factor	Score[a] 0	1	2	4
Age (yr)	≤ 39	> 39		
Antecedent pregnancy	Hydatidiform mole	Abortion	Term	
Interval (mo)[b]	< 4	4–6	7–12	> 12
hCG (IU/L)	< 10³	10³–10⁴	10⁴–10⁵	> 10⁵
ABO groups (female × male)		O × A or A × O	B or AB	
Largest tumor	< 3 cm	3–5 cm	> 5 cm	
Site(s) of metastases	Lung	Spleen, kidney	GI tract, liver	Brain
Number of metastases		1–3	4–8	> 8
Prior chemotherapy			One drug	Two or more drugs

[a] The total score for a patient is obtained by adding the individual scores for each prognostic factor: 4 = low risk; 5–7 = intermediate risk; > 7 = high risk.

[b] Time between end of antecedent pregnancy and start of chemotherapy

Adapted, with permission, from Sugarman SM, Kavanagh JJ: Gestational trophoblastic tumors, in Pazdur R (ed): Medical Oncology: A Comprehensive Review. Huntington, NY, PRR Inc, 1993.

ria depend on the tumor duration, volume, and location as well as on essential patient characteristics. Although several staging systems have been proposed, there is currently no uniform system for staging metastatic GTT. The World Health Organization (WHO) and the International Federation of Gynecology and Obstetrics (FIGO) have devised commonly used staging classifications.[1,2]

The FIGO staging system is a straightforward system based on anatomic criteria. In GTT, stage-0 tumor is a molar pregnancy limited to the uterine cavity; stage-I tumor is confined to the uterine body; and stage-II tumor includes local metastases to the pelvis and vagina. Stage-III tumor involves pulmonary metastases, whereas stage-IV tumor consists of distant metastatic disease. The WHO classification scheme (Table 2) is based on a scoring system to identify patients at high risk for treatment failure. With the WHO scoring system, patients are classified as being at low, middle, or high risk for treatment failure. A total score of up to 4 is considered low risk, 5 to 7 middle risk, and 8 or greater high risk.

Several factors have been associated with a poor prognosis.[1,22] One important predictor of poor outcome is

a large tumor volume at the time of diagnosis, manifesting as a high serum beta-hCG level (greater than 100,000 mIU/mL) or as bulky disease (mass greater than 5 cm in diameter). The number of metastatic sites is inversely related to prognosis. Patients with metastatic sites in the brain and liver have a worse outcome than patients with metastases to other sites. Women are at greater risk if the disease persists longer than 4 months after the antecedent pregnancy. Previous failure of chemotherapy, age older than 39 years, and maternal/paternal blood type also define a poor outcome.

TREATMENT

Although the treatment strategy for GTT must be individualized for each patient, Figure 1 summarizes the general diagnostic and therapeutic approach used at The University of Texas M. D. Anderson Cancer Center.[73] The stratification of risk groups enables physicians to direct an appropriate treatment strategy. Low-risk disease responds readily to single-agent chemotherapy and is virtually 100% curable. High-risk disease is not likely to be cured with single-agent therapy and therefore requires multidrug regimens.

Molar Pregnancy

For patients with complete or partial hydatidiform mole, evacuation of the mole by suction and sharp curettage should be performed.[74] Oxytocics also are given to produce uterine involution and to control bleeding. However, these agents should be used judiciously as they may cause hyponatremia and fluid overload. A baseline chest x-ray and beta-hCG measurement should be obtained prior to surgery. If curettage is performed after 16 weeks' gestation, an increased incidence of uterine perforation, hemorrhage, and pulmonary complications arises. In this situation, cardiopulmonary functions should be closely monitored, with surgical and critical care facilities available.[75]

If the patient is older than age 40 or desires sterilization, hysterectomy is a possible alternative. Approximately 25% of patients with molar pregnancy will have a prominent theca-luteal cyst; because these cysts will regress spontaneously, the uterine adnexa need not be removed during the hysterectomy unless adnexal metastases are seen. The safety and low toxicity of another alternative, a methotrexate/leucovorin regimen, make hysterectomy less appealing. Nevertheless, hysterectomy significantly decreases the risk of malignancy (3.5% vs 20%)[76] and is the preferred treatment in patients with placental site tumors because they are usually resistant to chemotherapy.

FIGURE 1

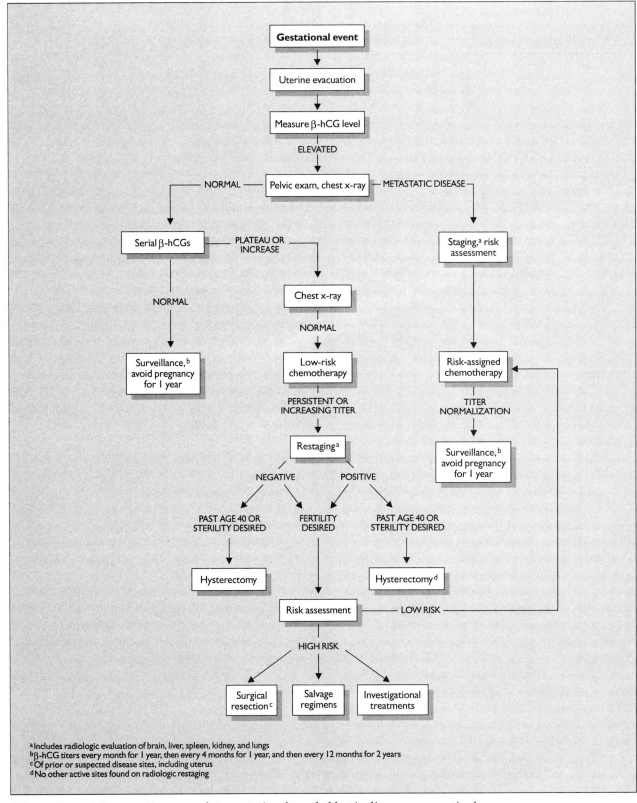

Diagnostic and therapeutic approach to gestational trophoblastic disease, as practiced at the M. D. Anderson Cancer Center

After molar evacuation, 80% of patients will need no further intervention.[5,6,34] However, these patients' weekly serum beta-hCG levels must be diligently monitored until they return to normal. Although normal beta-hCG levels typically return within 8 weeks of surgery, in a minority of patients, normal levels return at 14 to 16 weeks. Sometimes transient plateaus are observed before the beta-hCG level returns to baseline; however, an increased or prolonged plateau of beta-hCG titers implies persistent trophoblastic disease or metastatic spread and requires additional therapy.

Chemotherapy is indicated when there is a plateau or increase in beta-hCG levels on consecutive measurements, failure to reach normal titers by 16 weeks, or metastatic disease. Such patients are usually at low risk and will respond to single-agent chemotherapy. Methotrexate is the most commonly initiated single agent (Table 3). Other agents used successfully in this setting include dactinomycin (Cosmegen), fluorouracil, and etoposide (VePesid).[77,78] Therapy is continued for one to two courses after a normal beta-hCG level is achieved.

Prophylactic Chemotherapy: The use of prophylactic chemotherapy after molar evacuation remains controversial. Although short courses of dactinomycin and methotrexate after molar evacuation reduce the incidence of persistent or recurrent disease in patients at high risk, the effectiveness of chemoprevention in patients at low risk has not been proven. In 1965, a prospective study of the use of chemotherapy at the time of molar evacuation was conducted under the auspices of the National Cancer Institute to determine whether chemoprevention could reduce or eliminate the malignant sequelae of molar disease.[79] Of the 3 schedules evaluated, dactinomycin, 12 µg/kg/d intravenously for 5 days starting 3 days prior to molar evacuation, was found to be optimal in effectiveness and toxicity.

Goldstein randomized 200 patients to receive the same regimen or observation at the time of molar evacuation.[79] He found no cases of metastatic trophoblastic disease in the treated group, whereas four cases developed in patients who did not receive chemoprevention. Two of the four cases were hydatidiform moles, one was choriocarcinoma, and the pathology in the fourth was undetermined.[80] Because the disease remained treatable after progression or relapse, there was no overall survival benefit for the patients who received prophylactic chemotherapy.

In a prospective, randomized study of 71 patients, Kim et al found that chemoprophylaxis in patients with high-risk moles significantly reduced the incidence of persistent molar disease from 47% to 14%. However, among

TABLE 3

Chemotherapy Regimen for Low-Risk [a] Gestational Trophoblastic Disease

Drug	Administration	Cycle [b]
Methotrexate and	1 mg/kg (up to 70 mg) IM or IV days 1, 3, 5, 7	14 days
Folinic acid	0.1 mg/kg IM or IV days 2, 4, 6, 8	
Methotrexate	0.4 mg/kg IM or IV daily for 5 days	14 days
Methotrexate	30 to 50 mg/m² IM	7 days
Dactinomycin	10 µg/kg (up to 0.5 mg) IV daily for 5 days	14 days
Dactinomycin	1.25 mg/m² IV single dose	14 days

[a] Therapy based on WHO risk criteria (see Table 2).
[b] Withhold treatment for marrow recovery if necessary.

low-risk patients, there was no difference in the ability to achieve a complete response between the group receiving chemoprevention and the control group.[81] More courses of chemotherapy (2.5 vs 1.4) were required to produce a complete response in the group receiving chemoprophylaxis, implying that it induced tumor resistance. It thus seems reasonable to administer chemoprevention only if it is doubtful whether the patient will return for serial beta-hCG determinations.

Follow-up: As mentioned previously, all patients with molar disease should obtain a baseline chest x-ray. Serum beta-hCG levels should be obtained every 1 to 2 weeks until the level is normal for 3 consecutive assays. Complete remission is defined by three consecutive normal beta-hCG levels. Once this has occurred, beta-hCG levels should be checked monthly for 12 months, every 4 months for the following year, and then yearly for 2 years.

Although the use of oral contraceptives during the surveillance period remains controversial, strict contraception is required, because pregnancy would obviate the usefulness of beta-hCG as a tumor marker. In general, once a 12-month surveillance establishes a disease-free status, conception is acceptable, although these women are always at high risk for future molar disease and will require close observation during future pregnancies.[82] A pelvic ultrasound examination should be performed during the first trimester of all subsequent pregnancies to confirm that gestation is normal.[83]

Occasionally, women who undergo removal of a complete hydatidiform mole may develop the unusual complication of intermediate trophoblastic disease.[37] Such women usually present with vaginal bleeding and a slightly elevated hCG titer. Examination of the uterus reveals multiple nodules involving the endometrium and myometrium. These nodules do not readily respond to chemotherapy, and surgical intervention is therefore appropriate because progressive disease tends to develop.

Finally, physicians should maintain an awareness of the psychological, social, and sexual effects of GTT on patients and their partners. Most of these women experience a significant level of distress associated with GTT.[84] Many are likely to have fears of infertility despite physician reassurance. These women may also develop sexual dysfunction and lack of sexual desire, which may be attributed, in part, to a fear of future pregnancy. Psychosocial support should be provided, especially for patients undergoing treatment of metastatic disease.

Low-Risk Metastatic Disease

In more than 30 years of experience, single-agent chemotherapy with methotrexate has produced a high cure rate in patients with low-risk GTT.[80] Likewise, methotrexate plus leucovorin induces remission in 90% of patients with low-risk metastatic disease and with low toxicity.[86,87] The use of dactinomycin in methotrexate-resistant patients increased the cure rate to more than 95%. Dactinomycin also has been used successfully as single-agent therapy for low-risk GTT.[88,89] Approximately 80% of patients experience toxic reactions with dactinomycin, the most common being nausea and vomiting. The toxicity of methotrexate is minimal and may result in mucositis and myelosuppression.

Suggested therapeutic regimens for low-risk GTT are outlined in Table 3.[80,84] At The University of Texas M. D. Anderson Cancer Center, the regimen of methotrexate plus leucovorin is preferred because it obviates intravenous access problems, allows the therapeutic administration at home or work, minimizes the interruption of the patient's life, and is the least toxic of the regimens listed. These patients are usually treated for two to three courses after attaining a normal beta-hCG level.

If single-agent therapy with methotrexate or dactinomycin fails, or both, to achieve remission, multidrug chemotherapy must be attempted. This is necessary in nearly 40% of patients with low-risk metastatic GTT. Despite resistance to first-line chemotherapy, a cure rate of almost 100% is achieved with further combination chemotherapy.[86]

High-Risk Metastatic Disease

Because single-agent therapy is inadequate for patients with high-risk GTT, intensive combination chemotherapy is mandatory. The most widely employed regimens include MAC (methotrexate, dactinomycin, and cyclophosphamide [Cytoxan, Neosar] or chlorambucil [Leukeran]), EMA-CO (etoposide, methotrexate, dactinomycin, cyclophosphamide, and vincristine [Oncovin]), and the modified Bagshawe regimen (Table 4).[90]

MAC has been the most widely used primary multidrug regimen and has produced cure rates ranging from 63% to 80%.[91–94] MAC dosages consist of methotrexate, 0.3 mg/kg intravenously (IV) or intramuscularly (IM); dactinomycin, 8 µg/kg IV; and cyclophosphamide, 3 mg/kg IV, or chlorambucil, 0.15 mg/kg PO. Each drug is given as a 5-day course for 3 to 4 courses, with a 9- to 14-day interval between each course. In middle- to high-risk GTT, MAC is most efficacious when used as initial chemotherapy (65% survival), as opposed to secondary chemotherapy (39% survival)[92] following failed single-agent therapy.

The CHAMOCA regimen (hydroxyurea [Hydrea], dactinomycin, methotrexate with leucovorin rescue, cyclophosphamide, vincristine, and doxorubicin [Adriamycin, Rubex]), introduced by Bagshawe in the mid-1970s, produced a remission rate of 82%[90] but was inferior to MAC in terms of toxicity and effectiveness in a trial sponsored by the Gynecologic Oncology Group.[96] The discovery that etoposide is an effective agent against trophoblastic disease led to the development of the EMA-CO regimen by Bagshawe, who reported a survival rate of 83% in patients with high-risk choriocarcinoma.[97] This regimen has been confirmed to be highly effective at several centers, including the Brewer Trophoblastic Disease Center, where a 100% cure rate has been achieved over the past 5 years.[94]

EMA-CO (Table 4) is the preferred regimen for high-risk GTT. We also utilize this regimen for patients with middle-risk GTT, as defined by the WHO criteria. EMA-CO is generally well tolerated, with no life-threatening toxic effects. Alopecia occurs universally, and anemia, neutropenia, and stomatitis are mild. Reproductive function is preserved in approximately 75% of patients.

Within hours of receiving chemotherapy, patients with a significant tumor burden are at risk of hemorrhage into tumors and surrounding tissues. Thus, any acute organ toxicity that begins shortly after the induction of chemotherapy should be considered as possibly related to this phenomenon; to minimize these sequelae, some researchers have advocated a reduction in dosage at the beginning of therapy in patients with large-volume disease.

Surgical resection of persistent sites of disease (including the uterus), with or without chemotherapy, is an important strategy for any patient with chemotherapy-resistant disease. Identifying the sites of active or inactive but radiologically apparent disease is a central problem in this strategy. It is hoped that improvements in monoclonal-antibody scanning techniques will help to overcome this problem.

Salvage Therapy

Unfortunately, about 25% of women with high-risk metastatic disease become refractory to EMA-CO and fail to achieve a complete remission. Currently, there is no standard salvage chemotherapy regimen with EMA-CO failures. However, salvage regimens consisting of combinations of cisplatin (Platinol), etoposide, vinca alkaloids, and bleomycin (Blenoxane) have been administered.

Because of significant nephrotoxicity, cisplatin-containing regimens are withheld as primary therapy for GTT. Early studies show cisplatin-based regimens to be an effective salvage therapy in GTT. Cisplatin in combination with vincristine and methotrexate achieved a 33% response rate as salvage therapy.[98] At The University of Texas M. D. Anderson Cancer Center, Gordon et al reported a sustained remission rate of 20% in 10 patients treated with PVB (cisplatin, vinblastine, and bleomycin) after failure to respond to MAC.[99] A recent dose-intensive regimen, EMA-CE, utilizes cisplatin (100 mg/m^2) and etoposide (200 mg/m^2) combined with EMA, with favorable results.[100]

Another alternative is to give cisplatin in the EMA-POMB regimen (cisplatin, vincristine, methotrexate, bleomycin). POMB is administered as vincristine, 1 mg/m^2 IV, and methotrexate, 300 mg/m^2 IV (day 1); bleomycin, 15 mg IV over 24 h by continuous infusion (CI), and folinic acid, 15 mg bid for four doses (day 2); bleomycin, 15 mg IV over 24 h CI (day 3); and cisplatin, 120 mg/m^2 IV (day 4).

A new PEBA regimen (cisplatin, etoposide, bleomycin, doxorubicin) was recently reported from China and was found to be effective in EMA-CO-resistant disease.[101] A complete remission (CR) was achieved in 96% of the women, and 73% had a sustained CR that lasted at least 1 year. In a small study, ifosfamide (Ifex) alone and in combination with etoposide and cisplatin (VIP) showed promise as being an effective salvage drug in GTT.[102]

Another consideration in the treatment of refractory GTT is the use of high-dose chemotherapy with autologous bone marrow transplantation. In this setting, Lotz et al treated five women with refractory GTT with high-dose ifosfamide, carboplatin (Paraplatin), and etoposide (ICE).[103] Only one of the five women attained a durable

TABLE 4

Chemotherapy Regimens for Middle- and High-Risk ^{a} Gestational Trophoblasic Disease

Drug regimen	Administration
EMA-CO ^{b} (preferred regimen)	
Course 1 (EMA)	
Day 1 Etoposide	100 mg/m^2 IV over 30 min
Methotrexate	100 mg/m^2 IV bolus
Methotrexate	200 mg/m^2 IV as 12-h continuous infusion
Dactinomycin	0.5 mg IV bolus
Day 2 Etoposide	100 mg/m^2 IV over 30 min
Leucovorin	15 mg IV IM PO every 12 h for 4 doses, beginning 24 h after start of methotrexate
Dactinomycin	0.5 mg IV bolus
Course 2 (CO)	
Day 8 Cyclophosphamide	600 mg/m^2 IV over 30 min
Vincristine	1 mg/m^2 (up to 2 mg) IV bolus
EHMMAC ^{c} (alternative for middle-risk patients)	
Course 1	
Etoposide	100 mg/m^2 IV daily for 5 days
Course 2	
Hydroxyurea	0.5 mg PO, repeat in 12 hours, day 1
Methotrexate	50 mg IM, repeat every 48 h, days 2, 4, 6, 8
Course 3	
Dactinomycin	0.5 mg IV daily for 5 days
Course 4	
Vincristine	1.0 mg/m^2 IV days 1 and 3
Cyclophosphamide	400 mg/m^2 IV days 1 and 3

^{a} Therapy based on WHO risk criteria (see Table 2).
^{b} Repeat each regimen in sequence every 14 days as toxicity permits.
^{c} Courses should be given 7 to 10 days apart as toxicity permits. The sequence of courses is 1, 2, 3, 4, 1, 2, etc. Alternatively, regimen 4 may be held in reserve, to be used if one of the other regimens proves ineffective or toxic. The preferred sequence is then 1, 2, 3, 1, 2, 3, etc.

CR (68+ months). The risk and benefits of high-dose chemotherapy in the treatment of GTT is still under investigation.

Pulmonary Metastases

At the time of diagnosis, pulmonary metastases can be extensive and may cause respiratory failure and death.[104] Kelly et al identified several prognostic factors for early respiratory death in patients presenting with GTT and dyspnea.[105] These factors included cyanosis, pulmonary hypertension, anemia, tachycardia, extensive lung opacification, and a high WHO prognostic score. Bakri and colleagues described similar associations with early respiratory failure in 75 patients with pulmonary metastases.[106] Their clinical and radiographic findings included dyspnea, anemia, clinical pulmonary hypertension, cyanosis, more than 50% lung opacification, mediastinal involvement, and bilateral pleural effusion. Patients with extensive lung opacification (particularly when associated with anemia), pulmonary hypertension, or cyanosis were at high risk for respiratory failure.

In patients with extensive pulmonary metastases, reduced doses of initial chemotherapy (eg, 50%) have been suggested to diminish the risk of respiratory failure.[107] However, reduction of the initial chemotherapy dose did not uniformly protect against pulmonary failure and death.[105] All 19 patients who required mechanical ventilation for early respiratory failure died.[105,106] Because of the increased risk of pulmonary decompensation, women with extensive pulmonary metastases should be observed in an intensive care setting during induction chemotherapy. In a rare experience at our institution, induction chemotherapy in a young woman with extensive pulmonary metastases resulted in an embolic phenomenon, leading to severe CNS morbidity (multiple cerebrovascular accidents), leading, in turn, to sudden brain death, despite the patient's having been free of CNS disease prior to therapy. Early detection and diligent follow-up in patients with molar disease are mandatory to improve survival.

CNS Choriocarcinoma

Brain metastases pose a significant threat to the survival of patients with GTT, especially if the metastases appear while the patient is receiving chemotherapy. Although cerebral disease is observed clinically in only 7% to 28% of patients with choriocarcinoma,[22,30,56,62] postmortem examinations demonstrate CNS involvement in as many as 40% of cases.[108] This subset represents a significant fraction of patients who die of the disease.

Several investigators have examined the use of multimodality therapy in this group of patients. Weed et al reported a survival rate of 50% in patients with CNS involvement by choriocarcinoma who received multimodality therapy; disease-free periods of 12 to 120 months were achieved.[109] In six of seven patients who survived, the interval from diagnosis to remission averaged 5.5 months. In the seven patients who died, the average duration of CNS involvement was 17 months.

The addition of whole-brain irradiation and a change in the chemotherapeutic regimen to agents that cross the blood-brain barrier were successful in eradicating the tumor in three of seven patients who developed brain lesions while receiving therapy or who had a recurrence.

In 1983, Athanassiou et al reported results of a 23-year experience with choriocarcinoma involving the CNS at Charing Cross Hospital.[69] Overall, 8.8% of 782 patients with choriocarcinoma who received chemotherapy had CNS metastases. Of these patients, 48% presented with CNS disease prior to treatment. Although 49% of patients who presented with CNS metastases enjoyed long-term survival, only 6% of the patients who developed CNS disease while on therapy survived. After 1974, the overall survival rate was 80% in patients who presented with CNS disease and 25% in patients who developed CNS disease after initiation of treatment. The improved outcome was attributed to early detection of CNS disease by measurement of the serum:CSF beta-hCG ratio, CT scans of the brain, CNS prophylaxis in patients identified as being at high risk for developing brain metastases, and the combination of systemic and intrathecal therapy used for CNS metastases. Radiotherapy did not appear to benefit patients whose disease was resistant to chemotherapy.

In 1987, Yordan et al reported a retrospective analysis of 70 cases of GTT involving the CNS.[110] Of the 70 patients, half died before therapy was initiated. Of the remaining patients, 24% of those given chemotherapy alone survived, and 50% of patients given concurrent chemotherapy plus whole-brain irradiation achieved long-term remission. In the chemotherapy-plus-radiation group, none of the deaths was attributed to CNS disease.

Two different doses of radiation therapy were analyzed for effectiveness and toxicity. Among 10 patients receiving 3,000 cGy or more, there were no CNS disease recurrences. Of the seven patients receiving 2,500 cGy or less, one developed CNS relapse and achieved remission after further treatment. Resolution of CNS disease was documented by brain scan or autopsy in 50% of patients receiving 3,000 cGy or more but in only one of seven patients receiving 2,500 cGy or less. Yordan et al concluded that at the time of diagnosis of CNS disease, irradiation of the brain with 3,000 cGy given over 10 fractions should be initiated simultaneously with the start of chemotherapy.

The introduction of MRI has led to the diagnoses of even smaller CNS lesions than found in the past. Accordingly, the optimal integration of irradiation and chemotherapy remains to be defined. Likewise, select patients who have isolated CNS lesions and are refractory to chemotherapy should be evaluated by a neurosurgeon for possible resection.

FUTURE DIRECTIONS

Although the majority of patients with metastatic GTT will be cured, there remains a subset of patients who demonstrate persistent or recurrent disease after aggressive multiagent chemotherapy. These patients require special strategies. It is hoped that new therapeutic agents, such as the emerging class of topoisomerase-I inhibitors (camptothecin and its derivatives), angiogenesis inhibitors (TNP-470), and microtubule agents (paclitaxel [Taxol] and docetaxel [Taxotere]), will have activity in this disease. Strategies involving dose intensification with the use of growth factors (granulocyte colony-stimulating factor [filgrastim, Neupogen] and granulocyte-macrophage colony-stimulating factor [sargramostim, Leukine]) are reasonable approaches for patients with high-risk disease who do not respond quickly to conventional treatment. Monoclonal antibody-based diagnostic and therapeutic modalities are ideally suited for the identification and treatment of metastatic disease, because the tumor uniformly expresses a unique paternal antigen and has a rich vascular supply. It is hoped that emerging insights into the molecular mechanisms of GTT will lead to genetically based therapeutic strategies.

REFERENCES

1. World Health Organization Scientific Group: Gestational Trophoblastic Disease. Technical Report Series No 692. Geneva, World Health Organization, 1983.

2. Lurain JR: Gestational trophoblastic tumor. Semin Surg Oncol 6:347–353, 1990.

3. Szulman AE, Surti U: The syndromes of hydatidiform mole: I. Cytogenic and morphologic correlations. Am J Obstet Gynecol 131:665–671, 1978.

4. Szulman AE, Surti U: The syndromes of hydatidiform mole: II. Morphologic evolution of the complete and partial mole. Am J Obstet Gynecol 132:20–27, 1978.

5. Lurain JR, Brewer JI, Torok EE, et al: Natural history of hydatidiform mole after primary evacuation. Am J Obstet Gynecol 145:591–595, 1983.

6. Miller JM, Surwit EA, Hammond CB: Choriocarcinoma following term pregnancy. Obstet Gynecol 53:207–212, 1979.

7. Driscoll SG: Placental site chorioma: The neoplasm of the implantation site trophoblast. J Reprod Med 29:821, 1984.

8. Goldstein DP: Worldwide controversies in gestational trophoblastic neoplasms. Int J Gynaecol Obstet 15:207–215, 1977.

9. Buckley JD: The epidemiology of molar pregnancy and choriocarcinoma. Clin Obstet Gynecol 27:153, 1984.

10. Bagshawe KD, Golding PR, Orr AM: Choriocarcinoma after hydatidiform mole: Studies related to the effectiveness of follow-up practice after hydatidiform mole. Br Med J 2:733, 1969.

11. Mazur MT, Kurman RJ: Choriocarcinoma and placental site trophoblastic tumor, in Szulman AE, Buchsbaum HJ (eds): Gestational Trophoblastic Disease, pp 45–68. New York, Springer-Verlag, 1987.

12. Wei PY, Ouyang PC: Trophoblastic diseases in Taiwan. Am J Obstet Gynecol 85:844, 1963.

13. Palmer JR: Advances in the epidemiology of gestational trophoblastic disease. J Reprod Med 39:155–162, 1994.

14. Yen S, MacMahon BB: Epidemiologic factors of trophoblastic disease. Am J Obstet Gynecol 101:126, 1968.

15. Hayashi K, Bracken MB, Freeman DH, et al: Hydatidiform mole in the United States (1970–1977): A statistical and theoretical analysis. Am J Epidemiol 115:67–77, 1982.

16. Martin PM: High frequency of hydatidiform mole in native Alaskans. Int J Gynaecol Obstet 15:395, 1978.

17. Matsuura J, Chui D, Jacobs PA, et al: Complete hydatidiform mole in Hawaii: An epidemiological study. Genet Epidemiol 1:171, 1984.

18. Graham IH, Fajardo AM: The incidence and morphology of hydatidiform mole in Abu Dhabi, United Arab Emirates. Br J Obstet Gynaecol 95:391, 1988.

19. Joint Project for the Study of Choriocarcinoma and Hydatidiform Mole in Asia: Geographic variation in the occurrence of hydatidiform mole and choriocarcinoma. Ann N Y Acad Sci 80:174, 1959.

20. Bagshawe KD, Dent J, Webb J: Hydatidiform mole in England and Wales, 1973–1983. Lancet II:673, 1986.

21. Teoh ES, Dagwood MY, Ratnam SS: Epidemiology of hydatidiform mole in Singapore. Am J Obstet Gynecol 110:415, 1971.

22. Bagshawe KD: Risk and prognostic factors in trophoblastic neoplasia. Cancer 38:1373–1385, 1976.

23. Berkowitz RS, Bernstein MR, Laborde O, et al: Subsequent pregnancy experience with gestational trophoblastic disease: New England Trophoblastic Disease Center, 1965–1992. J Reprod Med 39:228–232, 1994.

24. Acosta-Sison H: Statistical study of chorioepithelioma in the Philippine General Hospital. Am J Obstet Gynecol 58:125, 1949.

25. Bertini B: Epidemiology of hydatidiform mole in Israel: A study based on 113 patients. Int J Gynaecol Obstet 11:55, 1973.

26. Parazinni F, LaVecchia C, Mangili G, et al: Dietary factors and risk of trophoblastic disease. Am J Obstet Gynecol 158:93, 1988.

27. Berkowitz RS, Cramer DW, Bernstein MR, et al: Risk factors for complete molar pregnancy from a case-control study. Am J Obstet Gynecol 152:1016, 1985.

28. Bagshawe KD, Rawlings G, Pike MC, et al: The ABO group in trophoblastic neoplasia. Lancet I:553, 1971.

29. Cross JC, Werb Z, Fisher SJ: Implantation and the placenta: Key pieces of the development puzzle. Science 266:1508–1518, 1994.

30. Park WW, Lees JC: Choriocarcinoma: A general review with analysis of 516 cases. Arch Pathol 49:73–104, 205–241, 1950.

31. Hertig AT, Edmonds HW: Genetics of hydatidiform mole. Arch Pathol 30:260, 1940.

32. Driscoll SG: Trophoblastic growths: Morphologic aspects and taxonomy. J Reprod Med 26:2181, 1981.

33. Kajii T, Ohama K: Androgenetic origin of hydatidiform mole. Nature 268:633–655, 1977.

34. Morrow CP: Postmolar trophoblastic disease: Diagnosis, management, and prognosis. Clin Obstet Gynecol 27:211, 1984.

35. Lurain JR, Brewer JI: Invasive mole. Semin Oncol 9:174–180, 1982.

36. Kurman RJ, Main CS, Chen HC: Intermediate trophoblast: A distinctive form of trophoblast with specific morphological, biochemical, and functional features. Placenta 5:349–370, 1984.

37. Silva EG, Tornos C, Lage J, et al: Multiple nodules of intermediate trophoblast following hydatidiform moles. Int J Gynecol Pathol 12:324–332, 1993.

38. Lawler S, Fisher RA, Dent J: A prospective genetic study of complete and partial hydatidiform moles. Am J Obstet Gynecol 164:1270, 1991.

39. Jacobs PA, Wilson CM, Sprenkle JA, et al: Mechanisms of

origin of complete hydatidiform moles. Nature 286:714–716, 1980.

40. Yamashita K, Wake N, Araki T, et al: Human lymphocyte antigen expression in hydatidiform mole: Androgenesis following fertilization by a haploid sperm. Am J Obstet Gynecol 135:597–600, 1979.

41. Wake N, Fujino T, Hoshi S, et al: The propensity to malignancy of dispermic heterozygous mole. Placenta 8:319, 1987.

42. Wallace DC, Surti U, Adams CW, et al: Complete moles have paternal chromosomes but maternal mitochondrial DNA. Hum Genet 61:145 1982.

43. Ohama K, Kajii T, Okamoto E, et al: Dispermic origin of XY hydatidiform moles. Nature 292:551–552, 1981.

44. Fisher RA, Povey S, Jeffries AJ, et al: Frequency of heterozygous complete hydatidiform moles, estimated by locus-specific mini-satellite and Y chromosome-specific probes. Hum Genet 82:259, 1989.

45. Mutter GL, Pomponio R, Berkowitz RS, et al: Sex chromosome composition of complete hydatidiform moles: Relationship to metastasis. Am J Obstet Gynecol 168:1547, 1993.

46. McFadden DE, Kalousek DK: Two different phenotypes of fetuses with chromosomal triploidy: Correlation with parental origin of the extra haploid set. Am J Med Genet 38:535, 1991.

47. Roberts DJ, Mutter GL: Advances in the molecular biology of gestational trophoblastic disease. J Reprod Med 39:201–208, 1994.

48. Steller MA, Mok SC, Yeh J: Effects of cytokines on epidermal growth factor receptor expression by malignant trophoblast cells in vitro. J Reprod Med 39:209–216, 1994.

49. Guillemot F, Nagy A, Auerbach A, et al: Essential role of Mash-2 in extraembryonic development. Nature 371:333–336, 1994.

50. Cheung AN, Srivastava G, Pittaluga S, et al: Expression of c-myc and c-fms oncogenes in hydatidiform mole and normal human placenta. J Clin Pathol 46:204, 1993.

51. Sarkar S, Kacinski BM, Kohorn EI, et al: Demonstration of myc and ras oncogene expression by hybridization in situ in hydatidiform mole and in the BeWo chariocarcinoma cell line. Am J Obstet Gynecol 154:390, 1986.

52. Cameron B, Gown AM, Tamini HK: Expression of c-erb B2 oncogene product in persistent gestational trophoblastic disease. Am J Obstet Gynecol 170:1616–1621, 1994.

53. Sheridan E, Hancock BW, Goyns MH: High incidence of mutations of the p53 gene detected in ovarian tumours by the use of chemical mismatch cleavage. Cancer Lett 68:83, 1993.

54. Cheung AN, Srivastava G, Chung LP, et al: Expression of the p53 gene in trophoblastic cells in hydatidiform moles and normal human placentas. J Reprod Med 39:223–227, 1994.

55. Persaud V, Ganjei P, Nadji M, et al: Cell proliferation activity and mutation of p53 suppressor gene in human gestational trophoblastic disease. West Indian Med J 42:142–143, 1993.

56. Berkowitz RS, Goldstein DP: Pathogenesis of gestational trophoblastic neoplasms. Pathol Annu 11:391–411, 1981.

57. Yuen BH, Carron W, Benedet JL, et al: Plasma beta-subunit human chorionic gonadotropin assay in molar pregnancy and chorio-carcinoma. Am J Obstet Gynecol 127:711–712, 1977.

58. Amir SM, Osathanondh R, Berkowitz RS, et al: Human chorionic gonadotropin and thyroid function in patients with hydatidiform mole. Am J Obstet Gynecol 150:723, 1984.

59. Goldstein DP, Berkowitz RS: Current management of complete and partial molar pregnancy. J Reprod Med 39:139–146, 1994.

60. Mutch D, Soper JT, Baker ME, et al: Role of computed axial tomography of the chest in staging patients with nonmetastatic gestational trophoblastic disease. Obstet Gynecol 68:348–352, 1986.

61. Kumar J, Ilancheran A, Ratnam SS: Pulmonary metastases in gestational trophoblastic disease: A review of 97 cases. Br J Obstet Gynaecol 95:70, 1988.

62. Stilp TJ, Bucy PC, Brewer JI: Cure of metastatic choriocarci-noma of the brain. JAMA 221:276–279, 1972.

63. Bakri Y, Berkowitz RS, Goldstein DP, et al: Brain metastases of gestational trophoblastic tumor. J Reprod Med 39:179–183, 1994.

64. Pastorfide GB, Goldstein DP, Kosasa TS: The use of a radio-immunoassay specific for human chorionic gonadotropin in patients with molar pregnancy and gestational trophoblastic disease. Am J Obstet Gynecol 120:1025–1028, 1974.

65. Vaitukaitis JL, Braunstein GD, Ross GT: A radioimmunoassay which specifically measures human chorionic gonadotropin in the presence of human luteinizing hormone. Am J Obstet Gynecol 113:751–758, 1972.

66. Wehmann RE, Ayala AR, Birken S: Improved monitoring of gestational trophoblastic neoplasia using a highly sensitive assay for urinary human chorionic gonadotropin. Am J Obstet Gynecol 140:753–757, 1981.

67. Kenimer JG, Hershman JM, Higgins HP: The thyrotropin in hydatidiform moles is human chorionic gonadotropin. J Clin Endocri-nol Metab 40:482–491, 1975.

68. Koonongs PP, Schalerth JB: CA125: A marker for persistent gestational trophoblastic disease? Gynecol Oncol 49:240–242, 1993.

69. Athanassiou A, Begent RHL, Newlands ES, et al: Central nervous system metastases of choriocarcinoma: Twenty-three years' experience at Charing Cross Hospital. Cancer 52:1728–1735, 1983.

70. Bagshawe KD, Harland J: Immunodiagnosis and monitoring of gonadotropin-producing metastases in the central nervous system. Cancer 39:112, 1976.

71. Bagshawe KD: Choriocarcinoma: The Clinical Biology of the Trophoblast and Its Tumors. London, Edward Arnold, 1969.

72. Carter J, Fowler J, Carlson J, et al: Transvaginal color flow Doppler sonography in the assessment of gestational trophoblastic disease. J Ultrasound Med 12:595–599, 1993.

73. Dubuc-Lissoir J, Sweizig S, Schlaerth JB, et al: Metastatic gestational trophoblastic disease: A comparison of prognostic classi-fication systems. Gynecol Oncol 45:40–45, 1992.

74. Hammond CB, Weed JC Jr, Currie JL: The role of operation in the current therapy of gestational neoplastic disease. Am J Obstet Gynecol 136:844–858, 1980.

75. Soper JT: Surgical therapy for gestational trophoblastic dis-ease. J Reprod Med 39:168–174, 1994.

76. Curry SL, Hammond CB, Tyrey L, et al: Hydatidiform mole: Diagnosis, management, and long-term follow-up of 347 patients. Obstet Gynecol 45:1, 1975.

77. Song HZ, Wu PH: Reevaluation of 5-fluorouracil as a single therapeutic agent for gestational trophoblastic neoplasms. J Obstet Gynecol 150:69–75, 1984.

78. Wong LC, Choo YC, Ma HK: Primary oral etoposide therapy in gestational trophoblastic disease. Cancer 58:14–17, 1986.

79. Goldstein DP: Prophylactic chemotherapy of molar pregnancy. Obstet Gynecol 38:817–822, 1971.

80. Goldstein DP: Prevention of gestational trophoblastic disease by use of actinomycin D in molar pregnancies. Obstet Gynecol 43:475–479, 1974.

81. Kim DS, Hyung M, Kyung TK, et al: Effects of prophylactic chemotherapy for persistent trophoblastic disease in patients with complete hydatidiform mole. Obstet Gynecol 67:690–694, 1986.

82. Sand PK, Lurain JR, Brewer JI: Repeat gestational trophoblas-tic disease. Obstet Gynecol 63:140–144, 1984.

83. Walden PAM, Bagshawe KD: Pregnancies after chemotherapy for gestational trophoblastic tumors. Lancet II:1241, 1979.

84. Wenzel LB, Berkowitz RS, Robinson S, et al: Psychological, social, and sexual effects of gestational trophoblastic disease on

patients and their partners. J Reprod Med 39:163–167, 1994.

85. Lurain JR: Chemotherapy of gestational trophoblastic disease, in Deppe G (ed): Chemotherapy of Gynecologic Cancer, pp 273–301. New York, Alan R Liss, 1990.

86. Berkowitz RS, Goldstein DP, Bernstein MR: Ten years' experience with methotrexate and folinic acid as primary therapy for gestational trophoblastic disease. Gynecol Oncol 23:111–118, 1986.

87. Gleeson NC, Finan MA, Fiorica JV, et al: Nonmetastatic gestational trophoblastic disease: Weekly methotrexate compared with 8-day methotrexate-folinic acid. Eur J Gynaecol Oncol 14:461–465, 1993.

88. Schlaerth JB, Morrow CP, Nalick RH, et al: Single-dose actinomycin D in the treatment of postmolar trophoblastic disease. Gynecol Oncol 19:53–56, 1984.

89. Twiggs LB: Pulse actinomycin D scheduling in nonmetastatic gestational trophoblastic neoplasia: Cost-effective chemotherapy. Gynecol Oncol 16:190–195, 1983.

90. Jones WB: Management of low-risk metastatic gestational trophoblastic disease. J Reprod Med 26:213–217, 1981.

91. Hammond CB, Borchert LG, Tyrey L, et al: Treatment of metastatic trophoblastic disease: Good and poor prognosis. J Obstet Gynecol 115:451–457, 1973.

92. Lurain JR, Brewer JI: Treatment of high-risk gestational trophoblastic disease with methotrexate, actinomycin D, and cyclophosphamide chemotherapy. Obstet Gynecol 65:830–836, 1985.

93. Gordon AN, Gershenson DM, Copeland LJ, et al: High-risk metastatic gestational trophoblastic disease. Obstet Gynecol 65:550–556, 1985.

94. Berkowitz RS, Goldstein DP, Bernstein MR: Modified triple chemotherapy in the management of high-risk metastatic gestational trophoblastic tumors. Gynecol Oncol 19:173–181, 1984.

95. Begent RHJ, Bagshawe KD: The management of high-risk choriocarcinoma. Semin Oncol 9:198–203, 1982.

96. Curry SL, Blessing JA, Disaia PJ, et al: A prospective randomized comparison of methotrexate, actinomycin D, and chlorambucil (MAC) versus modified Bagshawe regimen in 'poor-prognosis' gestational trophoblastic disease. Obstet Gynecol 73:357–362, 1989.

97. Bagshawe KD: Treatment of high-risk choriocarcinoma. J Reprod Med 29:813–820, 1984.

98. Newlands ES: New chemotherapeutic agents in the management of gestational trophoblastic disease. Semin Oncol 9:230, 1982.

99. Gordon AN, Kavanagh JJ, Gershenson DM, et al: Cisplatin, vincristine, and bleomycin combination therapy in resistant gestational trophoblastic disease. Cancer 58:1407–1410, 1986.

100. Surwit EA, Childers JM: High-risk metastatic gestational trophoblastic disease: A new dose-intensive, multiagent chemotherapeutic regimen. J Reprod Med 36:45–48, 1991.

101. Li-Pai C, Shu-Mo C, Jian-Xuan F, et al: PEBA regimen (cisplatin, etoposide, bleomycin, and Adriamycin) in the treatment of drug-resistant choriocarcinoma. Gynecol Oncol 56:231–234, 1995.

102. Sutton GP, Soper JT, Blessing JA, et al: Ifosfamide alone and in combination in the treatment of refractory malignant gestational trophoblastic disease. Am J Obstet Gynecol 167:489–495, 1992.

103. Lotz JP, Andre T, Donsimoni R, et al: High dose chemotherapy with ifosfamide, carboplatin, and etoposide combined with autologous bone marrow transplantation for the treatment of poor-prognosis germ cell tumors and metastatic trophoblastic disease in adults. Cancer 75:874–885, 1995.

104. Dubeshter B, Berkowitz RS, Goldstein DP, et al: Analysis of treatment failure in high- risk metastatic gestational trophoblastic dieseease. Gynecol Oncol 29:199, 1988.

105. Kelly MP, Rustin GJS, Ivory C, et al: Respiratory failure due to choriocarcinoma: A study of 103 dyspneic patients. Gynecol Oncol 38:149, 1990.

106. Bakri YN, Berkowitz RS, Khan J, et al: Pulmonary metastases of gestational trophoblastic tumor: Risk factors for early respiratory failure. J Reprod Med 38:175–178, 1994.

107. Rustin GJS, Bagshawe KD: Gestational trophoblastic tumours. CRC Crit Rev Oncol Haematol 3:103, 1985.

108. Gilbert HA, Kagan AR: Incidence, detection, and evaluation without histologic confirmation, in Weiss L (ed): Fundamental Aspects of Metastases, pp 385–405. Amsterdam, North Holland, 1976.

109. Weed JC, Hammond CB: Cerebral metastatic choriocarcinoma: Intensive therapy and prognosis. Obstet Gynecol 55:89–94, 1980.

110. Yordan EL Jr, Schlaerth JB, Gaddis O, et al: Radiation therapy in the management of gestational choriocarcinoma metastatic to the central nervous system. Obstet Gynecol 69:627–630, 1987.

CHAPTER 24

Carcinoma of the Uterine Cervix

Arsenio Lopez, MD, Andrzej P. Kudelka, MD,
Creighton L. Edwards, MD, *and* John J Kavanagh, MD
Department of Breast and Gynecologic Medical Oncology and Department of Gynecologic Oncology
The University of Texas M. D. Anderson Cancer Center, Houston, Texas

Over the past four decades, the incidence and mortality rates for uterine cervical carcinoma have decreased in the United States by as much as 70% to 75%.[1] This improvement is among the largest seen for any cancer site and has been attributed to the use of cervical cytologic screening.[2] The Papanicolaou smear allows detection of the disease at a preinvasive stage, and about 65,000 cases of carcinoma in situ are found this way annually.[3] However, cervical cancer remains a significant problem, and it is the most common female cancer in some developing countries.[4] In the United States, it is the seventh most common cancer in females. It is estimated that, in 1995, 15,800 new cases will be found and 4,800 deaths will be caused by cervical cancer.[3]

PATHOLOGY

The majority of cervical cancers are squamous-cell carcinomas. These lesions arise from the squamocolumnar junction and may be keratinizing or nonkeratinizing. Various methods of histologic grading have been used for cervical squamous-cell carcinoma, but these have no significant impact on prognosis.[5,6]

Adenocarcinomas of the uterine cervix arise from the endocervical columnar cells and account for about 14% of cervical carcinomas.[7] Over the past few decades, the percentage of adenocarcinomas has increased because, compared with squamous-cell carcinomas, they are more difficult to detect at a preinvasive stage.[8] Although most clinical studies on cervical neoplasia have involved patients with squamous-cell carcinomas, patients with adenocarcinomas are generally treated similarly. It was reported that adenocarcinoma has a worse prognosis than squamous-cell carcinoma.[9] However, several recent investigations showed that long-term survival rates for these two histologic types of disease are not significantly different.[10,11]

Other types of epithelial carcinomas of the cervix are less common but have important clinical implications.[12] Adenosquamous carcinomas contain malignant squamous and glandular components in the same tumor. These tumors are associated with a higher risk of pelvic lymph-node metastasis than squamous-cell carcinomas

or adenocarcinomas, but this finding has not had any significant effect on survival rates.[10,13,14] Glassy-cell carcinoma is a poorly differentiated form of adenosquamous carcinoma that responds poorly to surgery and radiation therapy.[15] Verrucous carcinoma is an extremely well-differentiated variant of squamous-cell carcinoma. This tumor may invade the vagina or endometrium but usually does not metastasize to the lymph nodes. Small-cell carcinomas are distinctive and, collectively, have a very poor prognosis; the most aggressive tumors are those with neuroendocrine differentiation.[16] This group should be distinguished from the poorly differentiated squamous-cell carcinomas with small cells and the adenocarcinomas with carcinoid features.

Other cervical malignancies include sarcomas, malignant melanomas, lymphomas, mixed müllerian tumors, germ-cell tumors, and trophoblastic tumors.

ETIOLOGY

The association between cervical neoplasia and sexual activity is well established,[17,18] and current studies have identified the human papillomavirus (HPV) as the most important factor responsible for this association. HPV, therefore, may be a causal agent in cervical neoplasia. An epidemiologic study by Schiffman et al[19] showed that the increased risk of cervical intraepithelial neoplasia (CIN) previously associated with other factors, such as increased lifetime number of sex partners, earlier age at first intercourse, lower level of education, lower income, and smoking, is actually a result of HPV infection. The only risk factor studied that was noted to be independent of HPV status was increased parity. Schiffman et al concluded that HPV satisfied all the requirements that designate a cause of cervical neoplasia.

Many types of HPV have been isolated in the human genital tract; infection with HPV types 16, 18, 45, or 56 has a high correlation with cervical cancer. In a retrospective study by Lorincz et al,[20] these high-risk types of HPV were present in 74% of cases of invasive cervical cancer and in 53% of cases of moderate to severe dysplasia. HPV-16 is the most prevalent among these types. HPV types 31, 33, 35, 51, 52, and 58 were deemed intermediate-risk viruses and were present in 10% of cases of invasive carcinoma and in 24% of cases of moderate to severe dysplasia. Types 6, 11, 42, 43, and 44 were designated low-risk viral types; they were present in only 4% of cases with moderate to severe dysplasia and not at all in invasive cancer. HPV types 6 and 11 were previously shown to be responsible for 95% of vulvar, vaginal, and anal exophytic condylomas.[21]

The multistep process from HPV infection to carcinogenesis is not yet completely understood. HPV genetic sequences have been observed to be integrated into the host genome just as the cell develops invasive properties.[22] It is known that the E6 protein produced by high-risk HPV types 16 and 18 can combine with the p53 protein and cause the same functional consequence as a *p53* gene mutation.[23,24] In contrast, E6 protein expression from the low-risk HPV-6 does not produce any such effect. The E7 protein of HPV-16 was also shown to bind to the p105-RB protein encoded by the retinoblastoma gene (*RB1*).[25]

The p53 and pRb proteins participate in the activity at the G1-S cell-cycle checkpoint that normally causes cells with DNA damage to undergo either cellular arrest at G1 or apoptosis.[26] The E6 and E7 oncoproteins produced by HPV-16 cause decreases in p53 and pRb proteins, respectively, undermining this cell-cycle checkpoint.[27,28] The alteration of the G1-S checkpoint leads to the inappropriate survival of genetically damaged cells and, thus, may be a step in the development of a malignancy. Various cofactors are probably necessary for carcinogenesis to progress completely. Somatic mutations of the *p53* gene may also be present in cervical carcinoma, but they are uncommon.[29]

An increased risk of cervical neoplasia also results from immunosuppression.[30] Immunosuppression was associated with an increased rate of HPV infection in several studies[31–33] and allows neoplastic proliferation due to deficient host-regulatory mechanisms. Women who have the human immunodeficiency virus (HIV) have increased incidence and recurrence rates of CIN that correlate with their degree of immunosuppression.[34] Furthermore, women who were HIV positive and who developed invasive cervical carcinoma were noted to have more advanced disease at presentation, poorer response to therapy, and higher recurrence and death rates.[35,36] A direct molecular interaction between HIV and HPV has also been described, with HIV gene products causing transactivation of HPV proteins.[37]

Smoking has been reported to increase HPV infection rates,[38] and this may explain the previously noted association between smoking and cervical neoplasia. Conflicting data have been reported for other postulated risk factors for cervical neoplasia, including herpes simplex virus type 2 infection, vitamin A and vitamin C deficiencies, use of oral contraceptives, and prenatal exposure to diethylstilbestrol.

NATURAL HISTORY

Cervical Intraepithelial Neoplasia

The development of invasive cervical carcinoma traditionally has been viewed as a continuum that begins with mild dysplasia. The terminology used to classify the precursor lesions of cervical cancer reflected this view; mild dysplasia was designated as CIN-1 and moderate dysplasia as CIN-2. Severe dysplasia and carcinoma in situ were grouped together as CIN-3, based on data suggesting that both types of lesions should be managed similarly.[39] Cervical lesions with histologic features of HPV infection were usually referred to as flat condylomas.

With the current understanding of the pathogenesis of cervical squamous-cell neoplasia, Richart has suggested modified terminology for the histologic classification of CIN.[40,41] CIN-2 and CIN-3 lesions, generally associated with aneuploidy and infection from just one of the high-risk HPV types, are grouped together as high-grade CIN and have a high probability of transformation to invasive carcinoma if left untreated. Flat condylomas and CIN-1 lesions are both associated with multiple infections from a heterogeneous group of HPV types and are grouped as low-grade CIN. This group has uncertain oncogenic potential, because no histologic features distinguish the low-grade lesions that will progress to carcinoma from those that will remain stable or regress. This modified histologic classification conforms with the Bethesda system for reporting cervical cytologic diagnosis, which is discussed later in this chapter. Richart's classifiction also recognizes that these lesions may involve two separate disease processes instead of the continuum they were previously thought to represent.

CIN-1 lesions have a high spontaneous remission rate. Nasiell et al[42] reported a 62% regression rate for CIN-1 lesions over the course of a large prospective study. Progression to either CIN-3 or invasive carcinoma occurred in 16% of the cases, with an average time to progression of 48 months. In an earlier study of CIN-2 lesions, the subgroup of patients that did not undergo a biopsy for diagnosis had a 50% regression rate and a 35% progression rate (average time to progression was 51 months).[43] A biopsy can eradicate a lesion; therefore, studies on the natural history of CIN should not include patients who have undergone this procedure. It is generally agreed that most patients with CIN-3 will eventually develop invasive cancer. Varied estimates have been made regarding the length of time it takes carcinoma in situ to progress to invasive carcinoma. A range of 3 to 10 years was reported by Barron et al.[44]

Preinvasive lesions are usually confined to the transformation zone of the cervix. This is a region in the cervical mucosa that was originally composed of columnar epithelial cells that are being replaced by squamous epithelium through the normal physiologic process of metaplasia. The change occurs most actively during fetal development, during adolescence, and at the time of a first pregnancy.

Invasive Cervical Carcinoma

Invasive carcinoma develops when malignant epithelial cells break through the basement membrane and spread to the cervical stroma. As the malignancy grows, it may produce a visible ulceration or an exophytic mass, or it may extensively infiltrate the endocervix, causing the cervix to expand and harden. The tumor usually presents as vaginal bleeding, frequently postcoital; with further progression, a malodorous vaginal discharge becomes more pronounced. The tumor then extends into the paracervical tissue, vagina, and endometrium. Inflammatory changes or tumor necrosis may produce a dull pain in the pelvic region. Lateral extension of disease to the pelvic wall results in severe discomfort, and lumbosacral nerve or nerve root involvement causes pain resembling sciatica. Anterior tumor growth results in bladder involvement manifested by urinary frequency, hematuria, a vescicovaginal fistula, or obstructive uropathy. Posterior tumor growth causes rectal extension, which leads to tenesmus, rectal bleeding, or a rectovaginal fistula.

Lymphatic spread of the carcinoma occurs with sequential involvement of pelvic, para-aortic, mediastinal, and supraclavicular lymph nodes. Hematogenous dissemination usually occurs late in the course of the disease and most commonly involves the lungs, bones, and liver.[45]

SCREENING AND DIAGNOSIS

Cervical Cytologic Screening

The use of the Pap smear as a screening tool for cervical cancer was first endorsed by the American Cancer Society in 1945. Its efficacy has resulted in reductions in both incidence rates and mortality rates for invasive cervical cancer in areas where the test is widely used.[2] Currently, both the American Cancer Society and the American College of Obstetricians and Gynecologists recommend that "all women who are or have been sexually active or who have reached the age of 18 years should have an annual Pap smear and pelvic examination. After a woman has had three or more consecutive satisfactory normal annual examinations, the Pap smear may be performed less frequently at the discretion of her physician."[46]

The Pap smear has a reported false-negative rate of 20%,[47] and factors that may contribute to underdiagnosis include inadequate sampling by the physician as well as laboratory errors. Samples must be obtained from the cervical surface with an Ayre spatula and from the

TABLE I

Comparison of Cervical Cytologic and Histologic Terminologies

Cytologic			Histologic
Papanicolaou system	WHO system	Bethesda system	CIN classification
Class I	Normal	Within normal limits	—
Class II	Atypical	Reactive or reparative changes; ASCUS	—
Class III	Mild dysplasia	Low-grade SIL[a]	CIN-1
Class III	Moderate dysplasia	High-grade SIL	CIN-2
Class III	Severe dysplasia	High-grade SIL	CIN-3
Class IV	Carcinoma in situ	High-grade SIL	CIN-3
Class V	Invasive squamous-cell carcinoma	Squamous-cell carcinoma	Squamous-cell carcinoma
Class V	Adenocarcinoma	Adenocarcinoma	Adenocarcinoma

[a] Includes changes associated with human papillomavirus (HPV) infection.   ASCUS = atypical squamous cells of undertermined significance, CIN = cervical intraepithelial neoplasia, SIL = squamous intraepithelial lesion, WHO = World Health Organization.

endocervical canal using a cytobrush, and the collected cells must undergo rapid fixation.[48] It is important to realize that a cervical cytology study is a screening tool and not a diagnostic test; therefore, a biopsy should be done on any visible lesion.

The cytologic classification system originally proposed by Dr. George Papanicolaou[49] had five groups (class I to class V). However, these groups were difficult to correlate with biopsy results, so other methods of reporting cervical cytologic findings were created, such as the World Health Organization (WHO) classification and CIN-based terminology. Because no uniform reporting system existed for cervical cytology, the Bethesda system was developed in a workshop convened by the National Cancer Institute (NCI).[50] Table 1 correlates the various terminologies used in reporting Pap smear results with histologic (ie, CIN-based) terminology.

The Bethesda system introduces several changes in the way the results of Pap smears are reported. The term squamous intraepithelial lesion (SIL) is used to refer to the precursor lesions of invasive squamous-cell carcinoma. Low-grade SIL includes CIN-1 and cellular changes associated with HPV. High-grade SIL combines CIN-2 and CIN-3. This categorization is based on the similarity in etiology, behavior, and treatment of the lesions within each group.

Among cytologists, the lack of reproducibility encountered using the dysplasia-CIN terminology[51] may be corrected with the use of only two categories.[52] Atypical squamous cells of undetermined significance (ASCUS) is a term used strictly for changes that truly are of unknown significance. This term should not be used for inflammatory or atrophic changes that were also referred to as atypical in the previous terminology. Under the Bethesda system, the cytology report is regarded as a medical consultation, and recommendations for further patient evaluation are given when appropriate. A statement about the adequacy of the specimen is also part of the cytology report.

Management of Abnormal Smears/Preinvasive Lesions

The main objectives in the evaluation of abnormal Pap smears are to rule out invasive carcinoma and to determine the extent of noninvasive lesions. A colposcopy is usually performed first when further evaluation is required. The colposcopy involves the use of a stereoscopic microscope to examine the cervix. A 3% acetic acid solution applied to the cervix prior to the examination will cause epithelial lesions to turn white. The subepithelial vascular distribution is also closely examined because it

may be abnormal in the presence of CIN. The examination is considered adequate only if the transformation zone and any lesions that may be present are seen in their entirety. Otherwise, the presence of invasive cancer cannot be ruled out. Punch biopsies are done on areas with significant colposcopic abnormalities, and an endocervical curettage (ECC) is performed to evaluate the endocervical canal.

Certain patients may require a cervical cone biopsy (conization), which involves the removal of a cone-shaped section of the cervix, to rule out invasive carcinoma. This is done using either cold knife, electrosurgical, or laser techniques. Indications for conization include: (1) an inadequate colposcopic examination, (2) a positive ECC, (3) biopsy results showing microinvasive carcinoma or indicating possible invasive carcinoma, and (4) findings of a lesion in the Pap smear with a higher grade than that found with colposcopically directed biopsy.

Complications associated with the procedure include hemorrhage, cervical stenosis, or cervical incontinence. Laser conization is a technically more difficult procedure, but it may result in fewer complications than cold knife conization. However, laser conization may cause thermal damage to the margins of the specimen, making it difficult to determine whether the margins are involved with tumor. In such cases, subsequent cold knife conization may be necessary.

Because fewer than 5% of patients with ASCUS have high-grade SIL on colposcopy,[53] it is reasonable to defer this procedure initially and repeat a Pap smear in 4 to 6 months. However, a colposcopy is needed if malignancy is suspected or if the atypical findings persist.

Patients with a Pap smear showing low-grade SIL usually undergo an immediate colposcopy for further evaluation. However, some physicians may elect to manage these patients by repeating Pap smears in 4 months because most of these lesions spontaneously regress. Colposcopy can be reserved for persistent lesions. If a biopsy done with an adequate colposcopy confirms the finding of low-grade SIL, the lesion can be treated immediately or can be followed via repeat colposcopy every 6 months. Treatment is indicated for any lesion that progresses and for those that persist after 2 years of follow-up.

Patients whose cervical cytology reveals high-grade SIL require a colposcopy. If the colposcopy is adequate and a biopsy confirms the presence of a high-grade lesion, immediate treatment is indicated.

SIL can be treated with either ablative therapy (ie, laser ablation or cryosurgery) or by excisional methods (ie, shallow laser conization or a loop electrosurgical excision procedure [LEEP]). Although ablative therapy results in many fewer complications, excisional methods offer the advantage of obtaining tissue for further histologic evaluation. LEEP uses thin wire loop electrodes to excise the entire transformation zone and any lesions it may contain.[54] This procedure requires less expensive equipment and causes less morbidity than laser conization.

STAGING

When a diagnosis of invasive cervical carcinoma is histically confirmed, the disease should be staged prior to initiating treatment. The most widely used staging system is the one developed by the International Federation of Gynecology and Obstetrics (FIGO; see Table 2). The FIGO system uses the findings from the physical examination, colposcopy, biopsies, ECC, x-ray examination of the lungs and skeleton, intravenous pyelography (IVP), cystoscopy, and proctosigmoidoscopy to determine the clinical stage.

In difficult cases, the pelvic examination ideally should be performed by several examiners while the patient is under general anesthesia. An IVP is recommended for all patients to rule out ureteral obstruction. Cystoscopy should be performed for disease stage IB or higher, and proctosigmoidoscopy can be limited to cases of clinically suspected rectal involvement or a history of diverticulitis. Involvement by a tumor should be confirmed by a biopsy. When qualified examiners disagree on the stage of the disease, the lower stage should be assigned.

The results of other diagnostic examinations, together with the operative findings, may be used to plan treatment; however, they should not be used to assign the clinical stage. These diagnostic examinations include computerized tomography (CT) scanning, magnetic resonance imaging (MRI), lymphangiography, and laparoscopy. A CT scan is sometimes used in place of an IVP to evaluate whether obstructive uropathy is present. The technique is helpful in determining para-aortic node involvement and is sometimes used to guide needle biopsies of these nodes. An MRI provides more accurate information about stromal and parametrial infiltration. A lymphangiogram may help to assess whether pelvic or para-aortic lymph-node metastasis has taken place.

Stage IA tumors, as defined by FIGO, are sometimes referred to as microinvasive carcinoma. Nevertheless, this definition includes cases of stromal invasion ranging from 3.1 to 5.0 mm deep, with a significant risk of lymph-node metastasis (6.2%).[55] Prior to the introduction of the FIGO system, the Society of Gynecological Oncologists (SGO) proposed a more restrictive definition, stating that a microinvasive lesion is one that invades the stroma to

TABLE 2

FIGO Staging of Carcinoma of the Cervix Uteri

Preinvasive carcinoma

Stage 0 Carcinoma in situ, intraepithelial carcinoma (cases of stage 0 tumors should not be included in any therapeutic statistics)

Invasive carcinoma

Stage I Carcinoma is strictly confined to the cervix (extension to the corpus should be disregarded)

Ia: Invasive cancer identified only microscopically; all gross lesions, even with superficial invasion, are stage Ib cancers; invasion is limited to measured stromal invasion with a maximum depth of 5 mm and no wider than 7 mm [a]

Ia1: Measured invasion of stroma no greater than 3 mm in depth and no wider than 7 mm

Ia2: Measured invasion of stroma greater than 3 mm and no greater than 5 mm in depth and no wider than 7 mm

Ib: Clinical lesions confined to the cervix or preclinical lesions greater than Ia

Ib1: Clinical lesions no greater than 4 cm in size

Ib2: Clinical lesions greater than 4 cm in size

Stage II Carcinoma extends beyond the cervix but has not extended on to the pelvic wall; the carcinoma involves the vagina, but not as far as the lower third

IIa: No obvious parametrial involvement

IIb: Obvious parametrial involvement

Stage III Carcinoma has extended to the pelvic wall; on rectal examination, there is no cancer-free space between the tumor and pelvic wall; the tumor involves the lower third of the vagina; all cases with a hydronephrosis or nonfunctioning kidney should be included, unless they are known to be due to other cause

IIIa: No extension onto the pelvic wall, but involvement of the lower third of the vagina

IIIb: Extension onto the pelvic wall or hydronephrosis or nonfunctioning kidney

Stage IV Carcinoma has extended beyond the true pelvis or has clinically involved the mucosa of the bladder or rectum

IVa: Spread of the growth to adjacent organs

IVb: Spread to distant organs

FIGO = International Federation of Gynecologists and Oncologists

[a] The depth of invasion should not be more than 5 mm taken from the base of the epithelium, either surface or glandular, from which it originates. Vascular space involvement, either venous or lymphatic, should not alter the staging.

Adapted from Shepherd JH: Staging announcement—FIGO staging of gynecologic cancers; cervical and vulva. Int J Gyn Cancer 5:319, 1995.

TABLE 3

Worldwide 5-Year Actuarial Survival Rates for Cervical Carcinoma by FIGO Stage

Stage	Number of patients	5-year survival (%)
I	12,143	81.6
II	10,285	61.3
III	8,206	36.7
IV	1,378	12.1

FIGO = International Federation of Gynecology and Obstetrics

Adapted from Petterson F (ed): Annual report on the results of treatment in gynecological cancer. Int J Obstet 36 (suppl):35, 1991.

a maximum depth of 3 mm beneath the basement membrane, with no lymphatic or vascular involvement.[56] The SGO definition is more widely used because it identifies tumors with a very low potential for metastasis (0.2%).[55] In such cases, lymph-node dissection is not required.

A recent revision of the FIGO staging divides stage 1b disease into 1b1 and 1b2 based on the size of the tumor. This change reflects the significance of tumor size in the management and prognosis of early-stage disease.

PROGNOSIS

The disease stage is an important factor that affects long-term survival (see Table 3). Clinical stage correlates with tumor burden as well as with the risk for lymph node and distant metastases.[57] Other gross tumor characteristics that have been shown to affect survival include tumor size and volume,[58,59] endometrial extension,[60] and bilateral parametrial involvement.[58]

In surgically treated patients, Burghardt et al[59] reported that tumor volume, determined by MRI, was a better prognostic indicator than the FIGO disease stage. Five-year survival ranged from 91% in patients with tumors smaller than 2.5 cm³ to 48% for patients with tumors larger than 50 cm³. Grimard et al[60] reported that the decreased survival rate associated with endometrial extension of the tumor was seen only in patients with stage IB disease. Decreased survival rate for patients having bilateral parametrial extension, compared with patients having only unilateral involvement, was reported for stage IIB disease.[61]

The effect of histologic cell type on prognosis is discussed at the beginning of this chapter in the section on pathology. Other histologic features that have been correlated with a decrease in the disease-free interval in patients with stage IB disease include increasing depth of tumor invasion and lymph-vascular space involvement.[62,63]

The presence of periaortic and pelvic lymph-node metastases results in lower survival rates. Tanaka et al[64] reported a 10% 5-year survival for surgically treated patients with periaortic lymph-node metastasis, 49% for those with involved pelvic lymph nodes, and 92% for patients with negative lymph-node involvement. This study also revealed a correlation between the number of disease-positive pelvic nodes and survival. The 5-year survival rate was 62% for those with one node positive for tumor, 36% for two positive nodes, 20% for three or four positive nodes, and 0% for those with five or more positive nodes.

A higher rate of recurrence was seen in patients with an S-phase fraction greater than or equal to 20%.[65] The overexpression of the *HER-2/neu*[66] and c-*myc*[67] oncogenes has been found to be associated with a poor prognosis.

The effect of various patient factors on prognosis has also been investigated. The results of studies on the effect of age were variable. In patients treated with radiation therapy, both anemia (Hb < 12 g/dL)[68] and thrombocytosis (> 400,000/μL)[69] have been associated with decreased survival rates. A lower survival rate was also reported for patients whose oral temperatures were greater than 100°F. In this study, the etiology of the fever remained uncertain for the majority of patients.[70]

TREATMENT

General Principles

The primary therapy for most cases of cervical carcinoma consists of surgery and/or radiation therapy. Treatment should be individualized based on the extent of disease and patient characteristics.

Surgery: Primary surgical management for invasive cervical cancer can be curative for patients with stage I through stage IIA disease. Which procedure is appropriate depends on the extent of disease and can range from a cervical conization to a radical hysterectomy with bilateral lymphadenectomy.

Cervical conization is usually used for diagnostic purposes but may occasionally be adequate therapy for patients with microinvasive carcinoma. A total extrafascial hysterectomy entails the excision of the uterus and cervix plus a small vaginal cuff. A radical hysterectomy with pelvic lymphadenectomy requires a more extensive dissection, with the en bloc removal of the uterus, cervix, parametrium, pelvic lymph nodes, and the upper portion of the vagina.

Pelvic exenteration is an option in some patients who develop central disease recurrence following primary radiation therapy. A total exenteration is usually required, and this involves the removal of the vagina, cervix, uterus, fallopian tubes, ovaries, bladder, and rectum. An anterior exenteration spares the rectum and may be used when disease recurrence is confined to the anterior vagina, cervix, or bladder. A posterior exenteration spares the bladder and is indicated for recurrent disease to the posterior fornix and rectovaginal septum.

Radiotherapy: Radiation therapy may be used as primary treatment for all stages of cervical cancer. Careful planning of treatment is necessary to maximize the radiation dose to the tumor while minimizing the risk of complications to the surrounding tissues. A combination of external and intracavitary irradiation is used for most stages of disease, with the exception of stage IA, in which intracavitary treatment alone is adequate. The dose of radiation is reported using two reference points, with both external and intracavitary sources contributing to each point. Point A is located 2 cm lateral and superior to the external os of the cervix. This point is used to express the dose delivered to the paracervical tissues. Point B is located 3 cm lateral to point A and corresponds to the pelvic sidewall.

External pelvic irradiation (teletherapy) should be delivered by a linear accelerator using portals encompassing the whole pelvis with additional boosts to the parametrium. Daily doses range from 150 to 200 cGy. External irradiation will result in a decrease in the anatomic distortion resulting from the tumor, thus allowing a more effective dose delivery with subsequent intracavitary irradiation.

Brachytherapy is most often given through intracavitary irradiation. This is delivered using applicators consisting of an intrauterine tandem, together with vaginal ovoids placed beside the cervix. The positions of the applicators are verified by radiographs. The applicators are then loaded with the radioactive isotope (usually cesium 137). This "afterloading" is performed either manually or by remote control. Most patients require two separate brachytherapy insertions, which are given 1 to 3 weeks apart. Occasionally, interstitial implants are also used for brachytherapy.

Carcinoma In Situ: Patients with only ectocervical lesions can be treated with cryotherapy, LEEP, laser therapy, or conization. Patients with endocervical involvement are treated with cervical conization if preservation of fertility is desired. A total abdominal or vaginal hysterectomy is the treatment of choice for women past reproductive age, especially if the lesion involves the inner cone margin. If surgery is contraindicated, a single intracavitary radiation treatment delivering an average dose of 4,612 cGy to point A has been shown to be adequate therapy.[71]

Stage IA: The preferred treatment for stage IA cancer of the uterine cervix is surgery. In cases where tumor invasion is less than or equal to 3.0 mm without lymph-vascular space involvement (microinvasive carcinoma), a total extrafascial hysterectomy is recommended.

Conization alone may be adequate treatment for these patients (to preserve fertility), but they must be closely followed up. The risk of lymphatic involvement in microinvasive carcinoma is less than 1%; therefore, a lymph-node dissection is not required. If the tumor invasion is greater than 3.0 mm or if the tumor extends beyond the cone margins, then a radical hysterectomy with pelvic node dissection is recommended.

Patients with stage IA disease who are not surgical candidates can be treated with intracavitary radiation therapy alone,[71] receiving a dose to point A of 6,000 to 7,500 cGy.

Stages IB and IIA: Selected small-volume stage IB and early-stage IIA disease can both be managed by radical hysterectomy or radiation therapy. Patient survival rates for these stages have been equivalent with either modality.[72] Treatment choice can be affected by various factors. In premenopausal or sexually active patients, surgery may be preferred because ovarian function and vaginal pliability can be preserved. Patients with medical contraindications to extensive surgery can usually tolerate radiation therapy. Table 4 summarizes the sequelae from both modalities.

Patients with stage IB disease and a tumor size greater than 3.0 cm have been reported to have lower recurrence rates and fewer complications when treated with radiation therapy instead of surgery.[73] Patients with para-aortic node involvement and patients with stage IIA disease and extensive extracervical involvement should be treated with radiation therapy. Radiation therapy usually consists of both external beam and intracavitary irradiation with a dose of 6,500 to 8,500 cGy to point A, but higher doses may be required for those with bulky endocervical carcinoma (at least 6-cm-diameter barrel-shaped cervix). In patients found to have disease-positive lymph nodes after a radical hysterectomy, total pelvic irradiation is recommended.

Stages IIB, III, and IV: The treatment for stages IIB, III, and IVA disease is radiation therapy. The usual regimen consists of external beam irradiation to the whole pelvis with two or more intracavitary applications delivering a dose of 7,000 to 9,000 cGy to point A.

Studies by the Gynecologic Oncology Group (GOG) have indicated that the concomitant use of hydroxyurea

TABLE 4

Comparison of Surgery vs Radiation Therapy for Stage IB/IIA Cancer of the Cervix

Criterion	Surgery	Radiation therapy
Survival	85%	85%
Serious complications	Urologic fistulae in 1%–2%	Intestinal and urinary strictures and fistulae in 1.4%–5.3%
Vagina	Initially shortened, but may lengthen with regular intercourse	Fibrosis and possible stenosis, particularly in postmenopausal patients
Ovaries	Can be conserved	Destroyed
Chronic effects	Bladder atony in 3%	Radiation fibrosis of bowel and bladder in 6%–8%
Applicability	Best candidates are < 65 years old, < 200 lb, and in good health	All patients are potential candidates
Surgical mortality	1%	< 1% (arising from pulmonary embolism during intracavitary therapy)

Adapted from Hatch KD: Cervix cancer, in Berek JS, Hacker NF (eds): Practical Gynecologic Oncology, 2nd Ed, pp 243–283, Baltimore, Williams & Wilkins, 1994

as a radiosensitizer resulted in an improved complete response rate, a longer progression-free interval, and a better survival rate in patients with stage IIIB and IVA disease.[74,75] Hydroxyurea was given at a dose of 80 mg/kg twice weekly during radiation.

Patients with stage IVB disease are treated palliatively with radiation therapy or chemotherapy.

Recurrent Disease: The treatment of recurrent cervical cancer will depend on the previous primary therapy and the site of tumor recurrence. Local disease recurrence after radical surgery can be managed with a combination of external and intracavitary irradiation. Additional interstitial irradiation may also be required. A 25% 5-year survival rate has been reported for these patients treated with salvage radiotherapy.[76] Patients who develop locally recurrent disease after primary radiotherapy are candidates for pelvic exenteration if the tumor does not extend to the pelvic wall. A 6.3% operative mortality rate has been reported for this procedure with a 5-year survival rate of 50%.[77] Chemotherapy may also be used for palliation.

Management During Pregnancy: The treatment of cervical cancer diagnosed during pregnancy depends on the stage of the disease and the age of gestation. When cervical carcinoma is diagnosed during the first trimester, immediate treatment appropriate for the stage of disease is recommended, and this will result in the termination of the pregnancy. Patients in the second trimester who have stage I disease may delay treatment until fetal maturity is reached without compromising treatment outcome.[78] Women who have more advanced disease should undergo immediate treatment. Delayed treatment is an option for all stages of the disease if the diagnosis is made during the third trimester.

Invasive Carcinoma Found at Simple Hysterectomy: Cervical carcinoma diagnosed in patients after a simple hysterectomy requires further therapy if found at a stage beyond microinvasive disease. Treatment options include radiotherapy or a second operation, depending on the extent of the tumor. Surgery would involve radical excision of parametrial tissue, cardinal ligaments, and vaginal cuff and a pelvic node dissection.

Ureteral Obstruction: If an untreated patient presents with ureteral obstruction and has no evidence of distant disease, ureteral catheters should be placed and radiotherapy with curative intent should be started. In patients with metastatic disease, treatment options include ureteral stents, palliative radiotherapy, chemotherapy, or supportive care only.

The Role of Chemotherapy

Because surgery and radiation therapy have been highly effective in treating most cases of early cervical carcinoma, chemotherapy has traditionally been used for the palliative management of advanced or recurrent disease that can no longer be managed by the other two modalities. However, various factors complicate the use of chemotherapy in patients with such disease. Prior radiation treatment can affect the blood supply to the involved field, which may result in decreased drug delivery to the tumor site. Pelvic irradiation also reduces bone marrow reserves, thus limiting the tolerable dose of most chemotherapeutic agents. Radiation may produce some of its cytotoxic effects through the same mechanism as alkylating agents, and it is thus thought to result in cross-resistance with some chemotherapeutic agents. A significant number of patients with advanced disease may also have impaired renal function, further limiting the use of certain chemotherapeutic regimens.

Among the chemotherapeutic agents used for cervical cancer (see Table 5), the ones that have demonstrated the most consistent activity as single agents are cisplatin

(Platinol) and ifosfamide (Ifex).[79] Cisplatin has been the most extensively evaluated single agent for cervical carcinoma. A dose of 100 mg/m^2 has been shown to have a higher response rate (31%) than a dose of 50 mg/m^2 (21%), but the higher dose was associated with increased toxicity, and the overall survival rates for the two dose groups did not differ significantly.[80] A cisplatin infusion over 24 hours is better tolerated than a 2-hour infusion, with no significant change in efficacy.[81] Ifosfamide has been reported to produce response rates ranging from 33% to 50% in various dose schedules.[82] A dose of 1.5 g/m^2 over 30 minutes for 5 days (administered with mesna [Mesnex]) produced a 40% overall response rate and a 20% complete response rate. One of the more promising new agents is irinotecan (CPT-11), a semisynthetic camptothecin analog that causes inhibition of topoisomerase I. Takeuchi et al[83] reported a response rate of 24% for cervical cancer. Preliminary data from a phase II trial at The University of Texas M. D. Anderson Cancer Center showed a 27% response rate.[84] Paclitaxel (Taxol) has shown some activity in squamous-cell cancer of the cervix, producing response rates of 14% to 17% (personal communication, McGuire W and Kudelka AP, 1995). Lower response rates are generally seen in patients who have had prior chemotherapy. Responses are also decreased in previously irradiated sites. The duration of response with single agents is brief, usually ranging from 4 to 6 months with survival durations ranging from 6 to 9 months.

Various combination chemotherapy regimens have been evaluated in phase II trials, and high response rates (greater than 50%) were seen even in patients who had prior radiation therapy. The results of some of these trials are listed in Table 6.[85–88] In the study of Buxton et al,[85] a subset analysis showed a response rate of 72% for the combination of bleomycin (Blenoxane)/ifosfamide/cisplatin in patients with tumors located in previously irradiated sites. However, there has not been an adequate phase III trial to determine whether any of the combination regimens offer a significant survival benefit over single-agent cisplatin.

The use of chemotherapy in the neoadjuvant (primary) setting for cervical carcinoma has also been investigated. Four randomized trials, wherein cisplatin-based combination chemotherapy followed by radiation therapy was compared with radiation therapy alone for disease stages ranging from IIB to IVA, failed to show any survival benefit from chemotherapy.[89–92] The study by Souhami et al[89] even showed increased toxicity and decreased survival rate in the neoadjuvant arm. The trial by Tattersall et al[92] also reported significantly inferior local disease

TABLE 5

Single-Agent Chemotherapy for Cervical Carcinoma

	Response (%)
Alkylating agents	
Cyclophosphamide	38/251 (15)
Chlorambucil	11/44 (25)
Melphalan	4/20 (20)
Ifosfamide	25/84 (29)
Mitolactol	16/55 (29)
Heavy metal complexes	
Cisplatin	182/785 (23)
Carboplatin	27/175 (15)
Antitumor antibiotics	
Doxorubicin	33/205 (16)
Bleomycin	19/176 (11)
Mitomcin	5/23 (22)
Antimetabolites	
Fluorouracil	29/142 (20)
Methotrexate	17/96 (18)
Hydroxyurea	0/14 (0)
Plant alkaloids	
Vincristine	10/55 (18)
Vinblastine	2/20 (10)
Etoposide	0/31 (0)
Miscellaneous agents	
Altretamine	12/64 (19)
Irinotecan (CPT-11)	13/55 (24)
Paclitaxel	
CCOP [a]	3/21 (14)
GOG [b]	9/52 (17)
Docetaxel [a]	1/13 (8)

[a] Personal communication: A. P. Kudelka, Gynecologic Medical Oncology, M. D. Anderson Cancer Center, Houston, Texas, 1995.
[b] Personal communication: W. McGuire, Medical Oncology, Emory University, Atlanta, Georgia, 1995.

CCOP = Community Clinical Oncology Program
GOG = Gynecologic Oncology Group

Adapted from Thigpen T, Vance RB, Khansur T: Carcinoma of the uterine cervix: current status and future directions. Semin Oncology 21 (suppl 2):45, 1994, and from Vermorken JB: The role of chemotherapy in squamous cell carcinoma of the uterine cervix: A review. Int J Gynecol Cancer 3:130, 1993.

control and survival rates in the patients randomized to receive primary chemotherapy, compared with those who received radiotherapy alone.[92]

Theoretically, toxic effects from neoadjuvant chemotherapy may prevent the delivery of adequate doses of radiation, and the issue of cross-resistance between these

TABLE 6

Combination Chemotherapy for Advanced or Recurrent Cervical Carcinoma

Chemotherapy regimen	Number of patients	Prior radiation therapy (%)	Complete response rate (%)	Overall response rate (%)
Bleomycin/ifosfamide/cisplatin[85]	49	86	20	69
Bleomycin/ifosfamide/carboplatin[86]	21	49	23	60
Vinblastine/bleomycin/cisplatin[87]	33	66	18	67
Fluorouracil/doxorubicin/ vincristine/cyclophosphamide[88]	31	87	9	58

two modalities was mentioned earlier. Neoadjuvant chemotherapy may be more suitable when it is combined with surgery. Such therapy has been noted to result in a decrease in lymph-node involvement, compared with the rate seen in historical controls. However, a randomized trial by Sardi et al[93] of patients with stage IB bulky disease failed to show any benefit in overall survival for patients who received neoadjuvant cisplatin/vincristine (Oncovin)/bleomycin prior to surgery and radiation therapy, compared with patients who had surgery and/or postoperative radiation therapy only.

Adjuvant chemotherapy has not been proven to benefit patients found to have pelvic lymph-node involvement after a radical hysterectomy. A randomized trial by Tattersal et al[94] failed to show any improvement in survival and relapse rates when adjuvant cisplatin/vinblastine/bleomycin was given to this group of patients.

The use of intra-arterial chemotherapy theoretically offers the advantage of increased drug concentration at the tumor site as well as decreased systemic delivery of the drug if a first-pass effect is present. Most response rates obtained with various regimens have not been superior to systemic chemotherapy.[95-97] Furthermore, catheter-related complications have been encountered and drug-related toxicity is still significant with intra-arterial chemotherapy.

Biologic agents have recently been found to have activity in cervical cancer. Lippman et al[98,99] reported an overall response rate of 50%, with a 12% complete response rate, in 32 previously untreated patients who had locally advanced cervical squamous-cell carcinoma and were treated with a combination of 13-*cis*-retinoic acid, 1 mg/kg orally, and alpha interferon (IFN-α), 6 million units subcutaneously, administered daily for at least 2 months. Of the 16 patients who responded, 9 eventually had disease progression, after a median response duration of 3 months. It is notable that only minimal toxicity was noted with this regimen.

Interferons and retinoids both have antiviral as well as immunoregulatory properties and are known to modulate malignant cell differentiation and proliferation. Furthermore, they are known to inhibit angiogenesis. Results from serial biopsies of the responders in the Lippman study showed a significant reduction in the amount of blood vessels.[100] Preliminary data from an ongoing trial using an induction regimen consisting of 13-*cis*-retinoic acid and IFN-α followed by concomitant radiotherapy, compared with radiotherapy alone, show a 42% response rate after the induction regimen, thus confirming the results of the previous trial.[101] The use of these biologic agents together with cisplatin is also being investigated.

Posttherapy Surveillance

Tumor regression may continue for up to 3 months after a patient completes radiation therapy, so response must be confirmed by monthly examinations during this period. Because the majority of recurrences appear within the first 2 years after treatment, patients should be evaluated every 3 months during that interval and less frequently thereafter. The physical examination should include palpation of the supraclavicular and inguinal lymph nodes, a breast examination, and a rectovaginal examination. An annual Pap smear and chest x-ray are also recommended.

If there are no contraindications, low-dose estrogen (eg, Premarin, 0.3 or 0.625 mg/d) and a progestational agent (eg, medroxyprogesterone [Provera], 2.5 or 5.0 mg/d) should be used indefinitely. The progestational agent is omitted in patients who have had a hysterectomy. An estrogen-containing vaginal cream (eg, Premarin) may be helpful for patients who still have dryness and dyspareunia. Sexual activity may be resumed after the completion of radiation therapy. For sexually inactive patients, use of a vaginal dilator may help maintain vaginal patency and allow better posttherapy surveillance.

CONCLUSION

The detection of HPV as an etiologic agent in cervical neoplasia has greatly advanced the understanding of this disease process. Interventions such as immunizations aimed against high-risk HPV types may have a future role in the prevention of cervical neoplasia. HPV screening may also have a role in the management of CIN and is under investigation.

Although surgery and radiation therapy have been very successful in the treatment of early-stage cervical carcinoma, the prognosis for advanced and recurrent disease remains poor, mainly because there is no effective systemic therapy. Cervical cytologic screening should be promoted. Other priorities should include the evaluation of new therapeutic agents through phase II trials and comparisons of combination chemotherapy regimens to single agents in adequate phase III trials. The use of neoadjuvant systemic therapy, including the biologic agents, should be explored further.

REFERENCES

1. Devesa SS, Silverman DT, Young JL, et al: Cancer incidence and mortality trends among whites in the United States, 1947–84. J Natl Cancer Inst 79:701—770, 1987.

2. Guzick DS: Efficacy of screening for cervical cancer: A review. Am J Public Health 68:125–134, 1978.

3. Wingo PA, Tong T, Bolden S: Cancer Statistics, 1995. CA Cancer J Clin 45:8–30, 1995.

4. Parkin DM, Muir CS, Whelan SL, et al (eds): Cancer Incidence in Five Continents, Volume VI. Lyon, International Agency for Research on Cancer, 1992.

5. Zaino RJ, Ward S, Delgado G, et al: Histopathologic predictors of the behaviour of surgically treated stage IB squamous cell carcinoma of the cervix: A Gynecologic Oncology Group study. Cancer 69:1750–1758, 1992.

6. Goellner JR: Carcinoma of the cervix: Clinical pathologic correlation of 196 cases. Am J Clin Pathol 66:775–785, 1976.

7. Greer BE, Figge DC, Tamimi HK, et al: Stage IB adenocarcinoma of the cervix treated by radical hysterectomy and pelvic lymph node dissection. Am J Obstet Gynecol 160: 1509–1514, 1989.

8. Young RH, Scully RE: Invasive adenocarcinoma and related tumors of the uterine cervix. Semin Diagn Pathol 7:205–227, 1990.

9. Eifel PJ, Morris M, Oswald J, et al: Adenocarcinoma of the uterine cervix. Cancer 65:2507–2514, 1990.

10. Hale RJ, Wilcox FL, Buckley CH, et al: Prognostic factors in uterine cervical carcinoma: A clinicopathological analysis. Int J Gynecol Cancer 1:19–23, 1991.

11. Anton-Culver H, Bloss JD, Bringman D, et al: Comparison of adenocarcinoma and squamous cell carcinoma of the uterine cervix: A population based epidemiologic study. Am J Obstet Gynecol 186:1507–1514, 1992.

12. Kurman RJ, Norris HJ, Wilkinson E: Atlas of Tumor Pathology, series 3: Vol 4. Tumors of the cervix, vagina, and vulva. Washington, DC, Armed Forces Institute of Pathology, 1992.

13. Shingleton HM, Gor H, Bradley DH, et al: Adenocarcinoma of the cervix: I. Clinical evaluation and pathologic features. Am J Obstet Gynecol 139:799–814, 1981.

14. Yazigi R, Sandstad J, Munoz AK, et al: Adenosquamous carcinoma of the cervix: Prognosis in stage IB. Obstet Gynecol 75:1012–1015, 1990.

15. Maier RC, Norris HJ: Glassy cell carcinoma of the cervix. Obstet Gynecol 60:219–224, 1982.

16. Van Nagell JR, Powell DE, Gallion HH, et al: Small cell carcinoma of the uterine cervix. Cancer 62:1586–1593, 1988.

17. Harris RWC, Brinton LA, Cowdell RH, et al: Characteristics of women with dysplasia or carcinoma in situ of the cervix uteri. Br J Cancer 42:359–369, 1980.

18. Rotkin ID: Epidemiology of cancer of the cervix: III. Sexual characteristics of a cervical cancer population. Am J Public Health 57:815–829, 1967.

19. Schiffman MH, Bauer HM, Hoover RN, et al: Epidemiologic evidence showing that human papillomavirus infection causes most cervical intraepithelial neoplasia. J Natl Cancer Inst 85:958–964, 1993.

20. Lorincz AT, Reid R, Jenson AB, et al: Human papillomavirus infection of the cervix: Relative risk associations of 15 common anogenital types. Obstet Gynecol 79:328–337, 1992.

21. Reid R, Greenberg M, Jenson AB, et al: Sexually transmitted papillomaviral infections: I. The anatomic distribution and pathologic grade of neoplastic lesions associated with different viral types. Am J Obstet Gynecol 156:212–222, 1987.

22. Cullen AP, Reid R, Campion MJ, et al: Analysis of the physical state of different human papillomavirus DNAs in intraepithelial and invasive cervical neoplasms. J Virol 65:606–612, 1991.

23. Scheffner M, Werness BA, Hulbregtse JM, et al: The E6 oncoprotein encoded by human papillomavirus types 16 and 18 promotes the degradation of p53. Cell 63:1129–1136, 1990.

24. Hoppe-Seyler F, Butz K: Repression of endogenous p53 transactivation function in HeLa cervical carcinoma cells by human papillomavirus type 16 E6, human mdm-2, and mutant p53. J Virol 67:3111–3117, 1993.

25. Dyson N, Howley P, Münger K, et al: The human papillomavirus 16 E7 oncoprotein is able to bind to the retinoblastoma gene product. Science 243:934–937, 1989.

26. Hartwell LH, Kastan MB: Cell cycle control and cancer. Science 266:1821–1828, 1994.

27. Kessis TD, Slebos RJ, Nelson WG, et al: Human papillomavirus 16 E6 expression disrupts the p53-mediated cellular response to DNA damage. Proc Natl Acad Sci USA 90:3988–3992, 1993.

28. Demers GW, Foster SA, Halbert CL, et al: Growth arrest by induction of p53 in DNA damaged keratinocytes is bypassed by human papillomavirus 16 E7. Proc Natl Acad Sci USA 91:4382–4386, 1994.

29. Paquette RL, Lee YY, Wilczynski SP, et al: Mutations of p53 and human papillomavirus infection in cervical carcinoma. Cancer 72:1272–1280, 1993.

30. Schneider V, Kay S, Lee HM: Immunosuppression as a high-risk factor in the development of condyloma acuminatum and squamous neoplasia of the cervix. Acta Cytol 27:220–224, 1983.

31. Sillman F, Stanek A, Sedis A, et al: The relationship between human papillomavirus and lower genital intraepithelial neoplasia in immunosuppressed women. Am J Obstet Gynecol 150:300–308, 1984.

32. Halpert R, Fruchter RG, Sedlis A: Human papillomavirus and lower genital neoplasia in renal transplant patients. Obstet Gynecol 68:251, 1986.

33. Vermund SH, Kelley KF, Klein RS, et al: High risk of human papillomavirus infection and cervical squamous intraepithelial lesions among women with symptomatic human immunodeficiency virus infection. Am J Obstet Gynecol 165:392–400, 1991.

34. Schafer A, Friedmann W, Mielke M, et al: The increased frequency of cervical dysplasia-neoplasia in women infected with the

human immunodeficiency virus is related to the degree of immunosuppression. Am J Obstet Gynecol 164:593–599, 1991.

35. Maiman M, Fruchter RG, Serur E, et al: Recurrent cervical intraepithelial neoplasia in human immunodeficiency virus–seropositive women. Obstet Gynecol 82:170–174, 1993.

36. Maiman M, Fruchter RG, Guy L, et al: Human immunodeficiency virus infection and invasive cervical carcinoma. Cancer 71:402–406, 1993.

37. Verson SD, Hart CE, Reeves WC, et al: The HIV-1 tat protein enhances E2-dependent human papillomavirus 16 transcription. Virus Res 27:133–145, 1993.

38. Burger MPM, Hollema H, Gouw ASH, et al: Cigarette smoking and human papillomavirus in patients with reported cervical cytological abnormality. Br Med J 306:749–752, 1993.

39. Richart RM: Cervical intraepithelial neoplasia, in Somers S (ed): Pathology Annual, pp 301-329. East Norwalk, Connecticut, Appleton-Century-Crofts, 1973.

40. Richart RM: A modified terminology for cervical intraepithelial neoplasia. Obstet Gynecol 75:131–133, 1990.

41. Richart RM, Wright TC: Controversies in the management of low-grade cervical intraepithelial neoplasia. Cancer 71:1413–1421, 1993.

42. Nasiell K, Roger V, Nasiell M: Behaviour of mild cervical dysplasia during long-term follow-up. Obstet Gynecol 67:665–669, 1986.

43. Nasiell K, Nasiell M, Vaclavinková V: Behaviour of moderate cervical dysplasia during long-term follow-up. Obstet Gynecol 61:609–614, 1983.

44. Barron BA, Cahill MC, Richart RM: A statistical model of the natural history of cervical neoplastic disease: The duration of carcinoma in situ. Gynecol Oncol 6:196–205, 1978.

45. Carlson V, Delclos L, Fletcher GH, et al: Distant metastasis in squamous-cell carcinoma of the uterine cervix. Radiology 88: 961–966, 1967.

46. Fink DJ: Change in the American Cancer Society checkup guidelines for detection of cervical cancer. Cancer 38:127, 1988.

47. Gay JD, Donaldson LD, Goellner JR: False-negative results in cervical cytologic studies. Acta Cytol 29:1043–1046, 1985.

48. Wilkinson EJ: Pap smears and screening for cervical neoplasia. Clin Obstet Gynecol 33:817–825, 1990.

49. Papanicolaou GN, Trout HF: Diagnosis of uterine cancer by the vaginal smear. New York, The Commonwealth Fund, 1943.

50. National Cancer Institute Workshop: The 1988 Bethesda System for reporting cervical/vaginal cytological diagnoses. JAMA 262:931–934, 1989.

51. Ismail SM, Colclough AB, Dinnen JS, et al: Reporting cervical intraepithelial neoplasia (CIN): Intra- and interpathologist variation and factors associated with disagreement. Histopathology 16:371–376, 1990.

52. Sherman ME, Schiffman MH, Erozan YS, et al: The Bethesda System: A proposal for reporting abnormal cervical smears based on the reproducibility of cytopathologic diagnoses. Arch Pathol Lab Med 116:1155–1158, 1992.

53. Cox JT, Schiffman MH, Winzelberg AJ, et al: An evaluation of human papillomavirus testing as part of referral to colposcopy clinics. Obstet Gynecol 80:389–395, 1992.

54. Wright TC, Gagnon S, Richart RM, et al: Treatment of cervical intraepithelial neoplasia using the loop electrosurgical excision procedure. Obstet Gynecol 79:173–178, 1991.

55. DePriest PD, van Nagell JR, Powell DE: Microinvasive cervical carcinoma. Clin Obstet Gynecol 33:846–851, 1990.

56. Creasman WF, Fetter BF, Clarke–Pearson DL, et al: Management of stage IA carcinoma of the cervix. Am J Obstet Gynecol 153:164–172, 1985.

57. Fagundes H, Perez CA, Grigsby PW, et al: Distant metastases after irradiation alone in carcinoma of the uterine cervix. Int J Radiat Oncol Biol Phys 24:197–204, 1992.

58. Stehman FB, Bundy BN, DiSaia PJ, et al: Carcinoma of the cervix treated with radiation therapy: I. A multi-variate analysis of prognostic variables in the Gynecologic Oncology Group. Cancer 67:2776–2785, 1991.

59. Burghardt E, Baltzer J, Tulusan AH, et al: Results of surgical treatment of 1028 cervical cancers studied with volumetry. Cancer 70:648–655, 1992.

60. Grimard L, Genest P, Girard A, et al: Prognostic significance of endometrial extension in carcinoma of the cervix. Gynecol Oncol 31:301–309, 1988.

61. Coia L, Won M, Lanciano R, et al: The patterns of care outcome study for cancer of the uterine cervix: Results of the second national practice survey. Cancer 66:2451–2456. 1990.

62. Delgado G, Bundy B, Zaino R, et al: Prospective surgical-pathological study of disease-free interval in patients with stage IB squamous cell carcinoma of the cervix: A Gynecologic Oncology Group study. Gynecol Oncol 38:352–357, 1990.

63. Zaino RJ, Ward S, Delgado G, et al: Histopathologic predictors of the behavior of surgically treated stage IB squamous cell carcinoma of the cervix: A Gynecologic Oncology Group study. Cancer 69:1750–1758, 1992.

64. Tanaka Y, Sawada S, Murata T: Relationship between lymph node metastases and prognosis in patients irradiated postoperatively for carcinoma of the uterine cervix. Acta Radiol Oncol 23:455–459, 1984.

65. Strang P, Eklund G, Stendahl B, et al: S-phase rate as a predictor of early recurrence in carcinoma of the uterine cervix. Anticancer Res 7:807–810, 1987.

66. Berchuck A, Rodriguez G, Kamel A, et al: Expression of epidermal growth factor receptor and HER-2/neu in normal and neoplastic cervix, vulva, and vagina. Obstet Gynecol 76:381–387, 1990.

67. Bourhis J, Le MG, Barrios M, et al: Prognostic value of c-myc proto-oncogene overexpression in early invasive carcinoma of the cervix. J Clin Oncol 8:1789–1796, 1990.

68. Bush RS, Jenkin RDT, Allt WEC, et al: Definitive evidence for hypoxic cells influencing cure in cancer therapy. Br J Cancer 37 (suppl 3):302–306, 1978.

69. Hernandez E, Lavine M, Dunton CJ, et al: Poor prognosis associated with thrombocytosis in patients with cervical cancer. Cancer 69:2975–2977, 1992.

70. Van Herik M: Fever as a complication of radiation therapy for carcinoma of the cervix. Am J Roentgenol Radium Ther Nucl Med 43:104–109, 1965.

71. Grisby PW, Perez CA: Radiotherapy alone for medically inoperable carcinoma of the cervix: Stage IA and carcinoma in situ. Int J Radiat Oncol Biol Phys 21:375–378, 1991.

72. Pilleron JP, Durand JC, Lenoble JC: Carcinoma of the uterine cervix, stages I and II, treated by radiation therapy and extensive surgery (1,000 cases). Cancer 29:593–596, 1972.

73. Eifel PJ, Burke TW, Delclos L, et al: Early stage I adenocarcinoma of the uterine cervix: Treatment results in patients with tumors less than or equal to 4 cm in diameter. Gynecol Oncol 41:199–205, 1991.

74. Hreshchyshyn MM, Aron BS, Boronow RC, et al: Hydroxyurea or placebo combined with radiation to treat stages IIIB and IV cervical cancer confined to the pelvis. Int J Radiat Oncol Biol Phys 5:317–322, 1979.

75. Stehman FR, Bundy RN, Keys H, et al: A randomized trial of hydroxyurea versus misonidazole adjunct to radiation therapy in carcinoma of the cervix: A preliminary report. A Gynecologic Oncol-

ogy Group study. Am J Obstet Gynecol 159:87–94, 1988.

76. Krebs HB, Helmkamp BF, Sevin BU, et al: Recurrent cancer of the cervix following radical hysterectomy and pelvic node dissection. Obstet Gynecol 59:422–427, 1982.

77. Shingleton HM, Soong SJ, Gelder MS, et al: Clinical and histopathological factors predicting recurrence and survival after pelvic exenteration for cancer of the cervix. Obstet Gynecol 73:1027–1034, 1989.

78. Duggan B, Muderspach LI, Roman LD, et al: Cervical cancer in pregnancy: Reporting on planned delay in therapy. Obstet Gynecol 82:598–602, 1993.

79. Thigpen T, Vance RB, Khansur T: Carcinoma of the uterine cervix: Current status and future directions. Semin Oncol 21 (suppl 2):43–54, 1994.

80. Bonomi P, Blessing J, Stehman F, et al: Randomized trial of three cisplatin dose schedules in squamous-cell carcinoma of the cervix: A Gynecologic Oncology Group study. J Clin Oncol 3:1079–1085, 1985.

81. Thigpen T, Blessing JA, DiSaia PJ, et al: A randomized comparison of a rapid versus prolonged (24 hr) infusion of cisplatin in therapy of squamous cell carcinoma of the uterine cervix: A Gynecologic Oncology Group study. Gynecol Oncol 32:198–202, 1989.

82. Coleman R, Jarper P, Gallagher C, et al: A phase II study of ifosfamide in advanced and relapsed carcinoma of the cervix. Cancer Chemother Pharmacol 18:280–283, 1986.

83. Takeuchi S, Noda K, Yakushiji M, et al: Late phase II study of CPT-11, topoisomerase I inhibitor, in advanced cervical carcinoma (abstract). Proc Am Soc Clin Oncol 11:224, 1992.

84. Kavanagh JJ, Kudelka AP, Edwards CE, et al: CPT-11 (Irinotecan): Phase II study in refractory squamous cell carcinoma of the cervix (abstract). Proc Am Assoc Cancer Res 35:234, 1994.

85. Buxton EJ, Meanwell CA, Hilton C, et al: Combination bleomycin, ifosfamide and cisplatin chemotherapy in cervical cancer. J Natl Cancer Inst 81: 359–361, 1989.

86. Murad AM, Triginelli SA, Ribalta JCL: Phase II trial of bleomycin, ifosfamide, and carboplatin in metastatic cervical cancer. J Clin Oncol 12:55–59, 1994.

87. Friedlander M, Kaye SB, Sullivan A, et al: Cervical carcinoma: A drug-responsive tumor-experience with combined cisplatin, vinblastine, and bleomycin therapy. Gynecol Oncol 16:275–281, 1983.

88. Chan WK, Aroney RS, Levi JA, et al: Four-drug combination chemotherapy for advanced cervical carcinoma. Cancer 49:2437–2440, 1982.

89. Souhami L, Gil RA, Allan SE, et al: A randomized trial of chemotherapy followed by pelvic radiation therapy in stage IIIB carcinoma of the cervix. J Clin Oncol 9:970–977, 1991.

90. Chauvergne J, Rohart J, Heron JF, et al: Essai randomise de chimiotherapie initiale dans 151 carcinomes du col uterin localement

etendus. Bull Cancer (Paris) 77:1007–1024, 1990.

91. Tattersall MHN, Ramirez C, Coppelson M: A randomized trial comparing platinum-based chemotherapy followed by radiotherapy vs radiotherapy alone in patients with locally advanced cervical cancer. Int J Gynecol Cancer 2:244–351, 1992.

92. Tattersall MHN, Lorvidhaya V, Vootiprux V, et al: Randomized trial of epirubicin and cisplatin chemotherapy followed by pelvic irradiation in locally advanced cervical cancer. J Clin Oncol 13:444–451, 1995.

93. Sardi J, Sananes C, Giaroli A, et al: The results of a prospective randomized trial with neoadjuvant chemotherapy in stage IB bulky squamous cell carcinoma of the cervix. Gynecol Oncol 49:156–165, 1993.

94. Tattersall MHN, Ramirez C, Coppelson M: A randomized trial of adjuvant chemotherapy after radical hysterectomy in stage IB-IIA cervical cancer patients with pelvic lymph node metastases. Gynecol Oncol 46:175–181, 1992.

95. Swenerton KD, Evers JA, White GW, et al: Intermittent pelvic infusion with vincristine, bleomycin and mitomycin C for advanced recurrent carcinoma of the cervix. Cancer Treat Rep 63:1379–1381, 1979.

96. Chen HSG, Gross GF: Intra-arterial infusion of anticancer drugs: Theoretical aspects of drug delivery and review of response. Cancer Treat Rep 64:31–40, 1980.

97. Kavanagh J, Wallace S, Delclos L, et al: Update of the results of intra-arterial (IA) chemotherapy for advanced squamous cell carcinoma of the cervix. Proc Am Assoc Cancer Res 3:172, 1984.

98. Lippman SM, Kavanagh JJ, Paredes-Espinoza M, et al: 13-cis-retinoic acid plus interferon alpha-2a: Highly active systemic therapy for squamous cell carcinoma of the cervix. J Natl Cancer Inst 84:241–245, 1992.

99. Lippman SM, Kavanagh JJ, Paredes-Espinoza M, et al: 13-cis-retinoic acid plus interferon-alpha 2a in locally advanced squamous cell carcinoma of the cervix. J Natl Cancer Inst 85:499–500, 1993.

100. Ahn WS, Lippman SM, Kavanagh JJ, et al: Biological basis of response of cervical squamous cell carcinoma to alpha interferon and 13-cis-retinoic acid (abstract 446). Proc Am Assoc Cancer Res 34:75, 1993.

101. Kavanagh JJ, Lippman SM, Paredes M, et al: 13-cis-retinoic acid (13cRA), interferon-alpha 2a (IFN-alpha2a) with and without radiotherapy for carcinoma of the cervix (abstract). Int J Gynecol Cancer 3(suppl 1):6, 1993.

102. Kurman RJ (ed): Blaustein's Pathology of the Female Genital Tract, 4th ed. New York, Springer-Verlag, 1994.

103. Hatch, KD: Preinvasive cervical neoplasia. Semin Oncol 21:12–16, 1994.

104. Marcial VA, Marcial LV: Radiation therapy of cervical cancer. Cancer 71 (suppl):1438–1445, 1993.

CHAPTER 25

Tumors of the Uterine Corpus

Saraswati P. Reddy, MD, Andrzej P. Kudelka, MD, Cesar Gonzalez de Leon, MD,
Creighton L. Edwards, MD, *and* John J. Kavanagh, MD
Division of Medicine and Department of Gynecologic Oncology
The University of Texas M. D. Anderson Cancer Center, Houston, Texas

Carcinoma of the endometrium is the most common female pelvic malignancy and the fourth most common cancer in females, after breast, bowel, and lung carcinomas. In 1995, an estimated 32,800 new cases of endometrial carcinoma and 5,900 related deaths will occur in the United States.[1] The relatively low mortality for this cancer is probably due to the fact that in 80% of cases, the disease is diagnosed when it is confined to the uterus. The recent rise in the incidence of endometrial carcinoma may be related to the decreased incidence of cervical carcinoma, prolonged life expectancy, and earlier diagnosis. This disease occurs mostly (75%) in postmenopausal women (mean age, 60 years), and only 4% of women with endometrial cancer are younger than age 40 at diagnosis.[1,2] Tumors of the uterine corpus include adenocarcinomas and their variants and sarcomas.

UTERINE CARCINOMAS

Epidemiology

Several lines of epidemiologic and clinicopathologic evidence support the hypothesis that there are two pathogenetic forms of endometrial carcinoma,[3,4] designated type I (estrogen related) and type II (estrogen independent) (Table 1). The estrogen-related carcinomas are better differentiated and usually grade 1 and stage I. The estrogen-independent carcinomas are often poorly differentiated, present at an advanced stage, occur in older patients (mean age, 66 years), and are rarely associated with endometrial hyperplasia. Unfavorable subtypes, such as serous carcinoma, adenosquamous carcinoma, and clear-cell carcinoma, appear to be estrogen independent.

Clinical evidence indicates that conditions resulting in hyperestrinism predispose patients to endometrial carcinoma. Obesity increases the risk 3- to 10-fold, depending on the degree of weight excess (Table 2). Adipose tissue contains aromatase enzymes that convert the adrenal-derived androstenedione to estrone, which can be converted to estradiol (a more potent estrogen), resulting in endometrial proliferation, hyperplasia, and potentially carcinoma. Polycystic ovarian syndrome, characterized by obesity, anovulation, abnormal bleeding or amenorrhea, hirsutism, and polycystic ovaries, increases the risk of endometrial carcinoma secondary to anovulation. Anovulation results in prolonged periods of estrogen exposure unopposed by a progestational agent. Infertility also is associated with this carcinoma, probably related to anovulation with the resultant unopposed estrogen effect. Use of iatrogenic unopposed contraceptives is another recognized predisposing factor. Other possible factors, such as hypertension and diabetes, are unconfirmed and probably do not independently influence risk.[5]

Hyperplasia is an important characteristic that correlates with low tumor grade and lack of myometrial invasion. Hyperplasia is rated according to the degree of cytologic atypia and is divided into three types: simple, which progresses to carcinoma in 1% of cases; complex, which has a progression rate of 3%; and atypical hyperplasia, which carries a risk of malignant transformation of 10% to 30%.

TABLE I

Pathogenetic Forms of Endometrial Carcinoma

Characteristic	Type I	Type II
Unopposed estrogen	Present	Absent
Menopausal status	Pre- and perimenopausal	Postmenopausal
Hyperplasia	Present	Absent
Atrophy	Absent	Present
Race	White	Black
Grade	Low	High
Myometrial invasion	Minimal	Deep
Specific subtypes	Adenoacanthoma Secretory Ciliated	Adenosquamous Serous Clear cell
Behavior	Stable	Progressive

Adapted from Kurman RJ, Zaimo R, Norris HJ: Endometrial carcinoma, in Kurman RJ (ed): Blaustein's Pathology of the Female Genital Tract, pp 439–486. New York, Springer-Verlag, 1994.

TABLE 2

Risk Factors for Endometrial Carcinoma

Factor	Relative risk
Obesity	
10–21 lb overweight	2
21–50 lb overweight	3
> 50 lb overweight	10
Menopausal estrogen use	4.5–13.9
Oral contraceptives	0.5
Sequential oral contraceptives	Unknown
Diabetes mellitus	2.0
Nulliparity	2× that of a woman with one child 3× that of a woman with five children
Tamoxifen use	7.5
Late menopause	2.4
Early menarche (< 12 years)	1.6–2.4
Polycystic ovarian syndrome	Unknown
Smoking	0.7–0.9

Adapted from Baker TR: Endometrial carcinoma, in Piver MS (ed): Handbook of Gynecologic Oncology, p 142. Boston, Little, Brown, 1995.

The role of tamoxifen in endometrial carcinoma has become a focus of concern. Indeed, in view of the widespread use of tamoxifen as adjuvant therapy for breast cancer, reports of an increased risk of endometrial cancer in users vs nonusers of tamoxifen are worrisome.[6] The findings of some studies suggested not only an increased risk of endometrial cancer in all tamoxifen users (relative risk, 1.3; 95% CI, 0.7 to 2.4) but also an even greater risk for women who had used the drug for longer than 2 years (relative risk, 2.3; 95% CI, 0.9 to 5.9).[7,8] Other studies[9] have confirmed this finding, showing that the frequency of endometrial cancers increases significantly along with relative risk (6.4) if tamoxifen is used for longer than 2 years.[9] Women receiving tamoxifen also show an increase in benign proliferative lesions of the endometrium, endometrial thickening, and Papanicolaou smears with a higher proportion of endometrial cells with nuclear atypia.[10] Tamoxifen is thought to exert these and other effects on the uterus by its partial estrogenic agonist action.[9]

The National Cancer Institute's breast cancer preven-

tion trial is an ongoing landmark study to determine whether tamoxifen prevents breast cancer in women at increased risk of this disease. However, in light of the previous data, the National Cancer Institute is changing the protocol to increase the surveillance for endometrial cancer through endometrial aspiration and yearly pelvic examinations.[11] Of the 4,000 women in the trial, 25 who had taken tamoxifen have been diagnosed with endometrial cancer; of these 25 patients, 5 have died of their disease.[9]

Most studies confirm that tamoxifen may cause potentially malignant changes in the endometrium in postmenopausal women.[12] Consequently, transvaginal ultrasonography can be used to identify women with thickened endometrium who should undergo endometrial sampling for microscopic analysis, but at present, this is quite controversial.[13]

Interestingly, tamoxifen has been used with some success to treat patients with endometrial cancer. Tamoxifen and its metabolite 4-hydroxytamoxifen stimulate some endometrial carcinoma cell lines but inhibit others, as well as some primary cultures of human endometrial carcinoma cells.[9,14] Nevertheless, the possible connection between tamoxifen and endometrial cancer is being sought.

Diagnosis

Although mass screening for endometrial cancer is impractical, screening of high-risk subgroups is justified. These groups include postmenopausal women receiving exogenous estrogens, particularly if they are obese, underwent menopause after age 50, or have coexistent polycystic ovarian disease or a family history of breast, endometrial, or ovarian carcinoma. There is consistent evidence that a family history of breast cancer is associated with a two- to threefold increased risk of breast cancer and that a positive family history of ovarian cancer increases the risk of breast cancer by nearly 50%.[15–18] One other high-risk group also bears mention: women with a family history of hereditary nonpolyposis colorectal cancer, which confers an increased risk of cancer, especially colorectal cancer. It has been recommended that colorectal cancer control programs be expanded to include endometrial cancer, the most common extracolonic cancer observed in hereditary nonpolyposis colorectal cancer families.[18]

Approximately 50% of women with endometrial carcinoma have a positive Papanicolaou smear. Endometrial tissue on a Papanicolaou smear, whether the tissue is normal or abnormal, implies endometrial pathology, but the accuracy of the test for endometrial cancer is poor (25%). Fractional dilatation and curettage provides the maximum amount of tissue from the endometrial cavity, and its accuracy is 90%. All patients suspected of having endometrial carcinoma should undergo an endocervical curettage and an endometrial biopsy. However, if sampling techniques fail to provide sufficient diagnostic information, dilatation and curettage is mandatory. A diagnosis of endometrial hyperplasia on endometrial biopsy does not obviate the need for fractional curettage.[5,19]

Clinical Features

Abnormal vaginal bleeding occurs in 90% of patients, usually in the form of unusual peri- or postmenopausal bleeding. Signs and symptoms of more advanced disease include pelvic pain and leukorrhea. Physical examination commonly reveals an obese, hypertensive, postmenopausal woman, although 35% of patients are not obese. Abdominal examination is usually unremarkable, except in advanced cases, in which ascites or an enlarged uterus may be present. Occasionally, a hematometra will present as a large, smooth, midline mass arising from the pelvis. On pelvic examination, it is important to inspect and carefully palpate the genital area and perform a rectovaginal examination to evaluate the fallopian tubes, cul-de-sac, and ovaries.

Pathology

Usually, carcinoma of the endometrium is easily diagnosed. Occasionally, however, a well-differentiated carcinoma may be confused with atypical hyperplasia. The main feature that helps to differentiate them is an infiltrating cellular or glandular pattern that produces a desmoplastic reaction in the stroma.

Adenocarcinomas are usually classified into three grades, depending on the degree of architectural differentiation of the tumor.

Grade I: In well-differentiated lesions, the cells are rather uniform, and a gland-like pattern is maintained. Mitoses are present but are not very helpful in identifying neoplastic potential. Approximately 70% to 75% of adenocarcinomas are well-differentiated lesions.

Grade II: In this moderately differentiated carcinoma, the proliferation of epithelial cells is more pronounced, and the lumina of the glands are often almost completely obliterated.

Grade III: Grade III adenocarcinomas are poorly differentiated lesions in which the glandular pattern is essentially eliminated by overgrowth of the epithelium.[4]

Variants of Adenocarcinoma

Most endometrial carcinomas are pure adenocarcinomas (Table 3). Adenoacanthoma indicates the presence of

TABLE 3

Classification of Endometrial Carcinoma

Endometrioid adenocarcinoma
    Villoglandular (papillary)
    Secretory
    Ciliated cell
    Endometrioid adenocarcinoma with squamous
      differentiation

Serous carcinoma (papillary serous)

Clear-cell carcinoma

Mucinous carcinoma

Squamous-cell carcinoma

Mixed types of carcinoma

Undifferentiated carcinoma

Adapted from Modified World Health Organization and International Society of Gynecological Pathologists classifications, in Kurman RJ (ed): Blaustein's Pathology of the Female Genital Tract. New York, Springer-Verlag, 1994.

benign squamous epithelium within an adenocarcinoma. This is not unusual and carries no prognostic importance. Adenosquamous carcinoma is a truly mixed neoplasia in which the squamous element is malignant. However, it is the degree of differentiation of the adenocarcinoma and not the malignant squamous component that determines the prognosis. Five-year survival rates, grade for grade, are similar for adenocarcinoma, adenoacanthoma, and adenosquamous carcinoma.

Uterine papillary serous carcinoma is similar in its clinical behavior to ovarian papillary serous carcinoma. More than 50% of patients with stage I uterine papillary serous carcinoma suffer a relapse outside the pelvis in the abdomen. Uterine papillary serous carcinoma, for which treatment remains unknown, must be distinguished from papillary (villoglandular) endometrioid carcinoma, which may respond to hormone therapy. Papillary serous carcinoma of the uterus is a virulent subtype of adenocarcinoma of the endometrium characterized by a poor prognosis, a high relapse rate, a propensity for transperitoneal seeding, and the frequent finding of more advanced disease at initial laparotomy.[20]

The need for aggressive treatment of this disease has long been recognized. Surgery, including a thorough staging laparotomy, followed by adjuvant therapy, is considered by many to be the initial step in management. What constitutes optimal adjuvant therapy, however, remains unresolved. Both radiation and chemotherapy have been tried as adjuvant therapy, with varying results.

Adjuvant whole abdominopelvic irradiation may be considered in the management of uterine papillary se-

TABLE 4

FIGO Staging of Endometrial Cancer (Revised Surgical Staging, 1988)

Stage	Grades	Description
Ia	1, 2, 3	Tumor limited to endometrium
Ib	1, 2, 3	Invasion to ≤ 50% myometrium
Ic	1, 2, 3	Invasion > 50% myometrium
IIa	1, 2, 3	Endocervical glandular involvement only
IIb	1, 2, 3	Cervical stroma invasion
IIIa	1, 2, 3	Tumor invasion of serosa and/or adnexae, and/or positive peritoneal cytology
IIIb	1, 2, 3	Vaginal metastases
IIIc	1, 2, 3	Metastases to pelvic and/or para-aortic lymph nodes
IVa	1, 2, 3	Tumor invasion of bladder and/or bowel mucosa
IVb	1, 2, 3	Distant metastases, including intra-abdominal and/or inguinal lymph node

Unofficial designation: Stage II occult (cervical involvement noted by microscopic examination alone); for practical purposes, patients with stage I or stage II occult disease may be managed alike.

FIGO = International Federation of Gynecology and Obstetrics

Adapted from Beahrs OH et al: Manual for Staging of Cancer, p 162. Philadelphia, JB Lippincott, 1992.

rous carcinoma.[20] Patients who stand to benefit most have early disease by surgical staging with or without positive peritoneal cytologic findings.[20] However, a review of the literature indicates that radiotherapy results in a 55% survival rate of only 55%, with follow-up ranging from 3 to 9 months.[21–26] Chemotherapeutic combinations with cisplatin (Platinol), doxorubicin (Adriamycin, Rubex), and cyclophosphamide (Cytoxan, Neosar) have also been used but have produced only some single, temporary responses. In short, systemic cisplatin-based combination chemotherapy appears to be of limited value for uterine papillary serous carcinoma.[22–27]

Mucinous adenocarcinoma accounts for fewer than 1% of all endometrial carcinomas. However, it is usually associated with a good prognosis, because most cases are stage I. A primary intestinal malignancy with uterine metastasis should be ruled out in the presence of this histologic variant.

Mesonephroid carcinoma is similar to clear-cell carcinoma arising in the ovaries and the clear-cell carcinoma of children exposed to diethylstilbestrol (DES), although no association with DES has been described for the mesonephroid neoplasm. This uncommon lesion accounts for 2% to 3% of all adenocarcinomas of the endometrium and tends to be deeply invasive, with a poor prognosis at the time of discovery.[4]

Undifferentiated carcinoma has no glandular, squamous, or sarcomatous differentiation and has a poor prognosis. Some of these tumors are small-cell carcinomas, and most of them contain epithelial antigens detected by immunologic stains.

Squamous-cell carcinoma is diagnosed only if there is no coexisting adenocarcinoma and no connection between the tumor and the squamous epithelium of the cervix. Only 23 cases of squamous-cell endometrial cancer have been reported to date.

Cancers of an identical cell type may be discovered simultaneously in the endometrium and ovaries. Usually, in such cases, the area that has the largest tumor mass and most advanced stage is designated the primary site. The prognosis depends on the grade and extension of the neoplasia at diagnosis.[2,4]

Clinical Findings

In approximately 20% of cases, endometrial carcinoma is detected while the patient is still asymptomatic. An atypical Papanicolaou smear suggests an adenocarcinoma. When atypical glandular cells are seen on the Papanicolaou smear, the risk that an adenocarcinoma will be found is approximately 20%, but this risk increases to nearly 50% in women older than age 60. Postmenopausal bleeding is the presenting symptom in 90% of women. Endometrial carcinoma must be considered in any woman older than age 40 who has abnormal uterine bleeding and in younger women in whom abnormal bleeding is associated with infertility or anovulation. In these cases, cytologic evaluation of vaginal smears may be useful but cannot replace biopsy or fractional curettage for diagnosis in high-risk patients.[28] Currently, there is no recognized screening program for this disease. Tumor spread may be by direct extension to adjacent structures, transtubal passage of exfoliated cells, or lymphatic or hematogenous dissemination.[19,29]

Staging and Prognosis

Since 1988, staging has incorporated surgical information, such as extension, grade, depth, and uterine-wall invasion, and peritoneal cytology (Table 4). Pretreatment evaluation should also include an intravenous pyelogram and barium enema to rule out coexistent gastrointestinal and urologic disease. The routine use of computed tomography (CT) or magnetic resonance imaging (MRI) of the pelvis is not advocated. However, in select cases, these studies may help to plan radiotherapy. The distribution of patients by stage and their respective 5-year survival rates are presented in Table 5.

Staging, including grade, is the most important prognostic factor. Other factors that may influence prognosis include age and vascular space invasion, which occurs in 15% of adenocarcinomas. The risk of pelvic-node metastasis is increased fourfold if the vascular space has been invaded. Receptor status (estrogen and progesterone) is important, and its level is inversely proportional to tumor grade, stage, and depth of invasion.

Histologic tumor grade, steroid receptor content, in vitro responsiveness to hormones, data on ploidy or DNA replicating activity obtained by flow cytometry, and fraction of cells in S phase are commonly used indicators of prognosis and responsiveness to therapy.[26] Tumor grade/stage and invasiveness correlate with the expression of several oncogenes, particularly *fms*, *neu*, *fos*, *myb*, *erb-B*, and *myc* and the augmented production of growth factors, transforming growth factor (TGF)-alpha, TGF-beta, and epidermal growth factor receptor. The clinical course of the disease and response to treatment can be followed by analysis of markers recognized by monoclonal antibodies.[26]

Treatment

Stage I and Stage II Occult: All medically fit patients should undergo total abdominal hysterectomy and bilateral salpingo-oophorectomy. The adnexa should be removed, as they may be the site of microscopic metastases and patients with endometrial carcinoma may have synchronous ovarian cancer. Peritoneal washings are taken from the pelvis, paracolic gutters, and subdiaphragmatic region. The excised uterus is opened and the depth of myometrial penetration and presence or absence of cervical involvement is determined by clinical observation and/or microscopic frozen section. In the absence of gross residual intraperitoneal tumor, pelvic and para-aortic lymph nodes should be sampled only if any of the following is noted: a grade 3 lesion; adenosquamous, clear cell, or serous carcinoma; myometrial invasion greater than 50%; or cervical extension. Lymph nodes need not be sampled for tumors limited to the endometrium, regardless of grade, because fewer than 1% of patients with these lesions have disease that has spread to pelvic or para-aortic lymph nodes.

Adjuvant radiation has not been shown to improve survival but can reduce the chance of a pelvic recurrence. Patients with a grade 1 lesion confined to the inner third of the myometrium have a 96% 5-year survival rate, and

TABLE 5

Distribution of Patients by Stage at Presentation and Respective Survival Rates

Stage	Percent at diagnosis	Percent survival at 5 yr
I	74.8	76.3
II	11.4	59.2
III	10.7	29.4
IV	2.9	10.3
Unstaged	0.2	51.8
Overall	100.0	66.9

Adapted from Hacker NF: Uterine cancer, in Berek JS, Hacker NF (eds): Practical Gynecologic Oncology, 2nd ed, pp 285–326. Baltimore, Williams & Wilkins, 1994.

adjuvant radiation does not improve on this. Patients with superficially invasive grade 2 carcinoma may be treated with intravaginal radiation (colpostats, 55 to 60 Gy), which has been shown to reduce the vaginal recurrence rate from 14% to 1.7%. Patients with grade 3 disease, invasion of more than one third of the myometrium, cervical extension, positive lymph nodes, or extrauterine pelvic disease should receive external pelvic irradiation with a dose of 45 to 50 Gy or a dome cylinder or cesium applicator to the vaginal cuff. Patients with extrapelvic disease should be considered for systemic therapy.

Stage II endometrial carcinoma can be confused with stage IB adenocarcinoma of the cervix. In this situation, it is helpful to note that patients with endometrial cancer more frequently are obese, are elderly, and have a bulky uterus, whereas patients with cervical carcinoma are younger, have a normal-sized corpus, and have a bulky cervix. Pelvic lymph nodes are involved in one third of patients with stage II endometrial cancer.

Two therapeutic approaches are currently in use for stage II endometrial carcinoma: (1) radical hysterectomy, bilateral salpingo-oophorectomy, and bilateral pelvic lymphadenectomy or (2) preoperative external pelvic irradiation and intracavitary radium or cesium, followed in 6 weeks by total hysterectomy and bilateral salpingo-oophorectomy.

Stage III: Clinical stage III disease is uncommon, and treatment should be individualized. Rates of 5-year survival vary in this heterogeneous population. Parametrial involvement, determined surgically, carries an overall 5-year survival rate of 40%. Patients with adnexal involvement alone have a survival rate of 80%, as opposed to a rate of 15% if other extrauterine structures are involved.

TABLE 6

Effect of Progestin-Receptor (PR) Status on Response of Endometrial Adenocarcinoma to Progestin Therapy

Study	Responders		Nonresponders	
	PR +	PR −	PR +	PR −
Creasman et al	4	0	1	8
Martin et al	13	1	0	6
Benrad et al	6	2	1	5
Ehrlich et al	7	1	1	15
Schwartz and Naftolin	1	0	7	4
Total	31 (89%)	4 (11%)	10 (19%)	38 (81%)

Adapted from Schwartz PE, Naftolin F: Hormone therapy, in Berek JS, Hacker NF (eds): Practical Gynecologic Oncology, 2nd ed, pp 613–636. Baltimore, Williams & Wilkins, 1994.

Adjuvant therapy is of unproven value in stage III disease. Abdominal recurrence is common (80%), but the abdomen is rarely the sole site of recurrence. Accordingly, whole abdominal irradiation is not warranted.[2,16,27,28]

Stage IV: The treatment of stage IV disease is designed primarily for palliation. Surgery is palliative, but if tumor is removed, estrogen-receptor and progesterone-receptor assays should be obtained. In stage IVA disease, irradiation (45 to 50 Gy) of the whole pelvis, and, if technically feasible, brachytherapy, is a reasonable approach. In patients with stage IVB lesions, a similar dose of external radiotherapy may be helpful.

Endometrial Cancer Diagnosed After Hysterectomy

This situation is best avoided by routinely opening the excised uterus in the operating room so that the adnexa can be removed and appropriate staging performed. Grade 1 lesions with involvement of less than one half of the myometrium require no further treatment. In the event of a grade 3 lesion or a grade 2 lesion with extension to the outer third of the myometrium or to the cervix, a relaparotomy should be performed, with the removal of adnexa, surgical staging, and appropriate postoperative irradiation. All other cases should undergo external pelvic irradiation.[16]

Treatment of Recurrent Disease

Patients with recurrent disease have an anticipated survival of up to 12 months. Half of the recurrences have a distant component and three fourths, a local component. About 80% of recurrences will occur within 3 years of initial treatment. The patient with an isolated vaginal recurrence may benefit from surgery and/or irradiation; others may benefit from systemic therapy (hormones, chemotherapeutic agents,[30] or biological agents).

Hormonal Therapy: Recurrent or metastatic endometrial carcinoma is usually treated initially with a hormonal agent such as a progestational agent or an antiestrogen (tamoxifen). Progestational agents have been the mainstay of treatment of endometrial cancer.

Responses are short and are seen primarily in better differentiated tumors. Some studies have shown significant antitumor activity for gonadotropin-releasing hormone (GnRH) analogs like leuprolide (Lupron) or goserelin (Zoladex).[29] Response rates range from 15% to 40%.[26,31] However, recent trials have reported lower response rates for such treatment, probably due to more stringent response criteria and a smaller number of patients with well-differentiated carcinomas.

In view of the factors that predict a response to progestational agents, it can be argued that patients with progesterone-receptor-positive tumors should be given first-line treatment with medroxy progesterone acetate. If the receptor status is unknown but the original tumor is well differentiated or the interval from initial diagnosis to recurrence is more than 1 year, the treatment of choice is hormonal. Because at least 3 months must elapse before the results of hormonal therapy can be evaluated, the selected patients must have a life expectancy of at least 4 months. There is no obvious dose response with progestins, and oral therapy appears as effective as parenteral therapy. Patients with grade 3 tumors have a ≤ 10% response rate. Attempts to identify patients more likely to respond to hormonal therapy have met with limited success, but data suggest that tumors with positive progestin receptors are more likely to respond to hormonal therapy (Table 6). GnRH agonists also may be of benefit.[32,33]

Other factors that suggest an increased likelihood of response to hormonal therapy are a long disease-free interval, exceeding 2 to 3 years, and low-grade tumors. In summary, because of their low toxicity, hormones should be used initially in patients with recurrent endometrial cancer, particularly patients with positive receptors. Therapy should be started with megestrol acetate (Megace), 40 mg orally two to four times daily, and continued until progression occurs. If the patient had an initial response to progestins, then tamoxifen, 20 mg given orally twice daily until further progression, should be considered.

Adjuvant hormonal therapy with progestational agents in endometrial cancer is attractive but unproven. Such therapy is usually guided by the pathogenetic type of disease and morphology of tumor, ie, well-differentiated endometrial cancers usually have high levels of hormone receptors in relation to steroid hormones and seem to be more sensitive to hormonal therapy. Cytoplasmic receptors to progesterone are estrogen-dependent proteins which increase in number with administration of estrogen or tamoxifen.

For patients whose profile indicates a decreased likelihood of response to progestins (negative receptor status, poor condition, undifferentiated tumor) or when the tumor load does not allow delay to await the results of hormonal manipulation, the use of cytotoxic drugs can be considered as initial therapy.

Chemotherapy: Patients in whom hormonal therapy fails may be considered for chemotherapy with palliative intent.[20] Responses have been identified in the literature for cisplatin, doxorubicin, carboplatin (Paraplatin), cyclophosphamide, and hexamethylmelamine (altretamine, Hexalen) (Table 7). Response rates with combination chemotherapy range from 20% to 50%. Most of the responses are partial, with a median duration of 4 to 8 months and a median survival of less than 12 months.

There is no survival benefit to combination chemotherapy over single-agent cisplatin.[2,34,35] Still, it is not entirely certain that combinations are more effective than single agents. Combinations including both doxorubicin and cisplatin seem to improve the initial likelihood of a response. In general, if a response is obtained, chemotherapy is continued until progression or intolerable toxicity occurs. The addition of a progestin to chemotherapy does not appear to enhance the response. The most frequently used combination is cyclophosphamide, 500 mg/m²; doxorubicin, 50 mg/m²; and cisplatin, 50 mg/m². Single-agent cisplatin or carboplatin would be reasonable and less toxic alternatives in this patient population.[36] Doxorubicin, could be reserved for hormone- and platinum-resistant tumors.[37]

Studies at M. D. Anderson on cisplatin, doxorubicin, and cyclophosphamide treatment of metastatic or recurrent endometrial cancer have shown an overall response rate of 45%, a complete remission rate of 14%, and a median response duration of 4 to 8 months.

Anecdotally, patients with tumors refractory to hormonal therapy and chemotherapy may respond to a combination of alpha interferon (IFN-α), 13-*cis*-retinoic acid, and alpha-tocopherol.[38] Interferons are known to modulate the expression of receptors for estrogen (ER), progesterone (PR), and epidermal growth factor (EGFR)

TABLE 7

Response Rate of Endometrial Cancer to Single-Agent Chemotherapy

Drug	Response (%)
Doxorubicin	19–38
Cisplatin	4–42
Carboplatin	32
Cyclophosphamide	0–20
Ifosfamide	13
Fluorouracil	24
Hexamethylmelamine	9–30
Paclitaxel [a]	35

Adapted from Thigpen JT: Chemotherapy of cancers of the female genital tract, in Perry MC (ed): The Chemotherapy Source Book, 1st ed, pp 1039–1067. Baltimore, Williams & Wilkins, 1992, and Thigpen J et al: Cancer 60:2104–2116, 1987.

[a] Ball HG: Personal communication, Fifth Biennial Meeting of the International Gynecologic Cancer Society, September, 1995.

in women with endometrial cancer.[39] However, no significant improvement in survival was reported in one study by Scambia and associates. The role of adjuvant systemic therapy remains to be adequately explored but is thus far unproven.

Finally, there is currently considerable interest in the activity of the natural product paclitaxel (Taxol) not only in ovarian cancer but also in endometrial cancer. Taxol has a unique mechanism of cytotoxicity that involves the polymerization of microtubules. Another taxane of interest is docetaxel (Taxotere).[40] Recently, the Gynecologic Oncology Group has reported the results of a phase II study of paclitaxel in endometrial cancer. The objective response rate was 35% with a 15% complete response rate (Ball HG, personal communication, September, 1995).

UTERINE SARCOMAS

Uterine sarcomas are rare heterogeneous tumors that account for 3% of uterine malignant neoplasms in white women, 10% of uterine malignancies in black women. These tumors are not estrogen dependent and appear at a median age of 60 years. Prior radiation therapy to the pelvis has been implicated in the genesis of uterine sarcomas, but this is unproven. The incidence of uterine sarcomas is 1.7 per 100,000 women. Carcinosarcoma is the most common uterine sarcoma, followed by leiomyosarcoma and endometrial stromal sarcoma. These neoplasms are frequently associated with obesity, diabetes,

TABLE 8

Staging Classification of Uterine Sarcoma

Stage	Description
I	Sarcoma is confined to the corpus
II	Sarcoma is confined to the corpus and cervix
III	Sarcoma has spread outside the uterus but is confined to the true pelvis
IV	Sarcoma has spread outside the true pelvis

TABLE 9

Simplified Classification of Uterine Sarcoma

Type	Homologous	Heterologous
Pure	Leiomyosarcoma Stromal sarcoma 1. Endolymphatic stromal myosis 2. Endometrial stromal sarcoma	Rhabdomyosarcoma Chondrosarcoma Osteosarcoma Liposarcoma
Mixed	Mixed mesodermal tumor	Mixed mesodermal tumor

Adapted from Hacker NF, Moore JG (eds): Essentials of Obstetrics and Gynecology, p 42. Philadelphia, WB Saunders, 1986.

TABLE 10

Response Rate of Uterine Sarcoma to Chemotherapy

Agent	Response rate (%) for tumor type			
	LMS	MMT	ESS	Unspecified
Doxorubicin	15–35	0–10	?	6
Cisplatin	5	18–42	?	5
Ifosfamide	14	32	–	–
Etoposide	11	6	–	8
Methotrexate	–	–	–	6

ESS = endometrial stromal sarcoma, LMS = leiomyosarcoma, MMT = mixed mesodermal tumor   Adapted, in part, from Thigpen JT: Chemotherapy of cancers of the female genital tract, in Perry MC (ed): The Chemotherapy Source Book, pp 1039–1067. Baltimore, Williams & Wilkins, 1992.

and hypertension.[16,25,41,42] The peak age of incidence for carcinosarcoma (mixed müllerian tumor) is 55 to 65 years of age, whereas it is 45 to 55 years of age for leiomyosarcoma and endometrial stromal sarcoma.[43]

Natural History and Clinical Presentation

Generally, uterine sarcomas are characterized by an aggressive growth pattern with early hematogenous spread and lymphatic dissemination in about 35% of patients with disease clinically confined to the uterus. Overall survival is poor, in the range of 1 to 2 years after diagnosis. The 5-year survival for stage 1 tumors is 50% but falls to 20% for leiomyosarcoma if there is any spread beyond the uterus and to approximately 16% for endometrial stromal sarcoma (ESS) irrespective of stage. However, low-grade leiomyosarcomas, ESS, and endolymphatic stromal myosis are associated with better cure and survival rates. Prognosis depends on the extent of extrauterine spread and the number of mitotic cells per 10 high-power fields. In the case of leiomyosarcoma, more than 10 mitotic cells constitute a very aggressive, high-grade tumor, whereas fewer than five mitotic cells usually indicate a benign tumor. Cases with 5 to 10 mitotic cells per 10 high-power fields and significant cellular atypia are considered high grade.

Abnormal uterine bleeding is the most frequent presenting symptom for all histologic types and occurs in at least 80% of patients. Pelvic pain is present in about one third of patients with sarcoma. Other less common presentations include uterine enlargement, prolapsed neoplasm, and malodorous discharge. Because of this aggressive and nonspecific clinical picture, the early diagnosis of uterine sarcomas is rare. However, if the diagnosis of a sarcoma is made prior to a hysterectomy, more appropriate treatment planning can be done if a CT scan or MRI of the pelvis is obtained. The diagnostic yield of Papanicolaou smear is 46% for endometrial stromal sarcoma and 22% for leiomyosarcoma, whereas with endometrial biopsy it is 91% for mixed mesodermal sarcoma. Like endometrial carcinomas, uterine sarcomas infiltrate the myometrium.

Staging: No accepted staging system exists for uterine sarcomas because of their rarity. Usually, a modified staging based on the system developed by the International Federation of Gynecology and Obstetrics (FIGO) for endometrial cancer is used (Table 8).[25,27,43]

Pathology: Uterine sarcomas are classified as pure sarcomas if they contain only one recognizable element and mixed sarcomas if they contain at least two elements (Table 9). These elements may be homologous, when tissue is native to the uterus (eg, smooth muscle, endometrial stroma, vessels) or heterologous, when its components are tissues foreign to the uterus (bone, cartilage, striated muscle, fat).

Carcinosarcomas and adenosarcomas belong to a group

of mixed tumors. Carcinosarcoma contains histologically malignant epithelial and nonepithelial elements. An adenosarcoma is characterized by a benign epithelial component and a malignant stroma. In the current classification system, these are referred to as "malignant mixed mesodermal tumor" or "malignant mixed müllerian tumor."[42,44]

Treatment

The only treatment of any proven curative value for uterine sarcomas is surgical excision with total abdominal hysterectomy and bilateral salpingo-oophorectomy. Random biopsies of retroperitoneal lymph nodes rarely yield clinically useful information. In stage I patients, the average survival rate is 45% at 2 years.[16] Although radiation therapy is often administered, its value is controversial as it seems to reduce pelvic recurrence without influencing overall survival. There is a high incidence of distant failure, particularly in the lungs and upper abdomen.[44]

Systemic chemotherapy is part of the integrated treatment of uterine sarcomas. Chemotherapy recommendations vary according to histologic subtype, even though there are no well-controlled series for any histologic type owing to the rarity of these tumors. The most active agents are doxorubicin, cisplatin, and ifosfamide. Unfortunately, most responses are partial and short duration. Adjuvant chemotherapy after hysterectomy is an attractive concept; however, neither survival nor progression-free interval are prolonged by currently available adjuvant chemotherapy.[38] The potential value of hormonal agents in the management of uterine sarcomas awaits further evaluation, although there have been anecdotal reports of responses to progestins or GnRH agonists.[16,45]

As mentioned above, chemotherapy recommendations vary according to histologic subtype (Table 10). The most frequently used combinations are doxorubicin, dacarbazine (DTIC-Dome), dactinomycin (Cosmegen), and cyclophosphamide or cyclophosphamide, vincristine (Oncovin), doxorubicin, and dacarbazine. A partial response follows chemotherapy in 20% to 30% and a complete response in 10% to 15%, but there is no improvement in survival. In leiomyosarcoma, the recommended treatment is doxorubicin (50 to 90 mg/m²) as a single agent, with dose escalation as tolerated. The addition of dacarbazine adds little in terms of response but more in terms of toxicity. The addition of other drugs (cyclophosphamide, cisplatin, vincristine, dactinomycin, or ifosfamide [Ifex])[46] does not appear to contribute to response or survival but, again, increases toxicity. In any case, the dose of doxorubicin should not be reduced in order to add other drugs.

For carcinosarcoma and mixed mesodermal tumor, the drug of choice is ifosfamide (1.2 to 1.5 g/m²/d for 5 days)[47] or cisplatin (50 to 75 mg/m²).[45,48–52] There is no evidence that combining these two drugs results in a higher response rate, and the combination is clearly more toxic. Carboplatin has not been tested but may be used in patients with renal compromise or poor performance status.[41–43] However, patients who receive prior pelvic radiation may develop greater myelosuppression. Hematopoietins may be considered to allow the maintenance of dose intensity.[33]

In the case of endometrial stromal sarcoma, optimal therapy is undefined.[53] However, frontline treatment with the single agent doxorubicin is suggested. If no response is noted, a trial of cisplatin or ifosfamide, as for carcinosarcoma, may be attempted. Low-grade sarcomas may respond to progestational agents or GnRH agonists. Yet, given the rarity of these tumors, inclusion of patients in clinical trials should be considered. No current role for chemotherapy has been defined in the adjuvant setting. Clearly, further studies are needed to identify additional active agents. Radiotherapy as safe treatment should be considered in patients who are considered inoperable and in whom parametrial metastases are present.[54]

REFERENCES

1. Wingo PA, Tong T: Cancer statistics, 1995. CA Cancer J Clin 45:8–30, 1995.

2. Park R, Grigsby P, Muss H, et al: Corpus: Epithelial tumors, in Hoskins WI, Perez C, Young RC (eds): Principles and Practice of Gynecologic Oncology, 1st ed, pp 663–693. Philadelphia, JB Lippincott, 1992.

3. Bokhman JV: Two pathogenetic types of endometrial carcinoma. Gynecol Oncol 15:10–12, 1983.

4. Kurman RJ, Norris HJ: Endometrial carcinoma, in Kurman RJ (ed): Blaustein's Pathology of the Female Genital Tract, 3rd ed, pp 338–372. New York, Springer-Verlag, 1987.

5. Piver MS, Marchetti DL: Endometrial carcinoma, in Piver MS (ed): Manual of Gynecologic Oncology and Gynecology. Boston, Little, Brown & Co, 1989.

6. Seachrist L: Restating the risks of tamoxifen Science 263:910–911, 1994.

7. Sasiene P: Endometrial cancer during tamoxifen treatment. Lancet 23;343:1048, 1994.

8. Baum M, Odling-Smee W, Houghton J: Endometrial cancer during tamoxifen treatment. Lancet 343:1291, 1994.

9. Rayter Z, Sheperd J, Gazrt JC: Tamoxifen and endometrial lesions. Lancet 343:1124, 1993.

10. Love RR: Endometrial cancer in tamoxifen treated breast cancer patients. J Natl Cancer Inst 86:1025–1026, 1994.

11. Smigel K, Ulbrich S: Breast cancer prevention trial will resume (news). J Natl Cancer Inst 86:961–963, 1994.

12. Kedar RP, Bourne TH: Effects of tamoxifen on uterus and ovaries of postmenopausal women in a randomised breast cancer prevention trial. Lancet 343:1318–1321, 1994.

13. Chambers JT, Chambers SK: Endometrial sampling: When,

where, why, with what? Clin Obstet Gynecol 35:28–39, 1992.

14. Anzai Y, Holinka CF, Kuramato H: Stimulatory effect of 4-hydroxytamoxifen on proliferation of human endometrial adenocarcinoma cells (Ishikawa line). Cancer Res 49:2362–2365, 1989.

15. Parazzinni F, Lavecchlia C, Negri E: Family history of breast, ovarian, and endometrial cancer and risk of breast cancer. Int J Epidemiol 22:614–618, 1993.

16. Thompson WD, Schildkrant JM: Family history of gynecological cancers: Relationships to the incidence of breast cancer prior to age 55. Int J Epidemiol 20:595–602, 1991.

17. Kelsey JL, Fischer DB, Holford TR, et al: Exogenous estrogens and other factors in the epidemiology of breast cancer. J Natl Cancer Inst 67:327–333, 1981.

18. Watson P, Vasen HF: The risk of endometrial cancer in hereditary nonpolyposis colorectal cancer. Am J Med 96:516–520, 1994.

19. Hacker NF: Uterine cancer, in Berek JS, Hacker NF (eds): Practical Gynecologic Oncology, 1st ed, pp 285–326. Baltimore, Williams & Wilkins, 1989.

20. Mallipeddi P, Kapp DS: Long-term survival with adjuvant whole abdominopelvic irradiation for uterine papillary serous carcinoma. Cancer 71:3076–3081, 1993.

21. Christman JE, Kapp DS: Therapeutic approaches to uterine papillary serous carcinoma: A preliminary report. Gynecol Oncol 26:228–235, 1987.

22. Chambers JT, Merino M: Uterine papillary serous carcinoma. Obstet Gynecol 69:109–113, 1987.

23. Gallion HH, Van Nagell JR, et al: Stage 1 serous papillary carcinoma of endometrium. Cancer 63:2224–2228, 1989.

24. Walker AN, Mills SE: Serous papillary carcinoma of endometrium: A clinicopathologic study of 11 cases. Diagn Gynecol Obstet 4:261–267, 1982.

25. Sutton GP, Brill L: Malignant papillary lesions of the endometrium. Gynecol Oncol 27:294–304, 1987.

26. Frank AH, Tseng PC: Adjuvant whole abdominal radiation therapy in uterine papillary serous carcinoma. Cancer 68:1516–1519, 1991.

27. Greven K, Olds W: Isolated vaginal recurrences of endometrial adenocarcinoma and their management. Cancer 60:419–421, 1987.

28. Larson DM, Johnson KK: Prognostic significance of malignant cervical cytology in patients with endometrial cancer. Obstet Gynecol 84:399–403, 1994.

29. Berman ML, Berek JS: Uterine corpus, in Haskel C (ed): Cancer Treatment, 3rd ed, pp 338–350. Philadelphia, WB Saunders, 1990.

30. Thigpen JT, Vance R, Lambuth B, et al: Chemotherapy for advanced or recurrent gynecological cancer. Cancer 60:2104–2116, 1987.

31. Moore TD, Philips PH, Nerenstone SR, et al: Systemic treatment of advanced and recurrent endometrial carcinoma: Current status and future direction. J Clin Oncol 9:1071–1088, 1991.

32. Burke TW, Wolfson AH: Limited endometrial carcinoma: Adjuvant therapy. Semin Oncol 21:84–90, 1994.

33. Perl V, Schally AV, Comaru-Schally AM, et al: Use of D-Trp-6-LH-RH in endometrial adenocarcinoma. Proceedings from the XXII Congreso Chileno de Obstetrica y Ginecologia, Santiago, Chile 2:7, 1987.

34. De Saia PJ, Creasman WT (eds): Clinical Gynecologic Oncology, pp 167–213. St Louis, CV Mosby Co, 1989.

35. Martinez A, Schray M, Podratz K, et al: Postoperative whole abdominopelvic irradiation for patients with high risk endometrial cancer. Int J Radiat Oncol Biol Phys 17:371, 1989.

36. Burke TW, Munkarah A, Kavanagh JJ: Treatment of advanced or recurrent endometrial carcinoma with single agent carboplatin. Gynecol Oncol 51:397–400, 1993.

37. Vishnevsky AS, Tsyrlina EV, Sofroniy DF: Criteria of endometrial carcinoma sensitivity to hormone therapy: Pathogenetic type of the disease and the tumor reaction to tamoxifen. Eur J Gynaecol Oncol 14:139–143, 1993.

38. Kudelka AP, Freedman RS, Kavanagh JJ: Metastatic adenocarcinoma of the endometrium treated with 13-cis-retinoic acid plus interferon-alpha. Anticancer Drugs 4:335–337, 1993.

39. Muss HB: Chemotherapy of metastatic endometrial cancer. Semin Oncol 21:107–113, 1994.

40. Deppe G: Chemotherapy for endometrial cancer, in Deppe G (ed): Chemotherapy of Gynecologic Cancer, 2nd ed, pp 155–174. New York, Alan R Liss, 1990.

41. Thigpen JT: Chemotherapy of cancers of the female genital tract, in Perry MC (ed): The Chemotherapy Source Book, 1st ed, pp 1039–1067. Baltimore, Williams & Wilkins, 1992.

42. Neijt JP: Systemic treatment in disseminated endometrial cancer. Eur J Cancer 29:628–632, 1993.

43. Kudelka AP, Freedman RS, Edwards CL, et al: Verbal communication. January 1993.

44. Kavanagh JJ, Kudelka AP: Systemic therapy of gynecologic cancer. Curr Opin Oncol 5:891–899, 1993.

45. Ozols RF: Advances in the chemotherapy of gynecological malignancies. Hematol Oncol 10:43–51, 1992.

46. Sutton GP, Blessing JA, McGuire W, et al: Phase II trial of ifosfamide and mesna in leiomyosarcomas of the uterus. Gynecol Oncol 36:295, 1990.

47. Sutton GP, Blessing JA, Rosenheim N, et al: Phase II trial of ifosfamide and mesna in mixed mesodermal tumors of the uterus. Am J Obstet Gynecol 161:309, 1989.

48. Hannigan E, Curtin J, Silverberg S, et al: Corpus: Mesenchymal tumors, in Hoskins WJ, Perez C, Young RC (eds): Principles and Practice of Gynecologic Oncology, 1st ed, pp 695–714. Philadelphia, JB Lippincott, 1992.

49. Zlovdek CH, Norris HJ: Mesenchymal tumors of the uterus, in Kurman RJ (ed): Blaustein's Pathology of the Female Genital Tract, 3rd Ed, pp 373–408. New York, Springer-Verlag, 1987.

50. Hoskins WJ, Perez C, Young RC: Gynecologic tumors, in DeVita VT, Hellman S, Rosenberg SA (eds): Cancer: Principles and Practice of Oncology, 3rd ed, pp 1099–1161. Philadelphia, JB Lippincott, 1989.

51. Hacker NF, Moore JG (eds): Essentials of Obstetrics and Gynecology, 1st ed. Philadelphia, WB Saunders, 1986.

52. Gershenson DM, Kavanagh JJ, Copeland LJ, et al: Cisplatin therapy for disseminated mixed mesodermal sarcoma of the uterus. J Clin Oncol 5:618, 1987.

53. Meden H, Meyer-Rath D, Schauer A: Endometrial stromal sarcoma of the uterus. Anticancer Drugs 2:35–37, 1991.

54. Omura GA, Blessing JA, Major F, et al: A randomized clinical trial of adjuvant Adriamycin in uterine sarcomas: A Gynecologic Oncology Group study. J Clin Oncol 3:1240, 1985.

SECTION 7

GENITOURINARY CARCINOMAS

CHAPTER **26**   **Prostate Cancer**

CHAPTER **27**   **Testicular Cancer**

CHAPTER **28**   **Bladder Cancer**

CHAPTER **29**   **Renal-Cell Carcinoma**

Prostate Cancer

Philip Agop Philip, MB, ChB, PhD, MRCP, *and* Randall Millikan, PhD, MD
Department of Genitourinary Medical Oncology
The University of Texas M. D. Anderson Cancer Center, Houston, Texas

The incidence and mortality of prostate cancer continue to rise and will continue to pose a major public health problem, especially with the increased longevity of the Western population. Prostate cancer has become the most common newly diagnosed cancer in American men, largely because of mass screening of asymptomatic individuals. In 1995, about 244,000 men in the United States will be diagnosed with prostate cancer, and 40,400 will die of it, a mortality rate second only to that of lung cancer.[1] The increase in incidence of prostate cancer primarily represents an increase in the proportion of patients with localized disease. Many such patients are curable with local therapy, and local treatments continue to evolve to minimize morbidity.[2]

Despite progress in diagnosis and local therapy, fundamental questions remain with regard to the etiology, prevention, and treatment of prostate cancer. Most notably, treatment of metastatic disease is strictly palliative, and there is still no treatment for hormone-refractory disease that is demonstrated to improve survival. Significant breakthroughs await improved understanding of the biology of prostate cancer and development of novel therapeutic strategies built on that understanding.

EPIDEMIOLOGY

Prostate cancer incidence is strikingly related to age. The incidence of clinically diagnosed prostate cancer is also significantly affected by geographic and racial factors, ranging from 0.8 per 100,000 men in Shanghai, China, to 100.2 per 100,000 men among blacks in Alameda County, California.[3] Epidemiologic studies have shown that mortality rates among US whites and blacks continue to rise, with rates increasing more rapidly among males over 74 years old and reduced in nonwhite young males.[4]

Despite these variations in the incidence of clinically detected prostate cancer, the prevalence of latent prostate cancers is actually quite similar across ethnic groups.[5] This suggests that there may be differences in factors required to cause a latent cancer to progress to a clinically detectable stage. Identification of these progression factors would have obvious therapeutic implications. Some of these factors may be environmental in origin because there is an increased incidence of clinical prostate cancer in men who have emigrated from countries with a low incidence to those with a high incidence.[6-8]

Except for an association with chronic prostatitis, epidemiologic studies have found no association between prostate cancer and type of diet, prevalence of venereal disease, sexual habits, smoking, or occupational exposure.[9] Vasectomy is not a definite risk factor for the future development of prostate cancer, and individuals who have undergone this procedure should not be categorized as highrisk.[10] Although the role of benign prostatic hypertrophy in the development of prostate cancer remains unclear, it is generally believed that the benign, hypertrophic prostatic cells do not directly transform into malignant cells.[11] One possible contributory factor to the pathogenesis of prostate cancer is elevated serum testosterone concentrations. This hypothesis is supported by observations that prostate cancers are responsive to testosterone suppression, that black men have serum testosterone levels on average 15% higher than white men,[12] and that the incidence of detectable prostate cancer in vegetarians and eunuchs, who have below-average or negligible levels of testosterone, is low.[13]

The prevalence of latent or "incidental" tumors is characteristic of the prostate gland. Autopsies of men over the age of 50 years have revealed microscopic foci of well-differentiated adenocarcinoma in serial sections of prostate glands otherwise considered to be normal. Every decade of aging nearly doubles the incidence of microscopic prostate cancer: from 10% for men in their 50s to 70% for men in their 80s. It has been estimated that 9 out of 10 men who eventually develop clinically recognized prostate cancer had cancer that remained undetected for decades.[14]

Significant clustering of prostate cancer within families, along with breast and central nervous system tumors, suggests a role for genetic factors in the etiology of this disease.[15] It is estimated that men from families in which two or more first- or second-degree relatives have prostate cancer may have as much as eight times greater risk of developing prostate cancer than the average male.[16] As with other malignancies, an inherited susceptibility to prostate cancer may lead to much earlier onset.

PATHOGENESIS

Despite the increasing incidence of prostate cancer, our knowledge of the molecular and cellular biology of prostatic adenocarcinoma remains significantly less than that of most other neoplasms. Nevertheless, over the past few years several important advances have been made.[17] Loss of heterozygosity studies and, more recently, comparative genomic hybridization techniques have suggested that chromosomes 6q, 8p, 9p, 10q, 13q, 16q, and 18q are potential sites for genes associated with the initiation of prostate carcinoma.[18-20] In one study 74% of the primary prostatic tumors showed evidence of DNA sequence copy number changes.[20] Losses were five times more common than gains. The most common abnormalities affected 8p and 13q. Furthermore, the pattern of genetic changes seen in recurrent tumors, with the frequent gain of chromosomes 7, 8q, and X, suggests that the progression of prostatic cancer and development of hormone-independent growth may have a distinct genetic basis.[21]

Although several oncogenes (*ras, myc, sis*) are expressed with a higher frequency in prostatic cancer cell lines, their overexpression in localized (ie, early-stage) prostatic tumors is uncommon.[21] In contrast, loss of function of tumor-suppressor genes appears to play a significant role in prostatic carcinogenesis. The known tumor-suppressor genes, *Rb* on 13q and *p53* on 17p, may play an important role in the progression of prostate cancer.[22] Mutations in the *p53* gene are considered late events in prostatic carcinogenesis, associated with advanced stage, loss of differentiation, and conversion from a hormone-dependent to hormone-refractory state.[23] In contrast, loss of the *Rb* gene appears to be an early event in prostatic carcinogenesis.[24] Gao et al[25] found decreased expression of another tumor-suppressor gene, *dcc* (*d*eleted in *c*olon *c*ancer), in 12 of 14 radical prostatectomy specimens.

The abnormal expression of peptide growth factors and their receptors may contribute to the growth and development of both local and metastatic prostate cancer. There is enhanced expression of epidermal growth factor (EGF) and coexpression of the epidermal growth factor receptor (EGFR) in human prostatic tumors, consistent with in vitro data supporting autocrine growth regulation by EGFR-mediated pathways.[26] Tissue containing benign prostatic hypertrophy and several prostate cancer cell lines express higher-than-normal levels of transforming growth factor (TGF)-beta,[27] as well as TGF-alpha and EGFR.[28] The fibroblast growth factors (FGFs), which have been isolated from prostatic tissue, have also

been implicated in prostate cell growth.[29] Moreover, male transgenic mice expressing *int-2*, a member of the fibroblast growth factor peptide family, develop prostatic hypertrophy.[30] Other members of the tyrosine kinase growth factor receptor family related to EGFR include the *HER-2/neu* (c-*erbB-2*) and c-*erbB-3* oncogenes. The increased expression of *HER-2/neu* and c-*erbB-3* has also been demonstrated in prostatic intraepithelial neoplasia and in primary prostatic cancers and matching metastases from the same patients.[31] Within the group of primary prostate tumors, there is a positive correlation between stage and Gleason grade of tumor and the immunohistochemical expression of *HER-2/neu*.[32] The progression of prostatic tumors to a hormone-refractory state is frequently associated with the expression of the anti-apoptotic gene *bcl-2*.[33,34]

The expression of the surface adhesion molecule E-cadherin was absent in almost 50% of prostatic tumor,[35] which correlated with tumor grade and stage and overall survival.[36]

Tumor-induced angiogenesis is an essential step in the progression of malignant neoplasms and the development of metastases. Weidner et al[37] noted that the mean microvessel count in the invasive primary prostatic specimen was significantly higher for patients with metastases than for patients without metastases. The microvessel count was also noted to be increased at higher Gleason scores. In a multivariate analysis in 74 patients, microvessel count remained significant, and Gleason score did not add additional predictive value.[37] The therapeutic potential of angiogenesis inhibitors is under active investigation.

Both benign and malignant prostatic disease are influenced by interactions between cells in the stromal and epithelial compartments.[38] It has been shown that the in vivo and in vitro behaviors of prostatic epithelial cells are affected by the presence or absence of mesenchymal cells, particularly fibroblasts, and/or their paracrine-acting products. The frequent metastases of prostate cancer to the axial skeleton and the production of osteoblastic metastases suggest a bidirectional paracrine interaction between prostate cancer and bone cells.

Recognition of premalignant lesions in the prostate may permit the identification of a high-risk population that might benefit from early screening. Because prostatic intraepithelial neoplasia is much more common in prostate glands with invasive carcinoma than in those without, this type of growth has been designated as a premalignant lesion. Another premalignant condition in the prostate is atypical adenomatous hyperplasia, or prostatic adenosis.[39]

PATHOLOGY

Histologically, almost all prostate cancers are adenocarcinomas. Such entities as sarcomas and transitional cell, small-cell, and squamous cell carcinomas are rare. Nonetheless, it is important to recognize these pathologic subtypes because they have distinct clinical behaviors and require different therapy. For example, patients with unusual sites of metastases (such as liver, skin, or bone marrow), low or normal levels of serum prostate-specific antigen (PSA), and newly diagnosed tumors that display hormone resistance should be evaluated for possible anaplastic small-cell pathology. Such anaplastic tumors respond better to chemotherapy than to hormonal treatments.[40] Similarly, transitional cell carcinoma of the prostate does not respond to hormonal manipulations but is moderately sensitive to radiation and chemotherapy.

The Gleason system for histologic grading of prostate tumors, which is based solely on morphology, correlates with malignant potential. Low-power microscopic examination of biopsy specimens (not those obtained by fine-needle aspiration) usually reveals tumor patterns ranging from well-differentiated, small glands to poorly differentiated sheets or cords of malignant cells. Five distinct glandular patterns are graded progressively from most to least differentiated. The grades of the two predominant patterns present in a surgical specimen are added to yield the final Gleason score. Patients with well-differentiated lesions (ie, Gleason scores 2–4) usually have early-stage disease and a good prognosis. Gleason scores 8–10, however, are associated with a poor prognosis. Gleason score correlates well with other known prognostic factors, such as tumor size, presence of pelvic lymph-node metastasis, and PSA level. The M. D. Anderson Cancer Center grading system is a simpler method that depends only on the percentage of gland formation in the tumor. It also appears to reflect the biologic behavior of prostate cancer.[41]

The DNA ploidy and S-phase fraction of prostatic tumors may provide additional prognostic information. Flow cytometric assessment of both DNA content and S-phase fraction is possible using small quantities of prostatic tissue obtained at biopsy.[42] Detection of a high S-phase fraction in a primary tumor may indicate lack of hormonal responsiveness and poor prognosis.[43]

Diploid tumors are associated with improved survival.[44]

NATURAL HISTORY

Epidemiologic studies suggest that the probabilities of the early events leading to so-called histologic cancers are similar worldwide.[45] Low-grade tumors can grow very slowly and remain localized to the gland for relatively long periods of time, during which they remain clinically undetectable. Tumors that become clinically significant arise mainly (80% of the time) in the peripheral zone of the prostate gland and less frequently in the transitional zone (15%) or central zone (5%). Significantly, the latter two areas are also frequent sites of benign prostatic hypertrophy. Tumors in the peripheral zone are palpable during digital rectal examination (DRE) but are inaccessible to transurethral resection. In contrast, tumors in the transitional zone surrounding the prostatic urethra are not palpable but can be removed easily during transurethral resection of the prostate.

Prostate cancers typically grow peripherally through the capsule along perineural sheaths that perforate the capsule at the upper outer corner and at the apex. Such tumors often invade the seminal vesicles and the neck of the urinary bladder. Occasionally, a prostatic tumor may invade across the fascial planes into the rectal wall.

Distant metastatic spread is both lymphatic and hematogenous. Lymphatic spread is usually orderly, first affecting the obturator lymph nodes, then advancing contiguously into the external iliac and hypogastric nodes, and finally involving the common iliac and periaortic nodes. Hematogenous spread is also characteristically orderly. In general, the axial skeleton is involved as the first site of metastasis. This is followed by spread to the proximal appendicular skeleton. Only in advanced disease do pulmonary and hepatic metastases appear. Metastases to either liver or lungs, especially in the absence of extensive skeletal involvement, should alert the physician to the possibility of small-cell carcinoma of the prostate, for which therapy significantly differs from that for adenocarcinoma. Metastases to the brain and other visceral sites are uncommon. Characteristically, bone metastases are osteoblastic and readily detected by radionuclide bone scans. While metastatic bone disease is almost always present when the pelvic lymph nodes are involved, the converse is not always true; bone metastasis often occurs without evidence of nodal involvement. Spinal metastases may extend into the epidural space and cause extrinsic compression of the spinal cord and progression to paraplegia. It is therefore prudent to thoroughly evaluate patients with backache for impending spinal cord compression. Paraneoplastic syndromes have been associated with disseminated prostate cancer and include disseminated intravascular coagulopathy and neuromuscular abnormalities. It should be noted that hypercalcemia is very unusual with prostate cancer, and other causes should be explored when it occurs in the prostate cancer patient.

DIAGNOSIS

Transrectal Ultrasonography

Adenocarcinoma of the prostate usually appears as a hypoechoic lesion and can be detected in the apex of the prostate. Transrectal ultrasonography (TRUS) may detect lesions as small as 5 mm in diameter. In addition, a TRUS-guided biopsy permits a more precise sampling of areas suggestive of cancer.[46] Since this procedure is associated with minimal morbidity and complications, it can be performed easily on an outpatient basis. It is important to keep in mind that only 20% of hypoechoic areas are actually cancerous because the hypoechoic appearance of prostatic tumors reflects their high cellular density and overlaps considerably with that of nonmalignant tissue that may be affected by inflammation. In addition, up to 30% of prostate lesions that are easily palpable during DRE can be missed by ultrasonic scanning because they are isoechoic rather than hypoechoic. In addition, cancers arising in the transitional zone of the prostatic gland, an area that is also the origin of benign prostatic hypertrophy, cannot be detected as hypoechoic tumors because of the heterogeneous texture of this region of the gland.

The role of TRUS in screening for prostatic cancer remains to be established. Advocates emphasize its ease and reliability in serial examinations and the limitations of the DRE. Skeptics, however, point to the relatively marginal specificity of the procedure and to the lack of proof that detection of early lesions actually improves the clinical outcome of affected patients.

Prostate-Specific Antigen

Prostate-specific antigen is a glycoprotein produced by both normal and malignant prostate cells. Although specific to the prostate in benign tissues, recent studies have shown that other human malignancies, such as breast and ovarian cancer, may also express PSA, albeit at significantly lower levels.[47,48]

An enlarged prostate caused by benign prostatic hypertrophy, especially in older males, accounts for the majority of borderline PSA elevations encountered in community practice. However, levels above 10 ng/mL are unlikely to be due to benign prostatic hypertrophy alone, necessitating a proper urologic evaluation.[49] Hudson et al[49] showed that only 2% of patients with benign prostatic hypertrophy had PSA levels over 10 ng/mL and that 44% of patients with prostate cancer (including 36% of those with clinical stage A or B disease) had levels over 10 ng/mL. On the other hand, up to one third of patients with localized prostate cancers have normal PSA values.[49,50] Therefore, measurement of PSA should not replace DRE in the early detection of prostate cancers but rather should complement it. It should be noted that PSA assays from different manufacturers may yield discordant results.[51]

Attempts to refine the predictive value of PSA have been reported. One approach uses the ratio of PSA to the prostatic volume.[52] This refinement adjusts for the fact that the upper range of normal PSA levels rises with age, due partly to the increasing size of the prostate gland. Using the 95th percentile, the upper limit of the normal range for the serum PSA concentration increases from 2.5 ng/mL for a 45-year-old man to 6.5 ng/mL for a 75-year-old man.[50] Another consideration in improving the diagnostic yield of PSA measurement is the "PSA velocity," or slope. It has been observed that serum PSA increases more rapidly in prostate cancer than in benign prostatic hypertrophy.[45] Further, a rise in PSA compared with previous measurements may be highly predictive of prostate cancer even though the PSA remains in the "normal" range.[50]

The kinetics of PSA release and clearance are important for its proper incorporation into therapeutic decision making in patients with prostate cancer. Routine DRE should not cause a significant elevation in PSA.[53] This is in contrast to the level of prostatic acid phosphatase (PAP), which is affected by DRE. Nevertheless, it is generally recommended that baseline levels of PSA be measured before DRE or any other prostatic manipulation. After major traumas, however, such as transurethral resection or needle biopsy of the prostate, PSA rises significantly, sometimes up to 50 times over baseline values, and remains elevated for weeks.[54] A markedly elevated serum PSA level caused by bacterial prostatitis may cause confusion in the diagnosis of prostatic cancer. Thus, serum PSA determination should be repeated after complete clinical resolution of inflammation to exclude prostatic malignancy.[55] The half-life of PSA has been calculated to be approximately 4.6 days.[56]

Serum PSA levels are lowered in patients receiving finasteride, an inhibitor of 5-alpha-reductase, which is used in the treatment of patients with benign prostatic hypertrophy, and it is therefore prudent to exclude prostatic carcinoma before starting patients on this drug. Any persistent elevation of PSA levels while on finasteride should initiate the necessary workup to rule out prostate cancer. It is recommended that in patients taking finasteride, the age-adjusted reference range of normal serum PSA levels be reduced by 50%.[57]

Screening for PSA leads to the detection of more organ-confined prostate cancers than does the use of other diagnostic methods such as DRE. The incidence of lymph-node involvement has decreased from 20% in historical series to less than 10% in contemporary studies.[58] Earlier studies have also shown that serum PSA can detect twice as many cancers as DRE in a screening situation[59] and that DRE may not be adequate to detect tumors in early stages.[60] Current consensus is that elevated serum PSA levels that lead to further evaluation with a prostate biopsy do not identify clinically unimportant prostate cancers.[61]

Screening

At present, no adequately performed prospective study has demonstrated a reduction in mortality rate attributable to annual prostate cancer screening. Because of the slow doubling time of primary prostatic carcinoma, it is advisable to confine screening for prostate cancer to men with a life expectancy of greater than 10 years.[62] Preliminary reports have suggested that the proportion of men with organ-confined tumors increases with PSA-based screening and that a reduction in prostate cancer mortality by means of screening is feasible.[63] However, the adoption of widespread screening of men for prostate cancer will await further evidence, particularly from prospectively randomized studies. Currently an NCI-funded randomized trial is under way to determine the survival advantage of screening. In the meantime, current recommendations of the American College of Surgeons are that all men over age 50 years be screened for prostate cancer annually with a DRE and PSA test.[64] Moreover, it has been recommended that men in high-risk groups, including blacks and men with a family history of prostate cancer, be screened at an earlier age.[64]

With the advent of screening the general population by PSA measurements, the diagnostic approach in asymptomatic individuals has been steadily evolving. A reasonable summary of the current approach is that if the serum PSA level is less than or equal to the upper limit of the age-specific reference range and the DRE results are unremarkable, the patient should be followed with annual evaluations. If the serum PSA level is greater than the age-specific reference range and the DRE yields normal results, a TRUS should be performed and any visible lesion should be biopsied. In addition, a systematic sextant biopsy of the remaining prostate tissue should be carried out. If none of these cores contain tissue from the transitional zone, two additional specimens from the anterior part of the prostate, one from each side, should be taken in order to completely sample the gland. If the DRE results are abnormal, irrespective of the serum PSA level, the patient should undergo TRUS. Using ultra-sound guidance, the palpable abnormalities should be biopsied, as should all hypoechoic lesions. In addition, a systematic sextant biopsy of the remaining prostate gland should be performed.

STAGING

The most commonly used staging system for prostatic carcinoma is shown in Table 1. This system incorporates features of the A-B-C-D system originally introduced by Whitmore and later revised by Jewett, as well as features of the tumor-node-metastasis (TNM) staging system devised by the American Joint Committee on Cancer and the International Union Against Cancer.[61] In general, the disease-specific mortality for untreated patients who have stage A disease is less than 2%. Of those with stage B or C disease, one fourth will die within 15 years of diagnosis. Unfortunately, about 70% of patients present with stage C or D prostate cancer. The 5-year survival rate for patients with stage D prostate cancer remains less than 20%.

Patients with newly diagnosed, biopsy-proven prostate cancer are investigated to determine the presence or absence of locoregional and distant metastases. Nuclear bone scans are performed in most patients. A positive bone scan correlates with a high level of PSA and identifies patients with stage D2 disease, rendering elaborate local therapy unnecessary. If the bone scan is negative, computed tomography should be performed to look for involvement of the pelvic lymph nodes. The extent of local disease may be defined better by TRUS as an adjunct to the DRE because clinical staging of the primary tumor is relatively imprecise. To date, no single modality such as DRE, TRUS, PSA measurements, or magnetic resonance imaging can accurately predict which tumors are organ confined and presumably curable by local therapeutic modalities. Preoperative measurement of the prostatic acid phosphatase level is often done. If elevated, this suggests the presence of advanced disease, again obviating the need for prostatectomy.[65] Several studies are currently evaluating the role of molecular staging using an enhanced reverse transcriptase-polymerase chain reaction assay for the detection of prostatic tumor cells in the blood.[66] However, at present there is no evidence of whether the increased sensitivity in detecting micrometastases of prostate cancer has any bearing on the management of patients who are upstaged with this procedure.

Tumor volume in advanced disease appears to influence response to therapy. Investigators at M. D. Anderson Cancer Center have devised a stratification for patients with metastatic disease based on the extent of

TABLE I

1992 American Joint Committee on Cancer and International Union Against Cancer TNM Staging Classification for Prostate Cancer

Primary Tumor (T)

TX   Primary tumor cannot be assessed

T0   No evidence of primary tumor

T1   Clinically inapparent tumor not palpable or visible by imaging

        T1a   Tumor incidental histologic finding in 5% or less of tissue resected

        T1b   Tumor incidental histologic finding in more than 5% of tissue resected

        T1c   Tumor identified by needle biopsy (eg, because of elevated PSA)

T2   Palpable tumor confined within prostate [a]

        T2a   Tumor involves half of a lobe or less

        T2b   Tumor involves more than half of a lobe, but not both lobes

        T2c   Tumor involves both lobes

T3   Tumor extends through the prostatic capsule

        T3a   Unilateral extracapsular enlargement

        T3b   Bilateral extracapsular extension

        T3c   Tumor invades seminal vesicle(s)

T4   Tumor is fixed or invades adjacent structures other than seminal vesicles

        T4a   Tumor invades external sphincter and/or bladder neck and/or rectum

        T4b   Tumor invades levator muscles and/or is fixed to pelvic wall

Lymph Node (N)

NX   Regional lymph nodes cannot be assessed

N0   No regional lymph-node metastasis

N1   Metastasis in a single lymph node, 2 cm or smaller in greatest dimension

N2   Metastasis in a single lymph node, larger than 2 cm but not larger than 5 cm in greatest dimension, or multiple lymph nodes, none larger than 5 cm in greatest dimension

N3   Metastasis in a lymph node larger than 5 cm in greatest dimension

Distant Metastasis (M)

MX   Presence of distant metastasis cannot be assessed

M0   No distant metastasis

M1   Distant metastasis

        M1a   Nonregional lymph nodes

        M1b   Bone

        M1c   Other sites

PSA = prostate-specific antigen

[a] Tumor found in one or both lobes by needle biopsy, but not palpable or visible by imaging is classified as T1c. (Invasion into the prostatic apex or into (but not beyond) the prostatic capsule is classified not as T3, but as T2.

metastatic involvement. Osseous I (OI) is metastatic axial skeletal involvement only. Osseous II is axial disease plus extremity skeletal involvement. Visceral I (VI) is pulmonary metastases, and visceral II (VII) denotes metastases in other viscera.[67]

TREATMENT

Early-Stage Prostate Cancer (Stages A and B)

The optimal method for managing patients with early-stage prostate cancer remains controversial. Evaluating response is difficult because early detection may increase the interval between diagnosis and death, regardless of the effectiveness of treatment (lead-time bias). In addition, the diagnosis and treatment of latent, rather than clinical, prostate cancer may seemingly achieve therapeutic efficacy when, in fact, these tumors were intrinsically innocuous. There is rising use of radical prostatectomy to treat patients with early stage prostate cancer. Nevertheless, valid comparisons between radiation therapy, radical prostatectomy, and "watch and wait" approaches are lacking, and no final consensus exists on the most appropriate treatment for patients with newly diagnosed early-stage prostate cancer. Further confounding the problem, approximately 30% of patients with clinical stage B and 60% of patients with clinical stage C disease have positive lymph-node involvement upon staging lymphadenectomy.[68,69] Lymph-node involvement may even be higher in patients with higher grade tumors.

Watchful Waiting: Difficulties arise in prospectively identifying patients in whom a deferred-treatment approach can be safely employed without jeopardizing survival or adversely affecting quality of life. Several investigators have questioned whether definitive therapy is necessary for all men with clinically localized prostate cancer.[70,71] However, many of the observational studies that recommended a watchful-waiting strategy had patients with predominantly well-differentiated tumors of low volume. In addition, many such studies included patients over the age of 70 years. In contrast, series recommending radical prostatectomy or radiation involved a larger proportion of younger men with moderately or poorly differentiated tumors.

At present it seems reasonable to offer curative therapy to men judged to have a life expectancy of 10 years or more, though there is no compelling evidence that a close watchful-waiting policy, with treatment deferred until the time of clinical progression, would produce inferior results. Certainly, patients with stage A1 well-differentiated prostate cancer may be simply followed up clinically. For other patients, although local progression is common, if not inevitable, how it affects quality of life in patients managed by watchful waiting requires further study.

Surgery vs Radiation for Localized Disease: In patients with early-stage disease limited to the prostate (stage A2, B1, or B2), both radical prostatectomy and radiation therapy can be curative but are associated with considerable morbidity. In a prospective randomized study by the Veteran Affairs Oncology Group, in which patients were assigned to either radiation therapy or surgery after confirmation that lymph-node metastases were absent, a higher percentage of surgically treated patients were free of recurrence after 5 years.[72] On the other hand, the results of a retrospective analysis of the long-term outcome of radiation therapy were comparable with those of surgical treatment in the cohort prospectively studied by the Veteran Affairs group.[73] Thus, neither approach has proved statistically superior in efficacy.[74]

Since neither surgery nor radiation therapy is clearly preferable for treating localized prostate cancer, each patient's therapy must be individually chosen after consideration of the potential benefits and risks. Currently, patients with a 10- to 15-year life expectancy, good performance status, and clinically localized prostate cancer that is not of high Gleason grade nor associated with a PSA level above 15 ng/mL are considered ideal candidates for radical prostatectomy.

Radical Prostatectomy: Radical prostatectomy involves the removal of the entire prostate, including the capsule, a layer of surrounding connective tissue, and the attached seminal vesicles. Newer techniques have significantly reduced impotence and hemorrhage, but urinary incontinence may occur in a small proportion of patients. Using the nerve-sparing technique pioneered by Walsh,[75] potency returns in 50% to 80% of patients after 1 year. Whether this technical modification compromises the overall effectiveness of the surgery with regard to local tumor control awaits longer periods of follow-up. Only selected patients, those with tumors that do not involve the neurovascular bundle in the pelvic plexus and branches innervating the corpora cavernosa lateral to the prostate gland, are eligible for this procedure.[76] Prostate-specific antigen must become undetectable after curative radical prostatectomy, and its presence after this procedure indicates residual prostatic cancer cells.

Zincke et al[2] reported the experience using radical prostatectomy for clinically organ-confined disease at the Mayo Clinic. Of the 1,143 patients followed up after radical prostatectomy, the 10- and 15-year disease-specific survival rates were 90% and 83%, respectively.

Only the tumor grade was a significant predictor for disease outcome. For the more recent 1,000 patients, hospital mortality was 0% and severe urinary incontinence had declined so that it only affected 1.4% of patients.

Radiation Therapy: External beam radiation from high-energy linear accelerators is used in the treatment of patients with localized prostate cancer that may be encompassed within a radiotherapy field. The treatment involves up to 50 Gy of wide-field radiation that includes the pelvic lymph nodes, followed by an additional booster dose to the prostate and surrounding tissues, for a total dose of 70 Gy.[7] Complications such as delayed impotence occur in approximately 40% of patients. Urinary incontinence, however, is relatively uncommon. Radiation-induced rectal damage may also be a troublesome side effect of radiation therapy.

The presence of residual tumor after radiation therapy has been a cause for concern. Systematic biopsies of tissue from patients treated with radiation therapy have shown a 35% to 91% incidence of apparently viable tumor.[78,79] The detection of viable tumor 1 year after radiation therapy predicts for the subsequent development of distant metastases.[80,81] PSA levels should fall to normal within 6 to 12 months after radiation therapy, and persistence of elevated levels may indicate residual disease and poor prognosis.

The recent introduction of high-precision three-dimensional conformal radiation therapy (3D-CRT) in the treatment of prostate cancer provides a promising approach for overcoming the problems of local tumor failure after radiation therapy.[82] In addition, 3D-CRT attempts to circumvent the problems associated with exposure of normal pelvic tissues to external beam radiation. 3D-CRT uses sophisticated computer-aided treatment planning to accurately conform the distribution of a prescribed radiation dose to the anatomic boundaries of the prostatic target volume.

Stage C Prostate Cancer

Surgical cure is unlikely in patients with stage C prostate cancer given that over 50% of patients have pelvic lymph-node involvement, and there is a significant chance of leaving residual tumor behind.[83] Long-term disease-free survival is possible for some patients who only have capsular penetration (clinical stage C1). However, in most patients simply extending the surgical margin of resection has no impact on disease-free survival.[84]

The use of adjuvant radiation and/or endocrine therapy in stage C disease remains controversial. A retrospective analysis of patients treated at the Mayo Clinic revealed that adjuvant therapy with radiation or orchiectomy for high-risk men decreased both the local and systemic progression rates but had no impact on survival.[85] This study result provides additional support for a deferred-treatment approach.

Radiation therapy has been the primary mode of treatment for patients with stage C prostate cancer.[86] In a series of patients treated with radiation and followed up for 20 years, 44% died of intercurrent illnesses and 47% died of prostatic cancer.[87] Hormonal therapy has also been used in the treatment of patients with stage C disease with the aim of local tumor control and downstaging of the tumor. Conversion from stage C to stage B or A may allow curative resection of the primary prostate cancer. Macfarlane et al[88] reported on 22 patients with stage B2 and C cancers who received preoperative combined androgen blockade. Although the PSA level became normal in the majority, only 33% showed a decrease in tumor size, based on ultrasonography volumes, and only 15% showed a decrease in clinical stage. In another study of 30 patients with stage C disease treated with preoperative hormonal therapy, 47% were downstaged to clinical stage B after therapy.[89] Pathologic staging, however, revealed organ-confined disease in only 10% of the patients. It appears that survival is identical for patients treated initially with hormonal therapy and those treated first with radiation and subsequently with hormonal therapy at the time of tumor progression.

Metastatic Prostate Cancer

Antiandrogen Therapy: Androgen deprivation remains the primary therapy for patients with metastatic prostate cancer, including stage D1 disease (N1-N3 M0). Androgen ablation is not curative therapy in patients with metastases to lymph nodes or beyond but is usually associated with significant disease control. Nevertheless, the duration of response is variable and the effect on the overall survival unclear. Up to 80% of patients with metastatic disease will respond initially to androgen ablation, but within 1 to 2 years, most of them will develop hormone-refractory disease.[90] Antiandrogen therapy should take into account the two sources of androgens in humans. The testes produce most of the testosterone, which is converted in the target cells by 5-alpha-reductase to dihydrotestosterone (DHT). In addition, the adrenal cortex produces androstenedione and dehydroepiandrosterone, which constitute about 5% of the circulating androgens.

Bilateral orchiectomy remains the definitive and most effective antitestosterone treatment. The procedure can be performed in an outpatient setting under local anesthesia with minimal morbidity. Estrogenic preparations, such as diethylstilbestrol (DES), have also been used for several decades. They exert their antitestosterone effect by inhibiting the secretion of pituitary luteinizing hormone through a negative-feedback loop. Side effects of estrogen therapy include gynecomastia and thromboembolism. Because of concerns about these side effects, daily doses of DES should not exceed 3 mg/d. At this dosage, complete suppression of testosterone is typical. A dose of 1 mg/d has also been advocated and is widely used. Although this dose probably produces fewer side effects, it effectively suppresses testosterone to castrate levels in only 70% of patients. Gynecomastia due to estrogens may be prevented by superficial irradiation of the breast tissue at a dose of up to 15 Gy before the start of therapy.

Another class of antiandrogens includes the receptor antagonists, such as flutamide. The use of flutamide alone is associated with a rise in serum luteinizing hormone and testosterone concentrations as the negative feedback of androgens on the pituitary gland is inhibited. This secondary rise in circulating testosterone may decrease the efficacy of flutamide; it is not used as monotherapy because combination therapy with testicular suppression, described below, is more effective. It is also notable that there was no survival advantage for patients treated with luteinizing hormone-releasing hormone (LHRH) alone when flutamide was added at the time of disease progression.[91]

The most commonly used approach in antiandrogen therapy involves the use of hypothalamic LHRH analogs. These synthetic peptides (leuprolide, buserelin, and goserelin) are administered by parenteral injection. Through binding to the LHRH receptors in the pituitary, these agents initially stimulate the release of luteinizing hormone but then block the stimulation of LHRH receptors by the endogenous pulsatile secretion of LHRH. The eventual result is suppression of follicle-stimulating hormone and luteinizing hormone secretion by the pituitary gland. Depot preparations are now available that require only monthly injections to achieve castrate levels of testosterone. The advantages of LHRH analogs are that they avoid the minor trauma of orchiectomy and allow potentially reversible testicular suppression. The disadvantages include cost, the necessity for monthly injections, and the potential for rapid worsening of a patient's condition during the initial 2 weeks of therapy. In patients with involvement of the spinal column, LHRH analogs alone are strictly contraindicated because they can exacerbate spinal cord compression and precipitate paraple-

gia. This initial flare-up may be blocked by giving flutamide for several days before and for 2 weeks after the depot LHRH injection. The main disadvantage of these depot peptides is their high cost; they are much more expensive in the long term than orchiectomy.

Several studies have compared the efficacy of combined androgen blockade (LHRH agonists or orchiectomy plus antiandrogens) with that of antiandrogen therapy alone.[92] Several trials using an orchiectomy control arm showed a benefit for combined therapy. Janknegt et al[93] examined 433 patients and showed a 6-month advantage in median time to progression (20.8 vs 14.9 months), which was statistically significant, and an 8-month difference in the median time to death from prostate cancer (37.1 vs 29.8 months, $P = .04$). A study by the European Organization for Research Treatment of Cancer showed a longer time to progression (71 vs 41 weeks; $P = .002$), longer survival (median, 34 vs 27.1 months, $P = .02$), and longer prostate cancer-specific survival (43.9 vs 28.8 months; $P = .001$) for patients receiving combined therapy.[94] The modest survival advantage of total androgen blockade must be weighed against its side effects and considerable expense.

Hormone-Refractory Prostate Cancer

Patients with disease progression in the presence of proven castrate levels of testosterone pose a major therapeutic challenge to the practicing oncologist. Responses to second-line hormonal agents are typically poor, and the median survival of such patients remains less than 1 year.[95]

It is important to note that most patients whose disease progressed despite hormonal therapy paradoxically remain sensitive to additional stimulation of tumor growth by androgens. A retrospective multivariate analysis of survival data on 341 patients with hormone-refractory prostate cancer revealed that continued androgen suppression was an important predictor of longer survival, as were weight loss, age, performance status, and disease sites.[96] Therefore, patients with hormone-refractory disease who have not undergone orchiectomy must continue their therapy with estrogen or LHRH analogs. Otherwise, they are at risk of severe, symptomatic exacerbations of their already terminal disease.

Flutamide Withdrawal: Several studies have demonstrated a favorable response to flutamide withdrawal in patients who have experienced a lengthy remission on combined antiandrogen therapy. In a recently reported study, flutamide was discontinued in 36 consecutive patients with disease progression despite castrate levels of testosterone.[97] Twenty-nine percent of patients experienced a significant decline in PSA levels (more than or equal to 80% in seven patients and less than or equal to 50% in three) from baseline after flutamide was discontinued. The duration of PSA response ranged from 2 to 10 or more months, with a median duration of 5 or more months.[97] Decline in PSA was associated with improvement in symptoms in all patients, and one patient had a partial response in an epidural mass with improvement in neurologic symptoms. All patients who responded to flutamide withdrawal received combined androgen blockade as their initial therapy.

Ketoconazole: Ketoconazole is an antifungal drug that in sufficiently high doses inhibits the adrenal and testicular synthesis of androgens. An initial report showed that the level of PSA decreased on average by 49% from the pretreatment level in 12 (80%) of 15 patients treated with ketoconazole for a median duration of 4 months.[98] A larger study of 44 patients showed 1 complete and 5 partial responses (14% response rate) with a median response duration of 27 weeks.[99] Major side effects from ketoconazole include severe gastric intolerance and adrenal suppression, the latter requiring supplemental hydrocortisone to prevent hypoadrenocorticolism.

Chemotherapy: Interest in chemotherapy for hormone-refractory prostate cancer has been rekindled with the demonstration of significant antitumor activity of several drug-combination regimens. One of the most active agents against prostate cancer is doxorubicin.[100] It is frequently administered at a dose of 20 mg/m^2 intravenously weekly. While doxorubicin can produce significant subjective improvement, significant prolongation of survival remains elusive.[101] The combination of doxorubicin and ketoconazole has been assessed in 39 patients with hormone-refractory disease.[67] Based on serial PSA measurements, 55% of patients experienced significant responses. Based on reduction of tumor size, objective partial responses occurred in 58% of patients with measurable disease. The combination of oral etoposide (50 mg/m^2) and estramustine (15 mg/kg/d) given for 21 days and repeated every 28 days has resulted in significant antitumor activity in patients with hormone-refractory prostate cancer.[101] Of the 18 patients with measurable disease, 3 and 6 patients had complete and partial responses, respectively. Ten of 42 patients experienced a greater than 75% reduction in PSA levels; 23 had a greater than 50% reduction. In contrast, single-agent oral etoposide had minimal activity in hormone-refractory prostate cancer.[102]

Another approach in the therapy of hormone-refractory prostate cancer involves the use of cytotoxic drugs plus hormonal agents. A randomized trial of combined vs sequential endocrine therapy and chemotherapy evaluated the effect of chemotherapy given early in the course of the disease. Patients were randomized to receive doxorubicin and cyclophosphamide either at the time of initial hormonal therapy (combination arm) or at the time of tumor progression (sequential arm). Patients in the combination arm had a higher response rate than those in the sequential arm (63% vs 48%, respectively), but no significant difference in survival was observed.[103]

Strontium-89: Strontium-89 is a beta-emitting radionuclide that may be used to deliver systemic radiation therapy to bone metastases.[104] Strontium-89, being chemically similar to calcium, is preferentially localized in bone. Over the past few years it has become recognized as a viable treatment option in the palliation of bone metastases secondary to prostate cancer. Occasionally, a transient increase in bone pain occurs within a few days of administration. In general, the major side effects of therapy with strontium-89 appear to be limited to hematologic toxicity, particularly thrombocytopenia.

A randomized phase III trial was performed in Canada to evaluate the effectiveness of strontium-89 in combination with local-field radiotherapy.[105] Patients with progressive disease after hormonal therapy were randomly assigned to receive local external beam radiation combined with either strontium-89 or a placebo. After 3 months, patients treated with strontium-89 plus radiation had significantly fewer new painful metastases and an increased interval of time to further radiotherapy, and on quality-of-life surveys they had superior improvement in pain and physical activity compared with the placebo group. There was no significant difference in the overall survival, but the strontium-89 treatment group had a greater number of patients with a 50% decline in PSA than the control group did. Investigators at M. D. Anderson Cancer Center are currently evaluating the efficacy of combining cytotoxic therapy (doxorubicin) with strontium-89.

Future Directions

Basic and clinical research in prostate cancer represent very active areas of research. Over the past few years our understanding of the biology of prostate cancer has considerably increased. Some of the molecular changes during prostatic carcinogenesis may lend themselves to therapeutic interventions.

For patients with advanced hormone-responsive prostate cancer, a plateau has been reached with regard to antiandrogen therapy. One approach that may decrease the morbidity of androgen deprivation involves intermittent androgen suppression to induce multiple apoptotic regressions of prostate cancer.[106] For patients with hormone-refractory prostate cancer, cytotoxic therapy in various combinations is currently being actively investigated. However, in the absence of drugs with significant single-agent activity, this approach seems unlikely to produce significant improvements. Therefore, the search will continue for new drugs that target critical biochemical events involved in the progression of prostate tumors. One promising approach is to inhibit angiogenesis, a process that is crucial for disease progression and metastasis. TNP-470 is a semisynthetic analog of fumagillin with potent antitumor activity in animals bearing prostate tumors and is currently in early clinical trials.[107,108]

Assessment of tumor response by bidimensionally measuring metastatic lesions is notoriously difficult in the majority of patients with prostate cancer, who have predominantly bone-only metastases. As such, only 10% to 20% of patients with metastatic disease are eligible for clinical trials based on the presence of measurable disease. Such obstacles have been partly overcome by the use of PSA as a marker for disease activity. A specific objective response may be categorized by the extent of PSA decline, such as 50% to 80% from baseline, and the duration of such a decline. Initial studies assessing the degree of PSA decline and its correlation with survival in patients receiving systemic therapy for hormone-refractory disease have shown that the median survival of patients with at least a 50% decline from the baseline PSA level is 20 months, in contrast to 8 months in patients with less than a 50% decline in the PSA level.[109]

REFERENCES

1. Wingo PA, Tong T, Bolden S: Cancer statistics. CA Cancer J Clin 45:8–30, 1995.

2. Zincke H, Bergstralh EJ, Blute ML, et al: Radical prostatectomy for clinically localized prostate cancer: Long-term results of 1,143 patients from a single institution. J Clin Oncol 12:2254–2263, 1994.

3. Ross RK, Paganini-Hill A, Henderson BE: Epidemiology of prostate cancer, in Skinner DG, Leskovsky G (eds): Diagnosis and Management of Genitourinary Cancer, pp 40–45. Philadelphia, WB Saunders, 1988.

4. Hsing AW, Devesa SS: Prostate cancer mortality in the United States by cohort year of birth, 1865–1940. Cancer Epidemiol Biomarkers Prev 3:527–530, 1994.

5. Yatani R, Chigusa K, Akazaki K, et al: Geographic pathology of latent prostatic carcinoma. Int J Cancer 29:611–616, 1992.

6. Haenzel W, Kurihara M: Studies of Japanese migrants: I. Mortality from cancer and other diseases among Japanese in the United States. J Natl Cancer Inst 40:43–68, 1968.

7. Staszewski J, Hoaenzel W: Cancer mortality among the foreign born in the United States. J Natl Cancer Inst 26:37–132, 1961.

8. Isaacson C, Selzer G, Kaye V, et al: Cancer in the urban Blacks of South Africa. South African Cancer Bulletin 22:49–84, 1978.

9. Zaridze DG, Boyle P: Cancer of the prostate: Epidemiology and etiology. Br J Urol 59:493–502, 1987.

10. Healy B: From the National Institute of Health: Does vasectomy cause prostate cancer? JAMA 269:2620, 1993.

11. Carter HB, Coffey DS: The prostate: An increasing medical problem. Prostate 16:39–48, 1990.

12. Ross RK, Bernstein L, Judd H, et al: Serum testosterone levels in healthy young black and white men. J Natl Cancer Inst 76:45–48, 1986.

13. Hill PB, Wynder EL: Effect of a vegetarian diet and dexamethasone on plasma prolactin, testosterone and dehydroepiandrosterone in men and women. Cancer Lett 7:273–282, 1979.

14. Gittes RF: Carcinoma of the prostate. N Engl J Med 324:236–245, 1991.

15. Cannon L, Bishop D, Skolnick M, et al: Genetic epidemiology of prostate cancer in the Mormon genealogy. Cancer Surv 1:47, 1982.

16. Steinberg GD, Carter BS, Beaty TL, et al: The familial aggregation of prostate cancer: A case control study (abstract). J Urol 143:313A, 1990.

17. Ware JL: Prostate cancer progression. Implications of histopathology. Am J Pathol 145:983–993, 1994.

18. Bergerheim USR, Kunimi K, Collins VP, et al: Deletion mapping of chromosome 8, chromosome 10, and chromosome 16 in human prostatic carcinoma. Genes Chromosom Cancer 3:215, 1991.

19. Macoska JA, Trybus TM, et al: Fluorescence in situ hybridization analysis of 8p allelic loss and chromosome 8 instability in human prostate cancer. Cancer Res 54: 3824–3830, 1994.

20. Visakorpi T, Kallioniemi AH, Syvanen A-C, et al: Genetic changes in primary and recurrent prostate cancer by comparative genomic hybridization. Cancer Res 55:342–347, 1995.

21. Peehl DM. Oncogenes in prostate cancer. Cancer 71:1159–1164, 1993.

22. Linehan WM: Molecular genetics of tumor suppressor genes in prostate carcinoma: The challenge and the promise ahead. J Urol 147:808–809, 1992.

23. Navone NM, Troncoso P, et al: p53 protein accumulation and gene mutation in the progression of human prostate carcinoma. J Nat Cancer Inst 85:1657–1669, 1993.

24. Phillips SM, Barton CM, Lee SJ, et al: Loss of the retinoblastoma susceptibility gene (RB1) is a frequent and early event in prostatic tumorigenesis. Br J Cancer 70:1252–1257, 1994.

25. Gao X, Honn KV, et al: Frequent loss of expression and loss of heterozygosity of the putative tumor suppressor gene DCC in prostatic carcinomas. Cancer Res 53:2723–2727, 1993.

26. Ching KZ, Ramsey E, et al: Expression of mRNA for epidermal growth factor, transforming growth factor-alpha and their receptors in human prostate tissue and cell lines. Mol Cell Biochem 126:151–158, 1993.

27. Wilding G, Zugmaier G, Knabbe C, et al: Differential effects of transforming growth factor beta on human prostate cancer cells in vitro. Mol Cell Endocrinol 62:79, 1989.

28. Wilding G, Valverius E, Knabbe C, et al: Role of transforming growth factor alpha in human prostate cancer cell growth. Prostate 15:1, 1989.

29. Marengo SR, Chung LWK: An orthotopic model for the study of growth factors in the ventral prostate of the rat: Effects of epidermal growth factor and basic fibroblast growth factor. J Andrology 15:277–286, 1994.

30. Muller WJ, Lee FFS, Dickson C, et al: The int-2 gene product acts as an epithelial growth factor in transgenic mice. EMBO J 9:907, 1990.

31. Myers RB, Srivastava S, Oelschlager DK, et al: Expression of p160^{erbB-3} and p185^{erbB-2} in prostatic intraepithelial neoplasia and prostatic adenocarcinoma. J Natl Cancer Inst 86:1140–1145, 1994.

32. Sadasivan R, Morgan R, et al: Overexpression of Her-2/neu

may be an indicator of poor prognosis in prostate cancer. J Urol 150:126–131, 1993.

33. McDonnell TJ, Troncoso P, et al: Expression of the protooncogene BCL-2 in the prostate and its association with emergence of androgen-independent prostate cancer. Cancer Res 52:6940–6944, 1992.

34. Colombel M, Symmans F, et al: Detection of the apoptosis-suppressing oncoprotein bcl-2 in hormone-refractory human prostate cancer. Am J Pathol 143:390–400, 1993.

35. Umbas R, Schalken JA, Aalders TW, et al: Expression of the cellular adhesion molecule E-cadherin is reduced or absent in high-grade prostate cancer. Cancer Res 52:5104–5109, 1992.

36. Umbas R, Isaacs WB, et al: Decreased E-cadherin expression is associated with poor prognosis in patients with prostate cancer. Cancer Res 54:3929–3933, 1994.

37. Weidner N, Carrol PR, et al: Tumor angiogenesis correlates with metastasis in invasive prostate carcinoma. Am J Pathol 143:401–408, 1993.

38. Chung LWK, Gleave ME, Hsieh J, et al: Reciprocal mesenchymal-epithelial interactions affecting prostate tumor growth and hormonal responsiveness. Cancer Surv 11:91–121, 1991.

39. Gaudin PB, Epstein JI: Adenosis of the prostate. Histologic features in transurethral resection specimens. Am J Surg Pathol 18:863–870, 1994.

40. Amato RJ, Logothetis CJ, et al: Chemotherapy for small cell carcinoma of prostatic origin. J Urol 147:935–937, 1992.

41. Brawn PN, Ayala AG, von Eschenbach AC, et al: Histologic grading study of prostate adenocarcinoma: The development of a new system and comparison with other methods—a preliminary study. Cancer 49:525–532, 1982.

42. Centeno BA, Zietman AL, et al: Flow cytometric analysis of DNA ploidy, percent S-phase fraction, and total proliferative fraction as prognostic indicators of local control and survival following radiation therapy for prostate carcinoma. Int J Radiat Oncol Biol Phys 30:309–315, 1994.

43. Visakorpi T, Kallioniemi O-P, Koivula T, et al: Review of new prognostic factors in prostatic carcinoma. Eur Urol 24:438–449, 1993.

44. Forsslund G, Esposti PL, Nilsson B, et al: The prognostic significance of nuclear DNA content in prostatic carcinoma. Cancer 69:1432–1439, 1992.

45. Carter BS, Beaty TH, et al: Mendelian inheritance of familial prostate cancer. Proc Natl Acad Sci USA 89:3367–3371, 1992.

46. Terris MK, Haney DJ, Johnstone IM, et al: Prediction of prostate cancer volume using prostate-specific antigen levels, transrectal ultrasound, and systematic sextant biopsies. Urology 45:75–80, 1995.

47. Yu H, Diamandis EP, Sutherland DJA: Immunoreactive prostate specific antigen levels in female and male breast tumors and its association with steroid hormone receptors and patient age. Clin Biochem 27:75–79, 1994.

48. Yu H, Diamandis EP, Levesque M, et al: Expression of the prostate-specific antigen by a primary ovarian carcinoma. Cancer Res 55:1603–1606, 1995.

49. Hudson MA, Brahnson RR, Catalina WJ: Clinical use of prostate specific antigen in patients with prostate cancer. J Urol 142:1011–1017, 1989.

50. Oesterling JE, Jacobsen SJ, et al: Serum prostate-specific antigen in a community-based population of healthy men: Establishment of age-specific reference ranges. JAMA 270: 860–864, 1993.

51. Vessella RL, Lange PH: Issues in the assessment of PSA immunoassays. Urol Clin North Am 20:607–619, 1993.

52. Semjonow A, Hamm M, Rathert P, et al: Prostate-specific antigen corrected for prostate volume improves differentiation of benign prostatic hyperplasia and organ-confined prostatic cancer. Br J Urol 73:538–543, 1994.

53. Chybowski FM, Bergstralh EJ, Oesterling JE: The effect of digital rectal examination on the serum prostate specific antigen concentration: Results of a randomized study. J Urol 148:83–86, 1992.

54. Hodge KK, McNeal JE, Stamey TA: Ultrasound guided transrectal core biopsies of the palpably abnormal prostate. J Urol 142:66–70, 1989.

55. Yamamoto M, Hibi H, Miyake K: Prostate specific antigen levels in acute and chronic bacterial prostatitis. Hinyokika Kiyo 39:445–449, 1993.

56. van Straalen JP, Bossens MM, de Reijke TM, et al: Biological half life of prostate specific antigen after radical prostatectomy. Eur J Clin Chem Clin Biochem 32:53–55, 1994.

57. Guess HA, Heyse JF, et al: The effects of finasteride on prostate specific antigen in men with benign prostatic hyperplasia. Prostate 22:31–37, 1993.

58. Catalona WJ, Smith DS, et al: Detection of organ-confined prostate cancer is increased through prostate-specific antigen-based screening. JAMA 270:948–954, 1993.

59. Brawer M, Chetner M, et al: Screening for prostatic carcinoma with prostate-specific antigen. J Urol 147:841–845, 1992.

60. Gerber GS, Thompson IM, et al: Disease-specific survival following routine prostate cancer screening by digital rectal examination. JAMA 269:61–64, 1993.

61. Ohori M, Wheeler TM, Scardino PT: The new American Joint Committee on Cancer and International Union Against Cancer TNM classification of prostate cancer. Cancer 74:104–114, 1994.

62. Stenman U, Hakama M, et al: Serum concentrations of prostate specific antigen and its complex with α_1-antichymotrypsin before diagnosis of prostate cancer. Lancet 344:1594–1598, 1994.

63. Littrup PJ, Goodman AC, Mettlin CJ, et al: The benefit and cost of prostate cancer early detection. CA Cancer J Clin 43:134–149, 1993.

64. Mettlin C, Jones G, Averette H, et al: Defining and updating the American Cancer Society guidelines for the cancer-related checkup: Prostate and endometrial cancers. CA Cancer J Clin 43:42–46, 1993.

65. Burnett AL, Chan DW, Brendler CB, et al: The value of enzymatic acid phosphatase in the staging of localized prostate cancer. J Urol 148:1832–1834, 1992.

66. Katz AE, Olsson CA, Raffo AJ, et al: Molecular staging of prostate cancer with the use of an enhanced reverse transcriptase-PCR assay. Urology 43:765–775, 1994.

67. Sella A, Kilbourn R, et al: Phase II study of ketoconazole combined with weekly doxorubicin in patients with androgen-independent prostate cancer. J Clin Oncol 12:683–688, 1994.

68. Whitmore WF Jr: Natural history and staging of prostate cancer. Urol Clin North Am 11:205–220, 1984.

69. Donahue RE, Man JH, et al: Pelvic lymph node dissection: Guide to patient management in clinically locally confined adenocarcinoma of the prostate. Urology 20:559–565,1982.

70. Johanssen JE, Adami HO, et al: Natural history of localized prostate cancer: Population study in 223 untreated patients. Lancet 1:799–804, 1989.

71. Adolfsson J, Steineck G, Whitmore WF: Recent results of management of palpable clinically localized prostate cancer. Cancer 72:310–322, 1993.

72. Paulson DF: Randomized series of treatment with surgery versus radiation for prostate adenocarcinoma (NIH Publ 88–3005). Natl Cancer Inst Monogr 7:127–131, 1988.

73. Bagshaw MA, Cox RS, Ray GR: Status of radiation treatment

of prostate cancer at Stanford University (NIH Publ 88–3005). Natl Cancer Inst Monogr 7:47–60, 1988.

74. Lange PH: Controversies in management of apparently localized cancer of the prostate. Urology 34:13–18, 1989.

75. Walsh PC: Radical retropubic prostatectomy with reduced morbidity: An anatomic approach (NIH Publ 88-3005). Natl Cancer Inst Monogr 7:133–137, 1988.

76. Epstein JI, Carmichael MJ, Pizov G, et al: Influence of capsular penetration on progression following radical prostatectomy: A study of 196 cases with long-term follow-up. J Urol 150:135–141, 1993.

77. Hanks GE: External beam radiation therapy for clinically localized prostate cancer: Patterns of care studies in the United States (NIH Publ 88–3005). Natl Cancer Inst Monogr 7:75–84, 1988.

78. Freiha FS, Bagshaw MA: Carcinoma of the prostate: Results of post-irradiation biopsy. Prostate 5:19–25, 1984.

79. Scardino PT, Wheeler TM: Local control of prostate cancer with radiotherapy: Frequency and prognostic significance of positive results of postirradiaton prostate biopsy (NIH Publ 88-3005). Natl Cancer Inst Monogr 7:95–103, 1988.

80. Kiesling VJ, McAninch JW, Goebel JL, et al: External beam radiotherapy for adenocarcinoma of the prostate: A clinical follow-up. J Urol 124:851–854, 1980.

81. Leach GE, Cooper JF, Kagan AR, et al: Radiotherapy for prostatic carcinoma: Post-irradiation prostatic biopsy and recurrence patterns with long-term follow-up. J Urol 128:505–509, 1982.

82. Leibel SA, Zelefsky MJ, Kutcher GJ, et al: The biological basis and clinical application of three-dimensional conformal external beam radiation therapy in carcinoma of the prostate. Semin Oncol 21:580–597, 1994.

83. Zincke H, Utz DC, Taylor WF: Bilateral pelvic lymphadenectomy and radical prostatectomy for clinical stage C prostatic cancer: Role of adjuvant treatment for residual cancer and in disease progression. J Urol 135:1199–1205, 1986.

84. Frydenberg M, Oesterling JE: Therapeutic strategies for clinical stage C prostate cancer. Problems in Urology 7: 166–179, 1993.

85. Cheng WS, Frydenberg M, et al: Radical prostatectomy for pathologic stage C prostate cancer. Influence of pathologic variables and adjuvant treatment on disease outcome. Urology 42:283–291, 1993.

86. Hanks GE: Treatment of locally advanced prostate cancer with radiation therapy. Urology 33(suppl 5):37–41, 1989.

87. Del Regato JA, Trailins AH, et al: Twenty years follow-up of patients with inoperable cancer of the prostate (stage C) treated by radiotherapy: Report of a national cooperative study. Int J Radiat Oncol Biol Phys 26:197–201, 1993.

88. Macfarlane MT, Abi-Aad A, et al: Neoadjuvant hormonal deprivation in patients with locally advanced prostate cancer. J Urol 150:132–134, 1993.

89. Narayan P, Lowe BA, Carroll PR, et al: Neoadjuvant hormonal therapy and radical prostatectomy for clinical stage C carcinoma of the prostate. Br J Urology 73:544–548, 1994.

90. Hsieh W-S, Simons JW: Systemic therapy of prostate cancer. New concepts from prostate cancer tumor biology. Cancer Treat Rev 19:229–260, 1993.

91. McLeod DG, Benson RG Jr, Eisenberger MA, et al: The use of flutamide in hormone refractory metastatic prostate cancer. Cancer 72:3870–3873, 1993.

92. Crawford ED, Eisenberger MA, McLeod DG, et al: A controlled trial of leuprolide with and without flutamide in prostatic carcinoma. N Engl J Med 321:419–424, 1989.

93. Janknegt RA, Abbou CC, et al: Orchiectomy and nilutamide or placebo as treatment of metastatic prostatic cancer in a multinational double-blind randomized trial. J Urol 149:77–83, 1993.

94. Denis LJ, Carneiro De Moura JL, et al: Goserelin acetate and flutamide versus bilateral orchiectomy: A phase III EORTC trial (30853). Urology 42:119–130, 1993.

95. Logothetis CJ, Hoosein NM, Hsieh J-T: The clinical and biological study of androgen independent prostate cancer (AI Pca). Semin Oncol 21:620–629, 1994.

96. Taylor CD, Elson P, Trump DL: Importance of continued testicular suppression in hormone-refractory prostate cancer. J Clin Oncol 11:2167–2172, 1993.

97. Scher HI, Kelly WK: Flutamide withdrawal syndrome: Its impact on clinical trials in hormone-refractory prostate cancer. J Clin Oncol 11:1566–1572, 1993.

98. Gerber GS, Chodak GW: Prostate specific antigen for assessing response to ketoconazole and prednisone in patients with hormone refractory metastatic prostate cancer. J Urol 144:1177–1179, 1990.

99. Eisenberger T, Trachenberg J: Effects of high dose ketoconazole in patients with androgen-independent prostatic cancer. Am J Clin Oncol 11:104–107, 1988.

100. Scher HI, Yagoda A, Watson RC: Phase II trial of doxorubicin in bidimensionally measurable prostatic adenocarcinoma. J Urol 132:1099–1102, 1984.

101. Pienta KJ, Redman B, et al: Phase II evaluation of oral estramustine and oral etoposide in hormone-refractory adenocarcinoma of the prostate. J Clin Oncol 12:2005–2012, 1994.

102. Hussain MH, Pienta KJ, et al: Oral etoposide in the treatment of hormone-refractory prostate cancer. Cancer 74:100–103, 1994.

103. Osborne C, Blumenstein B, Crawford ED, et al: Combined versus sequential chemo-endocrine therapy in advanced prostate cancer: Final results of a randomized Southwest Oncology Group Study. J Clin Oncol 8:1675–1682, 1990.

104. Porter AT, Vaishampayan N: Strontium-89 in metastatic prostate cancer. Urology Symposium 44:75–79, 1994.

105. Porter AT, McEwan AJB, et al: Results of a randomized phase III trial to evaluate the efficacy of strontium-89 adjuvant to local field external beam irradiation in the management of endocrine resistant metastatic prostatic cancer. Int J Radiat Oncol Biol Phys 25:805–813, 1993.

106. Akakura K, Bruchovsky N, et al: Effects of intermittent androgen suppression on androgen-dependent tumors. Cancer 71: 2782–2790, 1993.

107. Yamaoka M, Yamamoto T, et al: Angiogenesis inhibitor TNP-470 (AGM-1470) potentially inhibits the tumor growth on hormone-independent human breast and prostate carcinoma cell lines. Cancer Res 53:5233–5236, 1993.

108. Wood DP, Banks ER, et al: Identification of bone marrow micrometastases in patients with prostate cancer. Cancer 74:2533–2540, 1994.

109. Kelly WK, Scher HI, Mazumdar M, et al: Prostate specific antigen (PSA) as a measure of disease outcome in hormone refractory stage D2 prostate cancer (abstract). Proc Am Soc Clin Oncol 11:609, 1992.

CHAPTER 27

Testicular Cancer

Chris B. Bringhurst, MD, *and* Robert Amato, DO

Division of Medicine, The University of Texas M. D. Anderson Cancer Center, Houston, Texas

M ost testicular tumors are malignant and of germ-cell origin. They constitute only 1% of cancers in males overall but are the most common malignant neoplasm in men aged 15 to 35 years. Testicular cancers frequently present at an early stage, are very sensitive to chemotherapy, and are variably sensitive to radiotherapy. These tumors are highly curable, and the success in treating testicular cancer has turned the focus of many studies to reducing toxicity in selected good-prognosis patients and identifying poor-prognosis patients who require more aggressive treatment. In this chapter, we review the epidemiology, etiology, pathology, diagnosis, and treatment of testicular cancers.

EPIDEMIOLOGY AND ETIOLOGY

In 1995, an estimated 7,100 new cases of testicular cancer will be diagnosed in the United States, with an associated 370 deaths. This represents an incidence of 2.1 cases per 100,000 males.[1,2] Testicular cancer is most common in white males, who have an incidence more than four times that of black males.[3,4] The risk is highest in northern Europe. For example, in Denmark, the incidence is reported to be 6.3 per 100,000 males.[5]

Several conditions have been associated with testis cancer. Abnormal testicular development and descent are strongly associated with cancer; males with cryptorchidism are 10 to 40 times more likely than males with normal testes to develop testicular carcinoma.[6] The risk appears to be greater if the testis is retained in the abdomen rather than in the inguinal canal.[7,8] Surgical placement of the undescended testis into the scrotum before the age of 6 years reduces the risk but not to a normal level.[9] The higher temperature the undescended testis is exposed to in cryptorchidism was held to play a role in the development of testicular cancer, but epidemiologic studies have not supported this hypothesis.[10] In patients with unilateral cryptorchidism, 25% of testis cancers occur in the normally descended testis.

Testicular feminization syndromes have been shown to increase the risk of cancer in the gonads by 40 times, and these tumors are often bilateral. Herniorrhaphy before age 15 years, exposure to diethylstilbestrol early in gestational life, disorders of sexual differentiation, and infertility constitute other risk factors.[11–14] In addition, trauma, torsion of the testis, testicular atrophy from mumps, orchitis, radiation, and exposure to dimethylformamide during leather tanning are possible risk factors.[15]

PATHOLOGY AND NATURAL HISTORY

Testicular cancer is a general term for several distinct but related neoplasms. The most commonly used classification in the United States is a modified version of the system described by Dixon and Moore in 1952 (Table 1).[16] Germ-cell neoplasms account for nearly 93% of all primary testicular malignancies. Testicular lym-

TABLE I

Pathologic Classification of Testicular Malignancies

Germinal neoplasms

1. Carcinoma in situ
2. Seminoma
   a. Classic
   b. Spermatic
3. Embryonal carcinoma
4. Yolk-sac tumor (endodermal sinus tumor)
5. Choriocarcinoma
6. Teratoma
   a. Mature
   b. Immature
   c. With malignant transformation
7. Mixed

Nongerminal neoplasms

1. Sex cord-stromal tumor
   a. Leydig-cell tumor
   b. Sertoli-cell tumor
   c. Granulosa-thecal-cell tumor
2. Gonadoblastoma
3. Lymphomas and leukemias
4. Rhabdomyosarcoma
5. Other rare tumors and tumorous conditions
   a. Carcinoid
   b. Adenocarcinoma of the rete testis
   c. Epidermoid cyst
   d. Malacoplakia

Metastatic neoplasms

phomas represent about 4% to 5% of testicular cancers, and sex cord-stromal tumors make up nearly 3%. A few other rare tumors are occasionally seen.

Carcinoma in situ

Carcinoma in situ was originally perceived as a curiosity. Though not malignant, it is now recognized as an important precursor to testicular cancer. In one study, incidence of progression to invasive cancer was estimated to be 70% at 7 years. In this study, no cases of regression were noted.[17] In 75% to 99% of testicular cancers, carcinoma in situ is found adjacent to the tumor.[18] It is unclear whether all germ-cell tumors go through this stage, but it must be regarded as a preinvasive lesion and not ignored.

Seminoma

Pure seminoma is the most common germ-cell tumor and accounts for approximately 45% of testicular cancers.[19] The distinction between seminoma and nonseminoma is important, because the natural histories of these tumor types and their responses to treatment modalities differ, and hence so do appropriate treatment strategies.

Seminomas are believed to arise from primordial germ cells and have distinct clinical and pathologic features. The metastatic potential is low, and most patients present with early-stage disease. Overall, 75% present with stage I disease, 20% with stage II disease, and 5% with stage III or IV disease.[20] Seminoma is generally divided into two types: classic seminoma, which accounts for about 90% of cases, and spermatic seminoma, which accounts for the rest.

Classic seminoma typically presents in the fourth or fifth decade as an enlarging, painless testicular mass, and 2% of the time, bilateral disease is present. The pattern of spread is predominantly via the lymphatics to the para-aortic lymph nodes and then to the mediastinal and supraclavicular lymph nodes. Hematogenous dissemination to lung, liver, bone, and adrenals occurs, but is generally a late finding.

Low levels of beta-human chorionic gonadotropin (beta-hCG) are seen in 10% to 25% of pure seminomas, but this characteristic does not appear to influence prognosis.[21] Seminomas do not secrete alpha-fetoprotein (AFP), and an elevated AFP level should alert the clinician to the presence of nonseminomatous elements.

Anaplastic seminoma used to be regarded as a separate category because it appears more aggressive under a microscope and tends to present at a later stage. However, when compared with classic seminoma on a stage-for-stage basis, the prognosis is no worse. For this reason, it

is no longer regarded as a distinct entity and is included with the classic variant.

Spermatic seminoma accounts for about 10% of seminomas. It differs from classic seminoma in that it typically appears after the age of 60 years, it is bilateral 10% of the time, and it has an extremely indolent course. Metastases are rare, and the prognosis is excellent.

Nonseminomatous Germ-Cell Tumors

Nonseminomatous germ-cell tumors are a heterogeneous group of tumors that are grouped in the same category largely because they are frequently found together. It is difficult to generalize about their collective behavior, so each will be discussed separately, but it should be remembered that several or all of the histologic types discussed below may be present in the same patient. Nonseminomatous tumors that contain elements of seminoma are also common; they behave like nonseminomas and should be treated as such.

Embryonal Carcinoma: Embryonal carcinoma is the second most common testicular malignancy and in its pure form accounts for 15% to 30% of nonseminomatous germ-cell tumors. It occurs most commonly in the second decade of life and is rare after the fifth decade. It is not found in infants or children. One third of patients present with metastases to the para-aortic lymph nodes, lungs, or liver. This tumor secretes both AFP and beta-hCG. Placental alkaline phosphatase and cytokeratin are usually elevated, but carcinoembryonic antigen (CEA) generally is not.[22,23]

Yolk-Sac Carcinoma (Endodermal Sinus Tumor): Yolk-sac carcinoma is the most common testicular neoplasm in children, accounting for 75% of testicular tumors in this population. It is associated with an excellent prognosis.[24] It is rare in its pure form in adults but is frequently seen next to other germ-cell elements. When it does appear as pure yolk-sac carcinoma in adults, it is a virulent neoplasm. It typically spreads via the lymphatics but frequently has hematogenous dissemination. It has particular affinity for metastasis to the liver. AFP levels are generally elevated, whereas beta-hCG levels are not.[24]

Choriocarcinoma: Choriocarcinoma is extremely rare in its pure form, accounting for fewer than 1% of all testicular tumors, but is commonly found as a component of other testis tumors.[22] This is the most aggressive variant in adults, with early hematogenous and lymphatic spread. The poor prognosis of these patients is probably related to the typically larger volume of disease at presentation rather than an intrinsic resistance to treatment. This tumor secretes high levels of beta-hCG but normal levels of AFP.

Teratoma: Teratoma is a common component of mixed

germ-cell tumors but in its pure form only represents 2% to 3% of all testicular malignancies. It has been referred to as benign in the past because, technically, no malignant tissue exists in these terminally differentiated tumors. Degeneration to a malignant form, however, is observed, and patients have died of associated metastases. Younger patients tend to have more mature tumors and older patients more immature forms. These tumors do not respond to chemotherapy and can manifest as an enlarging mass during chemotherapy in a serologically responding tumor. Surgery is the only effective therapy. Teratomas can secrete both beta-hCG and, more typically AFP, although usually neither is elevated.

Mature Teratoma: All three germ-cell elements (endoderm, mesoderm, and ectoderm) are presenting mature forms of teratoma, and elements such as skin, bone, teeth, and hair can sometimes be seen histologically.

Immature Teratoma: Immature tumors contain tissues that cannot be recognized as normal elements. The immaturity of the teratoma has not been shown to be an indicator of biologic aggressiveness. This behavior appears to be more related to the age of the patient, with aggressive disease more common in older patients.[25]

Teratoma With Malignant Transformation: A variant of teratoma containing malignant non-germ-cell elements, presumably derived from somatic tissue within the teratoma, has recently been described.[26] The presence of malignant non-germ-cell elements at diagnosis or after induction chemotherapy implies a poor prognosis.[27] Teratomas have been demonstrated to degenerate into a variety of poor-prognosis malignancies, including sarcomas, adenocarcinomas, and neuroepitheliomas.[28,29] AML also occurs in patients with a history of teratomas.[30–32]

Patients with one of these tumors who have had a germ-cell malignancy in the past should be evaluated for a duplication on the short arm of chromosome 12p, or i(12p). This duplication is a good indicator that the tumor is of germ-cell origin. Limited success has been reported using platinum based chemotherapy.[26]

Sex Cord-Stromal Tumors

Leydig (Interstitial)-Cell Tumors: Leydig-cell tumors account for 1% to 3% of all testicular neoplasms.[33] They can appear at any age, but the median age at which they develop is 60 years. Leydig cells secrete both androgens and estrogens, and the clinical symptoms are usually related to endocrine abnormalities. Testicular swelling, gynecomastia, and decreased libido are common in patients with these tumors. Only 7% to 10% metastasize.

Sertoli-Cell Tumors: Fewer than 1% of testicular neoplasms are Sertoli-cell tumors. They can occur at any age, but 30% appear in the first decade of life. Patients generally present with a scrotal mass and sometimes have gynecomastia. Only about 10% of these tumors are malignant and, as with Leydig-cell tumors, the primary treatment is surgical.

Granulosa-Cell Tumor: Granulosa-cell tumors have two distinct types: juvenile and adult. The juvenile variety is the most frequently seen non-germ-cell testicular tumor in infants, and no malignant behavior has been reported in this type. The adult form is the least common of the sex cord-stromal tumors.

Gonadoblastomas: Gonadoblastoma is a mixed germ-cell and sex cord tumor that generally occurs in dysgenetic gonads or undescended testes during the teenage years. It is bilateral about 30% of the time. These tumors are clinically benign, but pathologic analysis reveals that they are accompanied by foci of malignant germ-cell tumors in 10% to 50% of cases. The prognosis varies and appears to depend on the other germ-cell components present and their extent of invasion. For patients with pure gonadoblastoma, the outcome is excellent.[34]

Lymphomas and Leukemias

Primary malignant lymphomas of the testis are uncommon, accounting for only 5% of all testicular neoplasms. Lymphoma involves the testis more commonly as a late manifestation of disseminated disease. This occurs in about 20% of all cases of lymphoma. It is important to note that the frequency of primary testicular lymphoma increases with age, and in patients over 60 years old it is the most common malignant tumor of the testis.

Leukemic infiltration of the testis usually occurs when the disease is disseminated; it can be detected in autopsy in up to 5% of patients with acute leukemia and 30% of patients with chronic leukemia. Testicular involvement is especially common among children with acute lymphoblastic leukemia who have had relapses after therapy.[35]

Rhabdomyosarcomas

Rhabdomyosarcoma is the most common sarcoma in children and can originate in the testis. Ninety-five percent of these patients present with a scrotal mass. The testicular parenchyma is rarely involved, but the tumor is common in the spermatic cord and paratesticular tissue. After surgery, local recurrences are frequent, and the pelvic lymph nodes are a common site of metastases.

Metastatic Neoplasms

Testicular metastases occur in 2.5% of men with malignant tumors. The most common primary sites are the prostate, lung, skin (melanoma), colon, and kidney.[36]

Extragonadal Germ-Cell Tumors

Extragonadal germ-cell tumors account for about 2% to 4% of all germ-cell tumors.[37] They can be seminomas or nonseminomas and generally occur in midline structures in the retroperitoneum, mediastinum, or pineal gland. Historically, it was felt that extragonadal nonseminomas had a worse prognosis than tumors arising in the testis. This is certainly true for those arising in the mediastinum. However, recent data indicate that nonseminomas arising in the retroperitoneum behave similarly to comparably sized stage II nonseminomas in the testis.[37-40]

Extragonadal seminomas, regardless of their origin, do no worse than testicular seminomas of similar stage.[41] Many, if not most, germ-cell tumors arising in the retroperitoneum originate in the testis, so patients with retroperitoneal tumors should all be evaluated for an occult testicular malignancy. At least 40% will have an occult testis tumor or carcinoma in situ. This is not the case for germ-cell tumors arising in the mediastinum; testicular biopsies for individuals with such tumors are not indicated.[42,43]

DIAGNOSIS

Testicular cancer is the most common malignancy in young males and frequently occurs during a crucial developmental period of their lives. For a variety of psychological, social, and educational reasons, the average delay in diagnosis after symptoms appear is 4 to 6 months.[44] There are no early symptoms. About 65% of patients present with painless swelling or a nodule in one gonad. In another 20%, the testicular enlargement is painful because of bleeding or infarction in the tumor, and acute pain in a patient with a cryptorchid testis suggests torsion of a hidden mass. About 10% of patients present with symptoms from metastases, such as lumbar back pain, gastrointestinal disturbance, respiratory symptoms, or a neck mass. Gynecomastia is seen in about 5% of patients and occasionally infertility is the initial complaint. Exophthalmos and skin metastases can be the first manifestations of choriocarcinoma.

The physical examination should include bimanual examination of the testes. The normal testis has an even consistency, is freely movable, and is separable from the epididymis. Any nodule or firm fixed area or mass is suggestive of disease, and testicular cancer must be considered until this possibility is disproved.

The differential diagnosis includes testicular torsion, epididymitis, epididymal orchitis, hydrocele, hernia, hematoma, or spermatocele. High-resolution ultrasonography is a rapid, reliable tool for to excluding the possibility of hydrocele or epididymitis when a tumor is suspected. It can also demonstrate whether the mass is intratesticular or extratesticular. If it is extratesticular and does not involve the tunica albuginea, then conservative treatment can be elected.[44]

A suspected testicular tumor should be surgically explored and biopsied through an inguinal incision. Careful histologic examination will establish the diagnosis. Trans-scrotal biopsy is contraindicated because it alters the lymphatic drainage, and if a malignancy is found, a more extensive surgical procedure is required to remove the primary tumor.[45] After the diagnosis is made, clinical tests to stage the patient are performed. These include a computed tomography (CT) scan of the abdomen and pelvis, chest x-ray and beta-hCG, AFP, lactate dehydrogenase (LDH), and sometimes placental alkaline phosphatase. If clinically indicated, a magnetic resonance imaging (MRI) or CT scan of the brain and a bone scan may be done.

The diagnosis and staging evaluations for extragonadal germ-cell tumors are similar to those for testicular tumors. Those with a retroperitoneal presentation should be explored for an occult testicular primary, which is frequently present. Again, with a mediastinal tumor, this is not indicated.[42,43]

Tumor Markers and Cytogenetic Abnormalities

Our ability to accurately diagnoses, stage tumors, monitor response to treatment, and assess patients for early relapse has been greatly facilitated with the identification of tumor markers. These markers can be divided into three categories: (1) serum proteins, such as beta-hCG, AFP, placental alkaline phosphatase, and LDH, (2) cytogenetic or chromosomal markers, such as i(12p), and (3) molecular markers, including oncogenes and tumor suppressor genes. Serum protein markers are the best studied and the most clinically relevant to date.

Beta-hCG, first detected in 1930 in the urine of patients with advanced choriocarcinoma, was the first tumor marker associated with testis cancer.[46] Subsequent refinements in our ability to measure CG have taken us from detecting it only occasionally in advanced disease to precisely measuring it in patients who have no observable tumor. The CG protein is composed of 2 subunits, alpha and beta, and modern assays measure only the beta portion. Beta-hCG is elevated in 40% to 50% of patients with testis cancer, including all patients with choriocarcinoma, approximately 80% of patients with embryonal carcinoma, and 10% to 25% of patients with pure seminoma.[47,48] The degree of elevation has some correlation with the volume of disease, and recurrent elevation is an excellent marker of early relapse.[49,50] Beta-hCG has a half-life of 24 to 36 hours, and, after surgery, levels should fall in accordance with this half-life. If they do not, residual disease is likely present.

When using beta-hCG to monitor response to chemotherapy, a 90% decrease every 21 days should be seen. Less steep declines are associated with the emergence of drug resistance and a poorer outcome.[51] It is important to note that some beta-hCG assays cross-react with luteinizing hormone (LH).[52] When the treatment has resulted in testicular atrophy, the LH can be substantially elevated. If a falsely elevated beta-hCG level is suspected, a single 200-mg injection of testosterone cypionate can be given and the beta-hCG level rechecked after 2 weeks.[53] Beta-hCG can also be increased in patients who use tobacco or marijuana, and this possibility should be looked into if a minor elevation persists.

Alpha-Fetoprotein (AFP) was detected in adult germ-cell tumors in 1974.[54] It is an abundant serum-binding protein in the fetus, but only minimal amounts of AFP are normally detectable in individuals more than 1 year old. Fifty to seventy percent of patients with testis cancer have elevations of AFP, which are most often seen in patients who have elements of embryonal or yolk-sac carcinoma[47,49] and occasionally seen in patients with teratoma, but not seen in patients with pure choriocarcinoma or pure seminoma.[55] Seminoma with an elevated AFP behaves like nonseminoma and should be treated as such.

High levels of AFP correlate with bulky disease, and after treatment, rising levels are a good marker for early recurrence. Because of AFP's long half-life (5 to 7 days), its occasional production by teratomas, its frequent sequestration inside cysts, and the variety of benign liver conditions that can cause it to be elevated, caution should be used when monitoring its rate of decline to assess response to therapy.

LDH: Levels of LDH and, in particular, its isoenzyme 1 are elevated in approximately 80% of patients with advanced testis cancer. Though not as specific as beta-hCG or AFP, in some patients LDH is the only elevated marker, so it can have clinical utility. High levels correlate with tumor burden, risk for relapse, and a poorer survival.[51]

Placental Alkaline Phosphatase: Placental alkaline phosphatase is the fetal isoenzyme of adult alkaline phosphatase. It is detectable in 30% to 50% of patients with stage I seminoma and in nearly 100% of patients with advanced seminoma but is less commonly elevated in nonseminomatous tumors.[56-58] Clinical experience with this marker is more limited than with beta-hCG, AFP, or LDH, but when it is elevated, it can be useful in following the course of seminoma. Smoking can cause false elevations of this marker; thus, in patients who smoke, placental alkaline phosphatase monitoring is less reliable.[51]

Cytogenetics and Molecular Markers: Cytogenetic abnormalities in testicular tumors are beginning to be explored. Detailed karyotypic analysis has revealed nonrandom changes in chromosomes 1, 5, 6, 7, 9, 11, 12, 16, 17, 21, 22, and X.[59] Of these, a duplication on the short arm of chromosome 12p, or i(12p), is the best studied and the most characteristic. This marker was present in one or more copies in approximately 89% of seminomas and 81% of nonseminomas studied.[58] Most of the remaining patients had other abnormalities involving the 12p chromosome.[60] The i(12p) marker is also observed in extragonadal germ-cell tumors and occasionally in ovarian dysgerminomas but is rare in other tumors. It is a highly specific marker for germ-cell tumors and a useful diagnostic tool in cancers of unknown origin.[61]

How i(12p) participates in the development of testis cancer is unknown. The oncogene c-*ki-ras 2* resides on the short arm of chromosome 12,[62] but amplification of this gene as a transforming event has been difficult to show. Other oncogenes and their products have been investigated, but as yet their significance and roles in the pathogenesis of testis cancer remain to be demonstrated.

In summary, beta-hCG, AFP, LDH, and placental alkaline phosphatase have been shown to be of value in diagnosis by identifying patients who have histologic types other that those reported, in staging by identifying patients with high tumor volume that is not readily radiographically apparent, in monitoring response to treatment, and in detecting relapse early, when it is most curable. The presence of i(12p) is useful in identifying tumors of unknown origin. Molecular markers are at present still research tools but ultimately are expected to yield improved diagnostic and therapeutic strategies as well as provide a much better understanding of these diseases.

STAGING AND TREATMENT

Carcinoma in situ

Carcinoma in situ (CIS) is known to be a preinvasive lesion, and detecting and treating it early in patients at risk for testicular carcinoma could potentially prevent cancer development. The only reliable way to diagnose CIS is with a surgical biopsy after puberty.

The likelihood of eventually developing a testicular tumor where CIS is present is extremely high, so screening is useful in groups at high risk of developing CIS.[42] Estimates of individuals with increased risk show that men with a unilateral testicular tumor have a 6% incidence of CIS in the other testis,[63] and men with a history of cryptorchidism have a 2% to 3% incidence of CIS.[64] In patients with extragonadal germ-cell tumors of the retroperitoneum, the incidence is greater than 40%,[43] and in intersex patients as well as individuals with gonadal dysgenesis, a greater than 25% incidence has been reported.[65]

Orchiectomy is the treatment of choice in patients in whom one testis is normal and the other contains CIS. In men who have had a previous unilateral orchiectomy and now have CIS in the remaining testis, 20 Gy of radiation given in 10 doses of 2 Gy is sufficient to eradicate the CIS and still maintain adequate endogenous testosterone.[42] Fertility does not appear to be compromised by this degree of radiation, but men with a history of testicular cancer in one testis and CIS in the other frequently have impaired spermatogenesis prior to any therapy.

Screening is only recommended for patients with a history of unilateral testis cancer, extragonadal germ-cell tumors of retroperitoneal origin, or gonadal dysgenesis and for intersex patients. In patients with a history of cryptorchidism, a testicular biopsy can be considered. Newer methods that involve examining the semen are being developed that may expand the designation of reasonable candidates for screening.

Seminoma

The treatment of seminoma is gratifying to the oncologist because the disease is quite curable. The expected overall survival is approximately 97%.[66] This tumor is quite radiosensitive as well as very chemosensitive.

Seminoma is relatively indolent and follows a predictable pattern of progression. It starts in the testis and spreads via the para-aortic lymph nodes to the mediastinal nodes and then the supraclavicular nodes. It rarely metastasizes to distant organs such as the lungs or bones without first being seen at nodal sites. Overall, 75% of patients present with stage I disease (confined to the testis), 20% with stage II disease, and fewer than 5% with stage III or IV disease.[66] Several similar staging systems for seminomas have been devised (Table 2). The main differences are in the definition of stage II and in the way bulky and nonbulky retroperitoneal disease are divided.

The initial considerations when planning treatment are to confirm that the tumor is truly a pure seminoma and to determine its stage. Careful review of the histologic and pathologic features is mandatory. The AFP level must be normal for the tumor to be considered a pure seminoma; beta-hCG and LDH levels should be tested and potentially will be elevated. The initial staging evaluation should include a chest x-ray, CT of the abdomen and pelvis, bone scan if symptoms indicate, and CT or MRI of the brain if neurologic symptoms are present.

TABLE 2

Staging of Seminoma

Royal Marsden Hospital	M. D. Anderson Cancer Center	Memorial Sloan-Kettering Cancer Center	American Joint Committee on Cancer	Boden-Gibb Commission on Cancer
I: confined to testis	I: confined to testis	A: confined to testis	I: confined to testis	A: confined to testis
IIa: RPLN < 2 cm	IIa: RPLN < 5 cm		IIN1: microscopic disease in RPLN	B: RPLN involved
IIb: RPLN ≥ 2 cm and < 5 cm	IIb: RPLN ≥ 5 cm and ≤ 10 cm	B1: RPLN < 5 cm	IIN2: ≤ 5 LNs involved, all < 2 cm	
IIc: RPLN ≥ 5 cm < 10 cm	IIc: RPLN > 10 cm	B2: RPLN ≥ 5 cm and < 10 cm	IIN3: > 5 LNs involved or LN > 2 cm	
IId: RPLN ≥ 10 cm		B3: RPLN ≥ 10 cm	IIN4: unresectable LN	
III: LN above diaphragm involved	III: LN above diaphragm or visceral organs involved	C: LN above diaphragm or visceral organs involved		C: LN above diaphragm or visceral organs involved
IV: extradnodal disease				

RPLN = retroperitoneal lymph node, LN = lymph node

TABLE 3

Follow-up of Patients With Seminoma ᵃ Treated by Orchiectomy Only

Test ᵇ	Baseline	Years 1 & 2		Years 3 & 4		Year 5	
		Every 3 months	Every 4 months	Every 4 months	Every 6 months	6 months	Yearly
Histology/ pathology	X	X		X		X	
beta-hCG, AFP, LDH	X	X		X		X	
Chest x-ray	X	X	X		X		X
CT abdomen/ pelvis	X		X		X		X

AFP = alpha fetoprotein, CT = computed tomography, beta-hCG = beta-human chorionic gonadotropin, LDH = lactate dehydrogenase, MRI = magnetic resonance imaging
ᵃ Surveillance for nonseminomas should be identical except the indicated tests should be performed every 2 months for the first 2 years, rather than every 3 months.
ᵇ CT or MRI of brain should be performed only if neurologic symptoms are present and bone scan only if symptoms indicate.

Stage I Treatment: Treatment of stage I seminoma is somewhat controversial. The para-aortic lymph nodes are involved in approximately 15% of clinical stage I cases, and standard treatment has been orchiectomy plus radiotherapy to the para-aortic nodes, as well as the ipsilateral common iliac and external iliac nodes. If there has been a previous inguinal surgery or if an advanced local primary has invaded the scrotal skin, there is an increased risk of pelvic node spread, and the radiotherapy field is extended to include the ipsilateral inguinofemoral node region.[67]

The standard dose of radiation, 25 to 40 Gy, results in a disease-free survival of 98% to 99%. A dose of 40 Gy has not been shown to be more effective than 25 Gy, so the lower dose should be used.[68–71] Side effects of radiation include dyspepsia in 6% of patients and frank peptic ulceration in 3%.[4] The effects on fertility are unclear, but most patients experience a decrease in sperm count that usually resolves in 3 years.[72,73] The relative risk of developing a second cancer within the irradiated field seems to be increased, but this effect does not become evident until 15 years after treatment.[74–76]

Because salvage treatment in seminoma is so successful and most patients with stage I seminoma patients are cured with their initial surgery, close surveillance after orchiectomy is being reported as a viable option to radiation to reduce short- and long-term toxicity. The advantage of this approach is that it avoids radiation in the 85% of patients who are cured with orchiectomy. The disadvantage is that those who relapse will have an increased tumor volume and may be more difficult to cure.

The results in 583 patients treated with orchiectomy alone and followed by investigators from the Princess Margaret Hospital, the Royal Marsden Hospital, and the Danish National Study are encouraging.[65] At 3 years, the rate of relapse was 15.5%, with a median time to relapse of 12 to 15 months. The relapses were treated with salvage radiation or chemotherapy. Only 2 of the original 583 patients (0.3%) died with disease, producing a 99.7% disease-free survival.[66]

It must be remembered that the lack of a sensitive and reliable marker in addition to the slow natural history of a seminoma make the surveillance approach challenging. The follow-up schedule in Table 3 is recommended. It is imperative that the patient be dependable and available for frequent follow-up for an extended period of time.

Stage II Treatment: The treatment strategy for stage II disease differs with the size of the involved abdominal lymph nodes. Historically, radiotherapy was used for all stage II patients, and it is still the treatment of choice for early stage II disease (abdominal masses less than 5 cm).

The usual dose is 36 Gy, which yields a disease-free survival of about 95%.[68,70,77–81] Mason and Kearsley, in a review of the literature, found that the risk of relapse in stage II disease was directly related to tumor bulk. Abdominal masses between 5 and 10 cm had a risk of relapse of 8%, and for masses greater than 10 cm, the risk of relapse increased to 35%.[82] Prophylactic irradiation to the mediastinum for abdominal masses smaller than 10 cm should be avoided, because this strategy does not appear to improve survival but does cause an excess of cardiac, pulmonary, and marrow toxic effects.[83]

There is no consensus on the optimal treatment for abdominal masses between 5 and 10 cm in diameter. The kidneys generally tolerate only 15 to 20 Gy of fractionated radiotherapy, and with tumors greater than 5 cm, there is frequently a significant amount of tumor overlying the kidneys. For this reason, some centers now recommend chemotherapy for all tumors greater then 5 cm.[74] If, however, the tumor is less than 10 cm and the kidneys are not in the field of radiation, then radiotherapy is still a good choice. Stage II disease with an abdominal mass larger than 10 cm is treated with chemotherapy similar to that used for stage III disease.

Stage III Treatment: The development of effective chemotherapy for advanced seminoma has lagged behind that for nonseminoma, in part because advanced seminoma is so uncommon. In the era before platinum drugs, responses to chemotherapy were common but cures were not. Platinum-based therapy has dramatically improved our ability to cure advanced-stage seminoma.

In 1974, the activity of cisplatin (Platinol) in germ-cell tumors was first reported,[84] and this agent quickly became the backbone of testicular chemotherapy regimens. Improved results with the PVB (cisplatin, vinblastine, and bleomycin [Blenoxane]) regimen were first reported in 1981[85] and subsequently confirmed in a larger multicenter trial.[86] The most common variations on this regimen are the BEP (bleomycin, etoposide [VePesid], and cisplatin) regimen, in which etoposide is substituted for vinblastine,[87,88] and the VIP (vinblastine, ifosfamide [Ifex], cisplatin) regimen in which ifosfamide is used in place of bleomycin.[89] These have yielded comparable disease-free survivals, ranging from 75% to 85%.[74]

Recently, the combination of cisplatin and etoposide has been shown to be at least as effective as other standard regimens with less toxicity, and it is now the standard in some institutions. The role of bleomycin in the treatment of seminoma is uncertain. The drug appears to add little benefit, and the high frequency of fatal pulmonary side effects among patients with pure seminoma suggests that this population may have a unique sensitivity to bleomycin.[90]

A somewhat different approach employs the use of sequential weekly cisplatin and cyclophosphamide (Cytoxan, Neosar). In one study, this combination resulted in a 92% long-term continuous disease-free survival.[91] In another group of patients, cisplatin alone and carboplatin (Paraplatin) alone were less successful, but a high proportion of these patients did respond to cisplatin-based salvage regimens. In 1992, a cure rate of 97% was reported with the combination of carboplatin, ifosfamide, and selective consolidation with alternating non-cross-resistant chemotherapy agents.[92]

Residual Mass: A residual mass can be detected after chemotherapy for bulky metastatic seminoma in one half to two thirds of cases. Attempts to resect these masses have often revealed only densely fibrotic tissue that is adherent to major blood vessels, and severe operative and postoperative complications have been reported.[87,92] The relationship between the size of a residual mass and whether it contains viable tumor is unclear, with some studies showing that a mass greater than 3 cm correlates with residual disease[93,94] and other studies not demonstrating this relationship.[95,96] A practical policy is to monitor these masses closely and administer radiotherapy to those that do not continue to shrink.[97]

Nonseminomatous Germ-Cell Tumors

The natural history of nonseminomatous germ-cell tumors tends to be less indolent and less predictable than that of seminomas. Nonseminomas have a greater likelihood of dissemination via the blood to distant sites, sometimes while bypassing the retroperitoneal lymphatics. Although nonseminomas (except for teratomas) are probably equally as chemosensitive as seminomas, they are less radiosensitive. As a result of these differences, the staging, treatment, and follow-up recommendations for nonseminoma are somewhat different from those for seminoma.

Several staging systems for nonseminomas have been proposed, but most of them are similar. Table 4 lists some of the more common systems in use. The main distinctions are in how the stages are labeled rather than in the actual stages themselves. The full tumor-node-metastasis (TNM) staging system is shown in Table 5.

Stage I Treatment: Clinical stage I tumors represent approximately 50% of all nonseminomatous germ-cell tumors. About 30% of these patients will relapse with occult metastatic disease if not given some form of adjuvant therapy. Numerous treatment approaches for stage I nonseminoma have been tried, but there is no consensus on which is best. These approaches have included (1) retroperitoneal lymph-node dissection (RPLND) after orchiectomy, (2) close surveillance after orchiectomy (no adjuvant therapy), (3) adjuvant chemotherapy for all patients or for selected individuals with adverse prognostic features, (4) RPLND and adjuvant chemotherapy for pathologic stage II patients, and (5) adjuvant radiotherapy.

Most of these approaches have their advocates, but adjuvant radiotherapy has fallen out of favor. Nonseminomas are less radiosensitive than seminomas, and side effects from the increased doses of radiation required to treat nonseminomas are prohibitive. Also, nonseminoma is more likely than seminoma to relapse outside the radiation ports.[98]

Proponents of RPLND for all stage I nonseminomas list the following advantages: This technique provides more accurate staging, it may be curative in 60% to 75% of cases with early evidence of nodal metastases, and it can provide an indication for immediate adjuvant chemotherapy in cases with more extensive nodal disease.[99] The disadvantages of the procedure include the following: Retrograde ejaculation occurs in most patients who undergo traditional RPLND and in 10% to 15% of patients who have a nerve-sparing RPLND, even when performed by experienced urologists[99]; a major surgery is performed in the 70% of patients who were already cured by orchiectomy alone; and the rate of relapse in patients who undergo RPLND is only decreased from 30% to about 12%. Most of these relapses, however, occur in the lungs and are generally easily managed with chemotherapy.

Another approach, surveillance after orchiectomy was introduced at the Royal Marsden Hospital in 1979 and is currently the recommended treatment for most clinical stage I patients in Europe and some centers in the United States. In 1993, Sternberg[100] reported on 1,337 patients culled from published studies who were not given RPLND or other adjuvant therapy. The median follow-up was 40 months, and the relapse rate was 28% with a median time to relapse of 5 to 6 months. The rate of complete remission with chemotherapy after recurrence and the overall survival were 99%. If surveillance is chosen, the follow-up is similar to that for surveillance for stage I seminoma (Table 3).

Adjuvant chemotherapy after orchiectomy with two cycles of chemotherapy, either for all patients or for selected high-risk patients, is another choice. This option is only beginning to be studied, so there are few data on it. The extremely high rate of cure with observation and

chemotherapy at recurrence makes it difficult to justify giving adjuvant chemotherapy to all patients. However, if a group with a sufficient risk of developing metastatic disease could be identified and if these patients could be cured with less chemotherapy and less associated toxicity, then it would be a reasonable option.

The Medical Research Council recently reported on a group of 259 patients, of which 61 were felt to have a greater than 50% chance of relapse.[101–103] This assessment was based on the presence of three or all of the following four factors: tumor invasion of the testicular veins, tumor invasion of the testicular lymphatics, the

TABLE 4

Staging of Nonseminomatous Germ-Cell Tumors

Description	Stage MSKCC	Stage WR	Stage TNM
Confined to testis	A	I	N0
Microscopic nodal involvement only, ≤ 5 nodes involved, and all nodes < 2 cm	B1	IIA	N1 or N2A
Grossly positive nodes, or ≥ 6 nodes involved	B2	IIB	N2B
Bulky retroperitoneal involvement, unresectable	B3	IIC	N3
Metastases above the diaphragm or spread to solid visceral organs	C	III	M1

MSKCC = Memorial Sloan-Kettering Cancer Center, WR = Walter Reed, TNM = tumor-nodes-metastasis staging system

TABLE 5

Tumor-Node-Metastasis (TNM) Classification of Testicular Tumors

Tumor status [a]	Regional lymph-node status	Metastasis status
T2: Confined to body of testis	N0: No nodes involved	M1: Supradiaphragmatic or extralymphatic involvement
T2: Extending through the tunica albica	N1: Microscopic only	
T3: Involving the rete testis or epididymis ≥ 6 involved nodes	N2A: Largest node ≤ 2cm, and	
T4: Involving the scrotal wall	N3: Nodal extension into adjacent structures	
	N4: Gross tumor following RPLND	

RPLND = retroperitoneal lymph-node dissection   [a] The T value does not affect (enter into) stage but is of some prognostic value in stage I disease

presence of undifferentiated cells, or the absence of yolk-sac elements. These high-risk patients were given two cycles of adjuvant BEP chemotherapy, and after a median follow-up of 18 months, no relapses have been seen.

In summary, none of the above treatment options have been conclusively shown to be superior, and the best choice for a given patient will likely depend on the resources and experience of the treating institution as well as the preferences and reliability of the individual.

Stage II Treatment: The optimal management of stage II nonseminomas is no more settled than for stage I disease, but fortunately, several good options exist. Stage IIC (unresectable) should be treated with chemotherapy similar to that recommended for good-prognosis stage III patients. However, for stage IIA and IIB, the decision of whether to treat initially with chemotherapy or with RPLND with or without adjuvant chemotherapy is unsettled. In Europe and in a few centers in the United States, primary chemotherapy for stage II patients is becoming the standard. However, most large cancer centers in the United States still recommend that patients with resectable stage II disease be treated with RPLND first.

Drawing conclusions from the literature is challenging because comparative trials are not available, and it is likely that neither option is superior in every situation. The expected cure rate with either treatment is greater than 95%, and aggressive therapy is not likely to affect this rate significantly. Thus, the goal is to maintain this cure rate while minimizing morbidity. Opinions vary as to whether chemotherapy or RPLND is more toxic, but it is obvious that surgery and full-course chemotherapy together are associated with greater morbidity than either approach alone. The goal, therefore, is to select the therapy that is most likely to be curative by itself.

The traditional approach for stage IIA and IIB disease has been RPLND. The rationale is that it is effective therapy and the most accurate method of staging. In a large prospective trial reported by the Testicular Cancer Intergroup Study, the risk of recurrence after RPLND without adjuvant chemotherapy was 40% for patients with N1 disease using TNM staging, (Table 5), 55% for patients with N2A disease, and 60% for patients with stage N2B disease.[99] These results agree with those of other retrospective series in that about 50% of patients with pathologic stage II disease relapse after RPLND.[104,105] The risk of recurrence after RPLND correlates with the degree of nodal involvement. When lymph nodes are larger than 3 cm, the risk of relapse rises to greater than 70%, and the need for adjuvant chemotherapy should be considered.[106]

Patients who are treated initially with RPLND can either receive two cycles of adjuvant chemotherapy or be observed closely and, if relapse occurs, receive three to four cycles of chemotherapy and possibly a second surgery. The advantage of observation is that it avoids any chemotherapy in the 50% of patients who are cured with their surgery alone. The disadvantage is that more chemotherapy is required if a relapse occurs and a second surgery could be indicated should a residual mass remain after this treatment. Because the toxicity of bleomycin and cisplatin is cumulative, two cycles of chemotherapy are significantly less toxic than three or four.

In the Testicular Cancer Intergroup Study, greater chemotherapy-related toxicity was seen in the group assigned to observation with chemotherapy at relapse than in the group treated initially with adjuvant chemotherapy. However, fewer patients in the observation arm required chemotherapy.[107] Which therapy is selected should be based on the patient's risk factors for recurrence. Individuals with risk factors such as vascular or lymphatic invasion in the primary or abdominal lymph nodes larger than 3 cm should probably receive two cycles of adjuvant chemotherapy. If these factors are not present, then close observation is a reasonable option.

A more recent approach to the management of stage IIA and stage IIB disease is to treat with three to four cycles of chemotherapy initially and to reserve RPLND for radiographically persistent retroperitoneal disease. Several studies have shown the feasibility of this approach.[108–113] Although most of these studies included patients with stage IIC disease, the complete remission rates were between 95% and 100%. However, to achieve a complete remission, 15% to 30% of the patients required an RPLND because of a residual mass. In studies of this approach with sufficient follow-up, the overall survival is comparable to that obtained with primary RPLND.

The advantages of primary chemotherapy vs RPLND alone are that a major surgery is avoided in 70% to 85% of the patients and that less compliance in returning for follow-up is required from the patient because the incidence of relapse is much less. Also, nerve-sparing RPLND cannot generally be done in this setting, and as a result, absent or retrograde ejaculation occurs in 70% to 80% of the patients undergoing RPLND.[114] The disadvantages are that every patient receives three to four cycles of chemotherapy, rather than only the 50% of patients who eventually relapse after surgery, and that 15% to 30% of the patients who receive primary chemotherapy will still require RPLND for a residual mass.

In choosing appropriate therapy, the importance of histologic type in the primary tumor site is becoming more clear.[115] If embryonal carcinoma without teratoma predominates, then initial treatment with chemotherapy is appropriate, because (1) residual abdominal masses are uncommon, and (2) this tumor frequently recurs in the lungs, making patients treated with RPLND alone at high risk of recurrence. If teratoma is present, then there is a high likelihood that a residual mass will remain in patients treated with primary chemotherapy and a RPLND will be needed anyway. Such patients would probably benefit most from initial treatment with a RPLND. At RPLND, if only minimal disease is found, then surgery alone is likely sufficient and observation is appropriate.[116] If lymph nodes larger than 3 cm are found or if the primary had, in addition to teratoma, a predominant embryonal component, then adjuvant chemotherapy is indicated.[106]

Stage III Treatment: Significant progress in chemotherapy for patients with advanced nonseminomatous germ-cell tumors has been made in the past 20 years. Presently, with multimodality therapy, the majority of these individuals are cured. The development of chemotherapy for stage III (disseminated) nonseminoma has been fascinating and serves as an important model for the treatment of solid tumors in general. This evolution is reviewed in numerous publications and oncology textbooks and will not be discussed in detail here.

Patients with disseminated nonseminomatous germ-cell tumors differ widely in the volume of disease at presentation. Their prognoses and need for aggressive treatment vary and largely depend on tumor bulk at diagnosis.

Most studies divide patients into good- and poor-prognosis categories. The goal is to improve cure rates by identifying patients at increased risk of relapse and treating them more aggressively, while sparing patients with high probabilities of cure the side effects of intensive therapy when a milder approach would be as effective. Several groups have come up with different criteria for making this division, including the National Cancer Institute,[116] the European Organization for Research and Treatment of Cancer,[117] M. D. Anderson Cancer Center,[118] Memorial Sloan-Kettering Cancer Center,[119] the Southeastern Cancer Study Group,[119] the Danish Testicular Cancer Study group,[120] and the Medical Research Council.[121] There is no consensus on which system is best and whatever the treating physician is most familiar with is probably acceptable.

In the Medical Research Council System (Table 6) four adverse criteria were identified. Sixty-seven percent of patients studied had none of these features and were placed in the good-prognosis group. Their 3-year surviv-

TABLE 6

Medical Research Council Criteria for High-Risk Stage III Nonseminomatous Testicular Cancer Patients

More than 20 lung metastases
AFP > 1,000 kU/L
Beta-hCG > 1,000 IU/L
Mediastinal mass > 5 cm
Liver, osseous, or central nervous system metastasis

AFP = alpha fetoprotein, beta-hCG = beta-human chorionic gonadotropin
Adapted, with permission, from Mead GM et al.[121]

al was 93%. The remaining 33% of patients had one or more adverse features and had a 3-year survival of 68%.[121]

Chemotherapy for Stage III Good-Prognosis Disease: Regardless of the tumor classification used, a complete remission rate of greater than 90% should be achieved with appropriate treatment. The prognoses of stage IIC and good-risk stage III patients are similar and the two groups are generally treated in the same way. PVB was initially shown to have excellent activity in this group of patients.[122] Subsequent studies have shown the BEP regimen to give comparable results with less toxicity.[123–125] A randomized study that compared three vs four cycles of BEP chemotherapy did not show any benefit for four cycles in this group but did show increased toxicity, so three courses have been recommended.

Other options include the CISCA/VB (cisplatin, cyclophosphamide, daunorubicin [Cerubidine] or vinblastine, and bleomycin) regimen[115] or the POMB/ACE (cisplatin, vincristine [Oncovin], methotrexate, bleomycin or dactinomycin [Cosmegen], cyclophosphamide, etoposide) program.[123,125] These strategies use a variable number of cycles that is determined by the patient's response to therapy. Two cycles are given beyond the maximum response. Excellent results have been reported with all of these regimens, and none has been conclusively shown to be superior in randomized trials. Much of the focus of recent research has been on reducing treatment toxicity while maintaining current cure rates. Trials are currently underway to look at less toxic regimens.

Chemotherapy for Stage III Poor-Prognosis Patients: The treatment of poor-prognosis stage III disease has been less gratifying. The same regimens used for good-prognosis patients have been tried in poor-prognosis patients but with considerably less success. Long-term survival rates vary drastically from study to study, largely because of differences in how risk groups are defined, but the cure rate has generally been reported to be between 35% and 65%.

When three vs four cycles of BEP were compared in this population, three cycles were clearly inferior and are therefore not recommended. Attempts however, to escalate doses of cisplatin beyond 100 mg/m^2 have only increased toxicity and have not improved survival.[126] Except in clinical trials, standard doses of cisplatin should be employed. Regimens such as POMB/ACE and CISCA/VB that employ a variable number of cycles have shown promising results in poor-prognosis patients in nonrandomized trials, but appropriate randomized trials have not been done to confirm their superiority.[115,127]

Newer approaches using ifosfamide[128] and autologous bone marrow transplantation (ABMT) are currently being studied,[129,130] but as yet their efficacy is unproven. The only randomized trial comparing standard chemotherapy vs two cycles of chemotherapy followed by high-dose chemotherapy and ABMT failed to show any benefit for the ABMT arm. Thus, this approach cannot be recommended.[130] Other strategies using multiple courses of non-cross-resistant regimens such as BOP (bleomycin, vincristine, cisplatin), CISCA, and POMB/ACE with growth factors to decrease the time intervals between treatments are showing early promising results.[118]

RPLNDP After Chemotherapy: The recommendations on whether to perform surgery after chemotherapy vary. Some investigators recommend observation for all patients irrespective of any residual radiographic abnormality,[131] and others prefer surgical exploration in all patients.[132,133] The only commonly accepted contraindication to surgery is the presence of an elevated AFP or beta-hCG level, which would imply viable germ-cell tumor; these patients are better served with salvage chemotherapy.[134]

A review of the literature on patients with advanced germ-cell tumors suggests that, at surgery, about 45% of patients are found to have necrosis only, 35% have teratoma, and 20% have viable tumor.[135,136] Surgery in patients with a residual mass requires that a full RPLND be done because a nerve-sparing procedure gives an unacceptably high rate of relapse.[135]

Attempts have been made to identify patients in whom a RPLND can be avoided based on the following: normal levels of serum markers after chemotherapy, absence of teratoma in the primary, greater than 90% tumor shrinkage, and a residual mass smaller than 2 cm. Using these criteria, approximately 20% of patients will not require surgery, but of these, about 20% will still have residual teratoma or viable germ-cell tumor.[137,138] Surgery for any residual mass is probably the safest option because of the

poor results with other treatments for these patients, but if surgery is not chosen, close follow-up is mandatory.

When necrosis or mature teratoma only is found at surgery, no further therapy is indicated. However, studies consistently show that the majority of patients in whom viable tumor is found will relapse. Overall survival is better if adjuvant chemotherapy is given initially rather than waiting and treating with salvage therapy at relapse.[137,138] The current recommendation is to give two additional cycles of alternate chemotherapy.[138]

Salvage Chemotherapy

Germ-cell tumors are unusual among solid tumors because cure is still possible after relapse or even after failure to achieve a complete remission with initial therapy. Approximately 5% of good-prognosis and 35% of poor-prognosis stage III patients require salvage chemotherapy. Both standard salvage chemotherapy and high-dose chemotherapy with bone marrow support are toxic, and the majority of patients who undergo these treatments will not achieve a durable complete remission and will die from their cancer. The best predictor of who will relapse is the response to initial therapy as manifested by the rate of fall of AFP and beta-hCG.[139,140]

Standard salvage chemotherapy uses new agents in combination with cisplatin to treat patients at conventional or moderately increased doses.[141] More aggressive treatment involves either increasing the frequency and number of cycles of chemotherapy[142,143] or administering very high doses of chemotherapy with bone marrow rescue.[143]

The conventional approach for patients with a first relapse is to use salvage chemotherapy. Approximately 25% to 30% of patients treated in this manner will achieve a durable complete remission.[142] The prognosis is much worse for those who fail to achieve a complete remission at initial therapy. Only about 7% of these will be cured with standard salvage treatment.[142] The most common salvage regimens used are PVbI (cisplatin, vinblastine, ifosfamide) for patients who relapse after BEP, and PEI (cisplatin, etoposide, ifosfamide) for patients who relapse after PVB.[144,145]

For patients who do not respond to standard salvage therapy and possibly for those who do not achieve a complete remission with initial therapy, high-dose chemotherapy with bone marrow support is another approach. A review of the literature indicates that between 8% and 20% of these patients can still achieve a durable complete remission. In some of these studies, however, follow-up was short and a selection bias was likely present.[146–149] This remission rate is far from ideal, but in this setting it is the best evaluated option so far.

New strategies are being developed that involve novel chemotherapeutic agents, alternation of non-cross-resistant courses utilizing growth factors to shorten the interval of chemotherapy based on patient hematologic and non-hematologic recovery, induction with two or more courses of standard salvage chemotherapy followed by high-dose chemotherapy with bone marrow support, and two or more courses of high-dose chemotherapy with bone marrow rescue.

CONCLUSIONS

The treatment of testicular neoplasms is both rewarding and challenging—rewarding because of its high cure rate, and challenging because knowing which therapies to select and how to use them requires a thorough understanding of the literature and the disease. It is also challenging because patients with testis cancers frequently require aggressive treatment to provide the best opportunity for cure, yet expert management to avoid unnecessary morbidity and mortality. There are still many improvements to be made in finding ways to reduce both short-term and long-term toxicity as well as in the area of salvage treatment.

REFERENCES

1. Wingo PA, Tong T, Bolden S: Cancer Statistics, 1995. CA Cancer J Clin 41:19–36, 1991.

2. Mostofi FK: Testicular tumors: Epidemiologic, etiologic and pathologic features. Cancer 32:1186–1201, 1973.

3. Schottenfeld D, Warshauer ME, Sherlock S, et al: the epidemiology of testicular cancer in young adults. Am J Epidemiol 112:232–246, 1980.

4. Henderson BE, Ross RK, Pike MC, et al: Epidemiology of testis cancer, in Skinner DG (ed): Urological Cancer, pp 237–250. New York, Grune & Stratton, 1983.

5. Clemmensen J: A doubling of morbidity from testis cancer in Copenhagen, 1943–1962. Acta Pathol Microbiol Scand 72:348–349, 1968.

6. Patel SR, Kvols LK, Richardson RL: Familial testicular cancer: Report of six cases and review of the literature. Mayo Clin Proc 65:804–808, 1990.

7. Strader CH, Weiss NS, Daling JR, et al: Cryptorchism, orchiopexy, and the risk of testicular cancer. Am J Epidemiol 127:1013–1318, 1988.

8. Gilbert JB, Hamilton JB: Studies in malignant testis tumors: III. Incidence and nature of tumors in ectopic testes. Surg Gynecol Obstet 71:731–743, 1940.

9. Sumner WA: Malignant tumor of the testis occurring 29 years after orchiopexy: Case report and review of the literature. Trans West Sect Am Urol Assoc 25:20–24, 1958.

10. Kragas MR, Weiss NS, Strader CH, et al: Elevated intrascrotal temperature and the incidence of testicular cancer in noncryptorchid men. Am J Epidemiol 129:1104–1109, 1989.

11. Depue RH, Pike MC, Henderson BE: Estrogen exposure during gestation and risk of testicular cancer. J Natl Cancer Inst 71:1151–1155, 1983.

12. Loughlin JE, Robboy SJ, Morrison AS: Risk factors for cancer of the testis. N Engl J Med 303:112–113, 1980.

13. Morrison AS: Cryptorchidism, hernia, and cancer of the testis. J Natl Cancer Inst 56:731–733, 1976.

14. Pottern LM, Brown LM, Hoover RN, et al: Testicular cancer risk among young men: Role of cryptorchidism and inguinal hernia. J Natl Cancer Inst 74:377–381, 1985.

15. Mills PK, Newell GR, Johnson DE: Testicular cancer associated with employment in agriculture and oil and natural gas extraction. Lancet 1:207–209, 1984.

16. Dixon FJ, Moore RA: Tumors of the male sex organs, in Atlas of Tumor Pathology, fascicle 31b–32. Washington, DC, Armed Forces Institute of Pathology, 1952.

17. Skakkebaek NE, Berthelsen JG, Muller J: Carcinoma in situ of the undescended testis. Urol Clin North Am 9:377–385, 1982.

18. Gondos B, Berthelsen JG, Skakkeback NE: Intratubular germ cell neoplasms (carcinoma in situ): A preinvasive lesion of the testis. Ann Clin Lab Sci 13:185–192, 1983.

19. Ulbright TM, Rorth LM: Recent developments in the pathology of germ cell tumors. Semin Diagn Pathol 4:304–319, 1987.

20. Smith R: Management of testicular seminoma, in Skinner DG, deKernion JB (eds): Genitourinary Cancer, pp 460–468. Philadelphia, WB Saunders, 1978.

21. Swartz D, Johnson D, Hussey D: Should an elevated human chorionic gonadotropin titer alter therapy for seminoma? J Urol 131:63–65, 1984.

22. Ro JY, Dexeus FH, El-Negar A, et al: Intratubular germ cell neoplasia. Semin Diagn Pathol 4:59–87, 1991.

23. Drago J, Nelson R, Palmer J: Childhood embryonal carcinoma of the testis. Urology 12:499–503, 1978.

24. Talerman A: The incidence of yolk sac tumor (endodermal sinus tumor) elements in germ cell tumor of the testis in adults. Cancer 36:211–215, 1975.

25. Kooijman CD: Immature teratomas in children. Histopathology 12:491–502, 1988.

26. Ahmed T, Bosl G, Hajdu S: Teratoma with malignant transformation in germ cell tumors in men. Cancer 56:860–863, 1985.

27. Loehrer P, Hui S, Clark S, et al: Teratoma following cisplatin-based combination chemotherapy for nonseminomatous germ cell tumors: A clinicopathological correlation. J Urol 135:1183–1189, 1986.

28. Ulbright TM, Loehrer PJ, Roth LM, et al: The development of non-germ cell malignancies with germ cell tumors. Cancer 54:1824–1833, 1984.

29. Ahlgren A, Simrell R, Triche T, et al: Sarcoma arising is a residual testicular teratoma after cytoreductive chemotherapy. Cancer 54:2015–2108, 1984.

30. Chaganti RSK, Ladanyi M, Samaniego J, et al: Malignant hematopoietic differentiation of a germ cell tumor. Genes Chromosomes Cancer 1:83–87, 1989.

31. Nichols C, Roth B, Heerema N, et al: Hematologic neoplasm associated with primary germ cell tumors—An update. N Engl J Med 322:1425–1429, 1990.

32. Ladanyi M, Samaniego F, Reuler V, et al: Cytogenetic and immunohistochemical evidence for germ cell origin of a subset of acute leukemias associated with mediastinal germ cell tumors. J Natl Cancer Inst 82:221–227, 1990.

33. Azer P, Braustein G: Malignant Leydig cell tumor. Objective tumor response to o,p'-DDD. Cancer 47:1251–1255, 1981.

34. Hart WR, Burkons DM: Germ cell neoplasms arising in gonadoblastomas. Cancer 43:669–678, 1979.

35. Giuler RL: Testicular involvement in leukemia and lymphoma. Cancer 23:1290–1295, 1969.

36. Haupt HM, Maun RB, Trump DL, et al: Metastatic carcinoma

to the testis: Clinical and pathological distinction from primary testicular neoplasms. Cancer 54:709–714, 1984.

37. Childs WJ, Goldstraw P, Nicholls JE, et al: Primary malignant mediastinal germ cell tumours: Improved prognosis with platinum-based chemotherapy and surgery. Br J Cancer 67:1098–1101, 1993.

38. Gross PE, Schwertfeger L, Blackstein ME, et al: Extragonadal germ cell tumors. A 14-year Toronto experience. Cancer 73:1971–1979, 1994.

39. Gutierrez Delgado F, Tjulandin SA, Garin AM, et al: Long term results of treatment in patients with extragonadal germ cell tumours. Eur J Cancer 29A:1002–1005, 1993.

40. Gerl A, Clemm C, Kohl P: Primary extragonadal germ cell tumors. Clinical manifestations, differential diagnosis and therapy. Medizinsche Klinik 89:240–244, 1994.

41. Mencel PJ, Motzer RJ, Mazumdar M, et al: Advanced seminoma treatment results, survival, and prognostic factors in 142 patients. J Clin Oncol 12:120–126, 1994.

42. Giwercman A, Skakkeback NE: Carcinoma in situ of the testis: Biology, screening and management. Eur Urol 23 (suppl 2):19–21, 1993.

43. Dauguard G, Rorth M, von der Maase H: Management of extragonadal germ-cell tumors and the significance of bilateral testicular biopsies. Ann Oncol 3:283–289, 1992.

44. Richie JP: Advances in the diagnosis and treatment of testicular cancer. Cancer Invest: 11:670–675, 1993.

45. Pizzocaro G: Transscrotal surgery and prognosis in resected stage 1 and 2 nonseminomatous germ cell tumors of the testis. Presented in San Francisco at the Annual Meeting of the Societe Internationale d'Urologie. Sept. 5–10, 1982.

46. Zondek B: Versuch einer biologischen (hormonalen) Diagnostik beim malignen Hodentumor. Chirug 2:1072–1080, 1930.

47. Bosl G, Geller N, Cirricione C, et al: Serum tumor markers in patients with metastatic germ cell tumors of the testis: A 10-year experience. Am J Med 75:29–35, 1983.

48. Mumperow E, Harlmann M: Spermatic cord beta-human chorionic gonadotropin levels in seminoma and their clinical implications. J Urol 147:1041–1043, 1991.

49. Vugrin D, Friedman A, Whitmore WF: Correlation of serum tumor markers in advanced germ cell tumors with response to chemotherapy and surgery. Cancer 53:1440–1445, 1984.

50. Klein EA: Tumor markers in testis cancer. Urol Clin North Am 20:67–73, 1993.

51. Bates SE: Clinical applications of serum tumor markers. Ann Intern Med 115:623–638, 1991.

52. Saller B, Clara R, Spottl G, et al: Testicular cancer secretes intact HCG and its free beta subunit: Evidence that HCG levels are the most reliable in diagnosis and follow-up. Clin Chem 36:234–239, 1990.

53. Catalana WJ, Vaitukaitis JL, Fair WR: Falsely positive specific human chorionic gonadotropin assays in patients with testicular tumors: Conversion to negative with testosterone administration. J Urol 122:1226–1228, 1979.

54. Abelev GI: Alpha-fetoprotein as a marker of embryospecific differentiations in normal and tumor tissues. Transplant Rev 20:137–145, 1974.

55. Lange PH, Nochomovity LC, Rosai J, et al: Serum alpha-fetoprotein and human chorionic gonadotropin in patients with seminoma. J Urol 124:472–478, 1980.

56. Koshida K, Nishino A, Yamamoto H, et al: The role of alkaline phosphatase isoenzymes as tumor markers for testicular germ cell tumors. J Urol 146:57–60, 1991.

57. Richie JP: Neoplasms of the testis, in Walch PC, Retik AB, Stamey TA, et al (eds): Campbell's Urology, 6th ed, pp 1222–1263. Philadelphia, WB Saunders, 1992.

58. Horwich A, Tucker DE, Peckham MJ: Placental alkaline phosphatase as a tumor marker in seminoma using the HITE2 monoclonal antibody assay. Br J Cancer 51:625–629, 1985.

59. Samaniego F, Rodriquez E, Houldsworth J, et al: Cytogenetic and molecular analysis of human male germ cell tumors: Chromosome 12 abnormalities and gene amplification. Genes Chromosom Cancer 1:289–292, 1990.

60. Geurts van Kessel A, Seiykerbwjk RF, Sinke RJ, et al: Molecular cytogenetics of human germ cell tumors: i(12p) and related chromosomal anomalies. 3rd Copenhagen Workshop: Carcinoma-in-situ and Cancer of the Testis, p 2. November 1–4, 1992, Copenhagen, Denmark, 1992.

61. Bosl G, Dmitrovsky E, Reuter VE, et al: Isochromosome of chromosome 12: A clinically useful marker for male germ cell tumors. J Natl Cancer Inst 24:1874–1878, 1989.

62. Wang LC, Vass W, Gao C, et al: Amplification and enhanced expression of the c-ki-ras 2 proto-oncogene in human embryonal carcinomas. Cancer Res 47:4192–4198, 1987.

63. vor der Maase H, Walbom-Jorgensen M, et al: Carcinoma in situ of contralateral testis in patients with testicular germ cell cancer: Study of 27 cases in 500 patients. Br Med J 293:1398–1401, 1986.

64. Giwercman A, von der Maase H, Berlheken JG: Localized irradiation of testes with carcinoma in situ: Effects on Leydig cell function and eradication of malignant germ cells in 20 patients. J Clin Endocrinol Metab 73:596–603, 1991.

65. Muller J: Abnormal infantile germ cells and development of carcinoma-in-situ in maldeveloped testis: A sterological and densitometric study. Int J Androl 10:543–567, 1987.

66. Thomas GM: Refining the therapy of testicular cancer. Eur Urol 23(suppl 2):24–25, 1993.

67. Thomas GM: Surveillance in stage I seminoma of the testis. Urol Clin North Am 20:85–91, 1993.

68. Babaian RJ, Zagers GK: Testicular seminoma: The M. D. Anderson experience. An analysis of pathological and patient characteristics and treatment recommendations. J Urol 139:311–314, 1988.

69. Fossa SD, Aass N, Kaahluus: Radiotherapy for testicular seminoma stage I: Treatment results and long-term post-irradiation morbidity in 365 patients. Int J Radiat Oncol Biol Phys 16:383–388, 1989.

70. Hamilton C, Horwich A, Easton D, et al: Radiotherapy for stage I seminoma testis: Results of treatment and complications. Radiother Oncol 6:115–120, 1986.

71. Thomas GM: Controversies in the management of testicular seminoma. Cancer 55:2296–2306, 1985.

72. Lester SG, Morphis JG, Hornback NB: Testicular seminoma: Analysis of treatment results and failures. Int J Radiat Oncol Biol Phys 12:353–358, 1986.

73. Fossa SD, Abyholm T, Normann N, et al: Post-treatment fertility in patients with testicular cancer. III: Ifluence of radiotherapy in seminoma patients. Br J Urol 58:315–319, 1986.

74. Hahn EW, Feingold SM, Nisce L: Aspermia and recovery of spermatogenesis in cancer patients following incidental gonadal irradiation during treatment: A progress report. Radiology 119:223–225, 1976.

75. Horwich A, Dearnaley DP: Treatment of seminoma. Semin Oncol 19:171–180, 1992.

76. Gregory C, Peckham MJ: Results of radiotherapy for stage II testicular seminoma. Radiother Oncol 6:285–292, 1989.

77. Hay JH, Duncan W, Kerr GR: Subsequent malignancies in patients irradiated for testicular tumours. Br J Radiol 57:597–602, 1984.

78. Zagars GK, Babaian RJ: The role of radiation therapy in stage II testicular seminoma. Int J Radiat Oncol Biol Phys 13:163–170, 1987.

79. Dosoretz DE, Shipley WU, Blitzer PH, et al. Megavoltage irradiation for pure testicular seminoma: Results and patterns of failure. Cancer 48:2184–2190, 1981.

80. Willan BD, McGowan DG: Seminoma of the testis: A 22-year experience with radiation therapy. Int J Radiat Oncol Biol Phys 11:1769–1775, 1985.

81. Lederman GS, Sheldon TA, Dhaffer JT, et al: Cardiac disease after mediastinal irradiation for seminoma. Cancer 60:772–776, 1987.

82. Epstein BE, Order SE, Zinreich ES: Staging, treatment and results in testicular seminoma: A 12-year report. Cancer 65:405–411, 1990.

83. Mason BR, Kearsley JH: Radiotherapy for stage II testicular seminoma. The prognostic influence of tumor bulk. J Clin Oncol 6:1856–1862, 1988.

84. Hanks G, Peters T, Owen J: Seminoma of the testis: Long term beneficial and deleterious results of radiation. Int J Radiart Oncol Biol Phys 24:913–919, 1992.

85. Higby DJ, Wallace HJ, Albert DJ, et al: Diamminodichloroplatinum II: A phase I study showing response in testicular and other tumors Cancer 33:1219–1225, 1974.

86. Mendenhall WL, Williams SD, Einhorn LH, et al: Disseminated seminoma: Re-evaluation of treatment protocols. J Urol 126:493–496, 1981.

87. Van Oosterom AT, Williams SD, Cortes Tunes G, et al: The treatment of metastatic seminoma with combination chemotherapy, in Jones WG, Ward AM, Anderson CK (eds): Germ Cell Tumours II, pp 229–233. Oxford, England, Pergamon, 1986.

88. Fossa S, Borge L, Aass N, et al: The treatment of advanced metastatic seminoma: Experience in 55 cases. J Clin Oncol 5:1071–1077, 1987.

89. Clemm C, Hartenstein R, Willich N, et al: Vinblastine-ifosfamide-cisplatin treatment of bulky seminoma. Cancer 58:2203–2207, 1986.

90. Peckham MJ, Horwich A, Blackmore C, et al: Etoposide and cisplatin with or without bleomycin as first-line chemotherapy in patients with small-volume metastases of testicular nonseminoma. Cancer Treat Rep 69:483–488, 1985.

91. Logothetis CJ, Samuels ML, Ogden SL, et al: Cyclophosphamide and sequential cisplatin for advanced seminoma: Long-term follow-up in 52 patients. J Urol 138:789–794, 1987.

92. Amato R: High cure rate (97%) with carboplatin, ifosfamide and selective consolidation in advanced seminoma (abstract 623). Proc Am Soc Clin Oncol 11:A691, 1992.

93. Schuette J, Niederle N, Scheulen ME et al: Chemotherapy of metastatic seminoma. Br J Cancer 51: 467–472, 1985.

94. Motzer RJ, Bosl GJ, Geller NL, et al: Advanced seminoma: The role of chemotherapy and adjunctive surgery. An Intern Med 108:513–518, 1988.

95. Fossa SE, Aass N, Ous S, et al: Histology of tumor residuals following chemotherapy in patients with advanced nonseminomatous testicular cancer. J Urol 142:1239–1242, 1989.

96. Horwich A, Dearnaley DP, Duchesne GM, et al: Simple nontoxic treatment of advanced metastatic seminoma with carboplatin. J Clin Oncol 7:1150–1156, 1989.

97. Schultz SM, Einhorn LH, Conces DJJ, et al: Management of postchemotherapy residual mass in patients with advanced seminoma: Indiana University Experience. J Clin Oncol 7:1497–1503, 1989.

98. Fossa SD: Response evaluation in seminoma, in Horwich A (ed): Testicular Cancer-Clinical Investigation and Management, pp 252–268. New York, Chapman and Hall Medical, 1991.

99. Rorth M, Jacobsen GK, von der Maase H, et al: Surveillance alone versus radiotherapy after orchiectomy for clinical stage I nonseminomatous testicular cancer. J Clin Oncol 9:1543–1548, 1991.

100. Horwich A: Current controversies in the management of testicular cancer. Eur J Cancer 27:322–326, 1991.

101. Williams SD, Stablein DM, Einhorn LH, et al: Immediate adjuvant chemotherapy versus observation with treatment at relapse in pathological stage II testicular cancer. N Engl J Med 317:1433–1438, 1987.

102. Lochrer PJ, Williams SD, Einhorn LH: Testicular cancer: The quest continues. J Natl Cancer Inst 80:1373–1382, 1988.

103. Sternberg CN: Role of primary chemotherapy in stage I and low-volume stage II nonseminomatous germ-cell testis tumors. Urol Clin North Am 20:93–103, 1993.

104. Cullen MH, Stenning S, Fossa SD: Short course adjuvant chemotherapy in high-risk Stage I nonseminomatous germ cell tumors of the testis (NSGCTT): Preliminary report of an MRC study (meeting abstract). Br J Cancer: 65(suppl 16):8, 1992.

105. Donahue JP, Einhorn LH, Perez JM: Improved management of nonseminomatous testis tumors. Cancer 42:2903–2908, 1978.

106. Schmoll HJ, Waegener W: Adjuvant therapy in resectable stage II nonseminomatous testicular cancer, in Jones SE, Salmon SE (eds): Adjuvant Therapy of Cancer IV, pp 539–548. Orlando, Grune & Stratton, 1984.

107. Pizzocaro G, Zanoni F, Salvioni R, et al: Difficulties of a surveillance study omitting retroperitoneal lymphadenectomy in clinical stage I nonseminomatous germ cell tumors of the testis. J Urol 138:1393–1396, 1987.

108. Weiss RB, Stablein DM, Muggia FM, et al: Toxicity comparisons between two chemotherapy regimens as adjuvant or as salvage treatment in nonseminomatous testicular cancer. Cancer 62:18–23, 1988.

109. Peckham MJ, Hendry WF: Clinical stage II nonseminomatous germ cell testicular tumors: Results of management by primary chemotherapy. Br J Urol 57:763–768, 1985.

110. Socinski MA, Garnick MB, Stomper PA, et al: Stage II nonseminomatous germ-cell tumors of the testis: An analysis of treatment options in patients with low-volume retroperitoneal disease. J Urol 140:1437–1441, 1988.

111. Vugrin D, Whitmore WF Jr: The role of chemotherapy and surgery in the treatment of retroperitoneal metastases in advanced nonseminomatous testis cancer. Cancer 55:1874–1878, 1985.

112. Oliver RTD, Dhaliwal HS, Hope-Stone HF, et al: Short-course etoposide, bleomycin and cisplatin in the treatment of metastatic germ cell tumors: Appraisal of its potential as adjuvant chemotherapy for stage 1 testis tumours. Br J Urol 61:53–58, 1988.

113. Logothetis CJ, Swanson DA, Dexeus F, et al: Primary chemotherapy for clinical stage II nonseminomatous germ cell tumors of the testis: A follow-up of 50 patients. J Clin Oncol 5:906–911, 1987.

114. Norman A, Fisher C, Hendry WF: Primary chemotherapy for stage II nonseminomatous germ cell tumors of the testis. J Urol 151:72–77, 1994.

115. Logothetis CJ: The case for relevant staging of germ cell tumors. Cancer 65:709–717, 1990.

116. Ozols RF, Deisseroth AB, Javadpour N, et al: Treatment of poor prognosis nonseminomatous testicular cancer with a high-dose platinum combination chemotherapy regimen. Cancer 51:1803–1807, 1983.

117. Sloter G, Haye S, Sleyfer D, et al: Preliminary results of BEP (bleomycin, etoposide, cisplatin) versus an alternating regimen of BEP and PVB (cisplatin, vinblastine, bleomycin) in high volume metastatic testicular nonseminomas. An EORTC study (abstract). Proc Am Soc Clin Oncol 5:106, 1986.

118. Amato RJ, 1995: upublished data.

119. Bosl GJ, Geller NL, Cerrincione C, et al: Multivariate analysis of prognostic variables in patients with metastatic testicular cancer. Cancer Res 43:3403–3407, 1983.

120. Vaeth M, Schulty HR, von der Maase H, et al: Prognostic

factors in testicular germ cell tumours: Experiences from 1058 consecutive cases. Acta Radiol Oncol 23:271–285, 1984.

121. Mead GM, Stenning SP, Parkinson MC, et al: The second Medical Research Council study of prognostic factors in nonseminomatous germ cell tumors. J Clin Oncol 10:85–94, 1992.

122. Einhorn LH, Donohue J: Cis-diamminedichloroplatinum, vinblastine and bleomycin combination chemotherapy in disseminated testicular cancer. Ann Intern Med 87:293–298, 1977.

123. Newlands ES, Begent RHJ, Rustin GJS, et al: Further advances in the management of malignant teratomas of the testis and other sites. Lancet 1:948–951, 1983.

124. Williams SD, Birch R, Irvin L, et al: Disseminated germ cell tumors: Chemotherapy with cisplatin plus bleomycin plus either vinblastine or etoposide A trial of the South East Cancer Study Group. N Engl J Med 316:1435–1440, 1987.

125. Newlands ES, Bagshawe KD, Begent RHJ, et al: Current optimum management of anaplastic germ cell tumours of the testis and other sites. Br J Urol 58:307–314, 1986.

126. Ozols RF, Ihde DC, Linehan M, et al: A randomized trial of standard chemotherapy versus a high-dose chemotherapy regimen in the treatment of poor prognosis nonseminomatous germ-cell tumors. J Clin Oncol 6:1031–1040, 1988.

127. Hitchins RN, Newlands ES, Smith DB, et al: Long-term outcome in patients with germ cell tumours treated with POMB/ACE chemotherapy: Comparison of commonly used classification systems of good and poor prognosis. Br J Cancer 59:236–242, 1989.

128. Wheeler BM, Loehrer PJ, Williams SD, et al: Ifosfamide in refractory germ cell tumors. J Clin Oncol 4:28–34, 1986.

129. Droz JP, Pico JL, Kramer A: Role of autologous bone marrow transplantation in germ-cell cancer. Urol Clin North Am 20:161–171, 1993.

130. Droz JP, Pico JL, Biron P, et al: No evidence of a benefit of early intensified chemotherapy (HDCT) with autologous bone marrow transplantation (ABMT) in the first line treatment of poor risk nonseminomatous germ cell tumors (NSGCT): Preliminary results of a randomized trial (abstract). Proc Am Soc Clin Oncol 11:C-602, 1992.

131. Levitt MD, Reynolds PM, Sheiner HJ, et al: Nonseminomatous germ cell testicular tumours: Residual masses after chemotherapy. Br J Surg 72:19–22, 1985.

132. Fossa SD, Ous S, Lien HH, et al: Post-chemotherapy lymph node histology in radiologically normal patients with metastatic nonseminomatous testicular cancer. J Urol 141:557–559, 1989.

133. Toner GC, Panicek DM, Heelan RT, et al: Adjunctive surgery after chemotherapy for nonseminomatous germ cell tumors: Recommendations for patient selection. J Clin Oncol 8:1683–1694, 1990.

134. Bajorin DF, Herr HW, Motzer RJ, et al: Current perspectives on the role of adjunctive surgery in combined modality treatment of patients with germ cell tumors. Semin Oncol 19:148–158, 1992.

135. Sheinfeld J, Bajorin: Management of the postchemotherapy residual mass. Urol Clin North Am 20:133–143, 1992.

136. Donohue JP, Einhorn LH, Williams SD: Cytoreductive surgery for metastatic testis cancer: Considerations of timing and extent. J Urol 123:1111–1114, 1982.

137. Fox EP, Einhorn LH, Weathers T, et al: Outcome analysis for patients with persistent germ cell carcinoma in post-chemotherapy (PC) retroperitoneal lymph node dissections (retroperitoneal lymphadenectomy) (abstract). Proc Am Soc Clin Oncol 11:198, 1992.

138. Einhorn LH, Williams SD, Mandelbaum I, et al: Surgical resection in disseminated testicular cancer following chemotherapeutic cytoreduction. Cancer 48:904–907, 1981.

139. Murphy BA, Motzer RJ, Mazumder M, et al: Serum markers decline during ifosphamide chemotherapy predicts event-free and overall survival in germ cell tumor patients (abstract C-1230). Proc Am Assoc Cancer Res 33:205, 1992.

140. Toner GC, Geller NL, Tan C, et al: Serum tumor marker half-life during chemotherapy allows early prediction of complete response and survival in nonseminomatous germ cell tumors. Cancer Res 50:5904–5910, 1990.

141. Motzer RJ, Geller NL, Tan CC, et al: Salvage chemotherapy for patients with germ cell tumors. The Memorial Sloan-Kettering Cancer Center experience (1979–1989). Cancer 67:1305–1310, 1991.

142. Einhorn LH: Salvage therapy for germ cell tumors. Semin Oncol 21(suppl 7):47–51, 1994.

143. Ledermann JA, Holden ES, Newlands RHJ: The long-term outcome of patients who relapse after chemotherapy for non-seminomatous germ cell tumours. Br J Urol 74:225–230, 1994.

144. Einhorn LH, Weathers T, Loehrer P, et al: Second line chemotherapy with vinblastine, ifosfamide, and cisplatin, after initial chemotherapy with cisplatin, VP-16, and bleomycin (PVP16B) in disseminated germ cell tumors (GCT): Long term follow-up (abstract 599). Proc Am Soc Clin Oncol 11: 599, 1992.

145. Harstrick A, Schmoll H-J, Wilke H, et al: Cisplatin, etoposide, and ifosfamide salvage therapy for refractory or relapsing germ cell carcinoma. J Clin Oncol 9:1–7, 1991.

146. Motzer RJ, Bosl GJ: High-dose chemotherapy for resistant germ cell tumors: Recent advances and future directions. J Natl Cancer Inst 84:1703–1708, 1992.

147. Nichols CR, Anderson J, Lazarus HM, et al: High-dose carboplatin and etoposide with autologous bone marrow transplantation in refractory germ cell cancer: An Eastern Cooperative Oncology Group protocol. J Clin Oncol 10:558–563, 1992

148. Motzer RJ, Gulati SC, Crown J, et al: High-dose chemotherapy and autologous bone marrow rescue for patients with refractory germ cell tumors: Early intervention is better tolerated. Cancer 69:550–556, 1992.

149. Nichols C, Tricot G, Williams S, et al: Dose-intensive chemotherapy in refractory germ cell cancer—A phase I/II trial of high-dose carboplatin with autologous bone marrow transplantation. J Clin Oncol 7:932–939, 1989.

CHAPTER 28

Bladder Cancer

Yung-Chang Lin, MD, *and* Shi-Ming Tu, MD

Department of Genitourinary Medical Oncology, Division of Medical Oncology
The University of Texas M. D. Anderson Cancer Center, Houston, Texas

It is estimated that, in 1995, about 50,500 new cases of urinary bladder cancer will be diagnosed and that 11,200 patients will die of the diease. The most common malignant tumor of the urinary tract, bladder cancer accounts for 6.5% of all cancers annually. It is the fifth most common cancer among American men,[1] and approximately three quarters of all cases occur in men.

Seventy-five percent of bladder cancers are superficial (confined within the lamina propria) at diagnosis. About 50% to 80% of superficial cancers recur, but only 15% to 20% progress to invasive disease (ie, tumors spreading beyond the lamina propria). Despite aggressive surgery or radiation, 50% of patients with muscle-invasive disease ultimately die of cancer.[2] For patients with metastatic disease, cytotoxic chemotherapy is the only available option, and the chances of long-term survival are minimal.

Understanding the mechanism of tumor progression and improving the results of treatment remain the most important research and clinical management issues surrounding bladder cancer. This chapter will review the risk factors, molecular biology, pathology, diagnosis, and currently available options for and results of treatment of the disease.

EPIDEMIOLOGY AND ETIOLOGY

Bladder cancer is predominantly a disease of the elderly male. The peak age of incidence is the seventh decade, and the male-to-female ratio is 3 to 1.

The incidence is higher in American whites than American blacks, higher in Western industrialized countries than African and Asian nations, and higher in urban areas than rural areas. These trends suggest a role for industrial substances in the development of bladder cancer.[3] Chemical carcinogens that have been linked with bladder cancers, such as 2-naphthylamine, benzidine, and 4-aminobiphenyl, are associated with several occupations: aniline dye, rubber, and textile work; painting; leather processing; and hairdressing.[3–5]

Cigarette smoking is the single greatest risk factor for bladder cancer; it is responsible for at least 50% of the cases in men. Compared with the nonsmoker, the smoker has twice the risk of developing the disease. Moreover,

the risk is dose related; persons who stop cigarette smoking have an intermediate risk between those for the smoker and the nonsmoker. Among smokers, pipe and cigar smokers have a relatively low risk of developing the disease, and chewing tobacco does not predispose to bladder cancer at all.[3,6,7]

Phenacetin-containing analgesics have been implicated in the pathogenesis of urothelial neoplasms. The effect of these analgesics is cumulative; women who have been taking phenacetin or one of its derivatives for 20 years or longer have an increased risk of developing urothelial cancer.[8,9] Chronic bladder infections or irritations, such as bilharziasis, bladder stones, and conditions requiring chronic indwelling catheterization, are associated with the development of squamous-cell carcinoma of the bladder.[3,10,11] Evidence suggesting that dietary factors such as coffee and artificial sweeteners are carcinogenic has been inconsistent.[12–14] On the other hand, milk and vitamin A have been associated with a decreased risk of bladder cancer.[3]

Familial bladder cancer accounts for a very small population of the patients with bladder cancer. A large case-control study suggested that a combination of genetic and environmental factors contributes to the occurrence of bladder cancer in these families. The estimated relative risk of developing the disease is 1.45 for a person with a family member who developed bladder cancer before the age of 45 years.[15]

MOLECULAR BIOLOGY

Although information on genetic changes in bladder cancer has been emerging in recent years, it is still too early to routinely apply these biologic markers in clinical practice. However, the results are intriguing and have potential for facilitating the diagnosis and management of bladder cancer.

Chromosomal Aberrations

The chromosomal studies of bladder cancer, as for most of the solid tumors, are very complicated, and results have been inconsistent. Using molecular biologic techniques, investigators are able to examine structural and numerical chromosomal changes and allelic deletions. Deletion of part or all of chromosome 9 was found in all stages of bladder cancer, suggesting that these changes may be responsible for early bladder carcinogenesis.[16,17] An increasing copy number of chromosome 7 was found to correlate with high tumor grade and proliferation.[18] Deletions of 3p, 11p, and 17p occurred predominantly in tumors of advanced stage; genes lost at these areas might be associated with tumor progression.[19] However, despite the advances in genetic studies, most of the affected genes in bladder cancer and their biologic functions remain unknown. The potential clinical relevance of these altered genes should be further investigated.

Suppressor Genes

The gene most frequently changed in bladder cancer and probably the most important gene in the progression of the disease is *p53*. The incidence of *p53* mutations was 50% to 60% in the bladder tumors examined by DNA sequencing or by expression of the p53 protein.[20-22] Moreover, the presence of *p53* mutation correlated with high-grade, invasive tumors.[21-22]

A recent study conducted by Esrig et al showed that 42% of 243 cystectomy specimens containing bladder cancer of all stages had overexpression of the p53 protein; this overexpression independently predicted a significantly increased risk of disease recurrence and death in this population.[21] Another study revealed that 48% of patients with carcinoma in situ (CIS) of the bladder had overexpression of the p53 protein; 86.7% of those with p53 overexpression subsequently developed progressive disease, compared with only 16.7% of patients without overexpression.[23]

The presence of *p53* mutation is probably the cause of the biologically aggressive behavior of CIS of the bladder. In contrast, the incidence of *p53* mutation in low-grade, low-stage papillary bladder cancer is very low. Therefore, it has been hypothesized that there are dual molecular pathways in the tumor progression of superficial bladder cancer based on the presence of *p53* mutation.[24]

Allelic loss of the retinoblastoma (*Rb*) gene has been shown in 28 of 94 patients with transitional-cell carcinomas. *Rb* loss happened significantly more frequently in tumors of high grade and advanced stage.[25] Altered expression of the Rb protein (total or partial absence of Rb expression), which represents losing all or part of the *Rb* gene, was reported in 34% of one series of patients with muscle-invasive disease[26] and in 37% of another such series.[27] Altered Rb expression was associated with poor prognosis and shorter tumor-free survival.[26,27]

Oncogenes

The role of oncogenes in bladder cancer is not as significant as in other solid tumors. The incidence of overexpression of *HER-2/neu* in bladder cancer is one of the highest among all human malignancies, ranging from 9% to 34% of cancers tested.[28,29] It was more frequently found in tumors of high grade and advanced stage. About 7% to 20% of bladder tumors were reported to contain a *ras* mutation, but the clinical significance of this mutation is not known.[30,31] Expression of epidermoid growth factor receptor in bladder tumors has been associated with the progression of muscle-invasive disease.[32]

PATHOLOGY

The majority of bladder cancers originate in the urothelium, the characteristic transitional-cell epithelium lining the urinary tract from the renal pelvis to the proximal urethra. In the United States, 85% to 95% of bladder cancers are transitional-cell carcinomas. Mixed tumors containing squamous-cell carcinoma and adenocarcinoma elements are reported at various rates between 10% and 30%. Pure squamous-cell carcinoma occurs in less than 3% of bladder cancers in the United States, but in areas where bilharziasis is epidemic (eg, Egypt), squamous-cell carcinoma of the bladder is the most common malignancy.[10] Adenocarcinoma accounts for 2% of bladder cancers; most occurs on the trigone of the bladder. A particular subset of adenocarcinomas arising from the urachus remnant locate over the dome of the bladder. About 70% to 80% of bladder cancers occur on the lateral or posterior walls of the bladder, and 20%, on the trigone. Thirty percent of tumors are multifocal at diagnosis.[33,34]

The grading of transitional-cell carcinoma is based on the cellular atypia, nuclear abnormalities, and number of mitoses. At M. D. Anderson Cancer Center, bladder tumors are classified according to World Health Organization criteria into three categories: grades 1, 2, and 3. Low-grade (grade 1) tumors usually grow superficially with papillary patterns, whereas high-grade (grade 3) tumors are usually solid and invasive.[35]

Carcinoma in situ is a histologically and biologically distinct cancer of the bladder. The tumor, by definition, is a superficial, nonpapillary, noninfiltrating flat neoplasia characterized by cellular anaplasia and nonspecific inflammatory changes. Brunn's nests (outpocketings of epithelium into the lamina propria) are a characteristic feature of this type of neoplasm.[36] CIS frequently occurs in patients with other types of bladder tumors and can be close to the tumor (in 26% to 40% of cases) or remote from it.[37]

Primary bladder tumors with CIS have a high frequency of recurrence and progression.[38] A retrospective study showed that 40% of patients with CIS developed invasive disease within 5 years.[39] Diffuse CIS in the absence of another type of tumor is a distinct subset of CIS; it usually involves 50% to 85% of the bladder mucosa. Presentation with bladder-irritative symptoms but nonspecific inflammatory cystoscopic findings are its characteristic features. Because the adhesion molecule is lost in CIS, the anaplastic cells easily shed into the lumen of the urinary tract; urine cytology tests yield positive results in over 90% of cases.[40]

CLINICAL PRESENTATION

There are no pathognomonic symptoms or signs of bladder cancer. Painless intermittent gross hematuria or microscopic hematuria is the leading sign, occurring in over 75% of patients. About 30% of patients, particularly those with invasive disease or CIS, have irritative symptoms such as dysuria or urinary frequency. Pelvic pain and symptoms of rectal obstruction occur in locally advanced disease; flank pain often results from ureteral obstruction.

DIAGNOSIS AND STAGING

The standard procedure for diagnosis and staging of bladder cancer is cystoscopy and bimanual examination under anesthesia (EUA). All visible tumors should be removed, and multiple random biopsies of the bladder wall, including the trigone and prostatic urethra, should be performed to rule out the presence of CIS or dysplasia. Cold-cup biopsy is preferred to avoid the effects of cautery, and the biopsy should extend deep into the muscle layer to enable determination of the depth of tumor invasion. EUA should be performed immediately after cystoscopy to assess the extent of disease (the thickness of the tumor and its mobility) and to determine the clinical stage. However, the accuracy rate of staging by EUA is less than 50%, usually because the inflammatory reaction blurs the tumor margin.[41]

Urine cytologic analysis and flow cytometry are useful for screening high-risk populations and for follow-up after tumor resection and the histologic diagnosis of CIS. The clinical application of flow cytometry is limited to patients who are known to have aneuploid chromosome numbers. Nonetheless, in these patients, this technique is more sensitive than cytologic analysis in detecting minimal or recurrent disease. The cell yield for these studies may be increased by brisk bladder lavage with normal saline during each cystoscopic examination.

Complete cell counts, biochemical survey, and urinalysis should be done prior to treatment. There is no serologic marker specific to bladder cancer, although elevation of serum levels of carcinoembryonic antigen and beta-human chorionic gonadotropin is not uncommon in cases of the disease. Radiographic studies are selected according to the clinical indication. Computed tomographic scans help in evaluating the tumor extent and metastasis. Intravenous pyelography is useful in detecting synchronous urothelial tumors of the upper urinary tract. Plain chest x-rays are routinely performed to evaluate pulmonary metastasis. Bone scan is indicated in patients with clinical symptoms suggestive of bone metastasis.

There are two staging systems for bladder cancer: the American Joint Committee on Cancer/International Union Against Cancer Tumor-Node-Metastasis (TNM) system and the Jewett-Marshall staging system. The latter was originated from the observation by Jewett that the depth of tumor invasion correlated with the tumor's clinical behavior and progression.[41] The two systems are compared in Table 1. Generally, the TNM system is preferred and accepted universally. Table 2 summarizes the nodal classifications utilized in the TNM system.

TREATMENT

Most patients with superficial disease do not die of bladder cancer. The goals of management in this group

TABLE I

Comparison Between Jewett-Marshall and TNM Staging

Staging system		
Jewett-Marshall	TNM	Description
O	T0	No definitive tumor
	Tis	Carcinoma in situ
A	Ta	Papillary tumor without invasion
	TI	Lamina propria invasion
B-1	T2	Superficial muscle invasion
B-2	T3a	Deep muscle invasion
C	T3b	Perivesical fat invasion
D-1	T4	Prostate, vagina, uterus, or pelvis side wall invasion
D-2	N1-3	Pelvic lymph-node metastasis
D-3	M	Lymph-node metastasis beyond pelvis
D-4	M	Distant metastasis

TNM = tumor-node-metastasis

TABLE 2

Nodal Classification (TNM Staging System)

Stage	Description
N1	Metastasis in single node, < 2 cm
N2	Metastasis in bilateral lymph nodes, or single node > 2 cm but < 5 cm
N3	Metastasis in any node > 5 cm
M	Lymph-node metastasis beyond pelvis, or distant metastasis

TNM = tumor-necrosis-metastasis

are to reduce the morbidity from recurrence and to prevent progression in the patients who are potentially at risk. In contrast, patients with invasive disease have a grave prognosis despite aggressive surgery or radiotherapy. The aims of management in this group are to improve the fraction of patients who achieve remission and to assure the best possible quality of life.

Superficial Disease

Transurethral bladder resection is the treatment of choice for superficial disease, which includes stages Ta, T1, and Tis (CIS). Other modalities include fulguration and photodynamic therapy. More than 80% of lesions can be controlled locally by surgery alone, but 30% to 80% of them will recur. Patients with the following conditions tend to have recurrences: high-grade tumor, multiple primary tumors, presence of cellular atypia, more than three previous recurrences, and endoscopically observed residual tumor.[42]

A retrospective study of patients with low-grade tumors showed that 80% of the recurrences happened within 3 months of the first resection.[43] The frequency of progression in stage and grade of the recurrences varied, ranging from 4% to 30% for stage and 10% to 30% for grade. Tumor stage and grade correlated with the incidence of recurrence and with survival. The NBCCGA study showed frequencies of progression of 4% for stage Ta tumors, 30% for stage T1 tumors, 2% for grade 1 tumors, and 45% for grade 3 tumors. The 10-year survival rates were 95% for patients with stage Ta, grade 1 tumors and only 50% for patients with stage T1, grade 3 tumors.[44]

Carcinoma In Situ

Local CIS can be controlled by resection only. For multifocal or diffuse CIS, surgical resection and fulguration of the mucosal lesions plus intravesical therapy is the treatment of choice. Prognostic factors that indicate whether a patient is better suited for endoscopic resection or for cystectomy include the extent of disease, association with irritative symptoms, and a history of prior disease. Cystoprostatectomy is indicated when the lesions are not controlled by endoscopic resection, the bladder is severely contracted, intravesical therapy has been unsuccessful, or there is histologic evidence of persistent CIS of the prostatic duct or of stromal invasion.[2] Panurothelial CIS, which involves the whole epithelium of the urinary tract, frequently recurs in either the upper urinary tract or the distal urethra despite radical surgery. The prognosis for patients with panurothelial CIS is dismal.

Intravesical therapy—the administration of cytotoxic agents or an immunomodulator through a catheter into the urinary bladder—has been empirically tried in patients with superficial disease as either primary or adjuvant treatment. The indications for intravesical therapy include a T1 tumor, multiple Ta tumors or a high-grade (grade 2 or 3) Ta tumor, CIS, and positive cytologic results after bladder tumor resection.[45] Complete removal of all gross tumor is required before intravesical therapy to improve treatment results. The currently available agents for this type of therapy are doxorubicin (Adriamycin, Rubex), thiotepa, mitomycin (Mutamycin), and bacillus Calmette-Guérin (BCG); tumors that fail to respond to a full course of one drug often respond to another drug. Patients should receive follow-up with cystoscopic examination and urinary cytologic analysis every 3 months for 1 year, then every 6 months for the next 2 years, and then annually.

In patients with superficial disease, adjuvant intravesical mitomycin administration has been proven to decrease recurrence rates from 51% to 10% at 1.5-year follow-up.[46] BCG was thought better than doxorubicin and thiotepa and at least as good as mitomycin in preventing recurrence and possibly in prolonging disease-free survival and avoiding the need for cystectomy.[45] Although the optimal preparation, dose, and schedule of intravesical BCG therapy are not clear, 6-week consecutive therapy is preferred by most clinicians. In one study, maintenance therapy for longer than 6 weeks did not improve response and resulted in more complications than 6-week therapy.[47] Schellhammer et al reported a complete response rate of 71% in 28 patients with superficial disease using a 6-week BCG schedule.[48] A randomized study comparing transurethral bladder resection with resection followed by intravesical BCG showed significant differences in complete response rate (8% vs 65%) and in frequency of subsequent salvage cystectomy

(35% vs 7%).[49] At Memorial Sloan-Kettering Cancer Center, long-term results in CIS patients who received BCG showed a 54% disease-free survival at 10 years; 33% of these patients retained a functional bladder.[50]

The toxic effects of intravesical therapy include myelosuppression, local irritative symptoms, and systemic toxic effects. Mitomycin is associated with the least systemic toxicity because of its large molecule, but thiotepa has the highest incidence of myelosuppression. BCG induces local granulomatous inflammation over the bladder wall and results in irritative symptoms. Fever occurs in 20% to 30% of patients, and other systemic side effects, including pneumonitis, hepatitis, arthritis, arthralgia, skin rash, and sepsis, have been reported in 5% of patients. Only a small proportion of these patients need antituberculous treatment.[51]

Invasive Disease

The treatment of choice for muscle-invasive disease is radical cystectomy with urinary diversion and bilateral pelvic lymph-node dissection. Many investigators have been attempting to preserve a functional bladder by limiting the extent of surgery when possible without compromising the results.

Conservative Management: For patients with superficial solitary muscle-invasive disease, a simple endoscopic resection may be curative. In a study at Memorial Sloan-Kettering Cancer Center, patients underwent secondary endoscopic resection after primary endoscopic resection of muscle-invasive bladder tumor. Those whose secondary resection showed no evidence of recurrence had a 65% disease-free survival rate (with a functioning bladder) and an 82% overall survival rate at 5 years.[52]

For patients who have only one muscle-invasive tumor without CIS or dysplasia elsewhere, partial cystectomy is another alternative for attaining long-term disease control with less morbidity. The tumor should preferably be located on the dome or posterior wall of the bladder and should have at least a 2-cm surgical margin. Some surgeons also suggest preoperative radiotherapy to offer better regional control and prevent intraoperative seeding. However, the patients who are candidates for radiotherapy account for less than 5% of the total population of those with muscle-invasive bladder tumors.[53]

Radical Surgery: Radical cystectomy with urinary diversion or construction of an internal reservoir and bilateral pelvic lymph-node dissection provide optimal control of muscle-invasive disease. This method enables the surgeon to prevent most local recurrences. Thus, the majority of recurrent tumors are distant metastases. Those patients who have multifocal primary tumors, diffuse CIS, or tumor in the prostatic urethra have significantly higher local recurrence rates. The overall survival rate of patients with muscle-invasive disease is about 50%; survival correlates with the depth of tumor invasion. The 5-year survival rate of patients with pathologic stage P2 and P3a tumors ranges from 60% to 80%. In patients with stage P3b or more advanced tumors, the 5-year survival rate drops to below 30%.[2,54,55]

Other Treatment Modalities: Primary radiotherapy (usually 5,000 to 7,000 cGy) with or without salvage surgery has been used mostly in Great Britain and Canada. The complete response rate to this treatment is approximately 40% to 50%, and the 5-year survival rate ranges from around 30% to 45%.[56,57] In the United States, most primary radiotherapy is given to patients who have intercurrent disease or unresectable tumor. Therefore, the different patient populations preclude definitive comparison between primary radiotherapy and surgery. Local disease recurrence remains the major problem after radiotherapy. In one series, 25% of the cancer-related deaths resulted from local recurrence.[56]

Preoperative radiotherapy (usually involving doses less than 4,000 cGy) followed by surgery has shown benefit in prolonging survival in both retrospective analyses and nonrandomized studies, but the only three prospective randomized trials have failed to confirm this result.[58] The optimal schedule and dose of preoperative radiotherapy are undetermined, and the potential advantage remains controversial.

Neoadjuvant and Adjuvant Chemotherapy: The fact that the majority of recurrences of locally advanced bladder tumors are in the form of distant metastases suggests that subclinical micrometastases were present in these cases at the time of surgery. Integrating systemic cytotoxic chemotherapy and primary surgery using various schedules to prevent distant metastasis and prolong survival has been increasingly studied. Most of the reported results are from phase II studies. Although the response rates are promising, a survival benefit has not been confirmed.[53]

Using the MVAC regimen (methotrexate, vinblastine, doxorubicin, and cyclophosphamide [Cytoxan, Neosar]) for preoperative chemotherapy, 27% of 71 patients (85% of whom had stage T3 or T4 tumors) had a complete response, and an additional 14% were downstaged to superficial in situ disease. With a median follow-up of 24 months, 58% of the complete responders remained free of disease.[59] Another randomized study has not shown a survival difference by using cisplatin (Platinol) as neoadjuvant therapy.[60] Currently there are several larger multi-institutional randomized neoadjuvant chemotherapy trials ongoing in North America and Europe.

Three single-institution trials have shown benefits of adjuvant chemotherapy. At M. D. Anderson Cancer Center, a three-arm trial compared low-risk patients who underwent surgery alone with high-risk patients (those with stage T3b or T4 tumor, nodal disease, and/or vascular and/or lymphatic invasion of primary tumor) who underwent surgery with or without adjuvant chemotherapy using the CISCA regimen (cisplatin, cyclophosphamide, and doxorubicin). The survival curve for high-risk patients receiving adjuvant chemotherapy was similar to that for low-risk patients. The 5-year survival rates for high-risk patients were 70% for the adjuvant group vs 35% for the nonadjuvant group.[61]

At the University of Southern California, a delay in time to progression was found in 71 patients with pathologic stage T3 or T4 disease and/or positive nodal metastases treated with three cycles of CISCA; 70% of patients who received CISCA were free of disease at 3 years compared with only 46% of patients who did not receive CISCA. The difference in median survival (4.3 years with CISCA vs 2.4 years without CISCA) was statistically significant.[62] Another trial using three cycles of MVAC as an adjuvant regimen was closed prematurely because of higher relapse rates in the nonadjuvant arm.[63] Despite the positive results of the three trials, several inadequacies preclude a definite conclusion.

In summary, although the general belief is that the promising results of combination chemotherapy for bladder cancer in the adjuvant setting should translate into prolonged survival, the role of chemotherapy as an adjunct to primary therapy is still undefined. The difficulties in evaluating these trials include the varied criteria in patient selection, the lack of an effective regimen and optimal dose schedule, and the lack of a large-scale multi-institutional trial. Currently the recommended criteria for patients entering adjuvant trials are as follows: locally advanced primary tumor (stage T3b or T4), nodal disease, and vascular or lymphatic invasion by the primary tumor. Any form of adjunctive chemotherapy should be considered experimental.

Bladder Preservation: Endoscopic resection of the primary tumor with concurrent or sequential chemoradiotherapy has been shown to obtain long-term disease control while allowing the patient to retain a functioning bladder or to delay the cystectomy. In a nonrandomized trial of cisplatin-based regimens, the complete response rates were about 70% to 80%, with a 70% 2-year survival rate. Seventy percent of these patients did not require cystectomy at 2 years.[64,65] The patient population met highly selective criteria: stage T2 or T3a tumor, no evidence of CIS, and an adequate bladder capacity.

In patients with advanced localized disease, the ability to sterilize tumors by combined modalities is questionable. Because of the potential risk of local recurrence, continuous surveillance is mandatory.[53] With the goal of maintaining a functioning bladder but not reducing long-term survival, primary treatment using combined modalities deserves further investigation in patients with superficial muscle-invasive disease.

Metastatic Bladder Cancer

Systemic cytotoxic chemotherapy remains the only option for treating patients with metastatic bladder cancer. With combination chemotherapy, a substantial frequency of tumor response has been achieved, including a significant proportion of complete responses. However, the disease continues to recur even with complete response, and long-term survival is rare. Further studies of new regimens or new modalities are urgent and ongoing.

Single-agent chemotherapy has been tested widely; complete response is uncommon, and responses last about 3 to 4 months. Cisplatin administered every 3 to 4 weeks is the most active regimen, producing an overall response rate of 30%. Methotrexate administered in a weekly or biweekly schedule has a pooled response rate of 29%. Response rates for other single agents are shown in Table 3.[66] A recent phase II trial of paclitaxel (Taxol) in 26 previously untreated patients showed an overall response rate of 42% and a complete response rate of 27%; the median response duration was 7 months.[67] Nevertheless, this promising result needs to be confirmed.

Combination chemotherapy is currently the most accepted modality for metastatic bladder cancer and has shown significant antitumor activity. The initial study at M. D. Anderson Cancer Center of CISCA in patients with transitional-cell carcinoma of the bladder revealed an overall response rate of 70% and a complete response rate of 39%. The median response duration in complete responders was 100 weeks.[68] Subsequently, other investigators have reported variable response rates to CISCA ranging from 13% to 70%, with a median rate of 46%.[53]

The cisplatin, methotrexate, and vinblastine (CMV) regimen, first studied at Stanford University, was reported to have a 28% complete response rate and an additional 28% partial response rate. The median survival in complete responders was 11 months, compared with 6 months in nonresponders.[69] The average response rates from other similar trials have ranged from 35% to 74%, with 20% to 30% complete response rates.[53] Although

TABLE 3

Response Rates of Patients With Single Chemotherapeutic Agents

Agent	Response rate (%)
Cisplatin	30
Methotrexate	30
Ifosfamide	28
Gallium nitrate	17
Doxorubicin	19
Vinblastine	16
Carboplatin	13
Fluorouracil	15
Epirubicin	15
Paclitaxel	40

Based on data from references 53, 66, and 67.

there has not been a comparative study with single-agent chemotherapy, both combination regimens were thought to be promising and to have acceptable side effects in the early 1980s.

MVAC, the four-drug combination regimen developed in 1983 by Memorial Sloan-Kettering Cancer Center,[70] has been the most popular regimen used in the United States. Response rates ranging from 40% to 72%, with approximately 25% to 30% complete responses, were reported.[53] The response duration was reported to be as long as 38 months in patients with complete responses but only 11 months in partial responders.[70] A randomized study comparing MVAC with cisplatin alone disclosed significant differences in terms of response rate (39% vs 12%) and median overall survival (12.5 vs 8.2 months).[71]

At M. D. Anderson Cancer Center, Logothetis et al conducted a prospective randomized study comparing MVAC with CISCA. The response rates were 65% and 46%, respectively, and median survivals were 48 and 36 weeks; thus, MVAC showed significant superiority over CISCA.[72] Overall, the majority of complete responses occurred in patients with lymph-node metastases. Patients with liver metastases had the worst result. Pure transitional-cell carcinomas had a significantly higher response rate than mixed tumors.[68, 70]

About 15% of patients with metastatic disease achieve durable remission with combination chemotherapy. Long-term follow-up in patients treated with MVAC has shown a 6-year survival of 32% for patients with nodal disease and 17% for those with advanced metastatic disease.[73]

The toxic effects of MVAC are significant; myelosuppression, sepsis, mucositis, nephrotoxicity, and neuropathy are not uncommon, and toxic death has been reported but is rare.[53,70,72] Patients with a long conduit or internal reservoir that can retain a significant amount of fluid may have decreased methotrexate clearance, leading to prolonged mucositis or myelosuppression.[2]

Several modified MVAC regimens have been proposed, such as eliminating vinblastine and methotrexate on days 15 and 22, replacing doxorubicin with epirubicin (Farmorubicin), and replacing cisplatin with carboplatin.[53] The purpose of these modifications is to reduce the toxicity without affecting the response rate. The results of phase II studies of these modified regimens are promising but still immature. Escalating the dose of MVAC with granulocyte-macrophage colony-stimulating factor rescue in 30 patients who had failed standard MVAC also produced a significant response rate of 40%.[74] However, the modest increase in dosage of MVAC did not produce a substantially different response rate from that of front-line therapy in the subsequent phase II study.[75]

Non-cisplatin-based regimens have increasingly been developed recently. A phase II study combining vinblastine, ifosfamide (Ifex), and gallium nitrite (Ganite) reported an overall response rate of 67%, with a 19% complete response rate.[76] Other regimens, such as those using as analogs of methotrexate and taxanes, have been studied in various stages of clinical trials. Preliminary results are promising, and further combination trials are under investigation.[53]

A biologic modifier combined with cytotoxic chemotherapy, ie, alpha interferon (IFN-α) plus flourouracil, produced a response rate of 30% in 32 patients who did not respond to previous cisplatin-based regimens.[77] Moreover, a current study in patients with metastatic disease is comparing standard MVAC with a new combination, consisting of fluorouracil, cisplatin, and IFN-α.

In summary, current front-line chemotherapy for metastatic bladder cancer remains MVAC and CMV. The MVAC regimen has produced better response rates and survival than single-agent cisplatin or CISCA. Modifications of MVAC are indicated for those who cannot tolerate standard MVAC or for use in clinical research. The new non-MVAC regimens, which have shown significant antitumor activity in some clinical trials, may be another reasonable alternative if their efficacy is confirmed. However, in light of the fact that most patients with metastatic bladder cancer ultimately die of the disease, the ideal regimen or strategy for treatment has not yet been determined and warrants further investigation.

REFERENCES

1. Wingo PA, Tong T, Bolden S: Cancer statistics, 1995. CA J Clin 45:8–30, 1995.

2. Fair WR, Fuks ZY, Scher HI: Cancer of the bladder, in Devita VT, Hellman S, Rosenberg SA (eds): Cancer: Principles and Practices of Oncology, 1052–1072. Philadelphia, JB Lippincott, 1993.

3. Silverman DT, Hartge P, Morrison AS, et al: Epidemiology of bladder cancer. Hematol Oncol Clin North Am 6:1–30, 1992.

4. Silverman DT, Levin LI, Hoover RN, et al: Occupational risk of bladder cancer in the United States: I. White men. J Natl Cancer Inst 81:1472–1480, 1989.

5. Hartge P, Harvey EB, Linehan MW, et al: Unexplained excessive risk for bladder cancer in men. J Natl Cancer Inst 82:1636–1640, 1990.

6. Augustine A, Hebert JR, Kabat GC, et al: Bladder cancer in relation to cigarette smoking. Cancer Res 48:4405–4408, 1988.

7. Burch JD, Rohan TE, Howe GR, et al: Risk of bladder cancer by source and type of tobacco exposure: A case-control study. Int J Cancer 44:622–628, 1989.

8. McCredie M, Stewart JH, Ford JM, et al: Phenacetin-containing analgesics and cancer of the bladder or renal pelvis in women. Br J Urol 55:220–224, 1983.

9. Piper JM, Tonocia J, Matanoski GM: Heavy phenacetin use and bladder cancer in women aged 20 to 49 years. N Engl J Med 313:292–295, 1985.

10. Tawfik HN: Carcinoma of the urinary bladder associated with schistosomiasis in Egypt: The possible causal relationship. International Symposium of the Princess Takamatsu Cancer Research Fund 18:197–199, 1987.

11. Kantor AF, Hartge P, Hoover RN, et al: Urinary tract infection and risk of bladder cancer. Am J Epidemiol 119:510–515, 1984.

12. Hartge P, Hoover RN, West PW, et al: Coffee drinking and risk of bladder cancer. J Natl Cancer Inst 70:1021–1026, 1983.

13. Auerbach O, Garfinkel L: Histologic changes in the urinary bladder in relation to cigarette smoking and use of artificial sweeteners. Cancer 64:983–987, 1989.

14. Risch HA, Burch JD, Miller AB, et al: Dietary factors and the incidence of cancer of the urinary bladder. Am J Epidemiol 126:1179–1191, 1988.

15. Kantor AF, Hartge P, Hoover RN, et al: Familial and environmental interaction in bladder cancer. Int J Cancer 35:703–706, 1985.

16. Miyao N, Tsai YC, Lerner SP, et al: Role of chromosome 9 in human bladder cancer. Cancer Res 53:4066–4070, 1993.

17. Orlow I, Lianes P, Lacombe L, et al: Chromosome 9 allelic loss and microsatellite alternations in human bladder cancer. Cancer Res 54:2848–2851, 1994.

18. Walman FM, Carroll PR, Kerschmann R: Centromeric copy number of chromosome 7 is strongly correlated with tumor grade and labeling index in human bladder cancer. Cancer Res 51:3807–3813, 1991.

19. Presti JC Jr, Reuter VE, Galan T, et al: Molecular genetic alternation in superficial and locally advanced human bladder cancer. Cancer Res 51:5405–5409, 1991.

20. Sidransky D, von Eschenbach A, Tsai YC, et al: Identification of p53 gene mutations in bladder cancers and urine samples. Science 252:706–709, 1991.

21. Esrig DE, Elamjian D, Groshen S, et al: Accumulation of nuclear p53 and tumor progression in bladder cancer. N Engl J Med 331:1259–1264, 1994.

22. Cordon-Cardo C, Dalbagni G, Saez GI, et al: p53 mutation in human bladder cancer: Genotypic versus phenotypic pattern. Int J Cancer 56:347–353, 1994.

23. Sarkis AS, Dalbagni G, Cordon-Cardo C, et al: Association of p53 nuclear overexpression and tumor progression in carcinoma in situ of the bladder. J Urol 152:388–392, 1994.

24. Spruck CH III, Ohneseit PF, Gonzalez-Zulueta M, et al: Two molecular pathways to transitional cell carcinoma of the bladder. Cancer Res 54:784–788, 1994.

25. Cairns P, Proctor AJ, Knowles MA: Loss of heterozygosity at the Rb locus is frequent and correlates with muscle invasion in bladder carcinoma. Oncogene 8:2305–2308, 1991.

26. Logothetis CJ, Xu H-J, Ro JY, et al: Altered expression of retinoblastoma protein and known prognostic variables in locally advanced bladder cancer. J Natl Cancer Inst 84:1256–1261, 1992.

27. Cordon-Cardo C, Wartinger D, Petrylak D, et al: Altered expression of the retinoblastoma gene product: Prognostic indicator in bladder cancer. J Natl Cancer Inst 84:1251–1256, 1992.

28. Sato K, Moriyama M, Mori S, et al: An immunohistologic evaluation of c-erbB-2 gene product in patients with urinary bladder carcinoma. Cancer 70:2493–2498, 1992.

29. Coombs LM, Pigott DA, Sweeney E, et al: Amplification and overexpression of c-erbB-2 in transitional cell carcinoma of the urinary bladder. Br J Cancer 63:601–608, 1991.

30. Knowles MA, Willamson M: Mutation of H-ras is infrequent in bladder cancer: Confirmation by single-strand conformation polymorphism and direct sequencing. Cancer Res 53:133–139, 1993.

31. Agnantis NJ, Constantinidou A, Poulios C, et al: Immunohistological study of the ras oncogene expression in human bladder endoscopy specimens. Eur J Surg Oncol 16:153–160, 1990.

32. Nguyen PL, Swanson PE, Jaszez W, et al: Expression of epidermal growth factor receptor in invasive transitional cell carcinoma of the urinary bladder: A multivariate survival analysis. Am J Clin Path 101:166–176, 1994.

33. Pode D, Fair WR: The development of bladder cancer. AUA Update, vol 7, lesson 40. Bellaire, Texas, American Urological Associates, Office of Education, 1987.

34. Melicow MM: Tumor of the bladder: A multifaceted problem. J Urol 68:467–478, 1974.

35. Mostofi FA, Sobin LH, Torloni M: Histological typing of urinary bladder tumor, in International Histological Classification of Tumor, No. 10. Geneva, World Health Organization, 1973.

36. Friedell GH, Soloway MS, Hilgar AG, et al: Summary of workshop on carcinoma in situ of the bladder. J Urol 136:1047–1048, 1986.

37. Cooper PH, Waisman J, Johanston WH, et al: Severe atypia of transitional epithelium and carcinoma of the urinary bladder. Cancer 31:1055–1060, 1973.

38. Althausen AF, Prout GR Jr, Daly JJ: Noninvasive papillary carcinoma of the bladder associated with carcinoma in situ. J Urol 116:575–579, 1976.

39. Tannenbaum M, Romas NA, Droller MJ: The pathobiology of early urothelial cancer, in Skinner DG, Lieskovsky G (eds): Genitourinary Cancer. Philadelphia, WB Saunders, 1988.

40. Farrow GM, Utz DC, Rife CC, et al: Clinical observation on sixty-nine cases of in situ carcinoma of the urinary bladder. Cancer Res 37:2794–2798, 1977.

41. Lieskovsky G: The staging and classification of bladder cancer and the management of superficial disease, in Skinner G (eds): Urological Cancer. New York, Grune & Stratton, 1983.

42. Heney NM, Ahmed S, Flanagan MJ: Superficial bladder cancer: Progression and recurrence. J Urol 130:1083-1086, 1983.

43. Fitzpatrick JM, West AB, Butler MR: Superficial bladder tumors (stage pTa, Grade 1 and 2): The importance of recurrence pattern following initial resection. J Urol 135:920–922, 1986.

44. Skinner DG: Current perspective in the management of high

grade invasive bladder cancer. Cancer 45:1886–1894, 1980.

45. Herr HW, Laudone VP, Whitmore WF Jr: An overview of intravesical therapy for superficial bladder tumor. J Urol 138:1363–1368, 1987.

46. Huland H, Otto U, Droese M, et al: Long-term mitomycin C instillation after transurethral resection of superficial bladder carcinoma: Influence on recurrence, progression and survival. J Urol 132:27–29, 1984.

47. Badalament RA, Herr HW, Wong GY, et al: A prospective randomized trial of maintenance versus nonmaintenance intravesical bacillus Calmette-Guérin for superficial transitional cell carcinoma of the bladder. J Clin Oncol 5:441–449, 1987.

48. Schellhammer PF, Ladaga LE, Fillion MB: Bacillus Calmette-Guérin for superficial transitional cell carcinoma of the bladder. J Urol 135:261–264, 1986.

49. Herr HW, Pinsky CM, Whitmore WF, et al: Long-term effect of intravesical bacillus Calmette-Guerin on flat carcinoma in situ of the bladder. J Urol 135:265–267, 1986.

50. Herr HW, Wartingu DD, Fair WR, et al: Bacillus Calmette-Guérin therapy for superficial bladder cancer: A 10-year follow up. J Urol 147:1020–1023, 1992.

51. Lamm DL, van der Meyden APM, Morales A, et al: Incidence and treatment of complications of bacillus Calmette-Guérin intravesical therapy in superficial bladder cancer. J Urol 147:596–600, 1992.

52. Herr HW: Conservative management of muscle-infiltrating bladder muscle: Prospective experience. J Urol 138:1162–1163, 1987.

53. Bosl GJ, Fair WR, Herr HW, et al: Bladder cancer: Advanced in biology and treatment. Crit Rev Oncol Hematol 16:33–70, 1994.

54. Skinner DG, Lieskovsky G: Contemporary cystectomy with pelvic node dissection compared to preoperative radiation therapy plus cystectomy in management of invasive bladder cancer. J Urol 131:1069–1072, 1984.

55. Montie JE, Straffon RA, Stewart BH: Radical cystectomy without radiation therapy for carcinoma of the bladder. J Urol 131:477–482, 1984.

56. Davidson SE, Symonds RP, Snee HP, et al: Assessment of factors influencing the outcome of radiotherapy for bladder cancer. Br J Urol 66:288–293, 1990.

57. Gospodarowicz MK, Hawkins NV, Rawlings GA, et al: Radical radiotherapy for muscle invasive transitional cell carcinoma of the bladder: Failure analysis. J Urol 142:1448–1453, 1989.

58. Parsons JT, Million RR: Planned preoperative irradiation in the management of clinical stage B-C (T3) bladder carcinoma. Int J Radiat Oncol Biol Phys 14:797–810, 1988.

59. Scher HI, Herr HW, Sternbery C, et al: Neo-adjuvant chemotherapy for invasive bladder cancer: Experience with the MVAC regimen. Br J Urol 64:250–256, 1989.

60. Matinez-Piniero JA, Jimenez-Leon J, Gonzalez-Martin M, et al: Neo-adjuvant cisplatin in locally advanced urothelial bladder cancer: A prospective randomized study of the group Cueto, in Splinter TAW, Scher HI (eds): Neoadjuvant Chemotherapy in Invasive Bladder Cancer, pp 95–103. Progress in Clinical and Biological Research. New York, Wiley-Liss, 1990.

61. Logothetis CJ, Johnson DE, Chong C, et al: Adjuvant cyclophosphamide, doxorubicin, and cisplatin chemotherapy for bladder cancer: An update. J Clin Oncol 6:1590–1596, 1988.

62. Skinner DG, Daniels JR, Russell CA, et al: The role of adjuvant chemotherapy following cystectomy for invasive bladder cancer: A prospective comparative trial. J Urol 145:459–464, 1991.

63. Stockle M, Meyenburg W, Wellek S, et al: Advanced bladder cancer (stage pT3b, pT4a, pN1 and pN2): Improved survival after radical cystectomy and 3 adjuvant cycles of chemotherapy. Results of a controlled prospective study. J Urol 148:302–307, 1992.

64. Shipley WU, Prout GR, Einstein AB, et al: Treatment of invasive bladder cancer by cisplatin and radiation in patients unsuited for surgery. JAMA 258:931–935, 1987.

65. Prout GR Jr, Shipley WU, Kaufman DS, et al: Preliminary results in invasive bladder cancer with transurethral resection, neoadjuvant chemotherapy and combined pelvic irradiation plus cisplatin chemotherapy. J Urol 144:1128–1134, 1990.

66. Yogoda A: Chemotherapy of urothelial tract tumor. Cancer 60:574–585, 1987.

67. Roth BJ, Dreicer R, Einhorn LH: Significant activity of paclitaxel in advanced transitional cell carcinoma of the urothelium: A phase II trial of the Eastern Cooperative Oncology Group. J Clin Oncol 12:2264–2270, 1994.

68. Logothetis CJ, Dexeus FH, Chong C, et al: Cisplatin, cyclophosphamide and doxorubicin chemotherapy for unresectable urothelial tumors: The M. D. Anderson experience. J Urol 141:33–37, 1989.

69. Harker WG, Meyers FJ, Freiha FS, et al: Cisplatin, methotrexate, and vinblastine (CMV): An effective chemotherapy regimen for metastatic transitional cell carcinoma of the urinary tract. A Northern California Oncology Group study. J Clin Oncol 3:1463–1470, 1985.

70. Sternberg CN, Yogoda A, Acher HI, et al: Methotrexate, vinblastine, doxorubicin and cisplatin for advanced transitional cell carcinoma of the urothelium: Efficacy and pattern of response and relapse. Cancer 64:2448–2458, 1989.

71. Loehrer PJ Sr, Einhorn LH, Elson PJ, et al: A randomized comparison of cisplatin alone or in combination with methotrexate, vinblastine and doxorubicin in patients with metastatic urothelial carcinoma: A cooperative study. J Clin Oncol 10:1066–1073, 1992.

72. Logothetis CJ, Dexeus FH, Finn F, et al: A prospective randomized trial comparing MVAC and CISCA chemotherapy for patients with metastatic urothelial tumor. J Clin Oncol 8:1050–1055, 1990.

73. Kantoff PW, Scher HI: Chemotherapy for metastatic bladder cancer. Hematol Oncol Clin North Am 6:195–203, 1992.

74. Logothetis CJ, Dexeus FH, Sella A, et al: Escalated therapy for refractory urothelial tumor: Methotrexate-vinblastine-doxorubicin-cisplatin plus unglycosylated recombinant human granulocyte-macrophage colony-stimulating factor. J Natl Cancer Inst 82:667–672, 1990.

75. Seidman AD, Scher HI, Gabrilove JL, et al: Dose-intensification of MVAC with recombinant granulocyte-colony stimulating factor as initial therapy in advanced urothelial cancer. J Clin Oncol 11:408–414, 1993.

76. Einhorn LH, Roth BJ, Ansari R, et al: Phase II trial of vinblastine, ifosfamide and gallium combination chemotherapy in metastatic urothelial carcinoma. J Clin Oncol 12:2271–2276, 1994.

77. Logothetis CJ, Hossan E, Sella A, et al: Fluorouracil and recombinant human interferon alpha-2a in the treatment of metastatic chemotherapy-refractory urothelial tumors. J Natl Cancer Inst 83:285–288, 1991.

CHAPTER 29

Renal-Cell Carcinoma

Gustavo A. Fonseca, MD, *and* Julie Ellerhorst, MD

Department of Genitourinary Medical Oncology
The University of Texas M. D. Anderson Cancer Center, Houston, Texas

Renal-cell carcinoma (RCC) is curable only in patients presenting with resectable, early-stage disease. Advanced local or metastatic disease carries an approximate 15% 5-year survival rate. However, the natural history of metastatic RCC is heterogeneous, and aggressive palliative treatment is recommended, especially for patients with a solitary metastatic site and good performance status. Response rates to cytokine therapy remain generally less than 25%, and complete responses are rare. To improve these results, combinations of biologics with and without cytotoxic chemotherapy are being investigated. Important advances in understanding the molecular aspects of RCC have been made in recent years. Modulation of the expression of genes involved in RCC is an approach awaited with great interest.

In the following discussion, we review the natural history of RCC, current methods for diagnosis and treatment, and promising therapeutic agents for metastatic disease.

EPIDEMIOLOGY

In the United States, the age-adjusted incidence of RCC has been rising steadily, and 28,800 new cases are expected to be diagnosed in 1995.[1] The male-to-female ratio ranges from 2:1 to 3:1.[1] Renal-cell carcinoma occurs most commonly in adults over the age of 40 years,[2,3] but family clustering with younger ages at presentation has been reported.[4]

Etiology: Numerous investigators have attempted to link the occurrence of RCC to environmental factors, dietary patterns, and occupational or medical exposures. In general, strong associations have not been found, partly because RCC is a relatively rare disease, and many associations, therefore, fall short of statistical significance. These epidemiologic studies have been extensively reviewed[2,5] and will be briefly summarized here.

The most prominent risk factor, and the only one that has been firmly established, is tobacco use. Multiple cohort and case-control studies have found the relative risk of RCC in smokers to be at least 1.5.[2] Furthermore, the risk appears to increase with the level of cigarette smoking in a dose-dependent fashion.[6]

A number of other potential risk factors have been investigated. Results of studies to determine the roles of dietary fat, alcohol, and obesity have been inconsistent.[2] Occupational exposures to cadmium,[7] asbestos,[8] and petroleum products[9] have been implicated in disease development, but their involvement has not been demonstrated convincingly. RCC has been reported in several patients previously exposed to thorotrast contrast media.[10] There are also reports of RCC in association with various nephropathies, including acquired renal polycystic disease,[11] xanthogranulomatous pyelonephritis,[12] and phenacetin-related analgesic nephropathy.[13]

Several forms of dominantly inherited RCC have been described.[4,14,15] One of the earliest reported associations of cancer to a germline cytogenetic abnormality was in a family with kidney cancer who had a translocation at the p21 locus in the short arm of chromosome 3 (3p).[16] RCC is known to develop in 40% to 70% of patients with von Hippel-Lindau (VHL) disease[4,17]; these patients are also at risk of developing pheochromocytomas or cerebellar and retinal hemangioblastomas. Familial cases of RCC represent less than 5% of the total patient population, but their study has proven fruitful, as the same genetic mutations seen in germlines of affected families are being described in nonhereditary cases.[14,15]

Three tumor suppressor genes appear to reside on 3p: the *VHL* gene at 3p25-26 and two more proximal genes, at 3p14 (proposed name, nonpapillary renal carcinoma gene, or *NRC-1*) and 3p21.[15,18–22] The *VHL* gene was recently cloned, but its specific cellular function is still unknown.[20] The *NRC-1* gene has been postulated to control the growth of RCC cells by inducing apoptosis.[19] Further clarification of the function of these genes is expected to enable the development of specific therapeutics at the cellular level. Other described changes in RCC are abnormal expression of the *p53* gene and mutations in chromosomes 11p, 17q, and 5q.[23,24]

PATHOLOGY

On gross examination, RCC is characteristically a solid hemorrhagic and necrotic mass. Microscopic examination reveals numerous vessels and vascular channels. Histologically, RCC can be separated into three

TABLE I

Robson's Staging System

Stage I

Tumor confined within capsule of kidney

Stage II

Tumor invading perinephric fat but still contained within Gerota's fascia

Stage III

Tumor invading the renal vein or inferior vena cave (A), or regional lymph-node involvement (B), or both (C)

Stage IV

Tumor invading adjacent viscera (excluding ipsilateral adrenal) or distant metastasis

---

cellular types: clear, granular, and sarcomatoid.[25,26] Clear-cell carcinoma, the most common-cell type, is present in more than 90% of tumors. It is characterized by unusually clear cells with a cytoplasm rich in lipids and glycogen. Granular cells display an eosinophilic cytoplasm secondary to an abundance of mitochondria and organelles. Sarcomatoid, or spindle-type, cells resemble fibroblasts of mesenchymal origin and represent 1% to 2% of kidney tumors. Clinically, however, a sarcomatoid component is predictive of a more aggressive behavior.[26]

A further distinction can be made by the pattern of cellular arrangement, dividing RCCs into solid and papillary tumors. Most RCCs are solid. In this solid tumor pattern, sinusoidal vessels provide the blood supply, whereas in the papillary tumor pattern, cells aggregate in papillae supplied by a single fibrovascular stalk. Genetic analysis of the latter tumor pattern seems to indicate a different cellular origin, as mutations in chromosome 3p are absent.[14,19,27]

A grading scale for RCC based on nuclear size and shape is frequently used. The most commonly used system is that of Fuhrman et al, which classifies cells from grades 1 to 4.[28] Nuclear grade appears to provide prognostic information, particularly for grades 1 and 4 tumors.

CLINICAL PRESENTATION

Common presentations of RCC include hematuria, abdominal mass, weight loss, anorexia, or symptoms arising from metastatic sites. The classic triad of flank pain, hematuria, and a palpable mass occurs in only 10% to 15% of patients and suggests advanced disease.[29]

A unique aspect of RCC is the frequent occurrence of various paraneoplastic syndromes, including hypercalcemia, polycythemia, fever, cachexia, hypertension, and hepatic dysfunction (Stauffer's syndrome).[30,31] Resolution of symptoms or biochemical abnormalities frequently follows successful treatment (eg, excision) of the primary tumor or metastatic foci.

Metastatic disease is detectable in 25% to 30% of patients at the time of diagnosis.[30] Frequent sites include the lung (50% to 60%), bone (30%), lymph nodes (30%), liver (30%), and adrenal glands (20%). Metastases to the brain, contralateral kidney, pancreas, or skin are found in 5% to 15% of these patients.

RADIOGRAPHIC EVALUATION

Computed tomography (CT) is the most useful tool for the study of kidney masses.[32] The overall accuracy of CT in the staging of RCC is 90% to 95%.[32,33] Advantages of this method include the ability to more clearly define nodal disease, ability to detect caval thrombi under most circumstances, reproducibility of studies, and ease of interpretation. In addition, other sites of intra-abdominal metastasis, such as the liver, adrenal glands, or contralateral kidney, may be detected. Magnetic resonance imaging offers few advantages over CT[34]; based on availability of resources, overall staging accuracy, and expense, CT remains the modality of choice.

Renal arteriograms are occasionally still performed during evaluation of a solid renal mass. Renal-cell carcinoma characteristically appears as a hypervascular tumor. However, RCC with a predominantly papillary tumor pattern or a sarcomatoid component will appear as a hypovascular mass. Under these circumstances, renal arteriography may be misleading.

Imaging studies are also performed to detect metastases. Because a significant number of patients have pulmonary metastasis at presentation, a chest x-ray film should be obtained as part of the initial evaluation. Bone scans have been traditionally used as part of the staging workup; however, in the absence of bone pain or an elevated alkaline phosphatase level, abnormal bone scan findings are uncommon.[35] Of note, bone metastasis from RCC may be purely lytic and may produce a weak signal or no signal on bone scan. If clinical suspicion of bone metastasis is high, a negative bone scan should be confirmed by a plain radiograph of the site in question. Computed tomographic scans of the brain are usually reserved for patients with neurologic symptoms or for those entering clinical trials.

Renal-cell carcinoma is commonly associated with the development of reactive lymph nodes, particularly those draining the primary tumor. If the presence of local nodal metastasis has bearing on therapeutic decisions, enlarged nodes seen on CT scan should be sampled to confirm the presence of metastasis.

STAGING AND PROGNOSIS

One of the most popular staging systems is that of Robson et al, introduced in 1963, later updated in 1969, and still commonly used in clinical practice (Table 1).[29,36] This system was employed in early studies correlating stage at presentation with prognosis. More recent studies have used the tumor, nodes, and metastasis (TNM) system (Table 2),[37] thus making comparisons between early and recent studies somewhat difficult. One of the major advantages of the TNM system is that it clearly separates individuals with tumor thrombi from those with local nodal disease. These two groups are combined in Robson's stage III category. The presence of local nodal metastasis is associated with shorter survival, whereas this is not necessarily the case for an inferior vena cava thrombus.

The 5-year survival for surgically treated patients who present with Robson's stage I disease (T1 or T2 N0 M0) is greater than 90%; stage II disease (T3a N0 M0), 65% to 70%; stage III disease (T3b–d or N1–3 M0), 40%; and stage IV disease (T4a or M1), 15% to 20%.[29,36,38,39]

Regardless of the staging system, there is a general consensus that poor survival is associated with increasing tumor size, regional lymph node involvement, and distant metastasis. In addition to advanced disease stage, other predictors of poor outcome include high nuclear grade (particularly Fuhrman's grade 4),[27] sarcomatoid elements,[26] aneuploidy,[25,40,41] and an inferior vena cava thrombus extending into or above the hepatic veins.[42]

SURGICAL TREATMENT

Local Disease

Radical nephrectomy is the mainstay of treatment for localized RCC. The classic description of radical nephrectomy includes excision of the kidney with all of the Gerota's fascia and removal of the ipsilateral adrenal gland; regional lymphadenectomy may also be included in the surgery.[36] The actual benefit derived from adrenalectomy and lymphadenectomy has been debated,[43,44] and in some cases these procedures are omitted from the resection. When present, intracaval tumor thrombi are also resected during the operation.[45] Radical nephrectomy is associated with a mortality rate of 2%, with most deaths occurring in patients with advanced disease. Intraoperative and postoperative complication rates are each

TABLE 2

TNM Staging for Renal-Cell Carcinoma

Tumor (T)

T1: tumor ≤ 2.5 cm, confined to kidney

T2: tumor > 2.5 cm, confined to kidney

T3: extension into renal vein, infradiaphragmatic vena cava, adrenal gland, or perinephric fat

T4: extension beyond Gerota's fascia

Nodes (N)

N1: single node ≤ 2 cm

N2: single node > 2 cm and ≤ 5 cm or multiple nodes ≤ 5 cm

N3: any node > 5 cm

Metastasis (M)

M1: distant metastasis

approximately 20%. The most common complications are injuries to the spleen and large vessels.[46]

Partial nephrectomy or tumor enucleation is performed when RCC occurs in a patient with a solitary kidney, in both kidneys, or occasionally in the setting of significant renal insufficiency.[47] Long-term follow-up studies of these patients have suggested that the modified surgical procedures do not compromise survival for individuals with small, early-stage lesions.[48,49] However, beyond the indications mentioned above, the role of partial nephrectomy has not been established, and at present, the procedure cannot be recommended for patients with unilateral disease and a normal contralateral kidney.

Metastatic Disease

For patients with metastatic RCC, palliative nephrectomy is offered for intractable hematuria, severe pain, or compression of adjacent viscera. Radical nephrectomy in patients with unresectable local or distant metastasis does not improve survival. Spontaneous regression of metastatic lesions has occurred objectively in less than 1% of cases after nephrectomy.[50] Palliative resection of solitary metastatic lesions is indicated for patients with RCC and may provide excellent, durable symptom control.[51,52]

Whether control of the primary carcinoma determines the clinical response of the metastatic disease is unsettled. An improved response was initially suggested by clinical trials of biologic agents, and for this reason, many trials of investigational agents now include prior nephrectomy in the entry criteria. Randomized trials to clarify this issue are under way.

RADIOTHERAPY

Renal-cell carcinoma is generally radioresistant, and the indications for radiation therapy are limited.[53–55] The major indication for radiation therapy is for palliation of symptomatic metastatic disease, most commonly painful bone lesions and brain metastases.[56,57]

ANGIO-INFARCTION

The vascular nature of RCC lends itself to treatment with angio-infarction. This modality has two general applications. First, preoperative infarction of the primary tumor or metastatic focus may be performed to minimize the amount of intraoperative morbidity.[58] Second, embolization may be performed for palliation of symptoms from an unresectable primary tumor or metastasis.[59] Embolization of a large renal mass frequently produces a postinfarction syndrome consisting of pain, fever, and gastrointestinal disturbances, occurring immediately after the procedure. Symptoms are managed with supportive care and usually resolve after several days.

SYSTEMIC THERAPY

Hormonal Therapy: A number of hormonal agents, most commonly progestins such as medroxyprogesterone acetate (Depo-Provera), have been used both in the adjuvant setting and for treatment of metastatic disease. There appears to be no benefit from the use of progestins as adjuvant therapy,[60] and in metastatic disease the objective response rate is at best 5%.[61,62]

Cytotoxic Chemotherapy: Renal-cell carcinoma is refractory to most traditional chemotherapeutic agents,[63,64] a property currently hypothesized to be the result of the high cellular expression of the multidrug resistance (MDR1) phenotype.[64,65] Several studies of single-agent or combination cytotoxic chemotherapy have found marginal efficacy at best.[64] Only two drugs, vinblastine and floxuridine, have shown reproducible significant activity.

Most of the recent trials of vinblastine have used monthly, 5-day infusions of 0.75 to 1.9 mg/m²/d. Objective responses are usually partial and occur in approximately 15% of patients.[64]

Floxuridine was first reported to be an active agent for metastatic RCC by von Roemeling et al in 1988.[66] These investigators used programmable infusion pumps to deliver continuous floxuridine in such a way that most of the dose was given in the afternoon and evening, based on animal studies showing improved tolerance when the drug was administered in a circadian fashion. Compared with constant-rate (flat-rate) infusions, this schedule resulted in reduced toxicity and permitted dose escalations.[67] The overall response rate was 28%, and some responses were durable. The dose range was usually 0.15 to 0.20 mg/kg administered daily for 14 days and repeated in 28-day cycles.

According to the recommended circadian schedule, 68% of the floxuridine dose is given between 1500 and 2100 hours, 15% between 2100 and 0300 hours, 2% between 0300 and 0900 hours, and 15% between 0900 and 1500 hours. When administered according to this schedule, floxuridine is generally well tolerated, producing only occasional gastrointestinal side effects (abdominal cramping, diarrhea, or mucositis), which are manageable.

The logistic difficulties of delivering floxuridine with programmable pumps generated interest in studying infusion of floxuridine at a constant rate.[68] Usually, the flat-rate dose is started at 0.075 to 0.125 mg/kg/d and given for 14 days in 28-day cycles. Wilkinson et al reported a response rate of 21%, which is comparable to that in the literature on the circadian schedule.[68] Administration of floxuridine in circadian rhythms permits delivery of greater amounts of drug, but whether the larger amounts in turn induce greater antitumoral effect remains to be determined in ongoing phase III studies.[68]

IMMUNOTHERAPY

Among the biologic agents used in clinical trials to treat metastatic RCC, three have shown reproducible activity: alpha interferon (IFN-α), interleukin-2 (IL-2, aldesleukin [Proleukin]), and gamma interferon (IFN-γ [Actimmune]).

Alpha Interferon: IFN-α was the first biologic agent found to have significant activity in patients with metastatic RCC. The mechanism of antitumoral activity of IFN-α may result from immunomodulation, antiangiogenesis, or direct cytotoxicity.[69] Several studies have consistently demonstrated response rates of 15%.[70–73] Therapy is usually started at doses of 2 to 5 million U/m²/d by subcutaneous injection. Higher doses, ranging from 10 to 20 million U/m²/d, have been used, but toxicity at these dose levels usually results in poor patient compliance.

Initiation of IFN-α therapy produces flu-like symptoms in most patients, but tolerance usually develops after several days to several weeks of treatment. Common toxic effects of chronic IFN-α therapy include fatigue, depression, anorexia, weight loss, and mild leukopenia. At high doses, central nervous system toxic effects can occur. Side effects of IFN-α can often be ameliorated by changing to an every-other-day or three-times-weekly schedule or by giving breaks in therapy. Most responses to IFN-α are partial and not sustained.

Interleukin-2: IL-2 is a cytokine produced by helper T-cells. IL-2 activates natural killer cells and T-cells and transforms a population of peripheral blood mononuclear cells into lymphokine–activated killer (LAK) cells. The first reports of IL-2 administration to patients with cancer appeared between 1983 and 1985.[74,75] The product used was a purified preparation obtained from mitogen-stimulated peripheral blood leukocytes or cultured cells from the Jurkat T-cell line. Shortly thereafter, recombinant IL-2 became available, permitting treatment of a substantial number of patients in phase I and II clinical trials.

A consistent observation from these studies was the apparent sensitivity of metastatic RCC to IL-2 therapy. This sensitivity was confirmed in several phase II studies that reported response rates of 10% to 30%, with a number of complete responses that persisted after cessation of therapy. However, selection criteria for these studies favored inclusion of younger patients with good performance status, low tumor burden, and the lung as the only site of disease, factors that may represent an already favorable subgroup of patients with RCC.[76]

In 1992, IL-2 was approved by the Food and Drug Administration (FDA) for the treatment of metastatic RCC. In the United States, IL-2 is currently manufactured only by recombinant techniques and dispensed in international units (IU). In reviewing the literature, however, one must take careful account of the units used in different reports. (A value of 6 IU is equivalent to 2 Roche units and to 1 Cetus unit.)

Initial trials of IL-2 used variations of what is now considered high-dose therapy, administered either as a rapid intravenous bolus or a continuous infusion.[77–79] High-dose intermittent bolus therapy is recommended by the FDA because this dose and schedule has produced the greatest number of complete responses in clinical trials. When treating patients according to these recommendations, the physician should be prepared to manage significant toxic effects and should have an intensive care facility available. The extreme toxicity of high-dose IL-2 is mainly characterized by fever, hypotension, oliguria with marked fluid retention, pulmonary edema, mental confusion, and hepatic dysfunction. These side effects usually resolve within 24 to 48 hours of discontinuation of therapy.[77,78]

Published trials of low-dose IL-2 therapy administered by continuous infusion or subcutaneous injection show less toxicity than and response rates comparable to those obtained for high-dose bolus therapy.[80–83] Ongoing clinical trials continue to investigate various doses and schedules of IL-2 in order to minimize toxicity and expense and permit incorporation of other cytotoxic or biologic agents into the regimen. Other trials are attempting to modulate the side effects of the cytokines by administering additional novel compounds. Of these, encouraging early reports are available for two particular agents: CT1501R, a pentoxifylline analog that inhibits interleukin-1 and tumor necrosis factor signal transduction,[84] and N^G-methyl-L-arginine, a nitric oxide synthesis inhibitor that counteracts the hypotensive side effects of IL-2.[85,86]

Gamma Interferon: IFN-γ is also a product of activated T-cells. This cytokine is unique in its ability to activate macrophages. When this agent is used at the maximum tolerated dose, responses are rarely seen in RCC or in other tumors. However, using serologic markers of macrophage activation, Aulitzky et al found the biologically active dose to be considerably lower than the maximum tolerated dose.[87] Their subsequent trial of fixed low-dose IFN-γ, administered as a weekly subcutaneous injection of 100 mg, produced a 30% response rate in patients with metastatic RCC.[87] The activity of low-dose IFN-γ has been confirmed in a second study, which reported a 15% response rate.[88] A notable advantage of this drug is its complete lack of serious toxicity, making it an ideal candidate for combination therapy.

Combination Biochemotherapy

Experimental models of antitumor synergy induced by the combination of IFN-α and IL-2[89] prompted interest in developing combination protocols.[82,90] The initial studies attempted to deliver the maximally tolerated doses of IL-2 and IFN-α but encountered extreme toxicity.[90] Trials of "low-dose" schedules (IL-2 at 4 to 18 million IU/m^2 and IFN-α at 4 to 6 million U/m^2) were able to increase compliance because the side effects were less intense, but the antitumoral effects reported have fluctuated from 0% to 50%.[90,91]

With expectations of obtaining greater antitumor activity by altering the drug pharmacodynamics, more recent trials have added chemotherapeutic agents such as fluorouracil and floxuridine.[92–94] Response rates around 35% have been described.[92–94] Interest in the development of "combination" biochemotherapies for RCC continues to increase, but to date there is no consensus on whether this approach is clinically superior to single-agent treatment.

Adjuvant therapy is also under active clinical investigation, but no specific treatment has proven to be superior to close surveillance in the care of patients who undergo surgery.

CONCLUSION

In summary, patients with disseminated RCC represent a challenge for the oncologist. Patients with a good performance status should be offered the opportunity to participate in clinical trials until more effective and safe therapies can be widely adopted.

REFERENCES

1. National Center for Health Statistics: Vital Statistics of the United States, 1991. Washington, DC, Public Health Service, 1994.

2. Dayal H, Kinman J: Epidemiology of kidney cancer. Semin Oncol 10:366–377, 1983.

3. Broecker B: Renal cell carcinoma in children. Urology 38:54–56, 1991.

4. Lynch HT, Walzak MP: Genetics in urologic cancer. Urol Clin North Am 7:815–829, 1980.

5. Bennington JL: Cancer of the kidney: Etiology, epidemiology, and pathology. Cancer 32:1017–1029, 1973.

6. Weir JM, Dunn JE: Smoking and mortality: A prospective study. Cancer 25:105–112, 1970.

7. Kolonel LN: Association of cadmium with renal cancer. Cancer 37:1782–1787, 1976.

8. Maclure M: Asbestos and renal adenocarcinoma: A case-control study. Environ Res 42:353–361, 1987.

9. Thomas TL, Deconfle P, Moure-Eroso R, et al: Mortality among workers employed in petroleum refining and petrochemical plants. J Occup Med 22:97–103, 1980.

10. Kauzlaric D, Barmeir E, Luscieti P, et al: Renal carcinoma after retrograde pyelography with thorotrast. Am J Roentgenol 148:897–898, 1987.

11. MacDougall ML, Welling LW, Wiegmann TB: Renal adenocarcinoma and acquired cystic disease in chronic hemodialysis patients. Am J Kidney Dis 9:166–171, 1987.

12. Papadopoulos I, Wirth B, Wand H: Xanthogranulomatous pyelonephritis associated with renal cell carcinoma. Eur Urol 18:74–76, 1990.

13. Lornoy W, Becaus I, de Vleeschouwer M, et al: Renal cell carcinoma, a new complication of analgesic nephropathy. Lancet 1:1271–1272, 1986.

14. Gnarra JR, Glenn GM, Latif F, et al: Molecular genetic studies of sporadic and familial renal cell carcinoma. Urol Clin North Am 20:207–216, 1993.

15. Gnarra JR, Tory K, Weng L, et al: Mutations of the VHL tumour suppressor gene in renal carcinoma. Nat Genet 7:85, 1994.

16. Cohen AJ, Li FP, Berg S, et al: Hereditary renal-cell carcinoma associated with a chromosomal translocation. N Engl J Med 301:592–595, 1979.

17. Maher ER, Yates JRW: Familial renal cell carcinoma: Clinical and molecular genetic aspects (editorial). Br J Cancer 63:176–179, 1991.

18. Maher ER, Bentley E, Yates JEW, et al: Mapping of the von Hippel-Lindau disease locus to a small region of chromosome 3p by genomic linkage analysis. Genomics 10:957–960, 1991.

19. Sanchez Y, El-Naggar A, Pathak S, et al: A tumor suppressor locus within 3p14-p12 mediates rapid cell death of renal cell carcinoma in vivo. Proc Natl Acad Sci USA 91:3383–3387, 1994.

20. Latif F, Tory K, Gnarra J, et al: Identification of the von Hippel-Lindau disease tumor suppressor gene. Science 260: 1317–1320, 1993.

21. Carroll PR, Murty VV, Reuter V, et al: Abnormalities at chromosome 3p12-14 characterize clear cell renal carcinoma. Cancer Genet Cytogenet 26:253–259, 1987.

22. Yamakawa K, Morita R, Takahashi E, et al: A detailed deletion mapping of the short arm of chromosome 3 in sporadic renal cell carcinoma. Cancer Res 51:4707–4711, 1991.

23. Foster K, Crossey PA, Cairns P, et al: Molecular genetic investigation of sporadic renal cell carcinoma: Analysis of allele loss on chromosomes 3p, 5q, 11p, 17 and 22. Br J Cancer 69:230–234, 1994.

24. Reiter RE, Anglard P, Liu S, et al: Chromosome 17p and p53 mutations in renal cell carcinoma. Cancer Res 53:3092–3097, 1993.

25. O'Toole KM, Brown M, Hoffman P: Pathology of benign and malignant kidney tumors. Urol Clin North Am 20:193–205, 1993.

26. Ro JY, Ayala AG, Sella A, et al: Sarcomatoid renal cell carcinoma: Clinicopathologic. A study of 42 cases. Cancer 59:516–526, 1987.

27. Kovacs G, Frisch S: Clonal chromosome abnormalities in tumor cells from patients with sporadic renal cell carcinomas. Cancer Res 49:651–659, 1989.

28. Fuhrman SA, Lasky LC, Limas C: Prognostic significance of morphologic parameters in renal cell carcinoma. Am J Surg Pathol 6:655–663, 1982.

29. Sene AP, Hunt L, McMahon RFT, et al: Renal carcinoma in patients undergoing nephrectomy: Analysis of survival and prognostic factors. Br J Urol 70:125–134, 1992.

30. Holland JM: Cancer of the kidney: Natural history and staging. Cancer 32:1030–1042, 1973.

31. Altaffer LF, Chenault OW: Paraneoplastic endocrinopathies associated with renal tumors. J Urol 122:573–577, 1979.

32. Richie JP, Garnick MB, Seltzer S, et al: Computerized tomography scan for diagnosis and staging of renal cell carcinoma. J Urol 129:1114–1116, 1983.

33. Benson MA, Haaga JR, Resnick MI: Staging renal carcinoma: What is sufficient? Arch Surg 124:71–73, 1989.

34. Bosniak MA: Problems in the radiologic diagnosis of renal parenchymal tumors. Urol Clin North Am 20:217–230, 1993.

35. Blacher E, Johnson DE, Haynie TP: Value of routine radionuclide bone scans in renal cell carcinoma. Urology 26:432–434, 1985.

36. Robson CJ, Churchill BM, Anderson W: The results of radical nephrectomy for renal cell carcinoma. J Urol 101:297–301, 1969.

37. Hermanek P, Sobin LH (eds): TNM Classification of Malignant Tumors, 4th ed, pp 136–138. Berlin, Springer-Verlag, 1987.

38. Basil B, Dosoretz DE, Prout GR: Validation of the tumor, nodes, and metastasis classification of renal cell carcinoma. J Urol 134:450–454, 1985.

39. Golimbu M, Joshi P, Sperber A, et al: Renal cell carcinoma: Survival and prognostic factors. Urology 27:291–301, 1986.

40. Roos G, Ljungberg B: DNA content in renal cell carcinoma and its clinical significance. Eur Urol 18(suppl 2):29–30, 1990.

41. Ljungberg B, Roos G: Value of DNA analysis for treatment of renal cell carcinoma. Eur Urol 18(suppl 2):31–32, 1990.

42. Sosa RE, Muecke EC, Vaughan ED, et al: Renal cell carcinoma extending into the inferior vena cava: The prognostic significance of the level of vena caval involvement. J Urol 132:1097–1100, 1984.

43. Robey EL, Schellhammer PF: The adrenal gland and renal cell carcinoma: Is ipsilateral adrenalectomy a necessary component of radical nephrectomy? J Urol 135:453–455, 1986.

44. Pizzocaro G, Piva L: Pros and cons of retroperitoneal lymphadenectomy in operable renal cell carcinoma. Eur Urol 18(suppl 2):22–23, 1990.

45. Libertino JA, Zinman L, Walkins E: Long-term results of

resection of renal cell cancer with extension into inferior vena cava. J Urol 137:21–24, 1987.

46. Swanson DA, Borges PM: Complication of transabdominal radical nephrectomy for renal cell carcinoma. J Urol 129:704–707, 1983.

47. Licht MR, Novick AC: Nephron sparing surgery for renal cell carcinoma. J Urol 149:1–7, 1993.

48. Graber P: Partial nephrectomy for renal carcinoma. Urol Int 47:213–215, 1991.

49. Stephens R, Graham SD: Enucleation of tumor versus partial nephrectomy as conservative treatment of renal cell carcinoma. Cancer 65:2663–2667, 1990.

50. Freed SZ, Halperin JP, Gordon M: Idiopathic regression of metastases from renal cell carcinoma. J Urol 118:538–542, 1977.

51. O'Dea MJ, Zincke H, Utz DC, et al: The treatment of renal carcinoma with solitary metastasis. J Urol 120:540–542, 1978.

52. Golimbu M, Al-Askari S, Tessler A, et al: Aggressive treatment of metastatic renal cancer. J Urol 136:805–807, 1986.

53. Kjaer M, Iverson P, Hvidt V, et al: Radiotherapy versus observation in stage II and III renal adenocarcinoma. Scand J Urol Nephrol 21:285–289, 1987.

54. Juusela H, Malmio K, Alfthan O, et al: Preoperative irradiation in the treatment of renal adenocarcinoma. Scand J Urol Nephrol 11:277–281, 1977.

55. Finney R: An evaluation of postoperative radiotherapy in hypernephroma treatment: A clinical trial. Cancer 32:1332–1340, 1973.

56. Seitz W, Karcher KH, Binder W: Radiotherapy of metastatic renal cell carcinoma. Semin Surg Oncol 4:100–102, 1988.

57. Halperin EC, Harisiadis L: The role of radiation therapy in the management of metastatic renal cell carcinoma. Cancer 51:614–617, 1983.

58. Bracken RB, Johnson DE, Goldstein HM, et al: Percutaneous transfemoral renal artery occlusion in patients with renal carcinoma. Urology 6:6–10, 1975.

59. Swanson DA, Wallace S: Surgery of metastatic renal cell carcinoma and use of renal infarction. Semin Surg Oncol 4:124–128, 1988.

60. Pizzocaro G, Piva L, Di Fronzo G, et al: Adjuvant medroxy-progesterone acetate to radical nephrectomy in renal cancer: 5-year results of a prospective randomized study. J Urol 138:1379–1381, 1987.

61. Bloom HJG: Hormone-induced and spontaneous regression of metastatic renal cancer. Cancer 32:1066–1071, 1973.

62. Harris DT: Hormonal therapy and chemotherapy of renal-cell carcinoma. Semin Oncol 10:422–433, 1983.

63. Hrushesky WJ, Murphy GP: Current status of the therapy of advanced renal carcinoma. J Surg Oncol 9:277–288, 1977.

64. Yagoda A, Petrylak D, Thompson S: Cytotoxic chemotherapy for advanced renal cell carcinoma. Urol Clin North Am 20:303–321, 1993.

65. Fojo AT, Shen DW: Intrinsic drug resistance in human kidney cancer is associated with expression of a human multidrug-resistance gene. J Clin Oncol 5:1922–1927, 1987.

66. von Roemeling R, Rabatin JT, Fraley EE, et al: Progressive metastatic renal cell carcinoma controlled by continuous 5-fluoro-2-deoxyuridine infusion. J Urol 139:259–262, 1988.

67. Bjarnason GA, Hruskesky WJM, Diasio R, et al: Flat versus circadian modified 14 day infusion of FUDR for advanced renal cell cancer (RCC): A phase III study (abstract). Proc Am Soc Clin Oncol 13:247, 1994.

68. Wilkinson MJ, Frye JW, Small EJ, et al: A phase II study of constant-infusion floxuridine for the treatment of metastatic renal cell carcinoma. Cancer 71:3601–3604, 1993.

69. Gutterman JU: Cytokine therapeutics: Lessons from interferon alpha. Proc Natl Acad Sci USA 91:1198–1205, 1994.

70. Quesada JR, Swanson DA, Trindade A, et al: Renal cell carcinoma: Antitumor effects of leukocyte interferon. Cancer Res 43:940–947, 1983.

71. Quesada JR, Swanson DA, Gutterman JU: Phase II study of interferon alpha in metastatic renal-cell carcinoma: A progress report. J Clin Oncol 3:1086–1092, 1985.

72. Umeda T, Niijima T: Phase II study of alpha interferon on renal cell carcinoma. Summary of three collaborative trials. Cancer 58:1231–1235, 1986.

73. Muss HB: Interferon therapy for renal cell carcinoma. Semin Oncol 14(suppl 2):36–42, 1987.

74. Lotze MT, Frana LW, Sharrow SO, et al: In vivo administration of purified human interleukin 2. J Immunol 134:157–166, 1985.

75. Lotze MT, Chang AE, Seipp CA, et al: High-dose recombinant interleukin 2 in the treatment of patients with disseminated cancer. JAMA 256:3117–3124, 1986.

76. Lissoni P, Barni S, Ardizzoia A, et al: Prognostic factors of the clinical response to subcutaneous immunotherapy with interleukin-2 alone in patients with metastatic renal cell carcinoma. Oncology 51:59–62, 1994.

77. Rosenberg SA, Lotze MT, Muul LM, et al: A progress report on the treatment of 157 patients with advanced cancer using lymphokine-activated killer cells and interleukin-2 or high-dose interleukin-2 alone. N Engl J Med 316:889–897, 1987.

78. West WH, Tauer KW, Yannelli JR, et al: Constant-infusion recombinant interleukin-2 in adoptive immunotherapy of advanced cancer. N Engl J Med 316:898–905, 1987.

79. Fisher RI, Coltman CA, Doroshow JH, et al: Metastatic renal cancer treated with interleukin-2 and lymphokine-activated killer cells. Ann Intern Med 108:518–523,1988.

80. Sosman JA, Kohler PC, Hank J, et al: Repetitive weekly cycles of recombinant human interleukin-2: Responses of renal carcinoma with acceptable toxicity. J Natl Cancer Inst 80:60–63, 1988.

81. Atzpodien J, Korfer A, Menzel T, et al: Home therapy using recombinant human interleukin-2 and interferon-alpha-2b in patients with metastatic renal cell carcinoma (abstract). Proc Am Soc Clin Oncol 10:177, 1991.

82. Vogelzang NJ, Lipton A, Figlin RA: Subcutaneous interleukin-2 plus interferon alfa-2a in metastatic renal cancer: An outpatient multicenter trial. J Clin Oncol 11:1809–1816, 1993.

83. Atzpodien J, Kirchner H, Lopez Hanningen E, et al: European studies of interleukin-2 in metastatic renal cell cancer (abstract). Proc Am Soc Clin Oncol 13:247, 1994.

84. Thompson J, Nemunaitis J, Vogelzang NJ, et al: Phase I trial of CT1501R in cancer patients receiving high-dose interleukin-2 (IL-2) (abstract). Proc Am Soc Clin Oncol 13:299, 1994.

85. Fonseca GA, Griffith OW, Jones E, et al: Interleukin-2 mediated hypotension in humans is reversed by N^Gmonomethyl-L-arginine, an inhibitor of nitric oxide production (abstract). Proc Am Assoc Cancer Res 35:251, 1994.

86. Kilbourn RG, Fonseca GA, Griffith OW, et al: N^Gmethyl-L-arginine, an inhibitor of nitric oxide synthase that reverses interleukin-2-induced hypotension. Crit Care Med 23:1995 (in press).

87. Aulitzky W, Gastl G, Aulitzky WE, et al: Successful treatment of metastatic renal cell carcinoma with a biologically active dose of recombinant interferon-gamma. J Clin Oncol 7:1875–1884, 1989.

88. Ellerhorst J, Jones E, Kilbourn R, et al: Fixed low dose gamma interferon is active against metastatic renal cell carcinoma (abstract). Proc Am Soc Clin Oncol 11:220, 1992.

89. Iigo M, Sakurai J, Tamura T, et al: In vivo antitumor activity of multiple injections of recombinant interleukin-2, alone and in combination with three different types of recombinant interferon, on

various syngeneic murine tumors. Cancer Res 48:5810–5817, 1988.

90. Figlin RA, Belldegrun A, Moldaver N, et al: Concomitant administration of recombinant human interleukin-2 and recombinant interferon alfa-2A: An active outpatient regimen in metastatic renal cell carcinoma. J Clin Oncol 10:414–421, 1992.

91. Wirth MP: Immunotherapy for metastatic renal cell carcinoma. Urol Clin North Am 20:283–295, 1993.

92. Sella A, Logothetis CJ, Fitz K, et al: Phase II study of interferon-alpha and chemotherapy (5-fluorouracil and mitomycin C) in meta-static renal cell cancer. J Urol 147:573–577, 1992.

93. Flacone A, Cianci C, Ricci S, et al: Alpha-2B-interferon plus floxuridine in metastatic renal cell carcinoma. A phase I-II study. Cancer 72: 564–568, 1993.

94. Sella A, Zukiwski A, Robinson E, et al: Interleukin-2 (IL-2) with interferon-alpha (IFN-alpha) and 5-fluorouracil (5-FU) in patients with metastatic renal cell cancer (RCC) (abstract). Proc Am Soc Clin Oncol 13:237, 1994.

SECTION 8

MISCELLANEOUS TUMORS

CHAPTER **30**   **Brain Tumors**

CHAPTER **31**   **Endocrine Tumors**

CHAPTER **32**   **Malignant Melanoma:**
Biology, Diagnosis, and Management

CHAPTER **33**   **Soft-Tissue and Bone Sarcomas**

CHAPTER **34**   **Retrovirus-Associated Malignancies**

CHAPTER **35**   **Unknown Primary Carcinomas:**
Diagnosis and Management

Brain Tumors

Edward W. Soo, MD, Eugenio G. Galindo, MD, *and* Victor A. Levin, MD

Department of Neuro-Oncology, Division of Medicine
The University of Texas M. D. Anderson Cancer Center, Houston, Texas

While the majority of primary central nervous system (CNS) tumors occur in patients over the age of 45 years, they are also the most prevalent solid neoplasms of childhood. About 16% of patients with brain tumors have a family history of cancer, and evidence points to chromosomal and genetic abnormalities. Magnetic resonance imaging (MRI) is superior to computed tomography (CT) in localizing tumors and in evaluating edema, hydrocephalus, and hemorrhage. Surgery is the most effective treatment, with radiotherapy playing a central role in the management of malignant tumors. Chemotherapy is important in increasing patient survival in some but not all types of tumors. Treatment approaches to specific types of tumors are discussed. These tumors include gliomas, astrocytomas, oligodendrogliomas, ependymomas, medulloblastomas, pineal region tumors, primary CNS lymphomas, meningiomas, neurilemomas, cerebral metastases, and meningeal carcinomatosis.

In 1995, it is estimated that 17,200 new cases of cancerous primary brain tumors will occur, with 13,300 deaths.[1] Every year approximately 35,000 adult Americans develop primary or metastatic brain tumors.[2,3] Central nervous system tumors are the most prevalent solid neoplasms in children under 15 years old, the second (after leukemia) leading cancer-related cause of death in children, and the third leading cancer-related cause of death in adolescents and adults between the ages of 15 and 34 years.[1,2,4] The majority of intracranial tumors, however, occur in patients over the age of 45 years, and recent evidence suggests that the incidence of malignant gliomas among the elderly is increasing.[5] In this review, we describe the principal concepts pertaining to malignant, benign, and metastatic brain tumors and briefly discuss epidemiology and pathogenesis, clinical presentation, diagnosis, and treatment approaches.

EPIDEMIOLOGY AND PATHOGENESIS

About 16% of patients with brain tumors have a family history of cancer.[2] Various genetic disorders can predispose people to brain tumors. For instance, neurofibromatosis is associated with acoustic neuromas, meningiomas, and gliomas; tuberous sclerosis is associated with astrocytomas; von Hippel-Lindau disease is associated with hemangioblastomas; Turcot syndrome is associated with glioblastomas and medulloblastomas; and Li-Fraumeni syndrome, an autosomal dominant inherited disorder, is characterized by the occurrence of diverse tumors such as malignant glioma, breast cancer, soft-tissue sarcoma, osteosarcoma, leukemia, and adrenocortical carcinoma at a younger age. Patients with multifocal gliomas are more likely than other glioma patients to have germline cell *p53* mutations, to have a second malignancy, or to have other family members with cancer.[6,7]

Chromosomal abnormalities include an increased number of copies of chromosome 7 or 22, nonrandom losses associated with chromosomes 9p, 10p, 10q, and 17p,[8–11] and sex chromosome aneuploidy with autosomal abnormalities.[12] Loss of chromosome 17p with or without *p53* gene alteration is seen in lower grades of astrocytoma,[13,14] loss of 9p appears to represent an intermediate event that occurs in most higher-grade astrocytomas,[8] and loss of a portion of chromosome 10 is a late event seen primarily in glioblastoma multiforme tumors.[14–16] Multiple deletions of chromosome 22 have been associated with meningiomas.[12,17,18] It has been postulated that such chromosomal losses may result in the deletion of tumor suppressor genes that normally inhibit tumorigenesis. Conversely, proto-oncogenes such as c-*cis*, c-*erbB*, *gli*, c-*myc*, and N-*ras* can be overexpressed in some brain tumors.

In addition to chromosomal abnormalities, cytokine and receptor aberrations are also seen in brain tumors. For instance, cells that produce tumor growth factor-alpha are seen in all grades of astrocytoma, although they are more often demonstrated in high-grade and more aggressive disease. Likewise, increased levels of epidermal growth factor receptors are seen in high-grade astrocytomas.[16]

The following factors have been implicated as causes of some brain tumors: environmental exposure to vinyl chloride (glioma),[19] Epstein-Barr virus (primary CNS lymphoma),[20] head injury (meningioma),[21] cranial irradiation (astrocytoma and meningioma),[22] immunosuppression associated with organ transplantation (primary CNS lymphoma),[23] and acquired immunodeficiency syndrome,

TABLE I

Syndromes Associated With Cerebral Hemisphere Tumors

Tumor location[a]	Frontal lobe	Temporal lobe	Parietal lobe	Focal infratentorial
Dominant hemisphere	Nonfluent dysphasia, contralateral hemiparesis, apraxia, personality changes	Dysnomia, impaired perception of verbal commands, Wernicke-like aphasia, seizures	Alexia, apraxia, disgraphia, hemiparesis, seizures	–
Nondominant hemisphere	Contralateral primitive grasping and sucking reflexes, personality changes	Minor perception problems, spatial disorientation	Perception abnormalities anosognosia, apraxia hemiparesis, homonymous hemianopia, visual inattention seizures	–
Both frontal lobes	Bilateral hemiplegia, spastic bulbar palsy, intellect impairment, mood liability, dementia, primitive reflexes	–	–	–
Either lobe (temporal or parietal)	–	Homonymous quadrantanopia, auditory hallucinations, aggressiveness	Mild-to-severe sensory extinction	–
Brain stem	–	–	–	Lower cranial nerve palsies (VI–VII), hemisensory deficit or hemiplegia due to involvement of long tracts, ataxia, paraplegia
Midbrain/fourth ventricle	–	–	–	Gait imbalance, ataxia of limbs or trunk, signs and symptoms of increased intracranial pressure
Cerebellum	–	–	–	Signs and symptoms of increased intracranial pressure, stumbling, gait imbalance, prominent morning headaches, nystagmus, dizziness, visual symptoms due to papilledema
Midline lesions (vermis)	–	–	–	Truncal and gait ataxia
Cerebellar hemispheres	–	–	–	Appendicular ataxia
Medullary	–	–	–	Cranial nerve deficits (VI, VII, IX, X), personality changes

[a] Thalamic tumors can result in headache (due to hydrocephalus), sensory abnormalities, intention tremor, and hemiballistic-like movements.

TABLE 2

Clinical Manifestations of Spinal Tumors

Tumor/location	Clinical findings
Foramen magnum	XIth and XIIth cranial nerve palsies; early development of ipsilateral arm weakness; cerebral ataxia; neck pain
Cervical	Ipsilateral arm weakness, eventually spreading to leg and opposite arm; wasting and fibrillation of neck, shoulder girdle, and arm muscles on ipsilateral side; early reduction in pain and temperature sensation in upper cervical regions; pain in cervical nerve distribution
Thoracic	Weakness of abdominal muscles; sparing of arms; unilateral root pains; sensory level changes, ipsilateral at first and becoming bilateral with time
Lumbosacral	Root pain in groin region and/or sciatic nerve distribution; weakened proximal pelvic muscles; impotence; bladder paralysis and decreased knee jerk and brisk ankle jerk reflexes
Cauda equina	Unilateral pain in back and leg, becoming bilateral when the tumor grows large; bladder and bowel paralysis

or AIDS (primary CNS lymphoma).[24] Chemotherapy has also been implicated but not substantiated as a cause of brain tumors.[25,26]

CLINICAL FEATURES

Symptoms of intracranial tumors are produced primarily by the tumor mass itself, the surrounding edema, or the infiltration and destruction of normal tissue. The general signs and symptoms of a brain tumor are headache, nausea and vomiting, behavioral and personality changes, slowing of psychomotor function, visual changes, and speech disturbances. Seizures are the presenting symptoms in only about 20% of patients. These can be focal motor or sensory (complex partial) seizures or generalized seizures. Focal cerebral syndromes are summarized in Table 1.[4]

In most primary spinal axis tumors, signs and symptoms arise not from parenchymal invasion but from spinal cord and nerve root compression. Primary spinal cord tumors account for 10% to 19% of primary CNS tumors. Although most spinal axis tumors are extradural metastases, the majority of primary spinal axis tumors are intradural gliomas. Ependymomas, followed by low-grade astrocytomas, are the most frequent gliomas of the spinal axis.

Clinically, patients with spinal axis tumors present to physicians with sensorimotor spinal tract syndrome, a painful radicular spinal cord syndrome, or central syringomyelia. Sensorimotor signs and symptoms caused by spinal cord compression can gradually develop over weeks or months, or they may suddenly occur in just hours or days. Initial presentation is asymmetric, and motor weakness is dominant with impairment of function at the affected levels. Because of external compression, dorsal column involvement occurs with paresthesias and the loss of pain and temperature sensations contralateral to the motor weakness. Radicular spinal syndrome presents as a sharp "knife-like" pain in the distribution of a sensory nerve root.

Radicular pain is of short duration but may be associated with a long-term, persistent ache. Pain can be exacerbated by coughing, sneezing, or anything that increases intracranial pressure. Local paresthesia, impairment of sensations of pain and touch, weakness, and muscle wasting are common. These findings sometimes antedate cord compression by months.

Spinal tumors, particularly intramedullary tumors, can also produce syringomyelic dysfunction by destruction and cavitation within the central gray matter of the cord. This destroys lower motor neurons, resulting in segmental muscle weakness, wasting, and loss of reflexes. Pain and temperature sensations are lost, but the sense of touch is preserved. With extension of the lesions, however, touch, vibration, and position senses are affected. Table 2 summarizes the clinical findings useful in localizing a spinal cord tumor.

NEUROIMAGING

Magnetic resonance imaging has been shown to be superior to CT in localizing tumors and in evaluating edema, hydrocephalus, and hemorrhage.[27] Brain tumors occasionally bleed, and this bleeding can be insignificant or cause dramatic clinical consequences. Metastatic brain tumors that tend to bleed include melanoma, renal-cell carcinoma, choriocarcinoma, and thyroid carcinoma. Of the gliomas, glioblastoma and oligodendroglioma are more commonly associated with hemorrhage than ependymoma and the low-grade astrocytomas. Both CT and MRI can detect acute hemorrhage, but MRI is better for finding subacute hemorrhage.

The ability to produce high-quality coronal images without bone artifact makes MRI better than CT for evaluating the base of the skull and the posterior fossa. For intra- and extramedullary spinal cord lesions, high-quality MRI with gadolinium diethylenetetraminepenta-acetic acid (Gd-DTPA) as the contrast agent is the diagnostic study of choice. Such imaging can delineate the spinal cord contour, visualize virtually all intrinsic tumors, and facilitate the diagnosis of leptomeningeal disease.[28] Another important application of MRI is the use of the sagittal image in radiation treatment planning.

MRI angiography may be used to distinguish a vascular malformation or aneurysm from a neoplasm. MRI has gradually replaced myelography, which is now used only when MRI is contraindicated or unavailable. Stereotaxic biopsy is another possible diagnostic modality using CT or MRI. In the past, only peripheral cortical lesions allowed biopsy sampling. Now, lesions located almost anywhere in the brain can be safely biopsied using this technique.[29]

When CT or MRI is used to follow the treatment response, it is often difficult to distinguish postoperative changes from residual tumor. The use of a contrast medium to enhance an image obtained within the first 5 days after surgery allows greater accuracy in identifying residual tumor. Corticosteroids profoundly affect CNS tissues for as long as 2 weeks after their administration. Therefore, at the time of postoperative imaging, patients should be receiving the same or a lower dose of steroid as when pretreatment scans were made. Positron emission tomography (PET) is the most reliable noninvasive scanning method for differentiating radiation-induced necrosis from tumor recurrence. Sometimes a biopsy is needed to confirm the diagnosis.[30]

TREATMENT: GENERAL CONCEPTS

Surgery is the fastest way to reduce tumor bulk. The goal is complete resection and cure. If complete resection is not possible, the second choice is to reduce tumor bulk and to decompress the brain. When the tumor is inaccessible, a stereotaxic needle biopsy should be performed to make the diagnosis.

In the case of a supratentorial tumor, an anticonvulsant agent and corticosteroids should be given to the patient before surgery; the former prevents seizures, and the latter may help to reduce cerebral edema and facilitate cerebral retraction, allowing better exposure of the tumor. In addition, diuretics and osmotic agents can be given to control intracranial pressure if the patient becomes lethargic or when deteriorating motor and language functions are noted by the physician.

Radiation Therapy

Radiation therapy is central to the management of malignant tumors. Because most primary CNS neoplasms are focal, they are theoretically curable with effective local therapy. However, by the time of diagnosis, most gliomas and lymphomas have already infiltrated the surrounding normal CNS tissues, resulting in poorly demarcated borders. It is, therefore, often necessary to irradiate a substantial amount of normal tissue.

Using conventional radiation after surgical resection, the median surival time depends on tumor histology, with 3 to 4 years reported for anaplastic astrocytoma[31,32] and 10 to 13 months reported for glioblastoma multiforme.[33] Radiation treatment of gliomas is complicated, because these tumors often display radioresistance as well as because radiation is so toxic to the surrounding normal brain tissues.

The total radiation dose commonly given is 60 Gy, in 180- to 200-cGy fractions over a limited tumor field. Unfortunately, this dose is inadequate to eradicate most primary tumors.[34,35] Strategies used to augment local radiation delivery include interstitial brachytherapy with iodine 125 or iridium 192 and radiosurgery with three-dimensional conformational photoradiation therapy (3D-CRT). To amplify the effects of radiotherapy or interstitial brachytherapy, a variety of dose-modifying agents and techniques are used, including interstitial hyperthermia, halogenated pyrimidine analogs, hypoxic cell radiosensitizers, and cisplatin (Platinol) chemotherapy. However, as local tumor control improves with brachytherapy, peripheral and distant CNS tumor recurrences become more common.[36,37]

Adverse reactions associated with cranial irradiation can be classified according to their time of presentation. Acute reactions generally involve increased intracranial pressure caused by whole-brain irradiation or intensification of preexisting neurologic symptoms or signs when treatment is limited to the lesion. Symptoms are generally mild and self-limited. They can occur during or very shortly after radiation and are usually caused by demyelination and edema. These symptoms respond to corticosteroids.

Early delayed reactions are characterized by somnolence or exacerbation of preexisting signs and symptoms. These reactions are thought to stem from temporary demyelination caused by the effects of radiation on oligodendroglial cells[38] or on capillary permeability.[39] These clinical findings are usually reversible. They occur 1 to 3 months after irradiation, are associated with demyelination and edema, and may also require corticosteroids to alleviate symptoms. In addition, early vascular abnormalities or tumor necrosis may induce clinical and radiographic changes that are indistinguishable from tumor progression.[40]

Late delayed injuries are the most serious complications of therapeutic irradiation. Clinical features include seizure disorders and various degrees of neuropsychologic impairment. These injuries develop several months to years after treatment, are the result of direct damage to the brain and blood vessels, and may be fatal or cause permanent neurologic damage.[34]

Radiation Injury

The brain's tolerance of radiation depends on the size of the dose per fraction and the total dose administered. Total doses in excess of 60 Gy delivered in 30 fractions over approximately 6 weeks will probably increase the risk of CNS tissue injury. Sheline et al[41] suggested that the threshold doses for brain injury are approximately 35 Gy for 10 fractions, 60 Gy for 35 fractions, and 76 Gy for 60 fractions. Factors that decrease the brain's radiation tolerance include incomplete development of the CNS in children,[41] vasculopathy associated with endocrine disorders,[42] CNS infection,[43] and edema.[44]

Corticosteroids may improve or stabilize the neurologic symptoms associated with radiation injury. Surgical resection may also benefit patients with focal radiation-induced lesions who deteriorate neurologically and become dependent on corticosteroids. The spinal cord is less tolerant of radiation than the cerebrum. Radiation myelopathy may present as a transient early delayed reaction or as a more ominous late delayed reaction. Transient radiation myelopathy can present clinically as Lhermitte's sign (electrical-shock–like paresthesias or numbness radiating from the neck to the extremities) when the neck is flexed. The syndrome develops after 3 to 4 months and gradually resolves over the ensuing 3 to 6 months without the need for specific therapy.

Persistent radiation myelopathy can be more serious; approximately 50% of patients die of secondary complications.[45] In these more severe cases, onset is bimodal. The first peak occurs at 12 to 14 months and the second at 24 to 28 months after radiotherapy. This sequence of events may be explained by a dual mechanism of injury: The earlier peak may represent demyelination and white matter necrosis caused by the direct effects of radiation on oligodendroglia, whereas the later peak may reflect intramedullary microvascular injury. Damage that accompanies this form of radiation myelopathy may be irreversible. Sometimes it is partial, and sometimes there is progressive functional loss that becomes complete over a period of several months. Less commonly, radiation myelopathy is manifested by the acute onset of paraplegia or quadriplegia, resulting from infarction of the spinal cord, which evolves over several hours or a few days.

No laboratory tests or imaging studies can distinguish radiation myelopathy from other spinal cord lesions, and the diagnosis is frequently one of exclusion. The medical and legal consequences of radiation myelopathy are such that the radiation dose is often limited to a "safe" level. A dose of 50 Gy in 25 fractions over 5 weeks is generally considered to be safe, the risk of myelopathy being less than 0.5%.[46]

GLIOMAS/ASTROCYTOMAS

Gliomas include astrocytomas, oligodendrogliomas, ependymomas, and mixed-type neoplasms. Astrocytomas are the most common type of malignant brain tumor in adults, accounting for 75% to 90% of such lesions. Histologically, astrocytomas are categorized as low-grade astrocytoma, mid-grade anaplastic astrocytoma, or high-grade glioblastoma multiforme. With the exception of juvenile pilocytic astrocytomas, subependymomas, and the limited number of astrocytomas that can be completely resected, even low-grade astrocytomas are highly lethal.

Assessment

Traditionally, astrocytomas have been graded according to the four-tier system proposed by Kernohan and Sayre,[47] but because this scheme did not correlate well with prognosis, other grading systems have been reported. Today, three-tiered grading systems are commonly used.[48–51] Cell density, pleomorphism, anaplasia, nuclear atypia, mitoses, endothelial proliferation, and necrosis are used to grade astrocytomas. The presence of necrosis separates anaplastic astrocytomas from glioblastoma multiforme.[52] A broad range of anaplasia is seen in mid-grade anaplastic astrocytomas.

Cellular markers have been developed to assist the physician in assessing patient outcome. The Ki-67 antibody MIB-1 labels an antigen in all phases of the cell cycle except G_o and is correlated with astrocytoma grade and patient survival rate. Cellular incorporation of bromodeoxyuridine (BrdU) is another marker that correlates with the DNA synthesis phase of the cell cycle and patient survival rate.[52] BrdU is administered before surgery; MIB-1 can be applied to paraffin-fixed material.

When the three-tier grading system is used, initially each tumor grade is correlated with distinct and separate median survival curves.[48,49] However, a subsequent review of 251 cases at Massachusetts General Hospital found no statistical differences in rate of survival between grades II and III.[53] Necrosis was found to be a significant predictor of short survival time, in agreement with previous studies.[54]

Astroglial tumors may also be classified by anatomic location (ie, optic-nerve glioma, hypothalamic glioma, brainstem glioma, cerebellar astrocytoma, and corpus callosum glioma). The location of such a tumor may have important implications for treatment and prognosis, even if the tissue is histologically benign.

Treatment and Prognosis

Low-grade gliomas constitute about 10% to 20% of all adult primary brain tumors. The majority are astrocytomas; approximately 5% are oligodendrogliomas or mixed oligoastrocytomas. Pathologically, low-grade gliomas are well differentiated and lack all the cellular features (high cellularity, pleomorphism, mitoses, vascular endothelial proliferation, and necrosis) that characterize anaplastic glioma. In patients whose low-grade astrocytoma has been completely resected, radiation does not appear to increase survival rates. Incompletely resected tumors may benefit from radiotherapy,[55–58] although the timing of treatment delivery remains controversial.

It is generally agreed that patients with neurologic impairment, tumor progression, or malignant transformation after surgery should undergo radiotherapy. Some practitioners commonly defer treatment, although close clinical and radiologic observation is maintained in asymptomatic patients or in those whose seizures are medically controlled.[59] Proponents of this approach argue that CT and MRI allow diagnosis of the disease early in its natural history. It is uncertain whether early irradiation is better than delayed irradiation or whether radiotherapy alters the prognosis.[60] With standard radiation therapy, the survival rate is 50% to 60% at 5 years and 30% to 40% at 10 years.

At recurrence, all patients should be evaluated for another biopsy and possible resection. A repeated course of standard radiation is seldom feasible, but some patients can be considered for radiosurgery or brachytherapy. Currently, chemotherapy has little role in the management of these tumors.[59]

Maximal surgical resection improves the results of subsequent radiation therapy and chemotherapy. Clinically, the extent of resection was a significant independent variable for survival in patients treated for malignant glioma.[61,62] Other variables such as preoperative Karnofsky performance status, use of adjuvant chemotherapy, and volume of residual disease had a significant impact on the time to tumor progression.[61,63] Studies have also demonstrated that repeat surgery is effective against recurrent cerebral astrocytoma[64,65] but only if an additional treatment modality is implemented after the surgery. Response to such a regimen can be improved if the patient is young and has a good performance status.

In cases of high-grade astrocytoma, the prognosis for patients with anaplastic astrocytomas is superior to that for patients with glioblastoma multiforme, and the addition of radiotherapy confers a significant improvement in survival rates over those of surgery alone.[66–68] Irradiation of the tumor and the close adjacent margins appears as effective as whole-brain irradiation and results in less morbidity.

Chemotherapy: Astrocytomas have been the most extensively treated of the primary intracranial tumors. Carmustine (BiCNU), lomustine (CeeNU), procarbazine (Matulane), and eflornithine (DFMO [Ornidyl]) have shown good, long-lasting antitumor activity. Tumor histology, patient age and performance status, and extent of surgical resection at onset of therapy influence the likelihood and duration of response. Generally, younger patients are more likely to respond and to have longer remissions, patients with better performance status do best, and patients who have a more extensive original resection do better than those who do not have surgery or have a biopsy only.[64,69,70]

Adjuvant chemotherapy following surgery and radiotherapy increases both time to disease progression and length of survival for patients with anaplastic gliomas.[71] Reoperation may be needed following apparent tumor progression to differentiate between active tumor growth and radiation necrosis or to debulk a large tumor mass.[72–74]

Specific recommendations for chemotherapy can only be made tentatively. In a meta-analysis of 16 trials, published in 1993, Fine and colleagues reported a small (10%) but statistically significant increase in the 1-year survival of patients who received chemotherapy.[75] Some individual studies show far better results. However, nitrosourea-based drug combinations, including the PCV combination (procarbazine, lomustine [CCNU], and vincristine), appear to be superior to single-agent therapy, according to one controlled study by the Northern California Oncology Group. In that study, postirradiation carmustine was compared with the PCV combination.[71] The greatest benefit from chemotherapy, based on time to progression and length of survival, was seen in PCV-treated anaplastic astrocytoma (82 vs 157 weeks) but not in glioblastoma multiforme.

New agents such as topotecan and temozolomide, with CNS penetration properties, are undergoing clinical trials. High-dose chemotherapy with autologous bone marrow rescue and intraarterial chemotherapy have not been beneficial.[76] Osmotic blood-brain barrier disruption followed by intraarterial or systemic therapy showed activity in preliminary phase II trials but was associated with significant morbidity.

Interstitial therapy can provide local delivery of high concentrations of drugs, which minimizes systemic side effects, but its real benefit is yet to be proven in randomized phase III trials. For recurrent astrocytomas, single-agent nitrosoureas and the PCV regimen are most commonly used, but they generate only limited responses. Other drugs and drug combinations continue to be studied.[4] Nevertheless, current advances in surgery make it unlikely that radiation or chemotherapy alone will provide a cure for gliomas and astrocytomas.

OLIGODENDROGLIOMAS

Much less common than the astrocytic tumors, oligodendrogliomas have a somewhat even peak incidence in people between the ages of 25 and 49 years, accounting for approximately 6% of all intracranial neoplasms in this age group. These tumors are derived from oligodendrocytes or their precursors in the O2A cell lineage.[77,78] In general, they tend to infiltrate the cerebral cortex more than do astrocytomas.

Histologic features have been used for grading, but they correlate less well with prognosis and with survival. Clinically, these tumors present in the typical fashion of hemispherical astrocytomas in the frontal or temporal lobe. The slow-growing low-grade oligodendroglioma appears on CT or MRI scans as a hypodense, non–contrast-enhancing mass that is calcified in approximately 50% of cases.

Surgical resection remains the primary mode of treatment in symptomatic patients and those with progressive disease. Total removal of gross tumor, when consistent with good neurologic outcome, is the surgical goal. Patients with unresectable or incompletely resected large tumors should be treated with radiotherapy. However, no randomized prospective trials have evaluated surgery alone vs surgery plus radiation in the treatment of oligodendroglioma. As yet, chemotherapy has no established role in the treatment of low-grade oligodendrogliomas, but some investigators are interested in evaluating regimens such as PCV for controlling these tumors.

Both anaplastic oligodendroglioma and mixed oligoastrocytoma are chemosensitive tumors, but the benefit of adjuvant chemotherapy has not been proven in prospective trials. Ongoing cooperative trials are comparing focal irradiation alone with neoadjuvant PCV chemotherapy followed by radiation.

EPENDYMOMAS

Ependymomas are tumors arising from cells of ependymal lineage. Sixty percent of intracranial ependymomas are infratentorial and 40% are supratentorial.[47] The fourth ventricle is the most common infratentorial site. Extension into the subarachnoid space occurs in 50% of these cases, and encasement of the medulla and upper cervical cord can occur. Of supratentorial ependymomas, 50% are primarily intraventricular; the remainder are parenchymal, arising from ependymal nests. Frequent findings of chromosomal aberrations in patients with these tumors suggest that the deletion of tumor suppressor genes is involved in the development of ependymomas.[12,79,80]

Clinical presentation depends on tumor location. Intraventricular tumors frequently cause increased intracranial pressure and hydrocephalus. As a result, most patients present with headache, nausea, vomiting, papilledema, and ataxia.

Either MRI or CT is sufficient for preoperative anatomic diagnosis. Ependymomas are best treated by extirpation followed by radiation. Tumor grade has been considered the most important determinant of tumor behavior and prognosis. The 5-year survival rate for patients with low-grade tumors ranged from 60% to 80%, whereas for those with anaplastic ependymomas, it was 10% to 47%.[81] When spinal irradiation was delivered in addition to the cranial treatment, no improvement of outcome was observed.[82,83]

This approach is used by most radiation therapists when treating malignant ependymomas of the posterior fossa. In patients with spinal cord ependymomas who were treated with radiation or surgery plus radiation, overall 5- and 10-year survival rates of 83% and 75% were seen, respectively.[84]

MEDULLOBLASTOMAS

Medulloblastomas most likely originate from germinative neuroepithelial cells in the roof of the fourth ventricle.[85] Most medulloblastomas (50% to 60%) occur in children 1 to 10 years old, with a peak between ages 5 and 9 years. A second, lesser peak occurs in adults between 20 and 30 years old.

Childhood medulloblastoma typically arises in the cerebellum, mostly in the midline and posterior vermes. In adults, it typically arises in a cerebellar hemisphere. Regardless of location, the risk of metastasis within the craniospinal intradural axis is relatively high. At presentation, up to 30% of cases will have positive cytology or myelographic evidence of spinal metastasis.[86,87] Extra-CNS metastases occur in less than 5% of cases; most metastases are to long bones.[86]

The overall disease-free 5-year survival rate for medulloblastoma is approximately 50%.[86,88-91] However, the extent of disease at initial diagnosis defines risk. Poor risk is defined as a less than 75% tumor resection; invasion of the brainstem; metastasis to the spinal cord, cerebrum, leptomeninges, or cerebellum; positive cytology 2 weeks or longer after surgery; and patient age under 4 years.[88,90,92] The 5-year disease-free survival rate of poor-risk patients who receive craniospinal irradiation with or without chemotherapy is approximately 25% to 30%.[93] Good-risk patients, on the other hand, have a 5-year disease-free survival rate of 66% to 70%.[90]

Treatment consists of complete surgical resection, if possible, followed by craniospinal irradiation.[94] Chemotherapy with combined regimens is an important adjunct.[95,96] In children under 2 years old, such chemotherapy is increasingly used to postpone radiotherapy.

PINEAL REGION TUMORS

Fewer than 1% of intracranial tumors occur in the pineal region, although in children they constitute 3% to 8%.[97] About half are germ-cell tumors that most often occur in the second decade of a person's life; a few present after the third decade.[98] Increasingly, chemotherapy plus irradiation is used to manage these tumors. Gliomas account for about 25% of pineal tumors. The remaining are tumors of pineal parenchymal cells or benign cysts. Neurologic signs and symptoms result from obstructive hydrocephalus and involvement of ocular pathways. The major ocular manifestation is Parinaud's syndrome.

Histology, tumor size, and extent of disease at presentation determine prognosis. Typically, patients with mature teratoma fare well with surgery. Germinomas respond best to radiation, although preradiation chemotherapy may increase the cure rate and allow reduction of the total radiation dose. Gliomas respond to therapy in the manner discussed in earlier sections. The remaining tumors respond variably to chemotherapy and radiotherapy, with survival ranging from months to years before recurrence.

PRIMARY CNS LYMPHOMAS

Only about 1% of all non-Hodgkin's lymphomas are primary CNS lymphomas. The incidence of this disease has increased threefold over the last two decades, and this is not fully explained by the AIDS epidemic or the greater number of immunodeficient patients.[99] Increased incidence of CNS lymphoma is correlated with the disappearance of intermediate-grade histology, suggesting a shift in the biology of the neoplasms.[100]

Primary CNS lymphomas have been associated with inherited immunosuppression (ataxia telangiectasia, Wiskott-Aldrich syndrome, and severe combined immunodeficiency syndrome), acquired immunosuppression (systemic lupus erythematosus, tuberculosis, vasculitis, and AIDS), immunosuppressive therapy given to transplant patients,[23] and Epstein-Barr virus infection.[20]

Both AIDS-related and non–AIDS-related primary CNS lymphomas are frequently B-cell lymphomas of the histiocytic type (large-cell immunoblastic or small non-cleaved-cell lymphoma). If a corticosteroid is given to a patient before brain biopsy, severe regression may alter the morphologic appearance of the tumor.[101] Because of the AIDS-associated CNS lymphomas, the age for overall peak incidence is decreasing, with these tumors becoming more common in a person's third and fourth decades. CNS lymphomas most often occur in men. The literature review by Murray et al[102] found that 52% of cases were supratentorial, 34% were multiple, 12% were cerebellar, 2% were in the brainstem, and less than 0.5% were spinal.

The average time from onset of symptoms to diagnosis is approximately 1 to 2 months. The pattern of presentation varies, with four broad categories: (1) Some lymphomas cause increased intracranial pressure; (2) some are associated with deficits in higher cortical function, including personality change and dementia; (3) others are associated with focal neurologic deficits; and (4) still others cause seizures.

The contrast-enhanced CT and MRI appearance of these lesions is sometimes distinctive. Multiple lesions and homogeneous enhancement or signal is suggestive of CNS lymphoma. Sometimes the extent of disease appears disproportionate to the neurologic deficit.

Treatment

Because of the diffuse nature of primary CNS lymphoma, the role of surgery is limited to biopsy. Whole-brain radiotherapy is considered standard treatment, producing a median survival time of 12 to 16 months in patients who do not have AIDS but only 2 to 5 months in patients with AIDS. Several studies suggest a dose-response survival relationship in patients receiving more than 5,000 cGy.[103–105] Some investigators have advocated prophylactic spinal-axis radiation,[106] but this is not the treatment norm.

It is clear that systemic chemotherapy can induce significant responses in patients with either newly diagnosed or recurrent primary CNS lymphoma who do not have AIDS. Methotrexate and other agents have been used.[4] When combination chemotherapy was given prior to radiation treatment, an overall response rate up to 80% was seen in those who completed the treatments. The median survival time ranges from 7 months to 16.5 months. However, relapse is rapid and few patients experience prolonged survival.[107–110]

MENINGIOMAS

Meningiomas arise from arachnoidal cells in the meninges. Overall, they are the most common type of benign brain tumor. They occur twice as often in women as in men[111] and are more common in patients with breast carcinoma. Therefore, it is important to make a tissue diagnosis of an apparent single intracranial metastasis in patients with breast cancer.[112]

Histologically, the majority of meningiomas are differentiated, with low proliferative capacity and limited invasiveness. Less commonly, meningiomas are more anaplastic, have a higher proliferative capacity, and are invasive. On CT and MRI scans, meningiomas are well-defined lesions that are easily enhanced with an intravenous contrast agent.[113,114]

Surgery remains the primary mode of treatment. In a large series of surgically resected meningiomas, Simpson[115] reported that even when there was a perceived total resection, the disease recurrence rate was 9%. A review from Massachusetts General Hospital showed that a "total resection" is followed by 7%, 20%, and 32% recurrence rates at 5, 10, and 15 years, respectively.[116] Two variables used to predict recurrence are mitotic rate and Simpson grade of tumor resection.[117]

Approximately 75% of all meningiomas display some cytogenetic abnormalities. Frequent allele loss from chromosome 22 is found in 60% of cases. This loss of antioncogene may be the starting point for future studies of oncogene mechanisms and a tumor's potential for recurrence.[118]

In patients with partially resected tumors, fractionated radiation or radiosurgery can improve the overall outcome if the lesion is less than 35 mm or located 3 to 5 mm from the optic nerve or chiasm.[119,120] For meningiomas that are surgically unresectable, radiation may provide important adjuvant therapy.[121–124]

Currently, chemotherapy is not used for newly diagnosed and unirradiated meningiomas. In patients with histologically malignant meningiomas or recurrent surgically inaccessible tumors, little objective antitumor activity has been seen with cytotoxic chemotherapy. Clinical trials are needed to develop effective chemotherapies.

Progesterone receptors and androgen receptors may be potentially useful in devising therapeutic regimens.[118]

ACOUSTIC SCHWANNOMAS

The major tumors occurring in the cerebellopontine angle are the acoustic nerve tumors and meningiomas. Acoustic neuromas or neurilemomas can originate on the VIIIth cranial nerve, involving the vestibular division at the point where the nerve acquires its reticulin and Schwann-cell component. Because these tumors grow slowly, they can reach substantial size before being detected. Neurilemomas can compress the Vth, VIIth, IXth, and Xth cranial nerves alone or in various combinations. These tumors can also compress the medulla and obstruct the flow of cerebrospinal fluid (CSF), leading to hydrocephalus.

Acoustic schwannomas are more common among people in the fifth decade of life. However, when they are associated with familial neurofibromatosis, they occur earlier, in late childhood and adolescence, and they may be bilateral. In a series from the Massachusetts General Hospital,[123] auditory and vestibular branch involvement occurred in 98% of the cases, facial weakness with disturbances of taste in 56%, sensory loss over the face in 56%, gait abnormality in 41%, and appendicular ataxia in 20%.

The aim of surgery is complete resection. The surgical approach is chosen after consideration of the patient's age and residual hearing and the size and location of the tumor.[125] Mortality ranges from 2% to 4%, depending on the size of the tumor.[126] Radiation, especially stereotaxic radiotherapy, has been used as an alternative to surgery in selected patients. Use of conventional external-beam radiotherapy for partially resected tumors is not common practice.

CEREBRAL METASTASES

Brain metastases occur in 25% to 35% of all cancer patients, of which approximately 15% will be symptomatic. The peak incidence of brain metastasis is bimodal, occurring first in children under 10 years old and then in adults between 55 and 59 years old. Eighty percent of brain metastases are supratentorial.[127–129] Most cerebral metastases originate from lung, melanoma, kidney, colon, soft-tissue sarcoma, breast, and non-Hodgkin's lymphoma.[129] The signs and symptoms at presentation include progressive neurologic deficit, seizure, headaches, and hemorrhage. Intracerebral hemorrhage is more likely to be present with melanoma, renal-cell carcinoma, or choriocarcinoma.

Surgery is the best treatment for a single metastatic

lesion[129–131] and may be indicated under the following circumstances: (1) The primary site is unknown; (2) the primary site is known, but the nature of the intracranial mass is in doubt (eg, meningiomas in patients with breast carcinoma); (3) the primary tumor is a well-controlled tumor, and a single intracranial lesion is present; or (4) serious symptoms from an accessible site of metastasis are present, even with known tumors elsewhere.[132]

Radiation therapy also plays an important role when primary tumors are responsive to radiation, eg, small-cell carcinoma of the lung or lymphoma.

In patients with multiple metastases, the goal is to palliate neurologic symptoms and signs. Radiation therapy is the most common modality used, while surgery has a very limited role. Chemotherapy may be useful in some patients with persistent or recurrent cerebral metastases, eg, small-cell carcinoma, breast carcinoma, germ-cell tumor, and non-Hodgkin's lymphoma. Use of steroids can increase and/or improve survival.[133] If the tumor is left untreated, survival time is between 1 and 2 months.

MENINGEAL CARCINOMATOSIS

Meningeal carcinomatosis is found in 5% to 8% of patients with solid tumors.[134,135] The most common tumors to metastasize to the leptomeninges are lung tumors, breast tumors, non-Hodgkin's lymphoma, melanoma, and genitourinary carcinomas. Mode of spread is via hematogenous seeding of the arachnoid.

The most common signs and symptoms include headache, lower motor weakness, paresthesias, back and neck pain, diplopia, mental status change, reflex asymmetry, sensory loss, and cranial nerve paresis.[136]

Direct examination of the CSF for tumor cells is a reliable and common way to make the diagnosis. Often, repeat lumbar punctures are required to identify malignant cells. Myelography and MRI with gadolinium-DTPA may be helpful in the diagnosis.[137] Treatment is palliative and includes craniospinal axis radiation and intrathecal chemotherapy.[138] Currently used agents are methotrexate, cytarabine, and thiotepa (Thioplex).

REFERENCES

1. Wingos PA, Tong T, Bolden S: Cancer statistics, 1995. CA Cancer J Clin 45:8–30, 1995.

2. Mahaley MS Jr, Mettlin C, Natarajan N, et al: National survey of patterns of care for brain-tumor patients. J Neurosurg 71:826–836, 1989.

3. Walker AE, Robins M, Weinfeld FD: Epidemiology of brain tumors: The national survey of intracranial neoplasms. Neurology 35:219–226, 1985.

4. Levin VA, Gutin PH, Leibel S: Neoplasms of the central nervous system, in DeVita VT, Hellman S, Rosenberg SA (eds): Cancer: Principles and Practice of Oncology, 4th Ed. Philadelphia, JB Lippincott, 1993.

5. Greig NH, Ries LG, Yancik R, et al: Increasing annual incidence of primary malignant brain tumors in the elderly. J Natl Cancer Inst 82:1621–1624, 1990.

6. Kyritsis AP, Bondy ML, Xiao MI, et al: Germline p53 gene mutations in subsets of glioma patients. J Natl Cancer Inst 86:344–349, 1994.

7. Kyritsis AP, Yung WKA, Leeds NE, et al: Multifocal cerebral gliomas associated with secondary malignancies. Lancet 339:1229–1230, 1992.

8. Bigner SH, Mark J, Burger PC, et al: Specific chromosomal abnormalities in malignant human gliomas. Cancer Res 48:405, 1988.

9. Jenkins RB, Kimmel DW, Moertel CA, et al: A cytogenetic study of 53 human gliomas. Cancer Genet Cytogenet 39:253, 1989.

10. Steck PA, Hadi A, Cheong P, et al: Evidence of two tumor suppressive loci on chromosome 10 involved in human glioblastoma. Genes Chromosom Cancer (in press, 1995).

11. Pershouse MA, Stubblefield E, Hadi A, et al: Analysis of the functional role of chromosome 10 loss in human glioblastomas. Cancer Res 53:5043–5050, 1993.

12. Yamada K, Kasama M, Kondo T, et al: Chromosome studies in 70 brain tumors with special attention to sex chromosome loss and single autosomal trisomy. Cancer Genet Cytogenet 73:46–52, 1994.

13. James CD, Carlbom E, Nordenskjold M, et al: Mitotic recombination of chromosome 17 in astrocytomas. Proc Natl Acad Sci USA 86:2858, 1989.

14. Lang FF, Miller DC, Koslow M, et al: Pathways leading to glioblastoma multiforme: A molecular analysis of genetic alterations in 65 histocytic tumors. J Neurosurg 81:427–436, 1944.

15. James CD, Carlbom E, Dumanski JP, et al: Clonal genomic alterations in glioma malignancy stages. Cancer Res 48:5546, 1988.

16. Wong AJ, Zoltick PW, Moscatello DK: The molecular biology and molecular genetics of astrocytic neoplasms. Semin Oncol 21(2):126–138, 1994.

17. Collins VP: The molecular genetics of meningiomas. Brain Pathol 1:19, 1990.

18. Dumanski JP, Rouleau GA, Nordenskjold M, et al: Molecular genetic analysis of chromosome 22 in 81 cases of meningioma. Cancer Res 50:5863, 1990.

19. Moss AR: Occupational exposure and brain tumors. J Toxicol Environ Health 16:703, 1985.

20. Hochberg RH, Miller G, Schooley RT, et al: Central nervous system lymphoma related to Epstein-Barr virus. N Engl J Med 309:745, 1983.

21. Schoenberg BS: Epidemiology of primary intracranial neoplasms: Disease distribution and risk factors, in Saleman M (ed): Neurobiology of Brain Tumors, Concepts in Neurosurgery, vol 4, pp 3–18. Baltimore, Williams & Wilkins, 1991.

22. Sogg RL, Donaldson SS, Yorke CH: Malignant astrocytoma following radiotherapy of a craniopharyngioma. J Neurosurg 48:622, 1978.

23. Schneck SA, Penn I: De novo brain tumors in renal transplant recipients. Lancet 1:1983, 1971.

24. Payan MJ, Gambarelli D, Routy JP, et al: Primary lymphoma of the brain associated with AIDS. Acta Neuropathol 64:78, 1984.

25. Malone M, Lumley H, Erdohazi M: Astrocytoma as a second malignancy in patients with acute lymphoblastic leukemia. Cancer 57:979, 1986.

26. Poster DS, Bruno S: The occurrence of second primary neoplasms in patients with non-Hodgkin's lymphoma. IRCS Med Sci: Cancer 8:554, 1980.

27. Brant-Zawadski M, Badami JP, Mills CM, et al: Primary intracranial tumor imaging: A comparison of magnetic resonance and CT. Radiology 150:435, 1984.

28. Dillon WP, Norman D, Newton TH, et al: Intradural spinal cord

lesions: Gd-DTPA enhanced MR imaging. Radiology 170:229, 1989.

29. Apuzzo MLJ, Chandrasoma PT, Cohen D, et al: Computed imaging stereotaxy: Experience and perspective related to 500 procedures applied to brain masses. Neurosurgery 20:930, 1987.

30. Byrne TN: Imaging of gliomas. Semin Oncol 21(2):162–171, 1994.

31. Prado MD, Gutin PH, Phillips TL, et al: Highly anaplastic astrocytoma: A review of 357 patients treated between 1977 and 1989. Int J Radiat Oncol Biol Phys 23:3–8, 1992.

32. Levin VA, Prados MR, Wara WM, et al: Radiation therapy with bromodeoxyuridine followed by CCNU, procarbazine, and vincristine (PCV) chemotherapy for the treatment of anaplastic gliomas. Int J Radiat Oncol Biol Phys (in press, 1995).

33. Simpson JR, Horton J, Scott C, et al: Influence of location and extent of surgical resection on survival of patients with glioblastoma multiforme: Results of three consecutive radiation therapy oncology (RTOG) clinical trials. Int J Radiat Oncol Biol Phys 26:239–244, 1993.

34. Liebel SA, Sheline GE: Tolerance of the brain and spinal cord to conventional irradiation, in Gutin PH, Leibel SA, Sheline GE (eds): Radiation Injury to the Nervous System, p 239. New York, Raven Press, 1991.

35. Suit HD, Baumann M, Skates S, et al: Clinical interest in determinations of cellular radiation sensitivity. Int J Radiat Biol 56:725–737, 1989.

36. Loeffler JS, Alexander E, Hochberg FH, et al: Clinical patterns of failure following stereotactic interstitial irradiation for malignant gliomas. Int J Radiat Oncol Biol Phys 19:1455, 1990.

37. Liebel SA, Scott CB, Loeffler JS: Contemporary approaches to the treatment of malignant gliomas with radiation therapy. Semin Oncol 21(2):198–219, 1994.

38. Hoffman WF, Levin VA, Wilson CB: Evaluation of malignant glioma patients during the postirradiation period. J Neurosurg 50:624, 1979.

39. Delattre JY, Rosenblum MK, Thaler HT, et al: A model of radiation myelopathy in the rat: Pathology, regional capillary permeability changes and treatment with dexamethasone. Brain 111:1319, 1988.

40. Graeb DA, Steinbok P, Robertson WD: Transient early computed tomographic changes mimicking tumor progression after brain tumor irradiation. Radiology 144:813, 1982.

41. Sheline GE, Wara WM, Smith V: Therapeutic irradiation and brain injury. Int J Radiat Oncol Biol Phys 6:1215, 1980.

42. Bloom B, Kramer S: Conventional radiation therapy in the management of acromegaly, in Black P, et al (eds): Secretory Tumors of the Pituitary Gland, vol 1, p 179. New York, Raven Press, 1984.

43. Rottenberg DA, Chernick MD, Deck MDF, et al: Cerebral necrosis following radiotherapy of extracranial neoplasms. Ann Neurol 1:339, 1977.

44. Burger PC, Mahaley MS Jr, Dudka L, et al: The morphologic effects of radiation administered therapeutically for intracranial gliomas: A postmortem study of 25 cases. Cancer 44:1256, 1979.

45. Schulthesis TE, Stephens LC, Peters LJ: Survival in radiation myelopathy. Int J Radiat Oncol Biol Phys 12:1765, 1986.

46. Bloom HJG: Intracranial tumors: Response and resistance to therapeutic endeavors 1970–1980. Int J Radiat Oncol Biol Phys 8:1083, 1982.

47. Kernohan JW, Sayre GP: Tumors of the central nervous system, in Atlas of Tumor Pathology, section 10, fascicle 35. Washington, DC, Armed Forces Institute of Pathology, 1982.

48. Daumas-Duport C, Scheithauer BW, Kelly PJ: A histologic and cytologic method for the spatial definition of gliomas. Mayo Clin Proc 62:435, 1987.

49. Daumas-Duport C, Scheithauer B, O'Fallon J, et al: Grading of astrocytomas, a simple and reproducible method. Cancer 62:2152,

1988.

50. Burger PC, Vogel FS, Green SB, et al: Glioblastoma multiforme and anaplastic astrocytoma. Pathologic criteria and prognostic implications. Cancer 56:1106–1111, 1985.

51. Ringertz N: Grading of gliomas. APMIS 27:51–64, 1950.

52. Bruner JM: Neuropathology of malignant gliomas. Semin Oncol 21(2):126–138, 1994.

53. Kim TS, Halliday AL, Headley-Whyte ET, et al: Correlates of survival and the Daumas-Duport grading system for astrocytomas. J Neurosurg 74:27, 1991.

54. Nelson JS, Tsukada Y, Schoenfeld D, et al: Necrosis as a prognostic criterion in malignant supratentorial, astrocytic gliomas. Cancer 52:550, 1983.

55. Leibel SA, Sheline GE, Wara WM, et al: The role of radiation therapy in the treatment of astrocytoma. Cancer 35:1551, 1975.

56. Fazekas JT: Treatment of grade I and II brain astrocytomas: The role of radiotherapy. Int J Radiat Oncol Biol Phys 2:661, 1977.

57. Shaw EG, Daumas-Duport C, Scheithauer BW, et al: Radiation therapy in the management of low grade supratentorial astrocytomas. J Neurosurg 70:853, 1989.

58. Wallner KE, Gonzales MF, Sheline GE, et al: Treatment results of juvenile pilocytic astrocytoma. Neurosurgery 69:171, 1988.

59. McDonald DR: Low-grade gliomas, mixed gliomas, and oligodendrogliomas. Semin Oncol 21(2):236–248, 1994.

60. Cairncross JG, Laperriere NJ: Low grade glioma: To treat or not to treat? Arch Neurol 46:1238, 1989.

61. Berger MS: Malignant astrocytomas: Surgical aspects. Semin Oncol 21(2):172–185, 1994.

62. Winger MJ, MacDonald DR, Cairncross JG: Supratentorial anaplastic gliomas in adults. J Neurosurg 71:487, 1985.

63. Ganju V, Jenkins RB, O'Fallon J, et al: Prognostic factors in gliomas. Cancer 74(3):920–927, 1994.

64. Salcman M: Malignant glioma management. Neurosurg Clin North Am 1:49, 1990.

65. Harsh GR IV, Levin VA, Gutin PH, et al: Reoperation for recurrent glioblastoma and anaplastic astrocytoma. Neurosurgery 21:615, 1987.

66. Sheline GE: Radiotherapy of primary tumors. Semin Oncol 2:29, 1975.

67. Marsa GW, Goffinet DR, Rubinstein LJ, et al: Megavoltage irradiation in the treatment of gliomas of the brain and spinal cord. Cancer 36:1681, 1975.

68. Walker MD, Alexander E, Hunt WE, et al: Evaluation of BCNU and/or radiotherapy in the treatment of anaplastic gliomas. J Neurosurg 49:333, 1978.

69. Byar DP, Green SB, Strike TA: Prognostic factors for malignant glioma, in Walker MD (ed): Oncology of the Nervous System, p 379. Boston, Martinus Nijhoff, 1983.

70. Salmon I, Dewitte O, Pasteels JL, et al: Prognostic scoring in adult histiocytic tumors using patient age, histopathologic grade, and DNA histogram type. J Neurosurg 80:877–883, 1994.

71. Levin VA, Silver P, Hannigan J, et al: Superiority of postradiotherapy adjuvant chemotherapy with CCNU, procarbazine and vincristine (PCV) over BCNU for anaplastic gliomas: NCOG 6G61 final report. Int J Radiat Oncol Phys Biol 18:321, 1990.

72. Salcman M: Resection and re-operation in neuro-oncology: Rationale and approach. Neurosurg Clin North Am 3:831–842, 1985.

73. Harsh GR IV, Levin VA, Gutin PH, et al: Reoperation for recurrent glioblastoma and anaplastic astrocytoma. Neurosurgery 21:615–621, 1987.

74. Moser RP: Surgery for glioma relapse: Factors that influence a favorable outcome. Cancer 62:381–390, 1988.

75. Fine HA, Dear KB, Loeffler JS, et al: Meta-analysis of radiation therapy with and without adjuvant chemotherapy for malignant glioma

in adults. Cancer 71:2585–2597, 1993.

76. Lesser GJ, Grossman S: The chemotherapy of high-grade astrocytomas. Semin Oncol 21(2):220–235, 1994.

77. Bishop M, de la Monte SM: Dual lineage of astrocytoma. Am J Pathol 135:517–527, 1989.

78. de la Monte SM: Uniform lineage of oligodendroglioma. Am J Pathol 135:529–540, 1989.

79. Sawyer JR, Sammartino G, Husain M, et al: Chromosome aberrations in four ependymomas. Cancer Genet Cytogenet 74:132–138, 1994.

80. Rogatto SR, Casartelli C, Rainho CA, et al: Chromosomes in the genesis and progression of ependymomas. Cancer Genet Cytogenet 69:146–152, 1993.

81. Liebel SA, Sheline GE: Radiation therapy for neoplasms of the brain. J Neurosurg 66:1, 1987.

82. Kovalic JJ, Flaris N, Grigsby PW, et al: Intracranial ependymoma long term outcome, patterns of failure. J Neurooncol 15:125–131, 1993.

83. Rousseau P, Habrand JL, Sarrazin D, et al: Treatment of intracranial ependymomas of children: Review of a 15-year experience. Int J Radiat Oncol Biol Phys 28:381–386, 1993.

84. Waldron JN, Laperriere NJ, Jaakkimalinen L, et al: Spinal cord ependymomas: A retrospective analysis of 59 cases. Int J Radiat Oncol Biol Phys 27:223–229, 1993.

85. Russell DJ, Rubinstein LJ: Pathology of Tumors of the Nervous System, 4th Ed. Baltimore, Williams & Wilkins, 1977.

86. Bloom HJG: Medulloblastoma in children: Increasing survival rates and further prospects. Int J Radiat Oncol Biol Phys 8:2023, 1982.

87. Deutsch M: The impact of myelography on the treatment results for medulloblastoma. Int J Radiat Oncol Biol Phys 10:999, 1984.

88. Jenkins D: Posterior fossa tumors in childhood: Radiation treatment. Clin Neurosurg 30:203, 1983.

89. Levin VA, Rodriguez LA, Edwards MSB, et al: Treatment of medulloblastoma with procarbazine, hydroxyurea, and reduced radiation doses to whole brain and spine. J Neurosurg 68:383, 1988.

90. Tait DM, Thornton-Jones H, Blood HJG, et al: Adjuvant chemotherapy for medulloblastoma: The first multi-center controlled trial of the International Society of Pediatric Oncology (SIOP I). Eur J Cancer 26:464, 1990.

91. Carrie C, Lasset C, Blay JY, et al: Medulloblastoma in adults. Survival and prognostic factors. Radiother Oncol 29:301–307, 1993.

92. Park TS, Hoffman HJ, Hendrick EB, et al: Medulloblastoma: Clinical presentation and management. Experience at the Hospital for Sick Children, Toronto, 1950–1980. J Neurosurg 58:543, 1983.

93. Lowery GS, Kimball JC, Patterson RB, et al: Extraneural metastases from cerebellar medulloblastoma. Am J Pediatr Hematol Oncol 4:259, 1982.

94. Tomita T, McLone DG: Medulloblastoma in childhood: Results of radical resection and low-dose neuraxis radiation therapy. J Neurosurg 64:238–242, 1986.

95. Packer RJ, Siegel KR, Sutton LN, et al: Efficacy of adjuvant chemotherapy for patients with poor-risk medulloblastoma: A preliminary report. Ann Neurol 24:503–508, 1988.

96. Finley F, August C, Packer R, et al: High dose chemotherapy with marrow "rescue" in children with malignant brain tumors (abstract). J Neurosurg Oncol 7(suppl):511, 1989.

97. Hoffman HJ: Pineal region tumors. Prog Exp Tumor Res 30:281, 1987.

98. Matsutani M, Takakura K, Sand K: Primary intracranial germ cell tumors: Pathology and treatment. Prog Exp Tumor Res 30:307, 1987.

99. Hochberg FH, Miller DC: Primary central nervous system lymphoma. J Neurosurg 68:835–853, 1988.

100. Miller DC, Hochberg FH, Harris NL, et al: Pathology with clinical correlations of primary central nervous system non-Hodgkin's lymphoma. The Massachusetts General Hospital Experience 1958–1989. Cancer 74(4):1383–1397, 1994.

101. Schwechhimer K, Braus DF, Schwarzkopf G, et al: Polymorphous high-grade B cell lymphoma is the predominant type of spontaneous primary cerebral malignant lymphoma. Am J Surg Pathol 18(9):931–937, 1994.

102. Murray K, Kun L, Cox J: Primary malignant lymphoma of the central nervous system. J Neurosurg 65:600, 1986.

103. Berry MP, Simpson WJ: Radiation therapy in the management of primary malignant lymphoma of the brain. Int J Radiat Oncol Biol Phys 7:55–59, 1981.

104. Cox JD, Koehl RH, Turner WM, et al: Irradiation in the local control of malignant lymphoreticular tumors. Radiology 112:179–185, 1974.

105. Ling SM, Roach M, Larson DA, et al: Radiotherapy of primary central nervous system lymphoma in patients with and without human immunodeficiency virus. Cancer 73(10):2570–2592, 1994.

106. Mendenhall NP, Thar TL, Agee OF, et al: Primary lymphoma of the central nervous system: Computerized tomography scan characteristics and treatment results for 12 cases. Cancer 52:1993–2000, 1983.

107. Lachance DH, Brizel DM, Gockerman JP, et al: Cyclophosphamide, doxorubicin, vincristine, and prednisone for primary central nervous system lymphoma. Neurology 44:1721–1727, 1994.

108. Forsyth PA, Yahalom J, DeAngelis LM: Combined modality the therapy in the treatment of primary central nervous system lymphoma in AIDS. Neurology 44:1473–1479, 1994.

109. Selch MT, Shimizu KT, DeSalles AF et al: Primary central nervous system lymphoma: Results at the University of California at Los Angeles and review of the literature. Am J Clin Oncol 17(4):286–293, 1994.

110. DeAngelis LM: Current management of primary central nervous system lymphoma. Oncology 9(1): 63–71, 1995.

111. Kepes JJ: Meningiomas: Biology, Pathology, and Differential Diagnosis. New York, Masson, 1982.

112. Rubinstein AB, Schein M, Reichenthal E: The association of carcinoma of the breast with meningioma. Surg Gynecol Obstet 169:334–336, 1989.

113. Maxwell RE, Chou SN: Pre-operative evaluation and management of meningiomas, in Schmidek HH, Sweet WH (eds): Operative Neurosurgical Technique, 2nd Ed, vol 1, pp 547–554. New York, Grune & Stratton, 1988.

114. Murtagh R, Linden C: Neuroimaging of intracranial meningiomas. Neurosurg Clin North Am 5(2):217–233, 1994.

115. Simpson D: The recurrence of intracranial meningiomas after surgical treatment. J Neurol Neurosurg Psychiatry 20:22, 1957.

116. Mirimanoff RO, Dosoratz DE, Linggood RM, et al: Meningioma: Analysis of recurrence and progression following neurosurgical resection. J Neurosurg 62:18, 1985.

117. Miller DC: Predicting recurrence of intracranial meningiomas. Neurosurg Clin North Am 5(2):193–200, 1994.

118. Smith DA, Cahill DW: The biology of meningiomas. Neurosurg Clin North Am 5(2):201–215, 1994.

119. Lunsford LD: Contemporary management of meningioma: Radiation therapy as an adjuvant and radiosurgery as an alternative to surgical removal. J Neurosurg 80:187–190, 1994.

120. Goldsmith BJ, Wara WM, Wilson CB, et al: Postoperative irradiation for subtotally resected meningiomas. J Neurosurg 80:195–201, 1994.

121. Forbes AR, Goldberg ID: Radiation therapy in the treatment of meningioma: The Joint Center for Radiation Therapy Experience,

1970 to 1982. J Clin Oncol 2:1139–1143, 1984.

122. Taylor BW, Marcus RB Jr, Friedman WA, et al: The meningioma controversy: Postoperative radiation therapy. Int J Radiat Oncol Biol Phys 15:299–304, 1988.

123. Adams RD, Victor M: Principles of Neurology, p 86. New York, McGraw-Hill, 1977.

124. DeMonte F: Current management of meningioma. Oncology 9(1):83–96, 1995.

125. Jackler RK, Pitts LH: Acoustic neuroma. Neurosurg Clin North Am 1:199, 1990.

126. Tator CH, Nedzelski JM: Preservation of hearing in patients undergoing excision of acoustic neuromas and other cerebellopontine angle tumors. J Neurosurg 63:168–174, 1985.

127. Ask-Upjmark E: Metastatic tumors of the brain and their localization. Acta Med Scand 154:1–9, 1956.

128. Posner JB, Chernik NL: Intracranial metastatic tumors. J Neurosurg 19:575–587, 1978.

129. Delattre JY, Krol G, Thaler HT: Distribution of brain metastases. Arch Neurol 45:741–744, 1988.

130. Sundaresan N, Galicich JH: Surgical treatment of brain metastases: Clinical and computerized tomography evaluation of the results of treatment. Cancer 55:1382–1388, 1985.

131. Patchell RA, Tibbs PA, Walsh JW, et al: A randomized trial of surgery in the treatment of single metastases to the brain. N Engl J Med 332:494–500, 1990.

132. Black PMcL: Brain tumors. N Engl J Med 324:1561–1562, 1991.

133. Horton J, Baxter DH, Olson DB, et al: The management of metastases to the brain by irradiation and corticosteroids. AJR Am J Roentgenol 111:344–336, 1971.

134. Patchell RA, Posner JB: Neurologic complications of systemic cancer. Neurol Clin 3:729–750, 1985.

135. Gonzalez-Vitale JC, Garcia-Bunuel R: Meningeal carcinomatosis. Cancer 1976:2906, 1976.

136. Wasserstrom WR, Glass JP, Posner JB: Diagnosis and treatment of leptomeningeal metastases from solid tumors: Experience with 90 patients. Cancer 49:759–772, 1982.

137. Sze G, Soletsky S, Broadnen R, et al: MR imaging of the cranial meninges with emphasis on contrast enhancement and meningeal carcinomatosis. AJNR Am J Neuroradiol 10:965–975, 1989.

138. Yap HY, Yap BS, Rasmussen S, et al: Treatment for meningeal carcinomatosis in breast. Cancer 50:219–222, 1982.

CHAPTER 31

Endocrine Malignancies

Ana G. Ruiz Allison, MD, *and* Rena Vassilopoulou-Sellin, MD
Section of Endocrinology, Department of Medical Specialties, Division of Medicine
The University of Texas M. D. Anderson Cancer Center, Houston, Texas

Endocrine neoplasms are relatively uncommon, but those that do occur are often difficult to detect and treat effectively. According to 1991 estimates, there were 13,900 cases of endocrine cancers in the United States, 12% of which will ultimately prove fatal. In this review, we discuss the epidemiology, etiology, pathology, diagnosis, and current treatment of the most common endocrine maligancies: thyroid carcinoma, parathyroid carcinoma, adrenal gland cancers, and malignant pheochromocytomas.

THYROID CARCINOMA

Epidemiology, Incidence, and Distribution

The incidence of thyroid cancer appears to have increased in recent decades (Figure 1), although this malignancy remains rare, with only 12,400 new cases reported in 1991.[1,2] The apparent increase in incidence is likely due to improved diagnosis and to the increased use of therapeutic irradiation. Certain thyroid cancers remain undiagnosed during a person's life; incidental thyroid cancers with or without metastases are found at autopsy in up to 10% of cases. Unsuspected or occult thyroid carcinomas are usually less than 0.5 cm in greatest dimension, papillary in nature, and are believed to follow an indolent course; they also have been noted to have a racial predilection. There is, for example, a higher prevalence of occult thyroid carcinoma among the Japanese than among the US population.[3]

Thyroid cancer constitutes about 1% of all malignant tumors, and the differentiated types account for 0.8% of all human malignancies. Although thyroid nodules are relatively common, only about 5% to 15% of clinically detectable, solitary, hypofunctioning (cold) thyroid nodules are found to be malignant. Thyroid tumors are rare in children, and increase in frequency with age. In children with thyroid nodules, the prevalence of cancer has been estimated at 15% to 20%. In particular, the risk of carcinoma in a dominant thyroid nodule in a child under 14 years old is approximately 50% (range, 20% to 73%), whereas the risk in an adult is less than 15%, with a slightly greater risk after age 60 years. Well-differentiated thyroid carcinomas account for over 90% of the malignant lesions, primarily papillary or follicular. Medullary thyroid carcinomas account for 4% to 10% of the thyroid carcinomas in children; teratomas, lymphomas, and anaplastic carcinomas of the thyroid occur rarely.

Medullary thyroid carcinomas represent 5% to 10% of all thyroid neoplasms.[4,5] About 80% of patients with medullary thyroid carcinoma have a sporadic form of the disease, and the remaining 20% inherit medullary thyroid carcinoma as an autosomal dominant trait, as part of the distinct clinical syndromes of multiple endocrine neoplasia (MEN) type IIA or IIB or familial medullary carcinoma of the thyroid. MEN IIA occurs in association with pheochromocytoma and parathyroid adenoma, while MEN IIB occurs in association with pheochromocytoma and mucosal neuromas or neurofibromas. The incidence of anaplastic thyroid carcinoma appears to be decreasing, but this is most likely because better techniques for differentiating other thyroid tumors from anaplastic disease have become available.

Etiology

External low-dose radiation therapy to the head and neck during infancy and childhood, used frequently from the 1940s to the 1960s to treat a variety of benign diseases, has been shown to predispose to thyroid cancer. The average time between irradiation and recognition of the tumor is 10 years but may be longer than 30 years.[6] Patients exposed to head or neck irradiation experience an increased frequency of benign tumors, but malignancy occurs in up to 30% of cases. Treatment of malignant diseases with higher x-ray doses (more than 2,000 cGy), especially at a young age, also has been associated with an increased risk of both benign and malignant neoplasms of the thyroid.

Besides radiation-induced thyroid cancer, there are only sparse data on the etiology of this malignancy.[7] Prolonged thyroid-stimulating hormone (TSH) stimulation has been implicated as a potential risk factor; however, patients with primary hypothyroidism do not appear to exhibit increased frequency of thyroid carcinoma.[8] Thyroid-stimulatory immunoglobulins present in patients with Graves' disease have also been implicated,[9] and associations between thyroid cancer and Hashimoto's

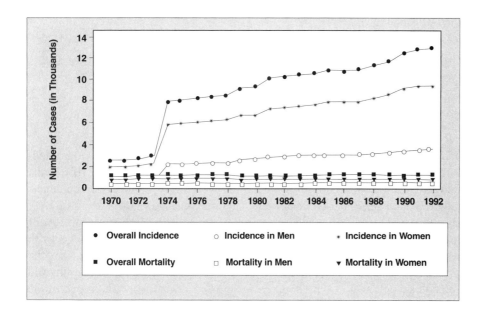

FIGURE I

Incidence and mortality rates for thyroid cancer. Data adapted from the National Cancer Institute's Surveillance, Epidemiology and End Results (SEER) database. Reprinted, with permission, from Vassilopoulou-Sellin.[1]

thyroiditis, Graves' disease, and multinodular goiter have been reported. However, any causative relationship between these diseases remains poorly documented.

The possible role of genetic factors is receiving a great deal of attention in familial cases of thyroid cancer. Two uncommon familial syndromes are associated with follicular thyroid carcinoma: Gardner's syndrome with polyposis of the large intestine, which is inherited as an autosomal dominant trait, and Cowden's disease, which is characterized by inherited multiple hamartomas. Genetic factors may also predispose people to radiation-induced thyroid neoplasms.

In a descriptive epidemiologic study of 7,696 patients with thyroid cancer in the United States between 1973 and 1981,[7] striking differences in incidence were noted among ethnic groups. Compared with white men and women, Puerto Rican Hispanics and blacks had significantly lower thyroid cancer rates. Conversely, New Mexican Hispanic men and Chinese, Japanese, Hawaiian, and Filipino men and women had significantly higher rates. Elevated thyroid cancer rates were also noted for residents of Hawaii, regardless of ethnic group, as well as for residents in areas bordering the Ring of Fire, such as Colombia, the Philippines, and Polynesia. An etiologic relationship between thyroid cancer and the presence of active volcanoes in this region has been postulated.

Pathology

Thyroid cancer is generally subdivided into a large group of well-differentiated neoplasms characterized by slow growth and high curability, and a small group of highly anaplastic tumors with a bleak outlook. The pathologic classification proposed by Woolner et al in 1961[4] was adopted by the American Thyroid Association with a few modifications, and in 1974 was accepted by the World Health Organization.

Thyroid cancer is classified into four main types, according to morphology and biologic behavior: papillary, follicular, medullary, and anaplastic. This classification has an advantage over systems based purely on histologic patterns, in that it relates morphology to methods of treatment and prognosis. Primary lymphoma of the thyroid, metastases from other primary sites, and other uncommon thyroid tumors are also encountered, though rarely (Table 1).[10]

Papillary tumors arise from thyroid follicular cells and are in most cases unilateral. They vary in size from microscopic to large cancers that may invade the thyroid capsule and infiltrate contiguous structures. Papillary tumors tend to invade the lymphatics, but they have little tendency to invade the blood vessels; psammoma bodies are common. Follicular tumors, although frequently encapsulated, commonly exhibit vascular and capsule invasion microscopically. Hürthle-cell carcinomas are considered a type of follicular cancer.

Many tumors have both papillary and follicular elements histologically; they are called follicular variants of papillary carcinoma, and are classified as papillary lesions because their clinical behavior is typically indistinguishable from that of pure papillary cancers. Occasionally, both papillary and follicular tumors occur as small lesions surrounded by a dense fibrotic reaction; they are called occult sclerosing lesions and may be associated with lymph-node metastases.

Medullary thyroid carcinoma is derived from C-cells (or calcitonin-secreting cells)[5] that are of ectodermal neural crest origin. Medullary carcinoma of the thyroid primarily arises in the upper two thirds of the gland where the C-cells are normally found. C-cells secrete a 32–amino acid peptide called calcitonin, which serves as a useful biochemical marker in patients with this cancer. Medullary carcinoma of the thyroid occurs as a solid mass or clusters of C-cell hyperplasia interspersed between normal-appearing thyroid follicles. These can be visualized with calcitonin immunostaining, which shows variable amounts of fibrosis and deposits of amyloid in 60% to 80% of tumors. Even the smallest visible tumors can be associated with metastases.

Anaplastic thyroid tumors[11] are derived from follicular cells. The presence of argyrophilic cytoplasmic granules distinguishes follicular from parafollicular origin, and thus can differentiate anaplastic follicular thyroid lesions from undifferentiated variants of medullary carcinoma. Thyroglobulin, normally synthesized in the follicular epithelium of the thyroid, is present in well-differentiated papillary and follicular carcinomas and infrequently in anaplastic carcinomas, but not in medullary carcinoma cells. Therefore, thyroglobulin immunoreactivity also is considered to be indicative of follicular epithelial origin.

The absence of thyroglobulin immunoreactivity in anaplastic carcinomas does not exclude follicular epithelial origin, because undifferentiated carcinoma cells may have lost the ability to synthesize this glycoprotein. Occasionally, it is possible to show that a case of anaplastic carcinoma arose from preexisting well-differentiated thyroid carcinoma.

Clinical Presentation and Course

Thyroid cancer is usually detected in a euthyroid patient as a dominant anterior neck mass that moves on deglutition and is "cold" on scintiscan. The diagnosis of medullary carcinoma of the thyroid can be made by measuring calcitonin levels after provocative pentagastrin and/or calcium administration. Because of the potentially familial nature of medullary cancer, consideration should be given to screening a patient's first-degree relatives after a positive diagnosis. Recent advances in molecular biology may allow for genetic detection of this disease in the near future.[12] Fine-needle aspiration of a nodule followed by immunohistochemical staining for thyroglobulin or calcitonin can lead to a correct diagnosis in most cases.

In adults with differentiated papillary thyroid cancer, up to 40% may present with regional lymph-node metas-

TABLE I

Classification of Unusual Thyroid Tumors

Primary thyroidal tumor

Thyroid epithelial-cell origin
  Anaplastic large (giant and spindle, osteoclastoma-like) cell carcinoma
  Anaplastic small (diffuse and compact) cell carcinoma[a]
  Squamous or adenosquamous carcinoma
  Mucinous carcinoma
  Clear-cell carcinoma

Lymphoid-cell origin
  Primary non-Hodgkin's lymphoma
  Plasmacytoma
  Hodgkin's lymphoma (rare)

Mesenchymal-cell origin
  Fibrosarcoma
  Osteogenic sarcoma
  Chondrosarcoma
  Hemangiosarcoma

Germ-cell origin
  Benign teratoma: infants
  Malignant teratoma: adults

Secondary (nonthyroidal) tumors

Distant spread by vascular or lymphatic routes
  Carcinomas: kidney, breast, lung, pancreas, melanoma, colon, ovary, bladder, vagina
  Lymphoproliferative: systemic nodal and extrathyroidal lymphomas, leukemia
  Sarcomas; Kaposi's sarcoma (AIDS); carcinosarcoma

Local extension from adjacent structures
  Larynx
  Esophagus
  Thyroglossal duct
  Parathyroid

---

[a] Most of the diffuse type are now recognized to be malignant lymphomas, and the remaining few are either compact medullary carcinomas or poorly differentiated insular follicular carcinomas.

Adapted, with permission, from Braverman LE, Utiger R (eds): The Thyroid: A Fundamental and Clinical Text, Philadelphia, JB Lippincott, 1991

tases; these are mostly ipsilateral, but bilateral and mediastinal lymph-node metastases may be encountered in a few patients. Distant metastases occur in less than 1% of patients at the time of presentation. The most common sites of metastasis, in decreasing order of frequency, are the lungs, bones, and other soft tissues.

Older patients have a higher risk for distant metastases. Most children and teenagers also present with a solitary nodule of the thyroid, but cervical node involvement is more common in this age group than in adults; up to 10% of children and adolescents may have lung involvement at the time of diagnosis.[13] The prognosis for patients who have received head and neck irradiation is similar to that of random cases, even though the former group may present with more extensive disease.[14]

Follicular thyroid carcinoma[15] occurs in older people, with peak incidence in the fifth decade of life. This disease occurs less often than papillary carcinoma, except perhaps in iodine-deficient areas or among patients with preexisting goiters. Follicular thyroid malignancies have a worse prognosis than papillary tumors, especially in patients with fixed/invasive lesions. Direct invasion of the strap muscles and trachea may occur and compromise resectability. Follicular tumors tend to metastasize to the lungs and bone (producing osteolytic lesions), often retain the ability to accumulate radioactive iodide, and can be treated with iodine.[13]

Invasion of the capsule and/or blood vessels is generally used to classify follicular neoplasms as malignant. Patient age over 50 years, tumor size larger than 3.9 cm, high tumor grade with high nuclear DNA content, presence of marked vascular invasion, adjacent tissue invasion, and distant metastases at diagnosis all are associated with increased cancer mortality.

The biology, natural history, and optimal therapy for Hürthle-cell carcinoma continues to generate debate because of persisting difficulties in the differentiation of benign from malignant lesions. While most lesions appear benign, without capsular invasion or vascular invasion, many are more aggressive, showing obvious invasion and having a pronounced tendency to recur in the neck years after the original resection. Therefore, aggressive surgery with thyroidectomy is generally recommended, especially for tumors greater than 2 cm, but controversy over this treatment approach remains.

Pulmonary metastases in differentiated thyroid carcinoma are often classified radiographically as either "micronodular" or "macronodular" disease. Micronodular metastases present a miliary, diffusely reticular pattern predominating in the lower lung fields, and tend to concentrate radioiodine diffusely. Macronodular (coarse) metastases with nodular masses of unequal size (varying between 0.5 cm and 3.0 cm) occur more frequently. Radioiodine incorporation is heterogeneous, but often not present. Transition from micro- to macronodular metastasis may occur during the course of the disease.

The most common clinical presentation of sporadic medullary thyroid cancer is a solitary thyroid mass found incidentally during routine examination. Most patients present in the fourth or fifth decades of life with a male:female ratio of 1.4:1.[5,16] Metastases to cervical and mediastinal lymph nodes are found in half of the patients and may be present at the time of initial presentation.

Distant metastases to the lungs, liver, bones, and adrenal glands most commonly occur late in the course of the disease. Secretory diarrhea, often severe, is the most prominent of the hormone-mediated clinical features of medullary carcinoma. Rarely, ectopic production of adrenocorticotropic hormone (ACTH) and/or corticotropin releasing hormone (CRH) may cause paraneoplastic Cushing's syndrome.

Anaplastic carcinoma, in sharp contrast to differentiated thyroid carcinomas, confers a dismal prognosis, with median survival time after diagnosis ranging from 4 to 12 months. Most studies show a 2-year survival rate close to 0%, and long-term survival of more than 5 years is rare. Anaplastic thyroid carcinoma is a locally and systemically aggressive disease, with better survival rates seen only in those patients with well-localized anaplastic tumors. Favorable prognostic features seem to be unilateral tumors, tumor size less than 5 cm, no invasion of adjacent tissue, and absence of nodal involvement. Anaplastic carcinoma most commonly presents as a rapid growth of a thyroid mass, frequently in a preexisting goiter. A history of a long-standing thyroid enlargement is noted in about 80% of the patients.

Therapeutic Options and Factors in Selecting Therapy

In patients with disease confined to the neck, surgical excision is the first treatment of choice. Postoperative examination with radioiodine scanning allows the identification of residual regional or distant foci of disease. Radioiodine can be used therapeutically to ablate such tumor deposits.[17] The thoroughness of thyroid resection and the optimal scheme for radioiodine surveillance and treatment remain subjects of discussion. In adults, cervical lymph-node metastases are associated with a higher incidence of recurrence but not with a diminished rate of survival.[18]

In a recent review of 101 patients with differentiated thyroid carcinoma and pulmonary metastases, Samaan et al analyzed potential prognostic factors and the efficacy of radioactive iodine treatment over time.[19] Uptake of radioactive iodine by lung metastases conferred a favorable prognosis, especially in patients with negative radiologic findings. The probability of radioactive iodine uptake was related to the degree of differentiation of the primary tumor. Pulmonary metastases were least common in patients with papillary carcinoma and most common in those with Hürthle-cell carcinoma. Patients less than 40 years old had a better prognosis than older patients. Patients under 20 years old with papillary and/or follicular thyroid cancer should have aggressive initial treatment because they tend to present with extensive regional disease and lymph-node metastases, and they have a high rate of tumor recurrence.[20]

For most patients with differentiated thyroid cancer, we recommend a near-total thyroidectomy with modified neck dissection as needed, followed by a postoperative iodine 131 scan and appropriate treatment. Following this initial program, thyroxine replacement therapy is prescribed, and patients are carefully followed up with regular physical examinations, chest radiographs, and serum thyroglobulin determinations. The optimal strategy for subsequent radioiodine scanning and/or therapy should be individualized. External irradiation has a limited role in this disease and should be reserved for locally invasive, carefully selected neoplasms that do not concentrate iodine. Systemic chemotherapy is required for certain cases of widespread disease, although available regimens have not been very effective to date.

In medullary thyroid carcinoma, the usual treatment is total thyroidectomy with careful cervical node examination and appropriate dissection. This approach is especially important for patients with familial disease, who are more likely to harbor bilateral disease. These patients should have a preoperative evaluation for possible coexisting pheochromocytoma; if the tumor is present, appropriate control of catecholamine hypersecretion should precede thyroid surgery.

For resectable lesions in anaplastic carcinoma, thyroid lobectomy with wide margins of adjacent soft tissue on the side of the tumor is appropriate. Total thyroidectomy and radical neck dissection result in an increased complication rate and are not likely to increase survival time in this disease. Radiotherapy and chemotherapy are important alternative approaches, but further evaluation is needed to optimize their effectiveness.[21]

PARATHYROID CARCINOMA

Incidence and Etiology

The prevalence of benign primary hyperparathyroidism has increased with the advent of multichannel autoanalyzers that permit the early detection of disease in asymptomatic patients. Nevertheless, the incidence of parathyroid carcinoma has not changed appreciably. This disease remains a rare cause of hypercalcemia; it is responsible for less than 2% of cases with primary hyperparathyroidism.[22] The etiology of parathyroid carcinoma is obscure. While regional head and neck irradiation is a significant factor in the genesis of parathyroid adenomas and benign hyperparathyroidism,[23] a similar association is not apparent for malignant parathyroid

disease.[24] Similarly, no association with prior iodine 131 exposure has been demonstrated.

Parathyroid carcinoma has rarely been reported in families with familial hyperparathyroidism. Thus, it may be prudent to screen the relatives of patients with parathyroid carcinoma for hypercalcemia to improve the chance of early diagnosis of parathyroid disease.

Clinical Presentation

Patients with parathyroid carcinoma tend to be younger than patients with benign hyperparathyroidism; the disease occurs with similar frequency in both sexes.[22] Most patients with malignant disease are symptomatic and have moderate to severe hypercalcemia (mean serum calcium level, 15 mg/dL; range, 10.0 to 24 mg/dL).[24] Parathyroid hormone levels are generally very elevated.

Involvement of peripheral target organs, such as kidneys or bone, is no longer considered characteristic of benign hyperparathyroidism, but is somewhat common in patients with functioning parathyroid cancer. Unlike patients with benign disease, patients with parathyroid carcinoma are more likely to have a palpable mass in the neck. Rare cases of nonfunctioning parathyroid carcinoma usually present as neck masses; their clinical course is similar to that in patients with functioning tumors.[25] Careful pathologic examination is needed to establish the diagnosis, but clinical concern about parathyroid cancer should be raised in patients with hyperparathyroidism who have a palpable neck mass and severe hypercalcemia, patients with recurrent hyperparathyroidism, or patients with associated unilateral vocal cord paralysis.

Parathyroid carcinoma is a slow-growing but tenacious malignancy, and the hypercalcemia it engenders may have catastrophic consequences.[26] The average time from initial surgery to the first recurrence is approximately 3 years but may be as long as 10 years. Local invasion of adjacent structures and lymph nodes can be present at initial operation. The thyroid gland is the most common site of involvement, followed by the recurrent laryngeal nerve, strap muscles, esophagus, and trachea. Distant metastases can be present at initial surgery; local spread to contiguous structures in the neck may be followed later by distant metastases to the lung, bone, and liver. Only 50% of patients are still alive 5 years after diagnosis. Death usually results from complications of the hypercalcemia rather than from the tumor burden.

Pathology

It is difficult to distinguish benign from malignant parathyroid tumors histologically. The principal features of this cancer include a trabecular pattern, mitotic figures, thick fibrous bands, and capsular or blood vessel invasion. Ultrastructural features of parathyroid carcinoma have been described, but these findings do not always help establish the diagnosis of malignancy. Other important features include lymphatic or hematogenous metastases and histologic evidence of tumor infiltration into the surrounding tissues (including macroscopic adherence or vocal cord paralysis).[27]

Although cytologic evidence of mitoses is necessary to confirm malignancy, mitotic activity alone is an unreliable indicator of such malignancy. On occasion, some highly differentiated tumors without distinct nuclear atypia are initially considered to be adenomas but are later reclassified when recurrence or metastases appear. On the other hand, a few parathyroid tumors may be classified as malignant because of their atypia, but neither metastasis nor relapse develops. One view is that the only reliable microscopic findings of malignancy are invasion of surrounding structures or metastasis to lymph nodes or other organs. Thus, ultimate diagnosis of parathyroid carcinoma can be made with confidence only after recurrence or metastatic spread occurs.

DNA aneuploidy determined by flow cytometry is a valuable adjunct marker in the diagnosis of malignancy and is associated with a poor prognosis.[28,29] Aneuploid parathyroid carcinomas are likely to show more malignant behavior than those with a diploid DNA pattern. It should be pointed out, however, that DNA aneuploidy may be found in some benign lesions. Therefore, this feature should be interpreted with caution.[30]

Adenomas can be subdivided into two groups—typical and atypical. If an atypical adenoma possesses one or more of the histologic features usually considered requisite for a diagnosis of parathyroid carcinoma or is grossly adherent to an adjacent structure at the time of operation, it might represent a case of low-grade parathyroid carcinoma. Patients with these tumors should be monitored more carefully than those with the typical benign form.

Treatment

Intraoperative identification of malignancy and appropriate initial surgery are critical in the therapy for parathyroid carcinoma. Because there is no evidence that preoperative localization studies shorten operating time or prevent surgical failures, these studies are not required during initial surgery.[31]

Resection of the tumor along with the ipsilateral lobe of the thyroid and abnormal central nodal tissue is indicated. A wide excision of locally recurrent tumor, an en bloc radical neck dissection and mediastinum dissection for lymphatic metastases, and an aggressive surgical resection of metastases whenever possible are recommended. Although these operations are not always curative, they usually offer palliation of the marked hypercalcemia for a considerable although variable period. Neck dissection is needed when there is evidence of regional node metastases.

After surgery, regular surveillance of serum calcium and parathyroid hormone (PTH) levels is essential. Thallium 201 isotope scanning has been used to aid in the localization of recurrent disease, but its reliability remains limited. Chest radiographs and computed tomographic (CT) scanning are useful for delineating pulmonary metastases. Isolated metastases may be resected to lengthen survival time and control hypercalcemia. As with benign, functioning parathyroid tumors, preoperative localization may be needed for patients who have had prior neck exploration.

Parathyroid carcinomas only rarely are located in the superior mediastinum or within the thymus. Putnam et al described a patient with mediastinal, nonfunctional parathyroid carcinoma that originated in the thymus and was treated with extended en bloc resection followed by prophylactic radiation therapy and chemotherapy.[32] Multiple metastases may not be amenable to surgical resection. Morbidity and mortality are generally caused by the effects of unremitting hypercalcemia rather than tumor growth. Medical treatments such as calcitonin, plicamycin (Mithracin), and bisphosphonates offer only temporary and palliative control of hypercalcemia.

Radiation therapy has not been very helpful in controlling primary and metastatic lesions,[22] nor has chemotherapy. In a case report of a patient who had parathyroid cancer metastatic to the lung and severe hypercalcemia (serum calcium level, 18.6 to 20.0 mg/dL), the combination of fluorouracil, cyclophosphamide (Cytoxan, Neosar), and dacarbazine resulted in complete remission for 5 months.[33] Because of the variable clinical course of this disease, it is important to individualize therapeutic strategies. Nevertheless, surgical resection where possible remains the most effective treatment for both local and metastatic disease.

ADRENAL GLAND NEOPLASMS

Adrenocortical Carcinoma

Epidemiology: Adrenocortical carcinoma is a rare and often highly malignant neoplasm that is usually diagnosed late in its course, resulting in short life expectancy for the patient. The etiology is unknown, but some cases have occurred in families with a hereditary cancer syndrome. The incidence is estimated at two per million population per year. Adrenocortical carcinoma accounts for about 0.2% of cancer deaths. Close to 50% of the tumors produce hormonal and metabolic syndromes that lead to their discovery.

Clinical Presentation: Approximately half of adrenocortical carcinomas are functioning and present with clinical features consistent with several syndromes of hormone hypersecretion (glucocorticoids, androgens, mineralocorticoids, and estrogens.[34] Thus, the symptoms and signs of Cushing's syndrome, virilizing or feminizing syndromes, and hyperaldosteronism may be the presenting features. The other 50% of the tumors are nonfunctioning, and are discovered as a result of metastases or when the primary tumor becomes large enough to produce abdominal symptoms. Smaller tumors may be discovered incidentally when unrelated abdominal complaints are investigated radiographically.[34,35] Nonfunctioning tumors occur predominantly in males and older patients, whereas functioning tumors are seen more frequently in women and younger patients.[36]

Cushing's syndrome is the most common clinical presentation for adults with functioning adrenocortical carcinoma. The clinical manifestations of excess cortisol are rapidly progressive and include weight gain, muscle weakness, easy bruising, irritability, insomnia, and centripetal obesity. The rare cases of Cushing's syndrome in children are often due to adrenal carcinoma. Obesity is the most common presenting sign, but it is more generalized than it is in adults because the effect on muscle tissue in the lower limbs is less evident in childhood.

Mixed syndromes, such as Cushing's and virilization, strongly suggest adrenal carcinoma. The combination of hirsutism, acne, amenorrhea, and rapidly progressing Cushing's syndrome in a young woman is a characteristic presentation. The androgen excess can moderate the severity of the catabolic effects of hypercortisolism. Skin and muscle atrophy, in particular, may not be as apparent in these patients.

In a male child who was normal at birth and who later develops precocious virilization, an adrenal carcinoma should be suspected. Similarly, in prepubertal girls, adrenocortical cancer represents a common cause of virilization. Feminization in the adult male, albeit rare, should immediately suggest adrenal carcinoma. In men, estrogen-secreting tumors are associated with gynecomastia, breast tenderness, testicular atrophy, impotence, and decreased libido. In women, estrogen-secreting tumors can cause tenderness and dysfunctional uterine bleeding; in prepubertal girls, precocious puberty may be seen.

Aldosterone-producing adrenocortical carcinomas are extremely rare, and the clinical manifestations are those of mineralocorticoid excess with hypertension and hypokalemia.

Treatment: Early diagnosis and complete surgical excision provide the best expectation for long-term survival, which is dismal overall. The survival rate for patients with adrenocortical cancer is 23% at 5 years and 10% at 10 years.[37] There is no significant difference between functioning and nonfunctioning tumors.

Since 1960, mitotane (o,p'-DDD [Lysodren]) has been one of only a few agents effective against adrenocortical carcinoma. Mitotane exerts a specific cytolytic effect on adrenocortical cells, and has been used to treat unresectable or metastatic adrenocortical carcinomas, both functioning and nonfunctioning. While reduction of hormone production can be obtained in two thirds of patients with functioning tumors, only 15% to 30% of patients have objective tumor regression, with a median duration of about 7 months.[38] Tumor regression is a more accurate indicator of clinical benefit, as steroid response merely reflects the action of mitotane on steroid biosynthesis. Because of the frequent recurrence of adrenal carcinoma, mitotane has been advocated for all patients after apparent complete surgical excision. However, the efficacy of adjuvant mitotane remains disappointing.[35,39] Although some patients achieve tumor regression with mitotane levels of 10 μg/mL, serum levels above 14 μg/mL are more often required; drug toxicity remains a difficult problem with such high doses.

Doxorubicin (Adriamycin, Rubex) has been of benefit in a limited number of patients. Innovative programs are clearly needed for this disease. Suramin, a sulfonated drug that is cytotoxic to human adrenocortical carcinoma cell lines, has been used with some benefit in the treatment of metastatic and inoperable adrenocortical cancer.[40] Postoperative irradiation of the tumor bed with wide margins has been found useful by some but not all investigators.[41] Effective palliation of metastatic disease, especially painful bone lesions, may be obtained with radiotherapy. Hormone hypersecretion can be controlled medically in most cases. The antifungal agents ketoconazole (Nizoral), aminoglutethimide (Cytadren), and metyrapone (Metopirone) are very effective in reducing steroid production and in palliating the often debilitating associated clinical symptoms. These drugs may be used alone or in conjunction with mitotane.

Adrenal Medulla Pheochromocytoma

Epidemiology and Incidence: Pheochromocytomas are catecholamine-secreting tumors that arise from chromaffin cells in the adrenal medulla or extra-adrenal sympathetic ganglia. They most commonly present with intermittent, episodic, or sustained hypertension and constitute a surgically correctable cause of hypertension in 0.1% to 1% of hypertensive persons.[42] The condition occurs in all age groups, but the peak incidence is the third to fifth decades. There is no sex predilection in adults, but in children, the disease is slightly more common in boys.

Approximately 10% of cases are inherited as an autosomal dominant trait, either independently or as a part of MEN type II; bilateral tumors are more common in this setting. In children, pheochromocytomas are rare but tend to be bilateral, because they are more likely to arise from inherited syndromes. Pheochromocytomas can be associated with other neuroectodermal disorders, such as neurofibromatosis, von Hippel-Lindau disease, cerebellar hemangioblastoma, Sturge-Weber's syndrome, and tuberous sclerosis.

Clinical Features: Pheochromocytomas can cause life-threatening cardiovascular disturbances by the release of excessive amounts of catecholamines. Patients with pheochromocytomas can present with a range of symptoms, from mild labile hypertension to a hypertensive crisis, myocardial infarction, or cerebral vascular accident,[43] any of which can result in sudden death. Hypertension is the most common manifestation of pheochromocytoma. The classic pattern of paroxysmal hypertension occurs in 30% to 50% of cases. Sustained hypertension, resembling essential hypertension, may also occur. In some cases, extreme fluctuations in blood pressure may be superimposed on sustained hypertension. In children with pheochromocytomas, the hypertension is most often sustained.

A characteristic presentation in adults includes "spells" of sudden intense headaches, pallor or flushing, tremors, apprehension, palpitations, hypertension, and diaphoresis. The paroxysms may last for a few minutes to several hours and may occur several times a day or much less frequently. The attacks can be precipitated by a particular body position, straining at stool, exercise, emotional distress, or anxiety. In the rare cases of pheochromocytoma of the urinary bladder, the paroxysm may be provoked by voiding and may be associated with micturition syncope. Some patients may present with angina pectoris or acute myocardial infarction caused by coronary artery spasm and increased myocardial oxygen demand. Orthostatic hypotension can result from diminished plasma volume and blunted sympathetic reflexes. Atrial and ventricular arrhythmias can be encountered. Congestive heart failure due to catecholamine cardiomyopathy and persistent hypertension, although rare, may occur.

The majority of patients with pheochromocytomas have mild weight loss, but obesity does not rule out the condition. Patients may have symptoms of hypermetabolism, such as heat intolerance, increased caloric requirements, or diaphoresis. Basal metabolic rate may be elevated, but thyroid function is normal. Some patients may have impaired glucose tolerance or deterioration of diabetic control; the altered carbohydrate metabolism is thought to be caused in part by the alpha-adrenergic effect of norepinephrine and epinephrine.

Patients may have cholelithiasis or severe constipation and abdominal distension caused by the inhibitory effect of catecholamines on gut motility. Paraneoplastic syndromes are occasionally present; Cushing's syndrome is seen most often and results from ectopic production of ACTH.[44] Other peptides of less clinical significance are produced, including somatostatin, calcitonin, oxytocin, and vasopressin. Polycythemia can be caused by excessive erythropoietin production or contraction of blood volume.

Diagnosis: The diagnosis of pheochromocytoma relies on an appropriate medical history and documentation of excessive catecholamine production.[45] Measurement of 24-hour urinary catecholamines and their metabolites, vanilmandelic acid (VMA) and metanephrine, is commonly used[46]; current methodology provides highly sensitive and reliable quantification of catecholamines. The metanephrine level is considered the most specific single test. Catecholamine measurements are very useful both for the initial diagnosis and for postoperative surveillance of patients with pheochromocytoma. It is important to remember that false-positive results may be caused by increased catecholamine excretion from severe physical or mental stress, or by certain medications. The VMA assay is the least specific and most susceptible to interfering substances.

Serum catecholamine measurements are more susceptible to false elevations due to stress-related physiologic fluctuations. The evaluation of serum catecholamines after clonidine suppression, however, provides a very useful diagnostic tool that is more convenient than urine collections. Dynamic provocative tests are very rarely indicated at this time.

Almost all pheochromocytomas are localized in the abdomen, mostly in the adrenal medulla. Other tumors tend to be localized in the posterior mediastinum, although they may occur in any distribution of the sympathetic ganglia. After the diagnosis is established biochemically, radiologic methods are used for preoperative localization of the lesion. At the present time, CT and magnetic resonance techniques are the most widely used.

Iodine 131 methyliodobenzylguanidine (^{131}I-MIBG) scintigraphy has recently become available and provides a "functional" image. This technique is most helpful in the detection of occult contralateral or extra-adrenal lesions. Positron emission tomography with hydroxyephedrine is a promising newer approach under investigation.[47]

Preoperative Medical Management: Patients undergoing surgical excision of pheochromocytoma must be adequately prepared to prevent hypertensive crises during the induction of anesthesia and manipulation of the tumor.[46] Phenoxybenzamine (Dibenzyline), an oral, long-acting, noncompetitive alpha-adrenoceptor-blocking agent, is a widely used, very helpful first drug. Propranolol, a beta-adrenoceptor blocker, is usually added after a few days to prevent tachycardia or arrhythmias. The tyrosine hydroxylase inhibitor metyrosine (Demser) may be added in patients whose hypertensive responses are not well controlled with alpha and beta blockers alone. It is important to remember that the use of beta blockers alone is hazardous, because they may precipitate a paradoxic rise in blood pressure. For inoperable tumors, a similar program with alpha-adrenoceptor and beta-adrenoceptor blockers as well as metyrosine can be used for chronic medical control.

Malignant Pheochromocytoma

Pheochromocytomas are rare tumors that are almost always benign. Only about 10% of these tumors are considered malignant. The histologic differentiation between benign and malignant lesions is extremely difficult and often impossible. Thus, specific diagnosis often must await the development of lymph node, hepatic, bone, or other distant metastases. Recurrent symptoms of pheochromocytoma, often many years after the original diagnosis, suggest the possibility of malignancy. Biochemical confirmation of recurrent catecholamine hypersecretion and localization of metastatic lesions with ^{131}I-MIBG scan constitute diagnostic proof.

The treatment of choice for malignant pheochromocytoma remains problematic. Chemotherapy using streptozocin (Zanosar)-based regimens or combined cyclophosphamide, vincristine, and dacarbazine programs have yielded promising responses.[48,49] Treatment with ^{131}I-MIBG has met with only limited success.[50] Radiotherapy can achieve significant palliation, especially for painful bone lesions. In most cases, uncontrolled catecholamine hypersecretion eventually escapes biochemical blockade, and fatal hypertensive crisis ensues. In those rare cases in which limited and resectable lesions can be identified, surgery can effect complete and lasting remission of the disease. Clearly, improved strategies for control of malignant pheochromocytoma are needed.

REFERENCES

1. Vassilopoulou-Sellin R: Management of papillary thyroid cancer. Oncology 9(2):145–151, 1995.

2. Boring G, Squires T, Tang T: Epidemiology of cancer, 1991. CA Cancer J Clin 41:19–36, 1991.

3. Fukunaga FH, Yatani R: Geographic pathology of occult thyroid carcinomas. Cancer 36:1095–1099, 1975.

4. Woolner LB, Beahrs OH, Black BM, et al: Classification and prognosis of thyroid carcinoma: A study of 885 cases observed in a thirty-year period. Am J Surg 102:354–394, 1961.

5. Bergholm U, Adami HO, Bergstrom R, et al: Clinical characteristics in sporadic and familial medullary thyroid carcinoma: A nationwide study of 249 patients in Sweden from 1959 through 1981. Cancer 63:1196–1204, 1989.

6. De Groot LJ, Paloyan E: Thyroid carcinoma and radiation, Chicago epidemic. JAMA 225:487–491, 1973.

7. Spitz MR, Sider LG, Newell GR: Ethnic patterns of thyroid cancer incidence in the United States 1973–1981. Int J Cancer 42:549–553, 1988.

8. Cooper DS, Axelrod L, De Groot LJ, et al: Congenital goiter and the development of metastatic follicular carcinoma with evidence for a leak of nonhormonal iodide: Clinical, pathological, kinetic, and biochemical studies and a review of the literature. J Clin Endocrinol Metab 52:294–306, 1981.

9. Ingbar SH, Filletti N, Vigneri R, et al: Role of the thyroid-stimulating antibodies of Graves' disease in the pathogenesis and course of thyroid cancer. Clin Res 35:646A, 1987.

10. Walfish PG, Rosen IB: Miscellaneous tumors of the thyroid in Braverman LE, Utiger RD (eds): The Thyroid, A Fundamental and Clinical Text, 6th Ed, pp 1184–1196. Philadelphia, JB Lippincott, 1991.

11. Nel CJC, Van Heerden JA, Goellner JR, et al: Anaplastic carcinoma of the thyroid: A clinicopathologic study of 82 cases. Mayo Clin Proc 60:51–58, 1985.

12. Gagel RF, Cote GJ: Decision making in multiple endocrine neoplasia type 2. Adv Endocrinol Metab 5:1–23, 1994.

13. Vassilopoulou-Sellin R, Klein MJ, Smith T, et al: Pulmonary metastases in children and very young adults with differentiated thyroid cancer. Cancer 71:1348–1352, 1993.

14. Samaan NA, Schultz PN, Ordonez NG, et al: A comparison of thyroid carcinoma in those who have and have not had head and neck irradiation. J Clin Endocrinol Metab 64:219–223, 1987.

15. Brennan MD, Bergstrahl EJ, Van Heerden JA, et al: Follicular thyroid cancer treated at the Mayo Clinic 1946 through 1970: Initial manifestations, pathologic findings, therapy and outcome. Mayo Clin Proc 66:11–22, 1991.

16. Saad MF, Ordonez NG, Rashid RK, et al: Medullary carcinoma of the thyroid: A study of the clinical features and prognostic factors in 161 patients. Medicine 63:319–342, 1984.

17. Samaan NA, Schultz PN, Hickey RC, et al: The results of various modalities of treatment of well-differentiated thyroid carcinoma: A retrospective review of 1599 patients. J Clin Endocrinol Metab 75:714–720, 1992.

18. McHenry CR, Rosen IB, Walfish PG: Prospective management of nodal metastases in differentiated thyroid cancer. Am J Surg 162:353–356, 1991.

19. Samaan NA, Schultz PN, Haynie TP, et al: Pulmonary metastasis of differentiated thyroid carcinoma: Treatment results in 101 patients. J Clin Endocrinol Metab 65:376–380, 1985.

20. Frankenthaler RA, Vassilopoulou-Sellin R, Cangir A, et al: Lymph node metastasis from papillary-follicular thyroid carcinoma in young patients. Am J Surg 160:341–343, 1990.

21. Ventatesh YSS, Ordonez NG, Schultz PN, et al: Anaplastic

carcinoma of the thyroid. Cancer 66:321–330, 1990.

22. Shane E, Bilezikian JP: Parathyroid carcinoma: A review of 62 patients. Endocrinol Rev 3:218–226, 1982.

23. Cohen J, Gierlowski TC, Schnider AB: A prospective study of hyperparathyroidism in individuals exposed to radiation in childhood. JAMA 264:581–584, 1990.

24. Obara T, Fujimoto Y: Diagnosis and treatment of patients with parathyroid carcinoma: An update and review. World J Surg 15:738–744, 1991.

25. Anderson BJ, Samaan NA, Vassilopoulou-Sellin R, et al: Parathyroid carcinoma: Features and difficulties in diagnosis and management. Surgery 94:906–915, 1983.

26. Sandelin K, Amer G, Bonderson L, et al: Prognostic factors in parathyroid cancer: A review of 95 cases. World J Surg 16:724–731, 1992

27. Altenahr E, Saeger W: Light and electron microscopy of parathyroid carcinoma: Report of three cases. Virchows Arch A Pathol Anat Histol 360:107–122, 1973.

28. Obara T, Fujimoto Y, Hirayama A, et al: Flow cytometric DNA analysis of parathyroid tumors with special reference to its diagnostic and prognostic value in parathyroid carcinoma. Cancer 65:1789–1793, 1990.

29. Obara T, Fujimoto Y, Kanaji Y, et al: Flow cytometric DNA analysis of parathyroid tumors: Implication of aneuploidy for pathologic and biologic classification. Cancer 66:1555–1562, 1990.

30. Joensuu H, Klemi PJ: DNA aneuploidy in adenomas of endocrine organs. Am J Pathol 132:145–151, 1988.

31. Doppman JL, Miller DL: Localization of parathyroid tumors in patients with asymptomatic hyperparathyroidism and no previous surgery. J Bone Miner Res 6:153–158, 1991.

32. Putnam JB, Schantz ST, Pugh WC, et al: Extended en bloc resection of a primary mediastinal parathyroid carcinoma. Ann Thorac Surg 50:138–140, 1990.

33. Bukowski RM, Sheelen L, Cunningham J, et al: Successful combination chemotherapy for metastatic parathyroid carcinoma. Arch Intern Med 144:399–400, 1984.

34. Luton JP, Cerdas S, Billand L, et al: Clinical features of adrenocortical carcinoma, prognostic factors, and the effect of mitotane therapy. N Engl J Med 322:1195–1201, 1990.

35. Vassilopoulou-Sellin R, Guinee VF, Klein MJ, et al: Impact of adjuvant mitotane on the clinical course of patients with adrenocortical cancer. Cancer 71:3119–3123, 1993.

36. Pommier RF, Brennan MF: An eleven-year experience with adrenocortical carcinoma. Surgery 112:963–971, 1992.

37. Venkatesh S, Hickey RC, Vassilopoulou-Sellin R, et al: Adrenal cortical carcinoma. Cancer 64:765–769, 1989.

38. Icard P, Chapnis Y, Andreassian B, et al: Adrenocortical carcinoma in surgically treated patients: A retrospective study of 156 cases by the French Association of Endocrine Surgery. Surgery 112:972–980, 1992.

39. Haak HR, Hermans J, Van de Velde CJH, et al: Optimal treatment of adrenocortical carcinoma with mitotane: Results in a consecutive series of 96 patients. Br J Cancer 69:947–951, 1994.

40. La Rocca RV, Stein CA, Danesi R, et al: Suramin in adrenal cancer: Modulation of steroid hormone production: Cytotoxicity in vitro and clinical antitumor effect. J Clin Endocrinol Metab 71:497–504, 1990.

41. Markoe AM, Serber W, Micaily B, et al: Radiation therapy for adjunctive treatment of adrenal cortical carcinoma. Am J Clin Oncol 14(2):170–174, 1991.

42. Beard CN, Sheps SG, Kurland LT, et al: Occurrence of pheochromocytoma in Rochester, Minnesota, 1950 through 1979. Mayo Clin Proc 58:802–804, 1983.

43. Bravo EL, Gifford RW: Pheochromocytoma: Diagnosis, localization, and management. N Engl J Med 311:1298–1303, 1984.

44. Spark RF, Connolly PB, Gluckin DS, et al: ACTH secretion from a functioning pheochromocytoma. N Engl J Med 301:416–418, 1979.

45. Stein PP, Black HR: A simplified diagnostic approach to pheochromocytoma: A review of the literature and report of one institution's experience. Medicine 70:46–66, 1990.

46. Samaan NA, Hickey RC, Shutts PE: Diagnosis, localization, and management of pheochromocytoma. Cancer 62:2451–2460, 1988.

47. Shulkin BL, Wieland DM, Schwaiger M, et al: PET scanning with hydroxyephedrine: An approach to the localization of pheochromocytoma. J Nucl Med 33:1125–1131, 1992.

48. Auerbuch SD, Steakley CS, Young RC: Malignant pheochromocytoma: Effective treatment with a combination of cyclophosphamide, vincristine, and dacarbazine. Ann Intern Med 109:267–273, 1988.

49. Schlumberger M, Gicquel G, Lumbroso J: Malignant pheochromocytoma: Clinical, histologic and therapeutic data in a series of 20 patients with distant metastases. J Endocrinol Invest 15:631–642, 1992.

50. Krempf M, Lumbroso J, Mornex R, et al: Use of [^{131}I] iodobenzylguanidine in the treatment of malignant pheochromocytoma. J Clin Endocrinol Metab 72:455–461, 1961.

CHAPTER 32

Malignant Melanoma: Biology, Diagnosis, and Management

Clay M. Anderson, MD, Jacques Tabacof, MD, *and* Sewa S. Legha, MD

Department of Melanoma/Sarcoma Medical Oncology
The University of Texas M. D. Anderson Cancer Center, Houston, Texas

Cutaneous malignant melanoma is a relatively common neoplasm. In the United States in 1995, an estimated 34,000 cases of melanoma will be diagnosed, and 7,200 persons will die of melanoma.[1] Early primary melanoma is highly curable, but once the disease becomes disseminated, it is nearly always fatal. The overall survival rate has more than doubled from 40% in the 1960s to more than 80% today, but this increase is attributable to earlier diagnosis rather than to treatment advances.[2] Treatment for locally advanced or metastatic melanoma has been largely unsatisfactory despite ongoing basic science research and innovative clinical approaches such as biotherapy, vaccines, and regional perfusion therapy. However, several new treatment strategies do show promise. This chapter reviews current epidemiologic and biologic aspects of melanoma, briefly describes the commonly used staging systems, and outlines therapeutic approaches for the different stages of disease, including metastatic melanoma.

EPIDEMIOLOGY

The lifetime incidence of malignant melanoma in the United States increased from 1 in 1,500 persons in 1935 to 1 in 105 persons in 1991, an increase greater than that for any other major cancer.[3] Malignant melanoma is currently the eighth most prevalent cancer in the United States.[1] It is a disease affecting persons of all ages, with a median age at diagnosis in the mid-40s.

Exposure to sunlight is an important risk factor for the development of malignant melanoma. Intermittent exposure, especially early in life, seems to be more important than simple cumulative exposure.[4] It is speculated that increased recreational exposure to the sun has contributed to the rising incidence of melanoma.

Epidemiologic studies have identified certain phenotypic factors consistently associated with increased risk for the development of malignant melanoma. These factors include blue, green, or gray eyes; blond or red hair; light complexion; freckles; sun sensitivity; and the tendency to burn rather than tan. Other significant risk factors include a family history of melanoma, a personal history of nonmelanoma skin cancer, an increased number of melanocytic nevi, and xeroderma pigmentosum.

Patients who have had one malignant melanoma are at increased risk for developing another; their risk is about 5%, compared with the approximately 1% lifetime risk of malignant melanoma in whites.[5]

Some malignant melanomas arise in "precursor" pigmented lesions, while others arise in normal-appearing skin. Two types of pigmented lesions have been reported to be precursors for malignant melanoma: congenital melanocytic nevi and dysplastic nevi, better known today as *atypical moles*.

Congenital melanocytic nevi contain nevus cells and are present at birth. They occur in 1% of newborns and are usually small (less than 1.5 cm) or medium-sized (1.5 to 19.9 cm). Whether small or medium congenital melanocytic nevi are associated with an increased risk for melanoma is still controversial. On the other hand, large congenital melanocytic nevi (20 cm or greater) are associated with a 6% lifetime risk of developing melanoma.[6]

Dysplastic nevi, or atypical moles, are acquired pigmented lesions of the skin that can occur in familial[7] and nonfamilial[8] settings. Patients with the dysplastic nevus syndrome have more than 100 moles, some of which have melanoma-like features (ie, asymmetry, border irregularity, and color variegation), and at least one mole larger than 8 mm in diameter.[9] The risk of malignant melanoma in people with this syndrome has been shown to be between 7- and 140-fold higher than that in the general population, with a family history of melanoma accounting for the higher figures.[10] Prospective close monitoring and early diagnosis may improve outcome in these high-risk individuals.

GENETICS

As the epidemiologic evidence indicates, there is definitely a genetic predisposition to malignant melanoma. In addition to polygenetic influences, there are also several syndromes of mendelian inheritance of a predisposition to melanoma. These syndromes include the classic familial atypical multiple mole melanoma (FAMMM) syndrome, non-FAMMM familial cutaneous malignant melanoma, xeroderma pigmentosum, and congenital nevocytic nevus syndrome.[11] Cannon-Albright et al demonstrated in a 1992 study that a series of kindreds with inherited malignant melanoma shared an abnormal genetic locus at the 9p13-p22 chromosomal region.[12] This same chromosomal region is frequently deleted or involved in translocations in sporadic melanomas. The locus has been mapped to the 9p21 area, cloned, and given the name multiple tumor-suppressor 1 (*MTS1*) gene.[13] This appears to be the same locus as a recently identified tumor-suppressor gene, *p16*.[14] The search is ongoing for other single or multiple "melanoma susceptibility genes."

Also of interest is work done to determine the genetic underpinnings of melanoma antigen expression. A recent article describes the mapping of the human melanoma antigen (*MAGE*) gene family to the chromosome region Xq27-qter. This finding raises the question of whether deletion of this gene in advanced melanoma might lead to resistance to immunotherapy.[15] It is hoped that research into the genetic determinants of melanoma will lead to advances in earlier diagnosis, targeted therapy, and gene therapy.

BIOLOGY

Melanocytes are cells of neural-crest origin that migrate to the skin and several other peripheral sites early during fetal development. They reside primarily in the basal layer of the epidermis and synthesize the pigment melanin, which is an important protective factor against the damaging effects of B-range ultraviolet light. Melanocyte-stimulating hormone is a pituitary hormone that supports the growth of melanocytes and causes increased production of melanin by the cells. The other major factor regulating melanocyte function is melatonin, an indole molecule that originates in the pineal gland and suppresses melanocyte function under conditions of decreased ambient light. Melanocytes respond to other paracrine growth factors as well, and malignant melanocytes produce growth factors themselves that may function in short autocrine loops to stimulate melanoma growth.[16] The neoplastic transformation of melanocytes gives rise to malignant melanoma.

A better understanding of melanoma biology was made possible in recent years by the development of tissue culture techniques and the establishment of cell lines from normal epidermal melanocytes and melanomas at different stages of progression.[17] It has been demonstrated that normal melanocytes require at least four mitogens to grow in culture media: insulin or insulin-like growth factor, fibroblast growth factor-alpha, melanocyte-stimulating hormone, and phorbol esters. In contrast, cell lines derived from intermediate stages of melanoma show successive loss of growth factor require-

ments, and metastatic melanomas proliferate in the absence of any exogenous proteins or phorbol esters.[16] These findings support the hypothesis that tumor cells produce autocrine growth factors and develop growth autonomy.

The importance of the microenvironment and cellular interactions in malignant melanoma biology has recently been recognized. Inhibition of growth of early-stage melanoma cell lines was observed when they were cocultured with dermal fibroblasts, whereas stimulation of growth was seen when cell lines derived from metastatic melanoma were cocultured with fibroblasts under the same conditions.[18] Identification of the factor or factors involved in modulating the growth of melanomas is an important area for research.

The mechanisms involved in melanoma invasion are being studied by several groups. Albelda et al[19] showed expression of the beta-3-integrin subunit by melanomas in vertical growth phase and by metastatic melanomas but not by benign melanocytes and radial-growth-phase melanomas. These data suggest the importance of integrin molecules in tumor invasion and their potential use as markers of melanoma cells entering the metastatic phase of tumor progression. Meissauer et al,[20] utilizing specific inhibitors of the fibrinolytic system, provided evidence that urokinase-type and tissue-type plasminogen activators also play a role in malignant melanoma invasion in vitro. Besides integrins and plasminogen-activating factors, other membrane-bound proteases[21] and oligosaccharidic structures[22] have been shown to participate in tumor invasion and are potential targets for new therapeutic modalities.

IMMUNOLOGY

Clinicians and researchers have long known that the interaction between the host immune system and melanoma is unique among human malignancies. The rare but intriguing phenomenon of spontaneous regression in malignant melanoma suggests an important role of the immune system in this disease. Histopathologic examination of primary (and sometimes metastatic) melanoma often reveals an active mononuclear inflammatory infiltrate and fibrosis. When these cells are invading within the melanoma mass, they are called *tumor infiltrating lymphocytes* (TIL). This phenomenon of an inflammatory infiltrate is sometimes called *pathologic regression*, and the prognostic importance of this finding is not yet clearly defined. Some evidence indicates that the presence of TIL may be a favorable prognostic factor in primary melanoma.[23]

A very important issue in tumor immunology concerns the mechanisms of immune response and tumor strategies to escape the immune system's surveillance, and much of the important work in these areas has been carried out in melanoma models. Elegant experiments by Pandolfi et al demonstrated loss of expression of HLA-A2 antigens in two melanoma cell lines accompanied by a lack of immunologic recognition by autologous lymphocytes.[24] Transfection of HLA-A2 complementary DNA partially restored the ability of autologous lymphocytes to destroy the corresponding melanoma cells. This work illustrates one of the mechanisms by which malignant melanoma may escape the immunologic system of the host.

In animal models, the role of cytotoxic T lymphocytes and natural killer (NK) cells in preventing the establishment of metastatic disease has been well defined.[25] However, the role of these cells in the natural history of human melanoma is less certain. NK cells seem to be present in metastatic melanoma specimens more frequently than in primary lesions.[26] Defects in NK activity in patients with metastatic disease have been described,[27] but a lack of correlation between NK activity and prognosis in melanoma patients also has been reported.[28] While HLA class I coexpression with cellular antigens is required for cytotoxic T-cell killing of melanoma cells, the ability of NK cells to kill melanoma is enhanced when down-regulation of class I antigens is induced by c-*myc* overexpression in melanoma cell lines.[29,30] Further investigation into the targets of both cellular and antibody-mediated immune responses to melanoma should lead to more sophisticated and less toxic treatment options.

TYPES OF MELANOMA

Major Subtypes

Malignant melanoma has four major subtypes with unique clinical features.[31]

Superficial spreading melanoma, which constitutes approximately 70% of melanomas, generally arises in a preexisting nevus. Early in its development, superficial spreading melanoma is a flat lesion with mixtures of deeply pigmented areas and amelanotic foci. As the lesion grows, the surface may become irregular, and the perimeter may show indentation.

Nodular Melanoma: The second most common pattern of growth (15% to 30%) is nodular melanoma. The lesion is typically blue-black and raised or dome-shaped, and it generally begins in uninvolved skin on the trunk, head, and neck areas. Nodular melanomas are more common in men and tend to arise in middle age. Five percent are amelanotic, and such lesions are frequently misdiagnosed. Nodular melanomas lack the radial growth phase typical of other melanomas and therefore have sharply demarcated borders. They are more aggressive and usually develop more rapidly than do superficial spreading melanomas.

Lentigo maligna melanoma, the third subtype, constitutes 4% to 10% of all melanomas and is typically located on the faces of older white women. The lesion's propensity to metastasize is small. In general, lentigo maligna melanomas are large (more than 3 cm), tan, flat lesions and are always associated with sun-related changes in the dermis and epidermis.

Acral Lentiginous Melanoma: The fourth type of malignant melanoma is the acral lentiginous variety. It occurs on the palms or soles or beneath the nail beds. However, not all plantar or solar melanomas are acral lentiginous lesions; a minority are superficial spreading or nodular melanomas. Acral lentiginous melanomas represent only 2% to 8% of melanomas in whites. In dark-skinned patients, such as blacks, Asians, and Hispanics, however, they account for 35% to 60% of melanomas. Acral lentiginous melanoma is primarily seen in older patients. Ulceration is commonly observed in this type of melanoma.

Of the four major subtypes of malignant melanoma, superficial spreading and lentigo maligna melanoma have the best survival rates, whereas nodular melanoma has the worst. However, when rates are adjusted for tumor thickness, there is no difference in 10-year survival rates between superficial spreading melanoma and nodular melanoma. The better prognosis associated with superficial spreading melanomas, therefore, seems to be related to the fact that they are thinner at the time of diagnosis. Lentigo maligna melanomas, on the other hand, have a better prognosis than the other growth patterns, even when matched by thickness.[32]

Less Common Subtypes

Three less common types of malignant melanoma deserve mention here because of their distinctive clinical presentations and poor prognoses.

Desmoplastic Melanoma: The first is desmoplastic melanoma, a melanocyte-derived neoplasm of the skin involving the epidermis but with a predominantly dermal tumor focus. Desmoplastic melanoma lesions are frequently amelanotic, involve deeper structures of the dermis, and have a tendency to track along peripheral nerve sheaths.[33] Survival is worse than for the common cutaneous melanomas, because dissemination occurs early in the natural history of desmoplastic melanomas.

Uveal Melanoma: Another special type of melanoma

TABLE I

Staging Systems for Melanoma

WHO stage	Extent of disease	AJCC stage	Extent of disease
I	Limited to the skin	IA	Localized lesion < 0.75 mm
		IB	Localized lesion 0.76–1.5 mm
II	Involved regional lymph nodes	IIA	Localized lesion 1.6–4.0 mm
		IIB	Localized lesion > 4.0 mm
III	Distant metastases present	III	Involved regional nodes or in-transit metastases
		IV	Distant metastases present

AJCC = American Joint Committee on Cancer
WHO = World Health Organization
Based on data from references 31 and 41.

TABLE 2

Ten-Year Survival Rates for Melanoma Patients by AJCC Stage

AJCC stage	10-year survival rate
I	85%
II	60%
III	20%
IV	< 5%

AJCC = American Joint Committee on Cancer
Based on data from reference 31.

is uveal (ocular) melanoma, a rare and clinically peculiar type of melanoma arising from the melanocytes of the pigmented uvea. This melanoma is curable when detected at an early stage. It may be observed when quite small, but at this stage is difficult to distinguish clinically from a benign nevus. Nonetheless, current opinion regards lesions greater than 2-mm thick as worrisome, and the smaller uveal melanoma lesions can be treated with local excision, photocoagulation, external-beam radiotherapy, or radioiodide plaque brachytherapy.[34] Enucleation is still recommended for larger lesions or when an increase in size or rate of growth is seen. Appropriate management of uveal nevi and small suspicious lesions

requires frequent follow-up by a qualified ophthalmologist or ocular oncologist. Unfortunately, most of the time, uveal melanoma presents at a more advanced stage, has an extremely poor prognosis, and has a propensity to metastasize to the liver.[35]

Mucosal Melanoma: The third clinically distinctive type of melanoma is the mucosal variant, which can arise in the mouth, anus, external or internal genital tract, upper respiratory tract, or elsewhere in the gastrointestinal tract. It also tends to present as advanced local disease and has an aggressive natural history leading to death. Mucosal melanomas seem to be less responsive to therapy than are the standard cutaneous types.[36]

DIAGNOSIS AND STAGING

Malignant melanoma should be suspected in any pigmented skin or mucosal surface lesion that changes in color or size, begins to itch, or bleeds spontaneously. The clinical characteristics that suggest malignancy include variegation in color; acquisition of red, white, or blue color in a previously brown or black lesion; border irregularity; and surface elevation.[37]

An elliptical excisional biopsy with a 2-mm margin of normal-appearing tissue is usually indicated for diagnostic purposes. Larger margins may be excessive for a benign condition and insufficient for treatment of a melanoma. Incisional or punch biopsies should be performed only when the amount of skin removed is critical because of lesion size or anatomic location. Such specimens should be taken from the clinically suspicious areas and should include a full thickness of skin and subcutaneous fat for adequate microstaging.

After a histopathologic diagnosis of malignant melanoma is made, the tumor must be staged to determine prognosis and treatment. Microstaging allows prognostic categorization of risk of relapse and survival. Tumor thickness is the single most important prognostic factor for patients with malignant melanoma limited to the primary site.[38]

Clark's levels of microinvasion reflect increasing depth of tumor penetration into the dermal layers and the subcutaneous fat.[39] Clark's level I indicates melanoma in situ; level II, invasion of the papillary dermis; level III, invasion of the papillary-reticular dermal interface; level IV, frank invasion of the reticular dermis; and level V, invasion of the subcutaneous tissue. In Breslow's microstaging system, the thickness of the lesion is measured with an ocular micrometer to determine the maximal vertical thickness of the melanoma.[40] Both systems are predictive of the risk of metastasis, but data from several institutions have shown that Breslow's thickness is a relatively more accurate and reproducible parameter than is Clark's level of invasion.

Two staging systems are commonly used for malignant melanoma. A simple and widely used three-stage system developed by the World Health Organization (WHO) categorizes patients on the basis of nodal and distant metastasis.[41] Stage I applies to melanoma localized to the primary site, stage II indicates the presence of regional lymph-node metastases, and stage III indicates metastatic spread of disease to distant organs. However, this staging system, although easy to remember, does not take into account tumor thickness, which is an important prognostic factor in malignant melanoma. Another limitation is that 85% or more of newly diagnosed cases of melanoma fall into stage I.

In view of the limitations of the WHO staging system, the American Joint Committee on Cancer (AJCC) developed a four-stage system incorporating tumor thickness as part of the staging criteria and dividing clinically localized melanomas into two stages according to the microstaging information. This system allows for a better distribution of metastatic risk and survival among the defined groups.[31] Table 1 compares the WHO and the AJCC staging systems for malignant melanoma.

PROGNOSIS

Table 2 shows the published survival rates for the various AJCC stages of malignant melanoma.[31] Survival relates directly to the eventual occurrence of disseminated disease and is not as yet thought to be influenced by treatment beyond surgical management of the primary lesion itself. It is hoped that treatment of advanced disease will be shown to affect survival in the future.

Survival can be predicted best by primary lesion thickness and by the presence of nodal or distant metastases as noted above, but some evidence suggests that measures of primary lesion progression, such as high mitotic rate, lack of tumor-infiltrating lymphocytes, and evidence of pathologic regression may influence prognosis independently.[42] Other well-known negative prognostic factors include ulceration of the primary lesion; location of the lesion on the head, neck, or back; and to a lesser extent, male sex.

TREATMENT OF PRIMARY MELANOMA

Because surgical management of the primary lesion is the only treatment known to affect survival, proper local treatment is crucial. An important question in the management of primary cutaneous melanoma is the appropriate width of the margins of excision.

A randomized prospective study sponsored by the WHO Melanoma Programme showed similar rates of disease-free and overall survival for patients with melanomas thinner than 2 mm excised with narrow margins (1 cm) or wide margins (3 cm). However, 4 of 305 patients with tumors thicker than 1 mm treated with narrow margins had local recurrences. The authors concluded that narrow excision with 1-cm margins is safe for melanomas thinner than 1 mm.[43]

Margins of 2 cm for tumors thicker than 1 mm have been shown in a large study by Balch et al to be adequate to control local recurrence, revising the previously held belief that margins of 3 to 5 cm were required for intermediate-thickness melanomas.[44] In this study, 486 melanoma patients with primary lesions between 1 and 4 mm thick were assigned randomly to receive 2- or 4-cm surgical margins. The outcomes in terms of local recurrence rate and development of in-transit metastases were not significantly different between the groups (0.8% vs 1.7% local recurrence and 2.1% vs 2.5% in-transit metastases, respectively). The best surgical margins for primary lesions thicker than 4 mm have yet to be determined, but for now, margins of 2 to 3 cm are considered prudent.

The role of prophylactic or elective lymph-node dissection in the management of primary malignant melanoma is controversial. Theoretically, removal of clinically normal lymph nodes bearing microscopic metastatic foci would improve prognosis. However, it is believed that patients with thick melanomas (greater than 4 mm) do not benefit from elective regional lymph-node dissection in view of the high likelihood that systemic metastasis has already occurred.[45] For thin melanomas (less than 1 mm), the low incidence of nodal metastasis does not justify the morbidity associated with lymph-node dissection.[46] However, for intermediate-thickness lesions (1 to 4 mm), nonrandomized studies have suggested a benefit from elective lymph-node dissection.[47,48]

Prospective, randomized studies that included patients with all tumor thicknesses, however, have failed to demonstrate improved survival among patients treated with immediate prophylactic node dissection, compared with those who underwent therapeutic node dissection at the time of clinically evident nodal metastases.[49] Ongoing randomized trials of patients with stage I melanoma of intermediate thickness should clarify the role of elective lymph-node dissection.[50]

In the meantime, an interesting new tool is available to help with the management of regional lymph nodes. A technique called *sentinel lymph-node mapping and resection* has been described by Morton et al.[51] The draining lymphatic vessels from a high-risk primary melanoma are identified by injecting dyes such as isosulfan blue and patent blue-V. The "sentinel" (first) lymph node that takes up the dye is surgically removed and subjected to histologic analysis. If this node is not involved with melanoma, there is a less than 5% chance that any lymph nodes in that drainage site are pathologically involved. This technique, after further study, may prove to be the best way to determine optimal surgical management of intermediate- and high-risk primary melanomas of the extremities with clinically uninvolved draining lymph nodes.

ADJUVANT THERAPY

Patients with metastatic involvement of the regional lymph nodes are best treated with therapeutic lymphadenectomy. Unfortunately, 60% to 70% of these patients will eventually have relapses, mainly in distant sites. Several adjuvant strategies have been employed in an attempt to improve the prognosis of these and other high-risk melanoma patients. As yet, they have not proved successful.

Levamisole (Ergamisol), a nonspecific immunostimulant, has been studied in the adjuvant setting with conflicting results. A randomized trial sponsored by the National Cancer Institute of Canada compared this agent alone, oral bacillus Calmette-Guérin (BCG) alone, BCG alternating with levamisole, and a no-adjuvant-treatment control arm. Compared with the control arm, patients treated with adjuvant levamisole showed a 29% reduction in recurrence and death.[52] This result contrasts with a randomized study by Spitler involving similar categories of patients but indicating that levamisole was ineffective as an adjuvant to surgery in high-risk patients with malignant melanoma.[53]

Among many negative studies of adjuvant chemotherapy or immunotherapy, a large randomized trial by the WHO Melanoma Programme did not show a benefit in terms of disease-free or overall survival from adjuvant dacarbazine, BCG, or both when compared with surgery alone for WHO stage II melanoma of any anatomic location and stage I melanoma of the trunk.[54] One prospective, nonrandomized trial of adjuvant therapy with the investigational agent vindesine (Eldisine) demonstrated a benefit in terms of disease-free survival and median survival in those receiving the drug after surgical lymphadenectomy, but the outcome in control patients was worse than expected.[55] One prospective, controlled, nonrandomized study of adjuvant chemohormonal therapy with tamoxifen, dacarbazine, cisplatin (Platinol), and carmustine (BiCNU) in 18 patients with high-risk stage III or completely resected stage IV disease showed no survival advantage in the treated patients, but showed a trend toward longer median disease-free survival.[56]

A polyvalent melanoma vaccine has also been studied in the adjuvant setting,[57] where it was shown in 55 stage II and stage III patients to be safe and to induce an immune response, but numbers were not large enough to assess treatment efficacy.

The use of isolated regional limb perfusion with melphalan (Alkeran) has also been studied in the adjuvant setting with conflicting results.[58] Multiple studies using normothermic and hyperthermic techniques showed slightly better disease-free survival than in historical controls, but there have been no randomized studies. In recent years, this technique has been studied more frequently for local recurrence, with encouraging results.[59,60] There are still no randomized studies, however. Technical complexity and expense make this treatment difficult to recommend without better data on efficacy.

The role of alpha interferon (IFN-α) in patients with surgically resected locoregional melanoma is being studied in two prospective, controlled randomized trials. A trial undertaken by the Eastern Cooperative Oncology Group using IFN-α at a dose of 20 million U/m^2/d given intravenously 5 days a week for 1 month, followed by 10 million U/m^2/d given subcutaneously 3 days a week for 11 months in patients with resected stage II or stage III disease has shown preliminary evidence of a modest benefit.[61] However, toxicity has been high in this trial. In contrast, a WHO study using IFN-α at a dose of 3 million U given subcutaneously three times per week for 3 years in stage III patients has reported no significant toxicity.[62] Preliminary results of this study also show a modest benefit in prolonging the time to disease progression.

Until these studies are published in peer-reviewed journals, the standard of care for patients with high-risk locoregional disease after definitive surgical treatment is still observation alone, because no form of adjuvant systemic or regional treatment has been established to have a beneficial role in prolonging survival. Patients at high risk for relapse should be encouraged to participate in clinical trials.

MANAGEMENT OF METASTATIC DISEASE

Malignant melanoma can metastasize to almost any organ in the body. The survival time for patients with metastatic disease ranges from 6 to 9 months when metastases are detected in multiple organ sites. Patients with metastases to skin, subcutaneous tissue, or distant lymph nodes have the longest survival, averaging 12 to 15 months. After regional lymph nodes, the lungs are the second most frequent initial site of relapse; patients with lung metastases have a median survival of 11 months.

TABLE 3

Selected Two-Drug Combination Chemotherapy Regimens for Advanced Melanoma

Study	Regimen	Number of patients	CR (%)	CR + PR (%)	Median response duration (mo)
Costanza et al[65]	Dacarbazine + semustine	122	9 (7)	18 (15)	4
Costanza et al[83]	Dacarbazine + dactinomycin	103	7 (7)	22 (21)	9
Avril et al[82]	Dacarbazine + fotemustine	63	9 (14)	21 (33)	> 6 (CRs only)
Vorobiof et al[80]	Dacarbazine + vindesine	46	2 (4)	8 (17)	5
Fletcher et al[81]	Dacarbazine + cisplatin	30	2 (7)	11 (37)	8

CR = complete response, PR = partial response   Adapted from Tabacof J, Legha SS: Malignant Melanoma: Current Concepts and Therapeutic Approaches, in Pazdur R (ed): Medical Oncology: A Comprehensive Review, p 366. PRR Inc, Huntington, NY, 1993.

Patients with liver, brain, or bone metastases have a median survival of only 3 to 4 months.[31]

Surgical removal of metastatic deposits can play an important role in the management of disseminated melanoma. The goal of surgical excision may be to render a patient free of disease by removing a solitary mass after systemic therapy or to provide relief from symptomatic disease in the palliative setting. In several series, resection of isolated metastases to the brain, lungs, gastrointestinal tract, skin, or subcutaneous tissues has resulted in overall 2-year survival rates ranging from 15% to 30% in selected patients, with some long-term survivors, especially among patients with solitary lung metastases.[31]

Radiotherapy plays a limited role in the management of metastatic melanoma. It is used mainly for palliation of central nervous system metastases or painful bone metastases and for control of pain and bleeding from recurrent unresectable cutaneous or lymph-node masses. More recently, use of the cobalt-60 gamma unit ("gamma knife") has shown encouraging results for long-term local control of brain metastases smaller than 2.5 to 3.0 cm in diameter.[63]

Single-Agent Chemotherapy

The only single agent approved for the treatment of melanoma is dacarbazine, which provides response rates of 15% to 20% but results in complete remission in less than 5% of treated patients. Responses have been observed mainly in soft tissues, ie, skin, subcutaneous tissue, lymph-node, and lung metastases, which are more responsive than metastatic deposits in the bones, liver, or central nervous system (these respond in less than 10% of patients). The responses obtained with this agent are usually short-lived, ranging from 3 to 6 months. Consequently, patients treated with dacarbazine have not experienced a significant increase in survival, which has generally ranged between 4 and 6 months.[64–66]

The nitrosoureas also have a significant but low level of antitumor activity in melanoma, with response rates around 15%.[65,67] This group of drugs includes carmustine, lomustine (CeeNu), and semustine (MeCCNU). Patients previously exposed to dacarbazine have an even lower rate of response to the nitrosoureas than untreated patients.[65] Fotemustine, a new nitrosourea, has recently been studied in Europe. A multicenter phase II study of 153 evaluable patients showed a 30% response rate in previously untreated patients and 24% overall. Responses were also observed in patients with brain metastases from melanoma.[68]

Other classes of chemotherapeutic agents with a low level of activity—10% to 20%—include the vinca alkaloids[69,70] and platinum compounds such as cisplatin and carboplatin.[71–73] The chemoprotectant agent ethiofos (WR-2721) may enhance the therapeutic index of platinum compounds, accounting for the total response rate of 53% in one small study (which has not been confirmed).[74]

Paclitaxel (Taxol), a new agent that acts on the microtubule assembly, has recently been studied in phase II trials.[75,76] Three complete responses and four partial responses were observed among 53 melanoma patients. Further exploration of this agent for the treatment of malignant melanoma may be warranted.

TABLE 4

Results With Selected Multidrug Combination Chemotherapy Regimens for Advanced Melanoma

Study	Regimen	Number of evaluable patients	CR (%)	CR + PR (%)	Median response duration (mo)
Verschraegen et al[93]	Cisplatin + vindesine + dacarbazine	92	4 (4)	22 (24)	5
Costanzi et al[79]	Dacarbazine +carmustine + hydroxyurea (BHD)	89	7 (8)	24 (27)	17
Seigler et al[84]	Lomustine + vincristine + bleomycin + dacarbazine (BOLD)	72	7 (10)	29 (40)	15
Johnson et al[89]	Bleomycin + vinblastine + cisplatin	50	3 (6)	11 (22)	4
Legha et al[91]	Cisplatin + vinblastine dacarbazine	50	2 (4)	20 (40)	9
Ringborg et al[90]	Cisplatin + vindesine + dacarbazine	36	3 (8)	15 (42)	4
Stables et al[87]	Lomustine + vindesine + bleomycin + dacarbazine (BELD)	34	6 (18)	14 (41)	> 6 (CRs only)
Nathanson et al[88]	Bleomycin + vinblastine + cisplatin	34	3 (9)	16 (47)	> 6

CR = complete response, PR = partial response   Adapted from Tabacof J, Legha SS: Malignant Melanoma: Current Concepts and Therapeutic Approaches, in Pazdur R (ed): Medical Oncology: A Comprehensive Review, p 366. PRR Inc, Huntington, NY, 1993.

A new lipid-soluble dihydrofolate reductase inhibitor, piritrexim isethionate (taken orally), produced a response rate of 23% in 31 evaluable patients.[77] Interestingly, responses were seen in previously treated patients as well as in previously untreated patients. Piritrexim appears to be more active than methotrexate and deserves further investigation in the treatment of melanoma.

Combination Chemotherapy

Based on the independent activity of dacarbazine and the nitrosoureas, several studies combining the two types of agents were performed in the late 1970s. However, these studies failed to show superiority of the combination over dacarbazine alone.[65,78] Dacarbazine has also been combined with dactinomycin (Cosmegen),[79] vinca alkaloids,[80] cisplatin,[81] and fotemustine.[82] The observed response rates with the two-drug combinations have ranged from 20% to 25%, which are not significantly superior to the rate with dacarbazine alone. The exception is fotemustine, which produced a response rate of 33% when combined with dacarbazine. Table 3 summarizes the results with selected two-drug combination regimens that include dacarbazine.

Combinations of three or more drugs, with or without dacarbazine, have also been investigated. A three-drug combination regimen of carmustine, hydroxyurea, and dacarbazine tested by the Southwest Oncology Group produced an overall response rate of 27% in 178 patients, with response duration averaging 6 months.[83] A regimen combining bleomycin (Blenoxane), vincristine (Oncovin), lomustine, and dacarbazine (BOLD), developed in the late 1970s at Duke University, produced a 40% total response rate, with a 9% complete response rate in 91 previously untreated patients.[84] Subsequent studies of the BOLD regimen have had less impressive results, with total response rates ranging from 4% to 20%.[85,86] However, one European study that substituted vindesine for vincristine demonstrated a response rate of 41%.[87]

A number of combination chemotherapy regimens without dacarbazine were studied in the late 1970s and early 1980s. The most promising was a combination of bleomycin, vinblastine, and cisplatin, which produced response rates ranging from 22% to 43% in several trials.[88,89]

Most recently, several groups have reported activity with a combination of dacarbazine, cisplatin, and a vinca alkaloid (either vinblastine or vindesine).[90–93] The response rates achieved with this three-drug combination have ranged from 24% to 45%, which are superior to those reported with dacarbazine alone. However, formal prospective, controlled studies have not been performed to confirm the apparent superiority of this regimen. Results with selected multiagent chemotherapy regimens are summarized in Table 4.

Hormonal Therapy

Hormonal manipulation in melanoma has been studied since the 1970s. The role of tamoxifen in the treatment of melanoma is controversial. As a single agent, this nonsteroidal antiestrogen has produced an objective response rate of only 6%.[94] However, a recent Italian study[95] comparing dacarbazine alone with the combination of dacarbazine and tamoxifen for metastatic melanoma reported a superior response rate (28% vs 12%) and longer median survival (48 weeks vs 29 weeks) favoring the chemohormonal arm. The additional benefit of tamoxifen was seen primarily among women.

Similarly, a regimen of tamoxifen, dacarbazine, carmustine, and cisplatin first studied in 1984 showed a response rate of 55% and a complete response rate of 20% in 20 patients with metastatic disease.[96] In addition, a report from McClay et al[97] showed a higher response rate with this combination (51%) than with the chemotherapy agents alone (10%). However, the survival rates were not significantly different in this trial because of early relapse in the central nervous system in the responding patients. This regimen, initially developed at Dartmouth University (hence, the Dartmouth regimen), is used quite widely in the community because of its high response rate in the initial studies. It has also been shown to produce a high response rate (55%) in patients with metastatic disease that progressed after prior therapy with interleukin-2 (IL-2, aldesleukin [Proleukin]).[98]

Another trial assessed the effectiveness of tamoxifen added to high-dose cisplatin and dacarbazine but failed to show an additional benefit.[99] Trials of combination chemotherapy and tamoxifen are shown in Table 5.[100]

Megestrol acetate was added to the Dartmouth regimen in one trial and produced a total response rate of 47% in 19 patients.[101] The rationale for using megestrol in this trial was the possible abrogation of chemotherapy resistance and prevention of treatment-related cachexia.

Another hormonal maneuver that has been studied is daily oral melatonin, the melanocyte-suppressive hormone of pineal origin that has been shown to have growth-suppressive, immune-stimulatory, and oncostat-

TABLE 5

Results With Selected Combination Chemotherapy/Tamoxifen Regimens for Advanced Melanoma

Study	Regimen	Number of evaluable patients	CR (%)	CR + PR (%)	Median response duration (mo)
McClay et al[97]	Dacarbazine + carmustine + cisplatin + tamoxifen	45	5 (11)	23 (51)	--
Fierro et al[100]	Dacarbazine + carmustine + cisplatin + tamoxifen	32	5 (16)	15 (47)	7
Buzaid et al[99]	Dacarabazine + cisplatin + tamoxifen	23	2 (9)	3 (13)	4
Del Prete et al[96]	Dacarbazine + carmustine cisplatin + tamoxifen (Dartmouth regimen)	20	4 (20)	11 (55)	--
Richards et al[98]	Dacarbazine + carmustine cisplatin + tamoxifen	20	0	11 (55)	2

CR = complete response, PR = partial response

TABLE 6

Activity of Recombinant Alpha Interferon Against Advanced Melanoma

Study	Interferon type	No. of patients	CR (%)	CR + PR (%)
Creagan et al[111]	alfa-2a	96	4 (4)	21 (22)
Robinson et al[108]	alfa-2b	63	2 (3)	7 (11)
Legha et al[110]	alfa-2b	62	1 (2)	5 (8)
Kirkwood et al[109]	alfa-2b	23	3 (13)	5 (22)

CR = complete response, PR = partial response   Adapted from Tabacof J, Legha SS: Malignant Melanoma: Current Concepts and Therapeutic Approaches, in Pazdur R (ed): Medical Oncology: A Comprehensive Review, p 367. PRR Inc, Huntington, NY, 1993.

TABLE 7

Activity of Recombinant Interleukin-2 (IL-2) Against Advanced Melanoma

Study	Number of patients	CR (%)	CR + PR (%)
IL-2 alone			
Parkinson et al[113]	46	2 (4)	10 (22)
McCabe et al[114]	45	2 (4)	7 (16)
Rosenberg et al[112]	23	0	6 (26)
IL-2 + LAK cells			
McCabe et al[114]	49	3 (6)	6 (12)
Rosenberg et al[112]	34	3 (9)	6 (18)
Dutcher et al[115]	32	0	6 (19)

CR = complete recovery, LAK = lymphokine-activated killer, PR = partial response   Adapted from Tabacof J, Legha SS: Malignant Melanoma: Current Concepts and Therapeutic Approaches, in Pazdur R (ed): Medical Oncology: A Comprehensive Review, p 367. PRR Inc, Huntington, NY, 1993.

ic properties in animal models. Melatonin treatment produced a 15% response rate with no toxic effect except fatigue in 40 patients with metastatic disease.[102] This interesting drug deserves further investigation, especially as a modulator of chemotherapy response.

High-Dose Chemotherapy With Autologous Bone Marrow Transplantation

High-dose chemotherapy with either single or multiple agents followed by autologous bone marrow transplantation for metastatic melanoma has produced high rates of response, ranging from 20% to 81%.[103–105] Complete response rates have ranged from 0% to 6%, with some additional patients being rendered free of disease after surgical resection of isolated sites of disease. However, the responses have been short-lived, with very few long-term survivors, and the treatment is accompanied by severe toxic effects and even death.

This treatment strategy has also been used in the adjuvant setting after lymphadenectomy in a randomized trial of immediate treatment with high-dose cyclophosphamide (Cytoxan, Neosar), cisplatin, and carmustine with marrow rescue, compared with the same treatment at the time of relapse, in 39 patients with high-risk regional disease.[106] Median time to progression was prolonged in the immediate treatment group, but median survival did not differ between the two groups.

Use of growth factors may reduce the toxicity associated with high-dose chemotherapy treatment and also may support dose escalation without bone marrow transplantation.

Biologic Therapy

Nonspecific immunotherapy, including BCG and *Corynebacterium parvum* treatments, has been used for decades in the treatment of malignant melanoma, although it has had only minimal impact on the natural history of the disease. Recently, the availability of lymphokines, such as the interferons and IL-2, produced by means of recombinant DNA technology, has rekindled interest in biologic therapy (immunotherapy) for malignant melanoma and other neoplasms.

Interferons: Initial studies of partially purified human leukocyte-derived interferon showed that it stimulated T-helper/inducer subsets of lymphocytes and increased NK cell activity[107] but had only minimal activity against melanoma. Subsequently, several groups studied recombinant interferons alfa-2a (Roferon-A) and alfa-2b (Intron A) at different dosages and schedules for the treatment of advanced melanoma, and observed response rates of 10% to 20%.[78] Four large studies of interferon in patients with advanced melanoma are summarized in Table 6.[108,109] The response rates in untreated patients ranged from 8% to 22%, which is similar to the activity produced by dacarbazine. However, interferon's well-known systemic toxicity limits its use in patients already debilitated by cancer.

Studies from The University of Texas M. D. Anderson Cancer Center showed that more than half of patients cannot tolerate interferon doses larger than 20 million U/m²/d. Lower doses of 10 million U/m² given three times a week were shown to have equal activity but to be better tolerated.[110] The greatest antitumor effects of interferon were obtained with long-term administration on a daily or three-times-weekly basis, whereas very few patients responded to once-weekly doses or 5-day courses every 3 weeks.[78]

Interferon has been used with equal efficacy in previously untreated and previously treated patients, in whom alternative chemotherapy is rarely effective. In a small proportion of melanoma patients, the disease has been controlled with interferon for periods in excess of 2 to 3 years.[111] The frequency of response to interferon is somewhat higher for soft-tissue metastases than for disease at other distant sites. Nonetheless, responses have been observed in lung and liver metastases as well.

Interleukin-2: The second biologic agent to show activity against metastatic melanoma was IL-2, a cytokine also known as T-cell-derived growth factor, which mediates the activation and expansion of effector lymphocytes after antigen exposure. In initial studies performed at the National Cancer Institute, six partial responses were obtained among 23 patients treated with IL-2 alone.[112] The combination of IL-2 with lymphokine-activated killer (LAK) cells, which are autologous lymphocytes activated by IL-2 ex vivo, resulted in three complete responses and three partial responses among 34 patients with metastatic disease.[112] More recent trials using bolus doses of IL-2 obtained modest response rates of 16% to 22%, which are not superior to the activity of single-agent chemotherapy. Table 7 summarizes trials using IL-2 alone and in combination with LAK cells for advanced melanoma.[113–115]

The bolus administration of IL-2 in initial trials was accompanied by severe toxic effects. Constitutional symptoms, capillary leak syndrome, and deaths occurred.[113] Continuous infusion of IL-2 was associated with decreased toxicity, and apparently maintained IL-2's potent immunomodulatory effects and ability to induce clinical responses. The continuous infusion schedule is therefore preferred, and the usual dose is 12 to 18 million $IU/m^2/d$ for 5 days.

IFN-α and IL-2 have also been used in combination by some investigators. In 1992, Sznol et al reported on the use of combined IL-2/LAK cells and IFN-α as immunomodulation along with low-dose cyclophosphamide and doxorubicin (Adriamycin, Rubex) in 40 patients with metastatic disease. There were six responders, but only one response was long-term.[116]

Keilholz et al compared two dosing schedules of IFN-α followed by IL-2 in 54 patients.[117] They found an improved response rate (41% vs 18%) when the IL-2 infusion was "front-loaded," ie, given as a peaking high-dose infusion over the first 42 hours with very-low-dose infusion for the rest of the 5 days, as opposed to being given as a constant-dose 5-day infusion. The toxicity of IL-2 was also reduced when given in this fashion.

Home subcutaneous therapy with IL-2 and IFN-α has also been attempted, with quite mild toxic effects, but tumor responses in the heavily pretreated patients were disappointing.[118] A phase III randomized trial reported in 1993 compared high-dose bolus IL-2 alone with the same IL-2 dose combined with concurrent IFN-α. This trial demonstrated low response rates not improved by the addition of IFN-α (5% vs 10% in the IL-2 and IL-2-plus-IFN-α groups, respectively) in 85 patients with advanced melanoma.[119] Overall, the results with cytokine therapy for metastatic melanoma have not been significantly better than those with combination chemotherapy.

Biochemotherapy

The term *biochemotherapy* applies to the combined use of biologic and chemotherapeutic agents. This treatment strategy has been studied with the hope that the two treatments used sequentially or concurrently might improve the response rates achieved with either therapy alone, without excessive additional toxicity.

The initial studies of biochemotherapy for malignant melanoma combined the most active chemotherapy agent, dacarbazine, with IFN-α. In a trial reported by Bajetta et al, among 75 evaluable patients with metastatic melanoma, 8% complete responses and 17% partial responses were observed, suggesting improved activity with the combination.[120] In contrast, an international multicenter randomized trial comparing the combination of IFN alfa-2b and dacarbazine with either agent alone was not able to confirm the superiority of the combined treatment over dacarbazine alone. However, the trial was closed prior to full patient accrual.[121]

A recently reported Australian multicenter randomized trial also failed to show a superior response rate with the combination of dacarbazine and IFN-α over dacarbazine alone.[122] In contrast to these negative results, a trial conducted in South Africa by Falkson et al obtained a notable response rate of 53% with combined dacarbazine and IFN alfa-2b.[123] In this trial, IFN alfa-2b was given intravenously 5 days a week for 3 weeks prior to starting dacarbazine, and then subcutaneously three times a week along with dacarbazine at a standard dosage. Median time to treatment failure and median survival were significantly longer with the biochemotherapy combination than with dacarbazine alone. Most important, a recently published multicenter randomized trial with 236 patients compared dacarbazine alone with dacarbazine and two different doses of IFN-α.[124] The response rates, in the range of 25%, did not differ among the arms, but response duration was longer in the IFN-α groups.

Stoter et al[125] and Flaherty et al[126] used a similar

strategy with dacarbazine and IL-2, and demonstrated response rates of 24% in 25 patients[125] and 22% in 32 patients.[126] More disappointing results were seen in a Southwest Oncology Group study using this combination, which produced no responses in 13 patients,[127] and in a trial by Fiedler et al, which produced two responses in 16 patients.[128] LAK cells added to this treatment strategy did not produce a more favorable response rate.[129] However, a trial by Khayat et al combining IFN-α and IL-2 with cisplatin did achieve a better response rate in 39 patients, with a 12% complete response rate and a 54% total response rate.[130] Lastly, the addition of intravenous BCG or *C parvum* extract to combination chemotherapy also has failed to produce a greater benefit.[131,132]

In summary, inconsistent clinical results have been seen with the addition of immunotherapy to single-agent chemotherapy. Overall, no additive benefit has been demonstrated, especially in the one large randomized trial.[124]

Because of these less than satisfactory results, a more intensive approach incorporating IL-2 and IFN-α with multiagent chemotherapy has recently been studied by several groups. At M. D. Anderson Cancer Center, since October 1990 we have been studying IL-2 and IFN-α given alternately or concurrently with the combination of cisplatin, vinblastine, and dacarbazine (CVD) for patients with metastatic malignant melanoma. Although administration of IL-2 by continuous infusion requires

TABLE 8
Results of Selected Biochemotherapy Regimens for Advanced Melanoma

Study	Regimen	Number of patients	CR (%)	CR + PR (%)
Chemotherapy + IFN				
Thomson et al[122]	Dacarbazine + IFN alfa-2a	87	6 (7)	18 (21)
	Dacarbazine	83	2 (2)	14 (17)
Bajetta et al[120]	Dacarbazine + IFN alfa-2a	75	6 (8)	19 (25)
Falkson et al[123]	Dacarbazine + IFN alfa-2b	30	12 (40)	16 (53)
	Dacarbazine	34	0 (0)	6 (18)
Chemotherapy + IL-2				
Atkins et al[136]	Dacarbazine + cisplatin + tamoxifen + IL-2	38	3 (8)	16 (42)
Flaherty et al[137]	Dacarbazine + cisplatin + IL-2	32	5 (16)	13 (41)
Flaherty et al[125]	Dacarbazine + IL-2	32	1 (3)	7 (22)
Dillman et al[129]	Dacarbazine + IL-2 + LAK cells	27	2 (7)	7 (26)
Chemotherapy + IFN + IL-2				
Richards et al[135]	Carmustine + dacarbazine + cisplatin + tamoxifen + IL-2 + IFN alfa-2a	42	10 (24)	24 (57)
Khayat et al[132]	Cisplatin + IL-2 + IFN-α	39	5 (13)	21 (54)
Legha et al[134]	Cisplatin + vinblastine + dacarbazine (CVD) + IL-2 + IFN alfa-2a	155	26 (17)	85 (55)

CR = complete response, PR = partial response, IFN = interferon, IL = interleukin, LAK = lymphokine-activated killer   Adapted from Tabacof J, Legha SS: Malignant Melanoma: Current Concepts and Therapeutic Approaches, in Pazdur R (ed): Medical Oncology: A Comprehensive Review, p 368. PRR Inc, Huntington, NY, 1993.

hospitalization, the CVD chemotherapy can be given in the outpatient clinic. Among 30 evaluable patients, preliminary results were 6 complete responses and 11 partial responses, for an overall response rate of 56%.[133] Since that time, a total of 155 patients have been treated with either sequential or concurrent biochemotherapy, with a complete response rate of 17% and a total response rate of 55%.[134] This regimen has been accompanied by severe multisystem toxicity, including myelosuppression, capillary leak syndrome, and renal and gastrointestinal toxic effects, limiting its applicability only to patients who have good performance status.

Results of a similar approach using sequential chemotherapy and immunotherapy were reported by the University of Chicago group. The chemotherapy regimen comprised carmustine, dacarbazine, cisplatin, and tamoxifen. IL-2 was given on a bolus schedule along with IFN alfa-2a. The reported response rate in 42 consecutive patients was 57%, with a complete response rate of 24%.[135]

Another biochemotherapy regimen using cisplatin and dacarbazine with high-dose IL-2 given in the inpatient setting achieved a complete response rate of 8% and a total response rate of 42% in 38 patients,[136] and a strategy using the same chemotherapy and IL-2 given in an outpatient setting produced very similar results (response rate, 42%; complete response rate, 9%).[137] Lastly, the protocol of Khayat et al used in 39 heavily pretreated patients could be considered as aggressive as these regimens, with a similar high response rate.[132] These aggressive regimens seem to increase complete and overall response rates significantly with only moderate and mostly manageable additional toxic effects. However, a survival benefit has not yet been shown conclusively. Table 8 summarizes the results of the major biochemotherapy studies.

Melanoma Vaccines and Monoclonal Antibodies

Vaccine therapy can be categorized into several types, including autologous melanoma cell preparations, allogeneic cell fraction preparations, purified melanoma antigens, and anti-idiotypic antibodies, which mimic melanoma antigens. Another consideration is the carrier or adjuvant in which the vaccine is delivered. Vaccine development for melanoma and other malignant tumors has progressed steadily in recent years, but a definite clinical benefit has yet to be demonstrated.

Morton et al have published the results of their whole-cell, polyvalent, allogeneic melanoma cell vaccine with BCG as an adjuvant in 136 patients.[138] Among 40 patients with evaluable disease, there were nine responders. The treated patients had a longer median survival than did historical controls, and survival was correlated with measures of an immune response to the vaccine.

An autologous vaccine studied in 64 patients by Berd et al was given after a cyclophosphamide dose, with BCG used as an adjuvant.[139] The response rate was 12%, and response correlated with the development of a cellular immune response to the vaccine. Some patients responded after initial disease progression.

Mitchell et al used an allogeneic lysate vaccine and a novel adjuvant called DETOX in 20 patients with metastatic disease, and demonstrated a 16% response rate.[140]

Anti-idiotypic antibodies (monoclonal antibodies directed against the variable region of antimelanoma antigen antibodies, thereby mimicking the antigen itself) have also been used as vaccines, with little toxicity and demonstration of a humoral immune response, but low response rates.[141] In addition to the anti-idiotypic antibodies, other monoclonal antibodies have been used as well.[142] Most of these agents have been directed against glycolipid antigens, which are preferentially expressed on melanocytes and melanoma. Some responses have been seen, and toxicity has not been a major problem. Further work is in progress.

FUTURE PROSPECTS

Despite rapid advances in our understanding of melanoma, there are still many more questions than answers. There is still no standard adjuvant treatment for patients with high-risk primary melanoma or effective treatment of newly diagnosed metastatic disease. It is hoped that improved treatment options will come with continued basic science investigation and well-designed clinical trials to test the efficacy of new regimens and compare results of alternative therapies.

An important issue likely to be resolved by ongoing trials is whether adjuvant IFN-α will decrease relapse rates and increase survival for patients with intermediate- and high-risk locoregional melanoma. Another crucial question, currently being studied at M. D. Anderson Cancer Center, is whether aggressive neoadjuvant biochemotherapy will improve outcome for high-risk patients with locoregional disease. The appropriate role of vaccines and the tools to assess immunologic responses are still being defined. The development of new pharmacologic agents using the molecular-mechanistic approach holds promise. Finally, gene therapy for melanoma, though still in the early stages of development, may allow a less toxic, more specific alternative to today's cytotoxic and biologic treatments.

CONCLUSIONS

Despite substantial improvements in survival rates in recent decades, the incidence of malignant melanoma and the associated absolute mortality are rising. The increase in survival is attributable entirely to earlier diagnosis. Efforts to treat metastatic disease have had minimal impact on survival. Initial excitement created by the first results with biologic therapy has been tempered by associated severe toxicities. Ongoing clinical research in the areas of biochemotherapy, melanoma vaccines, and new cytotoxic drugs offers hope of better therapy in the near future.

Recent developments in the understanding of tumor biology may someday translate into a significant benefit for patients. For now, efforts should be focused on primary prevention—avoidance of excessive solar exposure and use of sun protection—and secondary prevention programs emphasizing the importance of early diagnosis. Patients with advanced disease should be encouraged to participate in clinical trials.

REFERENCES

1. Wingo P, Tong T, Bolden S: Cancer statistics, 1995. CA Cancer J Clin 45:8–30, 1995.

2. Sober A: Cutaneous melanoma: Opportunity for cure. CA Cancer J Clin 41:197–199, 1991.

3. Ries L, Hankey B, Miller B, et al: Cancer Statistics Review 1973–1988. Bethesda, Md, National Cancer Institute, 1991.

4. Lew R, Sober A, Cook N, et al: Sun exposure habits in patients with cutaneous melanoma: A case control study. J Dermatol Surg Oncol 9:981–986, 1983.

5. Friedman R, Rigel D, Silverman M, et al: Malignant melanoma in the 1990s: The continued importance of early detection and the role of physician examination and self-examination of the skin. CA Cancer J Clin 41:201–226, 1991.

6. Rhodes A, Wood W, Sober A, et al: Non-epidermal origin of malignant melanoma associated with a giant congenital nevocellular nevus. Plast Reconstr Surg 67:782–790, 1981.

7. Clark WJ, Reimer R, Greene M, et al: Origin of familial malignant melanoma from heritable melanocytic lesions: "The B-K mole syndrome." Arch Dermatol 114:732–738, 1978.

8. Elder D, Goldman L, Goldman S, et al: Dysplastic nevus syndrome: A phenotypic association of sporadic cutaneous melanoma. Cancer 46:1787–1794, 1980.

9. Tiersten A, Grin C, Kopf A, et al: Prospective follow-up for malignant melanoma in patients with the atypical-mole (dysplastic nevus) syndrome. J Dermatol Surg Oncol 17:44–48, 1991.

10. Hoffman S, Yohn J, Robinson W, et al: Melanoma: 1. Clinical characteristics. Hosp Pract 15:35–46, 1994.

11. Lynch H, Fusaro R: Hereditary malignant melanoma: A unifying etiologic hypothesis. Cancer Genet Cytogenet 20:301–304, 1986.

12. Cannon-Albright L, Goldgar D, Meyer L, et al: Assignment of a locus for familial melanoma, MLM, to chromosome 9p13-p22. Science 258:1148–1152, 1992.

13. Hussussain C, Struewing J, Goldstein A, et al: Germline p16 mutations in familial melanoma. Nat Genet 8:15–21, 1994.

14. Kamb A, Gruis N, Weaver-Feldhaus J, et al: A cell cycle regulator potentially involved in genesis of many tumor types. Science 264:436–440, 1994.

15. Oaks M, Hanson JJ, O'Malley D: Molecular cytogenetic mapping of the human melanoma antigen to chromosome Xq27-qter: Implications for MAGE immunotherapy. Cancer Res 54:1627–1629, 1994.

16. Rodeck U, Herlyn M: Growth factors in melanoma. Cancer Met Rev 10:89–101, 1991.

17. Menrad A, Herlyn M: Tumor progression, biology and host response in melanoma. Curr Opin Oncol 4:351–356, 1992.

18. Cornil I, Theodorescu D, Man S, et al: Fibroblast cell interactions with human melanoma cells affect tumor cell growth as a function of tumor progression. Proc Natl Acad Sci USA 88:6028–6032, 1991.

19. Albelda S, Mette S, Elder D, et al: Integrin distribution in malignant melanoma: Association of the beta-3 subunit with tumor progression. Cancer Res 50:6757–6764, 1990.

20. Meissauer A, Kramer M, Hofmann M, et al: Urokinase-type and tissue-type plasminogen activators are essential for in vitro invasion of human melanoma cells. Exp Cell Res 192:453–459, 1991.

21. Aoyama A, Chen W-T: A 170-kDa membrane-bound protease is associated with the expression of invasiveness by human malignant melanoma cells. Proc Natl Acad Sci USA 87:8296–8300, 1990.

22. Seftor R, Seftor E, Grimes W, et al: Human melanoma cell invasion is inhibited in vitro by swainsonine and deoxymannojirimycin with a concomitant decrease in collagenase IV expression. Melanoma Res 1:43–45, 1991.

23. Mackensen A, Carcelain G, Viel S, et al: Direct evidence to support the immunosurveillance concept in a human regressive melanoma. J Clin Invest 93:1397–1402, 1994.

24. Pandolfi F, Boyle L, Trentin L, et al: Expression of HLA-A2 antigen in human melanoma cell lines and its role in T-cell recognition. Cancer Res 51:3164–3170, 1991.

25. Markovic S, Murasko D: Role of natural killer and T-cells in interferon induced inhibition of spontaneous metastases of the B16F10L murine melanoma. Cancer Res 51:1124–1128, 1991.

26. Kornstein M, Stewart R, Elder D: Natural killer cells in the host response to melanoma. Cancer Res 47:1411–1412, 1987.

27. Muller C, Pehamberger H, Binder M, et al: Defective interferon-augmented natural killer cell activity in patients with metastatic malignant melanoma. J Cancer Res Clin Oncol 115:393–396, 1989.

28. Hersey P, Edwards A, Milton G, et al: No evidence for an association between natural killer cell activity and prognosis in melanoma patients. Nat Immun Cell Growth Reg 3:87–94, 1984.

29. Peltenburg L, Steegenga W, Kruse K, et al: c-myc-induced natural killer cell sensitivity of human melanoma cells is reversed by HLA-B27 transfection. Eur J Immunol 22:2737–2740, 1992.

30. Versteeg R, Peltenburg L, Plomp A, et al: High expression of the c-myc oncogene renders melanoma cells prone to lysis by natural killer cells. J Immunol 143:4331–4337, 1989.

31. Balch C, Houghton A, Peters L: Cutaneous melanoma, in DeVita VT Jr, Hellman S, Rosenberg SA (eds): Cancer: Principles and Practice of Oncology, 4th ed, pp 1612–1614. Philadelphia, JB Lippincott, 1993.

32. Urist M, Balch C, Soong S-J, et al: Head and neck melanoma in 536 clinical stage I patients: A prognostic factors analysis and results of surgical treatment. Ann Surg 200:769–775, 1984.

33. Jain S, Allen P: Desmoplastic malignant melanoma and its variants. Am J Surg Pathol 13:358–373, 1989.

34. Hungerford J: Uveal melanoma. Eur J Cancer 29A:1368–1372, 1993.

35. Shields J: Management of uveal melanoma: A continuing dilemma. Cancer 72:2067–2068, 1993.

36. Cooper P, Mills S, Allen M: Malignant melanoma of the anus: Report of 12 patients and analysis of 255 additional cases. Dis Colon Rectum 25:693–703, 1982.

37. Wick M, Sober A, Fitzpatrick T, et al: Clinical characteristics of early cutaneous melanoma. Cancer 45:2684–2686, 1980.

38. Balch C, Soong S-J, Shaw H, et al: An analysis of prognostic factors in 8500 patients with cutaneous melanoma, in Balch C, Houghton A, Milton G, et al (eds): Cutaneous Melanoma, 2nd ed, pp 165–187. Philadelphia, JB Lippincott, 1992.

39. Clark WJ, From L, Bernardino E, et al: The histogenesis and biologic behavior of primary human malignant melanomas of the skin. Cancer Res 29:705–726, 1969.

40. Breslow A: Thickness, cross-sectional areas and depth of invasion in the prognosis of cutaneous melanoma. Ann Surg 182:572–575, 1975.

41. Goldsmith H: Melanoma: An overview. CA Cancer J Clin 29:194, 1979.

42. Clark WJ, Elder D, DuPont GI, et al: Model predicting survival in stage I melanoma based on tumor progression. J Natl Cancer Inst 81:1893–1904, 1989.

43. Veronesi U, Cascinelli N: Narrow excision (1-cm margin): A safe procedure for thin cutaneous melanoma. Arch Surg 126:438–441, 1991.

44. Balch C, Urist M, Karakousis C, et al: Efficacy of 2-cm surgical margins for intermediate-thickness melanomas (1 to 4 mm): Results of a multi-institutional randomized surgical trial. Ann Surg 218:262–267, 1993.

45. Crowley N, Seigler H: The role of elective lymph node dissection in the management of patients with thick cutaneous melanoma. Cancer 66:2522–2527, 1990.

46. Balch C: The role of elective lymph node dissection in melanoma: Rationale, results, and controversies. J Clin Oncol 6:163–172, 1988.

47. Balch C, Soong S-J, Milton G, et al: A comparison of prognostic factors and surgical results in 1,786 patients with localized (stage I) melanoma treated in Alabama, USA, and New South Wales, Australia. Ann Surg 196:677–684, 1982.

48. Drepper H, Kohler C, Bastian B, et al: Benefit of elective lymph node dissection in subgroups of melanoma patients: Results of a multicenter study of 3616 patients. Cancer 72:741–749, 1993.

49. Sim F, Taylor W, Pritchard D, et al: Lymphadenectomy in the management of stage I malignant melanoma: A prospective randomized study. Mayo Clin Proc 61:697–705, 1986.

50. Cady B: "Prophylactic" lymph node dissection in melanoma: Does it help? J Clin Oncol 6:2–4, 1988.

51. Morton D, Wen D, Wong J, et al: Technical details of intraoperative lymphatic mapping for early stage melanoma. Arch Surg 127:392–399, 1992.

52. Quirt I, Shelley W, Pater J, et al: Improved survival in patients with poor-prognosis malignant melanoma treated with adjuvant levamisole: A phase III study by the National Cancer Institute of Canada clinical trial group. J Clin Oncol 9:729–735, 1991.

53. Spitler L: A randomized trial of levamisole versus placebo as adjuvant therapy in malignant melanoma. J Clin Oncol 9:736–740, 1991.

54. Veronesi U, Adamus J, Aubert C, et al: A randomized trial of adjuvant chemotherapy and immunotherapy in cutaneous melanoma. N Engl J Med 307:913–916, 1982.

55. Retsas S, Quigley M, Pectasides D, et al: Clinical and histologic involvement of regional lymph nodes in malignant melanoma: Adjuvant vindesine improves survival. Cancer 73:2119–2130, 1994.

56. Saba H, Cruse C, Wells K, et al: Adjuvant chemotherapy in malignant melanoma using dacarbazine, carmustine, cisplatin, and tamoxifen regimens: A University of South Florida and H. Lee Moffitt Melanoma Center study. Ann Plast Surg 28:60–64, 1992.

57. Bystryn J-C, Oratz R, Harris M, et al: Immunogenicity of a polyvalent melanoma vaccine in humans. Cancer 61:1065–1070, 1988.

58. Cumberlin R, De Moss E, Lassus M, et al: Isolation perfusion for malignant melanoma of the extremity: A review. J Clin Oncol 3:1022–1031, 1985.

59. Baas P, Schrafford Koops H, Haekstra H, et al: Isolated regional perfusion in the treatment of melanoma of the extremities. Reg Cancer Treat 1:33–36, 1988.

60. Hafstrom L, Rudenstam C, Blomquist E, et al: Regional hyperthermic perfusion with melphalan after surgery for recurrent malignant melanoma. J Clin Oncol 9:2091–2094, 1991.

61. Kirkwood J, Hunt M, Smith T, et al: A randomized controlled trial of high-dose IFN alpha-2b for high-risk melanoma: The ECOG trial EST-1684 (abstract). Proc Am Soc Clin Oncol 12:390, 1993.

62. Cascinelli N, Bufalino R, Morabito A, et al: Results of adjuvant interferon study in WHO Melanoma Programme (letter). Lancet 343:913–914, 1994.

63. Coffey R, Flickinger J, Bissonette D, et al: Radiosurgery for solitary brain metastases using the cobalt-60 gamma unit: Methods and results in 24 patients. Int J Radiat Oncol Biol Phys 20:1287–1295, 1991.

64. Carbone P, Costello W: Eastern Cooperative Oncology Group studies with DTIC (NSC-45388). Cancer Treat Rep 60:193–198, 1976.

65. Costanza M, Nathanson L, Schoenfeld D, et al: Results with methyl-CCNU and DTIC in metastatic melanoma. Cancer 40:1010–1015, 1977.

66. Nathanson L, Walter J, Horton J, et al: Characteristics of prognosis and response to an imidazole carboxamide in malignant melanoma. Clin Pharmacol Ther 12:955–962, 1971.

67. Ramirez G, Wilson W, Grage T, et al: Phase II evaluation of 1,3-bis(2-chloroethyl)-1-nitrosourea (BCNU, NSC-409962) in patients with solid tumors. Cancer Treat Rep 56:787–790, 1972.

68. Jacquillat C, Khayat D, Banzet P, et al: Final report of the French multicenter phase II study of the nitrosourea fotemustine in 153 evaluable patients with disseminated malignant melanoma including patients with cerebral metastases. Cancer 66:1873–1878, 1990.

69. Retsas S, Peat I, Ashford R, et al: Updated results of vindesine as a single agent in the therapy of advanced malignant melanoma. Cancer Treat Rev 7(suppl):87–90, 1980.

70. Quagliana J, Stephens R, Baker L, et al: Vindesine in patients with metastatic malignant melanoma: A Southwest Oncology Group study. J Clin Oncol 2:316–319, 1984.

71. Mechl Z, Krejci P: Cis-diaminedichloroplatinum in the treatment of disseminated malignant melanoma. Neoplasma 30:371–377, 1983.

72. Chang A, Hunt M, Parkinson D, et al: Phase II trial of carboplatin in patients with metastatic malignant melanoma: A report from the Eastern Cooperative Oncology Group. Am J Clin Oncol 16:152–155, 1993.

73. Evans L, Casper E, Rosenbluth R: Phase II study of carboplatin in advanced malignant melanoma. Cancer Treat Rep 71:171–172, 1987.

74. Glover D, Glick J, Weiler C, et al: WR-2721 and high-dose cisplatin: An active combination in the treatment of metastatic melanoma. J Clin Oncol 5:574–578, 1987.

75. Legha S, Ring S, Papadopoulos N, et al: A phase II trial of Taxol in metastatic melanoma. Cancer 65:2478–2481, 1990.

76. Einzig A, Hochster H, Wiernik P, et al: A phase II study of

Taxol in patients with malignant melanoma. Invest New Drugs 9:59–64, 1991.

77. Feun L, Gonzalez R, Savaraj N, et al: Phase II trial of piritrexim in metastatic melanoma using intermittent, low-dose administration. J Clin Oncol 9:464–467, 1991.

78. Legha S: Current therapy for malignant melanoma. Semin Oncol 16:34–44, 1989.

79. Costanzi J, Fletcher W, Balcerzak S, et al: Combination chemotherapy plus levamisole in the treatment of disseminated malignant melanoma. Cancer 53:833–836, 1984.

80. Vorobiof D, Sarli R, Falkson G: Combination chemotherapy with dacarbazine and vindesine in the treatment of metastatic malignant melanoma. Cancer Treat Rep 70:927–928, 1986.

81. Fletcher W, Green S, Fletcher J, et al: Evaluation of cisplatin and DTIC combination chemotherapy in disseminated melanoma: A Southwest Oncology Group study. Am J Clin Oncol 11:589–593, 1988.

82. Avril M, Bonneterre J, Delaunay M, et al: Combination chemotherapy of dacarbazine and fotemustine in disseminated malignant melanoma: Experience of the French Study Group. Cancer Chemother Pharmacol 27:81–84, 1990.

83. Costanzi J, Vaitkevicius V, Quagliana J, et al: Combination chemotherapy for disseminated melanoma. Cancer 35:342–346, 1975.

84. Seigler H, Lucas V, Pickett N, et al: DTIC, CCNU, bleomycin and vincristine (BOLD) in metastatic melanoma. Cancer 46:2346–2348, 1980.

85. York R, Foltz A: Bleomycin, vincristine, lomustine, and DTIC chemotherapy for metastatic melanoma. Cancer 61:2183–2186, 1988.

86. Franco E, for the Prudente Foundation Melanoma Study Group: Chemotherapy of disseminated melanoma with bleomycin, vincristine, CCNU, and DTIC (BOLD regimen). Cancer 63:1676–1680, 1989.

87. Stables G, Doherty V, MacKie R: Nine years' experience of BELD combination chemotherapy (bleomycin, vindesine, CCNU, and DTIC) for metastatic melanoma. Br J Dermatol 127:505–508, 1992.

88. Nathanson L, Kaufman S, Carey R, et al: Vinblastine infusion, bleomycin, and cis-dichlorodiammineplatinum chemotherapy in metastatic melanoma. Cancer 48:1290–1294, 1981.

89. Johnson D, Presant C, Einhorn L, et al: Cisplatin, vinblastine, and bleomycin in the treatment of metastatic melanoma: A phase II study of the Southeastern Cancer Study Group. Cancer Treat Rep 69:821–824, 1985.

90. Ringborg U, Jungnelius U, Hansson J, et al: DTIC-vindesine-cisplatin in disseminated malignant melanoma: A phase II study (abstract). Proc Am Soc Clin Oncol 6:212, 1987.

91. Legha S, Ring S, Papadopoulos N, et al: A prospective evaluation of a triple-drug regimen containing cisplatin, vinblastine, and dacarbazine (CVD) for metastatic melanoma. Cancer 64:2024–2029, 1989.

92. Pectasides D, Yianniotis H, Alevizakos N, et al: Treatment of metastatic malignant melanoma with dacarbazine, vindesine, and cisplatin. Br J Cancer 60:627–629, 1989.

93. Verschraegen C, Kleeberg U, Mudler J, et al: Combination of cisplatin, vindesine, and dacarbazine in advanced malignant melanoma: A phase II study of the EORTC Malignant Melanoma Cooperative Group. Cancer 62:1061–1065, 1988.

94. Nesbit R, Woods R, Tattersall M, et al: Tamoxifen in malignant melanoma. N Engl J Med 301:1241–1242, 1979.

95. Cocconi G, Bella M, Calabresi F, et al: Treatment of metastatic melanoma with dacarbazine plus tamoxifen. N Engl J Med 327:516–523, 1992.

96. Del Prete S, Maurer L, O'Donnell J, et al: Combination chemotherapy with cisplatin, carmustine, dacarbazine, and tamoxifen in metastatic melanoma. Cancer Treat Rep 66:1403–1405, 1984.

97. McClay E, Mastrangelo M, Berd D, et al: Effective combination chemo/hormonal therapy for malignant melanoma: Experience with three consecutive trials. Int J Cancer 50:553–556, 1992.

98. Richards J, Gilewski T, Ramming K, et al: Effective chemotherapy for melanoma after treatment with interleukin-2. Cancer 69:427–429, 1992.

99. Buzaid A, Murren J, Durivage H: High-dose cisplatin with dacarbazine and tamoxifen in the treatment of metastatic melanoma. Cancer 68:1238–1241, 1991.

100. Fierro M, Bertero M, Novelli M, et al: Therapy for metastatic melanoma: Effective combination of dacarbazine, carmustine, cisplatin and tamoxifen. Melanoma Res 3:127–131, 1993.

101. Nathanson L, Meelu M, Losada R: Chemohormone therapy of metastatic melanoma with megestrol acetate plus dacarbazine, carmustine, and cisplatin. Cancer 73:98–102, 1994.

102. Gonzales R, Sanchez A, Ferguson J, et al: Melatonin therapy of advanced human malignant melanoma. Melanoma Res 1:237–243, 1991.

103. Wolff S, Herzig R, Fay J, et al: High-dose thiotepa with autologous bone marrow transplantation for metastatic malignant melanoma: Results of phase I and II studies of the North American Bone Marrow Transplantation Group. J Clin Oncol 7:245–249, 1989.

104. Shea T, Antman K, Eder J, et al: Malignant melanoma: Treatment with high-dose combination alkylating agent chemotherapy and autologous bone marrow support. Arch Dermatol 124:878–884, 1988.

105. Thatcher N, Lind M, Morgenstern G, et al: High-dose, double alkylating agent chemotherapy with DTIC, melphalan, or ifosfamide and marrow rescue for metastatic malignant melanoma. Cancer 63:1296–1302, 1989.

106. Meisenberg B, Ross M, Vredenburgh J, et al: Randomized trial of high-dose chemotherapy with autologous bone marrow support as adjuvant therapy for high-risk, multi-node-positive malignant melanoma. J Natl Cancer Inst 85:1080–1085, 1993.

107. Karavodin L, Golub S: Systemic administration of human leukocyte interferon to melanoma patients: III. Increased helper:suppressor ratios in melanoma patients during interferon treatment. Nat Immun Cell Growth Reg 3:193–202, 1984.

108. Robinson W, Kirkwood J, Harvey H, et al: Effective use of recombinant human alfa 2 interferon (IFN alfa2) in metastatic malignant melanoma (MMM): A comparison of two regimens (abstract). Proc Am Soc Clin Oncol 3:60, 1984.

109. Kirkwood J, Ernstoff M, Davis C, et al: Comparison of intramuscular and intravenous recombinant alpha-2a interferon in melanoma and other cancers. Ann Intern Med 103:32–36, 1985.

110. Legha S, Papadopoulos N, Plager C: Clinical evaluation of recombinant interferon alfa-2A (Roferon-A) in metastatic melanoma using two different schedules. J Clin Oncol 5:1240–1246, 1987.

111. Creagan E, Ahmann D, Frytak S: Phase II trials of recombinant leukocyte alpha interferon in disseminated malignant melanoma: Results in 96 patients. Cancer Treat Rep 70:619–624, 1986.

112. Rosenberg S, Lotze M, Mule J: New approaches to the immunotherapy of cancer using interleukin-2. Ann Intern Med 108:853–864, 1988.

113. Parkinson D, Abrams J, Wiernik P, et al: Interleukin-2 therapy in patients with metastatic malignant melanoma: A phase II study. J Clin Oncol 8:1650–1656, 1990.

114. McCabe M, Stablein D, Hawkins M, et al: The modified group C experience-phase III randomized trials of IL-2 vs IL-2/LAK in advanced renal cell carcinoma and advanced melanoma (abstract). Proc Am Soc Clin Oncol 10:213, 1991.

115. Dutcher J, Creekmore S, Weiss G, et al: Phase II study of high dose interleukin-2 (IL-2) and lymphokine-activated killer (LAK) cells in patients with melanoma (abstract). Proc Am Soc Clin Oncol 6:246, 1987.

116. Sznol M, Clark J, Smith J, et al: Pilot study of interleukin-2 and lymphokine-activated killer cells combined with immunomodulatory doses of chemotherapy and sequenced with interferon alfa-2a in patients with metastatic melanoma and renal cell carcinoma. J Natl Cancer Inst 84:929–937, 1992.

117. Keilholz U, Scheibenbogen C, Tilgen W, et al: Interferon-alpha and interleukin-2 in the treatment of malignant melanoma: Comparison of two phase 2 trials. Cancer 72:607–614, 1993.

118. deBraud F, Biganzoli L, Bajetta E, et al: Subcutaneous low-dose interleukin-2 plus alpha interferon in advanced melanoma. Tumori 79:187–190, 1993.

119. Sparano J, Fisher R, Sunderland M, et al: Randomized phase III trial of treatment with high-dose interleukin-2 alone or in combination with interferon alfa-2a in patients with advanced melanoma. J Clin Oncol 11:1969–1977, 1993.

120. Bajetta E, Negretti E, Giannotti B, et al: Phase II study of interferon alpha-2a and dacarbazine in advanced melanoma. Am J Clin Oncol 13:405–409, 1990.

121. Kirkwood J, Ernstoff M, Giuliano A, et al: Interferon alpha 2a and dacarbazine in melanoma. J Natl Cancer Inst 82:1062–1063, 1990.

122. Thomson D, Adena M, McLeod G, et al: Interferon-alfa-2a does not improve response or survival when combined with dacarbazine in metastatic malignant melanoma: Results of a multi-institutional Australian randomized trial. Melanoma Res 3:133–138, 1993.

123. Falkson C, Falkson G, Falkson H: Improved results with the addition of interferon alfa-2a to dacarbazine in the treatment of patients with metastatic malignant melanoma. J Clin Oncol 9:1403–1408, 1991.

124. Bajetta E, Di Leo A, Zampino M, et al: Multicenter randomized trial of dacarbazine alone or in combination with two different doses and schedules of interferon alfa-2a in the treatment of advanced melanoma. J Clin Oncol 12:806–811, 1994.

125. Stoter G, Aamdal S, Rodenhuis S, et al: Sequential administration of recombinant human interleukin-2 and dacarbazine in metastatic melanoma: A multicenter phase II study. J Clin Oncol 9:1687–1691, 1991.

126. Flaherty L, Redman B, Chabot G, et al: A phase I-II study of dacarbazine in combination with outpatient interleukin-2 in metastatic malignant melanoma. Cancer 65:2471–2477, 1990.

127. Flaherty L, Liu P, Fletcher W, et al: Dacarbazine and outpatient interleukin-2 in treatment of metastatic malignant melanoma: A phase II Southwest Oncology Group trial. J Natl Cancer Inst 84:893–894, 1992.

128. Fiedler W, Jasmin C, De Mulder P, et al: A phase II study of sequential recombinant interleukin-2 followed by dacarbazine in metastatic melanoma. Eur J Cancer 28:443–446, 1992.

129. Dillman R, Oldham R, Barth N, et al: Recombinant interleukin-2 and adoptive immunotherapy alternated with dacarbazine therapy in melanoma: A National Biotherapy Study Group trial. J Natl Cancer Inst 82:1345–1349, 1990.

130. Khayat D, Borel C, Torani J, et al: Sequential chemoimmunotherapy with cisplatin, interleukin-2, and interferon alfa-2a for metastatic melanoma. J Clin Oncol 11:2173–2180, 1993.

131. Verschraegen C, Legha S, Hersh E, et al: Phase II study of vindesine and dacarbazine with or without non-specific stimulation of the immune system in patients with metastatic melanoma. Eur J Cancer 29A:708–711, 1993.

132. Thatcher N, Wagstaff J, Mene A, et al: Corynebacterium parvum followed by chemotherapy (actinomycin D and DTIC) compared with chemotherapy alone for metastatic malignant melanoma. Eur J Cancer 22:1009–1014, 1986.

133. Legha S, Plager S, Ring S, et al: A phase-II study of biochemotherapy using interleukin-2 (IL-2) + interferon alfa-2a (IFN) in combination with cisplatin (C), vinblastine (V), and DTIC (D) in patients with metastatic melanoma (abstract). Proc Am Soc Clin Oncol 11:343, 1992.

134. Legha SS, Ring S, Bedikian AY, et al: Combined biochemotherapy in the treatment of advanced melanoma, in Program and Abstracts: Advances in the Biology and Clinical Management of Melanoma, pp 32–33 (abstract). Houston, The University of Texas M. D. Anderson Cancer Center, 1995.

135. Richards J, Mehta N, Ramming K, et al: Sequential chemoimmunotherapy in the treatment of metastatic melanoma. J Clin Oncol 10:1338–1343, 1992.

136. Atkins M, O'Boyle K, Sosman J, et al: Multi-institutional phase II trial of intensive combination chemoimmunotherapy for metastatic melanoma. J Clin Oncol 12:1553–1560, 1994.

137. Flaherty L, Robinson W, Redman B, et al: A phase II study of dacarbazine and cisplatin in combination with outpatient administered interleukin-2 in metastatic melanoma. Cancer 71:3520–3525, 1993.

138. Morton D, Foshag L, Hoon D, et al: Prolongation of survival in metastatic melanoma after active specific immunotherapy with a new polyvalent melanoma vaccine. Ann Surg 216:463–482, 1992.

139. Berd D, Maguire H Jr, McCue P, et al: Treatment of metastatic melanoma with an autologous tumor-cell vaccine: Clinical and immunologic results in 64 patients. J Clin Oncol 8:1858–1867, 1990.

140. Mitchell M, Harel W, Kempf R, et al: Active-specific immunotherapy for melanoma. J Clin Oncol 8:856–869, 1990.

141. Mittelman A, Chen Z, Kageshita T, et al: Active specific immunotherapy in patients with melanoma: A clinical trial with mouse anti-idiotypic monoclonal antibodies elicited with syngeneic anti-high molecular weight melanoma-associated antigen monoclonal antibodies. J Clin Invest 86:2136–2144, 1990.

142. Steffens T, Bajorin D, Houghton A: Immunotherapy with monoclonal antibodies in metastatic melanoma. World J Surg 16:261–269, 1992.

CHAPTER 33

Soft-Tissue and Bone Sarcomas

Danai Daliani, MD,[1] *and* S.R. Patel, MD[2]

[1]Division of Medicine and [2]Section of Sarcoma, Department of Melanoma/Sarcoma, Division of Medicine
The University of Texas M. D. Anderson Cancer Center, Houston, Texas

Sarcomas are a heterogenous group of tumors originating from mesenchymal tissues. According to American Cancer Society estimates, approximately 8,070 new cases will be diagnosed in 1995, including 6,000 cases of soft-tissue sarcomas and 2,070 cases of bone tumors.[1]

SOFT-TISSUE SARCOMAS

Soft-tissue sarcomas are extremely rare tumors. They represent 0.7% of adult malignancies[1]; it is estimated that in the United States 6,000 new cases and 3,600 deaths will occur from this disease in 1995.[1] Soft-tissue sarcomas occur more frequently in children; they represent 6.5% of all cancers in children younger than 15 years of age[1] and are the fifth leading cause of cancer death in this age group.

Soft tissues are the extraskeletal tissues of the body that support, connect, and surround other discrete anatomic structures. These tissues contribute more than 50% of the body weight and include muscles and tendons as well as fibrous, adipose, and synovial tissues.

Soft-tissue sarcomas represent a histologically heterogeneous group of malignant tumors arising in the soft tissues. The majority of soft-tissue sarcomas are of mesodermal origin, but some sarcomas are derived from the ectoderm (eg, tumors of the connective tissues of the face and tumors composed of neurons). Although sarcomas are often thought to be exclusively mesenchymal in origin, some histologic subtypes (eg, synovial sarcoma and epithelioid sarcoma) share some epithelial features, and it is even speculated that they may be derived from epithelial tissue containing the cytokeratin type of intermediate filament.[2]

Epidemiology and Pathogenesis

The pathogenesis of soft-tissue sarcomas is not completely understood. Exposure to environmental toxins has been linked with the development of two specific sarcomas: mesothelioma (asbestos[3]) and hepatic angiosarcoma (thorotrast[4] and vinyl chloride[5]). In 1979, a Swedish report linked exposure to phenoxyacetic acids (herbicides) and chlorophenols (wood preservatives)[6] to an increased risk of developing soft-tissue sarcomas, but this was not confirmed in later studies.[7-9] Ionizing radiation has been implicated as a cause of sarcomas arising in soft tissue and bone.[10] The latent period averages approximately 10 years but ranges between 2 and 30 years, and the prognosis is usually poor. The association of lymphedema and lymphangiosarcoma is well recognized, as in Stewart-Treves syndrome,[11] and carries a very poor prognosis.

Despite anecdotal reports about clusters of sarcomas in some families, there is no clear genetic predisposition except in the Li-Fraumeni syndrome.[12] On the other hand, soft-tissue tumors are thought to occur more frequently in patients with a variety of genetically transmitted diseases, such as the basal cell nevus syndrome, tuberous sclerosis, Werner syndrome, intestinal polyposis, and Gardner's syndrome.[13-18] Sarcomas rarely develop from preexisting benign soft-tissue tumors.[19] The exceptions are neurofibromas in type-I Recklinghausen's disease, which have an increased risk for degeneration into malignant schwannomas. Patients with this disease have a 15% risk of developing neurofibrosarcoma and should be carefully monitored.

Recent advances in molecular biology indicate that genetic mutations in mesenchymal stem cells within the soft tissues may be responsible for the development of sarcomas. Alterations in the retinoblastoma gene and *p53* gene have been found in a variety of soft-tissue sarcomas.[20,21] Germline mutations of these genes have been identified in familial retinoblastoma cases and in the Li-Fraumeni syndrome,[22,23] with soft-tissue sarcomas as manifestations of these disorders. In sarcomas, mutations of *p53* have been associated with specific tumor subtypes, high histologic grade, and a poor prognosis.[24]

Specific cytogenetic alterations have been associated with some sarcomas and appear to be pathognomonic. For example, t(11;22) is present in 90% of patients with extraskeletal Ewing's sarcomas,[25] and 50% of alveolar rhabdomyosarcomas show a t(2;13) translocation.[26,27] Myxoid liposarcomas have been found to have a t(12;16) translocation, clear-cell sarcoma a t(12;22) translocation, extraskeletal myxoid chondrosarcoma a t(9;22) translocation, and synovial sarcoma a t(x;18) translocation.[28] Neuroblastoma has been associated with structural abnormalities of chromosome 1p in 70% to 80% of cases, and these abnormalities appear to confer a poor prognosis.[29] The increasing availability of molecular biology techniques and the identification of specific DNA and RNA gene sequences as expressions of the gene product Myo D1 and oncogenes will help in the diagnosis of sarcomas.

Clinical Presentation

Soft-tissue sarcomas can occur in any anatomic region of the body because of the ubiquitous nature of connective tissue, but most sarcomas (60%) develop in the extremities. Three times as many sarcomas develop in the legs as in the arms. Other sites include the trunk (31%) and head and neck region (9%). The most common manifestations of sarcomas of the extremity are swelling and pain. Pain is usually mild and occurs later in the course of the disease. Thus, a patient might delay seeking medical attention, and a definitive diagnosis also might be delayed.[31] In children, the majority of soft-tissue sarcomas are rhabdomyosarcomas, arising in 20% of the cases in the extremities, in 37% in the head and neck region, and in 25% in genitourinary sites.[32] Patients with pelvic sarcomas might present with swelling of the leg that simulates primary iliofemoral thrombosis or with pain in the distribution of the femoral or sciatic nerve. Hypoglycemia is rare and is usually associated with large retroperitoneal sarcomas.

Evaluation

Imaging Techniques: Radiologic evaluation should include a chest x-ray and a computed tomography (CT) scan of the lungs, the most common sites of metastasis,[33] and a CT scan or, preferably, a magnetic resonance imaging (MRI) scan of the primary tumor-bearing area. MRI examination of the affected area using T1-weighted images, proton-density-weighted images, and T2-weighted images can maximize the contrast among soft-tissue neoplasm, muscle, fat, and vessels[34] and almost eliminates the need for an arteriogram.

If the lesion abuts bone, a bone scan should be obtained to help determine whether there is periosteal invasion or reaction.[35] A positive bone scan does not document bone involvement by the tumor, but it may represent periosteal reaction. The bone scan can serve as a guide to wide resection near the bone or to removal of the periosteum and/or part of the bone in patients treated with surgery alone.[36]

Biopsy: The biopsy of soft-tissue sarcomas is an important aspect of disease management. Needle biopsy is the preferred method because it is less invasive, less expensive, and easy to perform; however, a needle biopsy requires expertise in cytopathology for interpretation. Core biopsies can provide enough tissue for morphologic details, electron microscopy, DNA flow cytometry, cytogenetics, immunohistochemistry, and molecular studies, if necessary,[37] without compromising the definitive surgery.

If an open biopsy must be performed, the biopsy site should be removed at the time of definitive resection. Therefore, it is important for the biopsy incision not to compromise subsequent surgical excision. An excisional biopsy may be used for small or superficial lesions smaller than 2 cm in diameter. The tissues surrounding the tumor form a pseudocapsule that always contains invasive prongs of malignant tissue. Therefore, shelling out soft-tissue sarcomas is never curative. Local recurrence following such procedures occurs in approximately 80% of cases.

Pathology

There are approximately 70 different histologic types of soft-tissue sarcomas. Most sarcomas are classified according to the normal cell type they mimic, based on the system proposed by Enzinger and Weiss.[38] Even among experienced pathologists, significant disagreement often arises as to the cell of origin of an individual tumor.[39] The relative frequency of the various types of sarcomas differs according to a patient's age. In children, for example, the most common sarcoma is rhabdomyosarcoma, which represents 5% to 8% of all childhood cancers. It occurs primarily in infants and children and has a predilection for the head and neck region, urinary bladder, vagina, prostate, and retroperitoneum. In older children, it can also occur in the extremities.

Rhabdomyosarcoma may present as one of four subtypes: embryonal, botryoid, alveolar, and pleomorphic. Immunohistochemistry is very helpful in the differential diagnosis; rhabdomyosarcoma stains positive with antibodies to actin, desmin, myoglobulin, S-100 protein, vimentin, and Myo-D. Electron microscopy can also help by showing the characteristic Z-band pattern of skeletal muscle differentiation.[40,41] Along with the synovial, epithelioid, and clear-cell sarcomas, rhabdomyosarcoma has a higher tendency toward lymphatic dissemination to the regional lymph nodes,[42] in contrast to the generally low incidence (5%) of regional lymph-node metastases found in soft-tissue sarcomas.[43]

The embryonal subtype is the most frequent and constitutes 75% of all rhabdomyosarcomas. The differential diagnosis of this particular type includes some of the "small-cell tumors," such as lymphoma, neuroblastoma, oat-cell carcinoma of the lungs, Ewing's sarcoma, small-cell osteosarcoma, and mesenchymal chondrosarcoma.

Botryoid sarcoma is a subtype of embryonal sarcoma that has a polypoid or grapelike appearance. This tumor is commonly found in the urogenital tract of infants and children and rarely in the oral and nasal pharynges. The alveolar type—the second most common type of rhabdomyosarcoma—occurs in patients who are 10 to 25 years older and more frequently in the extremities. It is an aggressive tumor and has a poorer prognosis than the embryonal type. Pleomorphic rhabdomyosarcoma is the least common subtype. It occurs in adults, more commonly in the extremities, and should be differentiated from other pleomorphic sarcomas, pleomorphic lymphomas, pleomorphic melanomas, and carcinomas. Here again, electron microscopy and immunohistochemistry are very helpful.

In adolescents and young adults, the most common soft-tissue tumors are synovial sarcoma, epithelioid sarcoma, clear-cell sarcoma, and primitive neuroectodermal tumors. Synovial sarcoma occurs usually near the large joints of the lower extremities in patients 15 to 40 years of age and has a slightly higher incidence of lymph-node metastases.[44] Synovial sarcomas frequently calcify, which is rare for soft-tissue tumors; calcification may also occur in extraskeletal osteosarcoma, mesenchymal chondrosarcoma, and myositis ossificans.

In adults, the most common sarcoma is malignant fibrous histiocytoma (MFH), which accounts for 10% to 20% of all soft-tissue sarcomas.[45] This type of tumor is believed to be composed of neoplastic fibroblasts with acquired histiocytic features. MFH usually occurs in the thigh and retroperitoneum of adults 40 to 80 years old.[46] In general, the term refers to a high-grade sarcoma, with the exception of myxoid MFH, which is usually regarded as an intermediate-grade sarcoma.

Liposarcomas are the second most common adult sarcoma. They usually occur in the deep soft tissue of the extremities and retroperitoneum, rarely in the subcutaneous tissue, and almost never metastasize to the regional lymph nodes.[47] Liposarcomas occur slightly more frequently in men than in women (1.5:1) and can vary in behavior, ranging from low-grade, well-differentiated disease (also called atypical lipomatous tumor) to intermediate-grade myxoid liposarcoma to high-grade pleomorphic liposarcoma.

Leiomyosarcomas arise from smooth muscle and can occur anywhere in the body. They commonly arise in the retroperitoneum, where they behave very aggressively.

Neurofibrosarcomas originate from the neural sheath.

They are frequently associated with Recklinghausen's disease, where patients have a 15% risk of developing neurofibrosarcomas, either de novo or from malignant transformation of preexisting benign soft-tissue tumors.

Angiosarcomas include hemangiosarcomas and lymphangiosarcomas, which arise from blood vessels and lymphatic vessels, respectively. Although they are rare, representing only 2% of all soft-tissue sarcomas, they are almost always high-grade tumors, and the 5-year survival rate of patients is only 12% despite multimodality therapy.[48]

Alveolar soft-part sarcomas have no benign counterpart. These tumors evolve slowly, with most patients developing metastases that progress gradually over 5 to 15 years before death occurs. Five-year survival rates of 60% are common.[49] This subtype has a higher incidence of brain metastases.

Epithelioid sarcomas are very aggressive tumors of unknown origin. They occur almost exclusively in the extremities and have a tendency to spread to noncontiguous areas, including the skin, subcutaneous tissue, fat, bone, and draining lymph nodes, which are the most common sites of metastases for these tumors; the lungs are the second most common sites of metastases.[50]

Disease Grade and Staging

Sarcomas are classified according to their grade, which represents the most important prognostic factor.[51,52] Grade 1 describes well-differentiated disease, and, at the other extreme, grade 3 refers to poorly differentiated disease. The histopathologic grade of sarcomas is based on the degree of differentiation, cellularity, number of mitoses, pleormorphism, and amount of necrosis.

In multivariate analysis, necrosis has been shown to be the best parameter for predicting prognosis.[53,54] The next important prognostic factors are the size and location of the tumor. Sarcomas located in extremities generally have a better prognosis than those not in extremities, probably because they are diagnosed earlier, are more likely to be completely resected, and have a lower risk of dissemination. The staging system of the American Joint Committee on Cancer depends largely on grade and tumor-node-metastasis (TNM) classification (Table 1).[55] The lungs are the most frequent sites of metastasis (33%), followed by bone (23%) and the liver (15%).

Treatment

Local Disease: Most soft-tissue sarcomas are treated according to their grade, size, and location, except for Kaposi's sarcoma, extraskeletal Ewing's sarcoma, and

TABLE I

Staging System

T	Primary tumor
	T1: Tumor smaller than 5 cm
	T2: Tumor 5 cm or larger
G	Histologic grade of malignancy
	G1: Low
	G2: Moderate
	G3: High
N	Regional lymph nodes
	N0: No histologically proven regional lymph-node metastasis
	N1: Histologically verified regional lymph-node metastasis
M	Distant metastasis
	M0: No distant metastasis
	M1: Distant metastasis

Stage I:	IA G1T1N0M0	IB G1T2N0M0
Stage II:	IIA G2T1N0M0	IIB G2T2N0M0
Stage III:	IIIA G3T1N0M0	IIIB G3T2N0M0
Stage IV:	IVA G1-3T1-2N1M0	IVB G1-3T1-2N0-1M1

Adapted, with permission, from Bears OH, Henson DE, Hutter RVP, et al (eds): Manual for staging of cancer, American Joint Committee on Cancer, 4th ed, pp 145-149. Philadelphia, JB Lippincott Co, 1992.

rhabdomyosarcoma. In all grades of soft-tissue sarcomas, despite the presence of a pseudocapsule surrounding the tumor, extrusions of tumor extend through the capsule and form micro- and macronodules called satellites. High-grade sarcomas also have a significant incidence (almost 20%) of nodules found in normal tissue beyond the capsule—skip metastases—that are usually confined to the compartment of origin of the tumor. The goal of the treatment of local disease is local control followed by the preservation of optimal function.

The surgical margin achieved has a direct influence on the local recurrence rate.[38,56–59] Marginal en bloc excision through the pseudocapsule carries a risk of local recurrence of 70% to 90%. Wide en bloc excision through normal tissue has a local recurrence rate of 20% to 30% for low-grade lesions and as high as 50% for high-grade lesions. Radical resection involving removal of an entire compartment or amputation is associated with a risk of local recurrence of less than 50% but obvious limitations in function.

The results of combination radiotherapy (XRT) can influence decisions about proposed surgery. When properly designed XRT is coupled with surgery, narrow surgical margins with XRT have equivalent prognoses to those for wide surgical margins alone, and wide surgical margins coupled with XRT are equivalent to radical surgical margins for local control and survival.[60–62] Limb salvage should be considered when the oncologic margin is not compromised and the functional result is preferable to a prosthesis. Lymph-node dissection is not routinely recommended, even for the histologic types at high risk for lymph-node dissemination, unless clinical findings indicate that it should be performed.[38,42,57]

Pre- and postoperative XRT has been used in conjunction with surgery to improve local control of the tumor. If used postoperatively, a dose of 60 to 65 Gy is required to achieve local control.[60,63] If XRT is used preoperatively, the dose required is lower (ie, 50 to 54 Gy), and the radiation field is usually smaller.[64] This is because the postoperative radiation field should include the tumor site and all tissues handled during surgery, including the stab wound and drain tube sites. Also, preoperative XRT usually causes tumor shrinkage, so the tumor is smaller at the time of surgery and has significantly fewer viable cells. Thus, the surgical margins can be safely reduced and the likelihood of reseeding tumor cells during surgery is almost eliminated.

The advantages of postoperative radiation include the feasibility of immediate surgery and the avoidance of delay in wound healing caused by prior XRT. A study conducted at The University of Texas M. D. Anderson Cancer Center showed a local failure rate of 22% for patients receiving XRT postoperatively for grades 2 and 3 tumors larger than 5 cm vs a local failure rate of 10% for patients who received preoperative treatment.[65] Comparable results are reported by other investigators.[66] Wound morbidity after surgery and XRT is adversely affected by disease located in the lower extremity, advanced patient age, and a postoperative XRT boost with an interstitial implant, as shown by multivariate analysis.[67] Accelerated fractionation was of borderline significance, whereas high pathologic grade and a resection volume of more than 200 cm^3 were significant only on univariate analysis. Preoperative XRT is associated with more wound morbidity than postoperative XRT. Gentle handling of tissues during surgery with adequate hemostasis and drainage, sufficient immobilization, and omission of a postoperative boost XRT dose when possible (ie, negative histologic margins) can reduce wound morbidity.[68]

Investigators at the University of California at Los Angeles,[69] used intra-arterial chemotherapy with doxorubicin (Adriamycin, Rubex), 30 mg/d for 3 days as a continuous infusion, followed by preoperative XRT and wide resection, in patients with soft-tissue sarcoma. This strategy produced a local recurrence rate of less than 10%, which included an amputation rate of 5%. These results are comparable to those from more conventional surgery and radiation schemes.

Retroperitoneal sarcomas pose a complex problem, because complete resection is not often possible due to anatomic constraints.[70] In many cases, partial resection of a major organ is required, and even in completely resected sarcomas, a local recurrence rate of 50% to 70% is common.[71] XRT has been used as adjuvant therapy[72] and in unresectable disease.[73] Harrison et al reported the outcome of Yale University's experience with XRT in retroperitoneal sarcomas. All three patients who underwent a complete excision with negative margins and adjuvant XRT with more than 40 Gy survived free of disease for longer than 5 years. Among the 10 patients who underwent only a biopsy for unresectable retroperitoneal sarcomas, only 4 survived longer than 1 year, and the average radiation dose was 44 Gy. The remaining 6 patients received only an average of 27 Gy and did not survive for 1 year.[72]

These results agree with the results reported by Tepper et al from Massachusetts General Hospital.[73] Of the 13 patients who had a primary tumor treated with curative intent, seven patients underwent incomplete surgical resections, three of whom had a relapse of local disease when treated with radiation doses of less than 50 Gy; the four patients with good local disease control received radiation doses varying from 4,990 to 6,070 cGy. Of the three patients with unresectable disease, one treated with 62 Gy had good local control, whereas the other two treated with less than 50 Gy had local relapses. Due to the retrospective nature of the studies and the small number of patients, adjuvant XRT for retroperitoneal sarcomas remains controversial. XRT for unresectable disease, however, does have some potential for local control and palliation.

XRT has also been used with good results in the management of desmoid tumors. Desmoid tumors lack the capacity to metastasize, but they aggressively infiltrate locally and can be fatal.[74,75] Abdominal desmoid tumors usually occur in women postpartum.[76] Patients in whom a complete resection is possible have a good prognosis. Extra-abdominal desmoid tumors usually occur in the head and neck area, shoulder girdle, and inguinal region. Wide resection is often difficult or impossible in these areas, and the recurrence rate ranges between 50% and 75% for cases involving close or positive margins.[77]

XRT has been used by different investigators as an alternative treatment; it provided good local control in approximately 80% of cases when 60 Gy was given over 6 to 8 weeks.[77,78–82] A review of a 20-year experience at M. D. Anderson Cancer Center using XRT doses of 50 to 76 Gy to treat desmoid tumors revealed no evidence of a dose-control relationship, but a clear dose-complication relationship was seen. Therefore, the current recommended XRT dose at M. D. Anderson is 50 to 55 Gy at 1.8 Gy per fraction.[83] At the time of a patient's initial surgery, XRT is not routinely recommended.

A review of the M. D. Anderson experience with chemotherapy for desmoid tumors[84] identified 12 patients so treated; 10 with unresectable primary or recurrent disease and 2 treated preoperatively in an attempt to shrink the tumor and decrease surgical morbidity. Eleven patients received doxorubicin-plus-dacarbazine-based regimens; six of the nine patients whose responses could be evaluated had objective responses (two complete responses [CR] and four partial responses [PR]). With a response rate of more than 60%, chemotherapy is now recommended as primary therapy for inoperable/unresectable tumors.

Hormonal therapy with tamoxifen,[85] toremifene (Estrinex),[86] and progesterone[87] has been reported to achieve long-term remission of desmoid tumors. Indomethacin and ascorbic acid have been reported to cause regression of some desmoid tumors.[88] In addition, good responses have recently been reported with a combination of methotrexate and oral etoposide (VePesid).[89]

Adjuvant Chemotherapy: Adjuvant chemotherapy is considered standard therapy for rhabdomyosarcomas[32] and extraskeletal Ewing's sarcoma.[90] These two tumors are highly responsive to systemic chemotherapy, have a high incidence of systemic micrometastases, and are associated with a 5-year disease-free survival rate of less than 20%. The role of adjuvant chemotherapy in all other soft-tissue sarcomas remains controversial.

The most active single agents for soft-tissue-sarcomas are ifosfamide (Ifex, 30%),[91] doxorubicin (26%),[92] dactinomycin (Cosmegen, 17%),[93] and dacarbazine (16%).[94] The combination of dacarbazine and doxorubicin resulted in a response rate of 42%[95] and has been found to be superior to doxorubicin alone.[96,97] There was a dose-response relationship for doxorubicin, with regimens including doses of greater than 70 mg/m^2 having higher response rates than regimens using lower doses[84]; significantly less cardiotoxicity was seen when doxorubicin was administered as a prolonged infusion.[99,100] Ifosfamide (with mesna [Mesnex] for urothelial protection) resulted in a response rate of 25% to 30% in patients who did not respond to doxorubicin-based regimens.[101–103] A dose-response relationship was documented for ifosfamide in subsequent trials.[103,104]

Several prospective, randomized studies were conducted to evaluate the role of adjuvant chemotherapy in localized soft-tissue sarcomas (Table 2).[105–116] Several studies show a statistically significant improvement in disease-free survival; however, only one study (Bordeaux) showed a statistically significant difference in the rate of overall survival in favor of the adjuvant chemotherapy group. Despite criticism of the use of single-agent suboptimal-dose doxorubicin as adjuvant treatment in most of these cases and the inclusion of low-risk patients in some of the studies, results of a recent meta-analysis of 11 published prospective, randomized, adjuvant studies (that took into account only published information) revealed a disease-free survival advantage (68% vs 53%, $P < .00001$) and an overall survival advantage (81% vs 71%, $P = .0005$) for adjuvant chemotherapy for soft-tissue sarcomas.[117] A preferred approach is to provide preoperative chemotherapy to patients in a high-risk subset. This would help to identify patients who are more likely to benefit from aggressive systemic treatment while sparing the "nonresponders" from the morbidity of prolonged chemotherapy.

Recurrent Disease: The two most common types of disease recurrence are local recurrence and hematogenous spread that most commonly involves the lungs. Local recurrence should be treated with aggressive surgical resection or as a high-risk primary tumor, with preoperative chemotherapy followed by local therapy depending on the clinical situation. Eighty percent of local recurrences occur in the first 2 years after initial surgery, and all recurrences develop by 3 years.[118] Patients with isolated local recurrences have a 5-year survival rate of 45% to 85% when treated with aggressive local therapy.[119,120]

Resection of pulmonary metastases is indicated for patients with favorable prognostic factors—a tumor-doubling time of longer than 40 days, a disease-free interval of more than 1 year, fewer than three nodules, unilateral disease, and MFH tumor histology (rather than other histologies)[121–123]—yielding a 5-year survival rate of 10% to 30%, with little morbidity and very low mortality.

TABLE 2
Randomized Adjuvant Studies in Soft-Tissue Sarcomas

Study	Regimen	Follow-up	Number of patients	% Disease-free survival [a]	% Disease-free survival [b]	% Overall survival [a]	% Overall survival [b]
EORTC[105]	CVAD	44	468	61	61	68	71
Bordeau[106]	CVAD	40	59	37	65	43	93
MDA[107]	CVAAd	> 120	47	83	76	—	—
NCI[108]	ACM		85				
Extremity		60	67	28	54	60	54
Trunk		36	22	47	77	61	82
Retroperitneum		24	15	49	92	100	47
Mayo[109]	AVCAd	64	61	68	65	70	70
GOG[110]	A	60	156	45	60	47	60
Scandi[111]	A	22	139	44	40	55	52
UCLA[112]	A	28	119	52	56	70	80
ISC[113]	A	47	86	54	71	55	65
Rizzoli[114]	A	28	77	45	73	70	91
DFCI[115]	A	73	46	62	66	72	71
ECOG[116]	A	105	36	55	68	53	65

C = cyclophosphamide; V = vincristine, A = doxorubicin; D = dacarbazine; M = methotrexate; Ad = actinomycin
[a] Observation arm
[b] Chemotherapy arm

For patients with less favorable prognostic factors, chemotherapy is the only available treatment option, although CR rates range between 10% and 15% and only one third of patients achieve long-term disease-free survival. Doxorubicin and ifosfamide are the most active single agents, with response rates ranging from 15% to 40%. The combination of ifosfamide and doxorubicin with or without dacarbazine yielded variable results, with a CR rate of 5% to 10% and a PR rate of 25% to 48%.[124–129] Two prospective, randomized, cooperative group trials indicated better overall response rates with the ifosfamide/doxorubicin combination with or without dacarbazine but no significant improvement in CR rate or survival time.[130,131]

Attempts to use high-dose chemotherapy with or without total-body irradiation (TBI) have been disappointing. Responses were of short duration, and substantial treatment-related morbidity and mortality without improvement in the survival rate were seen.[132,133] The use of growth factors, such as granulocyte colony-stimulating factor (G-CSF) and granulocyte-macrophage colony-stimulating factor (GM-CSF) allows intensification of the chemotherapeutic regimens and reduces the morbidity related to neutropenia. The multilineage growth factor PIXY 321 (a fusion protein of GM-CSF and interleukin-3) or thrombopoietin with G-CSF or GM-CSF may allow an increase in the dose intensity by counteracting dose-limiting thrombocytopenia, which currently remains a significant consideration.

BONE SARCOMAS

Bone sarcomas account for 0.2% of all primary cancers in adults and approximately 5% of childhood malignancies. It is estimated that 2,070 new cases will be diagnosed in the United States in 1995 and that 1,280 deaths will be caused by bone sarcomas in the same year.[1]

Bone sarcomas are classified according to the tissue of origin: I, bone-forming tumors; II, cartilage-forming tumors; III, giant-cell tumors; IV, mesenchymal tumors; and V, vascular tumors.[134] The four most common types of bone sarcomas are osteosarcoma, chondrosarcoma, MFH of bone, and Ewing's sarcoma. A team at a specialized center, including an orthopedic surgeon with experience with bone tumors, a radiologist, an experienced pathologist, and a medical oncologist, is essential for the appropriate management of these tumors. As in the case of soft-tissue sarcomas, careful preoperative evaluation is necessary for patients with bone sarcomas.

Evaluation

Imaging Techniques: Staging requires plain films and CT scans of the involved area and the lungs. CT scanning of the area, including the entire bone and adjacent joint, helps to determine intraosseous and extraosseous extension.[135] CT scans of the lungs are required to evaluate for metastatic disease because the lungs are the most common sites of metastasis via hematogenous spread.[136] Bone scans can detect bone metastases and occasional multicentric primary lesions[137,138] or skip metastases.[139] MRI films of the area are very helpful in evaluating the extent of bone-marrow involvement and in detecting skip lesions. MRI can also help to evaluate a positive bone scan when findings on the corresponding plain radiograph are normal.[140,141] Some authors believe that MRI is the best single technique to use for preoperative evaluation,[142] whereas others prefer a baseline CT scan for better bony details and a preoperative MRI scan for surgical planning. As in the case of soft-tissue sarcomas, arteriograms are rarely necessary for surgical planning for bone sarcomas. However, they are very helpful in assessing the vasculature of the tumor preoperatively[143] and in determining chemotherapy response that manifests as a decrease in vascularity of the tumor.[144] After careful staging, a biopsy is performed, preferably by the same physician who will be involved in the patient's definitive treatment. The same principles apply for biopsy of bone sarcomas as for biopsy of soft-tissue sarcomas. The biopsy site should be removed during definitive resection.

Biopsy: Trephine or core biopsy under fluoroscopic visualization is recommended and in most cases (as with 89% of patients with suspected osteosarcoma at M. D. Anderson[145]) yields adequate material for diagnosis. Needle biopsy has the advantage of less tissue contamination than open biopsy. If the lesion extends to the extraosseous soft tissues, a biopsy of these components should be obtained. Intraosseous lesions require perforation of the cortex. In blastic lesions, tissue should be obtained from the least dense area.[146]

Staging of Bone Tumors

A surgical staging system proposed by the Musculoskeletal Tumor Society in 1980 is used for bone sarcomas (Table 3).[147] The system is based on the fact that bone sarcomas, regardless of their histologic type, behave similarly according to grade (G), location (T), and lymphnode involvement or distant metastases (M). Bone tumors metastasize almost exclusively through hematogenous spread, with pulmonary metastases usually occurring first followed by bony involvement.[148] Lymphatic involvement occurs rarely; it is found in 10% of cases at autopsy[136] and in 3% of patients with osteosarcoma undergoing amputation. Lymphatic involvement is considered a poor prognostic sign.[148]

TABLE 3

Surgical Staging of Bone Sarcomas

Stage	Grade	Site
IA	Low (G1)	Intracompartmental (T1)
IB	Low (G1)	Extracompartmental (T2)
IIA	High (G2)	Intracompartmental (T1)
IIB	High (G2)	Extracompartmental (T2)
III	Any G	Any T
		+ regional or distant metastases

Osteosarcoma

Epidemiology and Clinical Presentation: Osteosarcoma is the most common primary malignant bone tumor. It affects men more than women (ratio, 1.5:1).[1] There is a bimodal age distribution; the first peak occurs during childhood and adolescence and the second peak occurs during the sixth decade of life. It is a high-grade, malignant, spindle-cell tumor of the bone characterized by the production of osteoid by the malignant spindle-cell stroma.[149]

Genetic alterations of the retinoblastoma (*Rb*) gene have been identified in cases of osteosarcoma[150] in patients with hereditary retinoblastoma, who carry a risk for osteosarcoma of 7% in radiation ports and in nonirradiated long bones,[151] as well as in patients with sporadic osteosarcoma.[152] Loss of heterozygosity (LOH) and DNA alterations of the *Rb* gene in sporadic osteosarcomas indicate a poor prognosis.[153] During childhood and adolescence, 80% to 90% of osteosarcomas occur in a lower limb.[154] The disease's peak incidence during childhood/ adolescence and the predominance of the distal femur and proximal tibia as first sites of presentation in that age group indicate that osteosarcoma is associated with rapid growth of weight-bearing long bones.

In patients older than 40 years, the skull, pelvis, and mandible are frequent sites of osteosarcoma presentation. People with Paget's disease have a 10-fold risk of developing bone cancer.[155] Other conditions associated with an increased risk for bone sarcoma are hereditary multiple exostoses, enchondromatosis (Ollier's disease), enchondromatosis with skin hemangiomas (Maffucci's syndrome), polyostotic fibrous dysplasia, and osteogenesis imperfecta.[156] Ionizing radiation is the only environmental agent known to cause bone tumors. People who were exposed to radium and patients receiving radiation therapy are at increased risk for osteosarcoma.[157] Such risk is expected to decrease with the use of megavoltage therapy, which is not absorbed by bone as much as orthovoltage therapy is.

Fifty percent of all osteosarcomas occur in the knee joint area; the proximal humerus is the next most common site, with 25% of the cases. The axial skeleton is rarely involved.[154] The most common presenting symptom is pain, with a firm, palpable, soft-tissue mass fixed to the underlying bone with slight tenderness. There is no erythema or effusion in the adjacent joint, and range of motion is normal. Fewer than 1% of patients will have a pathologic fracture.

There are different types of osteosarcoma. Radiologically, the classic osteosarcoma may present as a lesion that can range from nearly normal to extremely dense or even involve complete destruction of the bone. In one series, purely lytic osteosarcoma was described in nearly 14% of patients.[158] Radiographically, purely lytic disease cannot be distinguished from a telangiectatic osteosarcoma, giant-cell tumor, aneurysmal bone cyst, or MFH of bone. The periosteal reaction classically described as "sunburst" is an important diagnostic feature; this is characteristically irregular and interrupted, which distinguishes malignancy from other benign conditions. A soft-tissue mass immediately adjacent to the bone lesion is usually present. Histologically, 75% of all osteosarcomas fall in the conventional category, which includes osteoblastic, chondroblastic, and fibroblastic subtypes. The survival rate is similar for all subtypes.[159]

In patients treated with surgery alone, the size of the tumor, the age of the patient, and the degree of malignancy did not correlate with the survival rate.[159] The most significant variable was anatomic site; patients with pelvic and axial lesions had lower survival rates than patients with tumors of the extremities, probably because of incomplete resection in the former group. The preoperative serum alkaline phosphatase level has been reported as a significant prognostic factor of survival time.[160] Tumor ploidy also has been shown to be a significant prognostic factor. Disease-free survival and overall survival times are significantly longer in patients with near-diploid cell lines.[161] However, a recent review of the published data on prognostic factors in the postadjuvant-chemotherapy era assessed age, anatomic location, tumor size, and tumor necrosis following neoadjuvant chemotherapy; only tumor necrosis maintained its significance as a predictor of disease-free survival in multivariate models.[162]

Treatment of Localized Disease: Prior to the 1970s, treatment of localized osteosarcoma consisted of amputation one joint above the tumor-containing bone or transmedullary amputation, with an overall survival rate of 5% to 20% at 2 years.[163] Pulmonary metastases usually occurred within 9 months and were responsible for the patient's death at 18 to 24 months after diagnosis.[164] The introduction of effective chemotherapeutic agents—high-dose methotrexate with leucovorin rescue,[165] doxorubicin,[166] cisplatin (Platinol),[167] and the alkylating agents ifosfamide[168] and high-dose cyclophosphamide (Cytoxan, Neosar)[169]—allowed a change in the approach to treatment of osteosarcomas.

The beneficial role of adjuvant chemotherapy in patients with osteosarcoma is now proven. A large multi-institutional study showed a 2-year disease-free survival rate of 66% for patients treated with surgery and adjuvant postoperative chemotherapy vs a 2-year disease-free survival rate of less than 20% for patients treated with surgery alone.[170] Moreover, the introduction of neoadjuvant chemotherapy allowed more conservative limb-salvage surgery in 50% to 80% of patients without compromising a patient's chance of survival by delaying surgery.[171]

Currently, limb-salvage surgery is preferred for a significant number of patients with osteosarcoma and other high-grade sarcomas. The risk of local recurrence (less than 5%) was shown to be the same or lower than that of patients treated with amputation in a carefully selected group of patients.[172] Contraindications for limb-salvage surgery include major neurovascular involvement, an inappropriate biopsy site, infection, a pathologic fracture with spread of tumor cells via hematoma, extensive muscle involvement, and immature skeletal age, especially for anticipated significant discrepancies in leg length. The latter is far less critical now with the development of expandable prostheses, but limb-sparing surgery is still usually not an option for children younger than 10 years old.[173]

A number of trials have evaluated the role of chemotherapy administered either preoperatively or postoperatively. Most of the chemotherapeutic regimens included combinations of doxorubicin, high-dose methotrexate, cyclophosphamide, cisplatin, and ifosfamide. Relapse-free survival rates of 48% to 77% have been reported with different regimens. The effectiveness of high-dose methotrexate, however, has not been universally accepted. Response rates ranging frp, 0% and 80% have been reported[174–178]; a dose-response relationship has been proposed.[179]

A study from the National Cancer Institute (NCI) evaluated the relationship of dose intensity to more than 90% tumor necrosis following neoadjuvant chemotherapy and suggested that large, highly concentrated doses of doxorubicin contribute to a favorable outcome in cases of Ewing's sarcoma and osteosarcoma. Cisplatin and high-dose methotrexate also revealed significant activity.[180] Doxorubicin and cisplatin-based adjuvant chemotherapy are now accepted as standard therapy for osteosarcoma in many institutions.

The role of chemotherapy prior to surgery (neoadjuvant) vs its role postoperatively (adjuvant) has not yet been established in a randomized trial. The rationale for neoadjuvant chemotherapy has been to institute early systemic therapy against micrometastases, to increase the chances for successful limb-salvage surgery, to decrease the risk of viable tumor cells being spread at the time of surgery, and, very importantly, to tailor treatment individually according to the patient's response.

Several systems have been proposed for grading the tumor response to neoadjuvant chemotherapy, all of which are based on the degree of cellularity and necrosis in the resected specimen.[181,182] Only grade 4 response, as determined by Huvos et al (absence of viable tumor within the entire specimen),[181] and more than 90% tumor necrosis, by the M. D. Anderson criteria,[182] predicted continuous disease-free survival.[183]

Both intra-arterial (IA) and intravenous (IV) chemotherapy have been administered preoperatively. A randomized trial using IA vs IV cisplatin combined with systemic doxorubicin and high-dose methotrexate showed a significantly higher histologic response (more than 90% tumor necrosis) in the group treated with IA cisplatin. No differences in the percentage of clinical/radiologic response or in the percentage of limb-salvage procedures performed were seen, and no differences in local or systemic side effects were observed.[184] IA cisplatin was compared with high-dose IV methotrexate at M. D. Anderson, and IA cisplatin was found to be more efficacious.[185] It should be noted that the IA technique requires excellent angiographic support facilities and experienced personnel to minimize complications.

At the present time, preoperative chemotherapy is standard at M. D. Anderson, with four cycles of systemic doxorubicin administered as a continuous infusion followed by cisplatin, preferably given IA where feasible, followed by limb-salvage surgery and the tailoring of postoperative therapy based on the tumor's response. Therapy is switched to ifosfamide and high-dose methotrexate for patients with less than 90% tumor necrosis. Patients with more than 90% tumor necrosis receive another six cycles of doxorubicin, with dacarbazine replacing cisplatin due to dose-limiting peripheral neuropathy.

Mature data from patients treated between 1980 and 1982 (cisplatin, 120 mg/m^2) have shown that patients with complete responses at the time of surgery had a 5-year continuous disease-free survival rate of 86%, compared with 13% for patients with partial and/or poor responses.[183,186] Patients treated later with intensified cisplatin (160 mg/m^2) showed a slight improvement in the overall survival rate, although this difference was not statistically significant. A significant improvement in the overall survival rate was observed for patients with less than 90% tumor necrosis (33%).[187] Late relapses, although rare, can occur; 1 of 37 patients treated at M. D. Anderson between 1980 and 1982 had a recurrence of disease more than 6 years after surgery. Therefore, careful long-term follow-up and reports of mature data are very important.

Recent studies[187a,187b] with muramyltripeptide phosphatidylethanolamine (MTP-PE), a synthetic, lipophilic analog of muramyldipeptide (MDP), the smallest component of a mycobacterium capable of stimulating the immune system, have shown that liposomes containing MTP-PE localize to the pulmonary microvasculature, resulting in activation of pulmonary macrophages. Animal studies revealed the efficacy of MTP-PE in canine osteosarcoma models.[188] A phase II study in humans documented histologic changes in the characteristics of the pulmonary nodules that recurred after treatment with MTP-PE[189]; peripheral fibrosis and inflammatory-cell infiltration with neovascularization were demonstrated as well as a change from high- to low-grade lesions after therapy. These changes indicated a potential role for MTP-PE in conjunction with surgery and chemotherapy in the treatment of osteosarcomas. A phase II trial of L-MTP-PE administered to patients with osteosarcoma who had pulmonary metastases that either developed during adjuvant chemotherapy or persisted despite chemotherapy showed a significant prolongation of disease-free survival in the patients who received treatment for 24 weeks.[190]

Treatment of Metastatic Disease: Metastatic osteosarcoma is a treatable and potentially curable disease when combined modality therapy is administered. The most frequent sites of metastasis are the lungs. Whether pulmonary metastasis is present at diagnosis or occurs after the primary tumor is treated, if the lungs are the only sites of metastatic disease, it should be resected aggressively. A 5-year postthoracotomy survival rate of nearly 40% has been reported by Putnam et al,[191] and similar results were reported by Skinner et al for patients treated with combined-modality therapy.[192] The number of nodules on preoperative lung tomograms, the disease-free interval, the resectability of the tumor, and the number of metastases resected at thoracotomy are prognostic factors influencing survival.[191] The completeness of the surgical resection is crucial to prolonged survival.[193] Variables such as preoperative chemotherapy vs immediate surgery, serum lactic dehydrogenase (LDH) level, alkaline phosphatase level, or the site of primary tumor did not affect the survival of patients who presented with metastatic disease.[194] Patients with unresectable metastatic disease have a poor prognosis. Ifosfamide (with mesna for urothelial protection), alone or in combination with etoposide, has shown activity in up to one third of patients with recurrent osteosarcoma.[194,195]

XRT was used as primary therapy for osteosarcoma in the 1950s and early 1960s, without good results.[196] High doses of radiation were required to sterilize only a small subset of tumors and were associated with significant necrosis of normal tissue. Preoperative XRT did not offer any survival advantage either compared with surgery alone.[197] XRT has been used successfully in facial lesions; when followed by wide surgical excision, XRT promotes a 5-year survival rate of 73%, compared with 35% to 45% with surgery alone.[198] For palliation of metastatic bone sarcomas and unresectable lesions in axial sites or the pelvis, XRT is useful, especially when combined with IA or IV radiosensitizers (5-bromodeoxyuridine or idoxuridine).[199,200]

Variants of Osteosarcoma

Parosteal and periosteal osteosarcomas are the most common variants of osteosarcoma. Parosteal osteosarcoma accounts for 4% of all osteosarcomas.[201] It usually occurs in older people, with a slightly higher incidence in women. The distal femur is involved in 75% of cases. Parosteal osteosarcoma arises from the cortex of bone. It presents as a mass that is occasionally associated with pain and grows slowly over months or years with late metastases. Overall survival rates range between 75% and 85%.[201,202]

Radiographically, parosteal osteosarcoma is characterized by a large, dense, lobulated mass broadly attached to the underlying bone without involvement of the medullary canal. However, such involvement can be present without being radiographically apparent. Parosteal osteosarcoma is treated surgically with wide excision alone. Dedifferentiated parosteal osteosarcoma and high-grade surface osteosarcoma have a much poorer prognosis and are treated with chemotherapy and surgery.

Periosteal osteosarcoma originates in the cortex, usually of the tibial shaft. A characteristic, small, radiolucent lesion, evidence of bone spicules on a plain radiograph, and a Codman's triangle are hallmarks of this disease.[203] Pathologically, periosteal osteosarcoma is usually a high-grade chondroblastic osteosarcoma. Treatment recommendations follow the same concepts as those for high-grade classic osteosarcoma.

Chondrosarcoma of Bone

Chondrosarcoma is the second most common primary malignant spindle-cell tumor of the bone, characterized by cartilaginous neoplastic tissue without direct osteoid formation. Occasionally, bone formation occurs from differentiated cartilage. There are five types of chondrosarcoma: central (arising within the bone), peripheral (arising from the bone surface), mesenchymal, dedifferentiated, and clear cell.[204] The most common variants are central and peripheral chondrosarcomas, which may arise as primary tumors or may be secondary to underlying benign neoplasms (multiple osteochondromas or enchondromas).[205–207] Chondrosarcomas usually present in patients older than 40 years of age. The most common sites are the pelvis (30%), femur (20%), and shoulder girdle (15%). Chondrosarcomas usually reach a significant size before symptoms, such as a palpable mass with pain or pressure and occasionally urinary symptoms (sometimes noted with pelvic tumors), are noted.

Chondrosarcomas are pathologically classified as grade I to grade III tumors. High-grade (grade III) tumors have the worst prognosis, with a risk of metastasis of 75%.[208] Surgical removal of the tumor is the treatment for chondrosarcoma. There is no effective chemotherapy for the central and peripheral types of the disease. Dedifferentiated chondrosarcoma, on the other hand, does respond to standard chemotherapy used against osteosarcoma, and such treatment should be employed.

Few reports document the efficacy of XRT in chondrosarcomas.[209–211] Five-year local control rates ranged between 45% and 82% and were directly related to the histology of the tumor. A review of a 15-year XRT experience with chondrosarcoma of bone at M. D. Anderson revealed that none of the four patients treated with a combination of neutron- and photon-beam XRT had disease recurrence locally.[211] One of the seven patients treated with conventional radiotherapy alone experienced local disease recurrence, suggesting a benefit from the mixed-beam technique.[211]

Clear-cell chondrosarcoma is the rarest type. This tumor grows slowly and locally recurs with some malignant potential. It is often confused with chondroblastoma. Treatment is wide surgical excision; systemic therapy is not required, and metastases occur only after multiple local recurrences.[212]

Mesenchymal chondrosarcoma is a rare, aggressive tumor that affects younger patients. It shows a predilection for flat bones and has high metastatic potential. Treatment is wide surgical excision with adjuvant chemotherapy. XRT is used when the tumor cannot be completely excised.[213,214]

Malignant Fibrous Histiocytoma of Bone

MFH is a high-grade tumor in bone as well as in soft tissues. It usually occurs during adulthood and commonly involves the metaphyseal ends of long bones, especially those of the knee joint.[215] MFH presents as a lytic, metaphyseal lesion with marked cortical disruption, minimal cortical or periosteal reaction, and no evidence of bone formation. Pathologic fractures are common.[216] The patient's alkaline phosphatase level is normal. MFH of bone disseminates rapidly to lung tissue, and lymph-node metastases have been reported in up to one third of cases with lung metastases.[217]

Although data are limited, it seems that MFH of bone is sensitive to chemotherapy.[218–220] In one study, patients treated with surgery and chemotherapy had a disease-free survival rate of 59%, compared with only 5% of patients treated with surgery alone.[218] In a recently updated study, 7 of 15 patients with MFH of bone treated with neoadjuvant chemotherapy at M. D. Anderson showed more than 90% tumor necrosis. The median continuous disease-free survival for patients who achieved more than 90% tumor necrosis was 43 months, compared with only 7 months for patients with less than 90% tumor necrosis ($P < .05$). A trend for better overall survival was documented (66 months vs 20 months, respectively), although it was not statistically significant.[221] MFH of bone should be treated as is osteosarcoma, with chemotherapy and surgery.

Ewing's Sarcoma

Ewing's sarcoma (ES) is a rare tumor that usually occurs in bone and presents most frequently during the second decade of life; it is an unusual occurrence before 5 or after 30 years of age. In patients up to 13 years old, ES occurs with equal frequency in girls and boys; after age 13, the disease is more common in males. ES is extremely rare in African and American blacks and Chinese populations but constitutes 12% of malignant primary tumors of bone in white persons. It was originally thought to arise from endothelial cells,[222] but mesenchymal, myeloid, reticular, pericystic, neuroepithelial, and primitive multipotential cells have been suspected to be the cells of origin.[223] The most widely accepted belief is that ES is of neuroectodermal origin.[224] ES is an undifferentiated, small, round-cell tumor that may be confused with other small, round, blue-cell tumors of childhood, among them small-cell osteosarcoma, mesenchymal and myxoid chondrosarcoma, rhabdomyosarcoma, lymphoma, neuroblastoma, and peripheral neuroepithelioma.

A careful review of light microscopy studies by an experienced pathologist is extremely important for the diagnosis of ES. Morphologic features may be indistinguishable from those of the peripheral primitive neuroectodermal tumors (pPNETs). Immunocytochemical staining is often positive for neuron-specific enolase (NSE),[225] although others believe that NSE is specific for pPNET and might be used to distinguish between the two entities.[226] The monoclonal antibody 5C11 has been reported to react exclusively with ES and not with pPNET,[227] whereas expression of the *MIC2* gene has been reported in both entities.[228] Electron microscopy studies may also assist the diagnosis, revealing dense core granules, neurites, neurotubules, and neurofilaments in prominent Golgi's complexes.[229] A chromosomal translocation t(11;22)(q24;q12) is a characteristic abnormality of ES,[230,231] but it has also been reported in pPNET.[232]

ES is associated with skeletal abnormalities (such as enchondroma and aneurysmal bone cyst) and genitourinary anomalies (hypospadias and duplicate collecting system).

Clinical Presentation, Prognostic Factors, and Staging: ES can affect any bone, although it most commonly presents in the femur and pelvis. The axial skeleton is often involved. In the long bones, ES usually localizes in the diaphysis, with frequent extension through the bone cortex into the soft tissues. It presents as a rapidly enlarging mass causing poorly localized pain. Constitutional symptoms, such as fatigue, weight loss, and fever, may be present, especially in metastatic disease. Leukocytosis and an elevated erythrocyte sedimentation rate (ESR) may mimic osteomyelitis. Metastases are present at the time of initial diagnosis in 15% to 50% of cases. The lungs are the most common sites of metastasis at presentation or relapse, followed by bone and bone-marrow sites. Metastases to the central nervous system occur in fewer than 1% of patients.[222]

Diagnostic and staging evaluations should include plain radiographs of the involved area and the lungs, CT or MRI scans of the primary tumor, a CT scan of the lungs, a bone scan, and bone-marrow biopsy and aspirate studies. There is no uniformly accepted staging system for ES, but a TNM system seems appropriate. Lymph-node (N) involvement is rare.

Central location of the tumor, systemic symptoms at diagnosis, elevated pretreatment LDH levels,[233] the presence of a gross extraosseous extension of the primary tumor,[234] metastatic disease at diagnosis,[235] and less-than-complete response to preoperative chemotherapy[236] are poor prognostic factors.

Treatment: ES is considered a systemic disease; even when a tumor is apparently localized, approximately 90% of the cases include occult metastatic disease. Before treatment with chemotherapy was available, local control was achieved in 50% to 85% of patients by means of surgery or radiation doses of more than 40 Gy to 50 Gy. However, only 10% of these patients survived for 5 years. Death was usually caused by distant metastatic disease.[237,238] Because XRT can establish good local control of Ewing's sarcoma,[222] the role of surgery has historically been limited to diagnostic biopsy and primary control of an expendable bone, such as a rib or clavicle.[239] Surgery can also be used to treat the primary tumor when XRT would jeopardize function. However, the higher rate of local control achieved with surgery or surgery plus XRT, compared with XRT alone,[240] and the desire for prevention of long-term side effects of XRT (growth failure, normal tissue damage, and development of second malignancies[241,242]) may broaden the indications for surgery.

The advent of chemotherapy significantly improved the disease-free survival rate (50% to 60%) at 2 to 3 years, compared with such rates when XRT or surgery was used alone.[243-249] The most active single agents are cyclophosphamide (50%),[250] doxorubicin (40%),[251] vincristine (Oncovin, 30%),[252] dactinomycin (33%), etoposide (30%), and high-dose melphalan (Alkeran, 80%).[253] Adjuvant chemotherapy is now accepted as standard therapy for ES. The combination of vincristine, dactinomycin, and cyclophosphamide has been evaluated alone or with doxorubicin or bilateral pulmonary XRT in a large intergroup study.[254] According to this study, the addition of doxorubicin significantly improved relapse-free survival and overall survival. A dose-intensity relationship exists between doxorubicin and ES.[180] A high-dose, intermittent method of chemotherapy delivery using the four drugs listed yielded significantly better disease-free survival (68%) and overall survival (77%) rates than a moderate-dose, continuous method (48% and 53%, respectively).[255] The high-dose, intermittent schedule also improved the relapse-free survival and overall survival rates of patients with ES of the pelvic or sacral bones, a group with a generally poor outcome.[256]

The combination of ifosfamide and etoposide has also shown activity in newly diagnosed[257] and previously treated[258] cases of ES, with response rates of 96% and 50% to 60%, respectively. Longer follow-up is needed to assess the duration of these responses and their effect on survival rates.

The prognosis for patients with recurrent or metastatic

disease is poor. Combination chemotherapy using doxo-rubicin, vincristine, cyclophosphamide, and dactinomy-cin has been the basis of treatment. Methotrexate, bleo-mycin (Blenoxane), and fluorouracil have been incorporated into some protocols,[244,259-261] with 5-year survival rates in the 30% range. XRT to the sites of metastatic disease (bone or soft tissue) in a dose of 45 to 50 Gy can be considered for palliation. Myeloablative therapy with high-dose etoposide, fractionated high-dose melphalan with or without carboplatin (Paraplatin), and total-body irradiation has yielded promising results (a projected relapse-free survival rate of 45% at 6 years, compared with a relapse-free survival rate of 2% in the historic control group). These patients have a poor prognosis (multifocal primary tumor and early or multiple relapses),[262] and the follow-up has been short.

In contrast, Horowitz et al[263] treated poor-risk patients with TBI and autologous bone marrow transplantation support after complete remission was reached with induction therapy. However, this study failed to show any benefit over nontransplantation protocols. Therefore, the role of high-dose chemotherapy with bone marrow transplantation support remains controversial.

REFERENCES

1. Wingo PA, Tong T, Bolden S: Cancer statistics. CA Cancer J Clin 44:8–30, 1995.

2. Leyvraz S, Costa J: Histological diagnosis and grading of soft-tissue sarcomas. Semin Surg Oncol 4:3–6, 1988.

3. McDonald AD, McDonald JC: Epidemiology of malignant mesothelioma, in Antman KH, Aisner J (eds): Asbestos-Related Malignancy, pp 31–55. Orlando, FL, Grune & Stratton, 1987.

4. DeSilva H, Abbott J, DaMotta L, et al: Malignancy and other effects following the administration of thorotrast. Lancet II:201–204, 1965.

5. Falk H: Vinyl chloride induced hepatic angiosarocma. Int Symp Princess Takamatsu Cancer Res Fund 18:39–46, 1987.

6. Hardell L, Sandstrom A: Case-control study: Soft-tissue sarcomas and exposure to phenoxyacetic acids or chlorophenols. Br J Cancer 39:711–717, 1979.

7. Wiklund K, Holm LE: Soft tissue sarcoma risk in Swedish agricultural and forestry workers. J Natl Cancer Inst 76:229–234, 1986.

8. Greenwald P, Kovaszway B, Collins DN, et al: Sarcomas of soft tissue after Vietnam service. J Natl Cancer Inst 73:1107–1109, 1984.

9. Kang H, Enzinger FM, Breslin P, et al: Soft tissue sarcomas and military service in Vietnam: A case-control study. J Natl Cancer Inst 79:693–699, 1987.

10. Robinson E, Nerget AZ, Wylie P: Review: Clinical aspects of postirradiation sarcoma. J Natl Cancer Inst 80:233–240, 1988.

11. Stewart FW, Treves NP: Lymphangiosarcoma in postmastectomy lymphedema: A report of six cases in elephantiasis chirurgica. Cancer 1:64–81, 1948.

12. Li FP, Fraumeni JF Jr: Soft tissue sarcomas, breast cancer, and other neoplasms: A familial syndrome? Ann Intern Med 71:747–752, 1969.

13. Fraumeni JF Jr, Vogel CL, Easton JM: Sarcomas and multiple polyposis in kindred: A genetic variety of hereditary polyposis? Arch Intern Med 121:57–61, 1968.

14. Schjweisguth O, Gerard-Marchant R, Lemerle J: Naevomatose baso-cellulaire association a un rhabdomyosarcome congenital. Arch Pediatr 25:1083–1093, 1968.

15. Heard G: Malignant disease in von Recklinghausen's neurofibromatosis. Proc R Soc Med 56:502–503, 1963.

16. Reed WB, Nickel WR, Campion G: Internal manifestations of tuberous sclerosis. Arch Dermatol 87:715–728, 1963.

17. Epstein CJ, Martin GM, Schultz AL, et al: Werner's syndrome: A review of its symptomatology, natural history, pathologic features, genetics, and relationship to the natural aging process. Medicine (Baltimore) 45:177–221, 1966.

18. Usui M, Ishii S, Yamawaki S, et al: The occurrence of soft tissue sarcomas in three siblings with Werner's syndrome. Cancer 54:2580–2586, 1984.

19. Huvos AG: The spontaneous transformation of benign into malignant soft tissue tumors. Am J Surg Pathol 9(suppl):7–20, 1985.

20. Seale KS, Lange TA, Monson D, et al: Soft tissue tumors of the foot and ankle. Foot Ankle Int 9:19–27, 1988.

21. Sallourn E, Slamant F, Cailland JM, et al: Diagnostic and therapeutic problems of soft tissue tumours other than rhabdomyosarcoma in infants under 1 year of age: A clinicopathological study of 34 cases treated at the Institut Gustave-Roussy. Med Pediatr Oncol 18:37–43, 1990.

22. Malkin D, Li FP, Strong LC, et al: Germ line p53 mutations in a familial syndrome of breast cancer, sarcomas, and other neoplasms. Science 250:1233–1238, 1990.

23. Mulligan LM, Matlashewski GJ, Scrable HJ, et al: Mechanisms of p53 loss in human sarcomas. Proc Natl Acad Sci U S A 87:5863–5867, 1990.

24. Kawai A, Nogushi M, Beppu Y, et al: Nuclear immunoreaction of p53 protein in soft tissue sarcomas: A possible prognostic factor. Cancer 73:2499–2505, 1994.

25. Callen D, Smith R, Bovine A: Chromosomal analysis in Ewing's sarcoma. Pathology 99:64–66, 1987.

26. Parham DM, Shapiro DN, Downing JR, et al: Solid alveolar rhabdomyosarcomas with the t(2;13): Report of two cases with diagnostic implications. Am J Surg Pathol 18:474–478, 1994.

27. De Chiara A, T'Ang A, Triche TJ: Expression of the retinoblastoma susceptibility gene in childhood rhabdomyosarcomas. J Natl Cancer Inst 85:152–157, 1993.

28. Angervall L, Kindblom LG: Principles for pathologic-anatomic diagnosis and classification of soft-tissue sarcomas. Clin Orthop 289:9–18, 1993.

29. Sainati L, Stella M, Montaldi A, et al: Value of cytogenetics in the differential diagnosis of the small round cell tumors of childhood. Med Pediatr Oncol 20:130–135, 1990.

30. Dias P, Dilling M, Houghton P: The molecular basis of skeletal muscle differentiation. Semin Diagn Pathol 11:3–14, 1994.

31. Lawrence W Jr, Donegan WL, Natarajan N, et al: Adult soft tissue sarcomas: A pattern of care survey of the American College of Surgeons. Ann Surg 205:349–359, 1987.

32. Maurer HM, Beltangady M, Gehan EA, et al: The Intergroup Rhabdomyosarcoma Study I: A final report. Cancer 61:209–220, 1988.

33. Potter DA, Glenn J, Kinsella T, et al: Patterns of recurrence in patients with high-grade soft-tissue sarcomas. J Clin Oncol 3:353–366, 1985.

34. Greenfield GB, Arrington JA: Magnetic resonance imaging of soft tissue tumors. Cancer Control 1:581–585, 1994.

35. Enneking WF: Preoperative staging of sarcomas. Cancer Treat Symp 3:67–70, 1985.

36. Yang JC, Rosenberg SA, Glatstein EJ, et al: Sarcomas of soft

tissues, in DeVita Jr VT, Hellman S, Rosenberg SA (eds): Cancer: Principles and Practice of Oncology, 4th ed, pp 1436–1488. Philadelphia, JB Lippincott Co, 1993.

37. Ball AB, Fisher C, Pittam M: Diagnosis of soft tissue tumors by Tru-cut biopsy. Br J Surg 77:756–758, 1990.

38. Enzinger FM, Weiss SW: Soft Tissue Tumors. 2nd ed. St. Louis, MO, CV Mosby Co, 1988.

39. Presant CA, Russell WO, Alexander RW, et al: Soft tissue and bone sarcoma histopathology peer review: The frequency of disagreement in diagnosis and the need for second pathology opinions: The Southeastern Cancer Study Group experience. J Clin Oncol 4:1658–1661, 1986.

40. Parham DM, Weber B, Holt H, et al: Immunohistochemical study of childhood rhabdomyosarcomas and related neoplasms: Results of the Intergroup Rhabdomyosarcoma Study Project. Cancer 67:3072–3080, 1991.

41. Dodd S, Malone M, McCulloch WM: Rhabdomyosarcoma in children: A histological and immunohistochemical study of 59 cases. J Pathol 158:13–18, 1989.

42. Weingrad DN, Rosenberg SA: Early lymphatic spread of osteogenic and soft-tissue sarcomas. Surgery 84:231–240, 1978.

43. Ruka W, Enwich LJ, Driscoll DL, et al: Prognostic significance of lymph node metastasis and bone, major vessel, or nerve involvement in adults with high-grade soft tissue sarcomas. Cancer 62:999–1006, 1988.

44. Germar R, Moore G: Synovial sarcoma. Ann Surg 131:22–25, 1975.

45. Ushigome S, Shimoda T, Nikaido T, et al: Histopathologic diagnosis and histogenetic problems in malignant soft tissue tumors: Reassessment of malignant fibrous histocytoma, epithelioid sarcoma, malignant rhabdoid tumor, and neuroectodermal tumor. Acta Pathol Jpn 42:691–706, 1992.

46. Pritchard DJ, Reiman HM, Turcotte RE, et al: Malignant fibrous histiocytoma of the soft tissues of the trunk and extremities. Clin Orthop 289:58–65, 1993.

47. Springfield D: Liposarcoma. Clin Orthop 289:50–57, 1993.

48. Holden C, Spittle M, Jones E: Angiosarcoma of face and scalp: Prognosis and treatment. Cancer 59:1046–1057, 1987.

49. Auerbach H, Brooks J: Alveolar soft part sarcoma: A clinicopathologic and immunohistochemical study. Cancer 60:66–73, 1987.

50. Chase DR, Enzinger FM: Epithelioid sarcoma. Am J Surg Pathol 9:241–263, 1985.

51. Trojani M, Contesso G, Coindre JM, et al: Soft tissue sarcomas of adults: Study of pathological prognostic variables and definition of a histopathological grading system. Int J Cancer 33:37–42, 1984.

52. Costa J, Wesley RA, Glatstein EJ, et al: The grading of soft tissue sarcomas: Results of a clinicopathologic correlation in a series of 163 cases. Cancer 53:530–541, 1984.

53. Lack EE, Steinberg SM, White DE, et al: Extremity soft tissue sarcomas: Analysis of prognostic variables in 300 cases and evaluation of tumor necrosis as a factor in stratifying higher-grade sarcomas. J Surg Oncol 41:263–273, 1989.

54. Kulander BG, Polissar L, Yang CY, et al: Grading of soft tissue sarcomas: Necrosis as a determinant of survival. Mod Pathol 2:205–208, 1989.

55. Bears OH, Henson DE, Hutter RVP, et al (eds): Manual for Staging of Cancer, American Joint Committee on Cancer, 4th ed, pp 145–149. Philadelphia, JB Lippincott Co, 1992.

56. Simon MA, Enneking WF: The management of soft tissue sarcomas of the extremities. J Bone Joint Surg (Am) 58:317–327, 1976.

57. Sugarbaker PH, Malawer MM: Musculoskeletal Survey for Cancer: Principles and Techniques. New York, NY, Thieme Medical Publishers, 1992.

58. Gerner R, Moore G, Pickren J: Soft tissue sarcomas. Ann Surg 181:803–808, 1975.

59. Contin J, McNeer G, Chu F, et al: The problems of local recurrence after treatment of soft tissue sarcomas. Ann Surg 168:47–53, 1968.

60. Suit HD, Russell WO, Martin RG: Sarcoma of soft tissue: Clinical and histopathologic parameters and response to treatment. Cancer 35:1478–1483, 1975.

61. Karakousis CP, Emrich LJ, Rao U, et al: Limb salvage in soft tissue sarcomas with selective combination of modalities. Eur J Surg Oncol 17:71–80, 1991.

62. O'Connor MI, Pritchard DJ, Gunderson LL: Integration of limb-sparing surgery, brachytherapy, and external beam irradiation in the treatment of soft-tissue sarcoma. Clin Orthop 289:73, 1992.

63. Suit HD, Mankin HJ, Wood WC, et al: Treatment of the patient with stage M0 soft tisuse sarcoma. J Clin Oncol 6:854–862, 1988.

64. Nielsen OS, Cummings B, O'Sullivan B, et al: Preoperative and postoperative irradiation of soft tissue sarcomas: Effect of radiation field size. Int J Radiat Oncol Biol Phys 21:1595–1599, 1991.

65. Barkley HT Jr, Martin RG, Romsdahl MM, et al: Treatment of soft tissue sarcomas by preoperative irradiation and conservative surgical resection. Int J Radiat Oncol Biol Phys 14:693–699, 1988.

66. Mansson E, Willems J, Aparisi T, et al: Preoperative radiation therapy of high malignancy grade soft tissue sarcoma. Acta Radiol 22:461–464, 1983.

67. Bujko K, Suit HD, Springfield DS, et al: Wound healing after preoperative radiation for sarcoma of soft tissues. Surg Gynecol Obstet 176:124–134, 1993.

68. Suit HD, Spiro IJ: The role of radiation in patients with soft tissue sarcomas. Cancer Control 1:592–598, 1994.

69. Eilber FR, Eckardt JJ, Rosen O, et al: Neoadjuvant chemotherapy and radiotherapy in the multidisciplinary management of soft tissue sarcomas of the extremity. Surg Oncol Clin North Am 2:611–620, 1993.

70. Jacques D, Coit D, Brennan M: Soft tissue sarcoma of the retroperitoneum, in Shiu MH, Brennan MF: Surgical Management of Soft Tissue Sarcoma, pp 157–169. Philadelphia, Lea & Febiger, 1989.

71. Jacques D, Coit D, Hadju S, et al: Management of primary and recurrent soft tissue sarcoma of the retroperitoneum. Ann Surg 212:51–59, 1990.

72. Harrison L, Gutierrez E, Fisher J: Retroperitoneal sarcoma: The Yale experience and review of the literature. J Surg Oncol 32:159–164, 1986.

73. Tepper J, Suit HD, Wood W: Radiation therapy of retroperitoneal soft tissue sarcoma. Int J Radiat Oncol Biol Phys 10:825–830, 1984.

74. Khorsand J, Karakousis CP: Desmoid tumors and their management. Am J Surg 149:215–218, 1985.

75. Posner MC, Shiu MH, Newsome JL, et al: The desmoid tumor: Not a benign disease. Arch Surg 124:191–196, 1989.

76. Brasfield RD, Das Gupta TK: Desmoid tumors of the anterior abdominal wall. Surgery 65:241, 1969.

77. Acker JC, Bossen EH, Halperin EC: The management of desmoid tumors. Int J Radiat Oncol Biol Phys 26:851–858, 1993.

78. Miralbell R, Suit HD, Mankin HJ, et al: Fibromatoses: From postsurgical surveillance to combined surgery and radiation therapy. Int J Radiat Oncol Biol Phys 18:535–540, 1990.

79. McCullough WM, Parsons JT, van der Griend R, et al: Radiation therapy for aggressive fibromatosis: The experience at the University of Florida. J Bone Joint Surg Am 735:717–725, 1991.

80. Karakousis CP, Mayordomo J, Zografos GC, et al: Desmoid tumors of the trunk and extremity. Cancer 72:1637–1641, 1993.

81. Bataini JP, Belloir C, Mazabraud A, et al: Desmoid tumors in adults: The role of radiotherapy in their management. Am J Surg 155:754–760, 1988.

82. Leibel SA, Wara WM, Hill DR, et al: Desmoid tumors: Local control and patterns of relapse following radiation therapy. Int J Radiat Oncol Biol Phys 9:1167–1171, 1983.

83. Sherman NE, Romsdahl MM, Evans HL, et al: Desmoid tumors: A 20-year radiotherapy experience. Int J Radiat Oncol Biol Phys 19:37–40, 1990.

84. Patel SR, Evans HL, Benjamin RS: Combination chemotherapy in adult desmoid tumors. Cancer 72:3244–3247, 1993.

85. Kinsbrunner B, Ritter S, Domingo J, et al: Remission of rapidly growing desmoid tumors after tamoxifen therapy. Cancer 52:2201–2204, 1983.

86. Brooks MD, Ebbs SR, Colletta AA, et al: Desmoid tumors treated with triphenylethylenes. Eur J Cancer 28A:1014–1018, 1992.

87. Lanari A: Effect of progesterone on desmoid tumors (aggressive fibromatosis). N Engl J Med 309:1523, 1983.

88. Waddell WR, Gerner RE: Indomethacin and ascorbate inhibit desmoid tumors. J Surg Oncol 15:85–90, 1980.

89. Weiss A, Lackman R: Chemotherapy of desmoid tumors and fibromatosis (abstract #1365). Proc Annu Meet Am Soc Clin Oncol 13:27, 1994.

90. Razek A, Perez CA, Tefft M, et al: Intergroup Ewing's sarcoma study: Local control related to radiation dose, volume, and site of primary lesion in Ewing's sarcoma. Cancer 46:516–521, 1980.

91. Klein HO, Wickramanayake PD, Coerper CL, et al: High dose ifosfamide and mesna as continuous infusion over five days—A phase I/II trial. Cancer Treat Rev 10(suppl A):167–173, 1983.

92. O'Bryan RM, Luce JK, Talley RW, et al: Phase II evaluation of Adriamycin in human neoplasia. Cancer 32:1–8, 1973.

93. Golbey R, Li MC, Kaufman RF: Actinomycin in the treatment of soft part sarcomas (abstract). James Ewing Society Scientific Program, 1968.

94. Buesa JM, Mouridsen HT, Oosterom ATV, et al: High dose DTIC in advanced soft tissue sarcomas in the adult: A phase II study of the EORTC Soft Tissue and Bone Sarcoma Group. Ann Oncol 2:307–309, 1991.

95. Gottlieb JA, Baker LH, Quagliana JM, et al: Chemotherapy of sarcomas with a combination of Adriamycin and dimethyltriazenoimidazole carboxamide. Cancer 30:1632–1638, 1972.

96. Omura GA, Major FJ, Blessing JA, et al: A randomized study of Adriamycin with and without dimethyltriazenoimidazole carboxamide in advanced uterine sarcomas. Cancer 52:626–632, 1983.

97. Borden EC, Amato DA, Rosenbaum C, et al: Randomized comparison of three Adriamycin regimens for metastatic soft tissue sarcomas. J Clin Oncol 5:840–850, 1987.

98. O'Bryan RM, Baker LH, Gottlieb JA, et al: Dose response evaluation of Adriamycin in human neoplasia. Cancer 39:1940–1948, 1977.

99. Zalupski M, Metch B, Balcerzak S, et al: Phase III comparison of doxorubicin and dacarbazine given by bolus versus infusion in patients with soft-tissue sarcomas: A Southwest Oncology Group Study. J Natl Cancer Inst 83:926–932, 1991.

100. Legha SS, Benjamin RS, Mackay B, et al: Reduction of doxorubicin cardiotoxicity by prolonged continuous intravenous infusion. Ann Intern Med 96:133–139, 1982.

101. Magrath IT, Sandlund JT, Rayner A, et al: Treatment of recurrent sarcomas with ifosfamide (abstract #C-528). Proc Annu Meet Am Soc Clin Oncol 4:136, 1985.

102. Antman KH, Ryan L, Elias A, et al: Response to ifosfamide and mesna: One hundred twenty-four previously treated patients with metastatic or unresectable sarcoma. J Clin Oncol 7:126–131, 1989.

103. Patel SR, Vadhan-Raj S, Trevino C, et al: Phase II study of high dose ifosfamide and G-CSF in patients with malignant bone tumors and metastatic soft-tissue sarcomas (abstract #1448). Proc Annu Meet Am Soc Clin Oncol 11:413, 1992.

104. Benjamin RS, Legha SS, Patel SR, et al: Single-agent ifosfamide studies in sarcomas of soft tissue and bone: The M. D. Anderson experience. Cancer Chemother Pharmacol 31(suppl 2):S174–179, 1993.

105. Bramwell V, Rouesse J, Steward W, et al: European experience of adjuvant chemotherapy for soft-tissue sarcoma: Interim report of a randomized trial of CyVADIC versus control, in Ryan JR, Baker LH (eds): Recent Concepts in Sarcoma Treatment, pp 157–164. Dordrecht, The Netherlands: Kluwer Academic, 1988.

106. Ravaud A, Nguyen BB, Coindre JM, et al: Adjuvant chemotherapy with CyVADIC in high-risk soft tissue sarcoma: A randomized prospective trial, in Salmon SE (ed): Adjuvant Therapy of Cancer VI, pp 556–566. Philadelphia, WB Saunders Co, 1990.

107. Benjamin RS, Terjanian TO, Fenoglio CJ, et al: The importance of combination chemotherapy for adjuvant treatment of high-risk patients with soft-tissue sarcomas of the extremities, in Salmon SE (ed): Adjuvant Therapy of Cancer V, pp 735–744. Orlando, FL, Grune & Stratton, 1987.

108. Chang AE, Kinsella TJ, Glatstein E, et al: Adjuvant chemotherapy for patients with high-grade soft-tissue sarcomas of the extremity. J Clin Oncol 6:1491–1500, 1988.

109. Edmonson JH, Fleming TR, Ivins JC, et al: Randomized study of systemic chemotherapy following complete excision of nonosseous sarcomas. J Clin Oncol 2:1390–1396, 1984.

110. Omura GA, Blessing JA, Major F, et al: A randomized clinical trial of adjuvant Adriamycin in uterine sarcomas: A Gynecologic Oncology Group study. J Clin Oncol 3:1240–1245, 1985.

111. Alvegard TA, Sigurdsson H, Mouridsen H, et al: Adjuvant chemotherapy with doxorubicin in high grade soft tissue sarcoma: A randomized trial of the Scandinavian Sarcoma Group. J Clin Oncol 7:1504–1513, 1989.

112. Eilber FR, Giuliano AE, Huth JF, et al: Adjuvant Adriamycin in high grade extremity soft tissue sarcomas: A randomized prospective trial. Proc Annu Meet Am Soc Clin Oncol 5:488, 1986.

113. Baker LH: Adjuvant therapy for soft tissue sarcoma, in Ryan JR, Baker LH (eds): Recent Concepts in Sarcoma Treatment, pp 144–148. Dordrecht, The Netherlands: Kluwer Academic, 1988.

114. Gherlinzoni F, Bacci G, Picci P, et al: A randomized trial for the treatment of high grade soft tissue sarcomas of the extremities: Preliminary observations. J Clin Oncol 4:552–558, 1986.

115. Antman KH, Ryan L, Borden E, et al: Pooled results from three randomized adjuvant studies of doxorubicin versus observation in soft tissue sarcomas: Ten-year results and review of the literature, in Salmon SE (ed): Adjuvant Therapy of Cancer VI, pp 529–544. Philadelphia, WB Saunders Co, 1990.

116. Antman KH, Amato D, Lerner H, et al: ECOG and Dana Farber Cancer Institute/MGH Study, in Salmon SE (ed): Adjuvant Therapy of Cancer V, pp 611–620. Orlando, FL, Grune & Stratton, 1987.

117. Zalupski M, Ryan J, Hussein M, et al: Defining the role of adjuvant chemotherapy for patients with soft tissue sarcoma of the extremities, in Salmon SE (ed): Adjuvant Therapy of Cancer VII, pp 385–392. Philadelphia, JB Lippincott Co, 1993.

118. Lindberg RD, Martin RG, Romsdahl MM, et al: Conservative surgery and postoperative radiotherapy in 300 adults with soft-tissue sarcomas. Cancer 47:2391–2397, 1981.

119. Giuliano AE, Eilber FR, Morton DL: The management of locally recurrent soft tissue sarcoma. Ann Surg 196:87–91, 1982.

120. Singer S, Antman KH, Corson JM, et al: Long term salvageability for patients with locally recurrent soft tissue sarcomas. Arch Surg 127:548–554, 1992.

121. Putman JB Jr, Roth JA, Wesley MN, et al: Analysis of prognostic factors in patients undergoing resection of pulmonary metastases from soft tissue sarcomas. J Thorac Cardiovasc Surg 87:260–268, 1984.

122. Jablons D, Steinberg SM, Roth JA, et al: Metastasectomy for soft tissue sarcoma: Further evidence for efficacy and prognostic indicators. J Thorac Cardiovasc Surg 97:695–705, 1989.

123. Casson AG, Putnam JB Jr, Natarajan G, et al: Five-year survival after pulmonary metastasectomy for adult soft tissue sarcoma. Cancer 59:662–668, 1992.

124. Bramwell V, Quirt I, Warr D, et al: Combination chemotherapy with doxorubicin and ifosfamide in advanced adult soft tissue sarcoma. J Natl Cancer Inst 81:1496–1499, 1989.

125. Shutte J, Mouridsen HT, Stewart W, et al: Ifosfamide plus doxorubicin in previously untreated patients with advanced soft tissue sarcoma. Eur J Cancer 26:558–561, 1990.

126. Loehrer PJ, Sledge GW, Nicaise C, et al: Ifosfamide plus doxorubicin in metastatic adult sarcomas: A multi-institutional phase II trial. J Clin Oncol 7:1655–1659, 1989.

127. Elias A, Ryan LM, Aisner J, et al: Mesna, doxorubicin, ifosfamide, dacarbazine (MAID) regimen for adults with advanced sarcoma. Semin Oncol 17(suppl 4):44–49, 1990.

128. Steward WP, Verzweij J, Somers R, et al: Doxorubicin plus ifosfamide with rh-GM-CSF in the treatment of advanced adult soft-tissue sarcomas: Preliminary results of a phase II study from the EORTC Soft Tissue and Bone Sarcoma Group. J Cancer Res Clin Oncol 117S:193–197, 1991.

129. Casali P, Pastorino V, Zuchinelli P, et al: Epirubicin plus ifosfamide and dacarbazine (EID) in advanced soft tissue sarcomas. Ann Oncol 3(suppl 2):S125–126, 1992.

130. Antman KH, Crowley J, Balcerzak SP, et al: An intergroup phase III randomized study of doxorubicin and dacarbazine with or without ifosfamide and mesna in advanced soft tissue and bone sarcomas. J Clin Oncol 11:1276–1285, 1993.

131. Edmonson JH, Ryan LM, Blevin RA, et al: Randomized comparison of doxorubicin alone versus ifosfamide plus doxorubicin or mitomycin, doxorubicin, and cisplatin against soft tissue sarcomas. J Clin Oncol 11:1269–1275, 1993.

132. Cheson D, Lacerna L, Leyland-Jones B, et al: Autologous bone marrow transplantation: Current status in future directions. Ann Intern Med 100:51–65, 1989.

133. Antman KH, Eder JP, Frei E: High dose chemotherapy with bone marrow support for solid tumors. Important Adv Oncol 221–235, 1987.

134. Ackerman LV, del Regato JA: Cancer Diagnosis, Treatment, and Prognosis, p 1028. St. Louis, MO, CV Mosby Co, 1954.

135. Rosenthal DI: Computed tomography in bone and soft tissue neoplasms: Application and pathologic correlation. Crit Rev Diagn Imaging 18:243–278, 1982.

136. Jeffree GM, Price CHG, Sissins HA: The metastatic spread of osteosarcoma. Br J Cancer 32:87–107, 1975.

137. Collins JD, Bassett L, Main GD, et al: Percutaneous biopsy following positive bone scans. Radiology 132:439–442, 1979.

138. McKillop JH, Etcubanas EL, Goris ML: The indications for and limitations of bone scintigraphy in osteogenic sarcoma: A review of 55 patients. Cancer 48:113–1138, 1981.

139. Malawer MM, Dunham WF: Skip metastases in osteosarcoma: Recent experience. J Surg Oncol 22:236–245, 1983.

140. Zimmer WD, Berquist TH, McLeod RA, et al: Bone tumors: Magnetic resonance imaging versus computed tomography. Radiology 155:709–718, 1985.

141. Sundaram M, McGuire MH, Herbold DR: Magnetic resonance imaging of osteosarcoma. Skeletal Radiol 16:23–29, 1987.

142. Bloem JL, Taminiau AHM, Eulderink FM, et al: Radiologic staging of primary bone sarcoma: MR imaging, scintigraphy, angiography, and CT correlated with pathologic examination. Radiology 169:805–810, 1988.

143. Hudson TM, Hass G, Enneking WF, et al: Angiography in the management of musculoskeletal tumors. Surg Gynecol Obstet 141:11–21, 1975.

144. Carrasco CH, Charnsangavel C, Raymond AK, et al: Osteosarcoma: Angiographic assessment of response to preoperative chemotherapy. Radiology 170:839–842, 1989.

145. Ayala AG, Raymond AK, Ro JY, et al: Needle biopsy of primary bone lesions: M. D. Anderson experience. Pathol Annu 24:219–251, 1989.

146. Ayala AG, Zornosa J: Primary bone tumors: Percutaneous needle biopsy: Radiologic-pathologic study of 222 biopsies. Radiology 149:675–679, 1983.

147. Enneking WF, Spanier SS, Goodman MA: A system for the surgical staging of musculoskeletal sarcoma. Clin Orthop 153:106–120, 1980.

148. McKenna RJ, Schwinn CP, Soong KY, et al: Sarcomata of the osteogenic series (osteosarcoma, fibrosarcoma, chondrosarcoma, parosteal osteosarcoma, and sarcomata) arising in abnormal bone: An analysis of 552 cases. J Bone Joint Surg Am 48:1–26, 1966.

149. Dahlin DC, Coventry MB: Osteosarcoma, a study of 600 cases. J Bone Joint Surg Am 49:101–110, 1967.

150. Togushida J, Ishizaki K, Sasaki MS, et al: Chromosomal reorganization for the expression of recessive mutation of retinoblastoma susceptibility gene in the development of osteosarcoma. Cancer Res 48:3939–3943, 1988.

151. Abramson DH, Ellsworth RM, Kitchin FD, et al: Second nonocular tumors in retinoblastoma survivors: Are they radiation-induced? Ophthalmology 91:1351–1355, 1984.

152. Togushida J, Ishizaki K, Sasaki MS, et al: Preferential mutation of paternally derived RB gene as the initial event in sporadic osteosarcoma. Nature 338:156–158, 1989.

153. Wadayama B, Togushida J, Shimizu T, et al: Mutation spectrum of the retinoblastoma gene in osteosarcomas. Cancer Res 54:3042–3048, 1994.

154. Wilner D: Osteogenic sarcoma (osteosarcoma), in Wilner D (ed): Radiology of Bone Tumors and Allied Disorders, pp 1897–2005. Philadelphia, W.B. Saunders Co, 1992.

155. Wick MB, Siegal GP, Unni KK, et al: Sarcomas of bone complicating osteitis deformans (Paget's disease), 50 years' experience. Am J Surg Pathol 5:47–59, 1981.

156. Fraumeni JF Jr, Boice JD Jr: Bone, in Schottenfeld D, Fraumeni JF Jr (eds): Cancer Epidemiology and Prevention, pp 814–826. Philadelphia, WB Saunders Co, 1982.

157. Huvos AG, Woodard HQ, Cahan WG, et al: Postradiation osteogenic sarcoma of bone and soft tissues: A clinicopathologic study of 66 patients. Cancer 55:1244–1255, 1982.

158. DeSantos LA, Edeiken B: Purely lytic osteosarcoma. Skeletal Radiol 9:1–7, 1982.

159. Lockshin MD, Higgins TT: Prognosis in osteogenic sarcoma. Clin Orthop 58:85–101, 1968.

160. Francis KC, Kohn H, Malawer MM: Osteogenic sarcoma. J Bone Joint Surg Am 55:754, 1976.

161. Look AT, Douglass EC, Meyer WH: Clinical importance of near-diploid tumor stem lines in patients with osteosarcoma of the extremity. N Engl J Med 318:1567–1572, 1988.

162. Davis AM, Bell RS, Goodwin PJ: Prognostic factors in osteosarcoma: A critical review. J Clin Oncol 12:423–431, 1994.

163. Sweetnam R: Surgical management of primary osteosarcoma. Clin Orthop 111:57–64, 1975.

164. Friedman MA, Carter SK: The therapy of osteogenic sarcoma: Current status and thoughts for the future. J Surg Oncol 45:482, 1972.

165. Jaffe N: Recent advances in the chemotherapy of metastatic osteogenic sarcoma. Cancer 30:1627–1631, 1972.

166. Cortes EP, Holland JF, Wang JJ, et al: Amputation and Adriamycin in primary osteosarcoma. N Engl J Med 291:998, 1974.

167. Ochs JJ, Freeman AI, Douglas HO Jr, et al: Cis-diamminedichloroplatinum (II) in advanced osteogenic sarcoma. Cancer Treat Rep 62:239–245, 1978.

168. Antman KH, Montella D, Rosenbaum C, et al: Phase II trial of ifosfamide with MESNA in previously treated metastatic sarcoma. Cancer Treat Rep 69:499–504, 1985.

169. Salh RA, Graham-Pole J, Cassano W, et al: Response of osteogenic sarcoma to the combination of etoposide and cyclophosphamide as neoadjuvant chemotherapy. Cancer 65:861–865,1990.

170. Link MP, Goorin AM, Miser A, et al: The effect of adjuvant chemotherapy in patients with osteosarcoma of the extremity. N Engl J Med 314:1600–1608, 1986.

171. Eilber FR, Eckardt JJ, Morton L: Advantages in the treatment of sarcomas of the extremity: Current status of limb salvage. Cancer 54:2695–2701, 1984.

172. Murray JA: Limb salvage surgery: An overview. Cancer Bulletin 42:332–337, 1990.

173. Rosen G, Caparos B, Huvos AG, et al: Preoperative chemotherapy for osteosarcoma. Cancer 49:1221–1230, 1982.

174. Jaffe N, Farber S, Traggis D, et al: Favorable response of metastatic osteogenic sarcoma to pulsed high dose methotrexate with citrovorum rescue and radiation therapy. Cancer 31:1367–1373, 1973.

175. Pratt C, Howarth C, Ransom J, et al: High dose methotrexate used alone and in combination for measurable primary and metastatic osteosarcoma. Cancer Treat Rep 64:11–20, 1980.

176. Jaffe N, Frei E, Traggis D, et al: Weekly high dose methotrexate-citrovorum factor in osteogenic sarcoma: Presurgical treatment of primary tumor and overt pulmonary metastases. Cancer 39:45–50, 1977.

177. Edmonson J, Creagan E, Gilchrist G: Phase II study of high dose methotrexate in patients with unresectable metastatic osteosarcoma. Cancer Treat Rep 65:538–539, 1981.

178. Grem J, King S, Wittes R, et al: The role of methotrexate in osteosarcoma. J Natl Cancer Inst 80:626–655, 1988.

179. Rosen G, Nirenberg A: Chemotherapy for osteogenic sarcoma. An investigative method, not a recipe. Cancer Treat Rep 66:1687–1697, 1982.

180. Smith MA, Ungerleider RS, Horowitz ME, et al: Influence of doxorubicin dose intensity on response and outcome for patients with osteogenic sarcoma and Ewing's sarcoma. J Natl Cancer Inst 83:1460–1470, 1991.

181. Huvos AG, Rosen G, Marcove RC: Primary osteogenic sarcoma: Pathologic aspects in 20 patients after treatment with chemotherapy, en bloc resection, and prosthetic bone replacement. Arch Pathol Lab Med 101:14–18, 1977.

182. Raymond AK, Chawla SP, Carrasco CH, et al: Osteosarcoma chemotherapy effect: A prognostic factor. Semin Diagn Pathol 4:212–236, 1987.

183. Benjamin RS, Chawla SP, Murray JA, et al: Preoperative chemotherapy for osteosarcoma: A treatment approach facilitating limb salvage with major prognostic implications, in Jones SE, Salmon SE (eds): Adjuvant Therapy of Cancer IV, pp 601-610. Orlando, FL, Grune Stratton, 1984.

184. Bacci G, Picci P, Arella M, et al: Effect of intra-arterial versus intravenous cisplatin in addition to systemic Adriamycin and high dose methotrexate on histologic tumor response of osteosarcoma of the extremities. J Chemother 4:189–195, 1992.

185. Jaffe N, Raymond AK, Ayala AG, et al: Analysis of the efficacy of intra-arterial cis-diamminedichloroplatinum II and high dose methotrexate with citrovorum factor rescue in the treatment of primary osteosarcoma. Cancer Treat Rep 2:157–163, 1989.

186. Benjamin RS, Chawla SP, Carrasco CH, et al: Primary chemotherapy for osteosarcoma-implications for limb salvage and ultimate prognosis, in Jacquillat C, Weil M, Khayat D (eds): Neo-Adjuvant Chemotherapy-First International Congress, pp 557–565. London, John Libby Eurotext, 1986.

187. Benjamin RS, Patel SR, Armen T, et al: Primary chemotherapy of osteosarcoma of the extremities—Long-term follow-up (abstract #1639). Proc Annu Meet Am Soc Clin Oncol 12:470, 1993.

187a. Sone S, Fidler IJ: In vitro activation of tumoricidal properties in rat alveolar macrophages by synthetic muramyldipeptide encapsulated in liposomes. Cell Immunol 57:42–50, 1981.

187b. Key ME, Talmadge JE, Fogler WE, et al: Isolation of tumoricidal macrophages from lung melanoma metastases of mice treated systemically with liposomes containing a lipophilic derivative of muramyldipeptide. J Natl Cancer Inst 69:1189–1198, 1982.

188. MacEwen EG, Kuzzman ID, Rosenthal RC, et al: Therapy for osteosarcoma in dogs with intravenous injection of liposome-encapsulated muramyltripeptide. J Natl Cancer Inst 81:935–938, 1989.

189. Kleinerman ES, Raymond AK, Bucana C, et al: Unique histological changes in lung metastases of osteosarcoma patients following therapy with liposomal muramyltripeptide (CGP 19835A lipid). Cancer Immunol Immunother 34:211–220, 1992.

190. Kleinerman ES, Gano J, Johnson D, et al: Efficacy of liposomal muramyltripeptide (L-MTP-PE) in relapsed osteosarcoma (abstract #1445). Proc Annu Meet Am Soc Clin Oncol 12:420, 1993.

191. Putnam JB Jr, Roth JA, Wesley MN, et al: Survival following aggressive resection of pulmonary metastases from osteogenic sarcoma: Analysis of prognostic factors. Ann Thorac Surg 36:516–523, 1983.

192. Skinner KA, Eilber FR, Holmes C, et al: Surgical treatment and chemotherapy for pulmonary metastases from osteosarcoma. Arch Surg 127:1065–1071, 1992.

193. Meyers PA, Heller G, Healey JH, et al: Osteogenic sarcoma with clinically detectable metastasis at initial presentation. J Clin Oncol 11:449–453, 1993.

194. Pratt CB, Douglas EC, Etcubanas EL, et al: Ifosfamide in pediatric malignant solid tumors. Cancer Chemother Pharmacol 24(suppl 1):524–527, 1989.

195. Miser JS, Kinsella TJ, Triche TJ, et al: Ifosfamide with mesna uroprotection and etoposide: An effective regimen in the treatment of recurrent sarcomas and other tumors of children and young adults. J Clin Oncol 5(8):1191–1198, 1987.

196. Cade S: Osteogenic sarcoma: A study based on 133 patients. J R Coll Surg Edinb 1:79–111, 1955.

197. Beck JC, Wara WM, Bovill EG, et al: The role of radiation therapy in the treatment of osteosarcoma. Radiology 120:163–165, 1976.

198. Chambers RG, Mahoney WD: Osteogenic sarcoma of the mandible: Current management. Am Surg 36:463–471, 1970.

199. Martinez A, Goffinet DR, Donaldson SS, et al: Intra-arterial infusion of radiosensitizer (BUDR) combined with hypofractionated irradiation and chemotherapy for primary treatment of osteogenic sarcoma. Int J Radiat Oncol Biol Phys 2:123–128, 1985.

200. Kinsella TJ, Glatstein EJ: Clinical experience with intravenous radiosensitizers in unresectable sarcomas. Cancer 59:908–915, 1987.

201. Ahuja SC, Villacin AB, Smith J, et al: Juxtacortical (parosteal) osteogenic sarcoma. J Bone Joint Surg Am 59:632–647, 1977.

202. Unni KK, Dahlin DC, Beaubout SW, et al: Parosteal osteogenic sarcoma. Cancer 37:2466–2475, 1976.

203. Unni KK, Dahlin DC, Beaubout SW: Periosteal osteogenic sarcoma. Cancer 37:2476–2485, 1976.

204. Shives TS, Wold LE, Dahlin DC, et al: Chondrosarcoma and its variants, in Sim FH (ed): Diagnosis and Treatment of Bone Tumors: A Team Approach, pp 211–217. Thorofare, NJ, Slack, 1983.

205. Marcove RC: Chondrosarcoma: Diagnosis and treatment. Orthop Clin North Am 8:811–819, 1977.

206. Garrison RC, Unni KK, Mcleod RA, et al: Chondrosarcoma arising in osteochondroma. Cancer 49:1890–1897, 1982.

207. Marcove RC, Mike V, Hutter RVP, et al: Chondrosarcoma of the pelvis and upper end of the femur: An analysis of factors influencing survival time in one hundred and thirteen cases. J Bone Joint Surg Am 54: 561–572, 1972.

208. Sanerkin NG: The diagnosis and grading of chondrosarcoma of the bone: A combined cytologic and histologic approach. Cancer 45:582–594, 1980.

209. Austin-Seymour M, Munzenrider J, Goitein M, et al: Fractionated proton radiation therapy of chordoma and low grade chondrosarcoma of the base of the skull. J Neurosurg 70:13–17, 1989.

210. Krochak R, Harwood AR, Cummings BJ, et al: Results of radical radiation for chondrosarcoma of bone. Radiother Oncol 1: 109–115, 1983.

211. McNaney D, Lindberg RD, Ayala AG, et al: Fifteen years' radiotherapy experience with chondrosarcoma of bone. Int J Radiat Oncol Biol Phys 8:187–190, 1982.

212. Unni KK, Dahlin DC, Beaubout SW, et al: Chondrosarcoma: Clear–cell variant: A report of 16 cases. J Bone Joint Surg Am 57:676–683, 1976.

213. Harwood AR, Krajbich JI, Fornasier VL: Mesenchymal chondrosarcoma: A report of 17 cases. Clin Orthop 158:144–148, 1981.

214. Huvos AG, Rosen G, Dabska M, et al: Mesenchymal chondrosarcoma: A clinicopathologic analysis of 35 patients with emphasis on treatment. Cancer 51:1230–1237, 1983.

215. McCarthy EF, Matsuno T, Dorfman HD: Malignant fibrous histiocytoma of bone: A study of 35 cases. Hum Pathol 10:57–70, 1979.

216. Huvos AG: Primary malignant fibrous histiocytoma of bone: Clinicopathologic study of 18 patients. N Y State J Med 76:552–559, 1976.

217. Spanier SS, Enneking WF, Enriquez P: Primary malignant fibrous histiocytoma of bone. Cancer 36:2084–2098, 1975.

218. Bacci G, Springfield D, Picci P, et al: Adjuvant chemotherapy for malignant fibrous histiocytoma in the femur and tibia. J Bone Joint Surg Am 67:620–625, 1985.

219. Heeten GJ, Koops HS, Kamps WA, et al: Treatment of malignant fibrous histiocytoma of bone: A plea for primary chemotherapy. Cancer 56:37–40, 1985.

220. Earl HM, Pringle J, Kemp B, et al: Chemotherapy of malignant fibrous histiocytoma of bone (MFHB). Ann Oncol 4:409–415, 1993.

221. Patel SR, Armen T, Carrasco CH, et al: Primary chemotherapy in malignant fibrous histiocytoma of bone—Updated UTMD Anderson Cancer Center Experience, in Banzet P, Holland JF, Khayat D, et al (eds): Cancer Treatment: An Update, pp 577–580. Paris, Springer-Verlag, 1994.

222. Ewing J: Diffuse endothelioma of bone. Proc N Y Path Soc 21:17–24, 1921.

223. Yunis EJ: Ewing's sarcoma and related small round cell neoplasms in children. Am J Surg Pathol 10:54–62, 1986.

224. Cavazzana AD, Magnani JL, Ross RA, et al: Ewing's sarcoma is an undifferentiated neuroectodermal tumor, in Evans AC, D'Angio GJ, Knudson AG, et al (eds): Advances in Neuroblastoma Research II, pp 487–498. New York, Alan R Liss, 1988.

225. Pinto A, Grant LH, Hayes FA, et al: Immunohistochemical expression of neuron-specific enolase and Leu7 in Ewing's sarcoma of bone. Cancer 64:1266–1273, 1989.

226. Tsokos M, Linnoila RI, Chandra RS, et al: Neuron-specific enolase in the diagnosis of neuroblastoma and other small, round-cell tumors in children. Hum Pathol 15:575–584, 1984.

227. Hara S, Ishii E, Tanaka S, et al: A monoclonal antibody specifically reactive with Ewing's sarcoma. Br J Cancer 60:875–879, 1989.

228. Ambros IM, Ambros PF, Strehl S, et al: MIC2 is a specific marker for Ewing's sarcoma and peripheral primitive neuroectodermal tumors. Cancer 67:1886–1893, 1991.

229. Ushigome S, Shimoda T, Takaki K, et al: Immunocytochemical and ultrastructural studies of the histogenesis of Ewing's sarcoma and putatively related tumors. Cancer 64:52–62, 1989.

230. Aurias A, Rimbaut C, Buffe D, et al: Chromosomal translocation in Ewing's sarcoma. N Engl J Med 309:496–497, 1983.

231. Tur Cavel C, Aurias A, Mugneret F, et al: Chromosomes in Ewing's sarcoma: An evaluation of 85 cases and remarkable consistency of t(11;22) (q24;q12). Cancer Genet Cytogenet 321:229–238, 1988.

232. Whang-Peng J, Triche TJ, Kuntsen T, et al: Cytogenetic characterization of selected small round cell tumors of childhood. Cancer Genet Cytogenet 21:185–208, 1986.

233. Johnson RE, Pomeroy TC: Prognostic factors for survival in Ewing's sarcoma. AJR Rad Ther Nucl Med 123:598–606, 1975.

234. Mendenhall CM, Marcus RB Jr, Enneking WF, et al: The prognostic significance of soft tissue extension in Ewing's sarcoma. Cancer 51:913–917, 1983.

235. Glaubiger DL, Makuch R, Schwarz J, et al: Determination of prognostic factors and their influence on therapeutic results in patients with Ewing's sarcoma. Cancer 45:2213–2219 1980.

236. Picci P, Rougraft BT, Bacci G, et al: Prognostic significance of histopathologic response to chemotherapy in nonmetastatic Ewing's sarcoma of the extremities. J Clin Oncol 11:1763–1769, 1993.

237. Phillips RF, Higinbotham NL: The curability of Ewing's endothelioma of bone in children. J Pediatr 70:391–397, 1967.

238. Wang CC, Schultz MD: Ewing's sarcoma. N Engl J Med 248:571–576, 1953.

239. Thomas PRM, Foulkes MA, Gilula LA, et al: Primary Ewing's sarcoma of the ribs. Cancer 51:1021–1027, 1983.

240. Bacci G, Toni A, Avella M, et al: Long-term results in 144 localized Ewing's sarcoma patients treated with combined therapy. Cancer 63:1477–1486, 1989.

241. Lewis R, Marcove RC, Rosen G: Ewing's sarcoma: Functional effects of radiation therapy. J Bone Joint Surg Am 59:325–331, 1977.

242. Teft M, Lattin P, Jereb B, et al: Acute and late effects on normal tissues following combined chemotherapy and radiation therapy for childhood rhabdomyosarcoma and Ewing's sarcoma. Cancer 37:1201–1223, 1976.

243. Rosen G, Wallner N, Tau C, et al: Disease-free survival in children with Ewing's sarcoma treated with radiation therapy and adjuvant four-drug sequential chemotherapy. Cancer 33:384–393, 1974.

244. Vietti TJ, Gehan EA, Nesbit ME: Multimodal therapy in metastatic Ewing's sarcoma: An intergroup study. Natl Cancer Inst Monogr 56:279–284, 1981.

245. Rosen G, Caparros B, Nirenburg A, et al: Ewing's sarcoma: Ten-year experience with adjuvant chemotherapy. Cancer 47:2204–2213, 1981.

246. Gasparini M, Lombardi F, Gianni C, et al: Localized Ewing's sarcoma: Results of integrated therapy and analysis of failures. Eur J Cancer 17:1205–1209, 1981.

247. Hayes FA, Thompson FL, Hustu HD, et al: The response of Ewing's sarcoma to sequential cyclophosphamide and Adriamycin induction therapy. J Clin Oncol 1:45–51, 1983.

248. Kinsella TJ, Glaubiger D, Deisseroth A, et al: Intensive combined modality therapy including low-dose TBI in high-risk Ewing's sarcoma patients. Int J Radiat Oncol Biol Phys 9:1955–1960, 1983.

249. Miser J, Kinsella TJ, Triche T, et al: Preliminary results of treatment of Ewing's sarcoma of bone in children and young adults: Six months of intensive combined modality therapy without mainte-

nance. J Clin Oncol 6:484–490, 1988.

250. Samuels ML, Howe CD: Cyclophosphamide in the management of Ewing's sarcoma. Cancer 20:961–966, 1967.

251. Oldham RK, Pomeroy TC: Treatment of Ewing's sarcoma with Adriamycin (NSC–123127). Cancer Chemother Rep 56:635–639, 1972.

252. Sutow WN: Vincristine (NSC-67574) therapy for malignant solid tumors in children (except Wilms' tumor). Cancer Chemother Rep 52:485–487, 1968.

253. Cornbleet MA, Corringham RET, Prentice HG, et al: Treatment of Ewing's sarcoma with high-dose melphalan and autologous bone marrow transplantation. Cancer Treat Rep 65:241–244, 1981.

254. Nesbit ME, Gehan EA, Burgert ED Jr, et al: Multimodal therapy for the management of primary, nonmetastatic Ewing's sarcoma of bone: A long-term follow-up of the First Intergroup Study. J Clin Oncol 8:1664–1674, 1990.

255. Burgert ED Jr, Nesbit ME, Garnsey LA, et al: Multimodal therapy for the management of nonpelvic localized Ewing's sarcoma of bone: Intergroup study: IESS-II. J Clin Oncol 8:1514–1524, 1990.

256. Evans RG, Nesbit ME, Gehan EA, et al: Multimodal therapy for the management of localized Ewing's sarcoma of pelvic and sacral bones: A report from the Second Intergoup Study. J Clin Oncol 9:1173–1180, 1991.

257. Meyer WH, Kun L, Marina N, et al: Ifosfamide plus etoposide in newly diagnosed Ewing's sarcoma of bone. J Clin Oncol 10:1737–1742, 1992.

258. Miser JS, Kinsella TJ, Triche TJ, et al: Ifosfamide with mesna uroprotection and etoposide: An effective regimen in the treatment of recurrent sarcomas and other tumors of children and young adults. J Clin Oncol 5:1191–1198, 1987.

259. Pilepich M, Vietti TJ, Nesbit ME, et al: Radiotherapy and combination chemotherapy in advanced Ewing's sarcoma: Intergroup Study. Cancer 47:1930–1936, 1981.

260. Hayes FA, Thompson EI, Parvey L, et al: Metastatic Ewing's sarcoma: Remission induction and survival. J Clin Oncol 5:1199–1204, 1987.

261. Cangir A, Vietti TJ, Gehan EA, et al: Ewing's sarcoma metastatic at diagnosis: Results and comparisons of two Intergroup Ewing's sarcoma studies. Cancer 66:887–893, 1990.

262. Burdach J, Jurgens H, Peters C, et al: Myeloablative radiochemotherapy and hematopoietic stem cell rescue in poor-prognosis Ewing's sarcoma. J Clin Oncol 11:1482–1488, 1993.

263. Horowitz ME, Kinsella TJ, Wexler LH, et al: Total-body irradiation and autologous bone marrow transplant in the treatment of high-risk Ewing's sarcoma and rhabdomyosarcoma. J Clin Oncol 11:1911–1918, 1993.

CHAPTER 34

Retrovirus-Associated Malignancies

Virginia Rhodes, MD, *and* Fredrick B. Hagemeister, MD

Department of Hematology, The University of Texas M. D. Anderson Cancer Center, Houston, Texas

Although investigators knew before 1980 that retroviruses could cause various forms of leukemia, lymphoma, and solid tumors in animals, not until then was the first human oncogenic retrovirus, human T-cell leukemia/lymphoma virus-I (HTLV-I), isolated.[1] Discovery of the human immunodeficiency virus (HIV) followed in l983.[2] These viruses are unique in being composed of single-stranded RNA, and they replicate by forming double-stranded DNA that is integrated into the host-cell genome. The enzyme reverse transcriptase is fundamental to the replication process.[3] Once the virus is incorporated into the host cell, a variety of proteins are produced that may activate or transform the normal cell into a malignant one. For example, retroviral genomes contain promoter and enhancer sequences that may activate adjacent host genes and trigger cell division (*cis*-activation). Expression of viral proteins may also contribute to activation of host genes (*trans*-activation). In addition, the viral genome may contain oncogenes that directly transform cells upon incorporation into the host cell genome.[3–5]

There are three families of retroviruses. Oncoviruses contain both direct transforming viruses and chronic transforming viruses that induce malignancy over long latency periods.[4] HTLV-I, -II, and -V are included in the oncovirus family.[4,6] Lentiviruses include HIV-1 and -2. The third family, spumaviruses, are not yet known to be associated with human diseases.[3,4]

HIV induces immune dysfunction in a variety of ways. Immune abnormalities observed in HIV infection include depletion and dysfunction of CD4-positive T-cells; polyclonal activation of B-cells (often associated with hypergammaglobulinemia and autoimmune phemomena); and diminished function of monocytes, macrophages, and natural killer cells (Table 1).[7] Patients exhibit impaired B-cell response to T-cell-dependent antigens, impaired cell-mediated immunity, delayed-type hypersensitivity, and abnormal cytokine expression. Collectively, these immune system defects provide multiple opportunities for malignant transformation on the molecular level and the maintenance of malignant cell growth once established.[4,7,8]

By the time the HIV epidemic was underway, investigators had already realized that transplant recipients develop atypical lymphomas involving extranodal sites or the central nervous system (CNS) at 25 to 50 times the expected rate, anogenital cancer at 100 times, Kaposi's sarcoma at 400 to 500 times, and squamous-cell cancers of the skin at 3 to 20 times the expected rate.[3,9,10] These patients present with malignancy within 2 to 8 years of the onset of immunosuppressive therapy and often exhibit particularly virulent tumors.[10] Similarly, HIV-infected patients present with malignancy at a higher than expected rate, at younger ages, and with a more virulent course than the general population.

Malignancy in patients with impaired immunity is the result of multiple factors. Immunosuppression itself can impair immune surveillance, which controls virally mediated cancers. Immunosuppressed patients often demonstrate chronic antigenic stimulation induced by an allograft or by repetitive acquired infections, which may increase the opportunity for random transforming mutations. Finally, dysregulation of the immune system, with a lack of the proper suppressor mechanisms, may result in malignant transformation.[9]

HIV-ASSOCIATED MALIGNANCIES

First described in 1983, HIV-1 is now recognized worldwide as a cause of the acquired immunodeficiency syndrome (AIDS). A second serotype, HIV-2, is confined primarily to West Africa. Since the onset of the AIDS epidemic, advances in therapy have prolonged the median life expectancy of patients with HIV infection to more than 12 years.[11] However, a consequence of this improved survival rate is a rising incidence of HIV-related malignancies. Levine has predicted that up to 40% of persons with AIDS will develop cancer[12]; therapy for these malignancies will thus pose a significant challenge to physicians caring for these patients in the future.

Although many malignancies have been reported in association with HIV infection, only three malignancies are conclusively associated with HIV infection and are considered AIDS-defining conditions. These include Kaposi's sarcoma (KS), intermediate or high-grade non-Hodgkin's B-cell lymphomas (including primary CNS lymphoma), and cervical carcinoma.[5,13,14] Other malig-

TABLE I

Abnormalities of CD4+ T-Lymphocytes, B-Lymphocytes, Monocytes, and Natural Killer Cells in HIV-Infected Individuals

Proposed mechanism	Pathophysiologic outcome	Symptoms
CD4+ lymphocytes		
Fusion of gp 120 with CD4	Syncytial formation/cell death	CD4+ T-cell depletion
Binding of secreted gp 120 to CD4	Immune-mediated cytolysis	CD4+ T-cell depletion
Binding of secreted gp 120 to CD4	T-cells with class II MHC molecules on antigen-presenting cells	
Binding of anti-CD4 antibodies to CD4	Cell death/defective antigen recognition	CD4+ T-cell depletion or dysfunction
Decreased expression of CD4 on the cell surface	Defective antigen recognition	CD4+ T-cell depletion or dysfunction
B-lymphocytes		
Defective T-cell helper function	Defective humoral immunity	Pyogenic infections
Infection with EBV, CMV, and double infection with HIV and EBV or HIV and CMV	Polyclonal B-cell proliferation	Hypergammaglobulinemia, autoimmune phenomena B-cell neoplasms
gp 120 binding to B-lymphocytes may imitate the binding of neuroleukin		
Monocytes/macrophages		
Defective T-cell helper function HIV infection of monocytes	Defective macrophage function Production of monokines (IL-1, TNF) Reservoir of infection in vivo	Fever, weight loss, interstitial pneumonitis, brain damage
Natural killer cells		
Defective inductive signals	Natural killer cells dysfunction in vivo	Tumor cell growth

CMV = cytomegalovirus, EBV = Epstein-Barr virus, HIV = human immunodeficiency virus, IL = interleukin, MHC = major histocompatibility complex, TNF = tumor-necrosis factor.   Adapted, with permission, from Lazo PA, Tsichlis PN: Biology and pathogenesis of retroviruses. *Semin Oncol* 17:269–294, 1990.

nancies (eg, Hodgkin's disease, anorectal carcinoma, pediatric smooth muscle tumors, noncervical gynecologic cancers, and nonmelanoma skin cancers) may be associated with AIDS but are probably underreported.[12]

KAPOSI'S SARCOMA

Prior to the AIDS epidemic, KS was seen mostly as an indolent, pigmented lesion involving the lower extremities in older men of Jewish, Eastern, or Mediterranean descent.[15,16] The disease rarely involved lymph nodes, mucous membranes, or visceral organs. Moreover, up to one third of these patients demonstrated a second primary malignancy, most frequently non-Hodgkin's lymphoma.[15,16]

An endemic form of KS also occurs in children and adults in tropical Africa. In adults, it is a benign nodular

form or a more aggressive local or visceral form with a median survival of 5 to 8 years.[15,16] In children, the disease involves visceral organs and lymph nodes with lymphedema. It is typically virulent and fatal in 2 to 3 years (Table 2).[15,16]

HIV-ASSOCIATED KAPOSI'S SARCOMA

Epidemiology

Aggressive KS is the most prevalent cancer among HIV-1-infected patients, with estimated attack rates as high as 30%.[17] The relative risk of KS in HIV-infected adult male homosexuals is 10,000- to 40,000-fold higher than in the general population.[3,18] However, this incidence has decreased over time. From 1981 to 1984, 50% of AIDS patients in San Francisco exhibited KS lesions during the course of their disease. By 1992, the rate had dropped to only 14%.[3,13,15,16,18] Yet despite this decrease, the overall incidence of AIDS-KS continues to rise along with the numbers of HIV-infected patients.[19]

The prevalence of KS varies among different categories of AIDS patients by the route of HIV infection and by geographic location (Figure 1).[8,16] Kaposi's sarcoma is six times more common in male homosexuals than in other risk groups, and 95% of AIDS-related KS cases in the United States and Europe are diagnosed in homosexual males.[15] Kaposi's sarcoma also occurs more often in San Francisco, New York, and Los Angeles, which have been centers of the AIDS epidemic.[14]

A history of anal-receptive intercourse or oral-fecal contact is linked to KS development, suggesting that a second infectious agent may be required for the development of KS.[12,14,16] This is supported by an observed decrease in the incidence of KS among homosexual males with changing sexual practices in the late 1980s; the occurrence of KS in homosexual males who are HIV seronegative; the nearly equal incidence of KS among males and females in Africa, where HIV is spread by heterosexual contact; and the incidence of KS in women with a history of sexual contact with bisexual men.[12] Despite extensive research, however, no "second agent" has been isolated. Other associations have not been

FIGURE 1

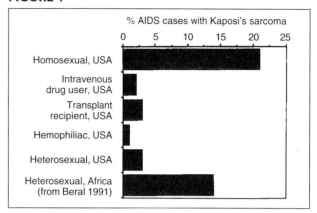

Prevalence of AIDS cases with Kaposi's sarcoma in different groups of HIV-infected patients. Reprinted, with permission, from Weiss RA: Retroviruses and human cancer. Semin Cancer Biol 3:321–328, 1992.

proven to cause KS but instead serve as markers of a population at risk for HIV infection and KS because of lifestyle.[12,16]

Pathology

All forms of KS are characterized by a proliferation of spindle cells in a background network of reticular and

TABLE 2

Kaposi's Sarcoma Variants

Type	Population	Clinical characteristics	Course
Classic	Older men (aged 50-80 yr) of Jewish and Mediterranean heritage	Usually confined to lower extremeties, often with venous stasis and lymphedema; M/F ratio 10-15:1	Indolent; survival 10-15 yr; 37% associated with other lymphoid malignancies
African	Young adult (aged 25-40 yr) black men in Central Africa	Localized nodular lesions (57%); large aggressive exophytic tumors or invasive to underlying bone (38%); M/F ratio 13:1	Indolent if nodular, otherwise slowly progressive and fatal within 5-8 yr
	Children (aged 2-13 yr)	Generalized lymphadenopathy, (5%); M/F ratio 3:1	Rapidly progressive; fatal within 2-3 yr
Renal transplant	Iatrogenically immunosuppressed patients	May be localized to skin or widespread with systemic involvement; M/F ratio 2.3:1	Can be indolent or rapidly progressive; may regress when immunosuppressive therapy is discontinued; fatal in 30%
Epidemic	AIDS patients; primarily homosexual men; few intravenous drug users and Africans	Disseminated mucocutaneous lesions often involving lymph nodes and visceral organs, especially gastrointestinal tract and lungs	Fulminant; less than 20% survival at 2 yr if associated with opportunistic infections

Adapted, with permission, from Krigel RL, Friedman-Kien AE: Epidemic Kaposi's sarcoma. *Semin Oncol* 17:350–360, 1990.

TABLE 3

AIDS Clinical Trials Group Staging Classification

	Good risk (All of the following)	Poor risk (Any of the following)
Tumor (T)	Confined to skin and/or lymph nodes and or minimal oral disease [a]	Tumor-associated edema or ulceration Extensive oral Kaposi's sarcoma Gastrointestinal Kaposi's sarcoma Kaposi's sarcoma in other nonnodal viscera
Immune system (I)	CD4 cells greater than or equal to 200/μL	CD4 cells less than 200/μL
Systemic illness (S)	No history of opportunistic infection or thrush No B symptoms [b] Performance status greater than or equal to 70 (Karnofsky)	History of opportunistic infection and/or thrush B symptoms present Performance status < 70 (Karnofsky)
		Other HIV-related illness (eg, neurologic disease, lymphoma)

AIDS = acquired immunodeficiency virus, HIV = human immunodeficiency virus
[a] Minimal oral disease is nonnodular KS confined to the palate.
[b] B symptoms are unexplained fever, night sweats, more than 100% involuntary weight loss, or diarrhea persisting more than 2 weeks.
Adapted, with permission, from Krigel RL, Friedman-Kien AE: Epidemic Kaposi's sarcoma. *Semin Oncol* 17:350–360, 1990.

collagen fibers; vascular and lymphatic proliferation, and the presence of mononuclear cells including macrophages, lymphocytes, and plasma cells. Lesions may involve only the reticular dermis (patch stage) or the full thickness of the dermis (plaque or nodular stage). As lesions evolve to the plaque and nodular stages, the number of interstitial cells increases. The abundance of cells is thought to reflect a cytokine-rich environment.[3,12,16,20]

The cell of origin of KS lesions is unknown, but the lesions are thought to originate from a pluripotent mesenchymal precursor cell. Endothelial (factor VIIIa) and spindle cell markers and expression of the gene for smooth muscle alpha-actin have been observed in vitro, implicating a vascular or lymphatic endothelial cell or vascular smooth muscle cell as the cell of origin.[3,13,16,20,21]

Pathogenesis of Kaposi's Sarcoma

Although KS lesions exhibit malignant behavior, it is unclear whether they are truly monoclonal malignant growths or benign, hyperplastic, polyclonal growths driven by continuous cytokine stimulation. No clonal cytogenetic abnormalities[12,17] and no oncogene rearrangements have been demonstrated in cell lines.[22] It is theorized that early KS lesions are hyperplastic and may progress or regress depending on the patient's immune status and extent of proliferative stimuli. Under continuous stimulation, however, some cells may undergo genetic changes and true malignant transformation.[20]

Kaposi's sarcoma cells maintained in culture can induce angiogenesis as well as produce cytokines that promote their own growth and the growth of normal endothelial cells, fibroblasts, and other mesenchymal cells.[20] Angiogenic cytokines include interleukin (IL)-1-beta, basic fibroblast growth factor, acidic fibroblast growth factor, and endothelial cell growth factor.[17,20] Other cytokines include IL-6, granulocyte-macrophage colony-stimulating factor (GM-CSF, sargramostim [Leukine]), transforming growth factor beta, and platelet-derived growth factor alpha. Kaposi's sarcoma cells also respond to exogenously produced cytokines originating from HIV-infected T-cells including IL-1, fibroblast growth factor, IL-6, and oncostatin M.[3,12,16,17,20,21] Oncostatin M acts directly to stimulate KS cells and induces KS cells to produce IL-6, which acts to sustain growth in an autocrine fashion.

The HIV virus itself may be responsible for transformation. When Vogel et al transfected fertilized eggs from mice with a recombinant HIV transactivating (*TAT*) gene with a long terminal repeat sequence, they observed the development of lesions resembling KS in 15% of male offspring.[23] The *TAT* gene product has also been shown to promote the growth of AIDS-associated KS cells.[12] The process of transformation may be associated with the expression of certain receptors, such as IL-6 and oncostatin M, that distinguish KS cells from their normal counterparts.

Immunosuppression supports the evolution of KS but

is not necessarily a prerequisite for KS development as KS can develop in HIV infection with normal or near-normal CD4 counts.[13,24] Other factors are likely involved in the pathogenesis of AIDS-associated KS. The distinct male predominance suggests a role for hormones in the pathogenesis of both classic and AIDS KS. Also, all forms of KS show a strong relationship to cytomegalovirus (CMV) exposure and a history of fecal-oral contact (the "second agent" theory).

Clinical Features

AIDS-associated KS may appear at any stage of HIV disease. Immune impairment is usually present: less than one sixth of HIV-infected patients have CD4-positive T-cell counts of less than 500/mm³.[16]

Typical lesions range from violaceous to brown and may be flat or raised and ulcerated. They are usually multicentric and symmetrical and may be in various stages of development. The lesions do not blanch and are usually not tender. A biopsy must be obtained to exclude bacillary angiomatosis or pyogenic granuloma, which may have a similar presentation in AIDS patients.[12,16] The tumor is often widespread, involving the skin, mucous membranes, gastrointestinal tract, lymph nodes, genitalia, oral cavity, conjunctiva, and/or lungs and airways.

Oral KS is a marker of more advanced HIV infection. Patients exhibit CD4 counts of less than 200/mm³ and

associated involvement of the gastrointestinal tract in 50% of cases. Gastrointestinal KS may be manifested by bleeding, diarrhea, or weight loss. Because barium enema may fail to demonstrate flat lesions, these patients should undergo endoscopy instead. Patients with pulmonary KS can present with shortness of breath, fever, cough, hemoptysis, or chest pain or be asymptomatic. Radiographic appearance is nonspecific and may demonstrate infiltrates, poorly defined nodules, or effusions. Effusions are exudative and often bloody.[12,25] Involvement of either the gastrointestinal (GI) tract or lung causes death in 10% to 20% of patients.[16] Patients may also present with disease limited to nodes, in which case lymph node biopsy is required to establish the diagnosis. Significant lymphedema may occur and is cytokine mediated.[12,15]

Staging and Prognostic Factors

The development of a universally accepted staging system for KS is complicated by the fact that the usual indicators of tumor burden in other metastatic cancers do not have the same prognostic significance in KS. However, Chachoua et al reported three adverse prognostic factors for survival in a cohort of epidemic KS patients: prior or coexistent opportunistic infection (OI), the presence of B symptoms (weight loss, fever, and night sweats), and an absolute CD4-positive T-cell count of

TABLE 4

Treatment Guidelines for Kaposi's Sarcoma

Status of KS	Status of HIV disease	Kaposi's sarcoma treatments [a]
Few, small cutaneous lesions, not in exposed areas	CD4 count < 200/µL Prior opportunistic infection or B symptoms [b]	No treatment Local treatment
	CD4 count > 200/µL No prior opportunistic infection or B symptoms	No treatment Local treatment of IFN + zidovudine
Cosmetically unacceptable lesions	Any	Local treatments or radiation therapy
Extensive cutaneous KS with or without asymptomatic visceral KS	CD4 count < 200/µL Prior opportunistic infection or B symptoms	Single- or multiagent chemotherapy or IFN + zidovudine
Localized bulky or painful KS	Any	Radiation therapy
Tumor-associated edema	Any	Radiation therapy or chemotherapy
Symptomatic visceral KS	Any	Multiagent chemotherapy

HIV = human immunodeficiency virus, IFN = interferon, KS = Kaposi's sarcoma
[a] In certain circumstances, different approaches may be combined for patients with multiple KS-related problems, eg, systemic chemotherapy with radiation to bulky disease sites.
[b] B symptoms: unexplained fever, night sweats, > 10% involuntary weight loss, or diarrhea persisting > 2 weeks.
Adapted, with permission, from Kraun SE et al: Kaposi's sarcoma. *Med Clin North Am* 76:235–252, 1992.

TABLE 5

Criteria for Defining Kapsosi's Sarcoma Response to Therapy

Complete response (CR)

No detectable residual disease, including tumor-associated edema or effusion, for at least 4 weeks. If residual pigmented lesions remain, biopsy of at least I representative lesion is required to document the absence of malignant KS cells. Restaging of known visceral disease with appropriate endoscopic or radiologic studies should be attempted. If such procedures are medically contraindicated (eg, invasive surgical restaging), the patient may be classified as having a clinical CR.

Partial response (PR)

A 50% or greater reduction in the number and/or size of previously existing lesions for at least 4 weeks without:

1. New skin or oral lesions or

2. New visceral sites of involvement or

3. The occurrence or worsening of tumor-associated edema or effusion or

4. An increase of 25% or more in the product of the bidimensional diameters of any indicator lesion

Patients with residual tumor-associated edema or effusion who otherwise meet the criteria for a CR will be classified as having a PR.

Stable disease

Any response not meeting the criteria for progression or PR

Progression

The presence of any of the following:

1. An increase of 25% or more in the size of previously existing lesions

2. The occurrence of new lesions or sites of disease

3. A change in the character of 25% or more of existing skin or oral lesions from macular to plaque-like or nodular

4. The development of new or increasing tumor-associated edema or effusion

Adapted, with permission, from Pluda JM et al: Therapy of AIDS and AIDS-related tumors. Cancer Chemother Biolog Response Mod Annual 12:395–429, 1991.

less than 300 cells/mm³.[26] The most important of these, OI, was associated with a median survival of only 7 months vs 20 months for those without prior OI. Other features, including the ratio of helper to suppressor cells and extent of disease, were not independent predictors of survival in this study.

Based on these findings, the AIDS Clinical Trials Group Oncology Committee of the National Institute for Allergy and Infectious Diseases proposed a KS staging system incorporating extent of disease, severity of immune dysfunction, and the presence of systemic B symptoms (Table 3). They also recommended the following staging methods for these patients: complete physical examination (including rectal and oral examination) biopsy of skin lesions and/or lymph nodes chest x-ray, gastroscopy and colonoscopy (bronchoscopy in patients with abnormal chest x-ray), CT scan of the abdomen, and laboratory studies (complete blood count, common serum chemistries, HIV serology, T4-T8 lymphocyte counts).[27]

Local Therapy

Therapy for KS patients is palliative and directed toward improving symptoms and overall quality of life since most patients with AIDS-associated KS die of opportunistic infections rather than KS.[16,18] Indications for treatment include cosmetic control, bulky oral lesions, lesions resulting in pain or significant edema, extensive cutaneous disease, or the presence of symptoms referable to viscera such as bleeding or obstruction (Table 4).[28,29] Criteria for defining the response of KS lesions to therapy are outlined in Table 5.[29]

Cryotherapy

Cryotherapy of KS lesions with liquid nitrogen may result in a complete or partial response in more than 85% of cases regardless of anatomic location or activity of underlying HIV infection,[30] although persistent KS can be demonstrated in the deep reticular dermis by biopsy. Patient candidates for cryotherapy include those with indolent KS and macular or papular lesions less than 1 cm in diameter. Two freeze-thaw cycles are recommended per treatment, to be repeated at 2- to 3-week intervals. The liquid nitrogen should be administered with a hand-held spray device rather than a cotton-tipped applicator to prevent transmission of HIV.[30] Advantages of cryotherapy are the short duration of treatment, minimal pain, ease of administration and repeat treatments, and potential combination with other modalities of treatment.

Laser and Surgical Therapies

Argon-laser photocoagulation has been preferentially used to treat vascular lesions owing to the specific uptake of laser energy by oxygenated hemoglobin in the tissues.[31] An argon laser is preferable to an Nd:YAG laser because of the Nd:YAG laser's tendency to cause bleeding. Laser photocoagulation therapy, which can be done on outpatients, can completely shrink smaller lesions, partially resolve larger lesions, lessen bleeding and pain, improve cosmetic appearance, and allow minimal wound care. However, like cryotherapy, it offers limited tissue penetration and is unlikely to resolve large, deep, or exophytic lesions.

Surgery has traditionally been reserved for lesions that cause visceral morbidity (bowel obstruction or bleeding) and for skin lesions that are large, are ulcerated, infiltrate underlying tissues or bone, or occur in areas that can cause morbidity, such as the face. Furthermore, the potential for HIV infection of the surgeon or laser operator remains a concern, and these modalities should be reserved for selected patients only.

Radiation Therapy

Radiation therapy does benefit most patients with KS lesions, as studies have shown. Tappero et al reported that more than two thirds of patients attained at least a partial response to radiation of KS lesions.[16] More recently, Berson et al achieved response rates of more than 80% with appropriate patient selection.[32] Current indications for radiotherapy include bleeding, pain, mass effect (large intraoral lesions, localized painful lymphadenopathy, localized lymphedema of extremities or genitalia), or cosmetically disfiguring lesions at selected sites (facial, ocular, or periorbital lesions or lesions of the feet) that fail to respond to intralesional or cryotherapy.[33]

Toxicities of radiotherapy include residual purple pigmentation, hyperpigmentation, desquamation, or ulceration in treated skin lesions; mucositis of the oral cavity, pharynx, and larynx (often ameliorated by prophylactic systemic antifungal and antiherpetic medication); and dry mouth or altered taste during treatment of oral lesions.[34-36] There is the suggestion that patients with oral lesions or lesions of the feet are especially sensitive to conventional doses of radiotherapy with enhanced toxicities that may limit the effectiveness of such therapy for these lesions.[35,36] Observed responses to radiotherapy vary by site of disease and the overall condition of the patient. Lesions treated to palliate pain or visceral symptoms are less likely to demonstrate objective responses and are more likely to recur locally than lesions treated for cosmetic reasons.[33,35] Lymphedema is also less likely to demonstrate a response: studies have shown only partial resolution in 40% of fields treated.[32]

Intralesional Therapy

Intralesional injections of vinblastine, vincristine, or bleomycin reportedly result in objective response rates of 60% to 88% with minimal or no systemic effects. As with cryotherapy, cosmetic response is often better than histo-logic response with residual disease by biopsy. Median duration of response vary from 4 to 6 months, with 40% of patients experiencing recurrent disease.[16]

Reported concentrations of intralesional vinblastine vary from 0.1 mg/mL to 0.6 mg/mL, with larger doses recommended for oral lesions or larger papulonodular lesions. Total doses administered at a treatment session are limited to 1 to 3 mg.[16,37-40] Patients are allowed a recovery time of 3 to 4 weeks before retreatment. Lesions may require two to three injections for maximal response. Pain at the injection site is the most common side effect, but hyperpigmentation, edema, blistering and ulceration, alopecia, and transient mononeuropathy are also reported. Biological therapeutic agents used intralesionally include alpha interferon (IFN-α), tumor-necrosis factor, and platelet factor 4, though all remain investigational at this time.[41-47]

Systemic Therapies

Patients with widely disseminated, progressive, or symptomatic disease are candidates for systemic therapy, including biologic-agent therapies, antiretroviral therapies, or single or multiagent chemotherapies. However, systemic therapies may be limited by severe toxicities or the intercurrent development of opportunistic infections.

Single-Agent Therapies

Single chemotherapeutic agents initially investigated in AIDS-associated KS include bleomycin (Blenoxane) and vincristine (Oncovin), both of which are minimally myelosuppressive. Responses with single agents are primarily partial responses and are measured in weeks.[48-53] The pulmonary toxicity resulting from use of bleomycin in AIDS-associated KS was evaluated by Ireland-Gill et al.[54] They retrospectively reviewed 28 patients treated with bleomycin plus vincristine (BV) or doxorubicin (Adriamycin, Rubex), bleomycin, and vincristine (ABV) who had undergone repeated pulmonary function testing of breathing capacity, diffusing capacity for carbon monoxide (DLCO), and lung volumes. A decline of more than 20% was considered clinically significant. The median bleomycin dose was 112 U (range, 10 to 313 U). Spirometry and lung volume tests showed no significant changes. A statistically significant difference in DLCO was observed for patients receiving cumulative bleomycin doses of more than 100 U vs those receiving less than 100 U.

Interferon is another single agent that has been tested in AIDS-associated KS. Its testing was prompted by its antiviral, antiproliferative, antiangiogenic, and immuno-regulatory activities. Like other biological-therapy agents, interferon offers the advantages of less myelosuppression and fewer systemic toxicities. Responses have been reported to differ depending on extent of disease, prior treatment with chemotherapy, prior or coexistent OI, and CD4-positive T-cell count. IFN-α therapy is the only biologic therapy approved by the US Food and Drug Administration (FDA) for AIDS-associated KS.[15]

A number of trials have confirmed the activity of single-agent interferon in AIDS-associated KS. Initial studies were designed to determine the optimal dose and schedule and whether a dose-response relationship exists for interferon.[55] In general, higher doses resulted in an improved response rate, with responses of 20% to 40% reported with doses of more than 20 million units (MU)/m^2.[55,56] Responders demonstrated improved survival over nonresponders. The most prominent toxicities included malaise and flu-like syndrome. Studies of combined interferon and cytotoxic chemotherapy demonstrated increased toxicity but not synergistic or additive activity.[55,56]

Factors predicting a poor response to interferon include extensive disease, constitutional symptoms, a CD4 count of less than 200/mm^3 at initiation of therapy, anemia, and current or prior OI.[56,57] Subsequent studies excluding patients with the worst prognostic indicators have resulted in improved response rates approaching 50%. Patients with CD4 counts of more than 200/mm^3 are almost four times more likely to respond than patients with CD4 counts of less than 200/mm.[3]

It has been suggested that IFN-α acts against HIV by suppressing the translation of its mRNA into protein, thus blocking the assembly of viral proteins into intact virions. Zidovudine (Retrovir), although not directly antiviral, acts by blocking the infection of previously uninfected cells.[57] When used in combination, these agents have demonstrated synergistic activity both in vivo and in vitro.

Trials combining interferon and zidovudine have been primarily phase I studies designed to establish the maximum tolerated dose of the combination. In one, Krown et al reported a maximum tolerated interferon dose of 18 MU with 100 mg zidovudine every 4 hours (an alternative schedule of 4.5 MU of interferon with 200 mg of zidovudine was also tolerated).[58] However, the excessive toxicity of lymphoblastoid interferon (IFN-α-N1) and zidovudine resulted in early closure of the third study arm.

Dose-limiting toxicities included neutropenia (defined as a cell count of 500 to 750/mm^3 and accounting for 10 of 17 dose reductions) as well as severe fatigue, malaise, and elevated transaminase levels. A decrease in hemoglobin concentration to 10 g/dL or lower was seen in all patients treated for 2 or more weeks. Although Krown's interferon-

zidovudine studies were not designed specifically to evaluate response, a response rate of 46% was demonstrated. Similar results are reported in studies by Fischl et al[59] and Kovacs et al.[60] The addition of GM-CSF to the combined regimen of interferon and zidovudine resulted in an improved absolute neutrophil count but not in an increased rate of tumor response, final CD4 count, or improvement in any other hematologic variable.[61]

Lymphoblastoid interferon has also been studied in AIDS-associated KS. Gelmann et al studied three schedules (7.5, 15, and 30 MU/m^2/d) for 28 days in 30 patients.[62] Responses were not dose dependent but correlated with high total lymphocyte count, high CD4 counts, absense of OI, and absence of endogenous acid-labile IFN-α in the circulation.

Other biologic response modifiers including beta interferon (IFN-β), gamma interferon (IFN-γ) and IL-2 (aldesleukin [Proleukin]) have been investigated as therapeutic agents in KS, with disappointing results. A phase II trial of IFN-β with a serine substitution at position 17 demonstrated a 16% response rate, with 42% of patients having stable disease. Toxicity included injection-site necrosis but rarely significant hematologic toxicity.[63] IFN-γ has demonstrated minimal activity with a response rate of less than 5%.[64] IL-2 as a single agent has failed to demonstrate significant activity in AIDS-associated KS and in combination with IFN-β, actually demonstrated disease progression in three of four patients.[65]

Combination Chemotherapy

Combination chemotherapeutic regimens are associated with higher reported overall response rates and complete response rates. Vincristine-, vinblastine-, and bleomycin-containing regimens are usually used as first-line therapy as they are well tolerated and produce minimal alopecia and bone marrow suppression. Etoposide (VePesid)- and doxorubicin-containing regimens are generally used when the disease becomes resistant to the less myelosuppressive agents. Advanced KS with pulmonary or other visceral involvement requires anthracycline-containing regimens.[66]

The optimal duration of chemotherapy is undefined and depends on both patient tolerance and response of KS lesions. Most combinations are administered every 2 weeks, and it is recommended that patients undergo approximately two cycles past best response. Attempts to prolong response with maintenance interferon therapy have resulted in only short responses (8 weeks), but this remains under investigation.[67]

The combination of bleomycin and vincristine has been investigated in AIDS-associated KS.[68–70] Gill et al studied 18 patients with compromised bone marrow function (defined as absolute granulocyte counts of less than 1,500/mm³, hemoglobin levels of less than 10 g/dL, or platelet counts of less than 100,000/mm³.[68] Patients previously exposed to myelosuppressive agents such as ganciclovir (Cytovene) or zidovudine or to previous single-agent chemotherapy were included. Patients received 10 mg/m² bleomycin and 1.4 mg/m² (2 mg maximum) vincristine biweekly. Objective responses were observed in 72% of patients. Response lasted 6 to 7 weeks in the two complete responders and a median of 8 weeks in the 11 partial responders.

Gompels et al retrospectively reviewed 46 patients who had received fixed doses of 2 mg vincristine as a bolus and 30 mg bleomycin as an infusion over 18 hours.[69] Vinblastine (2.5 to 5 mg) was administered instead of vincristine if peripheral neuropathy developed. Treatment was repeated every 3 to 4 weeks. Fifty-seven percent achieved a partial response, 34% had stable disease, and none had complete responses.

Rarick et al retrospectively studied the use of zidovudine with the combination of BV in an attempt to reduce the incidence of opportunistic infections.[70] All patients received 10 U/m² bleomycin and 2 mg vincristine in 2 week cycles but on different schedules of zidovudine. Patients were divided into two groups: Eight patients received a full dose of zidovudine (200 mg) every 4 hours; four patients received a half dose of zidovudine (100 mg) every 4 hours. The full-dose patients received a mean of 5.4 cycles of BV, while the half-dose group received a mean of 4.2 cycles of BV. In the full-dose group, 63% of patients achieved a complete response. In the half-dose group, no patients group achieved a complete response and 50% had a partial response. The overall response rate in both groups was 83%, with a median duration of response of 2 months. Only two patients developed infections while on therapy. However, the overall contribution of zidovudine to the response rate remains undetermined as this study was uncontrolled.

Doxorubicin-containing therapies have also been investigated. Gill et al compared the combination of ABV against doxorubicin alone in 61 patients with mucocutaneous KS.[49] The overall response rate for ABV was 88% vs 48% for doxorubicin alone; however, the median survival was the same (9 months) in both groups. A higher dose version of ABV was studied by Laubenstein et al.[50] In that study, the response rate was 84%, but 61% of patients developed OI and 44% required dose reductions to minimize hematologic toxicity.[50] The AIDS Clinical Trials Group is also studying the use of ABV plus zidovudine with growth factor support.

TABLE 6

Observed and Expected Incidence of Non-Hodgkin's Lymphoma in AIDS Patients

Age (yr)	Observed (n)	Expected (n) [a]	Observed/expected ratio
0-19	36	0.1	360
20-39	1,659	21.7	76
40-59	1,006	19.7	51
>60	123	6.3	20
Total	2,824	47.8	59

[a] Based on the US incidence of non-Hodgkin's lymphoma from 1981–1985. Adapted, with permission, from Northfelt DW, Kaplan LD: Clinical aspects of AIDS-related NHL. *Curr Opin Oncol* 3:872–880, 1991.

Future Therapies

Fumagillin analogs[71,72] and sulfated polysaccharide peptidoglycan compounds produced by bacteria[73,74] are potent inhibitors of angiogenesis and are currently being investigated for activity in AIDS-associated KS. Recombinant platelet factor 4 is also being investigated as an antiangiogenic agent.[45,46]

Because cytokines are so fundamental in the development and maintenance of AIDS-associated KS lesions, the use of inhibitors of cytokines or receptor antagonists is being investigated. Interleukin-4 is known to be a potent inhibitor of IL-6 in monocytes, and its activity in AIDS-related KS is now being studied.[42] Pentosan polysulfate, an inhibitor of basic fibroblast growth factor, is also being investigated.[75]

Other strategies under investigation include novel methods of chemotherapeutic drug delivery (liposomal doxorubicin[76–78]), photodynamic therapy,[79] use of differentiating agents such as all-*trans*-retinoic acid,[80] and the combined use of chemotherapy and biologicals with less myelosuppressive nucleoside analogs such as dideoxyinosine (ddI, didanosine [Videx]) and dideoxycytidine (ddC, zalcitabine [Hivid]).[42] New chemotherapeutic agents including paclitaxel (Taxol) are being investigated for efficacy and toxicity.[81]

NON-HODGKIN'S LYMPHOMA

Epidemiology

The Surveillance, Epidemiology, and End Results (SEER) program of the National Cancer Institute has demonstrated a more than 50% increase in non-Hodgkin's

TABLE 7

Incidence and Relative Risk of Non-Hodgkin's Lymphoma in AIDS Patients According to Mode of HIV Transmission [a]

HIV transmission group	Patients with any lymphoma, % [b]	Relative risk (95% CI) [c]
Hemophiliac or clotting disorder	5.2 (7/14/33)	1.66 [d] (1.07-2.56)
Homosexual or bisexual men	3.4 (420/468/1334)	1.13 (0.86-1.49)
Transfusion recipient	3.5 (17/15/58)	1.0
Children infected perinatally	1.3 (8/4/4)	0.90 (0.41-1.96)
Heterosexual contact, except those born in the Caribbean or Africa	1.9 (14/9/32)	0.77 (0.50-1.18)
Intraveneous drug user	1.6 (64/60/169)	0.6 [d] (0.43-0.85)
Heterosexual contact, born in the Caribbean or Africa	1.0 (2/4/9)	0.41 [d] (.19-.90)

[a] Does not include 79 patients with unknown HIV-transmission group
[b] Number of cases of primary brain/Burkitt's/immunoblastic lymphoma shown in parentheses
[c] Relative risk with reference to transfusion recipient, adjusted for age, sex, race, and year of AIDS diagnosis
[d] Significantly different from 1.0 ($P < .05$)
AIDS = acquired immunodeficiency syndrome, HIV = human immunodeficiency virus
Adapted, with permission, from Northfelt DW, Kaplan LD: Clinical aspects of AIDS-related NHL. *Curr Opin Oncol* 3:872–880, 1991.

lymphoma (NHL) cases from 1973 to 1987.[82,83] Although the factors contributing to this increase are not fully understood, the increased incidence of NHL in HIV-infected individuals has contributed in some part to this figure. AIDS-associated NHL is not entirely responsible for the increased incidence, however, as the increase predates the AIDS epidemic. The incidence of B-cell NHL has conclusively been demonstrated to be increased in HIV-infected individuals and as such is an AIDS-defining disease in approximately 3% of individuals newly diagnosed with AIDS.[82,84]

SEER data from 1973 to 1979 (pre-AIDS) revealed a steady rise in incidence of NHL with age, from 3.4/100,000 in men 20 to 24 years old to 68/100,000 in men more than 75 years old. The median age of diagnosis was 63 years for men and 68 years for women. Rates were one third lower for women than men at all ages, and the incidence in blacks was one third lower than in whites of both sexes. By 1987 (during the AIDS epidemic), the nationwide incidence of NHL in the 20- to 49-year age group rose from 6.3 to 11.7. In San Francisco, the incidence rose dramatically from 7.7 to 59.0.[83] By 1985, the incidence of NHL was approximately 60 times greater in persons with AIDS than in the general population (Table 6),[85,86] and Burkitt's lymphoma and primary CNS lymphoma were 1000 times more frequent in persons with AIDS.[85]

The SEER data for NHL also showed a concordance between geographic areas with high AIDS incidence and

high NHL incidence. Using marital status as a surrogate marker for homosexual behavior, significant increases in NHL were noted in geographic areas, such as New York, San Francisco, and Los Angeles, with the highest incidence of HIV infection.[83,84]

As the AIDS epidemic has evolved, it has become apparent that all HIV risk groups are at risk for the development of NHL. The World Health Organization European Region measured the frequency of NHL in all groups from children infected perinatally to hemophiliacs, intravenous (IV) drug abusers, and homosexual and bisexual men.[87] They noted a higher frequency of NHL in homosexual and bisexual men and hemophiliacs than in IV drug abusers, who exhibited a downward trend in NHL. This same pattern was recorded in the largest US study of AIDS-associated NHL (Table 7).[85] A bimodal distribution of NHL was observed, with a peak in adolescence (ages 10 to 19) and a second peak in middle age (ages 50 to 59).[88] It is suggested that the early age peak is attributable to Burkitt's lymphoma and that the second peak is attributable to immunoblastic and diffuse B-cell lymphomas.[85]

Non-Hodgkin's lymphoma can develop in HIV-infected patients at any time during the course of the illness. Northfelt et al examined the degree of immunodeficiency in terms of CD4 cell counts at the time of diagnosis of non-CNS AIDS-associated NHL.[89] Seventy-nine percent of patients had CD4 counts of more than 50, and 58% had counts of more than 100. The median CD4 count at diagnosis was 110. The authors concluded that the degree of immunodeficiency at diagnosis as measured by CD4 cells varies over a wide range and that no specific CD4 count is a useful marker for the development of non-CNS AIDS-associated NHL. These data contrast with those from a study by Pluda et al, which suggested that NHL is a late manifestation of HIV infection.[90] In this study, AIDS-associated NHL developed in 14.5% of patients after a median duration of 23.8 months of antiretroviral therapy. However, 50% of these patients had primary CNS lymphoma. There is evidence to suggest that primary CNS lymphoma is different from AIDS-associated NHL outside of the CNS and is indeed a late finding in HIV infection.[91] However, others have also suggested that lymphoma is a late manifestation of HIV infection since the incubation period between infection and the development of lymphoma in transfusion recipients is approximately 50 months, similar to that for the development of opportunistic infections.[86]

Pathologic Subtypes of Lymphoma

Most AIDS-associated lymphomas (80% to 90%) are high-grade B-cell neoplasms consisting of either immunoblastic or small noncleaved cell lymphomas. This is in contrast to the case in patients without HIV infection, in whom 10% to 15% are diagnosed with high-grade B-cell lymphomas.[83,84,92] Intermediate-grade large-cell, B-cell lymphomas are also observed with greater incidence in HIV-infected patients, although less commonly than high-grade lymphomas. In addition, Ioachim found that nearly twice as many extranodal lymphomas were of high-grade histology, whereas nodal lymphomas were equally divided between high-grade and intermediate-grade histology.[93]

Other B-cell malignancies, including low-grade small-cleaved-cell lymphoma, chronic lymphocytic leukemia,[94] and myeloma,[95] have been reported in HIV patients. T-cell neoplasms, including cutaneous T-cell lymphoma,[96,97] precursor T-cell lymphoma,[98] lymphoblastic lymphoma,[99] HTLV-I-associated T-cell leukemia,[100] peripheral T-cell lymphoma,[101] and Ki-1-positive anaplastic T-cell lymphoma,[102] have been described in HIV-infected individuals. These malignancies, however, have not increased in incidence and are not considered part of the AIDS epidemic.

Pathogenesis

Although the precise mechanisms of lymphoma development in AIDS have not been determined, host factors and not environmental factors are predominantly responsible for such lymphomas. HIV itself is not a transforming virus and thus is not directly involved in malignant B-cell transformation. HIV sequences are not uniformly detected in lymphoma tissue or in the reactive B-cell hyperplasia of persistent generalized lymphadenopathy which precedes the development of lymphoma in 30% of cases.[92] Polymerase chain reaction analysis reveals HIV present only in infiltrating T-cells. HIV infection thus does not appear to be an absolute prerequisite for the development of these lymphomas; in fact, more important than HIV infection itself is the immune dysregulation it causes.[92]

HIV-infected cells produce multiple cytokines, some of which serve as stimuli for B-cell proliferation and differentiation. These include IL-1, 2, 4, 6, 7, 10, IFN-γ, tumor-necrosis factor, lymphotoxin, and B-cell growth factor. In particular, IL-6 is an autocrine growth factor for B-cell malignancies such as multiple myeloma and chronic lymphocytic leukemia. HIV may also directly stimulate IL-6 from monocytes and macrophages, and elevated levels of IL-6 may predict the development of lymphoma in HIV infection.[92,103] Also, Epstein-Barr Virus (EBV)-positive B-cell lines from AIDS-associated Burkitt's lymphoma patients express large amounts of IL-10, suggesting this cytokine's role in B-cell growth and immortalization. In addition, HIV itself is capable of direct polyclonal activation of B-cells.

Ongoing B-cell proliferation and differentiation may result in an increased incidence of random mutations, which may in turn result in transformation.[82] The normally occurring DNA rearrangements involving the immunoglobulin heavy- and light-chain genes may provide vulnerable sites for mutation or translocations.[104] Molecular events may occur stepwise, with several molecular events required to induce transformation. Patients with reactive lymphadenopathy demonstrate multiple clonal rearrangements of immunoglobulin genes.[105] These lesions may be early precursor lesions, with additional molecular events required for transformation of a single malignant clone. The classic translocations of Burkitt's lymphoma—t(8;14), t(8;22), and t(8;2)—are all demonstrated in AIDS-associated Burkitt's lymphomas as well.

Rearrangements involving the c-*myc* oncogene have been observed and thus are also implicated, in AIDS-associated lymphomas.[82] Such rearrangements of c-*myc* imply a molecular mechanism similar to that in sporadic Burkitt's lymphomas. In addition, HIV infection of already immortalized B-cell lines can lead to up regulation of c-*myc* transcripts. C-*myc* activation in turn may result in altered phenotypic features that allow cells to escape immune surveillance by cytotoxic T-cells, including absence or low expression of class I major histocompat-

TABLE 8

Ann Arbor Staging Classification for Hodgkin's Disease

Stage	Characteristics
I	Involvement of a single lymph-node region (I) or a single extralymphatic organ or site (IE).
II	Involvement of two or more lymph-node regions on the same side of the diaphragm (II) or localized involvement of an extra-lymphatic organ or site (IIE).
III	Involvement of lymph-node regions on both sides of the diaphragm (III) or localized involvement of an extralymphatic organ or site (IIIE) or spleen (IIIS) or both (IIISE).
IV	Diffuse or disseminated involvement of one or more extralymphatic organs with or without associated lymph-node involvement. The organ(s) involved should be identified by a symbol: A, asymptomatic; B, fever, sweats, weight loss >10% of body weight.

Adapted, with permission, from DeVita Jr VT, Hellman S, Rosenberg S (eds): Cancer: Principles and Practice of Oncology, p 1886. JB Lippincott, Philadelphia, 1993.

ibilty complex antigens, insufficient expression of adhesion molecules required for effector-target cell interactions, and downregulation of EBV-coded antigens.[82] However, no consistent c-*myc* rearrangements occur in AIDS-associated lymphoma tissue, suggesting the presence of other operative mechanisms.[92]

The role of EBV in the development of AIDS-associated lymphoma has been suggested but is controversial. Collectively, data suggest that the virus is responsible for at least a portion of cases of AIDS-associated lymphomas and likely involved in all cases of primary CNS lymphoma in AIDS patients. A proportion (less than 50%) of systemic AIDS-associated lymphomas show signs of latent EBV infection and may also express combinations of EBV antigens not previously observed in B-cell lymphomas.[106] Lymphomas that are both EBV- and HIV-positive demonstrate evidence of clonal EBV infection, indicating that EBV integration occurs before clonal B-cell expansion and that EBV may play a role in lymphomagenesis.[107] In this study, approximately one third of patients with reactive generalized lymphadenopathy demonstrate EBV DNA, and the presence of EBV DNA correlates with development of lymphoma at a later time.[108]

Mutation or allelic loss of tumor suppressor genes has also been investigated in AIDS-associated NHL. For example, some smaller studies indicate that *p53* muta-

tions occur frequently in NHL (up to 37% in one study), especially in association with c-*myc* overexpression. In contrast, there is no evidence of retinoblastoma gene inactivation in AIDS-associated NHL.[109] The defect in tumor suppression and the deregulation of oncogene-induced growth may be central to the pathogenesis of these lymphomas. Also, viral proteins may bind to and inactivate p53, leading to dysregulation of cell growth.[104]

In summary, B-cell proliferation induced by HIV or EBV may foster mutations in critical oncogenes, or tumor suppressor genes may occur along with abnormal DNA rearrangements, leading to c-*myc* activation, clonal selection, and the development of a monoclonal B-cell lymphoma.

Clinical Presentation

Patients often seek medical attention for B symptoms (fever, night sweats, and weight loss of more than 10% of body weight) or for a rapidly growing mass lesion. Though these symptoms occur in approximately 75% of patients with AIDS-associated lymphomas, it is important to exclude other etiologies of these symptoms such as occult opportunistic infections.

Most patients with AIDS-associated NHL have advanced-stage disease at presentation and frequent involvement of extranodal sites. These features have been confirmed in multiple series. Between 64% to 83% of patients present with stage III or IV disease and between 65% and 91% with extranodal disease.[110,111] The most common extranodal sites in all reported series are bone marrow (25%), CNS parenchyma or meninges (32%), liver (12% to 48%), and gastrointestinal tract (26%).[112,113] Other reported sites include lung,[114] pleura,[115] rectum,[113] testis,[116,117] kidney,[118] spleen,[115] and heart.[119] The incidence of rectal NHL described in US series consisting largely of homosexuals is not duplicated in Italian series consisting largely of IV drug abusers.[120]

Staging and Prognostic Features

Besides routine chest x-ray and blood studies, patients with AIDS-associated NHL should undergo bone marrow biopsy and lumbar puncture. Computed tomography (CT) of the chest and abdomen, and CT or magnetic resonance imaging (MRI) of the brain or spinal cord, bone scans, and gastrointestinal contrast studies should be done as needed if symptoms suggest disease. Disease should be staged according to the Ann Arbor system (Table 8).

Although patients with AIDS-associated NHL are a diverse group, several common factors predicting for short survival have been identified. Levine et al retrospectively studied a group of 49 patients treated for systemic AIDS-associated lymphoma.[121] A Karnofsky performance status of less than 70%, history of AIDS before the diagnosis of lymphoma, and bone marrow involvement were independently associated with poor prognosis. In the absence of all three risk factors, median survival was 11.3 months; for the remaining patients, it was only 4 months. A complete response to therapy was associated with prolonged survival in the good-prognosis group (17.8 months vs 5 months in patients without complete response) but not in the poor-prognosis group. Patients in either group who attained a complete response (CR) to antilymphoma therapy remained at risk for dying of AIDS during lymphoma remission. Thus, attempts at prolonging survival must address both the neoplasm and the underlying HIV infection. The median survival for all patients with AIDS-associated NHL remains approximately 6.5 months.[88]

Therapy for AIDS-Related Non-Hodgkin's Lymphoma

Hematologic Effects of HIV Infection and HIV Therapies: The major factor limiting the use of chemotherapy in AIDS-related NHL either alone or with antiretroviral therapy is hematologic toxicity and poor bone marrow reserve at initiation of therapy. Infection with the HIV virus often results in bone marrow dysplasia, anemia, thrombocytopenia, and leukopenia. Both ineffective hematopoiesis and peripheral destruction of blood cells are responsible for cytopenias. Decreased survival of blood cells may be related to autoimmune phenomena as well as increased turnover driven by multiple infections[122] (Table 9).

Between 70% and 95% of AIDS patients are anemic at presentation, with mean hemoglobin levels ranging between 9.1 and 11.7 g/dL.[122,123] Less ill patients with HIV exhibit anemia in 5% to 16% of cases.[122] However, the incidence of anemia and other cytopenias increases with the degree of immunologic dysfunction and with progression from HIV seropositivity to frank AIDS.

Anemia in HIV disease is normochromic and normocytic. Seventy percent of patients receiving zidovudine demonstrate macrocytosis, with a mean corpuscular volume (MCV) of more than 100/fl after 2 weeks of therapy. Anemic HIV patients demonstrate an inappropriately low reticuloctye count, suggesting a hypoproliferative anemia or ineffective hematopoiesis. Patterns revealed by iron studies are consistent with chronic disease marked by an increased serum ferritin and decreased serum iron and total iron binding capacity. Serum ferritin levels parallel disease activity and are higher in AIDS than in

TABLE 9

Mechanisms Involved in the Peripheral Blood Cytopenias of Human Immunodeficiency Virus (HIV)-Seropositive Individuals

1. Opportunistic infections affecting the bone marrow (eg, cytomegalovirus, parvovirus, mycobacterium avium, or cryptococcus neoformans)

2. Deficiencies in vitamin B12, folate, and decreased production of erythropoietin

3. Presence of antiplatelet and anti-red blood cell antibodies or immune complexes

4. Neoplasms, in particular non-Hodgkin's B-cell lymphomas, spread to the bone marrow

5. Therapy with antiretroviral, antineoplastic, and chemotherapeutic agents

6. HIV infection

Adapted, with permission, from Zauli G, Dans BR: Role of HIV infection in the hematologic manifestations of HIV seropositive subjects. *Crit Rev Oncol Hematol* 15:271–283, 1993.

HIV seropositivity. Serum ferritin levels may also be elevated owing to the protein's role as an acute-phase reactant.[122]

A positive Coombs' test is observed in 20% of HIV-infected patients with hypergammaglobulinemia. Hemolytic anemia, however, is rarely observed. Nonspecific attachment of other antibodies to red cells is also frequently observed and is usually clinically silent.[122]

The incidence of thrombocytopenia also increases with increasing severity of immune dysregulation, ranging from 5% to 12% in HIV-seropositive patients and reaching as high as 30% in patients with AIDS.[122] Patients can exhibit classic immune thromocytopenic purpura (with increased numbers of megakaryocytes in the bone marrow) or may develop thrombocytopenia as a result of impaired thrombopoiesis, the toxic effect of medications, or a thrombotic thrombocytopenic purpura (TTP)-hemolytic uremia syndrome (HUS).[122] Furthermore, therapies in these patients vary in effect. Therapy with prednisone offers a durable response in only 10% to 20% of patients and may further worsen immune status. Zidovudine may increase platelet counts, though how it does so is unknown.[122] The most effective therapy seems to be intravenous gamma globulin (IVIG), which has a response rate of 88% but a median response duration of only 3 weeks.[122]

Leukopenia, encompassing both granulocytopenia and lymphocytopenia, is also observed in up to 75% of AIDS patients. Atypical lymphocytes, hyposegmented granu-

TABLE 10

Principal Toxicities of Dideoxynucleoside Agents

AZT (azidothymidine, zidovudine, 3′-azido-2′,3′ dideoxythymidine)

Bone marrow suppression; anemia with increased mean corpuscular volume is the most prominent feature; leukopenia and thrombocytopenia are often dose-limiting

Nausea and occasionally vomiting

Headaches

Malaise, fatigue, fever

Myalgias; myositis with increased creatinine kinase levels can be seen with chronic use

Seizures (rare, but reported to be fatal)

Confusion, tremulousness

Wernicke's-like encephalopathy (one case reported)

Bluish pigmentation of finger and toenails (especially in blacks)

Hepatic transaminase elevations

Stevens-Johnson syndrome (rare)

ddC (dideoxycytidine, 2′,3′-dideoxycytidine)

Painful peripheral neuropathy

Aphthous stomatitis

Maculopapular rash (occasionally pseudovesicular)

Fevers

Arthralgias, edema

Thrombocytopenia

ddI (dideoxyinosine, 2′,3′-dideoxyinosine)

Painful peripheral neuropathy

Sporadic pancreatitis (can be fatal)

Hyperamylasemia, hypertriglyceridemia

Headaches

Insomnia, restlessness

Hepatic transaminase elevations (occasional hepatitis)

Hyperuricemia (with high doses)

d4T (2′,3′-dideoxythymidinene, 2′,3′-dideoxy-2′,3′-didehydro-thymidine)

Painful peripheral neuropathy

Anemia

Hepatic transaminase elevations

Adapted, with permission, from Pluda JM et al: Hematologic effects of AIDS therapies. *Hematol Oncol Clin North Am* 5:229–248, 1991.

locytes, and vacuolated monocytes can be seen on peripheral smears. Phagocytosed pathogens may be demonstrated in neutrophils or monocytes.[122,123] Antibodies to granulocytes are also frequent in HIV disease, and though they do not necessarily correlate with the degree of neutropenia, they do correlate with progression to AIDS.[122]

Anemia, leukopenia, and pancytopenia are well-documented effects of treating HIV infection with zidovudine (Table 10).[124] Such treatment is also associated with lower mean hemoglobin levels and an increased need for red cell transfusions.[122] Up to 20% of patients may develop severe neutropenia (less than 500 cells/mm³). However, because zidovudine's toxicity is dose dependent, reducing the dose often ameliorates cytopenias.

In addition, zidovudine-related myelosuppression and synergistic effects may occur when zidovudine is combined with other drugs commonly administered to treat infections such as ganciclovir, pentamidine, trimethoprim-sulfamethoxazole, pyrimethamine, sulfadiazine, dapsone, and amphotericin B. Other retroviral drugs such as suramin, ribavirin, ddC, ddI, and interferon also produce hematologic toxicity. In particular, studies of the combined use of interferon and zidovudine in Kaposi's sarcoma have demonstrated significant hematologic toxicity.

Chemotherapy: The results of trials of therapeutic regimens for AIDS-associated NHL are summarized in Table 11.[94,111,125–144] Comparison of these regimens is limited, however, by the fact that various histologies are grouped together in each study, inclusion criteria vary among the studies, and trials have been both retrospective and prospective. However, several conclusions can be drawn from the experience to date in treating AIDS-associated NHL.

(1) The favorable results of dose escalation in non-AIDS-associated high-grade lymphomas do not translate to AIDS-associated lymphomas. This has been illustrated in studies by Gill et al,[127] Kaplan et al,[111] and Levine et al.[137] The study by Gill et al accrued patients sequentially on phase II studies of m-BACOD (methotrexate, leucovorin, bleomycin, doxorubicin, cyclophosphamide, vincristine, dexamethasone) and a newly developed regimen containing high doses of cytarabine and methotrexate as well as cyclophosphamide, vincristine, prednisone, bleomycin, and asparaginase (Elspar). The regimen was designed to expose patients to high-dose cytarabine and high-dose methotrexate early in the course of therapy to prevent the CNS relapse observed in two thirds of the earlier m-BACOD group. Complete remission was achieved in 54% of the m-BACOD group but in only 33% of the high-dose group, with significantly greater numbers of patients with OI and hematologic toxicity appear-

TABLE 11

Therapeutic Regimens for AIDS-Related Non-Hodgkin's Lymphoma

Regimen	CR rate	Median survival	Reference
Chemotherapy alone			
Cyclophosphamide, vincristine, methotrexate, and intrathecal methotrexate	7/25	3 months	125
ProMACE-MOPP	3/15	5 months	126
m-BACOD vs	7/13	11 months	127
High-dose methotrexate, high-dose cytarabine, plus cyclophosphamide, vincristine, bleomycin, prednisone, and asparaginase	3/9	6 months	127
Lomustine, etoposide, cyclophosphamide, and procarbazine	43%	7.5 months	128
Cyclophosphamide, doxorubicin, and etoposide	14/18	17.4 months	129
Various regimens including cyclophosphamide, doxorubicin, vincristine, methotrexate, bleomycin, prednisone, and chlorambucil	9/23	7 months	130
COMET-A vs	19/38	5.2 months	111
Multiple others	12/26	11.3 months	111
Various by histology			94
Small-noncleaved-cell	26%	5.5 months	
Immunoblastic/plasmacytoid	21%	2.0 months	
Large-noncleaved-cell	52%	7.5 months	
Chemotherapy plus antiretrovirals			
Cyclophosphamide, doxorubicin, teniposide, prednisone, vincristine, bleomycin plus zidovudine concurrent	4/29	4 months	131,132
Modified LNH regimen plus zidovudine in consolidation	88/136	9 months	133
12-week modified MACOP-B plus zidovudine in consolidation	10/30	8.1 months	134
CHOP plus zidovudine and alpha interferon	18/28	82 days to 641 days	135
Etoposide, vincristine, prednisone, cytarabine, mitoxantrone, cyclophosphamide plus antiretrovirals in consolidation	4/29	4.5 months	136
Low-dose m-BACOD plus zidovudine in consolidation	16/42	5.6 months	137
Chemotherapy plus growth factors			
CHOP vs	6/9	9 months	138
CHOP plus delayed GM-CSF	7/10	11.4 months	138
CHOP plus early GM-CSF	3/5	8 months	138
Cyclophosphamide, etoposide, doxorubicin, vincristine, methotrexate, plus daily zidovudine and GM-CSF	4/10	—	139
m-BACOD plus GM-CSF	8/16	14 months	140
LNH 84 or CHVmP / VCR-BLM plus G-CSF vs	78%[a]	—	141
without G-CSF	88%[a]	—	141
Cyclophosphamide, doxorubicin, etoposide, plus ddI and G-CSF	4/7	—	142
Novel regimens			
B4-blocked ricin	1/9	6.6 months	143
MGBG	2/10	4.3 months	144

CHOP = cyclophosphamide, doxorubicin, vincristine, prednisone, COMET-A = cyclophosphamide, vincristine, methotrexate, etoposide, and cytarabine, CR = complete response, ddI = dideoxyinosine, G-CSF = granulocyte colony-stimulating factor, GM-CSF = granulocyte-macrophage colony-stimulating factor, LNH = Lymphoma Non-Hodgkin's Study group, m-BACOD = CHOP plus methotrexate, bleomycin, MGBG = methyl-glycosaminoglycan, ProMACE-MOPP = prednisone, methotrexate, leucovorin, doxorubicin, cyclophosphamide, etoposide, VCR-BLM = vincristine-bleomycin. [a] Overall response rate

TABLE 12

Dose Levels for ACTG 074

	Level 0	Level 1	Level 2
Bleomycin	4 U/m^2 d 1		
Doxorubicin	25 mg/m^2 d 1	35 mg/m^2	45 mg/m^2
Cyclophosphamide	300 mg/m^2 d 1	450 mg/m^2	600 mg/m^2
Vincristine	1.4 mg/m^2 d 1		
Dexamethasone	6 mg/m^2 d 1-5		
Methotrexate	200 mg/m^2 day 15 followed at 24 h by leucovorin 25 mg q6h for six doses		
GM-CSF	20 micrograms/kg sc days 3-13 of the cycle		
Cytosine arabinoside	50 mg x four doses intrathecally in the first month		

Adapted, with permission, from Walsh et al Phase I trial of m-BACOD and Granulocyte Macrophage Colony Stimulating Factor in HIV-Associated NHL. Journal of Acquired Immune Deficiency Syndromes 6:265-271, 1993.

ing in the high-dose group. Median survival in the m-BACOD group was 11 months vs only 6 months in the high-dose group. The trial was terminated early because of the significant toxicity and high rate of OI.

The trial by Kaplan et al[111] employed a new chemotherapy regimen, COMET-A, consisting of cyclophosphamide, vincristine, methotrexate, etoposide, and cytarabine with CNS prophylaxis. This regimen was compared with standard therapies, including CHOP, m-BACOD, ProMACE-MOPP, COMLA, CVP, COMP,* and radiation therapy alone. Although the complete remission rate for COMET-A was 58%, 28% of patients developed OI and the median survival was only 5.2 months. Patients receiving "dose-intensive" regimens, defined as regimens having a cyclophosphamide dose of more than 1 g/m^2, had significantly shorter survival (median, 4.6 months) than patients receiving less intense regimens (median, 12.2 months).

Levine et al[137] have reported results for a regimen of low-dose m-BACOD with early CNS prophylaxis and the initiation of zidovudine at completion of chemotherapy. A complete remission rate of 46% was reported, with

---

* CHOP = cyclophosphamide, doxorubicin, vincristine, prednisone; COMLA = cyclophosphamide, vincristine, methotrexate, leucovorin, cytarabine; COMP = cyclophosphamide, vincristine, methotrexate, prednisone; CVP = cyclophosphamide, vincristine, prednisone; ProMACE-MOPP = prednisone, methotrexate, leucovorin, doxorubicin, cyclophosphamide, etoposide

long-term lymphoma-free survival in 75% of complete responders suggesting that low-dose therapy may be effective. No patient had an isolated CNS relapse; however, despite prophylaxis, OI developed in 20% of patients.

(2) Despite the advent of lower dose regimens designed to minimize toxicity, significant hematologic toxicities are still observed and often result in delays in therapy, dose reductions, or termination of therapy. The use of growth factors has been shown to ameliorate these toxicities and allow improved dose intensity. However, the clinical significance of the effects of growth factors on HIV replication are unknown.

Walsh et al and the AIDS Clinical Trials Group conducted a phase I study of m-BACOD with GM-CSF.[140] Three different doses of m-BACOD were used along with fixed doses of GM-CSF (Table 12).[140] Eight of 16 patients were able to be treated at the highest dose level, and none of these patients experienced dose-limiting hematologic toxicity. However, OI developed in one patient on dose level 1 and in one patient on dose level 2, and the level of p24 antigenemia increased in some patients given GM-CSF.

Kaplan et al also studied the use of GM-CSF with the CHOP regimen.[138] Patients receiving GM-CSF all had higher mean nadirs of absolute neutrophil count, shorter mean duration of chemotherapy, fewer chemotherapy cycles complicated by neutropenia and fever, fewer days hospitalized for fever and neutropenia, fewer reductions in chemotherapy doses, and less frequent delays in chemotherapy administration. However, these patients had a significant increase in p24 antigenemia (243%) baseline by week 3 after initiation of chemotherapy, suggesting stimulation of HIV activity.

(3) Opportunistic infections and recurrent lymphoma remain the primary causes of death in AIDS-associated NHL patients. Gisselbrecht et al treated non-CNS AIDS-associated lymphomas with a modified LNH 84 regimen consisting of three cycles of induction therapy with doxorubicin, cyclophosphamide, vindesine, bleomycin, and prednisone.[133] Patients who achieved a CR received consolidation therapy containing high-dose methotrexate, ifosfamide (Ifex), etoposide, asparaginase, and cytarabine. All patients received CNS prophylaxis. Sixty-five percent achieved complete remission after induction therapy, 22% had a partial remission or failed, and 15% died during induction therapy. The median survival was 9 months. The authors performed a concurrent prospective analysis of prognostic determinants and confirmed that a performance status more than 1, localized disease (stage I or II), absence of bone marrow involvement,

nonimmunoblastic histology, absence of B symptoms, no previous AIDS-defining diagnosis, and a CD4 count of more than 100/mm^3 were predictors of improved survival. They also found that 50% of patients having CD4 counts of more than 100, no B symptoms, a performance status of less than 2, and nonimmunoblastic histology had a 2-year survival, suggesting that factors that reflect the patient's underlying immunodeficiency are at least as important and perhaps more important determinants of survival than are factors intrinsic to the lymphoma itself.

Unresolved issues in the therapy for AIDS-associated NHL include the significance and influence on prognosis of pathologic subtype, the selection of therapy based on prognostic indicators, the contribution of antiretroviral therapy to overall survival, the contribution of dose-intensive therapy, and the effect of growth factors on retroviral replication and activity. The AIDS Clinical Trials Group is currently conducting a multi-institutional trial that stratifies patients to either the low-dose m-BACOD regimen or standard-dose therapy to determine if dose intensity improves survival. Growth factor support is being used in both groups to minimize toxicity.

PRIMARY CNS LYMPHOMA

Epidemiology

Prior to the AIDS epidemic, primary central nervous system (PCNS) lymphoma was a rare disorder accounting for 1% to 2% of all cases of NHL and fewer than 5% of all cases of primary intracranial neoplasms.[145] Increasing numbers of cases of PCNS lymphoma were reported in the 1970s, paralleling the increasing number of patients with congenital and iatrogenic immunosuppression. The incidence of PCNS lymphoma increased significantly in the 1980s with the onset of the AIDS epidemic and was designated an AIDS-defining disease early in the epidemic. As many as 6% of AIDS patients may develop PCNS lymphoma during their illness.[146]

Interestingly, there has been a simultaneous threefold increase in the incidence of PCNS lymphoma in patients who are immunocompetent. The cause of this increase is unknown. If the incidence continues to increase in both immunosuppressed and immunocompetent patients at the present rate, lymphoma will be the most common primary malignant neoplasm of the CNS by the year 2000.[145]

To learn more about PCNS lymphoma, Fine and Mayer retrospectively analyzed PCNS lymphoma in 792 immunocompetent and 315 AIDS patients (Table 13).[145] The mean age of patients with AIDS was significantly less than that of non-AIDS patients (30.8 vs 55.2), and the

TABLE 13

Patient Characteristics at Diagnosis

Characteristic	Immuno-competent patients	Patients with AIDS
Patients, n	792	315
Male:female (ratio)	442:328 (1.35)	118:16 (7.38)
Mean age, yr	55.2	30.8
History of opportunistic infection or Kaposi sarcoma, n (%)	Not available	115 of 143 (80)
Mean duration of symptoms before diagnosis, mo	2.8	1.8
Symptoms, %		
Neurologic deficits	56.4	51.0
Mental status changes	34.6	53.3
Seizures	11.2	26.7
Increased intracranial pressure	32.4	14.2

Adapted, with permission, from Fine HA, Mayer RJ: Primary central nervous system lymphoma. *Ann Intern Med* 119:1093–1104, 1993.

ratio of men to women with disease was altered in AIDS lymphomas, with men representing a greater proportion of AIDS PCNS lymphoma patients. Eighty percent of the AIDS patients had a history of OI, and 20% had PCNS lymphoma as their AIDS-defining illness.

Clinical Presentation and Diagnosis

The most common presenting symptoms of PCNS lymphoma are headache, cranial nerve palsies or focal neurologic deficits, new-onset seizures, hemiparesis, signs of increased intracranial pressure such as nausea and vomiting or papilledema, mental status changes, or subtle cognitive or personality changes (Table 13).[145]

The differential diagnosis of neurologic abnormalities in AIDS is long (Table 14),[147] and diligent evaluation including biopsy may be necessary to obtain the correct diagnosis. PCNS lymphoma is second only to toxoplasmosis as a cause of focal cerebral masses in AIDS. CT imaging reveals lymphomas to involve the cerebrum, brain stem, and cerebellum in decreasing order of frequency,[145,148] and lesions are often periventricular in location and necrotizing. Extension to the ventricles or subarachnoid space may allow cytologic diagnosis through the cerebrospinal fluid.[147]

Lymphoma lesions may appear as single or multifocal

TABLE 14

Neuropathic Abnormalities of AIDS

Primary or indirect effect of HIV-1

    AIDS-dementia complex

    HIV encephalitis/leukoencephalopathy

    Vacuolar myelopathy

    Myopathy

Opportunistic infections

    Parasites: toxoplasmosis

    Fungi, mycobacteria, and spirochetes

    Aspergillus, Candida, Cryptococcus, Mycobacterium avium-

    intracellulare, and *Treponema pallidum*

    Viral infection

    Cytomegalovirus (CMV), herpes simplex, herpes zoster,

    progressive multifocal leukoencephalopathy (PML)

Neoplasms

    Lymphoma

    Kaposi's sarcoma

Vascular

    Noninflammatory vasculopathy

    Granulomatous angiitis

Spinal cord and peripheral nervous system involvement

Pediatric

    Basal ganglia calcification

    Atrophy

    Corticospinal tract degeneration

    Microcephaly

AIDS = acquired immunodeficiency syndrome, HIV = human immunodeficiency virus. Adapted, with permission, from Davenport E et al: Neuroradiology of the immunosuppressed state. Radiol Clin North Am 30:611–637, 1992.

masses that are isodense, hyperdense, or hypodense, and thus difficult to distinguish from other mass lesions such as toxoplasmosis. However, lymphomas tend to exhibit larger and fewer (more than 3 cm) lesions than toxoplasmosis.[113] Ten percent of lesions may be radiographically occult.[145] In contrast to non-AIDS-associated lymphomas, which almost never exhibit ring enhancement, AIDS-associated lymphomas are twice as frequently multifocal and have ring (50% of cases) or solid enhancement.

PCNS lymphomas usually appear hypointense on T1-weighted MRI images and isointense or hyperintense on T2-weighted images.[145] Although the diagnosis can be suggested by CT or MRI, a definitive diagnosis by brain biopsy is recommended, especially in patients with negative toxoplasmosis titers and whose condition worsens on empiric antitoxoplasmosis therapy.[113,148] Although cerebrospinal fluid (CSF) analysis in these patients is frequently abnormal (pleocytosis, elevated protein, and decreased glucose), cytologic examination is diagnostic in less than one third of cases.[112,145] CSF may also be analyzed for markers of clonality such as B-cell gene rearrangement or kappa or lambda-light chain analysis.[145,148]

Immunophenotyping reveals all lymphomas to be of B-cell origin with intermediate- to high-grade histology. Sixty percent of AIDS patients exhibit high-grade histologies of small noncleaved cells or immunoblasts compared with only 22% of non-AIDS patients.[145,148]

Staging

Upon confirmation of a diagnosis of PCNS lymphoma, a full neurologic evaluation for staging should be performed including lumbar puncture, MRI of the spinal axis, and slit-lamp examination of the eye (7% to 18% of patients have ocular involvement at presentation).[146] The extent of systemic staging required is controversial. However, if physical examination, chest x-ray, and routine laboratory results are unremarkable, further imaging is rarely useful.[145] Other studies that may be done include bone marrow examination, abdomino-pelvic CT, chest CT, or gallium scanning.[146]

Pathogenesis

The detection of EBV in all cases of AIDS-associated PCNS lymphomas and the fact that these tumors are often polyclonal suggests a primary role for this virus in the pathogenesis of PCNS lymphomas. This is in contrast to the case in lymphomas in immunocompetent individuals and systemic lymphomas in patients with AIDS where EBV expression is variable and occurs in less than 50% of cases. It is theorized that EBV infection causes clonal expansion of B-cells that goes unchecked by the abnormal immunoregulatory mechanisms of a dysfunctional immune system. Oncogene activation (c-*myc* is implicated) may result in transformation of one clone and a selective growth advantage. In addition, these effects may be enhanced by the decreased immune surveillance normally found in the CNS.[145]

Prognostic Factors and Survival

The overall survival for patients with AIDS-associated PCNS lymphomas is 2 to 3 months vs 12 to 20 months for patients with non-AIDS-associated lymphomas.[145,146,150,151] The reasons for this difference are unclear, but several theories exist. It is possible that the tumors are biologically distinct and thus differ in their inherent responsiveness to chemoradiotherapy. Also, as Fine observed, trials have tended to use lower doses of radiotherapy in AIDS patients: 56% of patients with AIDS received less than 3,500 cGy vs only 12% of patients without AIDS.[145]

As with systemic AIDS-associated NHL, most patients die of sequelae of advanced HIV disease rather than lymphoma.[145,151] CNS lymphoma is a late manifestation of HIV disease, with most patients having CD4 counts less than 50/mm^3 and a well-established AIDS diagnosis manifested by prior or concurrent opportunistic infections. Twenty-five to 100% of autopsied AIDS patients with CNS lymphoma have coexisting CNS infections including HIV encephalitis, toxoplasmosis, cryptococcal meningitis, or cytomegalovirus encephalitis.[146] Patients who present with PCNS lymphoma as their AIDS-defining disease, however, live longer than patients with a prior history of opportunistic infections and represent the few cases, in the literature, of long-term survival.[145]

Therapy

Standard therapy consists of whole-brain radiation.[145,151] The optimal dose and fraction schedule are undefined, but doses of 2,200 to 6,000 cGy have been reported.[145,151,152] Radiation therapy can substantially improve the quality of life even if survival is not prolonged. Though there are minimal data regarding the use of chemotherapy, they do suggest that responses can occur and that survival is similar to radiotherapy.[146] Intracarotid chemotherapy has also been reported.[153]

HODGKIN'S DISEASE

Although several studies suggest an increased incidence of Hodgkin's disease in HIV patients,[154] it is still not considered an AIDS-defining malignancy.[155] However, there is evidence to suggest that concurrent HIV infection alters the natural history of Hodgkin's disease[156] and that Hodgkin's disease in individuals at risk for AIDS is a predictor of HIV positivity.

HIV-positive patients with Hodgkin's disease have been reported to have a high frequency of stage III and IV disease, B symptoms, and atypical patterns of disease spread with extranodal presentations.[155,157] In one series, two thirds of patients had extranodal disease and 48% had bone marrow involvement at diagnosis.

Histologically, patients present with a higher frequency of poor prognosis, mixed cellularity, and lymphocyte-depleted subtypes.[157-159] The survival of patients with concurrent HIV and Hodgkin's disease is much shorter than for those with Hodgkin's disease alone but better than for those with AIDS-associated non-Hodgkin's lymphomas.[160] A large series reviewed by Ames revealed a survival of only 30% at 1 year with a median survival of only 8 months.[155] As with AIDS-related NHL, patient deaths are primarily a consequence of advanced HIV infection and not Hodgkin's disease; in the Ames series, 70% of deaths were due to OI.[155] Standard therapies are employed but again are limited by severe cytopenias, which are often exacerbated by involvement of bone marrow by Hodgkin's disease.

It is currently recommended that all patients diagnosed with Hodgkin's disease be tested for HIV infection. Those found to be HIV positive may require modified treatment as it is cytopenias and OI, rather than uncontrolled Hodgkin's disease that worsens prognosis. A study designed to determine the natural history of Hodgkin's disease in HIV-positive individuals and to determine the efficacy and toxicity of ABVD alone (doxorubicin, bleomycin, vinblastine, dacarbazine) or with growth-factor support is currently planned by the AIDS Clinical Trials Group.[155]

CERVICAL NEOPLASIA

Epidemiology

HIV infection in women is the most rapidly increasing subtype of the disease, and women now account for 40% of all persons infected worldwide and 12% of all infected persons in the United States. The primary mode of transmission of the virus is now through heterosexual contact. An association between cervical cancer and AIDS is anticipated on the basis of common sexual risk factors. Also, immunosuppressed women such as transplant recipients have long been known to be at increased risk for lower genital tract neoplasia.[161] Furthermore, both transplant patients and AIDS patients are at increased risk for human papillomavirus (HPV) infection, long known to be involved in the pathogenesis of cervical cancer.[161]

The association between HPV infection and cervical dysplasia and carcinoma is well established; in fact HPV subtypes are divided by their ability to cause genital tract neoplasia. The risk of genital tract neoplasia by HPV subtype is low for subtypes 6, 11, and 42; intermediate for

FIGURE 2

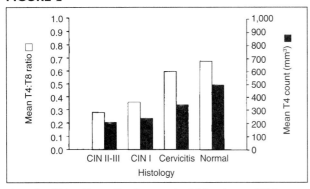

Graph of T-cell studies by cervical histology. CIN = cervical intraepithelial neoplasia. Reprinted, with permission, from: Maiman M et al: Colposcopic evaluation of human immundeficiency virus-seropositive women. Obstet Gyncecol 78:84–88, 1991.

subtypes 31, 33, 35, and 51 and high for subtypes 16, 18, 45, and 56.[161] Once contracted, the infection is lifelong and places the patient at continued risk of cervical dysplasia. Immunosuppression induced by HIV infection can result in reactivation of HPV infection. Coinfection with multiple HIV subtypes may be demonstrated in up to 13% of histologic specimens.[161] It is unknown, however, whether other viral infections such as genital herpes modify the incidence or clinical course of cervical neoplasia in HIV-infected women.[161]

The increased incidence of cervical neoplasia in women with HIV infection was only recently recognized as an AIDS-defining illness (January 1993) since few women have been included in clinical trials (only 6.7% of participants in AIDS Clinical Trials Group are women)[162] and no gender-specific trials have been done. The relationship between HIV infection and other gynecologic cancers (ie, ovarian or vulvar) remains to be determined. Vulvar cancer is reported with a rapidly progressive course.[163]

The incidence of HIV infection in women under age 50 presenting with cervical cancer is approximately 19%.[164] Most women with coexistent HIV and cervical cancer are asymptomatic for HIV disease and die of advanced cervical cancer rather than AIDS. Consequently, the Gynecologic Oncology Group is currently conducting a study involving HIV testing among women with cervical cancer to better define the incidence and pathogenesis of the disease.[162]

Gynecologic Manifestations of HIV Disease

Owing to the varying manifestations of gynecologic diseases in HIV-positive women, interpreting Papanico-

laou (Pap) smears for malignancy is often difficult. HIV-infected women tend to have recurrent and refractory vaginal candida infections, which tend to occur earlier in the course of HIV infection than oral or systemic fungal infections. HIV-infected women also demonstrate increased rates of sexually transmitted diseases including syphilis, trichomoniasis, gonorrhea, pelvic inflammatory disease, and genital ulcer disease. HIV-infected women show more consistent cytologic evidence of HPV infection than HIV-negative women.[162,164] For instance, in a study by Maiman et al 97% of HIV-positive patients versus only 50% of HIV-negative patients had evidence of HPV infection.[164] Other studies confirm these results.[165] HIV-infected women have as much as an 18-fold increased risk for the development of genital condylomata, which are resistant to primary therapy with failure rates as high as 40%.[166] Furthermore, HIV prevalence rates in women presenting for prenatal care or for treatment of sexually transmitted disease vary from 2% to 13%.[162] In light of such data, women presenting for gynecologic illness should be considered for HIV testing.[162]

Cervical Cytology

HIV-infected women demonstrate a wide range of cytologic abnormalities including inflammatory changes, hyperkeratosis, parakeratosis, trichomoniasis, herpetic changes, HPV-related changes, and varing degrees of cervical neoplasia. HIV-positive women show cytologic abnormalities in 30% to 60% of Pap smears and cervical dysplasia in 15% to 40% of smears.[161,162,167] The prevalence of these abnormalities increases as the immunodeficiency becomes more severe (Figure 2),[168] with patients with cervical intraepithelial neoplasia (CIN) demonstrating lower absolute CD4 counts and CD4:CD8 ratios.

A disturbing feature of cervical dysplasia in HIV-infected women is the inaccuracy of cytologic examination (Pap smear) in predicting CIN on biopsy.[162,168] A study by Maiman et al compared results of Pap smears with those of colposcopy plus biopsy and revealed that cytology alone correctly predicted CIN in only one of 13 patients;[168] conversely, 12 (39%) of 31 patients with normal smears had CIN on biopsy. In a more recent study, Wright et al[167] reported a 19% false-negative rate for Pap tests in HIV-seropositive patients, yet, even though this rate fell within the range for such tests in the general population (10% to 40%), the authors still recommended repeat Pap screening to reduce the risk of missing CIN on Pap smears. In addition, higher rates of concomitant vaginal infections may further obscure smears. As a result of these studies, it is recommended that HIV-positive women undergo more frequent cytologic screening (every 6 months) and undergo baseline colposcopy regardless of previous cytology.[162,169]

Cervical dysplasia in HIV-infected women is more often of higher grade (CIN II to III) with extensive cervical involvement as well as involvement of other sites (vulva, vagina, perianus) and the endocervix.[162,164] In addition, there is no association between CIN grade and age in HIV-positive women as there is in young HIV-negative women with high-grade lesions.

HIV-positive patients with invasive cervical cancer more frequently present with higher stage disease, as demonstrated in a study by Maiman et al in which 71% of HIV-positive patients had clinical stage II or higher disease versus 37% of HIV-negative patients.[164] Disease stage is also more likely to be revised upward based on surgical findings. In the study by Maiman et al, the mean CD4 cell count in HIV-infected patients with invasive cancer was 362/mm^3 vs 775/mm^3 in HIV-negative patients.[164] One hundred percent of the treated HIV-positive patients had persistent or recurrent disease vs 58% in the HIV-negative patients. The median time to recurrence was 1 month in the HIV-positive patients and 9 months in the HIV-negative patients, with a median time to death of 10 months in HIV-positive patients and 23 months in HIV-negative patients.

Therapy

Preinvasive Lesions: HIV-infected patients with intraepithelial neoplasia have been treated with therapies including laser therapy, cryotherapy, cone biopsy, hysterectomy, and topical therapies.[170] Yet overall results have been disappointing, with high recurrence rates of 40% to 60%.[161,162] Recurrence has been directly linked to the extent of immune deficiency: rates of more than 50% occur in patients with CD4 counts of less than 500/mm^3. Although the actual rate of progression of these lesions to invasive cancer is unknown, it is known that untreated lesions are more likely to progress in HIV-positive women.[162] Patients require repetitive treatments and close surveillance to avoid progression of lesions. The AIDS Clinical Trials Group is currently investigating topical fluorouracil plus ablative therapy as prophylaxis against recurrent CIN. In that study, patients are randomized to receive ablative therapy alone vs ablative therapy plus 2 g of fluorouracil vaginally every 2 weeks for 6 months.

Invasive Cervical Carcinoma

Management of HIV-positive patients with invasive cervical cancer is complicated by the fact that patients present with more advanced stages of disease, present with metastatic disease at uncommon sites, and demonstrate a significantly poorer prognosis. Unlike patients with other AIDS-related malignancies, most patients die from advanced cervial carcinoma rather than from HIV disease.[162] Again, patients with CD4 counts of more than 500/mm^3 fare better than patients with lower CD4 counts.

Therapies for invasive cervical carcinoma include surgery, radiation, and chemotherapy.[170] The usual indications for surgery are early disease with curative intent or complications of advanced disease such as bowel obstruction. Pelvic irradiation is often complicated by significant lymphopenia and worsening of overall immune status. Chemotherapy regimens include cisplatin, bleomycin, and vincristine and are complicated by high rates of hematologic toxicity. Antiretroviral agents may be used in combination with these modalities but often exacerbate hematologic toxicities. The effect of zidovudine on the development or recurrence of cervical dysplasia or neoplasia is unknown.[161]

ANORECTAL CARCINOMA

Epidemiology

Epidemiologic data confirm an increasing incidence of anal cancer in both men and women that predates the AIDS epidemic.[171] Suspected reasons for this increase include changing sexual habits and, more probably, increased exposure to HPV. Men with a history of homosexual activity are at highest risk. This is supported by a study of single, never-married men aged 20 to 49 in San Francisco between 1973 and 1989,[171] which showed a sevenfold increase in cases of squamous-cell carcinoma of the anus reported in that group. Other studies have reported incidences of anal cancer among homosexual men up to 40 times that expected in the general population.[171]

Pathogenesis

As in cervical cancer, HPV is also strongly associated with the development of anal cancer. The same subtypes of HPV are implicated in malignant transformation in anal cancer.[171] However, other factors probably contribute as well to cervical and anal cancer as not all cancers are HPV positive. Many HPV-negative anal and cervical cancers have been shown to contain *p53* mutations and it is known that HPV E6 protein transforms epithelial cells by inactivating *p53*. It is likely that *p53* mutation or inactivation represents the final common pathway of malignant transformation for these epithelial cells. In addition, c-*myc* activation occurs in approximately 30%

of HPV-16-associated anal cancers and in premalignant anal lesions.[171]

Disease Features

Like HIV-infected cervical cancer patients, HIV-infected anorectal cancer patients demonstrate a higher incidence of precancerous lesions, a higher incidence of high-grade lesions, lower CD4 counts, and a higher overall incidence of HPV infection, often with multiple subtypes present simultaneously. Patients with lower CD4 counts (and frank AIDS) demonstrate more severe disease than do patients with asymptomatic HIV infection.[170–172] Furthermore, the natural history is one of rapid progression to invasive and morbid lesions.

Screening

Screening for anal intraepithelial neoplasia or anal cancer involves routine Pap smears and anoscopy with biopsy of any suspicious lesions. Anal Pap smears have a reported sensitivity of approximately 70% (equivalent to that of cervical smears) and, as in cervical cancer, tend to underestimate the grade and incidence of neoplasia.[170] There are currently no standard recommendations regarding the optimal type and frequency of screening tests for anal cancer.[170] In any case, screening should be vigilant in patients who complain of abnormal discharge, bleeding, pruritus, bowel irregularity, or rectal or pelvic pain and in patients with previous preinvasive lesions or abnormal Pap smears. Other patients who should be considered for screening include HIV-negative men with a history of anal-receptive intercourse, HIV-positive men and women with CD4 counts less than 500/mm^3, and HIV-positive or HIV-negative women with a history of high-grade cervical intraepithelial neoplasia.[171]

Therapy

Patients with high-grade intraepithelial anorectal lesions (grade II or III) should be considered for ablative therapy (Table 15).[170] Patients with grade I lesions can be followed up every 6 months as these lesions may spontaneously regress or progress slowly enough to allow detection before invasive cancer develops.[170,171] Invasive lesions are treated with combined modality therapy with chemotherapy and external beam radiotherapy. Anecdotal experience suggests that HIV-infected patients have a decreased tolerance to full pelvic radiotherapy with increased myelotoxicity and mucositis, thus limiting the size of treatment fields.[173] No studies comparing the efficacy of different therapeutic modalities or the time course and incidence of recurrence have been published.

OTHER HIV-ASSOCIATED MALIGNANCIES

Many other solid tumors reportedly occur in conjunction with HIV infection. However, information about such tumors is found only in small series or case reports, and not enough epidemiologic evidence exists to demonstrate conclusively the increased incidence of these tumors. Collectively, however, these tumors do have some traits in common: often atypical and aggressive presentations, onset at an earlier than expected age, and absence of commonly defined risk factors. Other reported tumors include head and neck malignancies, skin cancers, lung cancers, gastrointestinal malignancies, testicular germ cell tumors, melanomas, thymomas, gliomas, and leiomyosarcomas.[174]

NON-HIV RETROVIRAL MALIGNANCIES: ADULT T-CELL LEUKEMIA/LYMPHOMA

Etiologic Agent

Adult T-cell leukemia is caused by the HTLV-I discovered by Poiesz in 1980. As with all retroviruses, HTLV-I replicates in lymphocytes by integrating its DNA into the host genome. Infection causes an antibody response, which can be detected by screening with commercially available enzyme-linked immunoassay kits. Infection should be confirmed by western blot analysis, radioimmunoprecipitation, or assays to document antibody to core or envelope antigens. These tests, however, do not reliably distinguish between HTLV-I and HTLV-II and can result in false-positives.[175] HTLV-II, although isolated from a cell line from a patient with hairy-cell leukemia and detected with increased frequency in IV drug abusers, is not known to be responsible for malignant disease.[175] Polymerase chain reaction (PCR), although more costly and difficult to perform, can distinguish between HTLV-I and HTLV-II and is becoming the diagnostic test of choice.[175,176] Another member of this retroviral family, HTLV-V, is suspected to be the etiologic agent of mycosis fungoides.[175]

Epidemiology

The epidemiologic patterns of HTLV-I and adult T-cell leukemia/lymphoma have distinct geographic distributions. The virus is endemic to Japan, the Caribbean, equatorial Africa, and Central and South America. In the United States, seropositive individuals are concentrated in the Southeast. Within these regions, the incidence of HTLV-I infection also clusters in particular ethnic subpopulations, notably persons of African descent in the Caribbean and Central and South American regions[176] and persons of black, Hispanic, or Native American descent in the United States.[175]

The virus can be transmitted horizontally through sexual transmission (both heterosexual and homosexual), parenterally through infected blood products or IV drug abuse, and vertically from mother to child through infected breast milk. Breast feeding especially can result in a significant rate of seroconversion: in one Japanese study, 20% of breast-fed infants seroconverted vs only 1% of bottle-fed infants.[176]

The risk of infection after receiving seropositive blood products is strong, approximately 63% of patients become infected after transfusion. In contrast to HIV, however, HTLV-I cannot be transmitted by plasma derivatives. This is supported by the fact that hemophiliacs do not have an increased risk of HTLV-1 infection.

Programs for screening of HTLV-I antibodies are in use in Japan and the United States. In Japan the program has significantly reduced the rate of HTLV-I transmission. However, the impact of screening in the United States, where the prevalence of the disease in the population is low, is at present unknown.[175]

The patterns of transmission are manifest in the population as an increase in seropositivity with age. Breast feeding is responsible for seropositivity in children, and the incidence of seropositivity rises dramatically with the onset of sexual activity in adolescent years. Once contracted, infection is lifelong. Approximately 1% to 5% of infected individuals will develop one form of adult T-cell leukemia-lymphoma.

Pathogenesis

Although HTLV-I preferentially infects CD4-positive cells, it does not have to bind to the receptor to enter the cell. Infection of circulating cells does require, however, cell-to-cell contact with an infected T-cell, though the exact mechanism of infection is unknown. Once infected, cells are activated, as manifested by their increased expression of the IL-2 receptor and major histocompatibility complex class II antigens. The *tax* gene of HTLV-I then *trans*-activates cellular genes for IL-2, the alpha chain of the IL-2 receptor, and the c-*fox* proto-oncogene, which serve as the preliminary events of T-cell transformation. The infected cells can then be maintained in continuous long-term culture.

Although the exact events of transformation have not been elucidated, a stepwise model of transformation begins with early tax-induced polyclonal T-cell proliferation mediated by deregulated expression of IL-2 and the IL-2 receptor. Additional molecular events are then required for transformation and selective monoclonal

TABLE 15

Standard Treatment Approaches for Anal Neoplasia

For anal intraepithelial neoplasia (AIN-2, AIN-3)

Ablative therapy after four-quadrant biopsy to rule out invasive cancer; electrocautery, cryoablation, or laser ablation may be performed at the discretion of the treating physician

For invasive anal cancer

Surgical excision ± local radiotherapy may be considered for small, localized cancers with minimal depth of invasion, or

Combined modality therapy (external beam radiotherapy + fluorouracil/mitomycin or fluorouracil/cisplatin chemotherapy)

Adapted, with permission, from Northfelt DW: Cervical and anal neoplasia and HPV infection in persons with HIV infection. *Oncology* 8:33–40, 1994.

growth. Though the transforming events are unknown, the tax gene is capable of impairing DNA repair by suppressing the expression of beta-polymerase. Consequently, karyotypic abnormalities (trisomy of chromosomes 3, 7, or 21) and chromosomal abnormalities (deletions of 6q21, 10p13, and 14q11; translocations; and loss of the X chromosome) are described, although no consistent genetic abnormalities are noted. The virus does not carry oncogenes and is not known to activate cellular oncogenes by insertional mutation.[177]

How the transformed phenotype is maintained is unknown since HTLV-I infection does not involve chronic viremia or expression of viral genes.[178] The role of cytokines in maintenance of the transformed clone is also unknown, although HTLV-I-transformed T-cells do produce a variety of cytokines including IL-1-alpha, IL-1-beta, IL-2, IL-3, IL-5, IL-6, platelet-derived growth factor, interferon-gamma, lymphotoxin, tumor-necrosis factor, and transforming growth factor beta.[177]

Clinical Features and Diagnosis

Adult T-cell leukemia/lymphoma has a long incubation period (20 to 30 years) from the time of infection to development of clinical disease.[177] In that time, patients may exhibit a premalignant form of the disease, which may or may not progress into a true malignant clone. This premalignant phase is characterized by the presence of atypical lymphocytes with lobulated nuclei and lymphadenopathy with HTLV-I seropositivity and monoclonal integration of HTLV-I. Clinically, patients show involvement of the skin, an absence of visceral involvement, normal white blood cell counts, and a minority of circulating leukemic cells. Approximately 50% of patients will progress to overt malignancy with either the chronic or acute forms of the disease. Structural genes in the integrated viral DNA may be abnormal, but no abnormalities in the transforming region have been noted.[179]

Patients whose lymph node biopsy shows abnormalities may exhibit lobular, atypical, Ki-1-positive cells, which may mimic the appearance of Reed-Sternberg cells. Consequently, patients have been misdiagnosed with atypical Hodgkin's disease in the past. But PCR analysis now demonstrates integration of HTLV-I DNA, and serial follow-up of these patients demonstrates transformation to overt T-cell leukemia/lymphoma over time.[179] Therefore a diagnosis of adult T-cell leukemia/lymphoma should be considered in all cases of atypical Hodgkin's disease.

The median age of onset of T-cell leukemia/lymphoma is 56 years, with a male-to-female ratio of 1.5:1. Approximately 25% of seropositive patients will present with lymphoma and no peripheral blood involvement. The acute form of the disease is characterized by lymphadenopathy, hepatospenomegaly, and skin lesions. Less commonly (in 50% of cases), patients may demonstrate hypercalcemia and lytic bone lesions. This is considered a paraneoplastic manifestation and is caused by activation of the gene coding for parathyroid hormone—related protein by the viral tax protein.[177] Patients also demonstrate increased lactate dehydrogenase and hyperbilirubinemia levels.

The lymphadenopathy involves all peripheral areas, the retroperitoneum, and the pulmonary hila but notably spares the mediastinum. The leukemia is characterized by circulating lobulated T-cells, mild or no anemia or thrombocytopenia, and mild involvement of the bone marrow. Skin involvement can vary from patches and papules to nodules and tumor formation.

Patients with the acute disease also demonstrate abnormalities of the immune system, particularly an increased incidence of OI, which cause death in approximately 50% of patients. The chronic form of the disease is characterized by visceral involvement, lymphadenopathy, and elevated leukocyte count but no hypercalcemia or hyperbilirubinemia.

Diagnosis

In adult T-cell leukemia/lymphoma immunophenotyping of peripheral blood cells or biopsy material from lymph nodes reveals terminal deoxynucleotide transferase (TdT)-negative T-helper cells (CD4 positive). It also reveals the expression of a mature phenotype (CD2, CD3, and CD5 positive) and the p55 chain of the IL-2 receptor, signs of cellular activation. Furthermore, the T-cells demonstrate rearrangement of the T-cell receptor V-beta gene and monoclonal integration of HTLV-I DNA.[177]

Prognostic Factors, Treatment, and Survival

Several factors predict poor response to therapy and short survival—the presence of leukemia, poor performance status, and elevated serum lactate dehydrogenase levels. So far, however, no specific therapy has been shown to consistently improve survival in these patients with adult T-cell leukemia/lymphoma. Standard chemotherapies produce poor responses and median survivals ranging from months to less than 1 year. Corticosteroids have been shown to benefit patients with myelopathy, but similar results have not been observed in leukemia/lymphoma patients. Nevertheless, promising new therapies include pentostatin and anti-IL-2-receptor (anti-Tac) antibodies.[177]

REFERENCES

1. Poiesz BJ, Ruscetti FW, Gazdar AF, et al: Detection and isolation of type C retrovirus particles from fresh and cultured lymphocytes of a patient with cutaneous T-cell lymphoma. Proc Natl Acad of Sci USA 77:7415–7419, 1980.

2. Barre-Sinoussi F, Chermann JC, Rey F, et al: Isolation of a T-lymphotropic retrovirus from a patient at risk for acquired immune deficiency syndrome (AIDS). Science 220:868–871, 1983.

3. Weiss RA. Retroviruses and human cancer. Semin Cancer Biol 3:321–328, 1992.

4. Lazo PA, Tsichlis PN: Biology and pathogenesis of retroviruses. Semin Oncol 17:269–294, 1990.

5. Gallo RC, Nerurkar LS. Human retroviruses: Their role in neoplasia and immunodeficiency. Ann NY Acad Sci 567:82–94, 1987.

6. McGrath MS, Ng VL: Human retrovirus-associated malignancy. Cancer Treat Res 47:267–284, 1989.

7. Zunich KM, Lane HC: Immunologic abnormalities in HIV infection. Hematol Oncol Clin North Am 5:215–228, 1991.

8. Valentine FT: Pathogenesis of the immunological deficiencies caused by infection with the human immunodeficiency virus. Semin Oncol 17:321–334, 1990.

9. Appelbaum JW: The role of the immune system in the pathogenesis of cancer. Semin Oncol Nurs 8:51–62, 1992.

10. Levine AM: Cancer in AIDS: Editorial overview. Curr Opin Oncol 1:55–56, 1989.

11. Cremer KJ, Spring SB, Gruber J: Role of human immunodeficiency virus type 1 and other viruses in malignancies associated with acquired immunodeficiency disease syndrome. J Natl Cancer Inst 82:1016–1024, 1990.

12. Levine AM: AIDS-related malignancies: The emerging epidemic. J Natl Cancer Inst 85:1382–1397, 1993.

13. Safai B, Diaz B, and Schwartz J: Malignant neoplasms associated with human immunodeficiency virus infection. CA Cancer J Clin 42:74–95, 1992.

14. Bernstein L, Hamilton AS: The epidemiology of AIDS-related malignancies. Curr Opin Oncol 5:822–830, 1993.

15. Krigel RL, Friedman-Kien AE: Epidemic Kaposi's sarcoma. Semin Oncol 17:350–360, 1990.

16. Tappero JW, Conant MA, Wolfe SF: Kaposi's sarcoma. J Am Acad Dermatol 28:371–395, 1993.

17. Kaplan MH: Human retroviruses and neoplastic disease. Clin Infect Dis 17(suppl 2):S400–406, 1993.

18. Levine A. Cancer in AIDS: Editorial overview. Curr Opin Oncol 4:863–866, 1992.

19. Schwartz JJ, Dias BM, Safai B: HIV-related malignancies. Dermatol Clin 9:503–515, 1991.

20. Ensoli B, Barillari G, Gallo R: Pathogenesis of AIDS-associated Kaposi's sarcoma. Hematol Oncol Clin North Am 5:281–295, 1991.

21. Miles SA: Pathogenesis of human immunodeficiency virus-related Kaposi's sarcoma. Curr Opin Oncol 4:875–882, 1992.

22. Biggar RJ: Cancer in acquired immunodeficiency syndrome: An epidemiologic assessment. Semin Oncol 17:251–260, 1990.

23. Vogel J, Hinrichs SH, Reynolds RK, et al: The HIV tat gene induces dermal lesions resembling Kaposi's sarcoma in transgenic mice. Nature 335:606–611, 1988.

24. Gill PS: Pathogenesis of HIV-related malignancies. Curr Opin Oncol 3:867–871, 1991.

25. Judson MA, Sahn SA: Endobronchial lesions in HIV-infected individuals. Chest 105:1314–1323, 1994.

26. Chachoua A, Krigel R, Lafleur F, et al: Prognostic factors and staging classification of patients with epidemic Kaposi's sarcoma. J Clin Oncol 7:774–780, 1989.

27. Errante D, Vaccher E, Tirelli U, et al: Management of AIDS and its neoplastic complications. Eur J Cancer 27:380–389, 1991.

28. Krown SE, Myskowski PL, Paredes J: Kaposi's sarcoma. Med Clin North Am 76:235–252, 1992.

29. Pluda JM, Broder S, Yarchoan R: Therapy of AIDS and AIDS-related tumors. Cancer Chemo Biol Response Modif 12:395–429, 1991.

30. Tappero JW, Berger TG, Kaplan LD, et al: Cryotherapy for cutaneous Kaposi's sarcoma (KS) associated with acquired immune deficiency syndrome (AIDS): A phase II trial. J Acq Immune Defic Syndr 839–846, 1991.

31. Wheeland RG, Bailin PL, Norris MJ: Argon laser photocoagulative therapy of Kaposi's sarcoma: A clinical and histologic evaluation. J Dermatol Surg Oncol 11:1180–1185, 1995.

32. Berson AM, Quivey JM, Harris JW: et al: Radiation therapy for AIDS-related Kaposi's sarcoma. Int J Radiat Oncol Phys 19:569–575, 1990.

33. Cooper JS, Steinfeld AD, Lerch I: Intentions and outcomes in the radiotherapeutic management of epidemic Kaposi's sarcoma. Int J Radiat Oncol Biol Phys 20:419–421, 1991.

34. deWit R, Smit WGJM, Veenhof KHN, et al: Palliative radiation therapy for AIDS-associated Kaposi's sarcoma by using a single fraction of 800 cGy. Radiother Oncol 19:131–136, 1990.

35. Chak LY, Gill PS, Levine AM, et al: Radiation therapy for acquired immunodeficiency syndrome—related Kaposi's sarcoma. J Clin Oncol 6:863–867, 1988.

36. Cooper JS, Fried PR: Toxicity of oral radiotherapy in patients with acquired immunodeficiency syndrome. Arch Otolaryngol Head Neck Surg 113:327–328, 1987.

37. Serfling U, Hood AF: Local therapies for cutaneous Kaposi's sarcoma in patients with acquired immunodeficiency syndrome. Arch Dermatol 127:1479–1481, 1991.

38. Newman SB: Treatment of epidemic Kaposi's sarcoma (KS) with intralesional vinblastine injection (IL-VLB) (abstract). Proc ASCO 7:5. 1988.

39. Brambilla L, Boneschi V, Beretta G, et al: Intralesional chemotherapy for Kaposi's sarcoma. Dermatologica 169:150–155, 1984.

40. Boudreaux AA, Smith LL, Cosby CD, et al: Intralesional vinblastine for cutaneous Kaposi's sarcoma associated with acquired immunodeficiency syndrome. J Am Acad Dermatol 28:61–65, 1993.

41. Cho J, Chachoua A: Kaposi's sarcoma. Curr Opin Oncol 4:667–673, 1992.

42. Mitsuyasu RT: Clinical aspects of AIDS-related Kaposi's sarcoma. Curr Opin Oncol 5:835–844, 1993.

43. Kahn JO, Kaplan LD, Volberding PA, et al: Intralesional recombinant tumor necrosis factor alpha for AIDS-associated Kaposi's sarcoma: A randomized double-blind trial. J Acq Immune Defic Syndr 2:217–223, 1989.

44. Aboulafia D, Miles SA, Saks SR, et al: Intravenous recombinant tumor necrosis factor in the treatment of AIDS-related Kaposi's sarcoma. J Acq Immune Defic Syndr 2:54–58, 1989.

45. Kahn J, Ruiz R, Kerschmann R, et al: A phase 1/2 study of recombinant platelet factor 4 (rPF4) in patients with AIDS related Kaposi's sarcoma (KS) (abstract). Proc ASCO 12:50, 1993.

46. Staddon A, Henry D, Bonnem E: A randomized dose finding study of recombinant platelet factor 4 (rPF4) in cutaneous AIDS-related Kaposi's sarcoma (KS) (abstract). Proc ASCO 13:50, 1994.

47. Sulis E, Floris C, Sulis ML, et al: Interferon administered intralesionally in skin and oral cavity lesions in heterosexual drug addicted patients with AIDS-related Kaposi's sarcoma. Eur J Clin Oncol 25:759–761, 1989.

48. Esplin JA, Levine AM: HIV-related neoplastic disease: 1991. AIDS 5:S203–210, 1991.

49. Gill PS, Rarick M, McCutchan JA, et al: Systemic treatment of AIDS-related Kaposi's sarcoma: Results of a randomized trial. Am J Med 90:427–433, 1991.

50. Laubenstein LJ, Krigel RL, Odajnyk CM, et al: Treatment of epidemic Kaposi's sarcoma with etoposide or a combination of doxorubicin, bleomycin, and vinblastine. J Clin Oncol 2:1115–1120, 1984.

51. Lassoued K, Clauvel JP, Katlama C, et al: Treatment of the acquired immune deficiency syndrome—related Kaposi's sarcoma with bleomycin as a single agent. Cancer 66:1869–1872, 1990.

52. Volberding PA, Abrams DI, Conant M, et al: Vinblastine therapy for Kaposi's sarcoma in the acquired immunodeficiency syndrome. Ann Intern Med 103:335–338, 1985.

53. Klein E, Schwartz RA, Laor Y, et al: Treatment of Kaposi's sarcoma with vinblastine. Cancer 45:427–431, 1980.

54. Ireland-Gill A, Espina BM, Akil B, et al: Treatment of acquired immunodeficiency syndrome—related Kaposi's sarcoma using bleomycin-containing combination chemotherapy regimens. Semin Oncol 19:32–37, 1992.

55. Abrams DI, Volberding PA: Alpha interferon therapy of AIDS-associated Kaposi's sarcoma. Semin Oncol 14:43–47, 1987.

56. deWit R: AIDS-associated Kaposi's sarcoma and the mechanisms of interferon alpha's activity: A riddle within a puzzle. J Intern Med 231:321–325, 1992.

57. Safai B, Bason M, Friedman-Birnbaum R, et al: Interferon in the treatment of AIDS-associated Kaposi's sarcoma: The American experience. J Invest Dermatol 95:166–169S, 1990.

58. Krown SE, Gold JWM, Niedzwiecki D, et al: Interferon-alpha with zidovudine: Safety, tolerance, and clinical and virologic effects in patients with Kaposi sarcoma associated with the acquired immunodeficiency syndrome (AIDS). Ann Intern Med 112:812–821, 1990.

59. Fischl MA, Uttamchandani RB, Resnick L, et al: A phase I study of recombinant human interferon-alpha 2A or human lymphoblastoid interferon-alpha N1 and concomitant zidovudine in patients with AIDS-related Kaposi's sarcoma. J Acq Immune Defic Syndr 4:1–10, 1991.

60. Kovacs JA, Deyton L, Davey R, et al: Combined zidovudine and interferon-alpha therapy in patients with Kaposi's sarcoma and the

acquired immunodeficiency syndrome (AIDS). Ann Inter Med 111:280–287, 1989.

61. Scadden DT, Bering HA, Levine JD, et al: Granulocyte-macrophage colony-stimulating factor mitigates the neutropenia of combined interferon alpha and zidovudine treatment of acquired immune deficiency syndrome-associated Kaposi's sarcoma. J Clin Oncol 9:802–808, 1991.

62. Gelmann EP, Preble OT, Steis R, et al: Human lymphoblastoid interferon treatment of Kaposi's sarcoma in the acquired immune deficiency syndrome. Clinical response and prognostic parameters. Am J Med 78:737–741, 1985.

63. Miles SA, Wang H, Cortes E, et al: Beta-interferon therapy in patients with poor-prognosis Kaposi sarcoma related to the acquired immunodeficiency syndrome (AIDS). Ann Intern Med 112:582–589, 1990.

64. Krigel RL, Odajnyk CM, Laubenstein LJ, et al: Therapeutic trial of interferon-gamma in patients with epidemic Kaposi's sarcoma. J Biol Response Modif 4:358–364, 1985.

65. Krigel RL, Padavic-Shaller KA, Rudolph AR, et al: Exacerbation of epidemic Kaposi's sarcoma with a combination of interleukin-2 and beta-interferon: Results of a phase 2 study. J Biol Response Modif 8:359–365, 1989.

66. Milliken S, Boyle MJ: Update on HIV and neoplastic disease. AIDS 7(suppl 1):S203–209, 1993.

67. Gill PS, Rarick MU, Bernstein-Singer M, et al: Interferon-alpha maintenance therapy after cytotoxic chemotherapy for treatment of acquired immunodeficiency syndrome—related Kaposi's sarcoma. J Biol Response Modif 9:512–516, 1990.

68. Gill P, Rarick M, Bernstein-Singer M, et al: Treatment of advanced Kaposi's sarcoma using a combination of bleomycin and vincristine. Am J Clin Oncol 13:315–319, 1990.

69. Gompels MM, Hill A, Jenkins P, et al: Kaposi's sarcoma in HIV infection treated with vincristine and bleomycin. AIDS, 6:1175–1180, 1992.

70. Rarick MU, Gill PS, Montgomery T, et al: Treatment of epidemic Kaposi's sarcoma with combination chemotherapy (vincristine and bleomycin) and zidovudine. Ann Oncol 1:147–149, 1990.

71. Ingber D, Fukita T, Kishimoto S, et al. Synthetic analogues of fumagillin that inhibit angiogenesis and suppress tumour growth. Nature 348:555–557, 1990.

72. Pluda JM, Wyvill K, Figg WD, et al: A phase I study of an angiogenesis inhibitor, TNP-470 (AGM-1470), administered to patients (PTS) with HIV-associated Kaposi's sarcoma (KS) (abstract). Proc ASCO 13:51, 1994.

73. Nakamura S, Sakurada S, Salahuddin SZ, et al: Inhibition of development of Kaposi's sarcoma—related lesions by a bacterial cell wall complex. Science 255:1437–1440, 1992.

74. Eckhardt SG, Burris HA, Eckardt JR, et al: Phase I assessment of the novel angiogenesis inhibitor DS4152 (tecogalan sodium) (abstract). Proceedings of ASCO 13:55, 1994.

75. Schwartsmann G, Sander E, Prolla G, et al: Phase II trial of pentosan polysulfate (PPS) in patients (PTS) with AIDS-related Kaposi's sarcoma (KS) (abstract). Proceedings of ASCO 12:54, 1993.

76. Northfelt DW, Martin FJ, Kaplan LD, et al: Pharmacokinetics (PK), tumor localization (TL), and safety of Doxil (liposomal doxorubicin) in AIDS patients with Kaposi's sarcoma (AIDS-KS) (abstract). Proceedings of ASCO 12:51, 1993.

77. Northfelt DW: Stealth liposomal doxorubicin (SLD) delivers more doxorubicin (dox) to AIDS-Kaposi's sarcoma (AIDS-KS) lesions than to normal skin. Proceedings of ASCO 13:51, 1994.

78. Thommes J, Northfelt D, Rios A, et al: Open-label trial of stealth liposomal doxorubicin (D-SL) in the treatment of moderate to severe AIDS-related Kaposi's sarcoma (AIDS-KS) (abstract). Proceedings of ASCO 13:55, 1994.

79. Bernstein ZP, Wilson D, and Mang TS: Pilot study—photodynamic therapy (PDT) for treatment of AIDS-associated Kaposi's sarcoma (AIDS/KS) (abstract). Proceedings of ASCO 13:51, 1994.

80. Von Roenn J, von Gunten C, Mullane M, et al: All-trans-retinoic acid (TRA) in the treatment of AIDS-related Kaposi's sarcoma (Kaposi's sarcoma: A phase II Illinois cancer center study) (abstract). Proceedings of ASCO 12:51, 1993.

81. Saville MW, Lietzau J, Wilson W, et al: A trial of paclitaxel (Taxol) in patients with HIV-associated Kaposi's sarcoma (KS) (abstract). Proceedings of ASCO 13:54, 1994.

82. Pluda JM, Yarchoan R, Broder S: The occurrence of opportunistic non-Hodgkin's lymphomas in the setting of infection with the human immunodeficiency virus. Ann Oncol 2(suppl 2):191–200, 1991.

83. Biggar RJ and Rabkin CS: The epidemiology of acquired immunodeficiency syndrome—related lymphomas. Curr Opin Oncol 4:883–893, 1992.

84. Levine AM: AIDS-associated malignant lymphoma. Med Clin North Am 76:253–268, 1992.

85. Northfelt DW, Kaplan LD: Clinical aspects of AIDS-related non-Hodgkin's lymphoma. Curr Opin Oncol 3:872–880, 1991.

86. Beral V, Peterman T, Berkelman R, Jaffe H: AIDS-associated non-Hodgkin lymphoma. Lancet 337:805–809, 1991.

87. Serraino D, Salamina G, Franceschi S, et al: The epidemiology of AIDS-associated non-Hodgkin's lymphoma in the World Health Organization European region. Brit J Cancer 66:912–916, 1992.

88. Irwin D, Kaplan L: Clinical aspects of HIV-related lymphoma. Curr Opin Oncol 5:852–860, 1993.

89. Northfelt DW, Volberding PA, Kaplan LD: Degree of immunodeficiency at diagnosis of AIDS-associated non-Hodgkin's lymphoma (abstract). Proceedings of ASCO 11:45, 1991.

90. Pluda JM, Yarchoan R, Jaffe ES, et al: Development of non-Hodgkin lymphoma in a cohort of patients with severe human immunodeficiency virus (HIV) infection on long-term antiretroviral therapy. Ann Intern Med 113:276–282, 1990.

91. Baumgartner JE, Rachlin JR, Beckstead JH, et al: Primary central nervous system lymphomas: Natural history and response to radiation therapy in 55 patients with acquired immunodeficiency syndrome. J Neurosurg 73:206–211, 1990.

92. Levine AM: Acquired immunodeficiency-syndrome related lymphoma. Blood 80:8–20, 1992.

93. Ioachim HL: Lymphoma: An opportunistic neoplasia of AIDS. Leukemia 6(suppl 3):30–33S, 1992.

94. Knowles DM, Chamulak GA, Subar M, et al: Lymphoid neoplasia associated with the acquired immunodeficiency syndrome (AIDS). Ann Intern Med 108:744–753, 1988.

95. Voelkerding KV, Sandhaus LM, Kim HC, et al: Plasma cell malignancy in the acquired immune deficiency syndrome. Am J Clin Pathol 92:222–228, 1989.

96. Janier M, Katlama C, Flageul B, et al: The pseudo-sezary syndrome with CD8 phenotype in a patient with the acquired immunodeficiency syndrome (AIDS). Ann Intern Med 110:738–740, 1989.

97. Goldstein J, Becker N, Del Rowe J et al: Cutaneous T-cell lymphoma in a patient infected with human immunodeficiency virus type 1. Use of radiation therapy. Cancer 66:1130–1132, 1990.

98. Ruff P, Bagg A, Papadopoulos K: Precursor T-cell lymphoma associated with human immunodeficiency virus type 1 (HIV-1) infection. Cancer 64:39–42, 1989.

99. Ciobanu N, Andreeff M, Safai B, et al: Lymphoblastic neoplasia in a homosexual patient with Kaposi's sarcoma. Ann Intern Med 98:151–155, 1983.

100. Shibata D, Byrnes RK, Rabinowitz A, et al: Human T-cell lymphotropic virus type I (HTLV-I)-associated adult T-cell leukemia-lymphoma in a patient infected with human immunodeficiency virus

type 1 (HIV-1). Ann Intern Med 111:871–875, 1989.

101. Sternlieb J, Mintzer D, Kwa D, et al: Peripheral T-cell lymphoma in a patient with the acquired innumodeficiency syndrome. Am J Med 85:445, 1988.

102. Gonzales-Clemente JM, Ribera JM, Campo E, et al. Ki-1 plus anaplastic large-cell lymphoma of T-cell origin in an HIV-infected patient. AIDS 5:751–755, 1991.

103. Emilie D, Coumbaras J, Raphael M, et al: Interleukin-6 production in high-grade B lymphomas: Correlation with the presence of malignant immunoblasts in acquired immunodeficiency syndrome and in human immunodeficiency virus-seronegative patients. Blood 80:498–504, 1992.

104. Karp JE and Broder S: The pathogenesis of AIDS lymphomas: A foundation for addressing the challenges of therapy and prevention. Leuk Lymphoma 8:167–188, 1992.

105. Pelicci P, Knowles DM, Arlin ZA, et al: Multiple monoclonal B cell expansions and c-myc oncogene rearrangements in acquired immune deficiency syndrome—related lymphoproliferative disorders. J Exp Med 164:2049–2076, 1986.

106. Shibata D, Weiss LM, Hernandez AM, et al: Epstein-Barr virus-associated non-Hodgkin's lymphoma in patients infected with the human immunodeficiency virus. Blood 81:2102–2109, 1983.

107. Neri A, Barriga F, Inghirami G, et al: Epstein-Barr virus infection precedes clonal expansion in Burkitt's and acquired immunodeficiency syndrome-associated lymphoma. Blood 77:1092–1095, 1991.

108. Shibata D, Weiss LM, Nathwani BN, et al: Epstein-Barr virus in benign lymph node biopsies from individuals infected with the human immunodeficiency virus is associated with concurrent or subsequent development of non-Hodgkin's lymphoma. Blood 77:1527–1533, 1991.

109. Knowles DM: Biologic aspects of AIDS-associated non-Hodgkin's lymphoma. Curr Opin Oncol 5:845–851, 1993.

110. Ziegler JL, Beckstead JA, Volberding PA, et al: Non-Hodgkin's lymphoma in 90 homosexual men. Relation to generalized lymphadenopathy and the acquired immunodeficiency syndrome. N Engl J of Med 311:565–570, 1984.

111. Kaplan LD, Abrams DI, Feigal E, et al: AIDS-associated non-Hodgkin's lymphoma in San Francisco. JAMA 261:719–724, 1989.

112. Freter CE: Acquired immunodeficiency syndrome-associated lymphomas. J Natl Cancer Inst 10:45–54, 1990.

113. Levine AM: Epidemiology, clinical characteristics, and management of AIDS-relatd lymphoma. Hematol Oncol Clin North Am 5:331–342, 1991.

114. Heitzman ER: Pulmonary neoplastic and lymphoproliferative disease in AIDS: A review. Radiology 177:347–351, 1990.

115. Dodd GD III, Greenler DP, Confer SR: Thoracic and abdominal manifestations of lymphoma occurring in the immunocompromised patient. Radiol Clin North Am 30:597–610, 1992.

116. Sokovich RS, Bormes TD, and McKiel CF: Acquired immunodeficiency syndrome presenting as testicular lymphoma. J Urol 147:1110–1111, 1992.

117. Green ST, Nathwani D, Goldberg DJ, et al: Urological manifestations of HIV-related disease. A case of AIDS-associated testicular seminoma, Kaposi's sarcoma, and possible intracranial lymphoma. Brit J Urol 67:188–190, 1991.

118. Tsang K, Kneafsey P, Gill MJ: Primary lymphoma of the kidney in the acquired immunodeficiency syndrome. Arch Pathol Lab Med 117:541–543, 1993.

119. Holladay AO, Siegel RJ, Schwartz DA: Cardiac malignant lymphoma in acquired immune deficiency syndrome. Cancer, 70:2203–2207, 1992.

120. Monfardini S: Malignant lymphomas in patients with or at risk for AIDS in Italy. Recent Results Cancer Res 112:37–45, 1988.

121. Levine AM, Sullivan-Halley J, Pike MC, et al: Human immunodeficiency virus-related lymphoma. Prognostic factors predictive of survival. Cancer 68:2466–2472, 1991.

122. Aboulafia DM, Mitsuyasu RT: Hematologic abnormalities in AIDS. Hematol Oncol Clin North Am 5:195–214, 1991.

123. Calenda V, Chermann JC: The effects of HIV on hematopoiesis. Eur J Hematol 48:181–186, 1992.

124. Pluda JM, Mitsuya H, Yarchoan R: Hematologic effects of AIDS therapies. Hematol Oncol Clin North Am 5:229–248, 1991.

125. Odajnyk C, Subar M, Dugan M, et al: Clinical features and correlation with immunopathology and molecular biology in a large group of patients with AIDS-associated small non-cleaved cell lymphoma (SNCL), Burkitt's and non-Burkitt's type (abstract). Blood 68:131a, 1986.

126. Dugan M, Subar M, Odajnyk C, et al: Intensive multiagent chemotherapy (chemo) for AIDS-related diffuse large cell lymphomas (LCL) (abstract). Blood 68:124a, 1986.

127. Gill PS, Levine AM, Krailo M, et al: AIDS-related malignant lymphoma: Results of prospective treatment trials. J Clin Oncol 5:1322–1328, 1987.

128. Remick S, McSharry J, Wolf B, et al: Novel oral combination chemotherapy (CT) in the management of AIDS-related non-Hodgkin lymphoma (NHL): Longer follow-up (abstract). Proceedings of ASCO 11:48, 1992.

129. Sparano JA, Wiernick PH, Strack M, et al: Infusional cyclophosphamide, doxorubicin, and etoposide (CDE) in HIV- and HTLV-I-related non-Hodgkin's lymphoma (NHL): A highly active regimen (abstract). Proceedings of ASCO 12:50, 1993.

130. Bermudez MA, Grant KM, Rodvein R, et al: Non-Hodgkin's lymphoma in a population with or at risk for acquired immunodeficiency syndrome: Indications for intensive chemotherapy. Am J Med 86:71–76, 1989.

131. Errante D, Tirelli U, Oksenhendler E, et al: Prospective study with combined low-dose chemotherapy and zidovudine for 37 patients (pts) with poor prognosis HIV-related non-Hodgkin's lymphoma (HIV-NHL) (abstract). Proceedings of ASCO 11:44, 1992.

132. Tirelli U, Errante D, Oksenhendler E, et al: Prospective study with combined low-dose chemotherapy and zidovudine in 37 patients with poor-prognosis AIDS-related non-Hodgkin's lymphoma. Ann Oncol 3:843–847, 1992.

133. Gisselbrecht C, Oksenjendler E, Tirelli U, et al: Non-Hodgkin's lymphoma associated with human immunodeficiency virus: Treatment with LNH 84 regimen in a selected group of patients. Leukemia 6(suppl 3):10–11S, 1992.

134. Sawka CA, Shepherd FA, Brandwein J, et al: Treatment of AIDS-related non-Hodgkin's lymphoma with a twelve week chemotherapy program. Leuk Lymphoma 8:213–220, 1992.

135. Huhn D, Weiss R, Nerl C, et al: HIV-related non-Hodgkin's lymphoma: CHOP-induction and AZT/IFN-alpha-maintenance therapy (abstract). Proceedings of ASCO 12:52, 1993.

136. Sawka C, Shepherd F, Brandwein J, et al: Novel combination chemotherapy for HIV-related non-Hodgkin's lymphoma (HIV-NHL) (abstract). Proceedings of ASCO 13:53, 1994.

137. Levine AM, Wernz JC, Kaplan L, et al: Low-dose chemotherapy with central nervous system prophylaxis and zidovudine maintenance in AIDS-related lymphoma. JAMA 266: 84–88, 1991.

138. Kaplan LD, Kahn JO, Crowe S, et al: Clinical and virologic effects of recombinant human granulocyte-macrophage colony-stimulating factor in patients receiving chemotherapy for human immunodeficiency virus-associated non-Hodgkin's lymphoma: Results of a randomized trial. J Clin Oncol 9:929–940, 1991.

139. Hahn S, Pluda J, Shay L, et al: Treatment of AIDS-related non-Hodgkin's lymphoma with chemotherapy, AZT, and GM-CSF (abstract). Proceedings of ASCO 11:45, 1992.

140. Walsh C, Wernz JC, Levine A, et al: Phase I trial of m-BACOD and granulocyte macrophage colony stimulating factor in HIV-associated non-Hodgkin's lymphoma. J Acq Immune Defic Syndr 6:265–271, 1993.

141. Tirelli U, Errante D, Vaccher E, et al: Treatment of HIV-related non-Hodgkin's lymphoma (NHL) with chemotherapy (CT) and G-CSF: Reduction in the days of hospitalization and toxicity with concomitant overall reduction in the cost (abstract). Proceedings of ASCO 12:53, 1993.

142. Sparano JA, Wiernik PH, Dutcher JP, et al: A pilot trial of infusional cyclophosphamide, doxorubicin, and etoposide (CDE) plus didanosine (DDI) in HIV-related non-Hodgkin's lymphoma (NHL) (abstract). Proceedings of ASCO 13:51, 1994.

143. Tulpule A, Anderson LJJ, Levine AM, et al: Anti-B4(CD19) monoclonal antibody conjugated with ricin (B4-blocked ricin: B4BR) in refractory AIDS-lymphoma (abstract). Proceedings of ASCO 13:52, 1994.

144. Levine AM, Weiss G, Tulpule A, et al: MGBG: A highly active drug in relapsed or refractory AIDS-lymphoma (abstract). Proceedings of ASCO 13:52, 1994.

145. Fine HA and Mayer RJ: Primary central nervous system lymphoma. Ann Intern Med 119:1093–1104, 1993.

146. Deangelis LM: Current management of primary central nervous system lymphoma. Oncology 9:63–71, 1995.

147. Davenport C, Dillon WP, and Sze G: Neuroradiology of the immunosuppressed state. Radiol Clin North Am 30:611–637, 1992.

148. Xerri L, Gambarelli D, Horschowski N, et al: What's new in primary central nervous system lymphomas? Pathol Res Pract 186:809–816, 1990.

149. MacMahon EME, Glass JD, Hayward SD, et al: Epstein-Barr virus in AIDS-related primary central nervous system lymphoma. Lancet 338:969–973, 1991.

150. Remick SC, Diamond C, Migliozzi JA, et al: Primary central nervous system lymphoma in patients with and without the acquired immune deficiency syndrome. A retrospective analysis and review of the literature. Medicine 69:345–360, 1990.

151. Goldstein JD, Dickson DW, Moser FG, et al: Primary central nervous system lymphoma in acquired immune deficiency syndrome. A clinical and pathologic study with results of treatment with radiation. Cancer 67:2756–2765, 1991.

152. Formenti SC, Gill PS, Lean E, et al: Primary central nervous system lymphoma in AIDS. Results of radiation therapy. Cancer 63:1101–1107, 1989.

153. Madajewicz S, Fuhrer J, Chowhan N, et al: Intracarotid chemotherapy (ICCT) with etoposide and cisplatin in patients (pts) with poor prognosis HIV-related-CNS-non-Hodgkin's lymphoma (HIV-CNS-NHL) (abstract). Proceedings of ASCO 12:55, 1993.

154. Hessol NA, Katz MH, Liu JU, et al: Increased incidence of Hodgkin's disease in homosexual men with HIV infection. Ann Intern Med 117:309–311, 1992.

155. Ames ED, Conjalka MS, Goldberg AF, et al: Hodgkin's disease and AIDS. Twenty-three new cases and a review of the literature. Hematol Oncol Clin North Am 5:343–356, 1991.

156. Gold JE, Altarac D, Ree HJ, et al: HIV-associated Hodgkin's disease: A clinical study of 18 cases and review of the literature. Am J Hematol 36: 93–99, 1991.

157. Pelstring RJ, Zellmer RB, Sulak LE, et al: Hodgkin's disease in association with human immunodeficiency virus infection. Pathologic and immunologic features. Cancer 67: 1865–1873, 1991.

158. Serraino D, Carbone A, Franceschi S, et al: Increased frequency of lymphocyte depletion and mixed cellularity subtypes of Hodgkin's disease in HIV-infected patients. Eur J Cancer 29A:1948–1950, 1993.

159. Tirelli U, Vaccher E, Rezza G, et al: Hodgkin's disease in association with acquired immunodeficiency syndrome (AIDS). A report on 36 patients. Acta Oncol 28:637–639, 1989.

160. Newcom S, Ward M, Napoli V, et al: Treatment of HIV-associated Hodgkin's disease (HIV-HD): Is there a clue regarding the etiology of Hodgkin's disease (abstract)? Proceedings of ASCO 11:44, 1992.

161. Stratton P, Ciacco K: Cervical neoplasia in the patient with HIV infection. Curr Opin Obstet Gynecol 6:86–91, 1994.

162. Maiman M: Cervical neoplasia in women with HIV infection. Oncology 8:83–94, 1994.

163. Giorda G, Vaccher E, Volpe R, et al: An unusual presentation of vulvar carcinoma in a HIV patient. Gynecol Oncol 44:191–194, 1992.

164. Maiman M, Fruchter RG, Serur E, et al: Human immunodeficiency virus infection and cervical neoplasia. Gynecol Onco 38:377–382, 1990.

165. Vermund SH, Kelley KF, Klein RS, et al: High risk of human papillomavirus infection and cervical squamous intraepithelial lesions among women with symptomatic human immunodeficiency virus infection. Am J Obstet Gynecol 165:392–400, 1991.

166. Matorras R, Ariceta JM, Rementeria A, et al: Human immunodeficiency virus—induced immunosuppression: A risk factor for human papillomavirus infection. Am J Obstet Gynecol 164:42–44, 1991.

167. Wright TC, Ellerbrock TV, Chiasson MA, et al: Cervical intraepithelial neoplasia in women infected with human immunodeficiency virus: Prevalence, risk factors, and validity of Papanicolaou smears. Obstet Gynecol 84:591–597, 1994.

168. Maiman M, Tarricone N, Vieira J, et al: Colposcopic evaluation of human immunodeficiency virus-seropositive women. Obstet Gynecol 78:84–88, 1991.

169. Hankins CA, Lamont JA, Handley MA: Cervicovaginal screening in women with HIV infection: A need for increased vigilance? Can Med Assoc J 150: 681–686, 1994.

170. Northfelt DW: Cervical and anal neoplasia and HPV infection in persons with HIV infection. Oncology 8:33–40, 1994.

171. Palefsky JM: Anal human papillomavirus infection and anal cancer in HIV-positive individuals: An emerging problem. AIDS 8:283–295, 1994.

172. Lipsey LR, Northfelt DW: Anogenital neoplasia in patients with HIV infection. Curr Opin Oncol 5:861–866, 1993.

173. Holland JM, Swift PS: Tolerance of patients with human immunodeficiency virus and anal carcinoma to treatment with combined chemotherapy and radiation therapy. Radiology 193:251–254, 1994.

174. Cohen P: Miscellaneous cancers associated with AIDS. Curr Opin Oncol 1:68–71, 1989.

175. Hjelle B: Human T-cell leukemia/lymphoma viruses. Arch Pathol Lab Med 115:440–450, 1991.

176. McFarlin DE, Blattner WA: Non-AIDS retroviral infections in humans. Ann Rev Med 42:97–105, 1991.

177. Hollsberg P, Hafler DA: Pathogenesis of diseases induced by human lymphotropic virus type I infection. N Engl J Med 328:1173–1182, 1993.

178. Smith MR, Greene WC: Molecular biology of the type I human T-cell leukemia virus (HTLV-I) and adult T-cell leukemia. J Clin Invest 87:761–766, 1991.

179. Sausville EA: T-cell leukemia-lymphoma and mycosis fungoides. Curr Opin Oncol 4:829–839, 1992.

CHAPTER 35

Unknown Primary Carcinomas: Diagnosis and Management

Jean-Pierre M. Ayoub, MD, Kevin P. Hubbard, DO, *and* Renato Lenzi, MD

Department of Clinical Investigation
The University of Texas M. D. Anderson Cancer Center, Houston, Texas

Unknown primary carcinomas are a significant health problem, constituting 3% to 10% of all tumors diagnosed in the United States each year.[1,2] While the majority of patients with metastatic carcinoma of unknown primary origin have short survival times and disease resistant to treatment, recent findings suggest that certain subsets of patients have tumors that are responsive to chemotherapy. Others can be successfully treated with regional therapy.

In this chapter, concepts and guidelines regarding a directed evaluation of patients with unknown primary carcinomas are presented, and the clinical course and treatment of disease presenting at each major site are reviewed.

A practical definition of unknown primary carcinoma is a biopsy-proven carcinoma with no identifiable source as determined by medical history and physical examination, complete blood cell count, chemistries, urinalysis, chest x-ray, computed tomography (CT) scan of the abdomen, CT scan or sonogram of the pelvis, and mammogram (in women). Abnormalities detected in the initial testing should be pursued if possibly indicative of a primary tumor. In patients presenting with metastatic carcinomas that have no obvious source, the subsequent search for a primary tumor is unrewarding in approximately 75% of the cases, even after the most thorough evaluation.[1,3]

This fact has caused much consternation for both patients and physicians. The treatment of malignancy is traditionally based on the identification of the origin of the tumor, and treatment is chosen and initiated based upon the natural history and the most specific therapies available for a certain type of tumor. Without knowledge of the primary site, the oncologist is often hesitant to recommend therapy.

In addition, the physician may believe that he or she has somehow failed to serve the patient adequately by being unable to identify a primary malignancy. Further, in reviewing the literature, the oncologist is presented with an assortment of disparate clinical trials and retrospective studies that often arrive at contradictory conclusions and, in many cases, exclusively stress the overall poor prognosis of this disease.

EPIDEMIOLOGY

Unknown primary carcinomas affect males and females equally. The median age at presentation is 56 to 60 years, and 10% of patients with an unknown primary tumor have a history of an antecedent cancer.[4] Postmortem examination will identify the occult primary tumor in 60% to 80% of cases.[5,6] In an autopsy series on patients with unknown primary tumors reported by Nystrom, the most commonly identified primary sites were pancreas (20%) and lung (18%).[7] The poor prognosis of these malignancies reflects the overall poor prognosis of unknown primary tumors as a group. Although breast and prostate cancers represent the most common cancers in women and men, these accounted for only 4% and 2%, respectively, of the primary sites found in a recent series.[8]

About 60% of the patients who present with an unknown primary carcinoma will be diagnosed with metastatic adenocarcinoma. An additional 30% of patients will have undifferentiated or poorly differentiated carcinomas. The remaining patients will have one of a variety of carcinomas that include squamous-cell carcinomas, neuroendocrine tumors, and malignancies that upon more detailed study will be found to be sarcomas, lymphomas, germ-cell tumors, melanomas, and unclassifiable undifferentiated malignant neoplasms.

BIOLOGY

In 20% to 40% of cases of unknown primary tumors, the primary site will not be identified even after autopsy.[5] Unknown primary carcinomas therefore exhibit unique biologic behavior, with the development of clinically devious metastatic lesions in the absence of a detectable primary tumor. Certain cancers such as melanoma and renal cancer are known to exhibit spontaneous regression of the primary tumor in association with the host's immunologic response. It is clear that many of these tumors have acquired the capacity to metastasize even though a primary lesion is not clinically evident.

The exact mechanisms of these phenomena are unclear, but models in which genetic alterations result in early metastasis have been proposed for other tumors[9] and may be applicable to unknown primary carcinomas as well. The notion that a genetic alteration is responsible is supported by data that demonstrated a partial or complete loss of the short arm of chromosome 1 in 12 of 13 patients with unknown primary tumors.[10] This chromosomal aberration has been reported by others as being characteristic of the karyotype most often associated with advanced malignancy and confirms the concept that structural changes of chromosome 1 exist in most forms of advanced cancer.[11] Multiple other karyotypic abnormalities have been demonstrated in unknown primary malignancies.

Molecular studies have shown overexpression of c-myc, ras, and c-erbB-2 in unknown primary tumors.[12] Although these are highly metastatic advanced tumors that would have been expected to have a high incidence of p53 mutations, the frequency of p53 mutations in a series of such tumor biopsy samples was found to be lower than anticipated (26%).[13]

DIAGNOSTIC EVALUATION

Much has been written about the proper approach to diagnostic evaluation of unknown primary tumors. Some authors advocate the use of a minimal diagnostic analysis, its scope limited to separating treatable disease from untreatable disease.[14] Others have supported a more aggressive approach wherein a complete assessment of the extent of the disease as well as detection of the primary tumor site is attempted.

We believe that a pragmatic approach is best. Extensive evaluation of all patients presenting with metastases of unknown primary carcinoma is an expensive and wasteful extreme (particularly in this era of heightened consciousness over the costs of health care). One study reported the average cost of investigation of a patient with an unknown primary tumor to be $17,973.[15] In that study, patient survival time reflected the natural history of unknown primary tumors: Mean survival time was 8.1 months, with only 18% of patients surviving 1 year. However, a strictly minimalist approach may result in the oversight of treatable (and potentially curable) neoplasms.

An important determinant of the appropriate extent of evaluation for a given patient with an unknown primary carcinoma is whether the data obtained by a diagnostic test will influence treatment decisions. If the initial data point to a treatable or potentially curable cancer (eg, a germ-cell tumor or lymphoma), then further investiga-tion should proceed until a precise clinical diagnosis can be made. Clinical data support the belief that patients who have unknown primary tumors that are later proved to have originated from a given site or from unique histology have an overall prognosis similar to that of patients who present with a known primary tumor.[16] The recommended general approach is thus one of directed evaluation based upon the clinical presentation, the initial pathologic findings, and the characteristics of the individual patient.

CLINICAL EVALUATION

In each case, a thorough medical history should be obtained, and a physical examination including a digital prostate exam in men and a pelvic exam in women should be performed. Determination of the patient's performance status, nutrition, and the presence or absence of concomitant medical illnesses and malignancy-related complications (such as paraneoplastic syndromes, painful metastases, or spinal-cord compression) that may affect patient care is required.

Laboratory tests should include routine biochemical and hematologic surveys. Initial radiographic studies should include chest x-ray films, CT scans of the abdomen, and a CT scan or sonogram of the pelvis. The role of CT scanning of the abdomen or pelvis is documented in patients with unknown carcinoma; detection of the site of origin in 30% to 35% of these patients has been reported.[17,18] Not surprisingly, the tumors most often identified on CT scans are those that arise from the pancreas, kidney, hepatobiliary tract, and ovary. CT scans of the chest should be performed for patients who have abnormalities evident on their chest radiographs. A cytologic analysis of the sputum should be performed in any patient with a radiographically documented chest abnormality.

All women with unknown primary carcinoma should undergo mammography and a careful pelvic examination. In cases of suspicious findings on a breast examination and a negative mammogram, patients should have a breast sonogram and a biopsy as indicated. Imaging or endoscopy of the upper and lower gastrointestinal (GI) tract is indicated for patients with abdominal complaints, ascites, liver metastases, or other findings in the initial workup that point to a possible GI primary tumor.

Patients with upper or mid-cervical adenopathy should receive a thorough evaluation including endoscopy by a head and neck surgeon as well as CT scanning of the head and neck region. Lower cervical or supraclavicular adenopathy suggests a primary tumor arising from below the clavicle, most commonly from the lung. Patients who have a pathologic diagnosis of papillary carcinoma in the neck or chest region should undergo imaging studies of the thyroid. Patients with inguinal lymphadenopathy may have a detectable primary site in the perineal or anorectal area, and anoscopy and colposcopy should be performed.[1] Evaluation by a urologist may reveal a primary carcinoma of the distal urinary tract.

HISTOPATHOLOGIC EVALUATION AND USE OF SERUM TUMOR MARKERS

All pathologic material obtained at biopsy should be evaluated by an experienced pathologist who is familiar with the special diagnostic problems of unknown primary carcinomas. The pathologist should also be informed of the patient's pertinent history and clinical findings and may be able to recommend further analysis based upon this information.

Light microscopy will show that about 60% of patients with unknown primary tumors have adenocarcinoma and that another 5% have squamous-cell carcinoma. In the remaining patients, light microscopy is much less specific and identifies the tumor as a poorly differentiated neoplasm, a poorly differentiated carcinoma, or a poorly differentiated adenocarcinoma.[1]

Subsequent evaluation of this group of poorly differentiated lesions by means of special immunohistochemical techniques is warranted because some of these tumors are curable or very responsive to treatment. Many immunohistochemical reagents are at the disposal of the pathologist, making the histologic classification of the tumor easier. Especially useful are the antibodies to common leukocyte antigens present in lymphoma and the antibodies to the prostate-specific antigen (PSA) present in most prostate cancers.[19,20]

The use of cytogenetic analysis in the diagnosis of unknown primary tumors is still limited but holds promise. Specific chromosomal abnormalities have been identified in several types of lymphoma (8,14 translocation in small non-cleaved-cell non-Hodgkin's lymphoma),[21] germ-cell tumors i(12p),[22] and neuroendocrine tumors t(11,22).[23] Because these tumors require specific therapies, identification of the specific tumors and directed therapy is preferable to empirically treating all patients who have poorly differentiated neoplasms with a generic cisplatin (Platinol)-based regimen of chemotherapy.[24]

Recently, Motzer et al have used cytogenetic techniques to identify a treatable subset of patients with poorly differentiated carcinomas. Response to cisplatin-based therapy correlated with the finding of i(12p) in tumors by either molecular or cytogenetic studies.[25] Because i(12p) is a chromosomal marker that characterizes germ-cell tumors, cytogenetic studies will provide another way to identify this treatable subset of poorly differentiated carcinomas.

The role of tumor markers in the evaluation of patients with unknown primary tumors is unclear. Most tumor markers are nonspecific, and they may be most useful in monitoring a patient's response to therapy.[26] Tumor markers do not appear to be predictive of response to chemotherapy,[27] but their directed use seems valuable in complementing the overall evaluation of patients with unknown primary cancers.[28,29]

Men who present with adenocarcinoma should have PSA and prostatic acid phosphatase levels measured, even in the absence of bony metastases. When tumor histology is undifferentiated, beta-human chorionic gonadotropin and alpha-fetoprotein levels should be measured, especially if the clinical presentation suggests an extragonadal germ-cell tumor.[29] In patients with hepatic tumors, alpha-fetoprotein levels should also be measured. The adenocarcinoma markers (CEA, CA125, CA15-3, and CA19-9) are often elevated in patients with unknown primary tumors and cannot be reliably used to identify a specific primary site.

Using the diagnostic approach outlined, it is possible to detect a primary neoplasm in 20% to 30% of patients presenting with unknown primary malignancies. In a review of primary tumors identified by this approach, investigators at M. D. Anderson Cancer Center found that the most common sites of origin for epithelial histologies were the lung (15%), the pancreas (13%), the colon/rectum (6%), the kidney (5%), and the breast (4%). Melanomas, sarcomas, and lymphomas each made up 6% to 8% of the total. The remaining cases were primary tumors of the stomach (4%), ovary (3%), liver (3%), esophagus (3%), mesothelioma (2%), prostate (2%), and a variety of other histologies (19%).[8]

CLINICAL PRESENTATION AND TREATMENT RECOMMENDATIONS

Not surprisingly, patients with unknown primary carcinomas present with many of the same symptoms as patients with advanced malignancies of known origin. In one review, clinical presentation included general deterioration (73%), digestive symptoms (58%), liver enlargement (58%), abdominal pain (56%), respiratory symptoms (45%), ascites (26%), and node enlargement (16%).[30]

Approximately 50% of patients who have unknown primary tumors present with multiple sites of involvement. In those with a dominant (or sole) site, the most common sites are the liver (25%), bone (22%), lung

(20%), lymph nodes (15%), pleural space (10%), and brain (5%).

The clinical course of patients with unknown primary carcinomas varies widely. Although as a group, their median survival time is poor, there are certain prognostic variables that suggest longer survival, such as involvement of lymph nodes only, pathologic diagnoses of squamous carcinoma and neuroendocrine carcinoma, and disease limited to one organ site. On the other hand, variables suggestive of a poor prognosis include male sex, pathologic diagnosis of adenocarcinoma, and metastatic involvement of the liver, lung, bone, pleura, or brain.[31]

For the majority of patients with unknown primary carcinomas, chemotherapy has not been shown to favorably affect survival. A small number of patients within this heterogeneous group, however, are candidates for curative treatment.

Clinicopathologic Subgroups

Extragonadal Germ-Cell Syndrome: As a group, patients who have undifferentiated or poorly differentiated carcinoma, are less than 50 years old, and present with rapidly growing midline tumors involving the lymph nodes, mediastinum, or retroperitoneum have been found to have tumors that are very responsive to chemotherapy, particularly to platinum-containing regimens. It is believed that these individuals have poorly differentiated extragonadal germ-cell tumors. Investigators have referred to this disease entity as "extragonadal germ-cell syndrome" or "germ-cell equivalents."[32–34] These patients have response rates to chemotherapy of 35% to 50%, and those who achieve a complete response often enjoy a durable remission.

Disease Limited to the Lymph Nodes: Another important clinical subset is made up of patients who present with lymph-node involvement with no other apparent metastases. These patients usually do better than those who show evidence of visceral involvement. The favorable prognosis may be related to a low tumor burden at the time of diagnosis rather than to intrinsic sensitivity to treatment of the tumor.

Cervical and Supraclavicular Adenopathies: Patients presenting with involvement of the mid- or high-cervical nodes are believed to have an occult primary tumor in the head or neck. Both squamous-cell carcinomas and adenocarcinomas are encountered, but patients who present with adenocarcinoma appear to have a poorer prognosis.

Supraclavicular adenopathy is another fairly common presentation, affecting 15% of the unknown primary tumor patients in the M. D. Anderson Cancer Center

series,[31] and represents either an undiagnosed tumor in the head and neck region or, more often, far-advanced malignant disease from a distant site. The majority of these tumors are squamous-cell or undifferentiated carcinomas. Patients with disease in the supraclavicular nodes have a worse prognosis than do patients with disease in other lymph-node-bearing areas. Carcinoma affecting lymph nodes on the right side most commonly arises from occult primary tumors of the lung and breast. When disease affects the lymph nodes on the left side, spread from intra-abdominal malignancies by way of the thoracic duct (Virchow's node) is an additional possibility.

Most individuals with squamous-cell carcinoma or adenocarcinoma involving only the cervical or supraclavicular lymph nodes should receive regional therapy and careful follow-up. Patients whose disease is limited to the mid- or high-cervical nodes benefit from local and regional therapy. The 3-year survival rate after radical neck dissection and/or radical cervical irradiation ranges from 35% to 60%.[1] Within this group, patients with N1 disease (according to the tumor, nodes, and metastasis, or TNM, staging system) have the better prognosis; patients with N3 disease, regardless of the local treatment modality used (surgery, radiotherapy, or both), fail to achieve complete remission in 65% of cases.

Recently, investigators have tried to improve the outcome of patients with N3 disease by adding systemic chemotherapy to local treatment modalities. In one study, induction chemotherapy with cisplatin and fluorouracil was followed by radiation therapy. The rate of complete remission improved to 60% in patients with N3 disease, and although the study sample was small, these complete remissions appeared durable (median, 39 months).[35] Patients with low cervical or supraclavicular nodes have a much worse survival rate.

Axillary adenopathy is an additional disease subset with a favorable prognosis. Women who present with adenocarcinoma in the axillary lymph nodes should undergo mammography because the most likely primary is breast cancer. Lesions identified by mammography should be biopsied. Suspicious areas not well imaged by mammography should be evaluated by breast ultrasonography; biopsy can be performed using ultrasound guidance.

These patients are best treated as if they had stage II breast cancer, and they may enjoy a significant survival benefit. Modified radical mastectomy has been recommended in these patients even when physical examination and mammography studies fail to identify a primary breast cancer. A report by Ellerbroek et al documented actuarial disease-free survival rates of 71% at 5 years and

65% at 10 years.[36] Survival rates were higher in patients who received systemic chemotherapy plus radiation therapy. Local control was also enhanced by irradiating the affected breast and axilla.

The prognosis is not as favorable in men who present with axillary adenopathy only. In these patients, a reasonable therapeutic approach is to proceed with axillary node dissection in an attempt to remove all known disease and to add local radiation, if needed. Patients are then observed without further therapy. If the disease is rapidly growing or bulky, systemic chemotherapy is administered before surgery or radiation therapy.

Inguinal Adenopathy: A few patients with unknown primary tumors present with inguinal adenopathy. Undifferentiated (anaplastic) carcinoma is identified in at least half of these cases. Some of these anaplastic "carcinomas" appear to be melanomas with no obvious primary skin lesion. The remaining patients have adenocarcinomas arising from the skin, genitourinary tract, anus, or pelvis. A detailed investigation for primary lesions in these areas is warranted. In patients with adenocarcinomas and poorly differentiated carcinomas that are strictly confined to the groin nodes, a superficial groin dissection should be performed. Further treatment is often withheld in these cases, while the patients are monitored for recurrent disease.[4] Chemotherapy may be offered in the face of systemic disease, preferably in the context of a clinical trial.

Melanoma involving the lymph nodes is a fairly common occurrence. Most patients present with clinical stage II disease and have a 5-year survival rate of 27% to 33%.[4] Authorities have recommended radical lymph-node dissection for melanomas presenting as unknown primary tumors, because a 5-year survival rate of 40% to 50% was reported for patients who had been aggressively treated.[37]

Malignant Ascites: Patients with malignant ascites usually belong to one of two subsets, each with a very different natural history of disease. The first group consists of patients with mucin-producing adenocarcinoma, who may present with ascitic fluid that contains signet-ring cells. These patients often have multiple peritoneal implants. This group has a poor prognosis and responds poorly to currently available treatment regimens.

The second group is made up of women with papillary adenocarcinoma in the peritoneal fluid; this disease is often associated with pelvic adenopathy or masses. These patients may have elevated CA125 levels but do not have detectable ovarian cancer. Some investigators consider these patients to have true unknown primary ovarian tumors or primary serous carcinomas of the perito-neum.[38,39] This disease has not been documented in males. Disease management should be the same as that for women with ovarian carcinoma. Response rates ranging from 32% to 39% have been reported in patients who undergo cytoreductive surgery followed by cisplatin-based chemotherapy.[1]

Neuroendocrine Tumors: Patients with poorly differentiated neuroendocrine tumors may present with patterns of metastases strongly resembling those of extragonadal germ-cell tumors. It may be difficult to separate this subset of neoplasms from the germ-cell group. However, immunohistochemical stains for neuron-specific enolase and chromogranin A (markers of neuroendocrine differentiation)[40] and for alpha-fetoprotein, beta-human chorionic gonadotropin, and placental alkaline phosphatase (markers supporting a diagnosis of germ-cell tumors) may aid in differentiation. Neuroendocrine tumors can also be diagnosed by electron microscopy, which can reveal the neurosecretory granules characteristic of such tumors.[41]

Although the nature and course of this clinical entity is still being defined, the clinical data suggest that this type of anaplastic tumor is responsive to cisplatin-based chemotherapy, even when the primary site is unknown. Achievement of a reasonable duration of response is also supported by clinical data.[42,43]

Pulmonary Metastases and Pleural Effusions: Individuals with multiple pulmonary metastases constitute the largest group of patients with unknown primary tumors, and lung cancer is the most frequent primary diagnosis made in this group. The diagnosis is commonly based on the results of chest radiography, CT scans, and either sputum cytology or bronchoscopy. It is very unusual for patients with pulmonary metastases to be candidates for surgical resection; these patients most often receive systemic chemotherapy. With the exception of some young patients whose tumors fit the criteria of germ-cell equivalents, these patients usually do very poorly.

Malignant pleural effusions are relatively common, affecting about 10% of patients with unknown primary tumors. Most of these patients have adenocarcinomas, which may be difficult to differentiate from mesotheliomas. Therapy for this group of patients is conservative. After initial diagnostic thoracentesis, patients are monitored for fluid reaccumulation. If the effusion reaccumulates quickly, pleurodesis may be attempted to slow the rate of fluid reaccumulation. When the effusion reaccumulates over a longer period or if new sites of disease develop, systemic chemotherapy should be administered.

Bony Metastases: When metastasis to bone is detected, men should be evaluated for prostate cancer and women for breast cancer. Exclusion of these diagnoses leaves a group of patients with both a poor prognosis and a potentially painful condition. Patients with a single bony metastasis should be given local treatment with surgery and/or radiation and then monitored. Patients with multiple-site disease and those whose tumors progress after radiation therapy should be offered a trial of chemotherapy. Many experimental agents are currently available in ongoing clinical trials. Therapy with bone-seeking radioisotopes (eg, strontium 89) may be useful in the treatment of disseminated painful bone metastases.[44]

Hepatic Metastases: Patients with hepatic metastases constitute 20% to 30% of individuals with unknown primary tumors. The most important diagnostic considerations in this class are to distinguish primary liver tumors from cancers that have metastasized to the liver and to identify the subset of patients with neoplasms of a more indolent nature (eg, neuroendocrine tumors). A careful pathologic review of liver biopsy specimens is therefore essential. Once these histologies are excluded, the most common diagnoses are adenocarcinoma and undifferentiated carcinoma. Initial therapy for these patients is systemic chemotherapy; hepatic intra-arterial therapy is an option for patients who do not respond to intravenous chemotherapy. Surgery should be considered an option for patients with resectable disease.

Brain Metastases: The important factor in treating patients who have brain lesions is to distinguish individuals with metastatic disease from those with primary brain tumors. Once this distinction has been made, patients with single metastatic lesions should be considered for surgery and those with multiple lesions should receive radiotherapy. Following treatment, patients should be monitored for recurrence or the appearance of a primary tumor, which in one report occurred most often in the lung.[45]

Other Sites

Single Sites Discovered Incidentally on Resection: Unknown primary tumors are notorious for unusual isolated presentations. Such lesions may appear on the skin, in single isolated lymph nodes removed during surgery for benign conditions, and at other, even more unusual sites. Patients should be examined for primary tumors and other sites of metastasis as described earlier. If no primary tumor and no additional sites of metastases are found, complete removal of the lesion must be ensured; this often requires additional excision with wider margins. The patient should then be monitored

without therapy, regardless of the tumor histology involved. Many such patients enjoy a prolonged survival time. Patients with isolated skin lesions may have an undifferentiated primary integumentary tumor with potential for cure after adequate local surgical treatment.

Multiple-Site Visceral Disease: Developing a strategy to care for patients with unknown primary carcinoma with metastases involving the viscera has proven exceedingly difficult. As noted previously, some subsets of patients in this category have disease that is responsive to therapy (eg, those with germ-cell tumors and their equivalents, women with papillary abdominal carcinomatosis, and patients with neuroendocrine tumors). In these patient subsets, the durations of remission and survival are considerable if complete remission is achieved with appropriate therapy.[46] Such patients should be treated aggressively with platinum-based chemotherapy regimens and may have overall response rates as high as 50% and complete response rates ranging from 20% to 35%.[32,33]

CHEMOTHERAPY

Data from chemotherapy trials enrolling patients with unknown primary carcinomas have historically been difficult to interpret. Many early studies were done prior to the era of controlled clinical trials, and the methods used in interpreting the results of these studies have been questioned. Additionally, combination regimens using newer chemotherapeutic agents have consistently demonstrated greater benefit than did older single-agent therapies.

Several difficulties arise when survival and response rates reported in different chemotherapy trials are compared. For example, histologic criteria for patient selection often varied from study to study. Moreover, in older studies, immunohistochemical methods were not used in the evaluation of pathologic specimens.

Patients who present in one of the subsets discussed previously should be managed as described in the appropriate section. For example, women with axillary adenopathy should receive local therapies in addition to chemotherapy with a combination regimen typically used for breast cancer. Such a protocol might be the FAC regimen (fluorouracil, doxorubicin [Adriamycin, Rubex], and cyclophosphamide [Cytoxan, Neosar]).[47] However, some generalizations can be made regarding the use of chemotherapy for patients with unknown primary tumors:

• In patients with widespread metastases and poor performance status, systemic chemotherapy is likely to be more harmful than beneficial, and only supportive therapy is usually indicated.

- Whenever possible, patients with unknown primary carcinoma who do not belong in the previously defined subgroups should be treated within the context of a clinical trial.
- Patients with moderately differentiated or well-differentiated adenocarcinomas who do not fit into one of the subsets previously discussed and who require chemotherapy have response rates of about 20% to 30%, and their median survival time ranges from 7 to 11 months when they are treated with combinations of doxorubicin and mitomycin (Mutamycin), with or without additional agents.[48] More recently, a cisplatin-based regimen has generated similar response rates.[49]
- Patients with undifferentiated or poorly differentiated adenocarcinomas other than those fitting in the extragonadal germ-cell or neuroendocrine tumor groups have traditionally been given a trial of a cisplatin-based regimen. Although most of these patients have a poor prognosis, Hainsworth and Greco have identified 5% to 15% as potentially curable by cisplatin-based chemotherapy.[50] A recent study, however, found that patients with a diagnosis of poorly differentiated carcinoma or poorly differentiated adenocarcinoma had similar survival rates whether they were treated with a combination of vincristine, doxorubicin, and cyclophosphamide or with a cisplatin-based regimen.[51]
- Patients with squamous-cell carcinomas who require chemotherapy are also often effectively treated using a cisplatin-based regimen. Investigators have discussed the merits of a combination of fluorouracil and cisplatin in squamous-cell carcinomas of the head and neck.[35]
- Patients with the extragonadal germ-cell syndrome or germ-cell equivalent and women with papillary abdominal carcinomas should be treated with a cisplatin-based regimen.
- Two recent studies examined the effectiveness of oral etoposide (VePesid) in unknown primary tumors. The drug was shown to have limited or no activity.[52,53]

CONCLUSION

It is clearly inappropriate to think of all patients with unknown primary neoplasms as having an untreatable disease and a poor outlook. Significant benefit may be achieved by administering regional or specific systemic therapies, and many of these patients can expect a prolonged survival. All patients should undergo a directed diagnostic evaluation for the primary tumor.

Some subsets of patients defined by clinical criteria (eg, axillary nodes with adenocarcinoma in women or peritoneal carcinomatosis with a papillary or serous histology), histologic criteria (eg, neuroendocrine, small-cell, or germ-cell tumor), or a combination of clinical and histologic criteria (eg, undifferentiated tumors with a midline presentation in patients less than 50 years old) may benefit significantly from aggressive treatment with platinum-containing regimens.

For the majority of patients who present with advanced unknown primary tumors, however, the prognosis remains poor and no treatment of established efficacy is available. For those patients, enrollment into a clinical trial of an experimental therapeutic approach appears appropriate. To effect significant improvement in the treatment and survival rate of patients with unknown primary malignancies, new insights into the biology of the disease and the development of new agents active against adenocarcinomas are critical.

REFERENCES

1. Hainsworth JD, Greco FA: Treatment of patients with cancer of an unknown primary site. N Engl J Med 329:257–263, 1993.
2. Wingo P, Tong T, Bolden S: Cancer statistics, 1995. CA Cancer J Clin 45:8–30, 1995.
3. Raber MN, Abbruzzese JL, Frost P: Unknown primary tumors. Curr Opin Oncol 4:3–9, 1992.
4. Casciato DA, Tabbarah HJ: Metastases of unknown origin, in Haskell CM (ed): Cancer Treatment, 3rd Ed, pp 798–814. Philadelphia, WB Saunders, 1990.
5. Daugaard G: Unknown primary tumours. Cancer Treat Rev 20:119–147, 1994.
6. Maiche AG: Cancer of unknown primary. Am J Clin Oncol 16:26–29, 1993.
7. Nystrom JS, Weiner JM, Heffelfinger-Juttner J, et al: Metastatic and histologic presentations in unknown primary cancer. Semin Oncol 4:53–58, 1977.
8. Abbruzzese JL, Abbruzzese MC, Lenzi R, et al: Analysis of a diagnostic strategy for patients with suspected tumors of unknown origin. J Clin Oncol 1995 (in press).
9. Fearon ER, Vogelstein B: A genetic model for colorectal tumorigenesis. Cell 61:759–767, 1990.
10. Bell CW, Pathak S, Frost P: Unknown primary tumors: Establishment of cell lines, identification of chromosomal abnormalities, and implications for a second type of tumor progression. Cancer Res 49:4311–4315, 1989.
11. Atkin NB: Chromosome 1 aberrations in cancer. Cancer Genet Cytogenet 21:279–285, 1986.
12. Pavlidis N, Briassoulis E, Bai M, et al: The expression of c-myc, ras, and c-erbB-2 in patients with carcinoma of unknown primary. Proc Am Soc Clin Oncol 13:1374, 1994.
13. Bar-Eli M, Abbruzzese JL, Lee-Jackson D, et al: p53 Gene mutation spectrum in human unknown primary tumors. Anticancer Res 13:1619–1624, 1993.
14. Stewart JF, Tattersall MHN, Woods RL, et al: Unknown primary adenocarcinoma. Br Med J 1:1530–1533, 1979.
15. Schapira DV, Jarret AR: Cost of diagnosis and survival of patients with unknown primary cancer. Proc Am Soc Clin Oncol 13:481,1994.
16. Horning SJ, Carrier EK, Rouse RV, et al: Lymphomas presenting as histologically unclassified neoplasms: Characteristics and response to treatment. J Clin Oncol 7:1281–1287, 1989.

17. Darsell PR, Sheedy PF II, O'Connell MJ: Computed tomography in search of cancer of unknown origin. JAMA 9:427–433, 1982.

18. McMillan JH, Levine L, Stephens RH: Computed tomography in the evaluation of metastatic adenocarcinoma of unknown origin. Radiology 143:143–146, 1982.

19. Warnke RA, Gatter CK, Falini B, et al: Diagnosis of human lymphoma with monoclonal antileukocyte antibodies. N Engl J Med 309:1275–1281, 1983.

20. Allhoff EP, Proppe KH, Chapman CM, et al: Evaluation of prostate specific acid phosphatase and prostate specific antigen in identification of prostate cancer. J Urol 129:315–318, 1983.

21. Arnold A, Cossman J, Bakhshi A, et al: Immunoglobulin gene rearrangements as unique clonal markers in human lymphoid neoplasms. N Engl J Med 309:1593–1599, 1983.

22. Bosl GJ, Dmitrovsky E, Reuter V, et al: i(12p): A specific karyotypic abnormality in germ cell tumors. Proc Am Soc Clin Oncol 8:131, 1989.

23. Whang-Peng J, Triche TJ, Knutsen T, et al: Chromosome translocations in peripheral neuroepithelioma. N Engl J Med 311: 584–585, 1984.

24. Ilson DH, Motzer RJ, Rodriguez E, et al: Genetic analysis in the diagnosis of neoplasms of unknown primary tumor site. Semin Oncol 20:229–237, 1993.

25. Motzer RJ, Rodriguez E, Reuter VE, et al: Molecular and cytogenetic studies in the diagnosis of patients with poorly differentiated carcinomas of unknown primary site. J Clin Oncol 13:274–282, 1995.

26. Bates SE: Clinical applications of serum tumor markers. Ann Intern Med 115:623–638, 1991.

27. Pavlidis N, Kalef-Ezra J, Briassoulis E, et al: Evaluation of six tumor markers in patients with carcinoma of unknown primary. Med Pediatr Oncol 22:162–167,1994.

28. Shahangian S, Fritsche HA: Serum tumor markers as diagnostic aids in patients with unknown primary tumors. Cancer Bulletin 41:152–156, 1989.

29. Abbruzzese JL, Raber MN, Frost P: The role of CA125 in patients with unknown primary tumors. Proc Am Soc Clin Oncol 10:39, 1991.

30. Mayordomo JI, Guerra JM, Guijarro C, et al: Neoplasms of unknown primary site: A clinicopathological study of autopsied patients. Tumori 79:321–324, 1993.

31. Abbruzzese JL, Abbruzzese MC, Hess KR, et al: Unknown primary carcinoma: Natural history and prognostic factors in 657 consecutive patients. J Clin Oncol 12:1272–1280, 1994.

32. Richardson RC, Schoumacher RA, Fer MF, et al: The unrecognized extragonadal germ cell syndrome. Ann Intern Med 94:181–186, 1981.

33. Greco FA, Vaughn WK, Hainsworth JD: Advanced poorly differentiated carcinoma of unknown primary site: Recognition of a treatable syndrome. Ann Intern Med 104:533–547, 1986.

34. Van der Gaast A, Verweij J, Henzen-Logmans SC, et al: Carcinoma of unknown primary: Identification of a treatable subset? Ann Oncol 1:119–122, 1990.

35. Jeremic B, Zivic DJ, Matovic M, et al: Cisplatin and 5-fluorouracil as induction chemotherapy followed by radiation therapy in metastatic squamous cell carcinoma of an unknown primary tumor localized to the neck. A phase II study. J Chemother 5:262–265, 1993.

36. Ellerbroek N, Holmes F, Singletary E, et al: Treatment of patients with isolated axillary nodal metastases from an occult primary carcinoma consistent with breast origin. Cancer 66:1461–1467, 1990.

37. Chang P, Knapper WH: Metastatic melanoma of unknown primary. Cancer 49:1106–1111, 1982.

38. Gershenson DM, Silva EG: Serous ovarian tumors of low malignant potential with peritoneal implants. Cancer 65:578–585, 1990.

39. Strand CM, Grosh WW, Baxter J, et al: Peritoneal carcinomatosis of unknown primary site in women: A distinguishing subset of adenocarcinomas. Ann Intern Med 111:213–217, 1989.

40. Heitz PU: Neuroendocrine tumor markers. Curr Rev Pathol 23:279–306, 1987.

41. Garrow GC, Greco FA, Hainsworth JD: Poorly differentiated neuroendocrine carcinoma of unknown primary tumor site. Semin Oncol 20:287–291, 1993.

42. Moertel CG, Kvols LK, O'Connell MJ, et al: Treatment of neuroendocrine carcinomas with combined etoposide and cisplatin: Evidence of major therapeutic activity in the anaplastic variants of these neoplasms. Cancer 68:227–233, 1991.

43. Hainsworth JD, Greco FA: Poorly differentiated carcinoma and germ cell tumors. Hematol Oncol Clin North Am 5:1223–1231, 1991.

44. Porter AT, McEwan AJ, Powe JE, et al: Results of a randomized phase III trial to evaluate the efficacy of strontium-89 adjuvant to local field external beam irradiation in the management of endocrine resistant metastatic prostate cancer. Int J Radiat Oncol Biol Phys 25:805–813, 1993.

45. Moser RP, Johnson ML, Yung WKA: Clinical presentations of unknown primary tumors: IV. Metastatic brain cancer in patients with no known primary site. Cancer Bulletin 41:173–177, 1989.

46. Hainsworth JD, Dial TW, Greco FA: Curative combination chemotherapy for patients with advanced poorly differentiated carcinoma of unknown primary site. Am J Clin Oncol 11:138–145, 1988.

47. Legha SS, Buzdar AU, Smith TL, et al: Complete remissions in metastatic breast cancer treated with combination drug therapy. Ann Intern Med 91:847–852, 1979.

48. Sporn, JR, Greenberg BR: Empiric chemotherapy in patients with carcinoma of unknown primary site. Am J Med 88:49–55, 1990.

49. Lenzi R, Raber MN, Frost P, et al: Phase II study of cisplatin, 5-FU, and folinic acid in patients with carcinoma of unknown primary origin. Eur J Cancer 29A:1634, 1993.

50. Hainsworth JD, Greco FA: Poorly differentiated carcinoma and poorly differentiated adenocarcinoma of unknown primary tumor site. Semin Oncol 20:279–286, 1993.

51. de Campos ES, Menasce LP, Radford J, et al: Metastatic carcinoma of uncertain primary site: A retrospective review of 57 patients treated with vincristine, doxorubicin, cyclophosphamide (VAC) or VAC alternating with cisplatin and etoposide (VAC/PE). Cancer 73:470–475, 1994.

52. van der Gaast A, Henzen-Logmans SC, Planting AS, et al: Phase II study of oral administration of etoposide for patients with well- and moderately-differentiated adenocarcinomas of unknown primary site. Ann Oncol 4:789–790, 1993.

53. Akerley W, Thomas A, Miller M, et al: Phase II trial of oral etoposide for carcinoma of unknown primary. Proc Am Soc Clin Oncol 13:1386, 1994.

SECTION 9

THERAPEUTIC MODALITIES & SUPPORTIVE CARE

CHAPTER 36   Biologic Therapy: Interferons, Interleukin-2, and Adoptive Cellular Immunotherapy

CHAPTER 37   Biologic Therapy: Hematopoietic Growth Factors, Retinoids, and Monoclonal Antibodies

CHAPTER 38   Current Treatment of Infection in the Neutropenic Patient

CHAPTER 39   Management of Fungal and Viral Infections in Cancer Patients

CHAPTER 40   Management of Cancer Pain

CHAPTER 41   Management of Nausea and Vomiting

CHAPTER 42   Oncologic Emergencies

CHAPTER 43   Epidemiology of Cancer and Prevention Strategies

Biologic Therapy: Interferons, Interleukin-2, and Adoptive Cellular Immunotherapy

Jorge E. Cortes, MD, John F. Seymour, MBBS, and Razelle Kurzrock, MD

Section of Biologic Studies, Department of Medical Oncology
The University of Texas M. D. Anderson Cancer Center, Houston, Texas

Biologic therapy for cancer may be defined as the use of compounds, or their derivatives, that can be found within the body to treat malignancy. The recent era of biologic therapy began with the identification and isolation of interferon (IFN)[1] and has been expanded with interleukin-2 (IL-2, aldesleukin [Proleukin]), the hematopoietic growth factors, and the retinoids. The technique of gene cloning has brought an increasing number of potentially useful compounds to the clinic. As we increase our understanding of the mechanisms of action of these and conventional cytotoxic drugs, it is likely that chemotherapy and biologic therapy will become less sharply differentiated. In this chapter, the IFNs, IL-2, and adoptive cellular immunotherapy will be reviewed. The hematopoietic growth factors and retinoids will be covered in a separate chapter.

THE INTERFERONS

The interferons constitute a family of naturally occurring proteins that were first recognized for their ability to confer on cells resistance to viral infection.[1] Although a multitude of other functions have been subsequently described, the property of viral interference remains necessary for classification as an interferon.

As listed in Table 1, the IFNs are designated alpha interferon (IFN-α), beta interferon (IFN-β [Betaseron]), and gamma interferon (IFN-γ [Actimmune]). The genes encoding these proteins and their receptors have been sequenced and cloned. IFN-α and IFN-β are class I (virus-induced) IFNs. These molecules share many biologic and structural properties and compete for binding to the same receptor. Both are acid stable, have cysteine-cysteine disulfide bonds necessary for biologic activity, and lack introns in their encoding genes. It is likely that their genes diverged from a common ancestor. Gene transcription is increased in response to the same inducers, and the molecular control of gene expression may be under control of the same promoter/enhancer sequences.

Alpha Interferon: At least 24 distinct species of IFN-α have been recognized. They are structurally similar, share 80% to 90% nucleotide sequence homology, and are coded for by genes located on chromosome 9. They are produced in vivo by leukocytes in response to viruses or double-stranded RNA. They differ subtly in biologic activity, but the exact roles of the numerous species are unknown. Most are nonglycosylated.

Two recombinant human IFN-α molecules are licensed for clinical use in the United States, IFN alfa-2a (Roferon-A) and IFN alfa-2b (Intron A). Each has a bioavailability of at least 80% when given by intramuscular or subcutaneous injection.

Beta Interferon: There is only one known species of IFN-β. It shares 25% amino acid homology with IFN-α,

TABLE I

Characteristics of Interferons

Type	Number of species	Amino acids [a]	Source	Glycosylation	Chromosome location Interferon	Receptor
Alpha	24+	166	Leukocytes	≥ 3 species	9p21	21q21
Beta	1	166	Fibroblasts	Yes	9p21	21q21
Gamma	1	146	T cells	Yes	12q24	6q

[a] Number of amino acids in the functional protein

and the encoding gene is located on chromosome 9. It is normally produced by fibroblasts and epithelial cells in response to the same inducers as IFN-α.

Gamma Interferon: The one known species of IFN-γ is a class II IFN (mitogen induced). Distinct from the other IFNs both structurally and functionally, it is encoded by a gene with three introns located on chromosome 12. The gene product lacks disulfide bonds and is acid labile. T lymphocytes can be induced to produce IFN-γ in vivo in response to soluble microbial antigen stimulation or by nonspecific mitogens such as IL-2.

Biologic Activity

The broad classes of action currently recognized for interferons are characterized as (1) antiviral, (2) antiproliferative, (3) regulator of differentiation, (4) modulator of lipid metabolism, (5) inhibitor of angiogenesis, (6) antitumoral, and (7) immunoregulator, with effects that include monocyte/macrophage activation, enhanced major histocompatibility complex (MHC) class I expression (IFN-α and IFN-β), enhanced MHC class II expression (IFN-γ), augmentation of natural-killer (NK) cell activity, stimulation of proliferation and differentiation of B-cells, and increased cytotoxic T-cell activity. In general, IFN-γ is a much more potent immunomodulator and IFN-α a more effective antitumor agent in vivo.

Cell-Surface Receptors: All biologic activities of the IFNs require binding to specific high-affinity cell-surface receptors. The two distinct receptor classes, type I and type II, correlate with the classes of IFNs that are bound (reviewed in Rubinstein and Orchansky).[2] All species of IFN-α and IFN-β bind only to type I receptors, with similar affinity. IFN-γ has no affinity for type I receptors, binding only to type II receptors.

Interferon Antibodies: Although IFNs are products of human cells, they usually act in a paracrine fashion and are not present in high concentrations in the circulation. Perhaps it is the difference in serum concentration or subtle differences in structure that have made the recombinant proteins immunogenic. In general, antibodies to recombinant IFN-α can be detected in up to two thirds of patients receiving the material, although only half of them are neutralizing antibodies.[3,4] Development of neutralizing antibodies is often accompanied by the loss of IFN-related side effects. Administration of nonrecombinant IFN-α may restore responsiveness in patients whose disease has relapsed after the development of neutralizing anti-IFN-α antibodies.[5] The antibodies cross-react with several natural IFNs, but the specificity is different in each patient. In some patients, the antibodies may disappear despite continuation of therapy.

Toxicity

In general, IFN-related side effects resolve shortly after treatment is discontinued. The common side effects are either acute (arising after the first few doses) or subacute or more chronic (arising beyond 1 week of therapy).[6]

Acute Effects: Patients who receive initial IFN-α therapy at doses above 2 million units almost always experience an acute first-dose effect. The symptom complex has been described as an influenza-like syndrome and classically consists of fever, chills, myalgia, tachycardia, and headache.

These symptoms are more common and more intense in older patients, especially at higher doses, and can be alleviated by premedication with acetaminophen. In addition, many patients tolerate IFN better with evening administration. If these simple measures are not successful, a nonsteroidal anti-inflammatory medication can provide relief. With daily dosing these symptoms lessen, usually disappearing within 7 to 10 days.

Chronic Effects: Beyond the first week of therapy, the pattern of toxicity changes. The most troublesome chronic complaint is profound fatigue, sometimes accompanied by anorexia. This is most prominent in patients receiving daily doses or doses above 10 million units and is more frequent in older patients and patients with poor pretreatment performance status. Neurologic effects (encephalopathy with somnolence, confusion, and memory loss) also occur at high doses.[7] These side effects, however, may be more common in patients with preexisting organic brain abnormalities.

The white blood cell and platelet counts usually fall to about 50% of pretreatment values during IFN therapy. These effects are readily reversible on withdrawal of IFN and are not associated with a high risk of infection or bleeding. In patients with compromised marrow function, neutropenia is more prominent. Autoimmune hemolytic anemia and thrombocytopenia have been documented in rare instances.[8,9]

Dose-related elevations of hepatic transaminases are seen in 20% to 30% of patients but are usually not dose limiting. Although acute renal failure has been reported, it is very uncommon. Proteinuria (less than 1 g/d) is the most frequently encountered renal side effect, affecting 15% to 20% of patients. The proteinuria is not associated with azotemia. Impotence and loss of libido can also occur in men undergoing IFN treatment.

Autoimmune phenomena can complicate the course of IFN therapy in approximately 5% of patients. Most commonly, patients will develop hypothyroidism, hemolytic anemia, or connective tissue disorders, but cardio-myopathy, porphyria, and glomerulonephritis are seen occasionally.

INTERLEUKIN-2

The interleukins are a family of polypeptides original-ly named for their ability to mediate interactions between leukocytes. Initially called T-cell growth factor, IL-2 was recognized as a product of activated T-cells that stimu-lates the proliferation and enhances the function of other T-cells and such immunocompetent cells as NK cells and B-cells. NK cells activated by IL-2 develop lymphokine-activated killer (LAK) activity. IL-2–activated B-cells generate secretory rather than membrane-associated IgM, and macrophages gain cytolytic maturation and elaborate transforming growth factor-beta (TGF-beta) upon stimu-lation with IL-2.

The *IL-2* gene, located on chromosome 4, has been cloned. The gene codes for a 153–amino acid protein and is structurally unrelated to the genes that encode the other interleukins and the IFNs. A 20–amino acid signal se-quence is cleaved, and two residues are *N*-glycosylated. This yields the mature single-chain IL-2 molecule, which has one disulfide bond necessary for biologic activity. Small concentrations of IL-2 can be detected in blood and follow a circadian variation.

In vitro, the major stimuli for IL-2 production are mitogen stimulation of T-cells and antigen recognition in combination with MHC. Costimulation of T-cells through CD28 is required for optimal synthesis of IL-2.

Biologic Activity

The interaction between IL-2 and effector cells is mediated through IL-2 binding to cell-surface receptors. The IL-2 receptor exists in three known forms with different affinities. The high-affinity receptor, which mediates much of the biologic activity of IL-2, is a trimeric protein representing 10% of IL-2–binding sites. Although it has been detected on large granular lymphocytes, mono-cytes, and B-cells, this receptor is located predominantly on activated T-cells. The intermediate affinity IL-2R is a heterodimer that is capable of signal transduction in the presence of large concentrations of IL-2. A circulating soluble form of the low-affinity single-chain IL-2 recep-tor has been associated with various disease states, in-cluding adult T-cell leukemia/lymphoma and hairy-cell leukemia. These soluble receptors are not involved in mediating the cellular effects of IL-2.

The rationale for exploring IL-2 as an anticancer agent relates to its immunomodulatory effects; T-cell stimula-tion; enhancement of NK-cell cytotoxicity; generation of

TABLE 2
Toxic Effects of Interleukin-2

Frequent (> 50% of patients given high doses)

Vascular leak syndrome
Fever and chills
Gastritis/vomiting/diarrhea
Erythroderma
Lethargy
Disorientation
Eosinophilia
Anemia
Thrombocytopenia
Cholestatic liver enzyme abnormalities

Other (< 20% of patients given high doses)

Hypothyroidism
Pruritus
Respiratory failure requiring intubation
Tachyarrhythmias
Myocardial ischemia/impaired systolic function

LAK-cell activity; induction of secretion of other lym-phokines such as IFN-γ, tumor necrosis factor-alpha (TNF-alpha), TGF-beta, IL-6, and IL-1; and stimulation of macrophage cytotoxic activity.[10]

Toxicity

The toxicity of IL-2 has hindered its widespread im-plementation as a therapeutic agent. As with other biolog-ic therapies, it is likely that the maximum tolerated dose is not the most immunologically effective dose, and it is probable that dose and schedule effects will differ among different tumor types. Much of the current investigation into IL-2 is directed toward development of effective schedules with a minimum of toxic side effects.

The common side effects of IL-2 are listed in Table 2. The most significant such effect is the vascular leak syndrome, which consists of weight gain, edema, ascites, pleural effusions, hypotension, and oliguric renal impair-ment. The mechanism by which the syndrome is created is unknown, but it is associated with high circulating levels of nitrogen oxides,[11] the stable metabolite of the endogenous vasodilator nitric oxide, and may be alleviat-ed by inhibitors of nitric oxide synthetase.[12] LAK-medi-ated damage of endothelial cells may also play a role. Hematologic toxicity is also frequent, with anemia and thrombocytopenia severe enough to require transfusion occurring in approximately 60% and 15% of patients, respectively. Transient oliguric renal dysfunction is also common.

ADOPTIVE CELLULAR IMMUNOTHERAPY

The aim of adoptive cellular immunotherapy is to enhance the immune recognition and destruction of a tumor by the administration of immunocompetent cells to the tumor-bearing host. It is a complex and expanding field of cancer treatment.[13] How these cells mediate antitumor activity is unclear, but the mechanism probably involves indirect cytokine-mediated effects as well as direct-contact tumor-cell killing.

Three broad classes of cells are being investigated: LAK cells, in vitro sensitized (IVS) lymphocytes, and tumor-infiltrating lymphocytes (TILs) (Table 3). Since these cells are often administered in combination with IL-2, the specific role of the adoptive cellular immunotherapy is difficult to determine. Current data are insufficient to conclude that adoptive cellular immunotherapy adds any benefit to IL-2 therapy alone.

THERAPEUTIC APPLICATIONS

Hairy-cell and chronic myelogenous leukemia (CML), severe thrombocytosis, multiple myeloma, Kaposi's sarcoma, various lymphomas, melanoma, and renal-cell carcinoma have been shown to respond to IFN or IL-2 treatment, with or without adoptive cellular immunotherapy.

Hairy-Cell Leukemia

Hairy-cell leukemia was the first cancer shown to be highly responsive to IFN.[14] This disease represents a malignant proliferation of mature B-lymphocytes. Approximately 500 new cases are diagnosed each year in the United States, accounting for 2% of adult leukemias. Clinical splenomegaly is present at diagnosis in 70% of patients, and the majority have some degree of bone marrow failure. Episodes of infection are common, and the risk is increased when the peripheral blood neutrophil count falls below 1×10^9/L. The hairy cells in peripheral blood and bone marrow have distinctive cytoplasmic projections and usually stain positively for tartrate-resistant acid phosphatase.

About 90% of patients with hairy-cell leukemia require treatment at diagnosis or during the course of the disease. The accepted criteria for treatment are hemoglobin values less than 10 g/dL or the need for transfusion, platelet counts less than 100×10^9/L, neutrophil counts less than 1×10^9/L or repeated infections, a leukemic phase with white blood cell counts more than 30×10^9/L and more than 50% hairy cells, symptomatic splenomegaly, bulky or painful lymphadenopathy (uncommon), bone lesions (uncommon), or autoimmune vasculitis (uncommon).[15]

Splenectomy: Before IFN was available, the median survival of patients with hairy-cell leukemia was 4 to 5 years, and most patients died of infection. Conventional chemotherapy was usually not beneficial. The mainstay of therapy was splenectomy.

Patients most likely to benefit from splenectomy are those who have cytopenias in the absence of extensive marrow replacement (less than 85% cellularity). Hematologic response is independent of the size of the spleen. In this setting, 40% of patients have normalization of peripheral blood counts, and a further 50% to 60% will have some improvement in at least one cell line after splenectomy.

However, most patients eventually require treatment for progressive disease. In the unfavorable group of patients with preoperative marrow cellularity of greater than 85%, the median time to progression was reported to be only 5 months.[16] Given the risks of splenectomy, the transience of many of the responses, and the fact that newer systemic therapies, including IFN, are highly effective in patients who have marked splenomegaly, the importance of splenectomy has diminished.

Interferon: Numerous investigators have confirmed the therapeutic efficacy of recombinant human IFN-alfa 2b and IFN-alfa 2a. Although few patients have been treated with IFN-β, this agent has also shown promising activity against hairy-cell leukemia, whereas IFN-γ is not active against this disease.

The standard dose of IFN-α is 3 million units given subcutaneously three times a week. Daily administration of IFN-α for the first 4 to 6 months may accelerate the response. Doses as low as 0.2 million U/m²/d have been investigated,[17] and although they maintain significant activity, the remission rates are inferior. However, in patients who suffer significant toxicity or who cannot tolerate the optimum dose, lower doses are useful.

In the first weeks of IFN therapy, many patients experience transient minor falls in blood counts. If these are significant or complicated by infection, the use of granulocyte colony-stimulating factor (G-CSF, filgrastim [Neupogen]) may reverse the neutropenia.[18] When a patient responds to treatment, a return to normal values is seen first in the platelet count (median, 2 months) and then in the neutrophil count and hemoglobin level (median, 4 to 5 months). Improvement in the peripheral blood precedes clearing of the bone marrow, which may take up to 10 months. Side effects usually are not dose limiting. While the optimal duration of IFN treatment is not clearly defined, most investigators recommend a minimum of 12 months.

Overall response rates are 80% to 90%, but most

TABLE 3

Characteristics of Lymphoid Cells Used for Adoptive Immunotherapy

Characteristic	Lymphokine-activated killer (LAK) cells	In vitro sensitized (IVS) cells	Tumor-infiltrating lymphocytes (TILs)
Source	Periperal blood lymphocytes or other lymphoid tissue	Peripheral blood lympho-cytes or lymph nodes	Tumor
Culture conditions			
Tumor stimulation	None	Inactivated autologous tumor	Tumor in initial culture
Duration	3–5 days	> 4 weeks	> 4 weeks
Effector phenotype (CD)	11b$^+$, 16$^+$, 56$^+$, 3$^+$ or 3$^-$	3$^+$, 8$^+$, or 4$^+$	3$^+$, 8$^+$, or 4$^+$

CD = cluster of differentiation antigen   Adapted from Topalian and Rosenberg [13]

responses are partial remissions. Previously untreated patients have a significantly higher response rate (complete response rate, 70%) than previously treated patients (complete response rate, 15%). Only 5% to 15% of patients do not show improvement in any parameter.

The time to relapse after cessation of therapy varies widely, with a median of 25 months reported.[19] Residual marrow hairy-cell infiltrate greater than 30% and post-treatment platelet count less than 160×10^9/L predict a shorter remission duration. However, reappearance of hairy cells in the bone marrow in the absence of abnormal peripheral blood counts is not a sufficient criterion to mandate therapy. High levels of soluble IL-2R at diagnosis may be predictive of response. Virtually all patients who relapse after treatment cessation remain sensitive to IFN and achieve a second remission of a duration comparable to the first (R. Kurzrock, unpublished data).

The postulated mechanisms of IFN activity in hairy-cell leukemia include a direct antiproliferative effect on the malignant clone, modification of oncogene expression, promotion of differentiation, suppression of responsiveness to B-cell growth factor, and modulation of effector cells including NK cells,[20] which are known to be functionally deficient in hairy-cell leukemia. Indeed, restoration of NK cell and T-helper activity as well as endogenous IFN-α production correlate with clinical response to IFN. TNF is elevated in patients with hairy-cell leukemia and is an autocrine growth factor for the malignant cells but an inhibitor of normal progenitors. IFN can decrease the serum levels of TNF and the autocrine growth stimulation of hairy-cell leukemia cells in vitro.

Purine Analogs: The purine nucleoside analogs also have significant activity in hairy-cell leukemia. Both pentostatin (Nipent) and cladribine (Leustatin) can elicit response rates of 90% or greater. Their main advantage is that the treatment period is shorter than that for IFN-α (3 months for pentostatin and 7 days for cladribine, vs 1 year for IFN-α).[21–25] However, in contrast to the immune effector-cell recovery that occurs with IFN-α) treatment, both pentostatin and cladribine cause a profound and prolonged lymphopenia with a reversal of the T4/T8 ratio and a reduction in absolute T4 counts to levels usually associated with severe immunosuppression. Patients must be monitored closely to detect any delayed effects of this immune dysregulation, although no increase in opportunistic infections or cancers has been reported.[26] One study of pentostatin used together with IFN-α achieved high partial response rates, but it is unclear whether this approach is superior to either drug alone.[27]

Given the range of effective therapies available, the goal for patients who have hairy-cell leukemia is a normal life expectancy.[23] To achieve this goal, neutropenic patients must be monitored carefully until their cytopenia responds to therapy. Infection remains the major cause of morbidity and mortality, and G-CSF may therefore be a useful supportive therapy.[18] In addition to gram-negative sepsis, these patients are at risk for unusual infections, including those due to disseminated atypical mycobacteria. Persistent fevers and night sweats without an obvious source should alert the physician to this possibility.

Chronic Myelogenous Leukemia

CML was the first human cancer found to be associated with a consistent chromosomal abnormality, the Philadelphia (Ph^1) chromosome, t(9;22)(q34;q11). Many chemotherapeutic agents can elicit complete hematologic responses in CML, although durable cytogenetic improvement is unusual. In the absence of durable cytoge-

TABLE 4

*Response to Alpha Interferon Therapy
in Early Chronic-Phase Chronic
Myelogenous Leukemia* [29]

Response	Patients (%)	Durable response (%)
Complete hematologic response	70–80	Not applicable
Cytogenetic response		
Minor	15–25	15
Partial	5–10	35
Complete	15–25	90

netic response, progression to blastic phase remains inevitable.

IFN-α can induce a complete hematologic remission in about 70% of patients with early chronic-phase disease (within 1 year from diagnosis). It is only in this patient subgroup that significant suppression of the Ph[1]-positive clone may be seen. Although 20% to 30% of patients with late chronic-phase CML (beyond 1 year from diagnosis) obtain complete hematologic remission, cytogenetic responses are minor and transient, and a long-term benefit is unlikely. Overall, about 40% to 50% of CML patients in early chronic phase achieve a cytogenetic improvement.

Approximately 15% to 25% of all patients treated achieve a complete cytogenetic response (100% diploid metaphases). Responses are durable in most of these patients, with a complete cytogenetic response persisting at a median follow-up of 3 years (Table 4).[28,29] Nevertheless, the *BCR/ABL* gene transcript remains detectable by the polymerase chain reaction,[30] which is capable of detecting 1 leukemic cell among more than 100,000 normal cells. Patients achieving a cytogenetic response have a survival advantage over those treated with conventional chemotherapy.[29]

Response to IFN-α is dose dependent. The recommended dose is 5 million U/m^2 daily, a considerably higher dose than that used in hairy-cell leukemia. Mild myelosuppression (white blood cell count, 2 to 4×10^9/L) is usually achieved with this dose. The median time to maximum hematologic response is 6 to 7 months. If patients have not shown a significant hematologic improvement by then, alternative therapy should be instituted. The median time to achieving a cytogenetic response is 12 months. Most patients develop tachyphylaxis to the early IFN side effects of fever, chills, and flu-like symp-

toms. However, at these higher doses, late neurologic effects (chronic fatigue and memory loss) and loss of libido in men may occur.

Because IFN is most active against small-volume disease, it has been used to treat recurrent CML after allogeneic bone marrow transplantation. Two studies[31,32] reported on a total of 12 patients with hematologic relapse after allogeneic bone marrow transplantation. Complete hematologic remission was obtained using IFN-α in eight patients, with a cytogenetic response seen in four. The use of IFN-α as maintenance therapy after bone marrow transplantation in Ph[1]-positive CML patients at high risk of relapse is, therefore, attractive.[33]

IFN-γ has been less extensively studied, but the rates of response achieved so far are inferior to those elicited by IFN-α.[34–36] Overall, hematologic responses (7 complete and 14 partial) occurred in 21 of 55 chronic-phase patients given IFN-γ, and only 7 attained any cytogenetic response.

Severe Thrombocytosis

Treatment of thrombocytosis in myeloproliferative disorders is one of the most promising new clinical applications of IFN-α. It was first observed that IFN-α lowers the platelet count in severe thrombocytosis complicating CML,[37] and this effect has been repeatedly demonstrated in essential thrombocythemia and other myeloproliferative disorders. Reports on more than 100 treated patients have been published.[37–44]

The induction dose of IFN-α in patients with severe thrombocytosis is generally 3 to 5 million U/d, and the maintenance dose, 2 to 3 million U/d. This approach has yielded an overall response rate (defined as a more than 50% reduction in platelet count) of greater than 80% (Table 5). Responses are achieved rapidly, with a median time to response of 1 to 3 weeks. Neutrophil counts do not drop below physiologic levels. Ongoing treatment is required, since the platelet count rises once IFN-α is withdrawn. Patients have received IFN-α therapy for more than 4 years with continuous response,[43,44] and virtually all initial thrombotic and hemorrhagic complications of thrombocytosis resolved during treatment and did not recur.

Multiple Myeloma

The first published report of IFN for multiple myeloma described a 100% response rate in four patients.[45] Since then the role of IFN has been explored in myeloma primarily in three situations—as a single agent in untreated or relapsed/refractory patients, as part of combined chemotherapy induction, and in the maintenance of a

TABLE 5

Response of Severe Thrombocytosis to Alpha Interferon

Number of patients	Disease	Interferon dose	Response (%)[a]	Reference
9	Chronic myelogenous leukemia	5×10^6 U/d	88	Talpaz et al [37]
8	6 Essential thrombocytosis 1 Polycythemia vera 1 Unclassified myeloproliferative disorder	5×10^6 U/d	75	Talpaz et al [39]
29	26 Essential thrombocytosis 3 Myelofibrosis	$1–4 \times 10^6$ U/d	84	Lazzarino et al [40]
15	3 Chronic myelogenous leukemia 5 Essential thrombocytosis 7 Polycythemia vera	$3.5–7 \times 10^6$ U/d	100	Ludwig et al [41]
18	Essential thrombocytosis	$3–5 \times 10^6$ U/d	88	Giles et al [42]
6	Essential thrombocytosis	4×10^6 U/d	100	Middelhoff et al [43]
31	5 Chronic myelogenous leukemia 9 Essential thrombocytosis 12 Polycythemia vera 5 Myelofibrosis	25×10^6 U/wk	71[b]	Gisslinger et al [38]

[a] Response defined as > 50% reduction in platelet count
[b] Defined as platelet count < 440×10^9/L for a minimum of 4 consecutive weeks

chemotherapy-induced or bone marrow transplantation-induced remission.

As with other tumor types, the exact mechanism of IFN's action against myeloma is unclear. However, it has been shown to have a direct cytotoxic effect on myeloma cells and growth-inhibitory effects (reviewed in Avvisati and Mandelli).[46]

Previously Untreated Patients: When IFN-α is used as a single agent in previously untreated patients, there is a distinct correlation between the dose of this agent and response at doses between 6 and 30 million U/m²/d.[47–49] However, the doses necessary to achieve high response rates are not tolerated, with severe central nervous system side effects occurring at doses over 6 million U/m²/d. Some reports describe a higher response rate in IgA myeloma.[48] Using tolerable doses, response rates in previously untreated patients are 10% to 40%, with a median time to response of 2 months and a median response duration of 14 to 20 months. In a randomized trial, however, IFN-α alone was inferior to standard melphalan (Alkeran) and prednisone chemotherapy.[48]

Relapsed Patients: In patients who relapse, IFN-α produces a response rate of 10% to 25%. This is similar to that achieved by standard chemotherapy. However, in patients who are refractory to chemotherapy, IFN-α as a single agent has produced an 18% response rate.[50] Simi-

larly, the addition of IFN-α to high-dose dexamethasone improved the response rate in patients for whom high-dose dexamethasone alone had failed.[51] In patients with relapsed disease that responds to conventional chemotherapy, the combination of IFN-α and dexamethasone may prolong disease-free survival.[52] The activity of this combination has been confirmed: Among 66 patients who had less than 75% tumor reduction with standard induction chemotherapy, 23 (35%) had further reductions in their monoclonal bands in response to IFN-α plus dexamethasone.[53]

Combination With Chemotherapy: The rationale for combining standard chemotherapeutic agents and interferon as induction treatment for myeloma is based on laboratory evidence of synergy.[54] Phase II studies have reported 75% response rates with interferon, melphalan, and prednisone[55] and 80% response rates with interferon, vincristine (Oncovin), carmustine (BiCNU), melphalan, cyclophosphamide (Cytoxan, Neosar), and prednisone.[56]

Results of large phase III trials conducted to confirm these promising response rates were recently published (Table 6).[57–63] One study showed a higher response rate with melphalan, prednisone, and IFN-α than with melphalan/prednisone alone (68% vs 42%, $P < .0001$),[57] whereas in a similar study, results were comparable for

TABLE 6

*Response Rates in Phase III Trials Comparing Chemotherapy Alone
With Combined Interferon (IFN) Therapy and Chemotherapy for Myeloma*

Reference	Number of patients	Chemotherapy	Response rate (%)		P value
			IFN + chemo	Chemo alone	
Preis et al [58]	48	Vincristine, melphalan, cyclophosphamide, and prednisone	57	41	> .20
Cooper et al [59]	272	Melphalan and prednisone	37	43	> .20
Galvez et al [60]	19	Vincristine, doxorubicin, carmustine, and prednisone	40	22	> .20
Montuoro et al [61]	50	Melphalan and prednisone	95	68	< .05
Corrado et al [62]	62	Melphalan and prednisone	45	48	> .20
Mellstedt et al [63]	185	Melphalan and prednisone	66	48	< .02
Osterborg et al [51]	335	Melphalan and prednisone	68	42	< .001

TABLE 7

*Results of Randomized Trials of Interferon (IFN) Maintenance Therapy in the
Plateau Phase of Myeloma*

Reference	Number of patients	Treatment arms	Response duration (median)	Survival (median)	P value
Peest et al [66]	71	5×10^6 U IFN-α 3×/wk Control	7 mo 7 mo	Not reported Not reported	> .2
Madelli et al [67]	101	3×10^6 U/m^2 IFN-α2b 3×/wk Control	26 mo 14 mo	52 mo 39 mo	.0002
Pestin et al [68]	314	5×10^6 U IFN-α2b 3×/wk Control	14 mo 6 mo	35 mo 36 mo	< .001
Salmon et al [53]	210	3×10^6 U IFN-α2b 3×/wk Control	Same	Not reported Not reported	.21

both groups (33% vs 44%, P = NS).[59] In no case, however, was there a difference in survival. Interestingly, there was a survival advantage for patients with IgA or Bence Jones myeloma who received IFN.[57] However, IFN has not been proved to add to the long-term outcome of standard chemotherapy. Also, the combination of IFN-α and dexamethasone has achieved results similar to those seen with dexamethasone alone in previously untreated patients.[64]

Maintenance Therapy: Once a "plateau phase" is reached in myeloma, ongoing chemotherapy is of no benefit. It may be that, at this time, the clonogenic cells are in the G_0 phase of the cell cycle and, therefore, are not sensitive to chemotherapeutic agents. Because IFN-α

has activity against these noncycling cells, it may be beneficial in prolonging the plateau phase.[65]

Results are available from four studies of IFN maintenance (Table 7).[53,66–68] Among the largest series, two showed a significant prolongation of remission duration and one an improved survival. A study from the Southwest Oncology Group using a lower dose of IFN failed to confirm the benefit of IFN,[69] but it is possible that the lower dose contributed to the negative finding.

Similarly, the use of maintenance IFN-α is being studied in remissions after autologous bone marrow transplantation. Preliminary results of the Medical Research Council trial suggest that IFN-α may prolong remission duration (reviewed in Jagannath and Barlogie).[70]

Kaposi's Sarcoma

Kaposi's sarcoma is a common tumor in persons infected with the human immunodeficiency virus (HIV). Clinical manifestations range from a single asymptomatic cutaneous lesion to a disseminated and life-threatening malignancy. In some cases, lesions are cosmetically unacceptable but do not threaten the function of vital organs. Since opportunistic infections remain the most common cause of death in people who have the acquired immunodeficiency syndrome (AIDS), the risks and benefits of treating Kaposi's sarcoma should be carefully considered for each individual.

Intralesional injection of IFN-α (3 to 5 million units three times a week for 4 weeks) is effective for isolated symptomatic lesions and causes minimal side effects.[71] Systemic IFN-α has been investigated as a single agent at low doses (1 to 7.5 million U/m^2, 3 to 7 days a week), intermediate doses (10 to 15 million U/m^2, 3 to 7 days a week), and high doses (20 to 50 million U/m^2, 3 to 7 days a week).

The high-dose schedules are poorly tolerated because of severe myelosuppression and neurotoxicity. Overall results from published series (reviewed in Krown)[72] show total (complete plus partial) response rates of 7%, 23%, and 32% with low-, intermediate-, and high-dose protocols, respectively. In patients who respond, regression is usually documented after 4 to 8 weeks of treatment, although maximal response may not occur for up to 6 or 8 months. Ongoing therapy is necessary to sustain responses, and the median response duration ranges between 4 and 18 months.[73,74]

Most series have determined that patients with relatively well preserved immunologic function are more likely to respond, suggesting an immunomodulatory action for IFN-α.[75] Patients without prior opportunistic infections or night sweats and a CD4 count above 200 to 400/mm³ are most likely to benefit from treatment.

Multiple trials have established that combination treatment with chemotherapeutic agents and IFN-α increases hematologic toxicity without improving results. When indicated on the basis of the CD4 count, zidovudine (Retrovir) can be combined with IFN in doses of less than 8 to 10 million U/d with an acceptable incidence of neutropenia.[76] The addition of granulocyte macrophage colony-stimulating factor (GM-CSF, sargramostim [Leukine]) to the regimen may allow further IFN dose escalation.[77]

Kaposi's sarcoma rarely affects patients without HIV, and so, IFN-α has not been adequately investigated in this small population.

TABLE 8

Response of Cutaneous T-Cell Lymphomas to Alpha Interferon (IFN)

Treatment	Response (%)	
	Complete	Overall
IFN alone [89,90]	17	52
IFN + retinoids [89]	11	60
IFN + PUVA [89,96,97,98]	58	92
IFN + nucleoside analogs [89,98,100]	6	43

PUVA = psoralen and ultraviolet A light

Hodgkin's Disease and Non-Hodgkin's Lymphomas

Hodgkin's Disease: Few data are available regarding IFN-α therapy for Hodgkin's disease. In the two largest reported series,[78,79] 8 of 44 heavily pretreated patients responded. If IFN is to have a role in this disease, it will likely be in conjunction with other treatment modalities.

Low-Grade Follicular Non-Hodgkin's Lymphoma: In non-Hodgkin's lymphoma, IFN-α has shown promising activity against low-grade follicular disease. A 40% to 50% response rate can be achieved using 3 to 50 million U/m^2 administered intramuscularly from three to seven times a week. Most responses are partial, and the median response duration is 8 months. Importantly, there does not appear to be cross-resistance between IFN and cytotoxic drugs. There might be a dose-response relationship, as many patients who responded received higher doses.

Three randomized studies using the combination of chemotherapy and IFN-α in follicular non-Hodgkin's lymphoma have been reported. Two large multi-institutional studies demonstrated an improved duration of remission when intermittent IFN-α was added to combination chemotherapy.[80,81] The third study, using single-agent chlorambucil for induction, did not demonstrate any improvement in remission rate from the addition of IFN-α.[82] Preliminary data show a median remission duration of 2 years in the chlorambucil-only arm, whereas no patients in the IFN-α arm have yet achieved a remission this long ($P = .013$). A survival advantage was documented in the two largest studies,[80,81] but not in an Eastern Cooperative Oncology Group study with longer follow-up.[83]

Maintenance Therapy: Several studies have explored low-dose (2 million U/m^2 three times a week) IFN-α maintenance therapy following remission induction in low-grade non-Hodgkin's lymphoma. McLaughlin et al[84] investigated IFN-α maintenance after remission induced by cyclophosphamide, doxorubicin (Adriamycin), vincristine, prednisone, and bleomycin (Blenoxane) in low-grade non-Hodgkin's lymphoma. The failure-free survival rate was 47% in the IFN-treated patients at 5 years. This result compared favorably with that for a previously treated control group, who had 29% failure-free survival at 5 years ($P = .01$).

A minor improvement in relapse-free survival was also reported in a smaller Italian study (reviewed in Gaynor and Fisher),[85] in which only 4 of 14 IFN-treated patients relapsed versus 10 of 25 patients given no maintenance therapy. An improved disease-free survival was also reported by the European Organization for Research and Treatment of Cancer.[86] Although promising, these results should be interpreted cautiously, since the patient numbers are small and no survival benefit has been demonstrated.

Intermediate- or High-Grade Disease: Aviles et al[87] reported that IFN maintenance may improve survival in patients with diffuse large-cell lymphoma who achieve a complete response after combination chemotherapy.

Cutaneous T-Cell Lymphoma

Cutaneous T-cell lymphomas are a heterogeneous group of malignancies of mature helper T-cells. They are characterized by primary skin involvement of several forms, from small papules to diffuse erythroderma or large skin tumors. Although the natural histories of these forms vary, patients with any of the forms usually die of advanced lymphoma or secondary infections. Despite predominant skin involvement initially, systemic spread occurs early in the course of the disease. Therefore, although local therapy can effectively control early stages of the disease, systemic therapy has been evaluated in an attempt to decrease the late progression of the disease. Chemotherapeutic agents can induce high response rates, but no survival advantage is obtained.[88,89]

Single-Agent Therapy With IFN-α: Bunn et al[90] first reported the activity of recombinant IFN-α in cutaneous T-cell lymphomas. Twenty patients with advanced stages of the disease refractory to two or more previous therapies were treated with IFN-α at a dose of 50 million U/m^2 intramuscularly, three times per week. Nine patients achieved partial remissions lasting a median of 5 months.[90] Numerous other reports[91–95] have confirmed these observations (Table 8), with response rates of 45% to 65% (reviewed in Bunn et al).[89] However, with IFN-α as a single agent, most of the responses were partial and not long lasting.

Combination Therapy With IFN-α: No studies are available for the combination of IFN-α with conventional chemotherapy. However, the agent has been used in combination with other therapeutic modalities. The combination of psoralen and ultraviolet A light (PUVA) is effective for the control of skin lesions in cutaneous T-cell lymphoma. Kuzel et al[96] used IFN-α at a dose of 12 million U/m^2 concurrently with PUVA in 39 patients and continued for 2 years. The overall response rate was 90%, with a complete responses in 62% and partial responses in 28%. The median response duration was 28 months.[96] Other smaller studies have confirmed these encouraging results (Table 8).[97,98]

Retinoids are also effective in the management of cutaneous T-cell lymphomas, with overall response rates of 58%, although responses are usually of short duration. IFN-α has been combined with retinoids, including isotretinoin (13-*cis*-retinoic acid, Accutane) and etretinate (Tegison). The response rate with this combination is approximately 60%, with 10% complete responses (Table 8). These results are similar to those achieved with IFN-α as a single agent, and so it is unclear whether the combination adds anything to IFN-α alone.[88]

Nucleoside analogs, including fludarabine (Fludara), 2-chlorodeoxyadenosine (2CdA), and pentostatin (Nipent), are a new group of chemotherapeutic agents with significant activity against lymphoid malignancies. They are effective as single agents, with pentostatin producing response rates of 40% to 60%; 2CdA, 20% to 30%; and fludarabine, 20%. IFN-α has been used in combination with fludarabine[99] and pentostatin,[100] and the overall response rate is 40% to 45%, with a complete response rate of 5% to 10% (Table 8). Therefore, these combinations do not seem to be superior to those of IFN-α alone.

Other Interferons: IFN-β and IFN-γ also have activity in cutaneous T-cell lymphomas, although they seem to be less effective than IFN-α. The overall response rates with these agents are 25% and 30%,[89] respectively.

Melanoma and Renal-Cell Carcinoma

Both melanoma and renal-cell carcinoma have shown some response to IFN-α and IL-2. It is important when reviewing the results, however, to remember that the natural histories of these tumors can be highly variable and that accurate prognostic indicators are not always available. Thus, interpretation of the results of small phase II trials in selected patients is very difficult.

Melanoma: In vitro, melanoma cells are among the most sensitive of all tumor cells to the antiproliferative effects of IFN-α.[101] This level of sensitivity has not been reproduced in vivo, however.

TABLE 9

Therapy With Dacarbazine (DTIC) Alone or With IFN-α for Metastatic Melanoma

Reference	Number of patients	Treatment	% response rate	Duration (median)	Survival
Kirkwood et al[104]	27	DTIC	19	Not reported	Not reported
	21	DTIC-IFN	19	Not reported	Not reported
Falkson et al[105]	31	DTIC	19	2.5 mo	9.6 mo
	30	DTIC-IFN	53	9.0 mo	17.6 mo
Thompson et al[106]	83	DTIC	17	286 d	269 d
	87	DTIC-IFN	21	258 d	229 d
Sertoli et al[107]	82	DTIC	20	2.6 mo	Not reported
	76	DTIC + high-dose IFN	28	6.6 mo	Not reported
	84	DTIC + low-dose IFN	23	9.0 mo	Not reported
Overall	223	DTIC	17		
	298	DTIC + IFN	27 *P* = .025		

As a single agent in metastatic disease, IFN-α reproducibly yields overall response rates of 5% to 30% (mean, 15%), based on 11 studies reporting on a total of 315 patients (reviewed in Kirkwood and Ernstoff).[102] The doses used ranged from 10 to 50 million U/m², usually given three times a week. There was no clear evidence of a dose-response relationship. Although the median response duration was only 4 months, some patients remained free of disease for many years. Indicators of likely response to interferon are low tumor burden and disease limited to the skin, lymph nodes, or soft tissue.[102] IFN-α has no activity against central nervous system disease and does not prevent metastasis to the central nervous system, even in responding patients.

In an attempt to improve these results, IFN-α has been used in combination with standard chemotherapeutic agents, although in vitro data fail to support claims of synergism against melanoma cells.[102] On the basis of an early report showing a 30% response rate for dacarbazine and IFN-α,[103] larger randomized studies were begun. The results from phase III studies published to date have shown mixed results (Table 9).[104–107]

Falkson et al[105] showed a significantly improved response rate, duration of response, and survival. Other studies, however, failed to detect any improvement in response rate or survival. If combination therapy imparts a survival benefit, it is likely to be smaller than that suggested by Falkson et al.[105] Two of the studies[105,107] reported prolonged remission duration among IFN-α–treated patients. IFN-α in conjunction with combination chemotherapy has not produced better results than combination chemotherapy alone.

If IFN-α can prolong remission duration, it would be reasonable to consider it as adjuvant treatment following complete resection of high-risk melanoma. Several studies of this approach are being carried out by cooperative groups. IFN-γ has also been investigated in this setting but has been found to offer no benefit.[108]

IL-2, alone or combined with adoptive cellular immunotherapy,[109] has also been investigated in melanoma. As a single agent, it has achieved a response rate of 10% to 20%.[110] The use of IL-2 in combination with chemotherapy has produced response rates of 13% to 42%, which are not clearly superior to those with chemotherapy alone.[111–114] Despite animal models suggesting synergistic activity of IL-2 with IFN-α, the response rates obtained with this combination are not superior to the results with either agent alone.[115]

More recently, chemotherapy has been given in combination with IL-2 and IFN-α (a schedule called biochemotherapy). With single-agent cisplatin (Platinol), the combination achieved a response rate of 54%. Using combination chemotherapy together with the biologic agents, the response rate has ranged from 33% to 63% (depending on the schedule, Table 10).[116–119] The impact on survival remains to be determined.[120]

Renal-Cell Carcinoma: Renal-cell carcinoma was one of the first tumors in which IFN activity was demonstrated.[121] Average response rates obtained using single-agent IFN-α are 10% to 15%, with most responses being partial. Long-term results, however, do not show prolongation of survival.[122,123] IFN-β and IFN-γ have no advantage over IFN-α.

On review, Muss[122] could find no evidence for a dose-

TABLE 10

Results of Biochemotherapy in Metastatic Melanoma

Reference	Treatment	% Response	
		Complete	Overall
Khayat el al[116]	Cisplatin/IL-2/IFN	13	54
Richards et al[117]	Cisplatin, carmustine, dacarbazine, tamoxifen/IL-2/IFN	24	57
Legha et al[118,119]	Cisplatin, vinblastine, dacarbazine/IL-2/IFN		
	Alternating	5	33
	Sequential	23	60
	Concurrent	12	63

IFN = interferon, IL-2 = interleukin-2

response relationship and recommended IFN-α, 5 to 10 million units three times a week, as the range of doses conferring the best therapeutic index. The median duration of response averages 6 to 10 months, and only 20% of responses are maintained beyond 12 months. Patients who have undergone prior nephrectomy and have had a long disease-free interval as well as those with metastatic disease confined to the lung are more likely to respond. The limited data available do not support adjuvant IFN-α treatment after complete resection of renal-cell carcinoma.[124]

IL-2 has proven activity in metastatic renal-cell carcinoma.[125] Both bolus and continuous-infusion IL-2 generate responses in 10% to 30% of patients, but the continuous-infusion protocol is better tolerated.[126] More recently, low-dose subcutaneous IL-2 has been used and produced similar results.[127] As in melanoma, the addition of adoptive cellular immunotherapy to IL-2 does not predictably improve response rates in metastatic renal-cell carcinoma. High pretreatment levels of C-reactive protein and IL-6 predict a diminished response to IL-2[128] and may be useful in selecting patients most likely to benefit from this therapy.

The combination of IL-2 and IFN has achieved higher response rates in some studies.[124] One preliminary report on this combination used together with fluorouracil achieved a response rate of 47%, but these results need further confirmation.[129]

CONCLUSIONS

With or without adoptive cellular immunotherapy, IL-2 remains an innovative treatment, but as currently administered it produces a low response rate in two relatively uncommon tumors (melanoma and renal-cell carcinoma) and significant toxicity. The feasibility of administering multidrug chemotherapy, IFN, and IL-2

has been established[130]; however, toxicity must be effectively managed and response rates improved significantly above those achievable with single-modality treatment before this approach gains a confirmed place in the treatment of patients with these cancers.

Although its mechanism of action is still incompletely understood, IFN-α is now firmly established as a powerful therapeutic compound in hairy-cell leukemia. IFN-α has also shown efficacy against other neoplasms, although these are mainly hematologic malignancies; it has less pronounced activity in solid tumors. In general, IFN-α is most effective against early or low-volume disease. Other strategies that merit exploration include synergistic combinations with retinoids, radiation potentiation, and augmentation of chemotherapy-induced cytotoxicity.[131]

REFERENCES

1. Isaacs A, Lindenmann J: Virus interference: I. The interferons. Proc R Soc Lond B Biol Sci 147:258–267, 1957.

2. Rubinstein M, Orchansky P: The interferon receptors. CRC Crit Rev Biochem 21:249–276, 1986.

3. Itri LM, Campion M, Dennin RA, et al: Incidence and clinical significance of neutralizing antibodies in patients receiving recombinant interferon alfa-2a by intramuscular injection. Cancer 59:668–674, 1987.

4. Spiegel RJ, Spicehandler JR, Jacobs SL, et al: Low incidence of serum factors in patients receiving alfa-2b interferon (Intron A). Am J Med 80:223–228, 1986.

5. Von Wussow P, Freund M, Jakschies D, et al: Natural IFN-alpha treatment of anti-recombinant IFN-alpha antibody positive patients with chronic myelogenous leukemia (CML). Blood 72(suppl):233a, 1988.

6. Quesada JR, Talpaz M, Rios A, et al: Clinical toxicity of interferons in cancer patients: A review. J Clin Oncol 4:234–243, 1986.

7. Mattson K, Niiranen A, Iivanainen M, et al: Neurotoxicity of interferon. Cancer Treat Rep 67:958–961, 1983.

8. Hui KS, Lichtiger B, Quesada JR: Cross-reactive red blood cell antigen-related substances in human leukocyte alpha interferon. Arch

Pathol Lab Med 110:128–130, 1986.

9. McLaughlin P, Talpaz M, Quesada JR, et al: Thrombocytopenia following α-interferon therapy in patients with cancer. JAMA 254:1353–1354, 1985.

10. Mule JJ, Rosenberg SA: Interleukin-2: Preclinical trials, in DeVita VT Jr, Hellman S, Rosenberg SA (eds): Biologic Therapy of Cancer, pp 142–158. Philadelphia, JB Lippincott, 1991.

11. Ochoa JB, Curti B, Peitzman AB, et al: Increased circulating nitrogen oxides after human tumor immunotherapy: Correlation with toxic hemodynamic changes. J Natl Cancer Inst 84:864–867, 1992.

12. Kilbourn RG, Griffith OW: Overproduction of nitric oxide in cytokine-mediated and septic shock. J Natl Cancer Inst 84:827–831, 1992.

13. Topalian SL, Rosenberg SA: Adoptive cellular therapy: Basic principles, in DeVita VT Jr, Hellman S, Rosenberg SA (eds): Biologic Therapy of Cancer, pp 76–101. Philadelphia, JB Lippincott, 1991.

14. Quesada JR, Reuben JR, Manning JT, et al: Alpha interferon for induction of remission in hairy cell leukemia. N Engl J Med 310:15–18, 1984.

15. Moormeier JA, Golomb HM: Diagnosis and treatment of hairy cell leukemia, in Wiernik PH, Canellos GP, Kyle RA, et al (eds): Neoplastic Diseases of the Blood, 2nd Ed, pp 111–121. New York, Churchill Livingstone, 1991.

16. Ratain MJ, Vardiman JW, Barker CM, et al: Prognostic values in hairy cell leukemia after splenectomy as initial therapy. Cancer 62:2420–2424, 1988.

17. Smalley RV, Anderson SA, Tuttle RL, et al: Randomized comparison of two doses of human lymphoblastoid interferon-alpha in hairy cell leukemia. Blood 78:3133–3141, 1991.

18. Glaspy JA, Souza L, Scates S, et al: Treatment of hairy cell leukemia with granulocyte colony-stimulating factor and recombinant consensus interferon or recombinant interferon-alpha-2b. J Immunother 11:198–208, 1992.

19. Ratain MJ, Golomb HM, Vardiman JW, et al: Relapse after interferon alfa-2b therapy for hairy cell leukemia: Analysis of prognostic variables. J Clin Oncol 6:1714–1721, 1990.

20. Vedantham S, Gamliel H, Golomb HM: Mechanism of interferon action in hairy cell leukemia: A model of effective cancer biotherapy. Cancer Res 52:1056–1066, 1992.

21. Grever M, Kopecky K, Head D, et al: A randomized comparison of deoxycoformycin (DCF) versus alpha-2a interferon (IFN) in previously untreated patients with hairy cell leukemia (HCL): An NCI-sponsored intergroup study (SWOG, ECOG, CALGB, NCCTG) (abstract). Proc Am Soc Clin Oncol 11:264, 1992.

22. Estey EH, Kurzrock R, Kantarjian HM, et al: Treatment of hairy cell leukemia with 2-chlorodeoxyadenosine (2-CdA). Blood 79:882–887, 1992.

23. Kurzrock R, Talpaz M, Gutterman JU: Hairy cell leukemia: Review of treatment. Br J Haematol 79(suppl 1):17–20, 1991.

24. Piro LD, Carrera CJ, Carson DA, et al: Lasting remissions in hairy cell leukemia induced by a single infusion of 2-chlorodeoxyadenosine. N Engl J Med 322:1117–1121, 1990.

25. Piro LD, Saven A, Ellison D, et al: Prolonged complete remissions following 2-chlorodeoxyadenosine (2-CdA) in hairy cell leukemia (HCL) (abstract). Proc Am Soc Clin Oncol 11:259, 1992.

26. Seymour JF, Kurzrock R, Freireich EJ, et al: 2-Chlorodeoxy-adenosine induces durable remissions and prolonged suppression of CD4 lymphocyte counts in hairy cell leukemia. Blood 83:2906–2911, 1994.

27. Martin A, Nerenstone S, Urba WJ, et al: Treatment of hairy cell leukemia with alternating cycles of pentostatin and recombinant leukocyte A interferon: Results of a phase II study. J Clin Oncol 8:721–730, 1990.

28. Talpaz M, Kantarjian H, Kurzrock R, et al: Interferon alpha produces sustained cytogenetic responses in chronic myelogenous leukemia Philadelphia chromosome-positive patients. Ann Intern Med 114:532–538, 1991.

29. Kantarjian H, Smith T, O'Brien S, et al: Prolonged survival following achievement of a cytogenetic response with alpha interferon therapy in chronic myelogenous leukemia. Ann Intern Med 122:254–261, 1995.

30. Dhingra K, Kurzrock R, Baine R, et al: Minimal residual disease in interferon-treated chronic myelogenous leukemia: Results and pitfalls of PCR-based analysis. Leukemia 6:754–760, 1992.

31. Arcese W, Mauro FR, Alimena G, et al: Interferon therapy for Ph[1] positive CML patients relapsing after T-cell depleted allogeneic bone marrow transplantation. Bone Marrow Transplant 5:309–315, 1990.

32. Higano CS, Raskind W, Durnam D, et al: Alpha interferon (IF) induces cytogenetic remissions in patients who relapse with chronic myelogenous leukemia (CML) after allogeneic bone marrow transplantation (BMT). Blood 74(suppl):83a, 1989.

33. Higano CS, Raskind WH, Singer JW: Use of alpha interferon for the treatment of relapse of chronic myelogenous leukemia in chronic phase after allogeneic bone marrow transplantation. Blood 80:1437–1442, 1992.

34. Kurzrock R, Talpaz M, Kantarjian HM, et al: Therapy of chronic myelogenous leukemia with recombinant interferon-gamma Blood 70:943–947, 1987.

35. Russo D, Fanin R, Zuffa E, et al: Treatment of Ph+ chronic myeloid leukemia by gamma interferon. Blut 59:15–20, 1989.

36. Silver RT, Benn P, Verma RS, et al: Recombinant gamma-interferon has activity in chronic myeloid leukemia. Am J Clin Oncol 13:49–54, 1990.

37. Talpaz M, Mavligit G, Keating M, et al: Human leukocyte interferon to control thrombocytosis in chronic myelogenous leukemia. Ann Intern Med 99:789–792, 1983.

38. Gisslinger H, Ludwig H, Linkesch W, et al: Long-term interferon therapy for thrombocytosis in myeloproliferative diseases. Lancet 1:634–637, 1989.

39. Talpaz M, Kurzrock R, Kantarjian H, et al: Recombinant interferon-alpha therapy of Philadelphia chromosome-negative myeloproliferative disorders with thrombocytosis. Am J Med 86:554–558, 1989.

40. Lazzarino M, Vitale A, Morra E, et al: Interferon alfa-2b as treatment for Philadelphia negative chronic myeloproliferative disorders with excessive thrombocytosis. Br J Haematol 72:173–177, 1989.

41. Ludwig H, Linkesch W, Gisslinger H, et al: Interferon-alpha corrects thrombocytosis in patients with myeloproliferative disorders. Cancer Immunol Immunother 25:266–273, 1987.

42. Giles FJ, Gray AJ, Brozovic M, et al: Alpha-interferon therapy for essential thrombocythaemia. Lancet 2:70–72, 1988.

43. Middelhoff G, Boll I: A long-term clinical trial of interferon alpha therapy in essential thrombocythemia. Ann Hematol 64:207–209, 1992.

44. Gisslinger H, Chott A, Scheithauer W, et al: Interferon in essential thrombocythaemia. Br J Haematol 79(suppl 1):42–47, 1991.

45. Mellstedt H, Ahre A, Bjorkholm M, et al: Interferon therapy in myelomatosis. Lancet 1:245–247, 1979.

46. Avvisati G, Mandelli F: The role of interferon-α in the management of myelomatosis. Hematol Oncol Clin North Am 6:395–405, 1992.

47. Quesada JR, Alexanian R, Hawkins M, et al: Treatment of multiple myeloma with recombinant α-interferon. Blood 67:275–278, 1986.

48. Ahre A, Bjorkholm M, Mellstedt H, et al: Human leukocyte interferon and intermittent high-dose melphalan-prednisone administration in the treatment of multiple myeloma: A randomized clinical

trial from the Myeloma Group of Central Sweden. Cancer Treat Rep 68:1331–1338, 1984.

49. Ahre A, Bjorkholm M, Osterborg A, et al: High doses of natural α-interferon (α-IFN) in the treatment of multiple myeloma: A pilot study from the Myeloma Group of Central Sweden (MGCS). Eur J Haematol 41:123–130, 1988.

50. Costanzi JJ, Cooper MR, Scarffe JH, et al: Phase II study of recombinant alpha-2 interferon in resistant myeloma. J Clin Oncol 3:654–659, 1985.

51. San Miguel JF, Moro M, Blade J, et al: Combination of interferon and dexamethasone in refractory multiple myeloma. Hematol Oncol 8:185–189, 1990.

52. Palumbo A, Boccadoro M, Garino LA, et al: Interferons plus glucocorticoids as intensified maintenance therapy prolongs tumor control in relapsed myeloma. Acta Haematol 90:71–76, 1993.

53. Salmon SE, Crowley J: Impact of glucocorticoids (GC) and interferon (IFN) on outcome in multiple myeloma (abstract). Proc Am Soc Clin Oncol 11:316, 1992.

54. Wellander CE, Morgan TM, Homesley HD, et al: Combined recombinant human interferon alpha2 and cytotoxic agents studied in a clonogenic assay. Int J Cancer 35:721–729, 1985.

55. Cooper MR, Fefer A, Thompson J, et al: Alpha-2-interferon/melphalan/prednisone in previously untreated patients with multiple myeloma: A phase I-II trial. Cancer Treat Rep 70:473–476, 1986.

56. Oken MM, Kyle RA, Greipp PR, et al: Chemotherapy plus interferon (rIFNa2) in the treatment of multiple myeloma (abstract). Proc Am Soc Clin Oncol 9:288, 1990.

57. Osterborg A, Bjorkholm M, Bjoreman M, et al: Natural interferon alpha in combination with melphalan/prednisone versus melphalan/prednisone in the treatment of multiple myeloma stages II and III: A randomized study from the Myeloma Group of Central Sweden. Blood 81:1428–1434, 1993.

58. Preis H, Scheithauer W, Fritz E, et al: VMCP chemotherapy with or without interferon-alpha-2 in newly diagnosed patients with multiple myeloma. Onkologie 12:27–29, 1989.

59. Cooper MR, Dear K, McIntyre OR, et al: A randomized clinical trial comparing melphalan/prednisone with or without interferon alfa-2b in newly diagnosed patients with multiple myeloma: A Cancer and Leukemia Group B study. J Clin Oncol 11:155–160, 1993.

60. Galvez CA, Bonamassa MA, Pire R: Multiple myeloma: Treatment with recombinant alfa-2b (Intron A) plus VABP vs VABP alone: A prospective randomized trial. J Cancer Res Clin Oncol 116(suppl):594, 1990.

61. Montuoro A, De Rosa L, De Blasio A, et al: Interferon/melphalan/prednisone versus melphalan/prednisone in previously untreated patients with myeloma. Br J Haematol 76:365–368, 1990.

62. Corrado C, Flores A, Pavlovsky S, et al: Randomized trial comparing melphalan-prednisone with or without recombinant alfa-2 interferon (rα2IFN) in multiple myeloma. Proc Am Soc Clin Oncol 10:304, 1991.

63. Mellstedt H, Osterborg A, Bjorkholm M, et al: Treatment of multiple myeloma with interferon alpha: The Scandinavian experience. Br J Haematol 79(suppl 1):21–25, 1991.

64. Dimopoulos MA, Weber D, Delasalle KB, et al: Combination therapy with interferon-dexamethasone for newly diagnosed patients with multiple myeloma. Cancer 72:2589–2592, 1993.

65. Horozewicz JS, Leong SS, Carter WS: Non-cycling tumor cells are sensitive targets for the antiproliferative activity of human interferon. Science 206:1091–1093, 1979.

66. Peest D, Deicher H, Coldeway R, et al: Melphalan and prednisone (MP) versus vincristine, BCNU, Adriamycin, melphalan and dexamethasone (VBAMDex) induction chemotherapy and interferon maintenance treatment in multiple myeloma: Current results of a multicenter trial. Onkologie 13:458–460, 1990.

67. Mandelli F, Avvisati G, Amadori S, et al: Maintenance treatment with recombinant interferon alfa-2b in patients with multiple myeloma responding to conventional induction chemotherapy. N Engl J Med 322:1430–1434, 1990.

68. Westin J: Interferon alfa-2b versus no maintenance therapy during the plateau phase in multiple myeloma: A randomized study. Br J Haematol 89:561–568, 1995.

69. Salmon SE, Crowley JJ, Grogan TM, et al: Combination chemotherapy, glucocorticoids, and interferon alfa in the treatment of multiple myeloma: A Southwest Oncology Group study. J Clin Oncol 12:2405–2414, 1994.

70. Jagannath S, Barlogie B: Autologous bone marrow transplantation for multiple myeloma. Hematol Oncol Clin North Am 6:437–449, 1992.

71. Sulis E, Flores C, Sulis ML, et al: Interferon administered intralesionally in skin and oral cavity lesions in heterosexual drug addicted patients with AIDS-related Kaposi's sarcoma. Eur J Cancer Clin Oncol 25:759–761, 1989.

72. Krown SE: Kaposi's sarcoma, in DeVita VT Jr, Hellman S, Rosenberg SA (eds): Biologic Therapy of Cancer, pp 346–353. Philadelphia, JB Lippincott, 1991.

73. Tirelli U, Vaccher E, Lazzarin A, et al: Epidemic Kaposi's sarcoma in Italy, a country with intravenous drug users as the main group affected by HIV infection. Ann Oncol 2:373–376, 1991.

74. Real FX, Oettgen HF, Krown SE: Kaposi's sarcoma and the acquired immunodeficiency syndrome: Treatment with high and low doses of recombinant leukocyte α-interferon. J Clin Oncol 4:544–551, 1986.

75. De Wit R: AIDS-associated Kaposi's sarcoma and the mechanisms of interferon alpha's activity: A riddle within a puzzle. J Intern Med 231:321–325, 1992.

76. Krown SE, Gold JWM, Niedzwiecki D, et al: Interferon-α with zidovudine: Safety, tolerance, and clinical and virological effects in patients with Kaposi sarcoma associated with the acquired immunodeficiency syndrome (AIDS). Ann Intern Med 112:812–821, 1990.

77. Krown SE, Paredes J, Bundow D, et al: Interferon-α, zidovudine, and granulocyte-macrophage colony-stimulating factor: A phase I AIDS Clinical Trials Group study in patients with Kaposi's sarcoma associated with AIDS. J Clin Oncol 10:1344–1351, 1992.

78. Redman J, Hagemeister F, McLaughlin P, et al: α-Interferon treatment of Hodgkin's disease (HD) (abstract). Proc Am Soc Clin Oncol 9:256, 1990.

79. Rybak ME, McCarroll K, Bernard S, et al: Interferon therapy of relapsed and refractory Hodgkin's disease: Cancer and Leukemia Group B study 8652. J Biol Resp Mod 9:1–4, 1990.

80. Solal-Celigny P, Lepage E, Brousse N, et al: Recombinant interferon alfa-2b combined with a regimen containing doxorubicin in patients with advanced follicular lymphoma. N Engl J Med 329:1608—1614, 1993.

81. Smalley RV, Anderson JW, Hawkins MJ, et al: Interferon alfa combined with cytotoxic chemotherapy for patients with non-Hodgkin's lymphoma. N Engl J Med 327: 1336–1341, 1992.

82. Price CGA, Rohatiner AZS, Steward W, et al: Interferon-α 2b in the treatment of follicular lymphoma: Preliminary results of a trial in progress. Ann Oncol 2(suppl 2):141–145, 1991.

83. Andersen JW, Smalley RV: Interferon alfa plus chemotherapy for non–Hodgkin's lymphoma: Five year follow-up. N Engl J Med 329: 1821–1822, 1993.

84. McLaughlin P, Cabanillas F, Hagemeister FB, et al: CHOP-Bleo plus interferon for stage IV low-grade lymphoma. Ann Oncol 4:205–211, 1993.

85. Gaynor ER, Fisher RI: Clinical trials of α-interferon in the

treatment of non-Hodgkin's lymphoma. Semin Oncol 18(suppl 7):12–17, 1991.

86. Hagenbeek A, Carde P, Somers R, et al: Maintenance of remission with human recombinant alpha-2 interferon (Roferon-A) in patients with stages III and IV low-grade malignant non-Hodgkin's lymphoma: Results from a prospective, randomized, phase III clinical trial in 331 patients. Blood 80:288A, 1992.

87. Aviles A, Diaz-Maqueo JC, Garcia EL, et al: Maintenance therapy with interferon alfa 2b in patients with diffuse large cell lymphoma. Invest New Drugs 10:351–355, 1992.

88. Kemme DJ, Bunn PA Jr: State of the art therapy of mycosis fungoides and Sezary syndrome. Oncology 6:31–42, 1992.

89. Bunn PA, Hoffman SJ, Norris D, et al: Systemic therapy of cutaneous T-cell lymphomas (mycosis fungoides and the Sezary syndrome). Ann Intern Med 121:592–602, 1994.

90. Bunn PA, Foon KA, Ihde DC, et al: Recombinant leukocyte interferon: An active agent in advanced cutaneous T-cell lymphomas. Ann Intern Med 101:484–487, 1984.

91. Kohn EC, Steis RG, Sausville ET, et al: Phase II trial of intermittent high-dose recombinant interferon alfa-2a in mycosis fungoides and the Sezary syndrome. J Clin Oncol 8:155–160, 1990.

92. Olsen EA, Rosen ST, Vollmer RT, et al: Interferon alfa-2a in the treatment of cutaneous T-cell lymphoma. J Am Acad Dermatol 20:395–407, 1989.

93. Vonderheid EC, Thompson R, Smiles KA, et al: Recombinant interferon alfa-2b in plaque-phase mycosis fungoides: Intralesional and low-dose intramuscular therapy. Arch Dermatol 123:757–763, 1987.

94. Tura S, Mazza P, Zinzani PL, et al: Alpha recombinant interferon in the treatment of mycosis fungoides (MF). Haematologica 72:337–340, 1987.

95. Papa G, Tura S, Mandelli F, et al: Is interferon alpha in cutaneous T-cell lymphoma a treatment of choice? Br J Haematol 79(suppl 1):48–51, 1991.

96. Kuzel TM, Roenigk HH Jr, Samuelson E, et al: Effectiveness of interferon alfa-2a combined with phototherapy for mycosis fungoides and the Sezary syndrome. J Clin Oncol 13:257–263, 1995.

97. Rook AH, Prystowsky MB, Cassin M, et al: Combined therapy for Sezary syndrome with extracorporeal photochemotherapy and low-dose interferon-alfa therapy. Arch Dermatol 127:1535–1540, 1991.

98. Mostow EN, Neckel SL, Oberhelman L, et al: Complete remissions in psoralen and UV-A (PUVA)-refractory mycosis fungoides-type cutaneous T-cell lymphoma with combined interferon alfa and PUVA. Arch Dermatol 129:747–752, 1993.

99. Foss F, Tingsgaard P, Jorgensen H, et al: Interferon treatment of cutaneous T-cell lymphoma. Eur J Haematol 51: 63–72, 1993.

100. Foss FM, Ihde DC, Breneman DL, et al: Phase II study of pentostatin and intermittent high-dose interferon alfa-2a in advanced mycosis fungoides/Sezary syndrome. J Clin Oncol 10:1907–1913, 1992.

101. Salmon SE, Durie BGM, Young L, et al: Effects of cloned human leukocyte interferons in the human tumor cell assay. J Clin Oncol 1:217–225, 1983.

102. Kirkwood JM, Ernstoff MS: Cutaneous melanoma, in DeVita VT Jr, Hellman S, Rosenberg SA (eds): Biologic Therapy of Cancer, pp 311–333. Philadelphia, JB Lippincott, 1991.

103. McLeod GRC, Thomson DB, Hersey P: Recombinant interferon alfa-2a in advanced malignant melanoma: A phase I-II study in combination with DTIC. Int J Cancer 40(suppl 1):31–35, 1987.

104. Kirkwood JM, Ernstoff MS, Giuliano A, et al: Interferon α-2a and dacarbazine in melanoma. J Natl Cancer Inst 82:1062–1063, 1990.

105. Falkson CI, Falkson G, Falkson HC: Improved results with the addition of interferon alpha-2b to dacarbazine in the treatment of patients with metastatic malignant melanoma. J Clin Oncol 9:1403–1408, 1991.

106. Thomson D, Adena M, McLeod GRC, et al: Interferon α-2a (IFN) does not improve response or survival when added to dacarbazine (DTIC) in metastatic melanoma: Results of a multi-institutional randomized trial QMP8704 (abstract). Proc Am Soc Clin Oncol 11:343, 1992.

107. Sertoli MR, Queirolo P, Bajetta E, et al: Dacarbazine (DTIC) with or without recombinant interferon alpha-2a at different dosages in the treatment of stage IV melanoma patients: Preliminary results of a randomized trial (abstract). Proc Am Soc Clin Oncol 11:345, 1992.

108. Meyskens FL Jr, Kopecky K, Samson M, et al: Recombinant human interferon-γ: Adverse effects in high-risk stage I and II cutaneous malignant melanoma. J Natl Cancer Inst 82:1071, 1990.

109. Rosenberg SA, Lotze MT, Muul LM, et al: A progress report on the treatment of 157 patients with advanced cancer using lymphokine-activated killer cells and interleukin-2 or high-dose interleukin-2 alone. N Engl J Med 316:889–897, 1987.

110. Rosenberg S, Yang J, Topalian S, et al: Treatment of 283 consecutive patients with metastatic melanoma or renal cell cancer using high-dose bolus interleukin-2. JAMA 271:907–912, 1994.

111. Flaherty L, Robinson W, Redman B, et al: A phase II study of dacarbazine and cisplatin in combination with outpatient administered interleukin-2 in metastatic melanoma. Cancer 71:3520–3525, 1993.

112. Atkins M, O'Boyle K, Sosman J, et al: Multiinstitutional phase II trial of intensive combination chemoimmunotherapy for metastatic melanoma. J Clin Oncol 12:1553–1560, 1994.

113. Stoter G, Aamdal S, Rodenhuis S, et al: Sequential administration of recombinant human interleukin-2 and dacarbazine in metastatic melanoma: A multicenter phase II study. J Clin Oncol 9:1687–1691, 1991.

114. Flaherty L, Liu P, Fletcher W, et al: Dacarbazine and outpatient interleukin-2 in treatment of metastatic malignant melanoma: A phase II Southwest Oncology Group trial. J Natl Cancer Inst 83:893–894, 1992.

115. Sparano J, Fisher R, Sunderland M, et al: Randomized phase III trial of treatment with high-dose interleukin-2 alone or in combination with interferon alfa-2a in patients with advanced melanoma. J Clin Oncol 11:1969–1977, 1993.

116. Khayat D, Borel C, Tourani J, et al: Highly active chemoimmunotherapy with cisplatin, interleukin-2, and interferon alfa-2a for metastatic melanoma. J Clin Oncol 11:2173—2180, 1993.

117. Richards J, Mehta N, Ramming K, et al: Sequential chemoimmunotherapy in the treatment of metastatic melanoma. J Clin Oncol 10:1338—1343, 1992.

118. Legha S, Ring S, Plager C, et al: Biochemotherapy using interleukin-2 + interferon alfa 2a in combination with cisplatin, vinblastine, and DTIC in advanced melanoma (abstract). Proc Am Soc Clin Oncol 10:293, 1991.

119. Legha S, Buzaid A, Ring S, et al: Improved results of treatment of metastatic melanoma with combined use of biotherapy and chemotherapy (abstract). Proc Am Soc Clin Oncol 1994; 13: 394.

120. Buzaid AC, Legha SS: Combination of chemotherapy with interleukin-2 and interferon-alfa for the treatment of advanced melanoma. Semin Oncol 21 (Suppl 14):23—28, 1994.

121. Quesada JR, Swanson DA, Trinidade A, et al: Renal cell carcinoma: Antitumor effects of leukocyte interferon. Cancer Res 43:940–947, 1983.

122. Muss HB: Renal cell carcinoma, in DeVita VT Jr, Hellman S, Rosenberg SA (eds): Biologic Therapy of Cancer, pp 298–311.

Philadelphia, JB Lippincott, 1991.

123. Minasian LM, Motzer RJ, Krown SE, et al: Interferon-α 2a (IFN-α) in 160 patients (PTS) with advanced renal cancer (RCC) (abstract). Proc Am Soc Clin Oncol 11:203, 1992.

124. Porzsolt F: Adjuvant therapy of renal cell cancer (RCC) with interferon alfa-2a (abstract). Proc Am Soc Clin Oncol 11:202, 1992.

125. Parkinson DR, Sznol M: High-dose interleukin-2 in the therapy of metastatic renal-cell carcinoma. Semin Oncol 22:61–66, 1995.

126. West WH, Tauer KW, Yannelli JR, et al: Constant-infusion recombinant interleukin-2 in adoptive immunotherapy of advanced cancer. N Engl J Med 316:898–905, 1987.

127. Stadler WM, Vogelzang NJ: Low-dose interleukin-2 in the treatment of metastatic renal-cell carcinoma. Semin Oncol 22:67–73, 1995.

128. Blay JY, Negrier S, Combaret J, et al: Serum level of interleukin-6 as a prognosis factor in metastatic renal cell carcinoma. Cancer Res 52:3317–3322, 1992.

129. Sella A, Zukiwski A, Robinson E, et al: Interleukin-2 with interferon-alpha and 5-fluorouracil in patients with metastatic renal cell cancer (abstract). Proc Am Soc Clin Oncol 13:237, 1994.

130. Legha S, Plager C, Ring S, et al: A phase II study of biochemotherapy using interleukin-2 (IL-2) + interferon alfa-2a (IFN) in combination with cisplatin (C) vinblastine (V) and DTIC (D) in patients with metastatic melanoma (abstract). Proc Am Soc Clin Oncol 11:343, 1992.

131. Borden EC: Interferons: Expanding therapeutic roles. N Engl J Med 326:1491–1493, 1992.

Biologic Therapy: Hematopoietic Growth Factors, Retinoids, and Monoclonal Antibodies

Mohammad Qasim, MD, Paula Marlton, MBBS, *and* Razelle Kurzrock, MD

Department of Hematology, The University of Texas M. D. Anderson Cancer Center, Houston, Texas

Biologic therapies are an increasingly important part of cancer treatment. In this chapter, we review the current status of studies of colony-stimulating factors (CSFs), erythropoietin (Epogen, Procrit), thrombopoietin, the retinoids, and monoclonal antibodies (MoAbs). The interferons, interleukin-2 (IL-2, aldesleukin [Proleukin]), and adoptive cellular immunotherapy are discussed in a separate chapter.

Further work in this field will include study of the normal physiologic functions of cytokines. Understanding how dysregulation of cytokine function participates in the development of pathologic states may lead to the identification of additional clinical applications. Combination therapies exploiting complementary actions and interactions among naturally occurring molecules promise an added dimension to biologic therapy. Testing of new molecules, particularly those belonging to the ever-enlarging interleukin family, will continue and may yield additional therapeutic opportunities.

HEMATOPOIETIC GROWTH FACTORS

Hematopoietic growth factors are a family of glycoproteins with important regulatory functions in the processes of proliferation, differentiation, and functional activation of hematopoietic progenitors and mature blood cells.[1] The concept of humoral control of hematopoiesis dates back to the work of Carnot and Deflandre in 1906, who demonstrated that erythropoiesis is stimulated by a humoral factor, much later called erythropoietin, present in the serum of anemic rabbits.[2] In the 1960s, Bradley and Metcalf[3] developed an in vitro bone marrow culture system and observed the formation of cell colonies from hematopoietic progenitors. This hallmark development ultimately facilitated the characterization of a variety of hematopoietic growth factors known as CSFs. The subsequent development of molecular techniques led to genetic cloning of these factors and a large supply of recombinant molecules.

As shown in Table 1, the hematopoietic growth factors include erythropoietin, the CSFs, various interleukins (IL-1 to IL-13), stem-cell factor (SCF) newly described thrombopoietin (c-*Mpl* ligand),[4] and *flt-3/flk-2*, a growth factor for early progenitor cells.[5] The CSFs include granulocyte CSF (G-CSF, filgrastim [Neupogen]), granulocyte-macrophage CSF (GM-CSF, sargramostim [Leukine]), multipotential CSF (multi-CSF, also known as IL-3), and monocyte macrophage CSF (M-CSF, also known as CSF-1). Substantial clinical data have accrued on the four CSFs and erythropoietin, and these molecules have already had a major impact on therapy for hematologic and oncologic disease.

Biology

The hematopoietic growth factors have pleiotropic effects on the proliferation, differentiation, and functional activation of blood cells. They interact at various levels of the hematopoietic differentiation cascade, from multipotent progenitors to mature cells.[6]

Each growth factor is encoded by a specific gene. The biologic effects of the growth factors are mediated through specific receptors on the surfaces of target cells. The receptor molecules are also encoded by specific genes, some of which have been cloned. The major cellular sources of the growth factors are monocytes, macrophages, T lymphocytes, endothelial cells, and fibroblasts. They are present and produce growth factors at multiple sites in the body. Erythropoietin production appears to be more restricted, however, with the predominant sources in the adult being the peritubular cells of the kidneys and the Kupffer cells of the liver.

Most growth factors stimulate more than one lineage. This ability to stimulate multiple cell lineages may be related to shared elements in receptor subunits. The receptors for GM-CSF, IL-3, and IL-5 are composed of a ligand-specific alpha chain and a common beta chain. Growth factors can be classified according to the level at which they act in hematopoiesis. Late-acting lineage-specific factors act on maturing cells. Erythropoietin, IL-5, and monocyte-macrophage CSF are examples of such factors. G-CSF regulates the proliferation and mat-

TABLE I

Hematopoietic Growth Factors and Their Actions

Factor	Target cell or activity [a]
Interleukin-1	Induces other growth factors
Interleukin-2	T-cell growth factor
Interleukin-3 (multi-CSF)	Multipotent progenitors
Interleukin-4	B-cell growth factor
Interleukin-5	Eosinophil differentiation factor
Interleukin-6	B-/T-cell growth and differentiation; mega karyocytes
Interleukin-7	B-/T-cell precursor growth
Interleukin-8	Neutrophil chemotactic factor
Interleukin-9	T-cell growth factor; megakaryocytes and burst-forming units-erythrocytes
Interleukin-10	Cytokine synthesis inhibition in natural-killer (NK) and T-cells
Interleukin-11	B-cells, multipotent progenitors, and mega-karyocyte growth
Interleukin-12	Stimulates natural-killer and cytotoxic T-cells
Granulocyte colony-stimulating factor (G-CSF)	Neutrophil growth and activation
Granulocyte-macrophage colony-stimulating factor (GM-CSF)	Growth and activation of neutrophils and macrophages
Erythropoietin	Erythroid growth and differentiation
SCF (c-*kit* ligand)	Stem-cell factor
Thrombopoietin	Thrombopoiesis

[a] Most hematopoietins have a wide array of functions. The functions listed reflect only one of the activities of interest for each of these factors.
Adapted, with permission, from Marlton P, Kurzrock R: Biologic therapy: Hematopoietic growth factors, retinoids, and monoclonal antibodies, in Pazdur R (ed): Medical Oncology: A Comprehensive Review, p 437. Huntington, NY, PRR Inc, 1993.

uration of neutrophil progenitors but also acts with other factors to support the proliferation of primitive, dormant progenitors. GM-CSF, IL-3, and IL-4 are examples of intermediate-acting lineage-nonspecific factors that support the proliferation of multipotential progenitors. IL-6, IL-11, IL-12, G-CSF, and SCF act synergistically with IL-3 to induce dormant primitive progenitors to enter the cell cycle.[7,8]

Erythropoietin promotes the proliferation and differentiation of committed erythroid progenitors. It may also interact with other hematopoietins to stimulate megakaryocytes in vitro. In vivo, erythropoietin produces consistent and sustained increases in erythropoiesis and hematocrit.

In addition to stimulating cell proliferation and differentiation, CSFs also affect cell survival and functional activation. GM-CSF sustains viability and potentiates the functions of neutrophils, eosinophils, and macrophages.[9] G-CSF also potentiates the function of mature neutrophils but, unlike GM-CSF, appears not to increase the neutrophil half-life.[10] M-CSF enhances monocyte production of other cytokines, such as interferon, tumor necrosis factor, and CSFs themselves.[11] Indeed, virtually every function of granulocytes and macrophages that has been studied is modulated to some degree by G-CSF, GM-CSF, or M-CSF. IL-3 may regulate the function of eosinophils and monocytes.[12] Erythropoietin does not appear to alter the function of erythrocytes.

Clinical Applications

The availability of large quantities of recombinant growth factors has facilitated the exploitation of their biologic properties in the treatment of disease. G-CSF, GM-CSF, and erythropoietin have all been approved for clinical use for specific indications. A list of these indications and some investigational uses are summarized in Table 2.

Abrogation of Myelosuppression After Chemotherapy: The concept of using growth factors to mitigate the myelosuppressive effects of chemotherapy has generated a great deal of excitement. The potential of CSFs to reduce the morbidity and mortality from chemotherapy and to allow dose escalation has been energetically explored.

Important studies have now established that G-CSF is able to abrogate or accelerate recovery from chemotherapy-induced neutropenia. For example, in a study of G-CSF following MVAC (methotrexate, vincristine [Oncovin], doxorubicin [Adriamycin, Rubex], and cisplatin [Platinol]) chemotherapy for urothelial tumors, the administration of therapy on schedule was possible in all patients receiving G-CSF but in only 29% of patients not receiving G-CSF.[13] The occurrence of mucositis was also diminished in the treated group.

In a study of patients with small-cell lung cancer, the duration of neutropenia was shorter and the number of

TABLE 2

Indications for Recombinant Hematopoietic Growth Factors

G-CSF

Approved indications

To decrease the incidence of infection, as manifested by febrile neutropenia, in patients with nonmyeloid malignancies receiving myelosuppressive anticancer drugs that are associated with a significant incidence of severe neutropenia with fever

GM-CSF

Approved indications

To accelerate myeloid recovery in patients with non-Hodgkin's lymphoma, acute lymphoblastic leukemia, and Hodgkin's disease who are undergoing autologous bone marrow transplantation

Indications under investigation for G-CSF and GM-CSF

To accelerate myeloid recovery in patients with myelodysplastic syndrome, AIDS (acquired immunodeficiency syndrome), marrow graft failure, peripheral blood stem-cell transplantation, congenital agranulocytosis, or malignancies not previously mentioned

ERYTHROPOIETIN

Approved indications

- Anemia of chronic renal failure (creatinine $\geq$ 1.8 mg/dL)

- Anemia with human immunodeficiency virus infection in patients undergoing treatment with zidovudine

- Anemia in cancer patients undergoing chemotherapy

Indications under investigation

- Anemia of chronic disease, including rheumatoid arthritis and cancer

- Donation of blood for autologous use

- Surgical bone loss

- Bone marrow transplantation

- Anemia of prematurity

- Myelodysplastic syndromes

- Sickle-cell anemia

G-CSF = granulocyte colony-stimulating factor, GM-CSF = granulocyte-macrophage colony-stimulating factor   Adapted, with permission, from Goodnough LT, Anderson KC, Kurtz S, et al: Indications and guidelines for the use of hematopoietic growth factors. Transfusion 33(11):944–959, 1993.

febrile neutropenic episodes was lower in the G-CSF-treated group than in the placebo group.[14] The treated patients also spent fewer days in the hospital and received

fewer antibiotics. Morstyn et al[15] confirmed the attenuation of neutropenia in patients treated with high-dose melphalan, even when the G-CSF was given as late as 8 days after chemotherapy.

GM-CSF has also produced encouraging results in the setting of chemotherapy-induced neutropenia. In comparisons with historic controls and in comparison between sequential courses of chemotherapy with and without GM-CSF, shorter durations of neutropenia and higher nadir neutrophil counts have been consistently observed in the treatment cycles with GM-CSF.[16,17] Despite the biologic data indicating that GM-CSF acts on early progenitors, no consistent enhancement of platelet recovery has been noted.

Autologous Bone Marrow Transplantation: Growth factors have been investigated for their ability to lessen myelosuppression associated with high-dose chemotherapy and autologous bone marrow rescue. G-CSF and GM-CSF have produced similar results in this setting. Studies have shown that time to neutrophil recovery in patients with Hodgkin's disease and lymphoid malignancies was reduced by these growth factors when compared with historic controls.[18,19] The number of febrile days and days in the hospital as well as the incidence of infection were also reduced. Toxic effects to organs were decreased, presumably as a result of shorter neutropenic periods. The ability of GM-CSF to enhance hematologic reconstitution has been confirmed in prospective, randomized trials.[20,21]

G-CSF treatment after allogeneic bone marrow transplantation (BMT) has been shown to reduce the duration of neutropenia. Patients who received G-CSF had fewer infections and required less antibiotic treatment and shorter hospitalization than patients who did not receive G-CSF.[22,23] Clinical trials of G-CSF use after BMT have also indicated quicker granulocyte recovery.[24–26]

Myelodysplastic Syndromes: The myelodysplastic syndromes (MDSs) are acquired primary or treatment-related neoplastic clonal stem-cell disorders characterized by ineffective hematopoiesis, dysplasia, and an increased propensity for leukemic transformation.[27] The French-American-British (FAB) classification identifies five MDS subtypes: refractory anemia, refractory anemia with ring sideroblasts, refractory anemia with excess blasts, refractory anemia with excess blasts in transformation, and chronic myelomonocytic leukemia. Chromosomal abnormalities are commonly associated with these disorders. Among the most frequent abnormality is the loss of the long arm of chromosome 5 (5q-), on which is located a cluster of growth factor-related genes, including those coding for GM-CSF, M-CSF, M-CSF receptor,

IL-3, IL-4, IL-5, and platelet-derived growth factor receptor. The significance of this association is under investigation. Because most patients with MDS die of infections and bleeding complications, therapy directed at increasing the number of circulating granulocytes and platelets and increasing red-cell mass appears very attractive.

Several studies have demonstrated a predictable increase in granulocyte count with GM-CSF and G-CSF in patients with MDS.[28-35] It is obvious from these studies that G-CSF or GM-CSF therapy can reduce the number of infections in patients with MDS who are neutropenic. Randomized trials comparing GM-CSF with placebo and G-CSF with observation have been reported. Most of these patients had fewer than 15% to 20% blasts in their bone marrow. There was no improvement in survival with either G-CSF or GM-CSF, and in the G-CSF study, overall survival of G-CSF-treated patients was shorter. The effect of GM-CSF on the cytopenias has been transient, disappearing in most cases with treatment cessation.

Studies of IL-3 in patients with MDS have been conducted in both Europe and the United States[36-38]; neutrophil responses occurred in 7 of 9 European patients and in 6 of 13 US patients. Reticulocyte and platelet responses were documented in a few patients. However, these responses rarely translated into a reduction in transfusion requirements. The modest improvements in the neutrophil count detected in these studies with IL-3 were not as substantial as those induced by G-CSF and GM-CSF. It is therefore likely that IL-3 will be most effective in combination with other growth factors, and such clinical trials are ongoing.

Acute Myeloid Leukemia: Estey et al[39] found no difference in the rate of infection or complete remission in patients with acute myeloid leukemia (AML) treated with fludarabine (Fludara), cytarabine, and G-CSF compared to historic controls treated with fludarabine and cytarabine alone. GM-CSF has been administered before chemotherapy in an attempt to induce leukemic blasts to enter the cell cycle, thus rendering them more susceptible to the drugs' cytotoxic effects. Despite evidence that blast production and ara-CTP (the active triphosphate derivative of cytarabine) incorporation into DNA are increased, the survival rate of patients receiving this therapy was inferior to that of historic controls.[40] Ongoing prospective, randomized trials are investigating the effect of GM-CSF before and during induction and consolidation and during the first two cycles of maintainence chemotherapy for newly diagnosed AML.[41] In an interesting study, Giralt et al[42] were able to obtain durable remissions in patients with AML who had relapsed after allogeneic BMT with G-CSF treatments.

Other Hematologic Disorders: Aplastic anemia is characterized by peripheral blood cytopenias and bone marrow hypoplasia, thus representing another potential target for CSF therapy. Vadhan-Raj et al[43] showed that leukocyte counts improved in all patients treated with GM-CSF. No significant effects were observed in other cell lineages. The increases in leukocyte counts, which were accompanied by enhanced granulocyte function, persisted only for the duration of the GM-CSF infusion. Other investigators demonstrated that GM-CSF therapy could not induce hematopoiesis in patients with the most severe form of aplastic anemia.[44] Very low doses of GM-CSF (5 to 20 µg/m²/d) have also successfully increased neutrophil counts in nearly 50% of patients with aplastic anemia.[45] Further investigation of GM-CSF in combination with other growth factors is warranted.

IL-3 has also been studied as a therapy for aplastic anemia. Ganser and co-workers[46] found increases in leukocyte counts in all nine patients treated. Platelet responses varied and included a transient decline in two patients. Kurzrock et al[36,47] have reported neutrophil responses in approximately one third of patients and platelet or reticulocyte responses in 10% of patients with aplastic anemia receiving IL-3. These effects were often modest and delayed in onset, although they persisted longer after cessation of IL-3 than did the effects of GM-CSF therapy. IL-3 combined with GM-CSF appears promising for increasing platelet counts as well as granulocyte counts in patients with aplastic anemia.[48]

G-CSF has revolutionized therapy for the chronic neutropenias. A number of reports on cyclic neutropenia, congenital neutropenia, and idiopathic neutropenia have confirmed neutrophil responses in virtually 100% of patients treated with G-CSF, and resolution of infectious complications has been observed.[47] GM-CSF produces less satisfactory results, with eosinophilia predominating over neutrophil responses; one report suggested, however, that very low doses (0.3 µg/kg/d) may be more effective than standard doses.[49]

Anemia: Erythropoietin was first used clinically in patients with anemia and chronic renal failure who were undergoing dialysis. It has shown consistent, sustained success in improving the hematocrit in this setting, presumably because the production of erythropoietin is impaired along with the impairment of other renal functions.[50] In contrast to the clinical settings in which CSFs are used, renal failure represents a true erythropoietin deficiency state.

Anemia frequently accompanies malignant disease, although endogenous erythropoietin production is not usually impaired in this setting. Miller et al[51] have shown, however, that the magnitude of the erythropoietin response in patients with cancer and anemia is blunted, compared with that of patients with iron-deficiency anemia. Patients with hematologic malignancies and anemia can have a wide range of endogenous erythropoietin levels, and a variety of contributory mechanisms of anemia probably exist.[47-52] Nonetheless, treatment of this group with erythropoietin has produced some encouraging data. In one study, 11 of 13 anemic patients with multiple myeloma responded to erythropoietin, with improvements in hemoglobin levels.[53] Less promising results were obtained in patients with MDS. Indeed, in our studies, only 2 of 16 patients with MDS responded.[52] Erythropoietin has been successful, however, in abrogating the anemia associated with therapy for acquired immunodeficiency syndrome (AIDS) therapy.[54]

Toxicity

The toxic effects of growth factors have been reviewed recently.[20] Unfortunately, no direct comparisons of G-CSF and GM-CSF have been performed. However, comparing their toxicities in different studies using equally effective doses in the same clinical settings reveals greater toxicity after GM-CSF administration.[20] The first dose of GM-CSF may be accompanied by flushing, tachycardia, hypotension, dyspnea, hypoxemia, musculoskeletal pain, and nausea in a small subset of patients. This first-dose effect is more common with intravenous administration. More important, GM-CSF can induce fever and chills, which are difficult to distinguish from the signs and symptoms of infection. Other complaints include lethargy, myalgia, bone pain, and anorexia, but they are usually mild. A capillary leak syndrome characterized by edema, effusions, and inflammation may develop. Other rare side effects of GM-CSF include exacerbation of thrombocytopenia and reactivation of autoimmune disorders. Doses lower than 5 µg/kg are usually reasonably well tolerated, whereas higher doses more frequently produce severe side effects.

The most frequent G-CSF toxicity is bone pain, which is more common with intravenous administration. Fever, rash, and arthralgia are uncommon. Mild splenomegaly may occur, particularly with long-term use of G-CSF. Thrombocytopenia also has been reported, albeit rarely. Doses between 1 and 20 µg/kg are usually well tolerated. At doses higher than 30 µg/kg, excessive leukocytosis typically occurs.

Interleukin-3 (IL-3) is well tolerated at doses lower than 1,000 µg/m^2/d, although low-grade fever and chills occur in a high percentage of patients. Headaches are more frequent at higher doses. Uncommon side effects include bone pain, edema, and nausea, all of which are generally mild.

Erythropoietin has caused very few side effects, even with long-term usage. Iron deficiency does occur, however, in patients with insufficient iron stores.

RETINOIDS

Retinoids are substances structurally or functionally related to vitamin A, or retinol. They exert profound effects on the growth, maturation, and differentiation of many cell types, both in vivo and in vitro.[55] Vitamin A is a vital factor in normal embryogenesis, and it influences limb development and growth pattern. The effects of retinoids are mediated by two classes of nuclear retinoic acid receptors, termed RAR and RXR. Each of these subclasses has subtypes designated alpha, beta, and gamma. These receptors are ligand-inducible, transcription-enhancer factors belonging to the nuclear receptor superfamily, which includes thyroid and steroid hormone receptors. Cytoplasmic retinoic acid-binding proteins are important in the mediation of some of the effects of retinoids. However, not all tissues responsive to retinoic acid possess this protein (eg, HL-60 cells).

Retinoids reportedly induce differentiation and/or suppression of proliferation of many cell lines, including embryonal carcinoma, leukemia, melanoma, neuroblastoma, and breast carcinoma. The best studied line is HL-60, which can be induced to differentiate to granulocytes expressing such functional characteristics as phagocytosis, complement receptors, chemotaxis, and the ability to reduce nitroblue tetrazolium. Synergy has been seen when retinoids were combined with vitamin D and its analogs as well as in combination with other cytokines.[56,57]

Clinical Applications

Chemoprevention: Sporn et al[58] were the first to use the term chemoprevention, which can be defined as the use of specific natural or synthetic chemical agents to reverse, suppress, or prevent carcinogenic progression to invasive cancer. This subject was recently reviewed by Lippman et al.[59]

A significant amount of data has accumulated over the past several years regarding the role of retinoids as chemopreventive agents, mainly in the setting of head and neck and lung cancers. Patients with a history of cancer of the head and neck and lungs are at a significantly increased risk of developing a second primary tumor. This is thought to be due to the "field cancerization" effect, in which diffuse injury to the epithelia results from the carcinogen exposure.

The ineffectiveness of current therapy for lung cancer also prompted studies evaluating the role of retinoids in preventing lung cancer development.[60] In a randomized, placebo-controlled trial, Hong and colleagues[61] have shown a significant decline in the incidence of second primary tumors with the use of isotretinoin 50 to 100 mg/m^2/d for 1 year in patients with treated head and neck cancers. Pastorino et al[62] evaluated retinyl palmitate (300,000 IU/d for 1 year) in patients with resected stage I lung cancer. There was a significant decline in the number of second primary tumors in patients who received retinyl palmitate, compared with a control group who received placebo. Bolla et al,[63] however, could not demonstrate any beneficial effects of etretinate, a synthetic retinoid, on the incidence of second primary tumors in patients with a history of squamous-cell carcinoma of the oral cavity or oropharynx. The role of retinoids as chemopreventive agents will be better defined upon completion of the large multicenter trials now under way (the North American Intergroup Lung Study and the European EUROSCAN study).[64]

In addition to their use in chemoprevention, retinoids have been used to treat various malignant diseases. Table 3 summarizes some of the data from these studies.

Acute Promyelocytic Leukemia: Classified as M3 in the FAB classification system, acute promyelocytic leukemia (APL) is a relatively uncommon leukemia. It is characterized by a propensity for coagulopathy and a high death rate from bleeding diatheses during induction. Morphologically, APL cells have abundant dense granules and Auer rods. Cytogenetic analysis reveals t(15;17) in the vast majority of patients. In instances in which no cytogenetic abnormality is present, more sensitive techniques, such as Southern blotting and reverse transcriptase-polymerase chain reaction amplification, reveal a characteristic RAR-alpha/PML gene rearrangement. The retinoic acid receptor RAR-alpha gene is located on the long arm of chromosome 17. The PML gene is located on chromosome 15. The t(15;17) translocation produces a recombinant gene, PML-RAR-alpha. The PML-RAR-alpha gene product is widely thought to be responsible for the differentiation block seen in APL blasts. The underlying mechanism or mechanisms of action of the block are still unknown.[65]

APL has traditionally been treated with anthracyclines with or without cytarabine. This treatment has a high complete remission rate, with a reported long-term survival of 30% to 40%.[66] Most treatment failures are due to early deaths from bleeding and infectious complications secondary to the aplastic state produced by induction chemotherapy.

TABLE 3
Retinoid-Responsive Diseases

Disease	Response rate (%)	Comment
Acute promyelocytic leukemia	80–100	Early relapse[70,82-86]
Juvenile chronic myelogenous leukemia	50	Small number of patients (10)[75]
Non-Hodgkin's lymphoma	40–50	Significant responses in T-cell lymphomas only[73,87,88]
Squamous-cell carcinoma of cervix	50–60	Treatment combined with alpha interferon[72]
Squamous-cell carcinoma of skin	60–70	Improved response in combination with alpha interferon[71,89]

All-*trans* retinoic acid (ATRA) has been successfully used to achieve complete remission in most patients with APL morphology and PML-RAR-alpha gene rearrangement.[67] ATRA therapy results in the terminal differentiation of APL blasts into functionally mature granulocytes. Furthermore, within the first 48 hours of treatment, ATRA therapy corrects the coagulopathy associated with APL. ATRA induces complete remission in 3 to 4 weeks of therapy in more than 90% of patients with APL.[68] De novo resistance to ATRA is very rare. ATRA therapy, unlike chemotherapy, does not produce an aplastic phase, thereby reducing the occurrence of infectious complications. ATRA therapy alone, however, has a high early (1 to 12 months) relapse rate, approaching virtually 100%. Recent studies have suggested that a combination of ATRA and chemotherapy may be better than either alone in terms of survival.[69,70] Patients whose disease relapses after ATRA therapy are generally resistant to retreatment with ATRA.

The mechanisms underlying ATRA sensitivity of APL blasts and the subsequent development of resistance are still not well defined. The PML-RAR-alpha gene product has been implicated in both leukemogenesis and response to ATRA. The development of resistance to ATRA is at least partly explained by the decline in drug levels due to the increased metabolism of ATRA during prolonged therapy.[65]

Other Malignancies: Using a combination of alpha interferon (IFN-α) and isotretinoin in patients with advanced squamous-cell carcinoma of the skin and cervix, Lippman et al[71,72] obtained significant responses. Cheng et al[73] investigated the use of 13-*cis* retinoic acid in patients with non-Hodgkin's lymphoma. In this study, T-cell lymphomas responded, but B-cell lymphomas did not. Kurzrock et al[74] demonstrated no benefit of ATRA treatment for patients with MDS. Castleberry et al[75] used ATRA to treat juvenile chronic myelogenous leukemia and obtained lasting remissions in 5 of 10 patients (two complete remissions and three partial remissions).

Toxicity

Retinoids are highly teratogenic compounds and therefore must be used with the utmost caution in women of child-bearing age. Apart from this serious side effect, retinoic acid toxicities are generally mild. Drying of the skin and mucous membranes occurs in virtually all patients. Arthralgias, hypertriglyceridemia, elevated liver function values, skin rashes, and mild hair loss occur in 10% to 25% of patients. More rarely, corneal opacities, exfoliation, pseudotumor cerebri, and proteinuria have occurred.

Retinoic Acid Syndrome

Retinoic acid syndrome (RAS), which is manifested as fever, respiratory distress, hyperleukocytosis, edema, pleural and pericardial effusions, hypotension, and renal failure, may occur in up to 20% of patients with APL treated with ATRA.[76] It occurs mainly within the first 3 weeks of treatment. Patients exhibiting hyperleukocytosis at the start of treatment have an increased risk of developing RAS. ATRA administered concomitantly with chemotherapy is beneficial in these patients.[77] High doses of corticosteroids given at the first sign of RAS were also beneficial.

MONOCLONAL ANTIBODIES

Hybridoma technology has provided a reliable system for the production of large quantities of antibodies of defined specificity (MoAbs). Hybridoma formation requires the fusion of B lymphocytes from immunized mice and myeloma cells, resulting in immortalized MoAb-producing cells.[78] Human B lymphocytes have also been used to create chimeric hybridomas; however, this technique remains difficult. Genetically engineered chimeric "humanized" MoAbs (MoAbs with a murine complementarity-determining region attached to a human immunoglobulin molecule) have been developed in an attempt to reduce the immunogenicity of murine MoAbs.

Antibodies are capable of binding with high affinity to specific determinants. The consequences of antibody binding vary and include (1) direct neutralization of the target (as in the case of certain viruses or toxins), (2) indirect mediation of immune damage by means of complement activation, and (3) activation of cellular cytotoxicity by other immunocompetent cells (antibody-dependent cell cytotoxicity). Variables influencing the outcome include the antibody isotype, binding affinity, and target epitope frequency.

The first step in monoclonal antibody therapy is to choose an appropriate target for antibody specificity. The optimum target is a tumor-specific surface antigen not expressed on normal tissue. For example, some B-cell malignancies demonstrate unique antigenic determinants by virtue of the clonal expression of immunoglobulin molecules on the malignant cells. Unique tumor determinants such as these are not found in most tumors, however, so other tumor-associated antigens have been targeted. They include differentiation antigens that are normally expressed only at specific stages of differentiation and on limited cell lineages (eg, common acute lymphoblastic leukemia antigen CD10 [CALLA], anti-T-activated cell antibody [anti-TAC]). Oncofetal antigens, including carcinoembryonic antigen (CEA) and alpha-fetoprotein, are alternative targets.

Many MoAbs do not adequately effect immune destruction of target cells alone. Thus, MoAbs have been conjugated with other agents that are cytotoxic, including toxins, chemotherapeutic agents, and radioisotopes. The resultant immunotoxins or immunoconjugates may have the potential to improve targeted cell therapy significantly. Potent protein toxins, such as ricin and diphtheria, have also been used, because they are active only after internalization into the cell. Common radioisotopes include iodine 131, yttrium 90, indium 111, and rhenium 186.

Another strategy for MoAb treatment involves targeting growth-factor receptors. Such antireceptor MoAbs compete with natural ligands functioning as autocrine growth factors, thus impairing tumor growth. Examples include anti-IL-2 receptor and antiepidermal growth factor receptor MoAbs. This strategy may also be used to deliver conjugated molecules via the cell receptor system.

Finally, MoAbs are being developed for use as diagnostic tools to locate residual tumor after treatment and to uncover occult tumors not localized by conventional methods.

Clinical Trials

The status of MoAb therapy for cancer was reviewed recently.[79-91] Table 4 summarizes some of the studies performed with MoAbs in various malignancies.[90-114] As is obvious at a glance, most of these studies were pilot or phase-I studies with small numbers of patients. The results generally have been disappointing. However,

TABLE 4

Monoclonal Antibodies (MoAbs) in Malignant Diseases

Study	MoAb	Disease	Number of responders/ number treated
Scheinberg et al[90]	M195 (CD33)	AML	0/10
Waldmann et al[91]	Anti-TAC (CD25)	T-ALL	6/19
Dyer et al[92]	CAMPATH	ALL	3/5
Caron et al[93]	Humanized M195	AML and blastic	—
Schwartz et al[94]	[131]I M195	ALL	—
Vitetta et al[95]	B-43-Pokeweed anti-CD-19 viral protein	ALL	—
Foon et al[96]	T101 (CD5)	CLL	0/13
Klien et al[97]	Anti-IL-6	Multiple myeloma	0/1
Hu et al[98]	Lym-1	B-cell lymphoma	0/10
Brown et al[99]	Anti-idiotype	B-cell lymphoma	9/17
Miller et al[100]	Leu-1 (CD5)	T-cell lymphoma	5/7
Dillman et al[101]	T101 (CD5)	T-cell lymphoma	0/12
Kaminski et al[102]	^{131}I-labeled anti-B1 (CD20)	B-cell lymphoma	6/9
Press et al[103]	^{131}I-labeled B1, 1F5,MB-1 + auto BMT	B-cell lymphoma	17/19
Ryan et al[104]	Several	Breast	0/10
Halpern et al[105]	Anti-PAP	Prostate	0/19
Goodman et al[106]	Anti-L6	Ovary	0/9
Jacobs et al[107]	[186]Relabeled NR-LU10 (intraperitoneal)	Ovary	4/17
Dillman et al[108]	Anti-CEA	Colorectal	0/30
Sears et al[109]	17-1A	Colorectal	1/60
Mellstedt et al[110]	17-1A	Colorectal	1/52
Takahashi et al[111]	A7-NCS	Colorectal	—
Halpern et al[112]	Anti-p97	Melanoma	0/24
Dillman et al[108]	Anti-p240	Melanoma	0/28
Houghton et al[113]	R24 (GD3)	Melanoma	4/21
Lynch et al[114]	N901-bR	Lung, small-cell	1/19

ALL = acute lymphocytic leukemia, AML = acute myeloid leukemia, BMT = bone marrow transplantation, CEA = carcinoembryonic antigen, PAP = prostatic acid phosphatase

these studies have demonstrated that MoAbs can be safely administered to humans with acceptable toxicity.

The initial failure of MoAb therapy may be attributable, at least in part, to the early development of human antimurine antibodies in recipients. These antibodies develop in 90% of patients after more than two treatments, greatly reducing the ability of the MoAbs to reach their target. Avascular tumor beds also prevent MoAbs from reaching the malignant tissue. Heterogeneity of tumor antigens and the mutation of antigens over time also abrogate the effectiveness of this target-specific therapy. Strategies to overcome these problems are being investigated and include the development of chimeric mouse/human MoAbs to reduce their immunogenicity.

Immunotoxins and immunoconjugates have met with modest success in vivo. Radionuclide conjugates have been used in the treatment of ovarian cancer, leukemia (anti-CD33 MoAb), non-Hodgkin's lymphoma, and brain tumors. Microscopic disease has proven more amenable to this therapy than has gross tumor. Immunotoxin therapy has most commonly used ricin. Encouraging results were observed when an anti-CD5 conjugate was administered to patients with chronic lymphocytic leukemia. Trials of ricin-linked MoAb therapy in patients with breast or colon cancer have been frustrated by the development of human antimurine antibodies and the consequent loss of MoAb efficacy. MoAbs have also been used after autologous BMT to purge tumor cells ex vivo in autologous bone marrow therapy or to select for progenitor cells in allogeneic BMT. In addition, MoAbs have been used to deplete the marrow of CD8+ cells to reduce the incidence of graft-vs-host disease.

MoAbs remain a conceptually logical approach to therapy. Further understanding of tumor immunology and advances in technology will facilitate the ongoing development of these strategies. Presently, clinical trials using chimeric "humanized" MoAbs, immunotoxins, and MoAbs conjugated to radioisotopes for diagnosis and therapy of malignant diseases are underway.

REFERENCES

1. Metcalf D: The granulocyte-macrophage colony-stimulating factors. Science 229:16–22, 1985.

2. Carnot P, Deflandre C: Sur l'activité hémpoiétique des différents organes au cours de la régénération du sang. CR Hebd Acad Sci 143:432–435, 1906.

3. Bradley TR, Metcalf D: The growth of mouse bone marrow cells in vitro. Aust J Exp Biol Med Sci 44:287–299, 1966.

4. Lok SI, Kanshansky K, Holly RD, et al: Cloning and expression of murine thrombopoietin cDNA and stimulation of platelet production in vivo. Nature 369:565–568, 1994.

5. Lyman SD, James L, Johnson L, et al: Cloning of the human homologue of the murine flt-3 ligand: A growth factor for early hematopoietic progenitor cells. Blood 83:2795–2801, 1994.

6. Groopman JE, Molina JM, Scadden DT: Hemopoietic growth factors. N Engl J Med 321:1449–1459, 1989.

7. Metcalf D: Hematopoietic regulators: Redundancy or subtlety? Blood 82:3515–3523, 1993.

8. Ogawa M: Differentiation and proliferation of hematopoietic stem cells. Blood 81:2844, 1993.

9. Metcalf D, Begley CG, Johnson GR, et al: Biologic properties in vitro of a recombinant human granulocyte-macrophage colony-stimulating factor. Blood 67:37–45, 1986.

10. Lord BI, Bronchud MH, Owens S, et al: The kinetics of human granulopoiesis following treatment with granulocyte colony-stimulating factor in vivo. Proc Natl Acad Sci USA 86:9499–9503, 1989.

11. Warren MK, Ralph P: Macrophage growth factor CSF-1 stimulates human monocyte production of interferon, tumor necrosis factor, and colony-stimulating activity. J Immunol 137:2281–2285, 1986.

12. Rothenburg ME, Owen WF Jr, Silberstein DS, et al: Human eosinophils have prolonged survival, enhanced functional properties, and become hypodense when exposed to human interleukin-3. J Clin Invest 81:1986–1992, 1988.

13. Gabrilove J, Jacubowski A, Scher H, et al: Effect of granulocyte colony-stimulating factor on neutropenia and associated morbidity due to chemotherapy for transitional cell carcinoma of the urothelium. N Engl J Med 318:1414–1422, 1988.

14. Crawford J, Ozer H, Stoller R, et al: Reduction by granulocyte colony-stimulating factor of fever and neutropenia induced by chemotherapy in patients with small-cell lung cancer. N Engl J Med 325:164–170, 1991.

15. Morstyn G, Campbell L, Souza LM, et al: Effect of granulocyte colony-stimulating factor on neutropenia induced by cytotoxic chemotherapy. Lancet 1:667–672, 1988.

16. Antman KS, Griffin JD, Elias A, et al: Effect of recombinant human granulocyte-macrophage colony-stimulating factor on chemotherapy-induced myelosuppression. N Engl J Med 310:593–598, 1989.

17. Morstyn G, Lieschke GJ, Cebon J, et al: Clinical experience with recombinant human granulocyte colony-stimulating factor and granulocyte-macrophage colony-stimulating factor. Semin Hematol 26:9–13, 1989.

18. Taylor KM, Jagannath S, Spitzer G, et al: Recombinant human granulocyte colony-stimulating factor hastens granulocyte recovery after high dose chemotherapy under autologous bone marrow transplantation in Hodgkin's disease. J Clin Oncol 7:1791–1799, 1989.

19. Nemunaitis J, Singer JW, Buckner CD, et al: Use of recombinant human granulocyte-macrophage colony-stimulating factor in bone marrow transplantation for lymphoid malignancies. Blood 72:834–836, 1988.

20. Grosh WW, Quesenberry PJ: Recombinant human hematopoietic growth factors in the treatment of cytopenias. Clin Immunol Immunopathol 62:S25–38, 1992.

21. Advani R, Chao NJ, et al: Granulocyte-macrophage colony-stimulating factor (GM-CSF) as an adjunct to autologous hematopoietic stem cell transplantation for lymphoma. Ann Intern Med 116:183–189, 1992.

22. Gisselbrecht C, Prentice HG, Barigalupo A, et al: Placebo controlled phase III trial of lenograstim in bone marrow transplantation. Lancet 343:696, 1994.

23. Schueing FG, Lilleby K, Clift RA, et al: Phase I study of rhG-CSF after marrow transplantation from HLA-identical siblings. Blood 82(S1):349a, 1993.

24. De Witte T, Gratwohl A, Van Der Lely N, et al: Recombinant human granulocyte-macrophage colony-stimulating factor accelerates neutrophil and monocyte recovery after allogeneic T-cell depleted bone marrow transplantation. Blood 79:1359–1365, 1992.

25. Anasetti C, Anderson G, Appelbaum FR, et al: Phase III study of rhGM-CSF in allogeneic marrow transplantation from unrelated donors. Blood 82:454a, 1993.

26. Nemunaitis J, Rosenfeld C, Ash R, et al: Phase III double-blind trial of rhGM-CSF (Sargramostin) following allogeneic bone marrow transplant (BMT). Blood 82(S1):286a, 1993.

27. Kouides PA, Bennet JM: Morphology and classification of myelodysplastic syndromes. Hematol Oncol Clin North Am 6:485–499, 1992.

28. Vadhan-Raj S, Keating M, Le Maistre A, et al: Effects of recombinant human granulocyte-macrophage colony-stimulating factor in patients with myelodysplastic syndromes. N Engl J Med 317:1545–1552, 1987.

29. Vadhan-Raj S, Hittleman WN, Ventura C, et al: GM-CSF and myelodysplastic syndromes. N Engl J Med 319:51–53, 1988.

30. Ganser A, Seipelt G, Eder M, et al: Treatment of myelodysplastic syndromes with cytokines and cytotoxic drugs. Semin Oncol 19(S4):95–101, 1992.

31. Greensberg P, Taylor K, Larson R, et al: Phase III randomized multicenter trial of G-CSF vs observation for myelodysplastic syndromes (MDS) (abstract). Blood 82(suppl 1):196a, 1993.

32. Schuster MW, Thompson JA, Larson R, et al: Randomized trial of subcutaneous GM-CSF versus observation in patients with myelodysplastic syndrome. J Cancer Res Clin Oncol 116(1):1079, 1990.

33. Willemze R, Van Der Lely H, Zwiersina H, et al: On behalf of EORTC leukemia cooperative group: A randomized phase I/II multicenter study of recombinant GM-CSF therapy for patients with myelodysplastic syndromes and relatively low risk of acute leukemia. Ann Hematol 64:173–180, 1992.

34. Estey EH, Kurzrock R, Talpaz M, et al: Effects of low dose recombinant human granulocyte-macrophage colony-stimulating factor (GM-CSF) on patients with myelodysplastic syndromes. Br J Haematol 77:291–295, 1991.

35. Greenberg P: Treatment of myelodysplastic syndromes with hemopoietic growth factors. Semin Oncol 19:106–114, 1992.

36. Kurzrock R, Talpaz M, Estrov Z, et al: Phase I study of recombinant human interleukin-3 in patients with bone marrow failure. J Clin Oncol 9:1241–1250, 1991.

37. Ganser A, Seipelt G, Lindemann A, et al: Effects of recombinant human interleukin-3 in patients with myelodysplastic syndromes. Blood 76:455–462, 1990.

38. Nimer SD, Paquette RL, Ireland P, et al: A phase I/II study of interleukin-3 in patients with aplastic anemia and myelodysplasia. Exp hematol 22(9):875–880, 1994.

39. Estey EH, Thall P, Andreef M, et al: Use of G-CSF before, during, and after fludarabine plus cytarabine induction therapy of newly diagnosed acute myelogenous leukemia or myelodysplastic syndromes: Comparison with fludarabine plus cytarabine without G-CSF. J Clin Oncol 12(4):671–678, 1994.

40. Estey EH, Thall P, Kantarjian H, et al: Treatment of newly diagnosed acute myelogenous leukemia with granulocyte-macrophage colony-stimulating factor (GM-CSF) before and during continuous-infusion high-dose ara-C and daunorubicin: Comparison to patients treated without GM-CSF. Blood 79:2246–2255, 1992.

41. Hiddemann W, Wormann B, Renter C, et al: New perspectives in the treatment of acute myeloid leukemia by hematopoietic growth factors. Semin Oncol 21(suppl 16):33–38, 1994.

42. Giralt S, Escudier S, Kantarjian H, et al: Preliminary results of treatment with filgrastim for relapse of leukemia and myelodysplasia after allogeneic bone marrow transplantation. N Engl J Med 329(11):757–761, 1993.

43. Vadhan-Raj S, Buescher S, Broxmeyer HE, et al: Stimulation of myelopoiesis in patients with aplastic anemia by recombinant human granulocyte-macrophage colony-stimulating factor. N Engl J Med 319:1628–1634, 1988.

44. Nissen C, Tichelli A, Gratwohl A, et al: Failure of recombinant human granulocyte-macrophage colony-stimulating factor therapy in aplastic anemia patients with very severe neutropenia. Blood 72:2045–2047, 1988.

45. Kurzrock R, Talpaz M, Gutterman J: Very low doses of GM-CSF administered alone or with erythropoietin in aplastic anemia. Am J Med 93:41–48, 1992.

46. Ganser A, Lindemann A, Seipelt G, et al: Effects of recombinant human interleukin-3 in patients with normal hematopoiesis and in patients with bone marrow failure. Blood 76:666–676, 1990.

47. Kurzrock R, Talpaz M, Estey EH, et al: Hematopoietic growth factors in bone marrow failure states. Cancer Bulletin 43:215, 1991.

48. Talpaz M, Patterson M, Kurzrock R: Sequential administration of IL-3 and GM-CSF in bone marrow failure patients: A phase I study (abstract). Blood 84(S1):28a, 1994.

49. Kurzrock R, Talpaz M, Gutterman J: Treatment of cyclic neutropenia with very low doses of GM-CSF. Am J Med 91:317, 1991.

50. Mohini R: Clinical efficacy of recombinant human erythropoietin in hemodialysis patients. Semin Nephrol 9:16–21, 1989.

51. Miller CB, Jones RJ, Piantadosi S, et al: Decreased erythropoietin response in patients with the anemia of cancer. N Engl J Med 322:1689–1692, 1990.

52. Kurzrock R, Talpaz M, Estey EH, et al: Erythropoietin treatment in patients with myelodysplastic syndrome and anemia. Leukemia 5:985–990, 1991.

53. Ludwig H, Fritz E, Kotzmann H, et al: Erythropoietin treatment of anemia associated with multiple myeloma. N Engl J Med 322:1693–1699, 1990.

54. Fischl M, Galpin JE, Levine JD, et al: Recombinant human erythropoietin for patients with AIDS treated with zidovudine. N Engl J Med 322:1488–1493, 1990.

55. Lotan R: Retinoids and squamous cell differentiation, in Hong WK, Lotan R (eds): Retinoids in Oncology, pp 43–72. New York, Marcel Dekker Inc, 1993.

56. Tanaka Y, Shima M, Yamoka K, et al: Synergistic effect of 1,25-dihydroxyvitamin D3 and retinoic acid in inducing U937 cell differentiation. J Nutr Sci Vitaminol (Tokyo) 38:415–426, 1992.

57. Bollag W, Peck R, Frey JR: Inhibition of proliferation by retinoids: Cytokines and their combination in four human transformed epithelial cell lines. Cancer Lett 62:167–172, 1992.

58. Sporn MB, Dunlop NM, Newton DL, et al: Prevention of chemical carcinogenesis by vitamin A and its synthetic analogs (retinoids). Fed Proc 35:1332–1338, 1976.

59. Lippman SM, Benner SE, Hong WK: Cancer chemoprevention. J Clin Oncol 12:851–873, 1994.

60. Benner SE, Pajak TF, Lippman SM, et al: Prevention of second primary tumors with isotretinoin in squamous cell carcinoma of the head and neck: Long term follow-up. J Natl Cancer Inst 86:140–141, 1994.

61. Hong WK, Lippman SM, Itri LM: Prevention of second primary tumors with isotretinoin in squamous cell carcinoma of the head and neck. N Engl J Med 323:825–827, 1990.

62. Pastorino V, Infante M, Maioli M, et al: Adjuvant treatment of stage I lung cancer with high dose vitamin A. J Clin Oncol 11:1216–1222, 1993.

63. Bolla M, Lefur R, Ton Van J, et al: Prevention of second primary tumors with etretinate in squamous cell carcinoma of oral cavity and oropharynx: Results of a multicentric, double-blind, randomized study. Eur J Cancer 30:767–772, 1994.

64. Benner SE, Lippman SM, Hong WK: Current status of retinoid chemoprevention of lung cancer. Oncology 9(3):205–210, 1995.

65. Grignani F, Fagioli M, Longo L, et al: Acute promyelocytic leukemia: From genetics to treatment. Blood 83:10–25, 1994.

66. Fenaux P: Management of acute promyelocytic leukemia. Eur J Haematol 50:65, 1993.

67. Degos L: Is acute promyelocytic leukemia a curable disease? Treatment strategy for long-term survival. Leukemia 8(S2):S6–8, 1994.

68. Warrel Jr RP, de The H, Wang ZY, et al: Acute promyelocytic leukemia. N Engl J Med 329:177, 1993.

69. Fenaux P, Chastang C, Degos L, et al: All-trans retinoic acid followed by intensive chemotherapy gives a high complete remission rate in prolonged remissions in newly diagnosed acute promyelocytic leukemia. Blood 80:2176–2181, 1993.

70. Kanamaru A, Takemoto Y, Tanimoto M, et al: All-trans retinoic acid for the treatment of newly diagnosed acute promyelocytic leukemia. Blood 85:1202–1206, 1995.

71. Lippman SM, Parkinson DR, Itri RS, et al: 13-Cis retinoic acid and interferon-2a: Effective combination therapy for advanced squamous cell carcinoma of the skin. J Natl Cancer Inst 84:235–240, 1992.

72. Lippman SM, Kavanagh JJ, Parades-Espinoza M, et al: 13-Cis retinoic acid plus interferon alpha-2a: Highly active systemic therapy

for squamous cell carcinoma of the cervix. J Natl Cancer Inst 84:241–245, 1992.

73. Cheng A, Su I, Chen C, et al: Use of retinoic acids in the treatment of peripheral T-cell lymphoma: A pilot study. J Clin Oncol 12:1185–1192, 1994.

74. Kurzrock R, Estey EH, Talpaz M: All-trans retinoic acid: Tolerance and biologic effects in myelodysplastic syndromes. J Clin Oncol 11:1489–1495, 1993.

75. Castleberry RP, Emanuel PD, Zuckerman KS: A pilot study of isotretinoin in the treatment of juvenile chronic myelogenous leukemia. N Engl J Med 331:1680–1684, 1994.

76. Frankel SR, Eardey A, Warrell Jr RP, et al: The 'retinoic acid syndrome' in acute promyelocytic leukemia. Ann Intern Med 117:292–296, 1992.

77. Dombret H, Sutton L, Degos L: Combined therapy with all-trans retinoic acid and high-dose chemotherapy in patients with hyperleukocytosis APL and severe visceral hemmorhage. Leukemia 6:1237–1242, 1992.

78. Koehler G, Milstein C: Continuous culture of fused cells secreting antibody of predefined specificity. Nature 256:495–496, 1975.

79. Dillman RO: Antibodies as cytotoxic therapy. J Clin Oncol 12(7):1497–1515, 1994.

80. Kuzel TM, Rosen ST: Antibodies in the treatment of human cancer. Curr Opin Oncol 6(6):622–626, 1994.

81. Caron PC, Scheinberg DA: Immunotherapy for acute leukemias. Curr Opin Oncol 6(1):14–22, 1994.

82. Warrell Jr RP, Frankel SR, Miller W, et al: Differentiation therapy of acute promyelocytic leukemia with tretinoin (all-trans retinoic acid). N Engl J Med 324:1385–1393, 1991.

83. Degos L, Chomienne C, Daniel MT, et al: Treatment of first relapse in acute promyelocytic leukemia with all-trans retinoic acid (letter). Lancet 336(8728):1440–1441, 1990.

84. Ohno R, Yoshida H, Fukutani H: Multi-institutional study of all-trans retinoic acid as a differentiation therapy of refractory acute promyelocytic leukemia. Leukemia 7:1722–1727, 1993.

85. Castaigne S, Chomienne C, Daniel MT: All-trans retinoic acid as a differentiation therapy for acute promyelocytic leukemias: I. Clinical results. Blood 76:1704–1709, 1990.

86. Huang ME, Yu-Chen Y, Shu-Rong C: Use of all-trans retinoic acid in the treatment of acute promyelocytic leukemia. Blood 72:567–572, 1988.

87. Kessler JF, Jones SE, Levine N: Isotretinoin and cutaneous helper T-cell lymphoma (mycosis fungoides). Arch Dermatol 123:201–204, 1987.

88. Hoting E, Meissner K: Arotinoid-ethylester: Effectiveness in refractory cutaneous T-cell lymphoma. Cancer 62(6):1044–1048, 1988.

89. Lippman SM, Meyskens FL: Activity of 13-cis retinoic acid (Accutane) in advanced squamous cell carcinoma of the skin. Ann Intern Med 107:449–501, 1987.

90. Scheinberg DA, Lovett D, Divgi CR, et al: A phase I trial of monoclonal antibody M195 in AML: Specific bone marrow targeting and internalization of radionuclide. J Clin Oncol 9:478–490,1991.

91. Waldmann TA, Goldmann CK, Bongiovanni KF, et al: Therapy of patients with human T-cell lymphotropic virus 1-induced adult T-cell leukemia with anti-tac, a monoclonal antibody to the receptor for IL-2. Blood 72:1805–1816, 1988.

92. Dyer MJS, Hale G, Hayhoe FGH, et al: Effects of CAMPATH-1 antibodies in vivo in patients with lymphoid malignancies: Influence of antibody isotype. Blood 73:1431–1439, 1989.

93. Caron PC, Co MS, Bull MK, et al: Biological and immunological features of humanized M195 (Anti-CD33) monoclonal antibodies. Cancer Res 52:6761–6767, 1992.

94. Schwartz MA, Lovett OR, Render A, et al: Dose-escalation trial of M195 labeled with iodine-131 for cytoreduction and marrow

ablation in relapsed or refractory myeloid leukemias. J Clin Oncol 11:294–303, 1993.

95. Vitetta ES, Thorpe PE, Uhr JW: Immunotoxins: Magic bullets or misguided missiles? Immunol Today 14:252–259, 1993.

96. Foon KA, Schroff RW, Bunn PA, et al: Effects of monoclonal antibody therapy in patients with chronic lymphocytic leukemia. Blood 64:1085–1093, 1984.

97. Klien B, Wijdenes J, Zhang XJ, et al: Murine anti-IL-6 monoclonal therapy for a patient with plasma cell leukemia. Blood 78:1198–1204, 1991.

98. Hu F, Epstein AL, Naeve GS, et al: A phase Ia clinical trial of Lym-1 monoclonal antibody serotherapy in patients with refractory B-cell malignancies. Hematol Oncol 7:155–166, 1989.

99. Brown SL, Miller RA, Horning SJ, ET al: Treatment of B-cell lymphomas with anti-idiotype antibodies alone and in combination with alpha interferon. Blood 73:651–661, 1989.

100. Miller RA, Oseroff AR, Stratte PT, et al: Monoclonal antibody therapeutic trials in seven patients with T-cell lymphoma. Blood 62:988–995, 1983.

101. Dillman RO, Shawler DL, Dillman JB, et al: Therapy of chronic lymphocytic leukemia and cutaneous lymphoma with T101 monoclonal antibody. J Clin Oncol 2:881–891, 1984.

102. Kaminski MS, Zasadny KR, Francis IR, et al: Radioimmunotherapy of B-cell lymphoma with [131I]anti-B1 (anti-CD20) antibody. N Engl J Med 329:459–465, 1993.

103. Press OW, Eary JF, Appelbaum FR, et al: Radiolabelled-antibody therapy of B-cell lymphoma with autologous bone marrow support. N Engl J Med 329:1219–1224, 1993.

104. Ryan KP, Dillman RO, DeNardo SJ, et al: Breast cancer imaging with In-111 human IgM monoclonal antibodies. Radiology 167:71–75, 1988.

105. Halpern SE, Dillman RO: Radioimmunodetection with monoclonal antibodies against prostatic acid phosphatase, in Winkler C (ed): Nuclear Medicine in Clinical Oncology, pp 164–170. Berlin, Springer-Verlag, 1986.

106. Goodman GE, Hellstrom I, Brodzinsky I, et al: Phase I trial of murine monoclonal antibody L6 in breast, colon, ovarian, and lung cancer. J Clin Oncol 8:1083–1092, 1990.

107. Jacobs AJ, Fer M, Su FM, et al: A phase I trial of rhenium 186-labeled monoclonal antibody administered intraperitoneally in ovarian carcinoma: Toxicity and clinical response. Obstet Gynecol 82:586–593, 1993.

108. Dillman RO, Beauregard J, Ryan KP, et al: Radioimmunodetection of cancer using indium-labeled monoclonal antibodies: International symposium on labeled and unlabeled antibodies in cancer diagnosis and therapy. Natl Cancer Inst Monogr 3:33–36, 1987.

109. Sears HF, Herlyn D, Steplewski Z, et al: Phase II clinical trial of a murine monoclonal antibody cytotoxic for gastrointestinal adenocarcinoma. Cancer Res 45:5910–5913, 1985.

110. Mellstedt H, Frodin J-E, Mascci G, et al: The therapeutic use of monoclonal antibodies in colorectal carcinoma. Semin Oncol 18:462–477, 1991.

111. Takahashi T, Toshiharu Y, Kitamura K, et al: Follow-up study of patients treated with antibody drug conjugate: Report of 77 cases with colorectal cancer. Jpn J Cancer Res 84:976–981, 1993.

112. Halpern SE, Dillman RO, Witztum KF, et al: Radioimmunodetection of melanoma utilizing 111-In-96.5 monoclonal antibody: A preliminary report. Radiology 155:493–499, 1985.

113. Houghton AN, Mintzer D, Cordon-Caro C, et al: Mouse monoclonal IgG3 antibody detecting GD3 ganglioside: A phase I trial in patients with malignant melanoma. Proc Natl Acad Sci U S A 82:1242–1246, 1985.

114. Lynch Jr TJ: Immunotoxin therapy of small-cell lung cancer. Chest 103:436–439S, 1993.

CHAPTER 38

Current Treatment of Infection in the Neutropenic Patient

Kenneth V.I. Rolston, MD

Section of Infectious Diseases, Department of Medical Specialties
The University of Texas M. D. Anderson Cancer Center, Houston, Texas

Neutropenia was recognized almost 3 decades ago as a major predisposing factor for the development of infection in patients with cancer.[1] The risk begins to increase when the neutrophil count drops below 1,000/mm³ and is greatest at counts of 100/mm³ or lower. At this level, approximately 20% of febrile episodes are caused by a bacteremic process.[2]

The increasing use of more intensive chemotherapeutic regimens to achieve maximal antitumor activity has produced severe and prolonged neutropenia in many patients. Some regimens used for remission induction in acute leukemia (eg, high-dose cytarabine) are associated with severe oropharyngeal mucositis and gastrointestinal toxicity, resulting in infection caused by enteric organisms and by organisms colonizing the oropharynx (eg, streptococci). The skin, which is often breached by vascular access devices and invasive procedures, serves as a portal of entry. The paranasal sinuses also have been recognized as important sites of infection in neutropenic patients.

PREDOMINANT BACTERIAL PATHOGENS AND CHANGING EPIDEMIOLOGY

Neutropenic patients are presumed to have developed an infection when they become febrile. However, it is not always possible to document an infection in these patients. Currently at The University of Texas M. D. Anderson Cancer Center, an infection can be documented in approximately 47% of patients with fever and neutropenia, whereas 53% are considered to have fever of undetermined origin.[3] The frequency of microbiologically documented infections differs from institution to institution and is influenced by factors such as the usage of prophylactic antibiotics in high-risk patients: Institutions that routinely use prophylactic antibiotics will probably have a lower incidence of microbiologically documented infections.

There have been several epidemiologic shifts in the types of microorganisms causing infection in neutropenic patients. Coagulase-negative staphylococci, *Staphylococcus aureus*, the enterococci, and the streptococci (particularly alpha-hemolytic [viridans] streptococci) are currently the most common gram-positive patho-

gens.[4] Most staphylococcal infections are cutaneous in origin, and most enterococcal infections arise in the gastrointestinal tract. However, some infections caused by *Staphylococcus epidermidis* are gastrointestinal in origin.[5] *Corynebacterium jeikeium* and *Bacillus* species are isolated less often but are capable of causing serious infections.

Although *Escherichia coli*, *Klebsiella* species, and *Pseudomonas aeruginosa* are still frequently isolated, heavy antibiotic use in neutropenic patients has led to the emergence of other, often resistant, gram-negative organisms in these patients (Table 1). While many institutions have reported a decreased incidence of *P aeruginosa* infections in recent years, it remains an important pathogen at some centers and is currently the third most frequently isolated gram-negative pathogen at M. D. Anderson.[3]

Gram-negative bacilli that have emerged as pathogens in recent times include *Acinetobacter calcoaceticus*; *Citrobacter*, *Enterobacter*, and *Serratia* species; and *Xanthomonas maltophilia*.[6–8] Other uncommon but significant gram-negative pathogens include *Alcaligenes* species, *Aeromonas hydrophila*, *Flavobacterium meningosepticum*, and *Flavimonas oryzihabitans*.[9–11]

INITIAL MANAGEMENT

Febrile neutropenic patients are often difficult to evaluate. Fever, which is occasionally low-grade (< 38°C), may be the only manifestation of a serious infection. As a result of an impaired inflammatory response, clinical signs of infection may be undetectable even on a thorough physical examination. Absence of evidence of infection on physical examination does not, however, exclude the possibility of infection.[12]

All appropriate sites (eg, blood, urine, stools) should be cultured prior to the administration of antibiotics. These procedures should be done as expeditiously as possible and should not cause a delay of more than 30 to 40 minutes in the administration of antibiotic therapy. Infections often develop and progress rapidly in neutropenic patients and can cause death if antibiotics are not administered promptly. A recent review of *P aeruginosa* infections from M. D. Anderson clearly demonstrated

TABLE I

Bacterial Pathogens in Neutropenic Patients

Common gram-positive pathogens

Staphylococcus aureus

Coagulase-negative staphylococci

 Staphylococcus epidermidis
 Staphylococcus haemolyticus
 Staphylococcus hominis

Enterococcus species

Streptococcus species

 Alpha hemolytic (viridans) streptococci
 Streptococcus pyogenes

Uncommon but significant gram-positive pathogens

 Corynebacterium jeikeium
 Bacillus species
 Streptococcus—Group G
 Streptococcus pneumoniae

Common gram-negative pathogens

 Escherichia coli
 Klebsiella species
 Pseudomonas aeruginosa
 Enterobacter species
 Citrobacter species
 Xanthomonas maltophilia
 Acinetobacter species

Uncommon but significant gram-negative pathogens

 Serratia marcescens
 Flavobacterium meningosepticum
 Alcaligenes species
 Flavimonas oryzihabitans
 Aeromonas hydrophila

the efficacy of prompt antibiotic therapy. The response rate was 74% when antipseudomonal therapy was given during the first 24 hours but fell to 46% if there was a delay of more than 24 to 48 hours.[13] Prompt, empiric, broad-spectrum antimicrobial therapy has, therefore, become standard.

Initial Antibiotic Regimens

Other properties of antibiotics that should be taken into consideration when selecting empiric regimens are listed in Table 2. A number of combination regimens have been proposed for the treatment of febrile episodes in neutropenic patients.[14] These regimens have been used successfully for many years and are modified to account for the availability of improved antibiotics that are less toxic, more potent, or more favorable pharmacokinetically.

Aminoglycoside-Containing Combinations: The combination of an antipseudomonal carboxypenicillin (ticarcillin [Ticar]) or ureidopenicillin (mezlocillin [Mezlin], piperacillin [Pipracil], azlocillin) with an aminoglycoside (gentamicin, tobramycin, amikacin) has for many years been considered standard initial therapy for the febrile neutropenic patient and has been widely used. More recently, aminoglycosides have been successfully employed in combination with extended-spectrum cephalosporins such as cefoperazone (Cefobid) and ceftazidime (Table 3).[15–17] These regimens produce response rates ranging from 71% to 76%.

The advantages of such combination regimens include a broad antimicrobial spectrum, minimal emergence of resistance during therapy, and the potential for synergistic activity against some gram-negative bacilli. Disadvantages include the toxicity generally associated with aminoglycosides (nephrotoxicity, ototoxicity) and lack of activity against many gram-positive organisms. Cancer patients are often elderly and are thus more susceptible to aminoglycoside toxicity. Many are already receiving other ototoxic and nephrotoxic drugs (amphotericin B [Fungizone], cisplatin [Platinol], cyclosporine [Sandimmune]), and administering aminoglycosides to these patients increases the risk of toxicity.

Double Beta-Lactam Combinations: Since beta-lactam antibiotics were found to have more consistent activity than aminoglycosides in neutropenic patients, regimens combining two beta-lactams were devised in an attempt to retain the advantages of combination therapy while avoiding aminoglycoside toxicity. Using a cephalosporin in combination with a carboxypenicillin (carbenicillin [Geocillin], ticarcillin) provided a broad-spectrum regimen with activity against organisms such as *Klebsiella* species, which were resistant to the carboxypenicillins. These broad-spectrum regimens were shown to be as effective as aminoglycoside-based regimens.[18]

With the availability of the ureidopenicillins (which are active against *Klebsiella* species) and the extended-spectrum cephalosporins (some of which can be used as single agents in neutropenic patients), the rationale for double beta-lactam combinations may need to be re-examined. Nevertheless, a large number of double beta-lactam combinations, including cefoperazone plus mezlocillin, cefoperazone plus piperacillin, ceftazidime plus piperacillin, ceftazidime plus ticarcillin/clavulanate (Timentin), and cefoperazone plus aztreonam (Azactam), have been found to be highly effective and well tolerated by patients.[19–21]

The limitations of double beta-lactam combinations include their relatively high cost, the rare possibility of antagonism, and the occasional emergence of resistant organisms such as *Enterobacter* and *Citrobacter* species. These combinations are also less than optimal against some currently prevalent gram-positive organisms (coagulase-negative staphylococci, methicillin-resistant staphylococci, and some viridans streptococci), but current evidence indicates that the addition of specific therapy (vancomycin) when such organisms are isolated or strongly suspected is almost always successful against the infections.

Vancomycin-Containing Combinations: Due to the resurgence of resistant gram-positive organisms in most cancer treatment centers, beta-lactam agents such as ceftazidime and aztreonam (with or without an aminoglycoside) have been evaluated in combination with vancomycin.[22–24] Although these regimens are effective, there are conflicting opinions regarding the initial use of vancomycin. Including vancomycin in the initial regimen may provide effective treatment for many gram-positive infections earlier in the course of a febrile episode, thus avoiding the need to wait for culture results or a clinical response. Vancomycin-containing regimens have been associated with shorter duration of fever (9 days vs 14 days) and quicker defervescence (61% within 24 hours vs 21% within 24 hours) in patients with gram-positive infections.[25] However, as a result, many patients receive vancomycin without a clear indication.

Another approach is to add vancomycin to the regimen

TABLE 2

Important Considerations for the Selection of Antibiotics in Neutropenic Patients

1. Antimicrobial spectrum

2. Bactericidal activity

3. Efficacy in neutropenic patients

4. Pharmacokinetic properties
   Tissue penetration
   Serum half-life
   Route of excretion

5. Toxicity

6. Cost

7. Potential for synergism/antagonism

8. Potential for emergence of resistance

9. Local prevalence/susceptibility pattern

TABLE 3

Overall Response Rates With Various Regimens in Febrile Neutropenic Patients

Regimen	% Response [a]
Amikacin + ceftazidime	71
Amikacin + cefoperazone	73
Amikacin + imipenem	76
Tobramycin + ceftazidime	71
Cefoperazone + aztreonam	77
Cefoperazone + piperacillin	75
Ceftazidime + piperacillin	74
Cefoperazone + mezlocillin	78 [b]
Vancomycin + aztreonam	
Vancomycin + ceftazidime	77
Vancomycin + ticarcillin/clavulanate	70
Cefoperazone	77
Ceftazidime	60
Ceftazidime	30
Ceftazidime	59
Imipenem	72
Imipenem	82

[a] All response rates shown are without modification of initial regimen
[b] Some patients were not neutropenic

only if gram-positive bacteria have been isolated and no clinical response has occurred after a few days of therapy. Several studies have shown that this approach is not associated with increased mortality and that its advantages include limiting the cost of therapy, avoiding vancomycin toxicity, and possibly reducing the potential for vancomycin resistance.

It is prudent to use vancomycin initially if an infection with methicillin-resistant staphylococci is strongly suspected or if these staphylococci are frequently isolated in the institution. There is also some evidence that infections caused by alpha-hemolytic (viridans) streptococci might respond better if treated initially with vancomycin. Otherwise, the addition of vancomycin to regimens is usually adequate if gram-positive organisms are isolated and the patient is not responding to existing therapy.

Monotherapy: The availability of broad-spectrum cephalosporins and carbapenems has made it possible to evaluate initial therapy with a single agent. Several recent studies have shown that single-agent therapy is safe and at least as effective as aminoglycoside-containing regimens or double beta-lactam combinations.[15,17,26] Winston and colleagues compared cefoperazone and ceftazidime, each combined with piperacillin, with imipenem alone in febrile neutropenic patients. The two double beta-lactam regimens were associated with response rates of 74% and

75%, respectively, while the response rate with imipenem alone was 82%.[19] Imipenem was also shown to be as effective as two aminoglycoside-containing combinations, ceftazidime plus amikacin and imipenem plus amikacin, in a study from M. D. Anderson.[17] This study also demonstrated that monotherapy with imipenem was superior to that with ceftazidime (72% vs 59% response rate).

The role of the extended-spectrum cephalosporins for single-agent therapy needs to be reexamined since they are only moderately active against many gram-positive organisms, and there are increasing reports of the emergence of resistance to these drugs among gram-negative bacilli such as *Enterobacter* and *Klebsiella* species. Patients on monotherapy need close monitoring for lack of response, emergence of resistance, or development of superinfections.

Other Approaches: The availability of newer broad-spectrum quinolones, such as ciprofloxacin (Cipro) and ofloxacin (Floxin) has made it possible to evaluate combinations of these agents with other antibiotics for febrile episodes in neutropenic patients. Ciprofloxacin has been combined with aminoglycosides, beta-lactam agents, and vancomycin and has also been used as a single agent.[27–31] Initial results with quinolone-containing combinations are promising, but further clinical experience will be necessary before they can be considered standard therapy. Currently available quinolones should not be used as single agents, because many staphylococci are now resistant to them and because they have limited activity against streptococci. The therapeutic use of quinolones also is limited by their widespread administration for prophylaxis against infection.

One approach to achieving maximal initial therapeutic effect and reducing toxicity is to initiate therapy with an aminoglycoside-containing combination and to discontinue the aminoglycoside after 72 to 96 hours. However, one study conducted by the European Organization for Research and Treatment of Cancer (EORTC) showed reduced efficacy in patients who were treated with a short-course combination regimen.[16] This approach needs further evaluation and should not be abandoned before a definitive study evaluating its role has been conducted.

Another approach is once-daily administration of the aminoglycoside rather than conventional (three-times-a-day) administration. This approach needs fuller evaluation in neutropenic patients.

Not all neutropenic patients have the same risk for developing infections or infection-related complications. Recently, investigators from the Dana-Farber Cancer Institute have developed a clinical model for predicting the medical risk of cancer patients with fever and neutropenia.[32,33] Using this model, four risk groups were identified. Patients in the highest risk group were those who had already been hospitalized when they developed fever. The incidence of serious complications in these patients was 34% and the mortality rate was 23%. At somewhat lower risk were outpatients with concurrent comorbidity (eg, hypotension, bleeding, altered mental status, hypercalcemia) or uncontrolled cancer. However, approximately 40% of febrile neutropenic patients were considered "low-risk." These were outpatients without comorbidity and with cancers that were responsive to antineoplastic therapy. Only 2% of these patients developed complications, and none died.

At M. D. Anderson, we have treated low-risk neutropenic patients with either an intravenous regimen (aztreonam plus clindamycin) or an oral regimen (ciprofloxacin plus clindamycin) without hospital admission.[34] Patients with significant infections and the elderly were not excluded, and in our initial trial 39% had microbiologically documented infections. The overall response rates were 88% for the oral regimen and 95% for the intravenous regimen, producing a combined response rate of 92% for outpatient antibiotic therapy. No patients developed hypotension or septic shock, and there were no infection-related deaths. Three patients on the oral regimen developed reversible acute renal failure.

In an ongoing follow-up trial of outpatient/home antibiotic therapy, a response rate of 90% was achieved using the same intravenous regimen or a slightly different oral regimen (ciprofloxacin plus amoxicillin/potassium clavulanate [Augmentin]). No serious complications and no infection-related deaths have occurred in this trial to date.[35]

Our experience indicates that with careful patient selection, appropriate antibiotic therapy, and close patient follow-up, low-risk febrile neutropenic patients can be treated safely without admission to the hospital. Although this approach is currently not considered standard practice and needs to be more thoroughly evaluated, it results in a considerable reduction in the cost of therapy, better utilization of resources, improved quality of life for patients and families, and the potential for reducing nosocomial superinfections caused by resistant bacteria and fungi.

Duration Of Therapy

The optimal duration of antibiotic therapy for febrile neutropenic patients continues to be debated. Some experts recommend continuation of therapy until the resolution of neutropenia, even if a prompt response renders the patient afebrile.[36] This approach requires prolonged administration of broad-spectrum antibiotics and probably increases the potential for the development of superinfections caused by resistant bacteria or fungi. It may also increase drug toxicity and the overall cost of therapy due to prolonged hospitalization.

Another approach is to discontinue antibiotic therapy in patients who have been treated for a minimum of 7 to 9 days, are clinically stable, have no evidence of active infection, and have been afebrile for 4 to 5 days but have persistent neutropenia. At M. D. Anderson, antibiotic therapy has been discontinued in stable, afebrile but neutropenic patients for the past 20 years, with resulting favorable response rates and low levels of superinfection and relapse.[3]

OTHER THERAPEUTIC MODALITIES

About 15% to 20% of infections in neutropenic patients fail to respond to antimicrobial therapy. In most cases, profound neutropenia persists, and patients remain febrile despite adjustments in antibacterial therapy and the addition of an antifungal agent. The role of granulocyte transfusions in such patients has been evaluated, with conflicting results. This approach has largely been abandoned due to technical problems, the incidence of reactions, failure to demonstrate a clear therapeutic benefit, and the potential for transmitting infections such as cytomegalovirus from the donor to the recipient.

The hematopoietic growth factors and other cytokines may yet play a significant role in the prevention and treatment of infections in neutropenic patients. These agents produce both quantitative and qualitative effects that could be beneficial. Granuloctye-macrophage colony-stimulating factor (GM-CSF, sargramostim [Leukine]) promotes the production of neutrophils and mononuclear cells. Granulocyte colony-stimulating factor (G-CSF, filgrastim [Neupogen]) and macrophage colony-stimulating factor (M-CSF) are narrower in their spectrum of activity, promoting the production of neutrophils or of mononuclear cells (ie, monocytes and macrophages) alone. The hematopoietic growth factors and other cytokines may act independently or in concert to improve the phagocytic functions of neutrophils and mononuclear cells against specific bacterial and fungal pathogens.[37]

A number of studies with GM-CSF and G-CSF in patients with solid tumors, leukemia, and autologous bone marrow transplantation following cytotoxic chemotherapy have shown that patients receiving these agents have a reduced period of neutropenia, decreased number of days with fever, and fewer defined infections.[38–44] These agents should not be used routinely in

TABLE 4

Infection Prevention in Neutropenic Patients

Suppression of endogenous flora

Nonabsorbable oral antibiotics
Absorbable oral antibiotics
Systemic antibiotics?

Prevention against acquisition of new organisms

Protected environments and other isolation techniques
Hand washing
Well-cooked foods with low bacterial content

patients who are neutropenic for less than 10 days, since the risk of infection in such patients is smaller and the response to conventional antibiotic therapy greater than in patients with more prolonged neutropenia.[45]

PREVENTION OF INFECTION

The high frequency of infection in cancer patients with myelosuppression has led to the development of programs for preventing infection. The two main strategies used are directed toward suppressing the endogenous microflora (from which up to 80% of infections in neutropenic patients arise) and preventing the acquisition of new organisms from environmental sources (Table 4). The former objective is usually achieved by administering prophylactic antibiotic regimens during periods of myelosuppression. The potential adverse effects of antimicrobial prophylaxis must be measured against its benefits. Many experts believe that the use of prophylactic antimicrobial regimens tilts the balance toward more resistant components of the bacterial and fungal flora, and these regimens generally have not been associated with a reduction in mortality.

The acquisition of new organisms from environmental sources can to some extent be prevented or reduced by various techniques, including strict hand-washing precautions, the use of well-cooked diets (which reduce contamination with gram-negative bacteria), and various isolation techniques or protected environments. In some instances, appropriate and effective prophylaxis against infection can obviate empiric therapy.[46,47]

SUMMARY

Infection continues to be a serious problem in patients with profound neutropenia. Advances in antibacterial therapy have enabled us to treat most common bacterial infections successfully. However, the spectrum of bacterial infection in these patients continues to change, requiring continued vigilance and the development of new strategies for infection prevention and therapy. The emergence of multidrug-resistant organisms will continue to challenge us for years to come. Generally, we need to focus more on infection prevention, as opposed to the treatment of established infections.

REFERENCES

1. Bodey GP, Buckley M, Sathe YS, et al: Quantitative relationships between circulating leukocytes and infections in patients with acute leukemia. Ann Intern Med 64:328–340, 1966.

2. Schimpff SC: Empiric antibiotic therapy for granulocytopenic cancer patients. Am J Med 80(suppl 5C):13–20, 1986.

3. Rolston KVI, Bodey GP: Infections in patients with cancer, in Holland JF, Frei E, Bast RC, et al (eds): Cancer Medicine, pp 2416–2441. Philadelphia, Lea & Febiger, 1993.

4. Koll BS, Brown AE: The changing epidemiology of infections at cancer hospitals. Clin Infect Dis 17(suppl 2):322–327, 1993.

5. Wade JC, Schimpff SC, Newman KA, et al: Staphylococcus epidermidis: An increasing cause of infection in patients with granulocytopenia. Ann Intern Med 97:503–508, 1982.

6. Rolston KVI, Guan Z, Bodey GP, et al: Acinetobacter calcoaeticus septicemia in patients with cancer. South Med J 78:647–651, 1985.

7. Bodey GP, Elting LS, Rodriguez S: Bacteremia caused by Enterobacter: 15 years of experience in a cancer hospital. Rev Infect Dis 13:550–558, 1991.

8. Elting LS, Bodey GP: Septicemia due to Xanthomonas species and nonaeruginosa Pseudomonas species: Increasing incidence of catheter-related infections. Medicine (Baltimore) 69:296–306, 1990.

9. Rolston KVI, Zandvliet SE, Rodriguez S, et al: Spectrum of Aeromonas and Plesiomonas infections in patients with cancer and AIDS. Experentia 47:437–439, 1991.

10. Rolston K, Tarrand J, Rubenstein EB, et al: Flavimonas oryzihabitans: An emerging pathogen in cancer patients (abstract 1134). 6th European Congress of Clinical Microbiology and Infectious Diseases. Seville, Spain, March 28–31, 1993.

11. Decker CF, Simon GL, Keiser JF: Flavimonas oryzihabitans (Pseudomonas oryzihabitans: CDC Group Ve-2) bacteremia in the immunocompromised host. Arch Intern Med 151:603–604, 1991.

12. Sickles EA, Greene WH, Wiernik PH: Clinical presentation of infection in granulocytopenic patients. Arch Intern Med 135:715–719, 1975.

13. Bodey GP, Jadeja L, Elting L: Pseudomonas bacteremia: Retrospective analysis of 410 episodes. Arch Intern Med 145:1621–1629, 1985.

14. Hughes WT, Armstrong D, Bodey GP, et al, for the Working Committee, Infectious Diseases Society of America: Guidelines for the use of antimicrobial agents in neutropenic patients with unexplained fever. J Infect Dis 161:381–396, 1990.

15. Fainstein V, Bodey GP, Elting L, et al: A randomized study of ceftazidime compared to ceftazidime and tobramycin for the treatment of infections in cancer patients. J Antimicrob Chemother 12(suppl A):101–110, 1983.

16. European Organization for Research and Treatment of Cancer (EORTC) International Antimicrobial Therapy Cooperative Group: Ceftazidime combined with a short or long course of amikacin for empirical therapy of gram-negative bacteremia in cancer patients with granulocytopenia. N Engl J Med 317:1692–1698, 1987.

17. Rolston KVI, Berkey P, Bodey GP, et al: A comparison of imipenem to ceftazidime with or without amikacin as empiric therapy in febrile neutropenic patients. Arch Intern Med 152:283–291, 1992.

18. Anaissie EJ, Fainstein V, Bodey GP, et al: Randomized trial of beta-lactam regimens in febrile neutropenic cancer patients. Am J Med 84:581–589, 1988.

19. Winston DJ, Ho WG, Bruckner DA, et al: Beta-lactam antibiotic therapy in febrile granulocytopenic patients: A randomized trial comparing cefoperazone plus piperacillin, ceftazidime plus piperacillin, and imipenem alone. Ann Intern Med 115:849–859, 1991.

20. Jones P, Bodey GP, Rolston K, et al: Cefoperazone plus mezlocillin for empiric therapy of febrile cancer patients. Am J Med 85(suppl 1A):3–8, 1988.

21. Bodey GP, Fainstein V, Elting LS, et al: Beta-lactam regimens for febrile neutropenic patients. Cancer 65:9–16, 1990.

22. Jones PG, Rolston KV, Fainstein V, et al: Aztreonam therapy in neutropenic patients with cancer. Am J Med 81:243–248, 1986.

23. European Organization for Research and Treatment of Cancer (EORTC) International Antimicrobial Therapy Cooperative Group: Vancomycin added to empirical combination antibiotic therapy for fever in granulocytopenic cancer patients. J Infect Dis 163:951–958, 1991.

24. Karp JE, Hick JD, Angelopulos C, et al: Empiric use of vancomycin during prolonged treatment-induced granulocytopenia. Am J Med 81:237–242, 1986.

25. Rubin M, Hathorn JW, Marshall D, et al: Gram-positive infections and the use of vancomycin in episodes of fever and neutropenia. Ann Intern Med 108:30–35, 1988.

26. Pizzo PA, Hathorn JW, Hiemenz J, et al: A randomized trial comparing ceftazidime alone with combination antibiotic therapy in cancer patients with fever and neutropenia. N Engl J Med 315:552–558, 1986.

27. Rolston KVI, Haron E, Cunningham C, et al: Intravenous ciprofloxacin for infections in cancer patients. Am J Med 87(5A):261S–265S, 1989.

28. Chan CC, Oppenheim BA, Anderson H, et al: Randomized trial comparing ciprofloxacin plus netilmicin versus piperacillin plus netilmicin for empiric treatment of fever in neutropenic patients. Antimicrob Agents Chemother 33:87–91, 1989.

29. Flaherty JP, Waitley D, Edlin B, et al: Multicenter, randomized trial of ciprofloxacin plus azlocillin versus ceftazidime plus amikacin for empiric treatment of febrile neutropenic patients. Am J Med 87(5A):278S–282S, 1989.

30. Smith GM, Leyland MJ, Farrell ID, et al: A clinical, microbiological and pharmacokinetic study of ciprofloxacin plus vancomycin as initial therapy of febrile episodes in neutropenic patients. J Antimicrob Chemother 21:647–655, 1988.

31. Meunier F, Zinner SH, Gaya H, et al: Prospective randomized evaluation of ciprofloxacin versus piperacillin plus amikacin for empiric antibiotic therapy of febrile granulocytopenic cancer patients with lymphomas and solid tumors. Antimicrob Agents Chemother 35:873–878, 1991.

32. Talcott JA, Finberg R, Mayer RJ, et al: The medical course of cancer patients with fever and neutopenia. Arch Intern Med 148:2561–2568, 1988.

33. Talcott JA, Siegel RD, Finberg R, et al: Risk assessment in cancer patients with fever and neutropenia: A prospective, two-center validation of a prediction rule. J Clin Oncol 10:316–322, 1992.

34. Rubenstein EBR, Rolston K, Benjamin RS, et al: Outpatient treatment of febrile episodes in low-risk neutropenic patients with cancer. Cancer 71:3640–3646, 1993.

35. Rolston K, Rubenstein E, Frisbee-Hume S, et al: Outpatient treatment of febrile episodes in low-risk neutropenic cancer patients (abstract). Proc Am Soc Clin Oncol 29:1505.

36. Pizzo PA, Robichaud KJ, Gill FA, et al: Duration of empiric

antibiotic therapy in granulocytopenic patients with cancer. Am J Med 67:194–200, 1979.

37. Roilides E, Pizzo PA: Perspectives on the use of cytokines in the management of infectious complications of cancer. Clin Infect Dis 17(suppl 2):385–389, 1993.

38. Nemunaitis J, Rainowe SN, Singer JW, et al: Recombinant granulocyte-macrophage colony-stimulating factor after autologous bone marrow transplantation for lymphoid cancer. N Engl J Med 324:1773–1778, 1991.

39. Antiman KS, GriffinJD, Elias A, et al: Effect of recombinant human granuloctye-macrophage colony-stimulating factor on chemotherapy-induced myelosuppression. N Engl J Med 319:593–598, 1988.

40. Lieschke GJ, Maher D, Cebon J, et al: Effects of bacterially synthesized recombinant human granulocyte-macrophage colony-stimulating factor in patients with advanced malignancy. Ann Intern Med 110:357–364, 1989.

41. Bronchud MH, Scarffe H, Thatcher N, et al: Phase I/II study of recombinant human granulocyte colony-stimulating factor in patients receiving intensive chemotherapy for small cell lung cancer. Br J Cancer 56:808–813, 1987.

42. Morystyn G, Campbell L, Souza LM, et al: Effect of granulocyte colony-stimulating factor on neutropenia induced by cytotoxic chemotherapy. Lancet 1:667–672, 1988.

43. Gabrilove JL, Jakubowski A, Scher H, et al: Effect of granulocyte colony-stimulating factor on neutropenia and associated morbidity due to chemotherapy for transitional-cell carcinoma of the urothelium. N Engl J Med 318:1414–1422, 1988.

44. Yoshida T, Nakamura S, Ohtake S, et al: Effect of granulocyte colony-stimulating factor on neutropenia due to chemotherapy for non-Hodgkin's lymphoma. Cancer 66:1904–1909, 1990.

45. Pizzo PA: Management of fever in patients with cancer and treatment-induced neutropenia. N Engl J Med 328:1322–1332, 1993.

46. Bodey GP: Current status of prophylaxis of infection with protected environments. Am J Med 76:678–684, 1984.

47. Verhoef J: Prevention of infections in the neutropenic patient. Clin Infect Dis 17(suppl 2):359–367, 1993.

CHAPTER 39

Management of Fungal and Viral Infections in Cancer Patients

Ricardo F. Garcia, MD, *and* Kenneth V.I. Rolston, MD

Section of Infectious Diseases, Department of Medical Specialties
The University of Texas M. D. Anderson Cancer Center, Houston, Texas

With the advent of modern therapeutic and prophylactic regimens, bacterial infections have become more effectively controlled, while fungal and viral infections have emerged as more prominent complications in the management of immuno-compromised patients. Now that newer antifungal and antiviral drugs are available, early diagnosis and treatment should result in a significant decrease in morbidity and mortality associated with these infections. However, because therapy is still suboptimal, primary prevention remains an important consideration.

FUNGAL INFECTIONS

Fungal infections have become a leading cause of morbidity and mortality in cancer patients.[1] One particular problem in the management of these infections is that early diagnosis is difficult, so treatment may be delayed, which often leads to a poor clinical outcome.[2]

Cancer patients commonly have neutropenia, cellular immune defects, and indwelling catheters, characteristics that make them an ideal target for the development of fungal infections (Table 1).

Candidiasis

Candidiasis is the most common nosocomial mycosis,[3] with *Candida albicans* representing half of all fungal isolates in cancer patients.[1] Recently, other species, such as *C tropicalis, C parapsilosis, C krusei,* and *C lusitaniae,* have emerged as important pathogens.[4] Possible explanations for the high incidence of candidal infections are mucosal damage resulting from chemotherapy, increased use of broad-spectrum antibiotics, prolonged neutropenia associated with more aggressive chemotherapy, use of corticosteroids, and the presence of central venous catheters.[1,5] Neutropenia is probably the most important of these factors.[6] Currently, it is believed that the majority of candidal infections in cancer patients originate from an endogenous source, such as the gastrointestinal tract. However, there are also exogenous sources. The intensive care unit is a typical setting for exogenous infection, where the transmission of infection through the hands of health-care workers has been demonstrated.[7] Candidiasis includes mucocutaneous candidiasis, candidemia,

acute disseminated candidiasis, and chronic disseminated candidiasis.[8] Treatment will depend on these distinctions (Table 2).

Mucosal Candidiasis: Oropharyngeal candidiasis is common in patients undergoing chemotherapy, especially if the regimen contains corticosteroids. Classically, the infection presents with creamy white patches and ulcers in the oral mucosa; however, the definitive diagnosis is based on a wet mount or gram stain and culture of the lesions. The initial treatment can be topical clotrimazole (Mycelex). For refractory or more severe cases, ketoconazole (Nizoral), 400 mg orally every day, and fluconazole (Diflucan), 100 mg orally every day, are equally effective.[9]

Esophageal candidiasis also is associated with cytotoxic chemotherapy and corticosteroids. Other important factors are mediastinal radiation and esophageal herpes. Clinically, the infection is manifested as dysphagia. Oral thrush may be absent in up to 30% of patients.[10] The definitive diagnosis is made by esophagoscopy with mucosal brushing or biopsy. In cases in which this procedure is contraindicated, empirical treatment with ketoconazole, 400 to 600 mg orally every day, or fluconazole, 100 to 400 mg orally every day, should be started.[8] Alternatively, amphotericin B (Fungizone), 0.3 to 0.4 mg/kg/d, may be used. Treatment should be continued for at least 2 to 3 weeks after symptoms resolve.

Candidiasis of the genitourinary tract usually starts as candiduria, which can be secondary to either upper or lower urinary tract infection. The presence of candiduria in the neutropenic patient frequently is associated with disseminated infection. Amphotericin B, at a dose of 0.5 to 1 mg/kg/d, is the treatment of choice for neutropenic patients.[8,9] Fluconazole is a good alternative because it concentrates well in the urine. If urinary catheters or stents are present, they should be removed when possible. Washout of the bladder with amphotericin B may be useful, but it is reserved for cases in which disseminated or renal infection has been ruled out.[11]

Candidemia: Candida spp in blood cultures from neutropenic patients are unlikely to be contaminants,[12] and in some cases they can be the manifestation of disseminated infection. Even non-neutropenic patients

TABLE I

Fungal and Viral Infections Associated With Defects in Host-Defense Mechanisms

Malignancy/intervention	Defects in host-defense mechanisms	Associated infection
Acute leukemia	Neutropenia	*Candida, Aspergillus*
Lymphoma	Cellular immune deficiency	*Cryptococcus,* VZV
Bone marrow transplantation	Increased activity of suppressor T-lymphocytes	CMV, VZV, HSV, adenovirus
Cancer chemotherapy	Mucositis, neutropenia, impaired cellular and humoral immunity	*Candida, Aspergillus*
Corticosteroids	Monocytopenia, lymphopenia, decreased inflammation, defective phagocytic function	Adversely affect all infections; predisposition to *Aspergillus*
Therapeutic irradiation	Impaired lymphocyte function, neutropenia, mucositis	VZV
Vascular catheter	Skin breakdown	*Candida*

VZV = varicella zoster virus, CMV = cytomegalovirus, HSV = herpes simplex virus   Adapted, with permission, from Lo W, Rolston KVI: Management of infections in cancer patients, in Pazdur R (ed): Medical Oncology: A Comprehensive Review, 1st ed, p 450. Huntington, NY, PRR Inc, 1993.

have an increased mortality rate if candidemia remains untreated. Thus, it is prudent to treat all infected patients with systemic antifungal agents.[13]

In neutropenic patients, the treatment of choice is amphotericin B at a dose of 0.5 to 1 mg/kg/d for 2 weeks or until neutropenia resolves. The drug can cause reversible renal failure (low glomerular filtration rate) and electrolyte abnormalities (hypokalemia and hypomagnesemia). Nephrotoxicity can be decreased with the administration of normal saline before and after infusion. Electrolytes should be monitored and replaced carefully. *C tropicalis* and *C parapsilosis* usually require higher doses of amphotericin B (0.75 to 1 mg/kg/d) in association with flucytosine.[8] *C lusitaniae* tends to be resistant to amphotericin B[14] but may respond to fluconazole and flucytosine. In-vitro susceptibility tests for fungi do not necessarily correlate with clinical results and so are not recommended as routine tests. However, they may aid in drug selection in patients who do not respond to initial treatment.[11,15]

A recent trial performed in non-neutropenic patients with candidemia showed that intravenous fluconazole, 400 mg/d, was as effective as amphotericin B, 0.5 to 0.6 mg/kg/d, and was better tolerated.[16] The most important side effects associated with fluconazole were nausea, vomiting, transient elevation of liver function tests, and skin rash.[17]

The management of candidemia in the presence of a vascular catheter is controversial. In some cases, the catheter may be the primary source of the fungemia, whereas in others it may be secondarily colonized, for example, from a gastrointestinal tract infection. Even in the latter situation, however, the chances of perpetuating the infection are greater if the catheter is not removed,[18] so removing it if possible would seem to be indicated.[8]

Acute Disseminated Candidiasis (ADC): ADC represents the acute involvement of two or more noncontiguous sites by *Candida* spp.[5] Clinically, it can manifest as a septic syndrome with hypotension, multiorgan failure, macronodular skin lesions, and endophthalmitis. The last symptom is usually absent during neutropenia, but in non-neutropenic patients, it is a reliable way to make the diagnosis. Persistent fungemia is not always present. The treatment of choice is amphotericin B, at a dose no lower than 0.6 mg/kg/d with or without flucytosine. The role of fluconazole has not been clearly established.[11]

Chronic Disseminated Candidiasis (CDC): Also known as hepatosplenic candidiasis, CDC is an indolent process that is established during neutropenia and becomes apparent after neutropenia resolves. Deep-seated abscesses are seen not only in the liver and spleen but also in other organs such as the kidneys, adrenals, and lungs. The clinical course is that of progressive debilitation,[5] and fungemia is rare. Abdominal pain and elevation of the alkaline phosphatase level after white blood cell counts recover should be cues for the diagnosis.[11] Computed tomography and biopsy and culture of the abscesses will provide a definitive diagnosis.[5] The initial treatment consists of amphotericin B with or without flucytosine; however, less than half of patients respond to this treatment.[19] Lipid formulations of amphotericin B are an attractive alternative because higher doses of the

TABLE 2

Treatment of Candidiasis and Aspergillosis in Cancer Patients

Infection	First choice	Alternative
Candidiasis		
Mucosal	Topical clotrimazole	Ketoconazole (400 mg PO qd) or fluconazole (100 mg PO qd)
Genitourinary tract	Amphotericin B (0.5–1 mg/kg/d)	Fluconazole (200 mg PO qd)
		Intravesical amphotericin B [a] (50 mg/L in D5W; infuse 1L/d)
Candidemia [b]	Amphotericin B (0.5–1 mg/kg/d) ± flucytosine (100–150 mg/kg/PO qd)	Fluconazole (400 mg IV qd)
ADC	Amphotericin B (no less than 0.6 mg/kg/d) ± flucytosine (100–150 mg/kg PO qd)	Fluconazole (400 mg IV qd)
CDC	Amphotericin B [c] (0.7–1 mg/kg/d) ± flucytosine (100–150 mg/kg PO qd)	Fluconazole (400 mg IV qd)
Aspergillosis		
Pulmonary	Amphotericin B [c] (1–1.5 mg/kg/d)	? Itraconazole (400 mg/d)
Extrapulmonary	Amphotericin B [c] (1–1.5 mg/kg/d) + flucytosine	? Itraconazole (400 mg/d)

ADC = acute disseminated candidiasis, CDC = chronic disseminated candidiasis
[a] Only used for cystitis or bladder colonization   [b] If central venous catheter present, remove when possible   [c] Lipid forms of amphotericin B should be considered

drug can be given with less nephrotoxicity.[20] Fluconazole also may be effective; it has been used in some refractory cases, with clinical response rates as high as 88%.[21]

Prophylaxis: It is very important to define the population of patients who may benefit from chemoprophylaxis of candidiasis. Patients with protracted (greater than 3 weeks) and profound (less than 100 cells/mL) neutropenia are at higher risk for invasive fungal infections. This situation usually is seen in patients undergoing bone marrow transplantation and induction therapy for acute leukemia.[2,22] Previous studies have shown that fluconazole, at oral doses of 200 to 400 mg/d, is effective at preventing superficial and disseminated candidiasis and at decreasing mortality directly related to systemic fungal infections in this population.[23–25] Furthermore, fluconazole (400 mg/d) has been compared with intravenous (IV) amphotericin B (0.5 mg/kg three times a week).[26] Both are equally effective, but fluconazole is better tolerated. Fluconazole is not active against *Aspergillus* spp, however, and it may select some resistant *Candida* spp, such as *C krusei* and *Torulopsis glabrata*.[5]

Aspergillosis

Invasive aspergillosis is a significant infection that usually develops in the presence of neutropenia and corticosteroid use.[27] Most commonly, it occurs in bone marrow transplantation (BMT) and leukemia patients, although patients with lymphoma or solid tumors also may be affected. The most common species causing invasive disease are *Aspergillus fumigatus* and *A flavus*.[5] Given this infection's high prevalence and poor outcome, a reduction in its incidence should greatly reduce the mortality in susceptible patients.

Invasive Pulmonary Aspergillosis: Invasive pulmonary aspergillosis is the most common form of aspergillosis seen in immunocompromised hosts.[28] Clinically, it may present as pleuritic chest pain, pulmonary hemorrhage, hemoptysis, and cavitation, all as a consequence of blood vessel infiltration.[29] Pulmonary infiltrates may be absent during the initial phase of the disease as a result of the lack of inflammatory response associated with neutropenia. The isolation of *Aspergillus* spp from respiratory secretions of susceptible patients should be considered evidence of disease because it is rarely a contaminant.[8] Bronchoalveolar lavages frequently is performed to establish the diagnosis, but the yield is quite low. Lung biopsy and culture of this tissue may be required for a definitive diagnosis. Noninvasive techniques, including assays for serum *Aspergillus* antigen, are currently under investigation.[13]

High doses of amphotericin B (1 to 1.5 mg/kg/d) are required for treatment. The addition of flucytosine may produce a synergistic response (Table 2). If they are combined, serum levels of flucytosine should be monitored and kept below 100 µg/mL to avoid major toxic reactions (mainly hematotoxicity). Lipid formulations of amphotericin B should be considered in protracted cases. Treatment should continue until the *Aspergillus* lesion disappears or stabilizes, which may take several months. The use of itraconazole (Sporanox) in neutropenic patients remains under investigation.[8] Its absorption may be erratic in patients with achlorhydria or patients receiving histamine (H_2) blockers. The drug should be taken with meals, and serum levels should be monitored.

An important cofactor for the treatment of invasive pulmonary aspergillosis is the reversal of immunosuppression. Sometimes, this can be achieved by the discontinuation of steroids and treatment with the granulocyte and macrophage colony-stimulating factors (G-CSF [Neupogen], M-CSF, and GM-CSF [Leukine]). In cases refractory to medical treatment that show a well-localized *Aspergillus* lesion, surgical excision may be indicated.[9]

Extrapulmonary Aspergillosis: Occasionally, *Aspergillus* infection may affect the paranasal sinuses and extend locally to the base of the skull and brain. In other cases, the central nervous system can be involved by direct hematogenous dissemination from a lung infection. Whatever the mechanism of infection, neurologic manifestations consist of focal neurologic deficits, including focal seizures, hemiparesis, and cranial nerve palsies.[30] Other possible extrapulmonary infections caused by *Aspergillus* are pericarditis, endocarditis, endophthalmitis, and cutaneous involvement. As in invasive pulmonary aspergillosis, treatment of extrapulmonary infections consists of high-dose amphotericin B in association with flucytosine (Table 2) and reversal of immunosuppression.[8]

Prophylaxis: The most common nosocomial sources of *Aspergillus* infection are contaminated air conditioners and construction sites. High-efficiency particulate air (HEPA) filters have been shown to be effective in decreasing the environmental source of infection.[31] Chemoprophylaxis for aspergillosis is not a well-established practice. Intranasal administration of amphotericin B decreases the colonization of the nasal mucosa but does not decrease the frequency of invasive pulmonary aspergillosis.[2] Itraconazole may play a role in the primary prevention of aspergillosis, but this has not been clearly defined. IV amphotericin B is effective as secondary prophylaxis, because it decreases the risk of relapse among patients who have a previous history of invasive

aspergillosis and are undergoing further cytotoxic chemotherapy.[32]

Other Fungi

Fungi considered to represent contamination or harmless colonization in immunocompetent individuals have been shown to be serious pathogens in the immunocompromised patient with cancer. *Trichosporon* spp, *Curvularia* spp, *Alternaria* spp, and *Fusarium* spp are some of the fungi reported with an increasing frequency.[33] In general, these infections are difficult to treat, and the final prognosis depends on the recovery of immune status. Successful treatment of disseminated fusariosis with amphotericin B in combination with granulocyte transfusions and GM-CSF has been reported.

Cryptococcus is another fungus that should be considered in cancer patients with defects in cellular immunity. Unlike the fungal infections previously described, neutropenia does not seem to be a risk factor. Cryptococcosis usually affects patients with acquired immunodeficiency syndrome (AIDS) or lymphomas or patients who have received bone marrow transplants or corticosteroids.[1,34] Commonly, it presents as fever and severe headache in cases of meningitis.

The diagnosis can be made by latex agglutination of cryptococcal antigen (from serum or cerebrospinal fluid) or by culture.[34] The treatment of choice for meningeal and disseminated cryptococcosis is amphotericin B in combination with flucytosine. In patients who have meningeal cryptococcosis and normal mental status, fluconazole, 400 mg/d, is considered safe as initial treatment. As long as the patient remains immunocompromised, as in patients with AIDS, chronic suppressive therapy is required. For this purpose, fluconazole seems to be superior to amphotericin B.[15]

Empirical Antifungal Treatment

The empirical use of antifungal treatment in neutropenic patients who remain febrile (usually for more than 7 days) in spite of broad-spectrum antibiotics has reduced invasive fungal infections and the morbidity and mortality associated with them.[35] In this circumstance, amphotericin B, at a dose of 0.5 mg/kg/d, is recommended. Triazoles such as fluconazole and itraconazole are potential alternatives, but further studies are needed to establish their efficacy as empirical treatments.[11]

Other Therapeutic Modalities

A reduction in the duration of neutropenia reduces the incidence of invasive fungal infections.[22] Use of cytokines such as G-CSF, GM-CSF, M-CSF, and gamma

TABLE 3

Management of Viral Infections in Cancer Patients

Infection	First choice	Alternative
Cytomegalovirus	Ganciclovir (10 mg/kg/d) ± IV IgG [a]	Foscarnet (40–60 mg/kg IV q8h)
Herpes simplex virus	IV acyclovir (5 mg/kg q8h)	Famciclovir (500 mg PO q8h)
		Foscarnet [b] (40–60 mg/kg IV q8h)
Varicella zoster virus	IV acyclovir (10 mg/kg q8h)	Famciclovir (500 mg PO q8h)
		Foscarnet [b] (40–60 mg/kg IV q8h)
Adenovirus	Not available	
Influenza A	Amantadine [c] (100 mg PO bid)	Rimantadine [c] (100 mg PO bid)
Parainfluenza	Not available	
Respiratory syncytial virus	Aerosolized ribavirin + IV IgG	

[a] Should be used if interstitial pneumonitis is present   [b] Indicated in cases of acyclovir-resistant strains   [c] Effective against influenza A only

interferon (IFN-γ [Actimmune]) may be beneficial. Previous studies using GM-CSF in combination with amphotericin B[36] have been encouraging, but significant side effects, such as the capillary leak syndrome, are possible limitations. The determination of monocyte and macrophage function and of circulating cytokine levels may identify patients likely to respond to this therapeutic modality.[37] Nevertheless, there is a need for randomized, placebo-controlled trials to determine the impact of these factors on the mortality rate.

The use of granulocyte transfusions from donors stimulated with G-CSF may be another strategy for increasing the levels of circulating granulocytes until endogenous recovery from granulocytopenia occurs.[38]

VIRAL INFECTIONS

Opportunistic viral infections are a significant cause of morbidity and mortality in immunocompromised patients such as BMT recipients and patients with hematologic malignancies.[39] The most common viruses isolated from these patients are the herpesviruses (especially cytomegalovirus [CMV], herpes simplex virus [HSV], and varicella zoster virus [VZV]. Their frequency is probably due to their ability to remain latent until they are reactivated when the patient is immunosuppressed. Infections by RNA respiratory viruses, such as respiratory syncytial virus (RSV) and influenza and parainfluenza viruses, usually occur in outbreaks and also are seen frequently.[40] At present, it is important to diagnose these infections correctly, because treatment is available for some of them[41] (Table 3).

Cytomegalovirus

Cytomegalovirus is a common cause of death in allogeneic BMT patients, ranking second after graft-vs-host disease (GVHD). CMV may be the result of primary infection (from donor bone marrow graft or blood products to a seronegative patient) or the reactivation of a latent infection.[39] The incidence of CMV infection is the same after autologous or allogeneic BMT; however, morbidity and mortality are lower in the autologous group.[42] Most commonly, infection appears 4 to 10 weeks after transplantation. Mild forms of the illness may manifest as fever, hepatitis, leukopenia, and thrombocytopenia.[34] Severe forms manifest as interstitial pneumonia (with a mortality rate of 80% to 90%) and gastroenteritis.[39]

The diagnosis can be established from the clinical presentation and the detection of CMV antigen or CMV cultures from buffy coat or urine. The development of effective, rapid techniques that utilize CMV-specific monoclonal antibodies has made possible the earlier diagnosis of this disease. In addition, DNA amplification using the polymerase chain reaction has made viral detection highly sensitive and should be useful for clinical diagnosis.[43] Occasionally, histopathologic diagnosis may be needed.

Treatment with acyclovir is not effective because the virus lacks thymidine kinase, an enzyme necessary for the activation of acyclovir.[44] Ganciclovir and foscarnet are active in vitro and in vivo against CMV. The initial treatments consist of IV ganciclovir at a dosage of 10 mg/kg/d (usually for 3 weeks) followed by a maintenance dosage of 6 mg/kg/d 5 days per week (for an additional 6 to 7 weeks).[45] Periodic blood cell counts should be measured, because the main toxicity of ganciclovir is hematologic.

In cases of CMV pneumonitis, CMV immunoglobulin G intravenous (CMV-IGIV) has been shown to improve survival,[46] probably because it blocks T-cell-mediated destruction of lung tissue.[47] To prevent CMV infection, seronegative allogeneic BMT recipients should receive seronegative blood products only. The prophylactic use of CMV-IGIV in BMT patients has decreased the incidence of CMV pneumonitis without significantly decreasing mortality.[48] The prophylactic use of ganciclovir for patients who were seropositive before transplantation[49] or as early treatment (as soon as CMV is detected in throat, urine, or blood cultures)[50] has reduced CMV infection and improved survival.

Herpes Simplex Virus

More than 80% of BMT patients will have reactivation of latent HSV residing in the neuronal ganglia. The same situation is true for patients with leukemia, lymphoma, or solid tumors who receive intensive chemotherapy.[46] This reactivation usually occurs within the first 3 weeks after transplantation or chemotherapy and is characterized by ulcerative oral lesions (in 85% of the cases) or genital lesions (in 15% of the cases).[51]

In immunocompromised patients, the herpetic lesions may be larger and deeper or may have another atypical aspect.[34] It is believed that several cases of chemotherapy-induced mucositis were actually due to HSV infection.[52] Other possible presentations of HSV infection in immunocompromised patients are esophagitis, tracheitis, pneumonitis, and, rarely, encephalitis. When pneumonitis occurs, it may present as a local infiltrate (usually originating from aspiration of the virus from the upper airways) or as a diffuse interstitial infiltrate (from viremia).[53]

The diagnosis of HSV infection is based on viral culture of suspected lesions. Treatment with acyclovir (Zovirax) has been effective by reducing the viral shedding, enhancing the resolution of pain, and shortening the time to healing.[54] The suggested dose is 5 mg/kg every 8 hours administered intravenously for a total of 7 days.

Alternatively, famciclovir (Famvir), a newly approved antiviral agent, has been shown to be effective against herpesviruses. It is the oral prodrug of penciclovir and has a considerably longer intracellular half-life than acyclovir. Side effects, which include headache, nausea, and diarrhea, are uncommon.[55]

Valacyclovir, the oral prodrug of acyclovir, is currently under investigation. Its oral administration results in plasma concentrations three to five times greater than those achieved with a comparable dose of oral acyclovir, and the intervals between valacyclovir doses can be longer. Strains of acyclovir-resistant HSV may develop. In such cases, foscarnet (Foscavir) is the treatment of choice.

Prophylaxis with acyclovir prevents the reactivation of the virus in patients undergoing BMT or cytotoxic chemotherapy. If the oral intake is inconsistent, the IV route is preferred. Doses as low as 250 mg/m^2 have been effective.[56]

Varicella Zoster Virus

VZV infection in cancer patients can present either as primary infection (chickenpox) or as reactivation (shingles). The latter infection can remain localized in a dermatomal distribution or can disseminate, causing extensive cutaneous and/or visceral involvement, which can prove fatal.[39] When visceral involvement occurs, the lungs are affected more commonly, followed by the liver and the central nervous system.[34] Patients with Hodgkin's disease or non-Hodgkin's lymphoma and patients undergoing BMT are at increased risk for VZV reactivation. Unlike HSV, VZV takes longer to reactivate (usually within the first 2 years).[41]

The treatment of choice is acyclovir, 10 to 12 mg/kg every 8 hours for no fewer than 7 days. This treatment decreases the time to full crusting and prevents the dissemination of the disease[57]; however, it does not have any significant impact on postherpetic neuralgia. Uncomplicated cases may be treated with famciclovir, at a dose of 500 mg orally every 8 hours.

Prophylaxis with acyclovir effectively prevents VZV reactivation; however, upon discontinuation of the drug, the rate of reactivation increases again.[58] VZV immunoglobulin has a role in the prevention of primary infection in the susceptible immunocompromised host.[59] A live, attenuated vaccine is under investigation.[60]

Adenovirus

Adenovirus affects patients with cellular immune defects. It is not clear whether the majority of infections are primary or a reactivation of latent viral infection. Pneumonia and hepatitis are the most common infections. Hemorrhagic cystitis occasionally occurs and has been associated with specific serotypes of the virus. No specific treatment is available[34]; however, in some anecdotal case reports, IV ribavirin (Virazole) has shown some efficacy.[61]

Respiratory RNA Viruses

Influenza virus is a known cause of annual epidemics of respiratory disease with significant morbidity and mortality, especially among cancer patients.[40] Clinically, this virus presents as fever, cough, coryza, myalgias, fatigue, and headache. Primary influenza pneumonia or secondary bacterial pneumonia may develop, especially in the immunocompromised host.[62]

Influenza A can be treated effectively with amantadine or rimantadine (Flumadine) during the early phases of disease. Measures should concentrate on prophylaxis; this can be accomplished with annual influenza vaccination for immunocompromised patients, their families, and hospital staff.[63] The efficacy of the vaccine is 60% to 90%,[64] but the rate may be lower in immunosuppressed patients. Chemoprophylaxis with amantadine (effective only for influenza A) should be administered for 2 weeks during nosocomial outbreaks when late immunization has been given.

Parainfluenza and RSV also can cause upper respiratory infection followed by severe viral pneumonia in susceptible hosts, such as BMT patients.[65,66] The diagnosis of parainfluenza can be difficult because the virus grows slowly in cell culture. The diagnosis of RSV can be made by culture or by detecting RSV antigen in respiratory specimens. Aerosolized ribavirin in association with IV immunoglobulins is effective in cases of RSV pneumonia.[67] There is, however, no well-established antiviral treatment of parainfluenza pneumonia.

REFERENCES

1. Koll BS, Brown AE: The changing epidemiology of infections at cancer hospitals. Clin Infect Dis 17(suppl 2):S322–328, 1993.

2. Walsh TJ, Lee JW: Prevention of invasive fungal infections in patients with neoplastic diseases. Clin Infect Dis 17(suppl 2):S468–480, 1993.

3. Anaissie E, Bodey GP: Nosocomial fungal infections: Old problems and new challenges. Infect Dis Clin North Am 4:867–882, 1989.

4. Horn R, Wong B, Kiehn TE, et al: Fungemia in a cancer hospital: Changing frequency, earlier onset, and results of therapy. Rev Infect Dis 7:646–655, 1985.

5. Anaissie E: Opportunistic mycoses in the immunocompromised host: Experience at a cancer center and review. Clin Infect Dis 14(suppl 1):S43–53, 1992.

6. Bodey GP: Fungal infections complicating acute leukemia. J Chron Dis 19:667–687, 1966.

7. Pfaller MA: Epidemiology and control of fungal infections. Clin Infect Dis 19(suppl 1):S8–13, 1994.

8. Walsh TJ: Management of immunocompromised patients with evidence of an invasive mycosis. Hematol Oncol Clin North Am 7:1003–1025, 1993.

9. Walsh TJ, De Pawn B, Anaissie E, et al: Recent advances in the epidemiology, prevention, and treatment of invasive fungal infections in neutropenic patients. J Med Vet Mycol 32(suppl 1):S33–51, 1994.

10. Grieve NWT: Case reports, Monilia oesophagitis. Br J Radiol 37:551–554, 1964.

11. Swerdloff JN, Filler SG, Edwards JE: Severe candidal infections in neutropenic patients. Clin Infect Dis 17(suppl 2):S457–467, 1993.

12. Wey SB, Mori M, Pfaller MA, et al: Hospital-acquired candidemia: The attributed mortality and excess length of stay. Arch Intern Med 148:2642–2645, 1988.

13. Meunier F, Wong B: Overview of management of fungal infections: Part 1. Clin Infect Dis 17(suppl 2):S492–493, 1993.

14. Merz WG: *Candida lusitaniae*: Frequency of recovery, colonization, infection, and amphotericin B resistance. J Clin Microbiol 20:1194–1195, 1984.

15. Graybill JR: Overview of management of fungal infections: Part 2. Clin Infect Dis 17(suppl 2):S513–514, 1993.

16. Rex JH, Bennett JE, Sugar AM, et al: A randomized trial comparing fluconazole with amphotericin B for the treatment of candidemia in patients without neutropenia. N Engl J Med 331:1325–1330, 1994.

17. Bennett JE: Overview of the symposium on fluconazole: A novel advance in the therapy for systemic fungal infections. Rev Infect Dis 12(suppl 3):S263, 1990.

18. Walsh TJ, Bustamante C, Vlahov D, et al: *Candida* suppurative peripheral thrombophlebitis: Prevention, recognition, and management. Infect Control 7:16–22, 1986.

19. Bodey GL: Azole antifungal agents. Clin Infect Dis 14(suppl 1):S161–169, 1992.

20. Lopez-Berestein G, Bodey GP, Frankel LS, et al: Treatment of hepatosplenic candidiasis with liposomal amphotericin B. J Clin Oncol 5:310–317, 1987.

21. Anaissie E, Bodey GP, Kantarjian H, et al: Fluconazole therapy for chronic disseminated candidiasis in patients with leukemia and prior amphotericin-B therapy. Am J Med 91:142–150, 1991.

22. Walsh TJ, Hiemenz J, Pizzo PA: Editorial response: Evolving risk factors for invasive fungal infections—All neutropenic patients are not the same. Clin Infect Dis 18:793–798, 1994.

23. Winston DW, Chandrasekar PH, Lazarus HM: Fluconazole prophylaxis of fungal infections in patients with acute leukemia: Results of a randomized, placebo-controlled, double-blind, multicenter trial. Ann Intern Med 118:495–503, 1993.

24. Goodman JL, Winston DJ, Greenfield RA, et al: A controlled trial of fluconazole to prevent fungal infections in patients undergoing bone marrow transplantation. N Engl J Med 326:845–851, 1992.

25. Ellis ME, Clink H, Ernst P, et al: Controlled study of fluconazole in the prevention of fungal infections in neutropenic patients with hematological malignancies and bone marrow transplant recipients. Eur J Clin Microbiol Infect Dis 13:3–11, 1994.

26. Anaissie E, Reuben A, Cunningham K, et al: Randomized trial of fluconazole vs intravenous amphotericin B for antifungal prophylaxis in neutropenic patients with leukemia (abstract 572). Program and Abstracts of the 30th Interscience Conference on Antimicrobial Agents and Chemotherapy. Washington, DC, American Society for Microbiology, 1990.

27. Schaffner A, Douglas H: Selective protection against conidia by mononuclear and against mycelia by polymorphonuclear phagocytes in resistance to *Aspergillus*. Observations on these two lines of defense in vivo and in vitro with human mouse phagocytes. J Clin Invest 69:617–631, 1982.

28. Walsh TJ, Pizzo PA: Treatment of systemic fungal infections: Recent progress and current problems. Eur J Clin Microbiol Infect Dis 7:460–475, 1988.

29. Walsh TJ: Invasive pulmonary aspergillosis in patients with neoplastic diseases. Semin Respir Infect 5:111–122, 1990.

30. Walsh TJ, Caplan LR, Hier DB: *Aspergillus* infections of the

central nervous system: Clinicopathological analysis. Ann Neurol 18:574–582, 1985.

31. Arnow PM, Sadigh M, Costas C, et al: Endemic and epidemic aspergillosis associated with in-hospital replication of *Aspergillus* organisms. J Infect Dis 164:998–1002, 1991.

32. Robertson MJ, Larson RA: Recurrent fungal pneumonias in patients with acute nonlymphocytic leukemia undergoing multiple courses of intensive chemotherapy. Am J Med 84:233–239, 1988.

33. Vartivarian SE, Anaissie EJ, Bodey GP: Emerging fungal pathogens in immunocompromised patients: Classification, diagnosis, and management. Clin Infect Dis 17(suppl 2):S127–135, 1993.

34. Rosenberg AS, Brown AE: Infection in the cancer patient. Dis Mon 39:510–569, 1993.

35. EORTC International Antimicrobial Therapy Cooperative Group: Empiric antifungal therapy in febrile granulocytopenic patients. Am J Med 86:668–672, 1989.

36. Bodey GP, Anaissie E, Gutterman J, et al: Role of granulocyte-macrophage colony-stimulating factor as adjuvant therapy for fungal infection in patients with cancer. Clin Infect Dis 17:705–707, 1993.

37. Neumanaitis J, Shannon-Dorcy K, Appelbaum FR, et al: Long-term follow-up of patients with invasive fungal disease who received adjunctive therapy with recombinant human macrophage colony-stimulating factor. Blood 82:1422–1427, 1993.

38. Strauss RG: Therapeutic granulocyte transfusions in 1993 (Editorial). Blood 81:1675–1678, 1993.

39. Holland HK, Wingard JR, Saral R: Herpesvirus and enteric viral infections in bone marrow transplantation: Clinical presentations, pathogenesis, and therapeutic strategies. Cancer Invest 8:509–521, 1990.

40. Whimbey E, Elting LS, Couch RB, et al: Influenza A virus infections among hospitalized adult bone marrow transplant recipients. Bone Marrow Transplant 13:437–440, 1994.

41. Meyers JD: Chemoprophylaxis of viral infection in immunocompromised patients. Eur J Cancer Clin Oncol 25:1369–1374, 1989.

42. Wingard JR, Chen DYH, Burns WH, et al: Cytomegalovirus infection after autologous bone marrow transplantation with comparison to infection after allogeneic bone marrow transplantation. Blood 71:1432–1437, 1988.

43. Chou S: Newer methods for diagnosis of cytomegalovirus infection. Rev Infect Dis 12(suppl 7):S727–736, 1990.

44. Whitley RJ, Gnann JW: Acyclovir: A decade later. N Engl J Med 327:782–789, 1992.

45. Bratanow NC, Ash RC, Turner PA, et al: Successful treatment of serious cytomegalovirus disease with 9(1,3-dihydroxy-2-propoxymethyl) guanine in bone marrow transplant patients. Blood 68:280a, 1986.

46. Gallagher J: Supportive care for viral infections in cancer patients. Curr Opin Oncol 3:643–647, 1991.

47. Winston DJ, Ho WG, Champlin RE: Current approaches to management of infections in bone marrow transplants. Eur J Clin Oncol 25(suppl 2):S25–35, 1989.

48. Winston DJ, Pollard RB, Ho WG, et al: Cytomegalovirus immune plasma in bone marrow transplant recipients. Ann Intern Med 97:11–18, 1982.

49. Schmidt GM, Horak DA, Niland JC, et al: A randomized, controlled trial of prophylactic ganciclovir for cytomegalovirus pulmonary infection in recipients of allogeneic bone marrow transplants. N Engl J Med 324:1005–1011, 1991.

50. Goodrich JM, Mori M, Gleaves C, et al: Early treatment with ganciclovir to prevent cytomegalovirus disease after allogeneic bone marrow transplantation. N Engl J Med 325:1601–1607, 1991.

51. Meyers JD: Treatment of herpesvirus infections in the immunocompromised host. Scand J Infect Dis 47:128–136, 1985.

52. Janmohamed R, Morton JE, Milligan DW, et al: Herpes simplex in oral ulcers in neutropenic patients. Br J Cancer 61:649–670, 1990.

53. Ramsey PG, Fife KH, Hackman RC, et al: Herpes simplex virus pneumonia. Clinical, virologic, and pathologic features in 20 patients. Ann Intern Med 97:813–820, 1982.

54. Meyers JD, Wade JC, Mitchell CD, et al: Multicenter collaborative trial of intravenous acyclovir for treatment of mucocutaneous herpes simplex virus infection in the immunocompromised host. Am J Med 73(suppl 1A):S229–235, 1982.

55. Jurewicz R, Boon R: Safety of famciclovir in patients with herpes zoster and genital herpes. Antimicrob Agents Chemother 38:2454–2457, 1994.

56. Shepp DH, Dandliker PS, Flournoy N, et al: Sequential intravenous and twice-daily oral acyclovir for extended prophylaxis of herpes simplex virus infection in marrow transplant patients. Transplantation 43:654–658, 1987.

57. Nyerges G, Meszner Z, Gyarmati E, et al: Acyclovir prevents dissemination of varicella in immunocompromised children. J Infect Dis 157:309–313, 1988.

58. Rand KH, Rasmussen LE, Pollard RB, et al: Cellular immunity and herpes virus infections in cardiac-transplant patients. N Engl J Med 296:1372–1377, 1976.

59. Groth KE, McCullough J, Marker SC, et al: Evaluation of zoster immune plasma. JAMA 239:1877–1879, 1978.

60. Hughes WT: Prevention of infections in patients with T cell defects. Clin Infect Dis 17(suppl 2):S368–371, 1993.

61. Liles WC, Cushing H, Holt S, et al: Severe adenoviral nephritis following bone marrow transplantation: Successful treatment with intravenous ribavirin. Bone Marrow Transplant 12:409–412, 1993.

62. Wright SA, Bieluch VM: Selected nosocomial viral infections. Heart Lung 22:183–187, 1993.

63. Centers for Disease Control: Prevention and control of influenza: Recommendations of the immunizations practices advisory committee. Morb Mortal Wkly Rep 41:1–17, 1992.

64. Graman PS, Hall CB: Epidemiology and control of nosocomial viral infections. Infect Dis Clin North Am 3:815–841, 1989.

65. Guidry GC, Black-Payne CA, Payne DK, et al: Respiratory syncytial virus infection among intubated adults in a university medical intensive care unit. Chest 100:1377–1384, 1991.

66. Whimbey E, Vartivarian SE, Champlin RE: Parainfluenza virus infection in adult bone marrow transplant recipients. Eur J Clin Microbiol Infect Dis 12:699–701, 1993.

67. Whimbey E, Bodey GP: Viral pneumonia in the immunocompromised adult with neoplastic disease: The role of common community respiratory viruses. Semin Respir Infect 7:122–131, 1992.

CHAPTER 40

Management of Cancer Pain

Sharon M. Weinstein, MD

Section of Pain and Symptom Management, Department of Neuro-Oncology
The University of Texas M. D. Anderson Cancer Center, Houston, Texas

The public fear that cancer is inevitably painful[1] is warranted: The majority of patients with advanced cancer and up to 60% of patients with any stage of disease will experience significant pain. The World Health Organization has estimated that 25% of all cancer patients die with unrelieved pain.[2]

Leading oncologic organizations have stated that the relief of pain and other symptoms should be a priority in the care of these patients.[3–6] The benefits of adequate pain control include facilitation of the diagnostic workup and treatment, improved functional status, and better quality of life.

It has been demonstrated that most cancer patients' pain can be relieved adequately with oral analgesics.[7,8] Despite this, cancer pain is undertreated for a multitude of reasons. The problem is not trivial, because unrelieved pain is known to be a risk factor for suicide in cancer patients.[9] The Eastern Collaborative Oncology Group 1991 survey of oncologists revealed that physicians attribute undertreatment to their own lack of education and poor clinical role models.[10] Hill and others have outlined other influences, such as physicians' fear of regulatory agency scrutiny and fear of patient addiction.[11,12] Current efforts are directed at standardizing pain treatment[13] and separating issues of pain treatment from those of substance abuse. It is encouraging to note that a dialogue between addiction specialists and cancer pain specialists has begun to address these issues.[14]

The effective management of cancer patients with pain is best accomplished in a multidisciplinary fashion with coordination of the services of oncologists, pain specialists, nurses, social workers, physiatrists, physical therapists, psychologists, psychiatrists, community health-care providers, clergy, and hospice workers.[15] Maintaining communication among members of the care-giving team is essential to providing optimal care.

DEFINITION OF PAIN AND ANATOMIC CORRELATES

Pain has been defined as "a sensory and emotional experience associated with tissue damage or described in terms of such damage."[16] In humans, parallel neural

FIGURE I

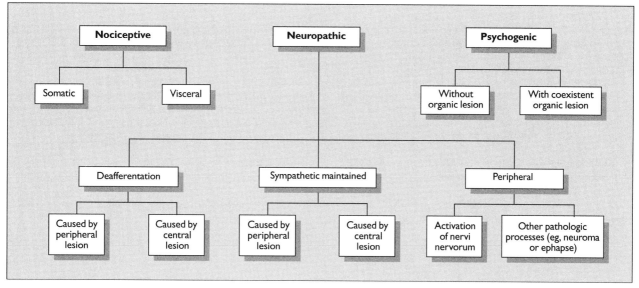

Proposed taxonomy of chronic pain, based on presumed pathophysiologic distinctions among nociceptive, neuropathic, and psychogenic pain. Adapted from Portenoy RK.[17]

TABLE 1

Cancer Pain Syndromes

Pain associated with direct tumor involvement

Due to invasion of bone
    Base of skull
        Orbital syndrome
        Parasellar syndrome
        Sphenoid sinus syndrome
        Clivus syndrome
        Jugular foramen syndrome
        Occipital condyle syndrome
    Vertebral body
        Atlantoaxial syndrome
        C-T syndrome
        L syndrome
        Sacral syndrome
    Generalized bone pain
        Multiple metastases
        Intramedullary neoplasm
Due to invasion of nerves
    Peripheral nerve syndromes
        Paraspinal mass
        Chest wall mass
        Retroperitoneal mass
    Painful polyneuropathy
    Brachial, lumbar, sacral plexopathies
    Leptomeningeal metastases
    Epidural spinal-cord compression
Due to invasion of viscera
Due to invasion of blood vessels
Due to invasion of mucous membranes

Pain associated with cancer therapy

Postoperative pain syndromes
    Postthoracotomy syndrome
    Postmastectomy syndrome
    Postradical neck dissection syndrome
    Postamputation syndrome
Postchemotherapy pain syndromes
    Painful polyneuropathy
    Aseptic necrosis of bone
    Steroid pseudorheumatism
    Mucositis
Postradiation pain syndromes
    Radiation fibrosis of brachial or lumbosacral plexus
    Radiation myelopathy
    Radiation-induced peripheral nerve tumors
    Mucositis
    Radiation necrosis of bone

Pain indirectly related or unrelated to cancer or its treatment

Myofascial pains
Postherpetic neuralgia
Osteoporosis

Adapted, with permission, from Portenoy RK.[2]

pathways transmit information about painful stimuli from the periphery, through the spinal cord, to multiple areas of the brain. Pain signals (nociceptive inputs) are localized and interpreted and the affective component assigned at the cerebral cortical level. Modulation of nociceptive input by opioid and nonopioid mechanisms occurs in the periphery, at the dorsal horn of the spinal cord, in the brain stem, and possibly in higher centers.

Pathophysiology

The pathophysiologic classification of pain forms the basis for therapeutic choices. Pain states may be broadly divided into those associated with ongoing tissue damage (nociceptive) and those resulting from nervous system dysfunction in the absence of ongoing tissue damage (non-nociceptive or neuropathic). The pathophysiologic schema proposed by Portenoy is shown in Figure 1.[17]

Damage to the nervous system may result in pain in an area of reduced sensation. Such pain is typically described as burning or lancinating. Patients may cite bizarre complaints, such as painful numbness, itching, or crawling sensations. The postamputation phenomenon of phantom pain (referred to the lost body part) may be disabling.

Care should be taken when considering the diagnosis of "psychogenic pain," or somatoform pain disorder,[18] because this type of pain is rare in cancer patients. More commonly, psychological factors affect the reporting of pain. It is also true that chronic unrelieved pain has psychological consequences, but this does not support a psychiatric basis for the pain complaint.

Pain Syndromes

Common cancer pain syndromes vary by tumor type and are related to patterns of tumor growth and metasta-

TABLE 2

Features of the Pain History

Location, pattern of radiation

Character

Temporal factors: onset, duration, time to maximum intensity, frequency, daily variation

Provocative factors

Palliative factors

Intensity (use pain-rating scales [Figure 3])

Adapted, with permission, from Colodney A, Weinstein SM.[21]

FIGURE 2

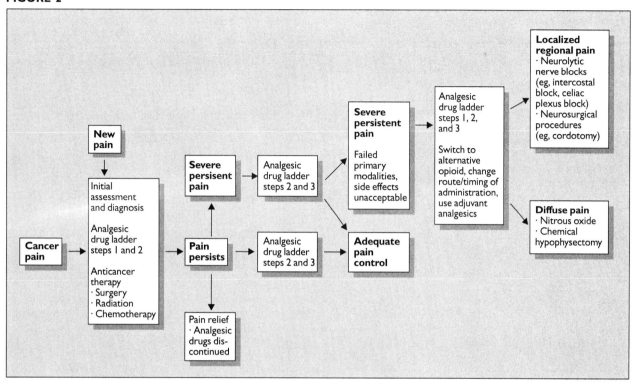

Algorithm for the integration of management approaches to cancer pain. Adapted from Foley KM, Arbit E.[19]

FIGURE 3

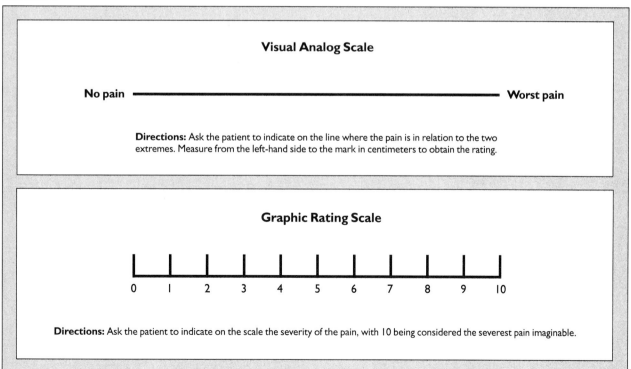

Pain rating scales used to establish a baseline against which treatment results are judged.

TABLE 3
Subgroups of Patients With Cancer Pain

Patients with acute cancer-related pain

Acute pain associated with the diagnosis of cancer

Acute pain associated with cancer therapy, including surgery, chemotherapy, and radiation therapy

Patients with chronic cancer-related pain

Chronic pain associated with cancer progression

Chronic pain associated with cancer therapy, including surgery, chemotherapy, and radiation therapy

Patients with preexisting chronic pain and cancer-related pain

Patients with a history of drug addiction with cancer-related pain

Actively involved in illicit drug use

In a methadone maintenance program

With a past history of drug abuse

Dying patients with cancer-related pain

Adapted, with permission, from Foley KM.[24]

FIGURE 4

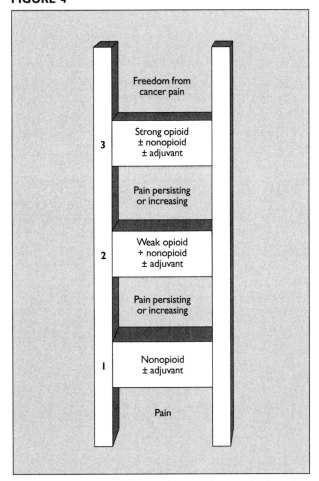

Analgesic ladder outlining the use of nonopioid analgesics, opioid analgesics, and analgesic adjuvants for progressively severe pain. Adapted from World Health Organization: Cancer Pain Relief and Palliative Care. Geneva, World Health Organization, 1990.

sis. Pain may be directly related to antineoplastic therapy and may be indirectly related or unrelated to either the neoplasm or its treatment (Table 1).[2]

MANAGEMENT

Elements of cancer pain management include a proper medical evaluation, psychosocial assessment, formulation of the pain "diagnosis," and consideration of pharmacologic and nonpharmacologic treatments. Ongoing care is needed to monitor the efficacy of analgesics and the evolution of different symptomatology during treatment or disease progression.

The steps in medical decision making are to: (1) determine whether primary antineoplastic therapy is indicated for palliation, (2) tailor pharmacologic analgesic therapy to individual needs, (3) consider concurrent nonpharmacologic analgesic methods, and (4) monitor the patient for response and modify treatment accordingly (Figure 2).[19] The patient remains the focus of care, although family members and other concerned individuals often participate in treatment decisions and require emotional support.

Patient Evaluation

The medical evaluation begins with a thorough history. Because there are no objective means with which to verify the presence of pain, one must believe a patient's complaint. The physiologic signs of acute pain—elevated blood pressure and pulse rate—are not reliable in verifying subacute or chronic pain. Most cancer patients report more than one site of pain.[20] A detailed history of each type of pain should be elicited (Table 2).[21] As the chief complaint resolves, what was initially considered a

TABLE 4

Nonopioid Analgesics and Nonsteroidal Anti-Inflammatory Drugs (NSAIDs) Useful for Treating Cancer Pain

Generic name	Usual dosage range	Maximum/ day	Adverse effects/ Comments
Acetaminophen	325–975 mg q4-6h	6,000 mg	Hepatic and renal impairment
Acetylsalicyclic acid (aspirin, ASA)	325–975 mg q4-6h	6,000 mg	Dyspepsia and GI ulceration, antiplatelet effect, bleeding
Choline magnesium trisalicylate	500–1,500 mg q8-12h	4,500 mg	Dyspepsia, reduced antiplatelet effect, hypermagnesemia in renal failure
Choline salicylate	435–870 mg q3-4h	5,220 mg	Dyspepsia, reduced antiplatelet effect
Magnesium salicylate	300–600 mg q4h	4,800 mg	Same as choline salicylate
Salsalate	1,000–1,500 mg q8-12h	4,000 mg	Same as choline salicylate
Sodium salicylate	325–650 mg q3-4h	5,200 mg	
Ibuprofen	200–800 mg q4-6h	3,200 mg	[a]; Dermatitis +
Ketoprofen	25–75 mg q6-8h	300 mg	[a]; Headache +++
Ketorolac tromethamine	Oral: 10 mg q4-6h	40 mg	[a]; Limit duration of therapy, headache +++, GI bleeding
	Parenteral: 60 mg, then 15–30 mg q6h	120 mg	[a]; Limit therapy to 5 days, headache +++, GI bleeding
Meclofenamate sodium	50–100 mg q4-6h	400 mg	[a]; Headache +, dermatitis +
Mefenamic acid	250 mg q6h	1,000 mg	[a]; Limit therapy to 7 days
Naproxen sodium	220–550 mg q8-12h	1,375 mg	[a]; Headache +
Naproxen	250–500 mg q8-12h	1,500 mg	[a]; Headache +

[a] Minor adverse reactions include dyspepsia, heartburn, nausea, vomiting, anorexia, diarrhea, constipation, flatulence, bloating, epigastric pain, abdominal pain, dizziness, and drowsiness. Major adverse reactions that may appear at any time include renal failure, hepatic dysfunction, bleeding, and gastric ulceration.
+ Each plus sign represents a 5% incidence of the reported adverse effect.
Adapted, with permission, from American Pain Society.[26]

secondary problem may require attention. Pain-rating scales should be used to establish a baseline against which the success of treatment may be judged (Figure 3). Behavioral observations may be used to assess patients who are unable to communicate. Although there are standardized tools for preverbal children,[22] they are not available for impaired adults. Therefore, it is sometimes necessary to treat pain presumptively.

The physical examination includes careful neurologic testing, especially if neuropathic pain is suspected. Pain in an area of reduced sensation, allodynia (ie, when normal stimuli are reported as painful), and hyperpathia or summation of painful stimuli support a neuropathic process.

The extent of disease and current medical conditions must be determined. Diagnostic tests should be reviewed and supplemented as necessary. Cancer treatment and prior analgesic interventions with their outcomes should be recorded. Psychological dependency on licit or illicit drugs, including alcohol, must be identified.

Psychosocial Assessment

To establish trust, the evaluating clinician should explore the significance of the pain complaint with the patient. The impact of pain and other symptoms on functional status must be understood to establish the goals of treatment. Suffering may be attributable to many factors other than physical complaints. The clinician should ask about such psychological factors as financial worries, loss of independence, family problems, social

TABLE 5

Guidelines for the Use of Opioid Analgesics

Start with an analgesic with the potential to provide relief

Know the essential pharmacology of the analgesic

Analgesic type

Pharmacokinetics

Influences of coadministered drugs, disease, or age on analgesic disposition and response

Equianalgesic starting dose for the drug and route to be used

Route of administration and a dosage form to fit the patient's needs

Individualize/titrate the dosage

Administer analgesics regularly after the initial titration of the dose

Use drug combinations that enhance analgesia

Recognize and treat adverse effects

Manage opioid tolerance

Manage opioid dependency (ie, prevent withdrawal)

Adapted, with permission, from Inturrisi C.[27]

isolation, and fear of death. Often cancer patients meet the diagnostic criteria for the psychiatric diagnosis of adjustment disorder, with anxiety and/or depressed mood.[23]

Patient Subgroups

It is useful to recognize distinct subgroups of patients (Table 3).[24] To help define the goals of therapy, age, prognosis, and history of drug or alcohol abuse may be considered. Adjustments in drug dosages are usually needed for elderly patients who are more sensitive to analgesics and their side effects. Children may require relatively larger doses of opioids.[25] The use of chronic opioid analgesics requires special consideration in patients who are in long-term remission. Patients with substance-abuse problems who are receiving opioids for pain demand careful attention.

Pharmacologic Treatment

The World Health Organization's three-step analgesic ladder outlines the use of nonopioid analgesics, opioid analgesics, and adjuvants for progressively severe pain (Figure 4). Nonopioid analgesics are associated with ceiling effects, and exceeding the maximum dose ranges can result in organ toxicity. Potential side effects, such as hematologic, renal, or gastrointestinal reactions, may be of clinical concern in cancer patients (Table 4).[26]

TABLE 6

Opioid Analgesics for Mild-to-Moderate Pain

Drug	Equianalgesic dose to 650 mg aspirin[a]	Dose interval	Half-life (hours)	Comments
Agonists				
Codeine	32–65 mg	q4-6h	2-3	[b,c]
Hydrocodone	—	q3-4h	4	[b]
Oxycodone	2.5 mg	q3-6h	—	[b]
Propoxyphene HCl	65–130 mg	q4h	6-12	[b]; Toxic metabolite (norpropoxyphene) accumulates with repetitive dosing
Propoxyphene napsylate	100–200 mg	q4h	6-12	[b]; Same as propoxyphene HCl
Mixed agonist-antagonist				
Pentazocine	30 mg	q4h	2-3	[d]

[a] The equianalgesic dose should not be interpreted as the starting, standard, or maximum dose, but a guide for switching drugs or changing routes of administration
[b] Doses of products containing aspirin or acetaminophen should be monitored for safety.
[c] Doses above 65 mg provide diminished incremental analgesia with increasing doses, but side effects may worsen.
[d] Can precipitate a withdrawal reaction in opioid-dependent patients; not recommended for treating cancer pain.
Adapted, with permission, from American Pain Society.[26]

TABLE 7

Opioid Analgesics for Severe Pain

Drug	Equianalgesic dose (mg) to 10 mg IV morphine		Half-life (hours)	Comments
	Oral	**Parenteral**		
Agonists				
Morphine sulfate, immediate release	30 mg q304h	10 mg q3-4h	3	[a]
Morphine sulfate, controlled release	90-120 mg q12h	N/A	3	[a]; Mg-for-mg conversion from immediate release; don't crush or chew tablets
Hydromorphone	7.5 mg q3-4h	1.5 mg q3-4h	2-3	[a]
Levorphanol	4 mg q6-8h	2mg q6-8h	12-15	[a]
Meperidine	300 mg q2-3h	100 mg q3h	2-3	[a]; [b]; CNS excitation/seizures due to normeperidine; contra-indicated in renal insufficiency
Methadone	20 mg q6-8h	10 mg q6-8h	15-36	[a]; Risk of delayed toxicity due to accumulation; reduce dose or lengthen dose interval if oversedation after 4-5 days; may schedule as prn initially
Oxycodone	30 mg q3-4h	N/A	—	[a]; [c]
Oxymorphone	N/A	1 mg	—	[a]
Fentanyl, transdermal	N/A	100 µg/h	—	[a]; [d]; Patch sizes of 25, 50, 75, 100 µg/h; slow onset to effect, necessitating "breakthrough" analgesics
Agonist-antagonist				
Butorphanol	N/A	2 mg	2.5-4	[a]; [b]; Intranasal formulation, 30 × pentazocine's antagonistic activity
Dezocine	N/A	10 mg	2-3	[a]; [b]; Greater antagonistic activity than pentazocine
Nalbuphine	N/A	10 mg	4-6	[a]; [b]; 10 × pentazocine's antagonistic activity
Pentazocine	180 mg	30 mg	2-3	[a]; [b]; Weak antagonistic activity; oral product combined with naloxone
Partial agonist				
Buprenorphine	N/A	0.3 mg	2-3	[a]; [b]; Equipotent to naloxone

[a] Common side effects include constipation, nausea, and sedation. Uncommon side effects include itching, dry mouth, and urinary retention. Rare side effects are hypotension and inappropriate antidiuretic hormone secretion.
[b] Not recommended for treatment of chronic cancer pain.
[c] Available alone and in combination with aspirin or acetaminophen; at higher doses, use as a single agent.

Adapted, with permission, from American Pain Society.[26]

[d] Patch duration = 72 hours but may be 48 hours for some patients.

Parenteral morphine dose (mg/24 h)	Transdermal fentanyl (µg/h)
8–22	25
23–37	50
38–52	75
53–67	100
68–82	125
83–97	150

TABLE 8

Adjuvant Drugs for Cancer Pain

Drug	Dosage	Therapeutic effects	Comments
Steroids			
Corticosteroids			
Prednisolone	10 mg tid PO	Potentiates analgesia	Effective for pain caused by compression
		Elevates mood	of nerves or spinal cord or from intra-
Dexamethasone	4 mg PO q6h or less	Improves appetite	cranial pressure; risk of GI bleeding
Progestin			
Medroxyprogesterone acetate	2–3 g/d for 10 days; 2 g for 3 weeks; 1 g thereafter	Potentiates analgesia Antitumor effects	Side-effects: nausea, vomiting, fluid retention → hypertension, edema, cardiac failure
Antidepressants			
Amitriptyline	Start 10–25 mg HS, increase gradually to 75–100 mg HS	Potentiates opioid analgesia Elevates mood Induces sleep	Effective for deafferentation pain (post-herpetic neuralgia, phantom limb pain, Pancoast's tumor)
Doxepin	Start 10–20 mg HS, increase gradually to 75–150 mg hs		
Imipramine	200 mg HS for severe depression	Antidepressant	High dose to treat severe depression as required
Anxiolytics			
Hydroxyzine	Start with 25 mg tid PO; increase to 50–100 mg q4–6h	Potentiates opioid analgesia Reduces anxiety Antiemetic Sedative	To potentiate analgesia, decrease anxiety, nausea, and vomiting Convulsions occur with more than 500 mg/d
Diazepam	5–10 mg PO, IV, or rectally bid or tid	Relief of acute anxiety and panic; also antiemetic and sedative	More antiemetic and fewer sedative effects than chlorpromazine; risk of orthostatic hypotension and hypotonia
Phenothiazines			
Methotrimeprazine	10–20 mg IM or 20–30 mg PO	Produces moderate analgesia without risk of tolerance or physical dependence	Used as alternative to narcotics if they are contraindicated
Chlorpromazine	10–25 mg q4–8h	Reduces anxiety Produces hypnosis	Risk of orthostatic hypotension; rarely causes jaundice and neurologic reaction
Prochloperazine	5-10 mg q4-8h	Antiemetic No analgesic effect	
Fluphenazine	1–3 mg every day	Reduces anxiety Antiemetic Analgesic	Combined with an antidepressant, useful in deafferentation pain (postherpetic neuralgia, postamputation pain, plexus neuropathy)
Haloperidol	Start 1 mg tid PO, increase to 2–4 mg tid PO	Decreases confusion Antiemetic	More potent antiemetic than chlor-promazine
Anticonvulsants			
Carbamazepine	Start 100 mg daily, increase by 100 mg q4 days to 500–800 mg/d	Anticonvulsant Decreases abnormal CNS neuronal activity	Useful for postherpetic neuralgia, de-afferentation pain; continuous hematologic monitoring required

Table 8 continues

TABLE 8 *continued*

Adjuvant Drugs for Cancer Pain

Drug	Dosage	Therapeutic effects	Comments
Anticonvulsants *continued*			
Phenytoin	Start 100 mg daily, increase by 25–50 mg q4 days to 250–300 mg/d		
Amphetamines			
Dextroamphetamine	2.5 mg tid or 5 mg/d PO in morning	Potentiate narcotic analgesia Elevate mood	For terminally ill patients with pain, depression, and lethargy
Methamphetamine	5 mg in morning	Decreases lethargy Increases physical activity	Tolerance develops rapidly

Adapted, with permission, from Bonica JJ[32] and Payne R.[33]

TABLE 9

Neurostimulatory and Neuroablative Procedures

Site	Procedure	Indications
Neurostimulatory procedures		
Peripheral nerve	Transcutaneous and percutaneous electrical nerve stimulation	Painful dysesthesias from tumor infiltration of nerve or trauma, eg, neuroma
Spinal cord	Dorsal column stimulation	Limited use in deafferentation pain in the chest, midline, and lower extremities
Brain stem	Periaqueductal stimulation	Used rarely to treat deafferentation pain in the chest, midline, or lower extremities
Thalamus	Thalamic stimulation	Used rarely to treat deafferentation pain in the chest, midline, or lower extremities
Neuroablative procedures		
Peripheral nerve	Neurectomy	Not indicated; neurolytic blocks are the procedure of choice
Nerve root	Rhizotomy	Somatic and deafferentation pain from tumor infiltration of the cranial and, rarely, intercostal nerves
Spinal cord	Dorsal root entry zone lesion	Unilateral deafferentation pain from brachial, intercostal, and lumbosacral plexopathy, and postherpetic neuralgia
	Cordotomy	Unilateral pain below the waist, often combined with local neurolytic blocks in perineal and bilateral lumbosacral plexopathy
	Myelotomy	Midline pain below the waist, but rarely employed because it involves extensive surgery
Brain stem	Mesencephalic tractotomy	Pain in the nasopharynx and trigeminal region
Thalamus	Thalamotomy	Unilateral deafferentation pain in the chest and lower extremities
Cortex	Cingulotomy; frontal lobotomy	Not commonly used for cancer pain
Pituitary	Transsphenoidal hypophysectomy	Bone metastases in endocrine-dependent tumors, eg, breast and prostate cancers

Adapted from Foley KM, Arbit E.[19]

TABLE 10

Anesthetic Procedures

Type of procedure	Most common indications
Nerve block	
Peripheral	Pain in discrete dermatomes in the chest and abdomen
Epidural	Unilateral lumbar or sacral pain; midline perineal pain; bilateral lumbosacral pain
Intrathecal	Midline, perineal pain; bilateral lumbosacral pain
Autonomic	
Stellate ganglion	Sympathetic-maintained pain; arm pain
Lumbar sympathetic	Sympathetic-maintained pain; lumbosacral plexopathy; vascular insufficiency of the lower extremities
Celiac plexus	Midabdominal pain
Continuous epidural infusion of local anesthetics	Unilateral and bilateral lumbosacral pain; midline perineal pain
Chemical hypophysectomy	Diffuse bone pain
Inhalation therapy	Generalized pain; incident pain
Trigger-point injection	Focal muscle pain

Adapted from Foley KM and Arbit E.[19]

General guidelines for opioid therapy are outlined in Table 5.[27] The rules of opioid use are to: (1) individualize the agent, route, dose, and schedule; (2) titrate to efficacy; (3) provide for breakthrough pain; (4) anticipate and treat side effects; and (5) make conversions from one route to another or one agent to another by using known equianalgesic doses. Opioid agonists do not exhibit ceiling effects. Dosing is guided by efficacy and limited by side effects (Table 6).[26] Dosages of tablets combining a nonsteroidal anti-inflammatory drug (NSAID) and an opioid are limited according to the NSAID.

The oral route of administration should be used when possible. If this is not feasible or systemic side effects are uncontrollable, alternative routes are indicated (Table 7).[26] Spinal routes,[28,29] both epidural and intrathecal, can be employed with internal delivery systems that allow patients to be fully ambulatory. Although in wide use, these methods have not been tested for cost-effectiveness. The spinal route should be considered if oral and other routes are unavailable or systemic therapy produces unacceptable side effects. Another advantage of spinal administration is that local anesthetic agents may be combined with the opioid to enhance analgesia at a lower total opioid dose.

The side effects of opioids can usually be anticipated and treated. In particular, laxatives should be prescribed with regular opioid dosing. Physical dependence and tolerance to some effects develop with chronic opioid use. Tolerance is likely to develop to respiratory depression, sedation, and nausea.[27] Tolerance to analgesia is not a major clinical problem and can usually be managed by changing the dose of an agent or substituting another agent.[24] Most current definitions of addiction imply a behavioral syndrome of compulsive, harmful use but do not require the existence of physical dependence or tolerance.[30] Iatrogenic addiction is not likely to occur in patients without a substance-abuse history.[31]

During chronic opioid therapy, certain precautions should be observed. Normeperidine is a toxic metabolite of meperidine that accumulates with repetitive dosing; thus, the use of meperidine for chronic pain is limited. Placebo use is discouraged, because it does not help to distinguish the pathophysiology of pain. Physical withdrawal symptoms can be avoided by tapering doses. A changed mental status should not be attributed to opioid therapy until medical and neurologic factors have been fully evaluated.

Neuropathic pain may be less responsive to standard analgesics alone. Adjuvants such as antidepressants, anticonvulsants, benzodiazepines, local anesthetics, neuroleptics, psychostimulants, antihistamines, corticosteroids, levodopa, calcitonin, and diphosphonates are useful for particular indications (Table 8).[32,33] These agents may be administered through oral and other routes.[34]

Nonpharmacologic Treatment

Many nonpharmacologic approaches are available for the treatment of cancer pain, but the indications for these forms of therapy have yet to be defined.

Stimulation and Ablation: The loss of normal sensory input, as occurs when a peripheral nerve is severed, may lead to deafferentation pain. Some patients obtain relief from electrical stimulation, which augments non-nociceptive input (Table 9).[19] Neurostimulation may be applied transcutaneously or via implanted devices to peripheral nerves, the spinal cord, or the brain. Carefully selected patients may benefit from surgical implantation of stimulation devices.[35,36]

Neuroablation, or destruction of nerve tissue, may be accomplished by chemical or surgical means. The goal of this technique is to isolate the site of somatic pain from the central nervous system. The efficacy of each procedure must be weighed against the risks. A significant percentage of patients who fail to respond to oral therapy may be helped with appropriate nerve blocks. It is not known which patients might benefit from earlier procedures.[37,38] Somatic nerve blocks may be diagnostic (ie, to determine the indication for permanent neurolysis of somatic nerves), facilitative, prophylactic, or therapeutic. Visceral blocks (such as the celiac plexus block) have been demonstrated to be effective for specific pain syndromes. Sympathetically maintained pain is suggested when signs of marked sympathetic dysfunction accompany typical diffuse burning or deep aching pain. Sympathetic blockade may then be diagnostic and therapeutic. In some cases of refractory generalized pain, pituitary adenolysis has been effective (Table 10).[19]

Surgical ablation[39] may be accomplished by rhizotomy (section of nerve root) or dorsal root entry-zone lesions. Spinal anterolateral tractotomy or cordotomy, mesencephalotomy, medullary tractotomy, and cingulotomy should be reserved for carefully selected cases.

Physical Therapy: Physical therapy modalities, such as massage, ultrasonography, hydrotherapy, electroacupuncture, and trigger point injection, are indicated for musculoskeletal pain and may enhance exercise tolerance in a patient undergoing rehabilitation.[40] Skillful soft-tissue manipulation is probably underutilized.

Psychological Techniques: Cancer patients may regain a much needed sense of control by using psychological techniques, such as imagery, hypnosis, relaxation, biofeedback, and other cognitive-behavioral methods.[41]

Ongoing Care

The goals of treatment must be frequently reviewed and integrated into the overall management plan.[42,43] Communication among the professional staff, patient, and family or other significant caregivers is essential. A sensitive, frank discussion with the patient regarding his or her wishes should guide medical decision-making during all phases of illness.

CONCLUSIONS

Control of cancer pain remains a challenge. A combination of pharmacologic and nonpharmacologic methods will relieve pain for the majority of cancer patients, yet a significant number of patients have pain that defies our best efforts to provide effective therapy. Current investigation into the pathophysiology of some forms of neuropathic pain holds promise for the development of new strategies. Advances in existing ambulatory-care technology may produce better systems for the long-term management of pain.

REFERENCES

1. Levin DN, Cleeland CS, Dar R: Public attitudes toward cancer pain. Cancer 56:2337–2339, 1985.

2. Portenoy RK: Cancer pain: Epidemiology and syndromes. Cancer 63:2298–2307, 1989.

3. World Health Organization: Cancer Pain Relief and Palliative Care. Geneva, World Health Organization, 1990.

4. Stjernsward J: Cancer pain relief: An important global public health issue, in Fields HL, et al (eds): Advances in Pain Research and Therapy, vol 9, pp 555–558. New York, Raven Press, 1985.

5. Bonica JJ: Treatment of cancer pain: Current status and future needs, in Fields HL, et al (eds): Advances in Pain Research and Therapy, vol 9, pp 589–616. New York, Raven Press, 1985.

6. American College of Physicians, Health and Public Policy Committee: Drug therapy for severe chronic pain in terminal illness. Ann Intern Med 99:870–873, 1983.

7. Ventafridda V, Tamburini M, Caraceni A, et al: A validation study of the WHO method for cancer pain relief. Cancer 59:850–856, 1987.

8. Walker VA, et al: Evaluation of WHO analgesic guidelines for cancer pain in a hospital-based palliative care unit. J Pain Symptom Management 3:145–149, 1988.

9. Breitbart W: Suicide, in Holland J, Rowland J (eds): Handbook of Psychooncology, pp 291–299. New York, Oxford University Press, 1990.

10. von Roenn JH, Cleeland CS, Gonin R, et al: Physician attitudes and practice in cancer pain management: A survey from the Eastern Cooperative Oncology Group. Ann Intern Med 119:121–126, 1993.

11. Hill CS, Fields HL (eds): Drug Treatment of Cancer Pain in a Drug-Oriented Society: Advances in Pain Research and Therapy, vol 11. New York, Raven Press, 1990.

12. Friedman D: Perspectives on the medical use of drugs of abuse. J Pain Symptom Management 5(suppl):S2–5, 1990.

13. Acute Pain Management Guideline Panel: Acute Pain Management: Operative or Medical Procedures and Trauma. Clinical Practice Guideline. AHCPR Publ No 92-0032. Rockville, Md, Agency for Health Care Policy and Research, Public Health Service, U.S. Department of Health and Human Services, 1992.

14. Portenoy RK, Payne R: Acute and Chronic Pain, in Lowinson JH, Ruiz P, Millman RB (eds): Substance Abuse: A Comprehensive Textbook, 2nd ed, pp 691–721. Baltimore, Williams & Wilkins, 1992.

15. NIH Consensus Development Conference Statement: The Integrated Approach to the Management of Pain, vol 6, no 3, 1986.

16. IASP Subcommittee on Taxonomy: Pain terms: A list with definitions and notes on usage. Pain 8:249–252, 1980.

17. Portenoy RK: Mechanisms of clinical pain: Observations and speculations. Neurol Clin 7:207, 1989.

18. American Psychiatric Association: Diagnostic and Statistical Manual of Mental Disorders, 3rd ed, Revised, pp 264–267. Washington, DC, American Psychiatric Association, 1987.

19. Foley KM, Arbit E: Management of cancer pain, in DeVita VT, Hellman S, Rosenberg SA (eds): Cancer: Principles and Practice of

Oncology, vol 2, 3rd ed, pp 2064–2087. Philadelphia, JB Lippincott, 1989.

20. Twycross RG, Fairfield S: Pain in far-advanced cancer. Pain 14:303–310, 1982.

21. Colodney A, Weinstein, SM, Multidisciplinary management of cancer pain. Pain Digest 1:221–229, 1991.

22. McGrath PJ, Unruh AM: Pain in Children and Adolescents: The Measurement and Assessment of Pain. New York, Elsevier Science Publishers, 1987.

23. Deragotis LR, Marrow GR, Fetting J, et al: The prevalence of psychiatric disorders among cancer patients. JAMA 249:754, 1983.

24. Foley KM: Pharmacologic approaches to cancer pain management, in Fields HL et al (eds): Advances in Pain Research and Therapy, vol 9, pp 629–653. New York, Raven Press, 1985.

25. McGrath PA: Pain in Children: Nature, Assessment, and Treatment. New York, Guilford Press, 1990.

26. American Pain Society: Principles of Analgesic Use in the Treatment of Acute Pain and Cancer Pain, 3rd ed. Skokie, Illinois, American Pain Society, 1992.

27. Inturrisi C: Management of cancer pain—pharmacology and principles of management. Cancer 63(suppl):2308–2320, 1989.

28. Plummer J, Cherry D, Cousins M, et al: Long-term spinal administration of morphine in cancer and non-cancer pain: A retrospective study. Pain 44:215–220, 1991.

29. Greenberg HS: Continuous spinal opioid infusion for intractable cancer pain, in Foley KM, Inturrisi C (eds): Advances in Pain Research and Therapy, vol 8, pp 351–359. New York, Raven Press, 1986.

30. Jaffe JH: Drug addiction and drug abuse, in Gilman AG, Goodman LS, Rall TW, et al (eds): The Pharmacologic Basis of Therapeutics, 8th ed, pp 532–581. New York, Macmillan Publishing Co, 1985.

31. Porter J, Jick H: Addiction rare in patients treated with narcotics. N Engl J Med 302:123, 1980.

32. Bonica JJ: The Management of Pain. Philadelphia, Lea & Febiger, 1990.

33. Payne R, Foley KM (eds): Cancer pain. Med Clin North Am 71:2, 1987.

34. Portenoy RK: Pharmacologic Management of Neuropathic Pain; A Neurology Alert Special Report. American Health Consultants, 1992.

35. Meyerson BA: Electrostimulation procedures: Effects, presumed rationale, and possible mechanisms, in Bonica JJ, et al (eds): Advances in Pain Research and Therapy, vol 5; pp 495–534. New York, Raven Press, 1983.

36. Duncan GH, Bushnell MC, Marchand S: Deep brain stimulation: A review of basic research and clinical studies. Pain 45:49–60, 1991.

37. Arner S: The role of nerve blocks in the treatment of cancer pain. Acta Anaesthesiol Scand Suppl 74:104–108, 1982.

38. Cousins MJ, Bridenbaugh PO (eds): Neural Blockade, 2nd Ed. Philadelphia, JB Lippincott, 1988.

39. Meyerson BA: The role of neurosurgery in the treatment of cancer pain. Acta Anaesthesiol Scand Suppl 74:109–113, 1982.

40. Travell J, Simons D: Myofascial Pain and Dysfunction. Baltimore, Williams & Wilkins, 1983.

41. Breitbart W: Psychiatric management of cancer pain. Cancer 63(suppl):2336–2342, 1989.

42. Coyle N, Adelhardt J, Foley KM: Changing patterns in pain, drug use, and routes of administration in the advanced cancer patient. Pain (suppl 4):S339, 1987.

43. Twycross RG, Lack SA: Therapeutics in Terminal Cancer, 2nd ed. London, Churchill Livingstone, 1990.

CHAPTER 41

Management of Nausea and Vomiting

Mary K. Crow, MD,[1] Habib M. Ghaddar, MD,[1] Richard Pazdur, MD,[2] *and* Giuseppe Fraschini, MD[3]

[1] Division of Medicine, [2] Department of Gastrointestinal Medical Oncology and Digestive Diseases, and
[3] Department of Breast and Gynecologic Medical Oncology
The University of Texas M. D. Anderson Cancer Center, Houston, Texas

The development of new and effective antiemetic agents has contributed to significant progress in the supportive care of cancer patients. Discoveries made in the last decade have changed our view of chemotherapy-induced nausea and vomiting from an inevitable problem or the norm to an exceptional and unacceptable occurrence.

In this chapter, we will review the types of chemotherapy-induced nausea and vomiting, their physiology, factors that affect emesis and its control, the antiemetic agents available—with a major emphasis on new advances—and an up-to-date approach to the management of this problem.

TYPES OF EMESIS

Chemotherapy causes three types of emesis. The first, most common, and best understood is acute emesis, arbitrarily defined as emesis occurring within the first 24 hours of chemotherapy. Despite major advances in its management, acute emesis still occurs in one third of patients receiving high doses of cisplatin (Platinol) and may cause patients to refuse further therapy.[1,2]

The second type of chemotherapy-related emesis is delayed emesis, defined as emesis occurring 24 hours or more after chemotherapy administration. The physiology of delayed emesis is poorly understood. Known risk factors for delayed emesis include female sex, a cisplatin dose exceeding 100 mg/m^2, and prior acute emesis following chemotherapy.[3] Delayed emesis has been reported in 20% to 50% of all cisplatin-treated patients and in up to 93% of patients treated with high-dose cisplatin.[4-6] This emetic syndrome may affect patients who do not have acute emesis and may be quite severe. In one study, delayed emesis necessitated hospital readmission in 11% of patients treated with high-dose cisplatin.[7] The occurrence and patterns of delayed emesis following non-cisplatin chemotherapy have not been well described.

The third type of chemotherapy-related emesis is anticipatory emesis, which begins prior to the administration of chemotherapy, usually in patients whose emesis was poorly controlled during a previous chemotherapy cycle. Anticipatory emesis affects nearly 25% of patients who have received several rounds of chemotherapy[8] and is believed to be a conditioned response to the hospital environment or other treatment-related associations.

PHYSIOLOGY

Neurologic structures involved in the chemotherapy-induced emetic reflex include the vomiting center, or emetic center, in the lateral reticular formation of the medulla; the chemoreceptor trigger zone (CTZ) in the area postrema of the medulla; the cerebral cortex; and the vagal and splanchnic afferents from the gut to the vomiting center and CTZ.[9]

The vomiting center is the final common pathway for vomiting stimuli and coordinates the act of vomiting. This reflex center receives stimuli from the vestibular areas, the pathway involved in motion sickness; from the cerebral cortex, the pathway believed to be involved in anticipatory vomiting; from the CTZ; and from the gut through vagal and greater splanchnic afferents.

Because the CTZ is in the area postrema, an area of the medulla characterized by the absence of an effective blood-brain barrier, this center may be directly stimulated by chemotherapeutic agents or their metabolites. Until recently, such stimulation was considered the fundamental emetogenic mechanism in patients receiving chemotherapy. However, evidence now shows that chemotherapeutic agents induce vomiting by stimulating neuroreceptors in the gastrointestinal tract as well.

Early research focused on dopamine receptors because of the therapeutic benefit obtained from two types of dopamine-receptor antagonists, the phenothiazines and metoclopramide. The histaminic and muscarinic receptors were also known to be involved.[10,11] However, because metoclopramide lacks activity as an antiemetic at low doses, despite adequate dopamine-receptor blockade, the role of dopamine receptors was questioned. At higher doses, metoclopramide becomes more effective and displays significant antagonism against serotonin receptors.[12]

Serotonin has since been identified as the principal mediator of chemotherapy-induced emesis. Subsequent investigations have allowed separation of efficacy, eg,

FIGURE I

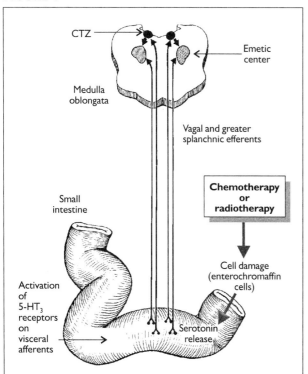

Pathogenesis of chemotherapy- and radiotherapy-induced emesis. Enterochromaffin cells of the GI tract, when damaged by chemotherapy or radiotherapy, release serotonin, which activates peripheral and/or central receptors for 5-hydroxytryptamine (5-HT$_3$), or serotonin type 3. CTZ = chemoreceptor trigger zone. Adapted from Cubeddu et al.[13]

FIGURE 2

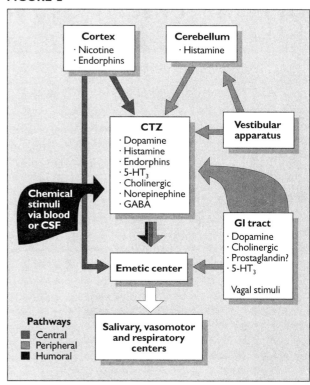

Central, peripheral, and humoral pathways of emesis and some of the neuroreceptors believed to be involved in the pathogenesis of chemotherapy-induced nausea and vomiting. Major physiologic pathways are indicated by the larger arrows. CTZ = chemoreceptor trigger zone; 5-HT$_3$ = 5-hydroxytryptamine; GABA = γ-aminobutyric acid.

serotonin-mediated effects, from toxicity, eg, dopamine-mediated effects. More recently, attention has shifted to the 5-hydroxytryptamine (5-HT$_3$), or serotonin type-3, receptor. Recent receptor-binding studies have identified four distinct receptors, some of which possess distinct subtypes.[10]

Figure 1 provides a new model of the pathogenesis of chemotherapy- and radiotherapy-induced emesis.[13] Enterochromaffin cells of the gastrointestinal tract, when damaged by chemotherapy or radiotherapy, release serotonin, which activates peripheral and/or central 5-HT$_3$ receptors. Receptors for 5-HT$_3$ have been found in vagal afferents from the upper gastrointestinal tract and in neurons of the area postrema.[14] Urinary 5-hydroxyindoleacetic acid (5-HIAA) is derived mainly from serotonin in the gastrointestinal tract, and 80% of total body serotonin is found in the enterochromaffin cells of the gastrointestinal tract close to the vagal afferents. In clinical studies, urinary 5-HIAA levels increased significant-

ly in patients treated with cisplatin, and these increases correlated with the number of vomiting episodes.[13]

Agents that block 5-HT$_3$ receptors control emesis caused by non-cisplatin chemotherapy and by abdominal irradiation. Research continues on 5-HT$_3$ and other neuroreceptors, such as the opiate μ receptors, which may be important in other emetogenic circumstances, as shown in Figure 2.

FACTORS INFLUENCING EMESIS

Factors that affect emesis and its control can be divided into those inherent to the patient and those related to the chemotherapeutic regimen or the antiemetic program, as shown in Table 1.[15] An appreciation of these factors should assist the clinician in selecting the appropriate antiemetic regimen and the investigator in interpreting and designing clinical studies.

Factors predisposing patients to emesis include younger age,[15] female sex,[15] and susceptibility to motion

TABLE 1

Factors Affecting Chemotherapy-Induced Emesis

Patient related

Prior exposure to chemotherapy
Age
Gender
History of alcohol abuse
History of motion sickness

Chemotherapy related

Emetic potential and pattern of each agent
Dose, route, schedule
Combination of agents

Antiemetic related

Efficacy and side effects
Dose, route, schedule
Combination of agents
Concomitant nonpharmacologic agents

Adapted, with permission, from Tonato et al.[15]

TABLE 2

Emetogenic Potential of Various Chemotherapeutic Agents

Agent	Onset (h)	Duration (h)
Very high (> 90% incidence)		
Cisplatin	1–6	24–48
Dacarbazine	1–3	1–12
Mechlorethamine	0.5–2	8–24
High-dose melphalan	3–6	6–12
High (60%–90%) incidence		
Carmustine	2–4	4–24
Cyclophosphamide	4–12	12–24
Procarbazine	24–27	Variable
High-dose etoposide	4–6	24+
Moderate (30%–60%)		
Doxorubicin	4–6	6+
Mitoxantrone	4–6	6+
Fluorouracil	3–6	24+
Carboplatin	4–6	12–24
Low (10%–30% incidence)		
Bleomycin	3–6	—
Cytarabine	6–12	3–5
Etoposide	3–8	—
Melphalan	6–12	—
Ifosfamide	1–2	Extended
Mercaptopurine	4–8	—
Methotrexate	4–12	3–12
Mitomycin	1–4	48–72
Vinblastine	4–8	—
Very low (< 10% incidence)		
Vincristine	4–8	—
Chlorambucil	48–72	—

sickness.[16] Prior chemotherapy, particularly with poor control of emesis, increases the likelihood of emesis with subsequent treatments, independent of the anticipatory component.[17] In one prospective and two retrospective studies, acute emesis was more easily controlled in chronic heavy drinkers (ie, those who consumed more than 100 mg of alcohol [five mixed drinks] daily) than in other patients.[18,19]

Age also influences the patient's predisposition to antiemetic side effects. Patients younger than 30 years have a 13-fold greater risk of extrapyramidal side effects from dopamine-receptor antagonists than do older patients (27% vs 2%).[20] When these drugs are used for several consecutive days, dystonic reactions are even more common.[21]

Chemotherapeutic agents differ in their emetic potential and cause different patterns of emesis onset and duration. Cisplatin tends to cause almost immediate acute emesis, whereas the acute emesis associated with cyclophosphamide tends to have a more delayed onset, usually 8 to 12 hours after drug administration.[22] Table 2 groups agents into four categories according to their emetogenic potential.

The emetogenic potential and pattern of any chemotherapeutic agent can vary, sometimes markedly, based on the dose, route, and schedule of administration. Melphalan (Alkeran), for example, has low emetogenic potential at standard doses but becomes intensely emeto-genic at high doses. When agents are given in daily, fractionated doses or by continuous infusion, the intensity of the emetic reactions is generally lowered, but emesis is more prolonged. Combinations of chemotherapeutic agents result in more intense emesis and more complex emetic patterns. Knowledge of the emetic intensity and pattern of a chemotherapeutic regimen (peak activity, duration, and delayed phase) is fundamental to the planning of appropriate antiemetic therapy.

Furthermore, the efficacy and adverse effects of antiemetics vary with the dose, route, and schedule of administration and with the other agents or nonpharmacologic therapeutic modalities with which they are combined. These things may also affect the pattern of emesis following chemotherapy.

METHODOLOGY OF ANTIEMETIC TRIALS

Because of the subjectivity of endpoints such as nausea and the multiplicity of potential variables, the most suitable type of study for assessing antiemetics is a prospective, randomized, double-blind, parallel group trial with stratification for established prognostic factors.[15,23,24] Crossover studies are complicated by the loss of participants on the second course, the influence of the first course outcome on the response to the crossover regimen, and the impossibility of assessing efficacy during subsequent courses. These limitations offset the advantages that crossover studies offer—namely, the requirement for smaller patient populations and the ability of participants to express their preference for one regimen. Trials with a placebo-controlled arm in highly emetogenic chemotherapy are unethical.

Close attention should be paid to trial design and the manner in which endpoints are chosen, defined, and evaluated. Ideally, trials should stratify participants for variables such as age, sex, prior chemotherapy, emetogenicity of chemotherapy, cancer type, and history of chronic alcohol abuse. Whether episodes of dry retching are included with vomiting episodes will affect the end result of the study and, eventually, how effective a drug is considered to be. The only objective endpoint in antiemetic trials remains complete absence of nausea and vomiting.

Assessment of response to antiemetic therapy is becoming more standardized[15] as descriptors such as "mild" or "severe" are being replaced with more objective definitions. "Complete response" is defined as no vomiting or dry retching episodes in 24 hours, and "major response" as only one or two such episodes. The assessment of nausea by means of visual analog scales also is more objective and reliable.

During the development of the 5-HT$_3$-receptor antagonists, control of vomiting, not of nausea, was the primary endpoint. Since strict criteria for rescue treatment were used, dose-finding studies usually established a partially effective dose rather than a completely effective dose. Also, these drugs were compared with cocktails containing corticosteroids, benzodiazepines, or diphenhydramine. Matching an antiemetic treatment that is given once a day, ie, granisetron (Kytril) or tropisetron, with a cocktail requires that the patients receive placebo injections or dummy drugs. This has been difficult to justify, and, thus, many trials have been unblinded.[25]

ANTIEMETIC AGENTS

In general, antiemetic therapy consists of a combination of agents. Table 3 summarizes the doses, schedules of administration, and side effects of the most commonly used agents.

Phenothiazines

Phenothiazines, which include prochlorperazine and chlorpromazine, were the first antiemetics to be used to control chemotherapy-induced emesis. However, at standard doses, they are clearly inferior to other available agents, including ondansetron (Zofran), granisetron, tropisetron, metoclopramide, dexamethasone, and tetrahydrocannabinol.[26–31] Phenothiazines prevent emesis by blocking dopamine type-2 receptors in the CTZ. The advantage of the phenothiazines is their convenience of administration: These agents can be given orally, intramuscularly, intravenously, or rectally. Like metoclopramide, phenothiazines may become more effective when given at higher doses,[32] but their adverse effects also are likely to become more pronounced. Side effects include extrapyramidal symptoms, dystonic reactions, akathisia, sedation, anticholinergic effects, and orthostatic hypotension.

Substituted Benzamides

Of the substituted benzamides, metoclopramide is the most frequently used for controlling chemotherapy-induced emesis. Its failure at low doses, as demonstrated by the lack of superiority over placebo,[33] called into question both the prominent role of dopamine receptors in chemotherapy-induced nausea and vomiting and the old theory that emesis was induced by decreased lower esophageal sphincter tone and delayed gastric emptying.

In the early 1980s, high-dose metoclopramide was demonstrated to be safe and effective in treating chemotherapy-induced emesis.[17] At a dosage of 1 to 3 mg/kg IV every 2 hours, metoclopramide was superior to placebo and to prochlorperazine in cisplatin-treated patients.[26] High-dose metoclopramide then became the gold standard for treatment, and comparative studies demonstrated its superiority over all other antiemetics available until the late 1980s. As a single agent, high-dose metoclopramide achieves complete control of emesis in up to 40% of patients receiving high-dose cisplatin.[26] Combined with dexamethasone, high-dose metoclopramide completely controls emesis in up to 60% of patients.[34,35]

Side effects such as extrapyramidal symptoms (especially dystonia in younger patients) and akathisia are a major problem.[20] These effects may be prevented by the addition of an antihistamine, such as diphenhydramine, or lorazepam.[36] Another disturbing side effect is diarrhea, which can be significantly reduced by the addition of dexamethasone.[34]

TABLE 3

Doses, Schedules, and Major Side Effects of Commonly Used Antiemetics

Agent	Dose	Route	Frequency	Major side effects
Granisetron	40 µg/kg 1 mg	IV PO	Daily Daily	Headache, constipation
Ondansetron	0.15 mg/kg 8–32 mg 8 mg (1 mg/h) 8 mg	IV IV IV PO	4–8 h Daily Continuous 8 h (tid)	Headache, constipation
Tropisetron	5 mg 5 mg	IV PO	Daily Daily	Headache, constipation
Metoclopramide	2–3 mg/kg 1–3 mg/kg 20 mg	IV PO PO	2–3 h 3–4 h 8 h (tid)	Dystonia, akathisia, hypotension, sedation, extrapyramidal reactions, diarrhea
Haloperidol	1–3 mg 1–2 mg	IV PO	2–6 h 3–6 h	Dystonia, akathisia, hypotension, sedation
Droperidol	0.5–2 mg	IV	4 h	Extrapyramidal reactions
Prochlorperazine	5–10 mg 10–20 mg 25 mg 10–20 mg	PO PO Rectal IM	3–4 h 8–12 h 4–6 h 3–6 h	Extrapyramidal reactions, sedation, dystonia, hypotension, anticholinergic effects, akathisia
Chlorpromazine	25–50 mg 25 mg	PO IM/IV	3–6 h 3–6 h	Same as prochlorperazine
Thiethylperazine	10 mg	PO/rectal	4 h	Same as prochloperazine
Dexamethasone	10–20 mg 4 mg	IV PO	Daily 4–12 h	Hyperglycemia, euphoria, insomnia, rectal pain
Methylprednisolone	250–500 mg	IV	Daily	Same as dexamethasone
Lorazepam	0.025 mg/kg 1–2 mg	IV PO	4–8 h 4–8 h	Sedation, amnesia, confusion, hypotension
Diphenhydramine	25–50 mg 25–50 mg	IV PO	6 h 6 h	Anticholinergic effects, sedation
Delta-9-tetrahydro-cannabinol (dronabinol)	5–10 mg/m²	PO	3–4 h	Dysphoria, confusion, ataxia, hypotension, tachycardia, hallucination
Nabilone	2 mg	PO	6–12 h	Same as dronabinol

High-dose oral metoclopramide appears to be safe and as effective as the intravenous form.[37–39] It is not approved by the US Food and Drug Administration (FDA) as an antiemetic, however. Oral metoclopramide, like all oral antiemetics, should be used only as a prophylactic measure or in patients who fully respond to this route of administration, since nausea and vomiting might preclude its intake. An intranasal preparation is under investigation.[40]

Serotonin-Receptor Antagonists

There are two FDA-approved 5-HT$_3$-receptor-selective antagonists available for the prevention and treat-

ment of chemotherapy-induced nausea and vomiting. Ondansetron and granisetron are available in the United States intravenously and orally. A third such drug, tropisetron, is available in both forms only in Europe. The pharmacologic profiles of these three agents are somewhat different,[41,42] but no clear difference has manifested in the available clinical experience. Their doses and schedules are given in Table 3.

Ondansetron: Ondansetron was the first serotonin-receptor antagonist to be approved by the FDA for chemotherapy-induced nausea and vomiting. With various intravenous schedules, ondansetron achieved complete control of emesis in 40% to 75% of patients receiving cisplatin-based chemotherapy, partial control in an additional 20% to 30%, and a significant delay in emesis.[13,43-46] Ondansetron was superior to metoclopramide for multiple-day, cisplatin-based regimens.[47] None of these early studies, however, demonstrated better control of delayed nausea and vomiting by either metoclopramide or ondansetron. Ondansetron has also been tested with the highly emetogenic dacarbazine and is very effective.[48-51]

In the United States, intravenous ondansetron has been approved for use at a dosage of 0.15 mg/kg every 4 hours for a total of three doses. This agent, however, is active at a broad range of doses and has marked flexibility. The most effective dose and schedule have not yet been determined. Single daily doses (8 or 32 mg) and continuous low-dose infusions have been found to be equally effective.[52]

In a recent multicenter, stratified, randomized, double-blind, parallel-group study evaluating 699 patients treated with cisplatin, a single 32-mg dose of ondansetron was somewhat more effective than a single 8-mg dose and at least as effective as the standard regimen of three 0.15-mg/kg doses.[53] However, a similarly designed European study did not show any significant difference among single 8- or 32-mg doses or an 8-mg dose followed by a continuous infusion.[54] Unfortunately, no study has evaluated a single intermediate dose of ondansetron. Single lower-dose schedules may be very cost effective if proved as efficacious as the 32-mg dose.

Ondansetron is also available in oral form (4- and 8-mg tablets). Since its efficacy by this route appears comparable to that of the injectable formulation, at least for non-cisplatin-induced emesis, intravenous administration is not needed in most instances if the oral form is started prior to chemotherapy. In breast cancer patients treated with cyclophosphamide (Cytoxan, Neosar), doxorubicin (Adriamycin, Rubex), and fluorouracil, dosages of 1, 4, and 8 mg three times daily were found effective, with dose-related efficacy and no dose-related increase in toxicity. All three ondansetron dosages were more effective than a conventional, partly intravenous antiemetic regimen given to a fourth group.[55]

A larger, multicenter randomized study assessing the same oral dosages in cancer patients who received non-cisplatin therapy showed similar efficacy for the 4- and 8-mg tablets and a dose-effect trend.[56] Two multicenter randomized trials have shown that 8 mg of oral ondansetron twice a day is as effective as 8 mg three times a day for the prevention of nausea and vomiting in cyclophosphamide-based chemotherapy.[57,58]

A major advantage of ondansetron is its lack of dys-

tonic reactions and the other extrapyramidal effects seen with dopamine-receptor antagonists such as metoclopramide, butyrophenones, and phenothiazines. The side effects of ondansetron include headache (which is easily controlled by nonnarcotic analgesics), constipation, mild sedation, and a transient increase in serum transaminases. Recent studies have indicated that combinations of ondansetron and prochlorperazine for emesis prophylaxis may increase clearance of cyclophosphamide and cisplatin.[59,60]

Granisetron: Dose-ranging studies of granisetron have established that 10 to 40 µg/kg as a single intravenous dose prior to cisplatin chemotherapy achieves complete control of emesis in 40% to 61% of patients, with one third of patients free of nausea, and also significantly delays time to first emetic episode.[61,62] Interestingly, granisetron in these studies also had a positive effect on appetite, with 50% of these patients able to eat within 24 hours of chemotherapy at granisetron doses greater than 10 µg/kg.[61]

A randomized, double-blind, phase III trial comparing granisetron (a single intravenous dose of 80 µg/kg) with the combination of metoclopramide, dexamethasone, and diphenhydramine showed equivalent complete control of emesis (46% vs 44%). However, delayed emesis and nausea were controlled slightly better by the cocktail.[63] Other studies comparing the efficacy of 40 µg/kg and 160 µg/kg reported no statistical difference in efficacy or safety between the doses but did document the efficacy of granisetron as a rescue treatment as well as the safety of dosing up to 240 µg/kg within a 24-hour period.[64]

While cisplatin produces profound emetogenic effects with 1 to 2 hours of administration, other agents, such as cyclophosphamide or carboplatin, have peak effects at 6 to 18 hours. A single intravenous dose of 40 µg/kg of granisetron given as prophylaxis prior to such moderately emetogenic chemotherapy achieves complete control of vomiting in 68% of patients vs 47% of patients receiving a chlorpromazine and dexamethasone cocktail as prophylaxis.[65,66] Combining granisetron with dexamethasone given intravenously prior to moderately emetogenic chemotherapy provided complete control of vomiting in a recent trial.[67]

Two single-blind studies have compared granisetron to various combinations of metoclopramide, dexamethasone, and alizapride (an investigational agent available in the European market), over a 5-day fractionated chemotherapy regimen containing cisplatin.[68,69] Initial complete control of vomiting was superior in the granisetron arm (87% vs 66%). Throughout the 5-day period, control of emesis was seen in 47% to 54% receiving granisetron vs

44% of patients receiving the combination. Extrapyramidal side effects were observed in 5% to 21% of patients receiving the combination therapy.

Two open-label studies have evaluated the efficacy of granisetron (40 µg/kg in a single intravenous dose) over multiple cycles of chemotherapy. Overall, 60% 87% of patients had either no vomiting or only one episode during eight or more cycles of cisplatin-containing chemotherapy, and the incidence of adverse events did not increase with multiple cycles.[70,71]

An oral formulation of granisetron was recently released in the United States. A double-blind study comparing the 1-mg oral dose of granisetron given twice a day with a 10-mg oral dose of prochlorperazine given twice a day in moderately emetogenic chemotherapy showed granisetron was significantly better in achieving total control (defined as no emetic episodes, no nausea of any severity, and no need for antiemetic rescue) in both genders and at 24 hours.[72] Moreover, oral granisetron (1 mg twice daily) with or without dexamethasone is as effective as high doses of metoclopramide and dexamethasone for cisplatin-induced emesis.[73,74]

Like that of ondansetron, the side effect profile of granisetron is favorable across many different chemotherapy regimens and patient populations.[75] Headache, mild to moderate in severity, has been seen in 15% of patients at doses of 2 to 160 µg/kg. Constipation has occurred in 7%, especially in patients receiving multiple-day therapy. No patients have reported extrapyramidal symptoms. Other adverse effects, such as hypertension, diarrhea, agitation, and somnolence, have been reported in less than 10% of patients.[75]

Tropisetron: Tropisetron is currently available only in Europe, where most of the clinical trials have been conducted. The first results reported were from an open-label trial of patients who had experienced severe nausea and vomiting during prior chemotherapy. Complete control of vomiting was seen in 66% of chemotherapy courses at a tropisetron dose of 20 mg (given in two 15-minute intravenous infusions).[76]

Several double-blind dose-finding studies have defined a single 5-mg intravenous or oral dose prior to chemotherapy as effective.[42,77] Other trials have evaluated tropisetron as a single 5-mg intravenous dose on day 1 of chemotherapy followed by 5 mg once daily on subsequent days and compared this with combinations of lorazepam and metoclopramide.[78,79] Complete control of vomiting was seen in 45% to 67% of patients receiving tropisetron vs 22% of patients receiving the cocktail, although the incidence of nausea was equal and delayed nausea and vomiting were not affected.

The efficacy of tropisetron during fractionated or multiple cycles of chemotherapy awaits formal study but can be inferred from many studies to be at least equivalent to that of the other 5-HT$_3$ receptor antagonists available.[42]

Comparative Trials: There are few trials comparing the three 5-HT$_3$-receptor antagonists. A recent randomized, double-blind study comparing single doses of granisetron, 10 µg/kg and 40 µg/kg IV, vs three 0.15-mg/kg IV doses of ondansetron in chemotherapy-naive patients receiving cisplatin did not demonstrate any significant differences between treatment groups in control of emesis, nausea, or side effects.[80,81]

In another open-label, prospective, randomized trial, no difference was seen between granisetron, 3 mg IV, ondansetron, 24 mg IV,[82] or tropisetron, 5 mg IV.[83] Two randomized, double-blind, parallel-group studies comparing granisetron in a single, daily 3-mg IV dose with ondansetron, 8 mg IV two[84] or three[85] times daily for patients receiving cisplatin-based chemotherapy also did not show a difference in efficacy (both greater than 88%). Cost comparisons of these agents with each other and with conventional antiemetics are needed.

Corticosteroids

The mechanism by which corticosteroids act as antiemetics is still unclear. The two corticosteroids most commonly used as antiemetics are dexamethasone and methylprednisolone. Neither has a known therapeutic advantage over the other. Although their role as single agents is minor but definite,[27,86] they are essential to some combination antiemetic regimens.

Dexamethasone, at intravenous doses of 10 to 20 mg, improved the efficacy of high-dose metoclopramide in cisplatin-treated patients by 20%.[34] Dexamethasone also improved the efficacy of ondansetron in a similar patient population by 27% (91% vs 64% with ondansetron alone).[87] However, dexamethasone may decrease the incidence of extrapyramidal side effects of dopamine-receptor antagonists as well as the incidence of diarrhea associated with metoclopramide administration.[34]

Dexamethasone and methylprednisolone are safe and well tolerated. Blood sugar monitoring is recommended when corticosteroids are used in diabetics. Acute transient rectal pain has been reported with rapid infusion.[40]

Benzodiazepines

The short-acting benzodiazepine lorazepam has a distinctive role in the management of chemotherapy-induced nausea and vomiting. It is a drug with documented antiemetic, amnesic, and anxiolytic effects.[88] When lorazepam was given before and after cisplatin, at doses of

0.025 mg/kg (not exceeding 4 mg), 46% of patients did not recall receiving chemotherapy, regardless of whether they vomited or not, and 80% had no significant anxiety following chemotherapy. These data support the use of lorazepam for the prevention of anticipatory vomiting, although it is not clear whether the prophylactic effect is related to the drug's amnesic properties.

As discussed earlier, lorazepam may also significantly decrease the incidence of dystonic reactions to metoclopramide.[36] Side effects of lorazepam include perceptual disturbances, urinary incontinence, hypotension, diarrhea, sedation, and amnesia.

Antihistamines

The most commonly used antihistamine, diphenhydramine, has modest antiemetic activity as a single agent. Its main use is in antiemetic combinations to reduce the extrapyramidal side effects of dopamine-receptor antagonists. Side effects of diphenhydramine include sedation and anticholinergic effects.

Butyrophenones

The butyrophenones, typified by haloperidol and droperidol, also work by blocking dopamine receptors in the CTZ. At dosages of 1 to 3 mg IV every 2 to 6 hours, haloperidol has definite antiemetic activity, although it is less effective than high-dose metoclopramide in controlling emesis.[5,89] Higher doses of haloperidol given intravenously and more frequently have been reported to achieve better results. Side effects of haloperidol include akathisia, dystonic and extrapyramidal reactions, and hypotension.

Cannabinoids

Tetrahydrocannabinol and nabilone are second-line antiemetics with limited efficacy.[28,29,90] Their mechanism of action is unclear. Side effects, which include euphoria, dizziness, paranoid ideation, and somnolence, are more common in older patients.

COMBINATION REGIMENS

Combining antiemetics can improve efficacy over that of a single agent or counteract the toxicity of one of the agents. The most effective combinations prior to the availability of the 5-HT$_3$-receptor antagonists generally included a dopamine type-2 neuroreceptor blocker, a glucocorticoid, and an antihistamine and/or a benzodiazepine. The number of agents used and their doses and schedule depended on the expected emetogenic potential and emetic pattern of the chemotherapeutic regimen employed. These antiemetic combinations are the standards against which newer agents have been evaluated. Table 4 lists commonly used antiemetic combinations, including those that employ 5-HT$_3$-receptor antagonists instead of dopamine-receptor antagonists.

The enhanced efficacy of combinations over single agents has been demonstrated by the improved management of acute and delayed emesis achieved by adding dexamethasone to high-dose intravenous metoclopramide (60% vs 40%),[34] oral metoclopramide (57% vs 35%),[91] and intravenous ondansetron (91% vs 64%)[87] and by the improved overall efficacy achieved by adding dexamethasone to the butyrophenones.[7] Amelioration of toxicity is exemplified by the decreased incidence of dystonic reactions to dopamine-receptor antagonists when diphenhydramine or lorazepam is added.[36] The incidence of diarrhea from metoclopramide is significantly reduced when it is combined with dexamethasone.[34]

Very encouraging early reports suggest that the efficacy of ondansetron may be increased when it is used in combination with other antiemetics. The combination of ondansetron and dexamethasone achieved complete emetic control in 91% of patients receiving cisplatin doses exceeding 50 mg/m^2, whereas ondansetron alone was completely effective in only 64% of patients.[87] The same combination was recently compared with a three-agent regimen of metoclopramide, dexamethasone, and diphenhydramine and found to be more effective and more tolerable.[92] In another study, the addition of a dopamine-receptor blocker in standard doses appeared to enhance the activity of ondansetron against moderately emetogenic chemotherapy.[93]

Tropisetron has been combined with dexamethasone or haloperidol to increase control of both acute and delayed nausea and vomiting in patients receiving cisplatin-based chemotherapy or high-dose alkylating agents.[94,95] Total control of acute nausea and vomiting was increased to 75% with tropisetron and dexamethasone, and delayed nausea and vomiting were also significantly controlled.[94] Haloperidol, 0.5 mg every 12 hours, given with tropisetron improved control of vomiting in the first 24 hours of chemotherapy.[95]

MANAGEMENT OF DELAYED EMESIS

Effective therapy for delayed emesis remains inadequate, probably because this problem is not well understood. Regimens with proven efficacy include the combination of oral metoclopramide and dexamethasone (Table 4), which in a double-blind, randomized trial proved to be superior to placebo (81% vs 61%).[90] Dexamethasone as a single agent has more limited efficacy.[91]

Based on the conflicting and inconclusive results of

TABLE 4

Combination Antiemetic Regimens for Emetogenic Chemotherapy

Antiemetic regimen	Schedule	Recommended use
Ondansetron, 0.15 mg/kg IV	30 min prior to chemotherapy, then every 4 h after chemotherapy is given, for a total of 3 doses	Acute emesis (highly emetogenic regimens)
+ dexamethasone, 20 mg IV	40 min prior to chemotherapy	
± lorazepam, 1.5 mg/m^2 IV	35 min prior to chemotherapy	
Ondansetron, 8–32 mg IV	30 min prior to chemotherapy	Acute emesis (cisplatin and non-cisplatin regimens)
+ dexamethasone, 10–20 mg IV	30–45 min prior to chemotherapy	
± lorazepam, 1.5 mg/m^2 IV	30–45 min prior to chemotherapy	
Granisetron, 1 mg IV	30 min prior to chemotherapy and daily during chemotherapy	Acute emesis (cisplatin and non-cisplatin regimens, multiple-day regimens)
+ dexamethasone, 20 mg IV	40 min prior to chemotherapy	
Tropisetron, 5 mg IV day 1, then 5 mg PO daily during chemotherapy	30 min prior to chemotherapy	acute emesis (cisplatin and non-cisplatin regimens, multiple-day regimens)
+ dexamethasone, 8 –20 mg, IV	40 min prior to chemotherapy	
Metoclopramide, 3 mg/kg IV	30 min prior to chemotherapy, followed by a second dose 90 min after chemotherapy is given	Acute emesis (high-dose cisplatin)
+ dexamethasone, 20 mg IV	40 min prior to chemotherapy	
+ lorazepam, 1.5 mg/m^2 IV	35 min prior to chemotherapy	
Metoclopramide, 2 mg/kg IV	30 min prior to chemotherapy, followed by a second dose 90 min after chemotherapy is given	Acute emesis (moderate-dose cisplatin, non-cisplatin regimens)
+ dexamethasone, 20 mg IV	40 min prior to chemotherapy	
+ lorazepam, 1.5 mg/m^2 IV, or diphenhydramine, 50 mg IV	35 min prior to chemotherapy	
Metoclopramide, 0.5 mg/kg PO	On 1st and 2nd day after chemotherapy is given, then as needed on 3rd and 4th day	Delayed emesis (cisplatin)
+ dexamethasone, 8 mg PO	On 1st and 2nd day after chemotherapy is given	
+ dexamethasone, 4 mg PO	On 3rd and 4th day after chemotherapy is given	

four trials, oral ondansetron alone does not appear promising for the management of delayed emesis.[45,96–98] In contrast, combinations of ondansetron with oral dexamethasone, especially starting 16 hours after chemotherapy administration, protected 86% of patients from acute emesis and 65% from delayed emesis.[99] However, in one randomized, double-blind, multicenter trial, the combination of granisetron and dexamethasone for delayed nausea and vomiting caused by high-dose cisplatin chemotherapy was not significantly different from that of dexamethasone alone.[100]

MANAGEMENT OF ANTICIPATORY EMESIS

Since anticipatory emesis is believed to be a conditioned response that usually occurs in patients in whom emesis was poorly controlled during previous chemo-

therapy, good control of emesis during the first chemotherapy course remains the most effective means of prevention. Although different approaches have been tried, including behavioral modification therapy, counseling, desensitization, and hypnosis, treating this problem once it has occurred is generally difficult. Pharmacologic therapy has been limited to lorazepam, as previously discussed. Other benzodiazepines, such as alprazolam, may be similarly effective.

OTHER MANAGEMENT CONSIDERATIONS

Table 5 lists various general principles for the management of chemotherapy-induced emesis. The rationale underlying most of these principles has been given earlier, along with specific examples and recommendations for putting them into practice.

TABLE 5

General Principles for Management of Chemotherapy-Induced Emesis

- Rule out other causes of nausea and vomiting, which may require appropriate and specific treatment.

- Be aware of chemotherapy- and patient-related factors that influence the patterns and intensity of emesis, and choose the antiemetic regimen accordingly.

- Combinations of antiemetic agents provide better protection; more agents may be required with more intensely emetogenic chemotherapy.

- Prevention is more effective than treating established emesis; initiating an appropriate antiemetic regimen before emetogenic chemotherapy will also reduce emesis and anticipatory emesis with subsequent chemotherapy administrations.

- Treat emesis for the expected duration with scheduled antiemetics rather than "as needed" administration.

- Nonpharmacologic antiemetic modalities may enhance the success of antiemetic therapy.

- Limit use of expensive antiemetics; however, control of nausea and vomiting should take precedence over cost.

When dealing with emesis in patients receiving chemotherapy, other causes of nausea and vomiting should always be kept in mind. Cancer patients may develop nausea and vomiting as a result of bowel obstruction, fecal impaction, brain metastasis, leptomeningeal disease, hypercalcemia and other metabolic problems, narcotic analgesics, autonomic neuropathy induced by vinca alkaloids or paraneoplastic syndromes, or advanced cancer itself, independent of other factors.[101,102] These possible causes are particularly relevant to delayed or anticipatory emesis.

Finally, the cost of antiemetic agents should be considered.[103,104] Although newer agents may have shown higher efficacy in selected groups of patients, these agents tend to be more expensive. Older agents with time-honored safety and efficacy may be considerably less expensive and sometimes of equal or better efficacy for specific indications, such as for delayed or anticipatory emesis or with less intensely emetogenic chemotherapy. Thus, as long as control of nausea and vomiting remains optimal, judicious use of the newer, more expensive agents is highly recommended.

REFERENCES

1. Bleiberg H: Antiemetic agents. Curr Opin Oncol 4:597–604, 1992.

2. Hoagland AC, Morrow GR, Bennett JM, et al: Oncologists' views of cancer patient noncompliance. Am J Clin Oncol 6:239–244, 1983.

3. Gandara DR, Harvey WH, Monaghan GG, et al: The delayed emesis syndrome from cisplatin: Phase III evaluation of ondansetron versus placebo. Semin Oncol 19(suppl 10):67–71, 1992.

4. Grunberg SM, Akerly WL, Krailo MD, et al: Comparison of metoclopramide and metoclopramide plus dexamethasone for complete protection from cisplatin-induced emesis. Cancer Invest 4:379–385, 1986.

5. Grunberg SM, Gala KV, Lampenfeld M, et al: Comparison of the antiemetic effect of high dose intravenous metoclopramide and high dose intravenous haloperidol in a randomized double-blind crossover study. J Clin Oncol 12:782–787, 1984.

6. Kris MG, Gralla RJ, Clark R, et al: Incidence, course and severity of delayed nausea and vomiting following administration of high dose cisplatin. J Clin Oncol 3:1397–1404, 1985.

7. Mason BA, Dambra J, Grossman B, et al: Effective control of cisplatin-induced nausea using high dose steroids and droperidol. Cancer Treat Rep 66:243–245, 1982.

8. Mitchell EP: Gastrointestinal toxicity of chemotherapeutic agents. Semin Oncol 19:566–579, 1992.

9. Borison HL, McCarthy LE: Neuropharmacology of chemotherapy-induced emesis. Drugs 25(suppl 1):8–17, 1983.

10. Andrews PLR, Davis CJ: The mechanism of emesis induced by anticancer therapies, in Andrews PLR, Sanger CJ (eds): Emesis in Anti-Cancer Therapy, Mechanisms and Treatment, pp 113–162. London, Chapman & Hall Medical, 1993.

11. Peroutka SJ, Snyder SH: Antiemetics: Neurotransmitter receptor binding predicts therapeutic action. Lancet 1:658–659, 1982.

12. Fozard JR, Mobarok Ali ATM: Blockade of neuronal tryptamine receptors by metoclopramide. Eur J Pharmacol 49:109–112, 1978.

13. Cubeddu LX, Hoffman IS, Fuenmayor NT, et al: Efficacy of ondansetron (GR 38032F) and the role of serotonin in cisplatin-induced nausea and vomiting. N Engl J Med 322:810–816, 1990.

14. Kilpatrick GJ, Jones BJ, Tyers MB: Binding of the 5-HT$_3$ ligand, 3H-GR65630, to rat area postrema, vagus nerve and the brains of several species. Eur J Pharmacol 159:157–164, 1989.

15. Tonato M, Roila F, Del Favero A: Methodology of antiemetic trials: A review. Ann Oncol 2:107–114, 1991.

16. Morrow GR: The effect of a susceptibility to motion sickness on the side effects of cancer chemotherapy. Cancer 55:2766–2770, 1985.

17. Gralla RJ, Braum TJ, Squillante A, et al: Metoclopramide: Initial clinical studies of high dosage regimens in cisplatin-induced emesis, in Poster E (ed): The Treatment of Nausea and Vomiting Induced by Cancer Chemotherapy, pp 167–176. New York, Masson, 1981.

18. D'Acquisto RW, Tyson LB, Gralla RJ, et al: The influence of a chronic high alcohol intake on chemotherapy-induced nausea and vomiting (abstract). Proc Am Soc Clin Oncol 5:257, 1986.

19. Sullivan JR, Leyden MJ, Bell R: Decreased cisplatin induced nausea and vomiting with chronic alcohol ingestion. N Engl J Med 309:796, 1983.

20. Kris MG, Tyson LB, Gralla RJ, et al: Extrapyramidal reactions with high-dose metoclopramide. N Engl J Med 309:433–434, 1983.

21. Allen JC, Gralla RJ, Reilly C, et al: Metoclopramide: Dose related toxicity and preliminary antiemetic studies in children receiving cancer chemotherapy. J Clin Oncol 3:1136–1141, 1985.

22. Cubeddu LX, Hoffman IS, Fuenmayor NT, et al: Antagonism of serotonin S3 receptors with ondansetron prevents nausea and emesis induced by cyclophosphamide containing chemotherapy regimens. J Clin Oncol 8:1721–1727, 1990.

23. Olver IN, Simon RM, Aisner J: Antiemetic studies: A methodological discussion. Cancer Treat Rep 70:555–563, 1986.

24. Olver IN: Methodology in anti-emetic trials. Oncology 49: 269–272, 1992.

25. McVie GJ, de Bruijn KM: Methodology of antiemetic trials. Drugs 43(suppl 3):1–5, 1992.

26. Gralla RJ, Itri LM, Pisko SE, et al: Antiemetic efficacy of high-dose metoclopramide: Randomized trials with placebo and prochlorperazine in patients with chemotherapy-induced nausea and vomiting. N Engl J Med 305:905–909, 1981.

27. Markman M, Sheidler V, Ettinger DS, et al: Antiemetic efficacy of dexamethasone: Randomized, double-blind, crossover study with prochlorperazine in patients receiving cancer chemotherapy. N Engl J Med 311:549–552, 1984.

28. Frytak S, Moertel CG, O'Fallon J, et al: Delta 9-tetrahydrocannabinol as an antiemetic in patients treated with cancer chemotherapy: A double-blind comparison with prochlorperazine and a placebo. Ann Intern Med 91:825–830, 1979.

29. Sallan SE, Cronin CM, Zelen M, et al: Antiemetics in patients receiving chemotherapy for cancer: A randomized comparison of delta-9 tetrahydrocannabinol and prochlorperazine. N Engl J Med 302:135–138, 1980.

30. Perez EA, Gandara DR: The clinical role of granisetron (Kytril) in the prevention of chemotherapy-induced emesis. Semin Oncol 21(suppl 5):15–21, 1994.

31. de Bruijn KM: Tropisetron. A review of the clinical experience. Drugs 43(suppl 3):11–22, 1992.

32. Carr BI, Blayney D, Goldberg DA, et al: High doses of prochlorperazine for cisplatin-induced emesis: A prospective, random, dose-response study. Cancer 60:2165–2169, 1987.

33. Gralla RJ: Metoclopramide: A review of antiemetic trials. Drugs 25(suppl 1):63–73, 1983.

34. Kris MG, Gralla RJ, Tyson LB, et al: Improved control of cisplatin-induced emesis with high dose metoclopramide and with combination of metoclopramide, dexamethasone, and diphenhydramine: Results of consecutive trials in 255 patients. Cancer 55:527–534, 1985.

35. Allen SG, Cornbleet MA, Warrington PS, et al: Dexamethasone and high-dose metoclopramide: Efficacy in controlling cisplatin-induced nausea and vomiting. Br Med J 289:878–879, 1984.

36. Kris MG, Gralla RJ, Clark RA, et al: Antiemetic control and prevention of side effects of anticancer therapy with lorazepam or diphenhydramine when used in combination with metoclopramide plus dexamethasone: A double-blind, randomized trial. Cancer 60:2816–2822, 1987.

37. Anthony LB, Krozely MG, Woodward NJ, et al: Antiemetic effect of oral versus intravenous metoclopramide in patients receiving cisplatin: A randomized, double-blind trial. J Clin Oncol 4:98–103, 1986.

38. Taylor WB, Bateman DN: Oral bioavailability of high-dose metoclopramide. Eur J Clin Pharmacol 31:41–44, 1986.

39. Edge SB, Funkhouser WK, Berman A, et al: High-dose oral and intravenous metoclopramide in doxorubicin/cyclophosphamide-induced emesis. Am J Clin Oncol 10:257–263, 1987.

40. Krasnow SH: New directions in managing chemotherapy-related emesis. Oncology 5(suppl):19–24, 1991.

41. Andrews PLR: The pharmacologic profile of granisetron (Kytril). Semin Oncol 21(suppl):3–9, 1994.

42. Lee RC, Plosker GL, McTavish D: Tropisetron. A review of its pharmacodynamic and pharmacokinetic properties, and therapeutic potential as an antiemetic. Drugs 46:925–943, 1993.

43. Marty M, Pouillart P, Scholl S, et al: Comparison of the 5-hydroxytryptamine$_3$ (serotonin) antagonist ondansetron (GR 38032F) with high dose metoclopramide in the control of cisplatin-induced emesis. N Engl J Med 322:816–821, 1990.

44. Hesketh PJ, Murphy WK, Lester EP, et al: GR 38032F (GR-C

507/75): A novel compound effective in the prevention of acute cisplatin-induced emesis. J Clin Oncol 7:700–705, 1989.

45. DeMulder PHM, Seynaeve C, Vermorken JB, et al: Ondansetron compared with high-dose metoclopramide in prophylaxis of acute and delayed cisplatin-induced nausea and vomiting. Ann Intern Med 113:834–840, 1990.

46. Hainsworth J, Harvey W, Pendergrass K, et al: A single-blind comparison of intravenous ondansetron, a selective serotonin antagonist, with intravenous metoclopramide in the prevention of nausea and vomiting associated with high-dose cisplatin chemotherapy. J Clin Oncol 9:721–728, 1991.

47. Sledge GW, Einhorn L, Nagy C: Phase III double-blind comparison of intravenous ondansetron and metoclopramide as antiemetic therapy for patients receiving multiple-day cisplatin-based chemotherapy. Cancer 70:2524–2528, 1992.

48. Bonneterre J, Chevallier B, Metz R, et al: A randomized double-blind comparison of ondansetron and metoclopramide in the prophylaxis of emesis induced by cyclophosphamide, fluorouracil, and doxorubicin or epirubicin chemotherapy. J Clin Oncol 8:1063–1069, 1990.

49. Legha SS, Hodges C, Ring S: Efficacy of ondansetron against nausea and vomiting caused by dacarbazine-containing chemotherapy. Cancer 70:2018–2020, 1992.

50. Kaasa S, Kvaloy S, Dicato MA, et al: A comparison of ondansetron with metoclopramide in the prophylaxis of chemotherapy-induced nausea and vomiting: A randomized double-blind study. Eur J Cancer 26:311–314, 1990.

51. Schmoll HJ: The role of ondansetron in the treatment of emesis induced by non-cisplatin containing chemotherapy. Eur J Cancer Clin Oncol 25(suppl 1):535-539, 1989.

52. Marty M, d'Hallens H: A single daily dose of ondansetron is as effective as a continuous infusion in the prevention of cisplatin induced nausea and vomiting. Ann Oncol 1(suppl 1):112, 1990.

53. Beck TM, Hesketh PJ, Madajewicz S: Stratified, randomized, double-blind comparison of intravenous ondansetron administered as a multiple-dose regimen versus two single-dose regimens in the prevention of cisplatin-induced nausea and vomiting. J Clin Oncol 10:1969–1975, 1992.

54. Seynaeve C, Schuller J, Buser K, et al, and the Ondansetron Study Group: Comparison of the anti-emetic efficacy of different doses of ondansetron, given as either a continuous infusion or a single intravenous dose, in acute cisplatin emesis: A multicenter, double-blind, parallel group study. Br J Cancer 66:192–197, 1992.

55. Fraschini G, Ciociola A, Esparza L, et al: Evaluation of three oral dosages of ondansetron in the prevention of emesis associated with doxorubicin-cyclophosphamide chemotherapy. J Clin Oncol 9:1268–1274, 1991.

56. Beck TM, Ciociola AA, Jones SE, et al: Efficacy of oral ondansetron in the prevention of emesis in outpatients receiving cyclophosphamide-based chemotherapy. Ann Intern Med 118:407–413, 1993.

57. DiBenedetto, J, Cubeddu L, Ryan T, et al: Twice daily oral ondansetron effectively prevents nausea and vomiting associated with cyclophosphamide-doxorubicin-based chemotherapy (abstract 1780). Proc Am Soc Clin Oncol 14:538, 1995.

58. Beck T, York M, Chang A, et al: Oral ondansetron 8 mg BID is as effective as 8 mg TID in the prevention of nausea and vomiting associated with cyclophosphamide-based chemotherapy (abstract 1781). Proc Am Soc Clin Oncol 14: 538, 1995.

59. Cagnoni PJ, Matthes S, Dufton C, et al: Ondansetron significantly reduces the area under the curve (AUC) of cyclophosphamide (CPA) and cisplatin (cDDP) (abstract 1489). Proc Am Soc Clin Oncol 14:462, 1995.

60. Gilbert CJ, Petros WP, Cavanaugh C, et al: Influence of

ondansetron (OND) on the pharmacokinetics (PK) of high dose cyclophosphamide (CPA) (abstract 931). Proc Am Soc Clin Oncol 14:316, 1995.

61. Navari RM, Kaplan HG, Gralla RT, et al: Efficacy and safety of granisetron, a selective 5-hydroxytryptamine-$_3$ receptor antagonist in the prevention of nausea and vomiting induced by high-dose cisplatin. J Clin Oncol 12:2204–2210, 1994.

62. Rivier A, on behalf of the Granisetron Study Group: Dose finding study of granisetron in patients receiving high-dose cisplatin chemotherapy. Br J Cancer 69:967–971, 1994.

63. Warr D, Wilan A, Venner P, et al: A randomized, double-blind comparison of granisetron and high-dose metoclopramide, dexamethasone and diphenhydramine for cisplatin induced emesis. Eur J Cancer 29A:33–36, 1993.

64. Soukop M: A comparison of two dose levels of granisetron in patients receiving high-dose cisplatin. Eur J Cancer 26(suppl 1):S15–29, 1990.

65. Marty M, on behalf of the Granisetron Study Group: A comparison of granisetron as a single agent with conventional combination antiemetic therapies in the treatment of cytostatic induced emesis. Eur J Cancer 28A(suppl 1):S12–16, 1992.

66. Marty M: A comparative study of the use of granisetron, a selective 5-HT$_3$ antagonist, versus a standard anti-emetic regimen of chlorpromazine plus dexamethasone in the treatment of cytostatic-induced emesis. Eur J Cancer 26(suppl 1):S28–32, 1990.

67. Roila F, and the Italian Group for Antiemetic Research: Dexamethasone, granisetron, or both for the prevention of nausea and vomiting during chemotherapy for cancer. N Engl J Med 332:1–5, 1995.

68. Bremer K, on behalf of the Granisetron Study Group: A single-blind study of the efficacy and safety of intravenous granisetron compared with alizapride plus dexamethasone in the prophylaxis and control of emesis in patients receiving 5-day cytostatic therapy. Eur J Cancer 28A:1018–1022, 1992.

69. Diehl, V, on behalf of the Granisetron Study Group: Fractionated chemotherapy—Granisetron or conventional antiemetics? Eur J Cancer 28A(suppl 1):S21–28, 1992.

70. Blijham GH, on behalf of the Granisetron Study Group: Does granisetron remain effective over multiple cycles? Eur J Cancer 28A(suppl 1):S17–S21, 1992.

71. de Wet M, Falkson G, Rapoport BL: Repeated use of granisetron in patients receiving cytostatic agents. Cancer 71:4043–4049, 1993.

72. Palmer R, Moriconi W, Cohn J, et al: A double-blind comparison of the efficacy and safety of oral granisetron with oral prochlorperazine in preventing nausea and emesis in patients receiving moderately emetogenic chemotherapy (abstract 1740). Proc Am Soc Clin Oncol 14:528, 1995.

73. Heron JF, Geodhals L, Jordaan JP, et al: Oral granisetron alone and in combination with dexamethasone: A double-blind randomized comparison against high-dose metoclopramide plus dexamethasone in prevention of cisplatin-induced emesis. Ann Oncol 5:579–584, 1994.

74. Hacking A, on behalf of the Granisetron Study Group: Oral granisetron—simple and effective: A preliminary report. Eur J Cancer 28A (suppl 1):S28–32, 1992.

75. Dilly S: Granisetron (Kytril) clinical safety and tolerance. Semin Oncol 21 (suppl 5):10–14, 1994.

76. Leibundgut U, Lancranjan I: First results with ICS 205-930 (5-HT$_3$ receptor antagonist) in prevention of chemotherapy-induced emesis. Lancet 1:1198, 1987.

77. Van Belle SJ-P, Stamatakis L, Bleiberg H, et al: Dose-finding study of tropisetron in cisplatin-induced nausea and vomiting. Ann

Oncol 5:821–825, 1994.

78. Sorbe BG, Hogberg T, Glimelius B, et al: A randomized, multicenter study comparing the efficacy and tolerability of tropisetron, a new 5-HT$_3$ receptor antagonist, with a metoclopramide-containing antiemetic cocktail in the prevention of cisplatin-induced emesis. Cancer 73:445–454, 1994.

79. Anderson H, Thatcher N, Howell A, et al: Tropisetron compared with a metoclopramide-based regimen in the prevention of chemotherapy-induced nausea and vomiting. Eur J Cancer 30A:610–615, 1994.

80. Ritter H, Hall S, Mailliard J, et al: A comparative clinical trial of granisetron and ondansetron in the prophylaxis of cisplatin-induced emesis (abstract 1739). Proc Am Soc Clin Oncol 14:528, 1995.

81. Navari R, Gandara D, Hesketh P, et al: Comparative trial of granisetron and ondansetron in the prophylaxis of cisplatin-induced emesis. J Clin Oncol 13:1242–1248, 1995.

82. Bonneterre J, Hecquet B: Granisetron IV compared with ondansetron IV plus tablets in the prevention of nausea and vomiting induced by moderately emetogenic chemotherapy regimen. A randomized cross-over study, pp 22–24. Presented at a satellite to the 7th ECCO meeting, Jerusalem, Israel, October 1993.

83. Jantunen IT, Muhonen TT, Kataja VV, et al: 5-HT$_3$ receptor antagonists in the prophylaxis of acute vomiting induced by moderately emetogenic chemotherapy—A randomized study. Eur J Cancer 29A:1669–1672, 1993.

84. Ruff P, Paska W, Geodhals L, et al: Ondansetron compared with granisetron in the prophylaxis of cisplatin induced acute emesis: A multicentre double-blind, randomized, parallel-group study. Oncology 51:113–118, 1994.

85. Noble A, Bremer K, Geodhals L, et al: A double-blind, randomized, crossover comparison of granisetron and ondansetron in 5-day fractionated chemotherapy: Assessment of efficacy, safety, and patient preference. Eur J Cancer (in press).

86. Aapro MS: Corticosteroids as antiemetics. Cancer Res 108:102–111, 1988.

87. Roila F, Tonato M, Cognetti F, et al: Prevention of cisplatin-induced emesis: A double-blind multicenter randomized crossover study comparing ondansetron and ondansetron plus dexamethasone. J Clin Oncol 9:675–678, 1991.

88. Laszlo J, Clark RA, Hanson DC, et al: Lorazepam in cancer patients treated with cisplatin: A drug having antiemetic, amnesic, and anxiolytic effects. J Clin Oncol 3:864–869, 1985.

89. Neidhart J, Gagen M, Wilson H, et al: Comparative trial of the antiemetic effects of THC and haloperidol. J Clin Pharmacol 21:385–390, 1981.

90. Sallan S, Zinsberg N, Frei EM: Antiemetic effect of delta-9-tetrahydrocannabinol in patients receiving cancer chemotherapy. N Engl J Med 293:795–797, 1975.

91. Tyson LB, Kris MG, Gralla RJ, et al: Double-blind, randomized trial for the control of delayed emesis: Comparison of placebo vs dexamethasone vs metoclopramide plus dexamethasone (abstract). Proc Am Soc Clin Oncol 6:267, 1987.

92. Roila F, Tonato M, Ballatori E, et al: Ondansetron + dexamethasone vs metoclopramide + dexamethasone + diphenhydramine in prevention of cisplatin-induced emesis: Italian Group for Antiemetic Research. Lancet 340:96–99, 1992.

93. Herrstedt J, Sisgaard T, Boesgaard M, et al: Ondansetron plus metopimazine compared with ondansetron alone in patients receiving moderately emetogenic chemotherapy. N Engl J Med 328:1076–1080, 1993.

94. Sorbe B, Hogberg T, Himmelmann A, et al: Efficacy and tolerability of tropisetron in comparison with a combination of tropisetron and dexamethasone in the control of nausea and vomiting

induced by cisplatin-containing chemotherapy. Eur J Cancer 30A:629–634, 1994.

95. Bregni M, Siena S, Di Nicola M, et al: Tropisetron plus haloperidol to ameliorate nausea and vomiting associated with high-dose alkylating agent cancer chemotherapy. Eur J Cancer 27:561–565, 1991.

96. Kris MG, Tyson LB, Clark RA, et al: Oral ondansetron for the control of delayed emesis after cisplatin. Cancer 70:1012–1016, 1992.

97. Gandara DR, Harvey WH, Monaghan GG, et al: Efficacy of ondansetron in the prevention of delayed emesis following high dose cisplatin (DDP) (abstract). Proc Am Soc Clin Oncol 9:328, 1990.

98. Roila F, Bracarda S, Tonato M, et al: Ondansetron (GR38032F) in the prophylaxis of acute and delayed cisplatin-induced emesis. Clin Oncol (R Coll Radiol) 2:268–272, 1990.

99. Rittenberg CN, Gralla RF, Lettow LA, et al: New approaches in preventing delayed emesis: Altering the time of regimen initiation and use of combination therapy in a 109 patient trial (abstract 1731).

Proc Am Soc Clin Oncol 14:526, 1995.

100. Johnston D, Latreille J, Laberge F, et al: Preventing nausea and vomiting during days 2-7 following high dose cisplatin chemotherapy (HDCP). A study by the National Cancer Institute of Canada Clinical Trials Group (NCIC CTG). Proc Am Soc Clin Oncol 14: 529, 1995 (abstract 1745).

101. Reuben DB, Mor V: Nausea and vomiting in terminal cancer patients. Arch Intern Med 146:2021–2023, 1986.

102. Bruera E, Catz Z, Hooper R, et al: Chronic nausea and anorexia in advanced cancer patients: A positive role for autonomic dysfunction. J Pain Symptom Manage 2:19–21, 1987.

103. Cunningham D, Gore M, Davidson N, et al: The real cost of emesis: An economic analysis of ondansetron vs metoclopramide in controlling emesis in patients receiving chemotherapy for cancer. Eur J Cancer 29A:303–306, 1993.

104. Goddard M: The real cost of emesis. Eur J Cancer 29A:297–298, 1993.

CHAPTER 42

Oncologic Emergencies

Virginia Rhodes, MD, *and* Ellen Manzullo, MD

Department of Medical Specialties, The University of Texas M. D. Anderson Cancer Center, Houston, Texas

An oncologic emergency may be defined as any acute potentially morbid or life-threatening event directly or indirectly related to a patient's tumor or its treatment. The differential diagnosis for a patient with cancer who presents with acute conditions includes medical emergencies not related to the patient's diagnosis of cancer. Occasionally, these emergent conditions may be the presenting symptom of a previously undiagnosed neoplasm.

Oncologic emergencies may be categorized by their system of origin, as metabolic, or as hematologic. The signs and symptoms of oncologic emergencies are often common problems experienced by individuals with cancer such as nausea, pain, headache, and fever. For prevention and early detection of oncologic emergencies, physicians must maintain a high degree of suspicion and must adequately educate patients about preventative measures and reporting of symptoms.

NEUROLOGIC EMERGENCIES

Spinal Cord Compression

Epidural spinal cord compression is devastating, and it is not an uncommon complication of malignancy. Spinal cord compression occurs in approximately 5% of patients with cancer, or 20,000 patients per year in the United States.[1] Untreated spinal cord compression will invariably progress to produce paralysis, sensory loss, or loss of anal sphincter control.

The majority of cases of spinal cord compression in adults arise from metastatic breast, lung, or prostate cancer. In children, the tumors most commonly metastatic to the spine include neuroblastoma, Ewing's sarcoma, osteogenic sarcoma, and rhabdomyosarcoma.[2] Other cancers that often cause spinal cord metastases include lymphoma, melanoma, renal cancer, sarcoma, and myeloma.

Compression usually results when an epidural tumor extends from an adjacent vertebral metastasis or from a pathologic vertebral compression fracture. In approximately 10% of cases, epidural compression results from direct paravertebral spread of tumor with epidural extension. Lymphoma and myeloma are the most common tumors of this type.[3]

The compression occurs at the thoracic level of the spinal cord in 70% of patients as this is the portion of the cord that is narrowest, and the dorsal kyphosis can enhance symptoms. Tumors may cause compression at multiple noncontiguous sites in 10% to 38% of patients. The neurologic deficit is determined by the level of involvement of the cord. Cervical compression results in quadriplegia, thoracic compression in paraplegia, upper lumbar involvement in bowel and bladder dysfunction and extensor plantar reflexes, and cauda equina involvement in loss of bowel and bladder function and lower motor neuron weakness with normal plantar reflexes. The corticospinal tracts, posterior columns, and spinocerebellar tracts are most susceptible to compression. The Brown-Séquard syndrome (a loss of vibratory and position senses on the side of compression and a contralateral loss of pain and temperature sensations) may be observed with lateral compression.[4]

In 95% of patients, the initial symptom of epidural spinal cord compression is progressive pain in an axial or radicular distribution. Cancer patients who present with new back pain should be considered to have impending cord compression until proven otherwise. Similar to that of degenerative joint disease (DJD), pain from compression is often aggravated by movement, Valsalva's maneuver, straight leg raise, and neck flexion. However, certain characteristics of pain originating from spinal cord compression distinguish it from that of DJD. The pain of spinal cord compression is often burning or dysesthetic in nature and is exacerbated by palpation or percussion over the spine. The pain can occur at any level, whereas that of DJD is often felt in the low cervical or lumbar regions. Spinal cord compression pain is progressive and unrelenting, whereas pain from DJD is often characterized by remissions and exacerbations. The pain of cord compression often worsens when a patient lies down. Weakness, sensory loss, and incontinence are later findings. Once a neurologic symptom develops, it can evolve rapidly to paraplegia over a period of hours or days.

The differential diagnosis of epidural spinal cord compression includes epidural abscess, subdural abscess, hematoma, herniated disc, hypertrophic arthritic changes, intramedullary cord metastases, leptomeningeal disease, radiation myelopathy, myelopathy secondary to intrathecal chemotherapy, or vascular malformation.[5] Evaluation often includes plain films of the spine, which may demonstrate lytic or blastic lesions or erosion of the pedicles. However, absence of these findings does not exclude cord compression.

Magnetic resonance imaging (MRI) has surpassed myelography as the diagnostic procedure of choice[2] for cases of spinal cord compression. Myelography should be reserved for patients (such as those with cardiac pacemakers) unable to undergo MRI. Use of contrast enhancement with MRI increases the ability to detect leptomeningeal and intramedullary disease. Patients should undergo full spinal imaging prior to definitive therapy to exclude unexpected epidural disease at other levels that may later become symptomatic.

The most important factor determining prognosis is the level of neurologic function at the beginning of therapy. Once a serious neurologic deficit develops, fewer than 10% of patients regain function despite aggressive therapy.[3] Immediate therapy involves the use of corticosteroids. Dexamethasone is the most commonly used steroid, but there is controversy regarding the optimal loading and maintenance doses. Commonly used doses of dexamethasone include a loading dose of 10 to 100 mg followed by 4 to 24 mg four times a day.[1] Higher doses may be administered to patients with rapidly progressive symptoms. Steroids are then slowly tapered throughout definitive therapy.

Radiotherapy alone is the definitive treatment for most patients. The recommended radiation field is two normal vertebral bodies above and below the margins of the epidural tumor.[6] There is no established optimal dose and fraction schedule.[7]

Radiotherapy plus laminectomy is of no benefit, and laminectomy may increase morbidity by producing spinal cord instability. Anterior spinal decompression with stabilization is an option for patients who are physiologically able to tolerate the surgery. The following are indications for surgery: histopathology is unknown; neurologic deterioration develops during or after radiation; metastases are radiation resistant; pathologic fracture causes compression by bone; or there is instability of the spine. Rarely, chemotherapy can be used as primary therapy in chemosensitive tumors, but it is often inadequate as a single modality of treatment.

Increased Intracranial Pressure

Involvement of the brain parenchyma with mass lesions or obstruction of the flow of cerebrospinal fluid (CSF) by tumor tissue may lead to increased intracranial pressure. If the pressure increase is severe enough, herniation may result. Patients may present with headache, cranial nerve symptoms, nausea and vomiting, or the onset of seizures.

Normal intracranial pressure is less than 10 mm Hg; when it increases to greater than 20 mm Hg, injury is likely and symptoms may develop. This is associated with loss of brain autoregulation and development of ischemia or herniation.

Three herniation syndromes have been described. Central herniation is characterized by slow deterioration in the level of consciousness, with associated headache and focal neurologic deficits. Progression results in global neurologic changes, Cheyne-Stokes respiration, and small reactive pupils. Central herniation is often difficult to distinguish from metabolic encephalopathy and is usually the result of a hemispheric mass.

Uncal herniation is characterized by rapid loss of consciousness, lateral pupillary dilatation, and ipsilateral hemiparesis. It is usually the result of a mass in the temporal lobe or the lateral fossa of the frontal lobe.

Tonsillar herniation is characterized by occipital headache, vomiting, and hiccups followed by decreasing level of consciousness and respiratory compromise. It usually results from a posterior fossa mass.[8]

Patients with early signs of increased intracranial pressure and herniation should be given intravenous corticosteroids. Usually, dexamethasone is given in doses similar to those used to relieve cord compression. Other temporizing measures include elevation of the patient's head to 30 degrees higher than the level of the heart, restriction of intravenous fluids, correction of hyperglycemia, and intubation with hyperventilation to maintain arterial P_{CO_2} at 25 to 30 mm Hg.[9]

Patients with impending herniation should also be treated with intravenous mannitol, 1 to 1.5 g/kg in a 20% solution. Mannitol can be repeated every 4 to 6 hours in doses adjusted to prevent excessive volume contraction and hypernatremia. Serum osmolality of greater than 320 mOsm/L should be avoided.[9] Surgical intervention with decompression or shunting should proceed as soon as possible.

Seizures

Seizures may be the presenting symptom in 15% to 30% of patients with brain metastases. Seizures can also be the result of complications of therapy, including infections, metabolic abnormalities, or medications.

Proper management of seizures acutely includes administration of diazepam (5 mg) or lorazepam for sus-

TABLE I

Paraneoplastic Syndromes of the Nervous System

Paraneoplastic syndromes	Associated neoplasms
Peripheral nervous system disorders	
Neuropathies	
Subacute sensory neuropathy (PSN)	Small-cell lung cancer
Symmetric sensimotor neuropathy	Carcinoma, lymphoma, myeloma
Motor neuropathy	Osteosclerotic myeloma
Guillain-Barré syndrome	Hodgkin's disease
Acquired amyloid neuropathy	Myeloma
Mononeuritis multiplex	Small-cell lung cancer
Intestinal pseudo-obstruction	Small-cell lung cancer
Neuromuscular junction disorders	
Myasthenia gravis	Thymoma
Lambert-Eaton myasthenic syndrome	Small-cell lung cancer
Muscle	
Polymyositis, dermatomyositis	Small-cell lung cancer, breast, ovary, lymphoma
Subacute necrotizing myopathy	Carcinoma, lymphoma
Central nervous system	
Encephalomyelitis (PEM)	Small-cell lung cancer, breast, ovary, lymphoma
Limbic	
Brain stem	
Subacute cortical degeneration (PCD)	
Opsoclonus, myoclonus	Neuroblastoma, ovary, lung
Necrotizing myelopathy	Small-cell lung cancer, breast
Cancer-associated retinopathy and uveomeningitis	Small-cell lung cancer, breast

PCD = paraneoplastic cerebellar degeneration, PEM = paraneoplastic encephalomyelitis, PSN = paraneoplastic sensory neuropathy
Adapted, with permission, from Schiller JH, Jones JC.[10]

tained seizures. Care must be taken to avoid injury to the patient and to maintain a patent airway. Patients should have a full diagnostic evaluation, including imaging, cultures, drug levels (if appropriate), and serum chemistries.

Patients with mass lesions should receive dexamethasone first and then definitive therapy. Sustained anticonvulsant therapy should then be initiated with phenytoin at a loading dose of 15 mg/kg and a maintenance dose of 300 mg/d.

Altered Mental Status

Altered mental status may take the form of confusion, decreased attentiveness, delirium, dementia, or coma. The condition may occur as a direct result of primary or metastatic lesions of the nervous system or secondarily from metabolic derangements, paraneoplastic syndromes, organ failure, infections, immune-mediated events, or iatrogenic causes. A full discussion of causes of altered mental status is beyond the scope of this chapter; however, several deserve mention.

Paraneoplastic neurologic syndromes can occur in the form of peripheral nervous system, muscular, neuromuscular, or central nervous system (CNS) disorders

(Table 1) and can be seen in a variety of malignancies.[10] Many of these syndromes are mediated by autoantibodies. For many, the etiology is still undefined. A paraneoplastic syndrome may be the initial presenting symptom of a malignancy or may occur at any time during the course of disease. These syndromes must be differentiated from the direct effects of cancer or therapy. The activity of the syndrome can parallel the course of the disease or exhibit an independent course. Specific therapy is often lacking and, therefore, is limited to treatment of the underlying malignancy.

Many chemotherapeutic agents produce neurologic toxicity. Among these are cytarabine, carmustine (BiCNU), etoposide (VePesid), fludarabine (Fludara), methotrexate, paclitaxel (Taxol), cisplatin (Platinol), ifosfamide (Ifex), vincristine (Oncovin), vinblastine, interleukin-2 (aldesleukin [Proleukin]), and interferon.

Leptomeningeal Disease

Leptomeningeal carcinomatosis is seen most commonly in the setting of advanced adenocarcinomas, with 4% to 15% of solid tumors demonstrating metastases to the leptomeninges. Lymphomas (7% to 15%) and leukemias (5% to 15%) as well as primary brain tumors (1% to 12%) also metastasize to the leptomeninges.[11]

Clinical presentation varies but is generally referable to three areas: the cerebral hemispheres, the cranial nerves, and the spinal cord and roots. Patients can present with symptoms in unusual neurologic distributions. Symptoms and signs include headache, changes in mental status , nausea or vomiting, focal weakness of an extremity, seizures, pain in an axial or radicular distribution, dermatomal sensory loss, and bladder and bowel dysfunction. Cranial nerve findings can include diplopia, hearing loss, facial numbness, loss of visual acuity, and ophthalmoplegia.

Patients should undergo a lumbar puncture, as CSF cytology is the diagnostic procedure of choice. Increased protein, decreased glucose, and pleocytosis are suggestive of leptomeningeal disease, but only CSF cytology is diagnostic. Imaging can also suggest the diagnosis if studding of the leptomeninges or clumped nerve roots are seen. Gadolinium enhancement can improve the image.

Therapy includes whole neuraxis radiation for radiosensitive tumors or, for less sensitive tumors, intrathecal chemotherapy with thiotepa (Thioplex), cytarabine, or methotrexate, with or without radiotherapy.[12]

CARDIOVASCULAR EMERGENCIES

Cardiac Tamponade

Malignant pericardial effusions are the most common cause of pericardial tamponade. It is important for the physician to recognize this condition because it can lead to the early death of a patient who had an otherwise treatable malignancy and a good short-term prognosis. The median survival time for untreated patients is approximately 4 months; only 25% survive 1 year. However, it is estimated that patients with breast cancer who are successfully treated can survive approximately 10 to 13 months, and patients with other tumors can survive 6 months or longer.[13]

Cardiac tamponade is rarely caused by primary tumors of the pericardium. Metastatic tumors including lung and breast tumors, lymphoma, leukemia, and melanoma are much more likely to cause the condition. Effusions and tamponade may also be caused by uremia, drugs, or radiation injury to the pericardium.

Presenting symptoms include dyspnea, cough, chest pain, fever, peripheral edema, hoarseness, hiccups, or nausea. Patients may also have no clinical symptoms. Physical examination will reveal hypotension, elevated jugular venous pressure, tachycardia, narrow arterial pulse pressure, and pulsus paradoxus greater than 10 mm Hg. A chest x-ray will show the characteristic large "water bottle" heart in slowly accumulating effusions; in rapidly accumulating effusions, the film may show a normal cardiac silhouette. Results of an electrocardiogram may demonstrate low electrical voltage with QRS complexes of less than 5 mV and electrical alternans.

The diagnostic test of choice is the echocardiogram. The functional significance of the effusion is demonstrated by the presence of collapse of the right atrium and right ventricle in diastole. Catheterization of the right side of the heart demonstrates increase and equalization of pressures of the right atrium, the right ventricle, the pulmonary artery in diastole, and the pulmonary capillary wedge pressure. The right atrial pressure tracing and the clinical jugular venous pulse demonstrate a prominent X descent.[14]

Therapy is directed at relief of acute symptoms and prevention of reaccumulation. Temporizing measures include intravenous fluids, pressors, and oxygen, although positive pressure ventilation is contraindicated, as it decreases venous return to the heart.

Pericardiocentesis is the preferred procedure for immediate relief of symptoms. The fluid that is removed should be sent for chemical and cytologic analysis. Modalities to prevent reaccumulation of fluid include systemic chemotherapy, catheter drainage and sclerosis, radiation therapy, or surgical intervention. Sclerosis is achieved with tetracycline or bleomycin (Blenoxane); minimal experience is also reported with instillation of cisplatin, mechlorethamine (Mustargen), teniposide (Vumon), fluorouracil, thiotepa, quinacrine hydrochloride (Atabrine), and radioisotopes.[13]

External beam radiation is often effective in leukemia- or lymphoma-induced effusions and may be administered in doses of 1 to 2 Gy/d over 3 to 4 weeks. A total dose of less than 35 to 40 Gy should prevent radiation pericarditis. Surgical procedures include pericardiectomy, pleuropericardial window, or subxiphoid pericardiotomy. Patients should be initiated on the appropriate systemic therapy concurrently if their performance status permits.

Superior Vena Cava Syndrome

Malignancy is also the most common cause of superior vena cava (SVC) thrombosis and the superior vena cava syndrome (SVCS). Lung cancer is the most common origin of the malignancy, leading to SVCS in 3% to 15% of patients. Other common causes include lymphoma and tumors metastatic to the mediastinum. A nonmalignant but cancer-associated cause of the syndrome is related to indwelling catheters for vascular access.

Superior vena cava syndrome develops as a result of diminished blood return to the heart. Clinical presentation varies, depending on the degree of obstruction of the SVC. Near total or complete obstruction results in the classic symptoms of the syndrome—facial edema, dyspnea, cough, orthopnea, and edema of the neck and upper extremities. Patients present less frequently with hoarseness, dysphagia, headache, dizziness, syncope, chest pain, lethargy, or alteration in mental status.[15] If SVCS is left untreated, increased intracranial pressure, intracerebral bleeding, and airway compromise can develop.

Patients presenting with overt SVCS may be diagnosed by physical examination alone. However, more subtle presentations require diagnostic imaging. A chest x-ray may reveal a widened mediastinum or a mass in the right side of the chest. Computed tomography (CT) and MRI scans are useful in that they define anatomic relation of structures, document the nature of obstruction as intrinsic or extrinsic, and can document collateral circulation. Invasive contrast venography is the most conclusive diagnostic tool. It precisely defines the etiology of obstruction and provides catheter access for thrombolytic therapy.

If a patient has not previously been diagnosed with malignancy, establishing a tissue diagnosis is critical. The choice of therapy in cases where the patient's life is not at acute risk is governed by the type of tumor causing the obstruction. Tests such as sputum cytology, thoracentesis, bronchoscopy, needle aspiration of a peripheral lymph node, or mediastinoscopy can be performed safely and provide a diagnosis. Thoracotomy should be performed only if the other studies are non-diagnostic.

Therapy is guided by the urgency of the presentation and the type of malignancy. Patients rarely require urgent radiotherapy prior to obtaining a diagnosis. Temporizing measures include head elevation, supplemental oxygen, limited intravenous fluids, and limited use of diuretics. Corticosteroids should also be initiated for symptoms of respiratory or CNS compromise.

Definitive therapy includes radiotherapy with increased dose fractions (300 to 400 cGy) on the first 3 days followed by full course radiation at conventional dose fractions (180 to 200 cGy) and up to 3,000 to 5,000 cGy, depending on tumor type. Chemotherapy may be used alone for small-cell bronchogenic carcinoma or in conjunction with radiotherapy for lymphomas.[15]

The role of thrombolytic therapy and invasive maneuvers involving stents and angioplasty are evolving. Thrombolytic therapy with streptokinase or urokinase may be useful if it is administered within 7 days of the onset of symptoms. Successful resolution of thrombosis is unlikely after 1 week. Suggested doses of urokinase and streptokinase, respectively, are a 4,400-U/kg bolus of urokinase followed by an infusion of 4,400 U/kg/h, and a 250,000-U bolus of streptokinase followed by an infusion of 100,000 U/h.[15] Patients are at increased risk for another thrombosis, including deep venous thrombosis, and should continue to receive anticoagulant drugs such as heparin or warfarin. Warfarin in low doses can also decrease the incidence of catheter-related thrombosis. Selected patients may benefit from expandable stents, angioplasty, or surgical bypass.

RESPIRATORY EMERGENCIES

Respiratory complications are commonly encountered in patients with cancer, either directly as a result of tumor growth and invasion (eg, obstruction, hemoptysis, lymphangitic spread, and leukostasis), or indirectly as a result of therapy (eg, infections, pulmonary edema, hypersensitivity reactions, and toxic injury from chemotherapy or radiation). Pulmonary infiltrates and infections are discussed elsewhere in this volume, in the chapters on infections in patients with cancer, and will not be further delineated here.

Airway Obstruction

Airway obstruction may occur as a result of endobronchial lesions or extrinsic compression from adjacent structures. Presentation may be acute or subacute. Patients present with complaints of cough, fullness in the neck, hemoptysis, dyspnea, dysphagia, or stridor. Common disease processes include bronchogenic cancer, head and neck cancers, lymphoma, thymoma, or thyroid malignancies.

Acute therapy for impending obstruction involves intubation or tracheostomy. Patients should receive supplemental oxygen and corticosteroids. Appropriate systemic or local therapy should be initiated, depending on tumor type. Subacute obstructing lesions may be palliated with neodymium-yttrium aluminum garnet (Nd:YAG) laser therapy or endobronchial stents or brachytherapy.

Massive Hemoptysis

Massive hemoptysis, defined as expectoration of 400 to 600 mL of blood within 24 hours, is a rare event. Patients more commonly have non-life-threatening hemoptysis with blood-streaked sputum or smaller amounts of expectorated blood. These episodes should not be dismissed, however, as they may herald more serious bleeding.

Malignancy is second to infection as the most common cause of hemoptysis. Massive hemoptysis is most often seen with tuberculosis, aspergillosis, lung abscesses, bronchiectasis, and bronchogenic carcinoma. Contributing to the risk of hemoptysis are abnormal clotting parameters or thrombocytopenia, which may be seen with cancer chemotherapy.

The physical examination should be directed toward determining the site of hemorrhage. A head and neck examination should always be included to rule out non-pulmonary sites of bleeding. Bronchoscopy, if possible during hemoptysis, is the diagnostic procedure of choice and allows iced-saline lavage. Sites of bleeding can be identified in 85% to 90% of cases, and the patient should be positioned with the site of hemorrhage dependent.

Management includes bed rest in a semi-erect position, sedation, humidified oxygen, blood and fluid replacement, and transfusion of platelets and correction of abnormal clotting parameters. Endobronchial tamponade may be used acutely as a temporizing measure until definitive therapy can be initiated. Definitive therapies include surgical resection, Nd:YAG laser ablation, and bronchial artery catheterization and embolization.

Toxic Lung Injury

Chemotherapy: The lung is uniquely susceptible to chemotherapy-induced injury, as it contains the largest vascular and endothelial surface area. The lung is the first capillary bed reached by intravenously (IV) administered chemotherapy and, thus, is the area of the highest concentration of these drugs. The lung also has the highest tissue oxygen content, which can enhance the toxicity of mitomycin (Mutamycin), bleomycin, cyclophosphamide (Cytoxan, Neosar), and carmustine. The primary mechanism of injury is mediated by oxygen free radicals on capillary endothelium and necrosis of pneumonocytes. Some agents also cause hypersensitivity reactions with acute respiratory distress.

Clinically, toxic injuries may affect the pulmonary parenchyma, vasculature, airways, or pleura.[16] Patients can present with a subacute process consisting of low-grade fevers, cough, and progressive dyspnea, or they can be acutely ill with high fevers, chills, and dyspnea suggestive of pneumonia. Physical examination demonstrates cyanosis, tachypnea, tachycardia, and use of accessory muscles of respiration. Depending on the etiology, auscultation may reveal diffuse crackles or clear lung fields.

Diagnostic evaluation is difficult, because symptoms and test results are often nonspecific. Toxic injury is a diagnosis of exclusion, and full evaluation is directed at excluding other common causes of respiratory decompensation including infection and parenchymal involvement by tumor. Patients should have arterial blood gas measurements, cultures, a chest x-ray, and ventilation/perfusion scans or angiography if such are clinically warranted. Bronchoscopy with samples for culture can increase the recovery of infectious agents. Occasionally, patients require open lung biopsy for definitive diagnosis.

Therapy involves stopping the toxic agent and administering corticosteroids. Supportive management with diuretics and mechanical ventilation may be required. Toxic injuries are reversible to varying degrees, and preventive measures should be routinely employed. Such measures include minimizing supplemental oxygen with bleomycin therapy and avoiding chest radiotherapy in these patients. Regular monitoring of gas exchange function with serial diffusion capacity of carbon dioxide (D_Lco) measurements is recommended as an early index of toxic lung injury.

Radiation: The toxic effects of radiotherapy on the lung are also mediated by oxygen free radicals on vascular endothelium. Radiation toxicity to the lung may be acute or chronic. Radiation pneumonitis is an acute syndrome characterized by dyspnea, cough, and fever associated with an infiltrate on the chest x-ray corresponding to the radiotherapy port. Factors predisposing a patient to the development of the syndrome include a high total dose of irradiation (greater than 6,000 cGy), a large volume of irradiated tissue, the fractionation schedule, and chemotherapy with bleomycin, mitomycin, or doxorubicin (Adriamycin, Rubex). Age and presence of chronic obstructive pulmonary disease are not independent risk factors.

Therapy involves use of oxygen and corticosteroids (prednisone in doses of 1 to 1.5 mg/kg, initially). Treatment is continued with a slow tapering of the steroids. Most patients present within several weeks to 3 months after receiving radiation, although symptoms can develop as late as 6 months.

Patients may also present with late radiation fibrosis in a radiotherapy port approximately 6 months to 2 years after receiving radiation. Fibrosis is a fixed lung injury and thus is poorly responsive to therapy with steroids. Long-term supplemental oxygen is often required.

GENITOURINARY EMERGENCIES

Hemorrhagic Cystitis

Hemorrhagic cystitis may be caused by certain chemotherapeutic agents (busulfan [Myleran], cyclophosphamide, ifosfamide, thiotepa), pelvic irradiation, some viruses, immune-acting agents (as in the penicillin family of antibiotics), and invasive urothelial tumors. The incidence of hemorrhagic cystitis, despite prophylactic measures with high-dose chemotherapy, can be as high as 40%, and mortality rates of 2% to 4% are reported with uncontrolled hemorrhage. Twenty percent of patients treated with pelvic irradiation also experience bladder complications.[17]

The toxic effects of oxazaphosphorine drugs on the bladder is mediated by the aldehyde metabolite acrolein. Prophylactic measures are aimed at minimizing the formation of acrolein and its contact with urothelium. These measures include vigorous hydration to encourage frequent urination, continuous bladder irrigation, and administration of the uroprotective agent mesna (Mesnex). Mesna is a sulfhydryl compound that, unlike N-acetyl cysteine, neutralizes acrolein without reducing the therapeutic effect of the oxazaphosphorine parent drug. Mesna is oxidized to an inactive disulfide after parenteral administration and is then excreted almost exclusively by the kidney. In the urine, mesna neutralizes acrolein as well as slowing its production by slowing degradation of 4-hydroxy metabolites of alkylating agents.[17]

The appropriate dose of mesna is controversial and recommended doses range from 60% to 160% of the cyclophosphamide dose.[18] It can be administered parenterally or orally. The half-life of mesna is shorter than that of cyclophosphamide (1.5 vs 6 hours). Therefore, it must be administered in repeated doses or as a continuous infusion throughout administration of the alkylating agent. The optimal schedule is not well defined, but administration should begin prior to or concurrent with alkylating agent administration. Patients should have regular urinalyses to evaluate microscopic hematuria that may herald significant bleeding.

Once hemorrhagic cystitis develops, initial conservative therapies include clot evacuation, continuous bladder irrigation with saline or hydrocortisone, cessation of anticoagulant therapy, control of factors that predispose a patient to bleeding diatheses, or systemic therapy with aminocaproic acid.[19] Second-line therapies include cystoscopy and fulguration, intravesical formalin administration,[19] intravesical prostaglandin administration (carboprost tromethamine [Hemabate]),[20] oral or parenteral conjugated estrogens,[21] or intravesical administration of silver nitrate, phenol, or aluminum hydroxide. Intractable cases may require urinary diversion, internal iliac artery ligation or embolization, or cystectomy.

Urinary Tract Obstruction

Urinary tract obstruction most commonly occurs in the ureters or the bladder neck. An obstruction may be intrinsic or extrinsic in nature. Retroperitoneal primary or metastatic tumors that commonly cause

TABLE 2

Tumors Causing Ureteral Obstruction

Primary Retroperitoneal Tumors

Benign neoplasms	Malignant neoplasms
Lipoma	Liposarcoma
Fibroma	Fibrosarcoma
Rhabdomyoma	Rhabdomyosarcoma
Hemangioma	Malignant hemangio-pericytoma
Neurilemoma	Malignant schwannoma
Lymphangioma	Lymphangiosarcoma
	Lymphosarcoma
	Hodgkin's disease
	Reticulum-cell sarcoma
	Non-Hodgkin's lymphoma
Myxoma	Myxosarcoma
Benign pheochromocytoma	Malignant pheochromocytoma
Nephrogenic cysts	Urogenital ridge tumor
Dermoid	Teratoma

Secondary Retroperitoneal Tumors
Cervix
Prostate
Urinary bladder
Colon
Ovary
Uterus
Stomach
Breast
Lymph nodes
Pancreas
Lung
Gallbladder
Testis
Small bowel

Adapted, with permission, from Greenfield A, Resnick MI: Genitourinary Emergencies. Semin Oncol 16(6):517, 1989.

this type of obstruction are outlined in Table 2.[4]

Ureteral obstruction may be unilateral or bilateral, depending on the etiology. Bladder outlet obstruction typically produces bilateral hydronephrosis. Prostate and cervical cancers as well as radiation fibrosis are common causes of bladder outlet obstruction.

Evaluation is directed at determining the site of obstruction. Useful imaging modalities include intravenous urogram, renal ultrasound, and CT of the abdomen and pelvis. Occasionally patients require invasive percutaneous procedures.

Therapies that relieve obstruction include percutaneous nephrostomy tubes, ureteral stents, suprapubic catheters, and transurethral resection of the prostate. Patients with obstruction also require antibiotic therapy to prevent pyelonephritis or systemic urosepsis.

TABLE 3

Causes of Renal Failure in Cancer Patients

Urinary obstruction

Severe volume depletion

Parenchymal disease
  Glomerulonephritis (eg, cryoglobulinemia)
  Vasculitis
  Hypercalcemic nephropathy
  Tumor replacement
  Tumor lysis syndrome
    Acute uric acid nephropathy
    Calcium phosphate nephropathy

Myeloma kidney

Drug nephrotoxicity
  Methotrexate
  Cisplatin
  Mitomycin
  Alpha interferon
  Interleukin-2
  Antibiotics

Adapted, with permission, from Arrambide K, Toto RD.[26]

GASTROINTESTINAL EMERGENCIES

Neutropenic Enterocolitis

Neutropenic enterocolitis (typhlitis) is a syndrome characterized by abdominal distension, tenderness on the right side of the abdomen, watery diarrhea, and fever observed in the setting of chemotherapy- or disease-induced neutropenia.[22] The syndrome is most often associated with hematologic malignancies, aplastic anemia, myelodysplastic syndromes, and rarely, solid tumors (as with aggressive chemotherapy of breast cancer).[23] The incidence of the syndrome is reported as 12% to 46% in autopsy studies.[24] Differential diagnosis includes appendicitis, pseudomembranous enterocolitis, and diverticulitis. The cause of death in these patients is usually sepsis, and mortality rates range from 50% to 100%.[24]

Pathologically, the syndrome is characterized by patchy inflammation involving the full thickness of the bowel wall. It is associated with well-demarcated ulcers and necrosis with minimal inflammatory infiltration of the ileum, cecum, or ascending colon. Factors that predispose a patient to this condition include prolonged ileus with bacterial invasion, direct damage to bowel mucosa, and hemorrhage into the bowel wall with necrosis. Nearly all patients presenting with this syndrome were treated previously with antibiotics that allowed the occurrence of fungal overgrowth and the selection of virulent organisms capable of invading the bowel wall.[22]

Typhlitis is a clinical diagnosis; laboratory and x-ray findings are nonspecific. Plain films of the abdomen reveal the pattern of ileus with a distended cecum. A CT scan is the test of choice and may reveal thickening of the bowel wall with pneumatosis. Invasive studies such as endoscopy or a barium enema should be avoided as patients are at high risk for perforation.

Therapy is controversial. The literature reports a higher survival rate with surgical treatment than with medical treatment alone. However, these data are complicated by the fact that these patients are critically ill and often have comorbid conditions that adversely affect their prognosis. Medical management can be successful if the condition is recognized early.

Medical management consists of bowel rest; nasogastric suction; broad-spectrum antibiotics including agents effective against anaerobic, gram-negative, and *Clostridium difficile* organisms; use of hematopoietic growth factor support; and total parenteral nutrition. Surgery is indicated for perforation, bleeding, abscess formation, or failure of medical management. Necrotic bowel should be resected, and bowel diversion should be performed; primary anastamoses are unlikely to be successful in leukopenic patients.

Gastrointestinal Bleeding and Perforation

After hemorrhagic gastritis and peptic ulcer disease, malignancy is the third leading cause of gastrointestinal bleeding in patients with cancer. Lymphoma is the most likely tumor to directly cause bleeding.[25] Perforation is a much less common complication with lymphomas, occurring in only 3% to 10% of cases. Patients with tumors likely to bleed when therapy is given (lymphomas, metastatic renal cell carcinomas) should have these resected prior to initiation of therapy, if possible.

Treatment modalities for hemorrhage include surgery and use of vasopressin, Nd:YAG laser, and arterial embolization for unresectable lesions. Evaluation should be vigilant to exclude other sites of bleeding.

METABOLIC EMERGENCIES

Tumor Lysis Syndrome

Rapid destruction of malignant cells can result in the release of cellular breakdown products and intracellular ions causing potentially lethal metabolic derangements. Tumor lysis syndrome is observed in tumors with a rapid proliferation index including Burkitt's lymphoma, acute lymphocytic leukemia, acute nonlymphocytic leukemia, and less frequently, solid tumors of small-cell type, breast cancer, and medulloblastoma. The syndrome usually follows induction chemotherapy but can also be seen after treatment with radiotherapy, corticosteroids, hormonal agents (such as tamoxifen, biologic agents (such as interferon), or spontaneously in patients with a high tumor burden.

Metabolically, the syndrome is characterized by hyperuricemia, hyperkalemia, hyperphosphatemia, and hypocalcemia. These can occur individually or in varying combinations. Unchecked, uric acid can precipitate in renal tubules and calcium-phosphate complexes can precipitate in the renal interstitium. These precipitates impair renal function, resulting in metabolic acidosis, which may worsen the syndrome. This constellation of metabolic findings can distinguish this syndrome from other causes of renal failure in patients with cancer (Table 3).[26]

High tumor burden, high serum lactate dehydrogenase (LDH), volume depletion, acid-concentrated urine, and excessive urinary uric acid excretion may predispose a patient to tumor lysis syndrome. Azotemia is often present before chemotherapy is initiated.[26]

Patients may be clinically asymptomatic in the early stages of the syndrome. Advanced electrolyte abnormalities, however, may result in cardiac rhythm disturbances, seizures, carpopedal spasm, neuromuscular irritability, or disturbances in level of consciousness. Prophylactic measures including alkalinization of the urine, vigorous hydration, and administration of allopurinol should be initiated prior to initiation of systemic therapy. These measures can also be effective in the early stages of the syndrome. Unfortunately, prophylactic measures are not always successful in averting the syndrome.

Therapy includes regular monitoring of electrolytes, blood-urea-nitrogen (BUN), creatinine, uric acid, phosphorus, and calcium levels, often several times a day. Hydration should exceed 3,000 mL/m^2/d (200 to 300 mL/h). Urinary flow can also be increased by use of a diuretic such as mannitol. Sodium bicarbonate can be added to IV fluids at 100 mEq/L for urinary alkalinization. Allopurinol should be administered in doses of 500 mg/m^2 on days 1 to 3, then reduced to 200 mg/m^2 throughout cytoreductive therapy. This regimen should be continued for at least 2 to 3 days after the completion of chemotherapy.[27]

Patients with hyperkalemia should be monitored continuously for cardiac rhythm disturbances. Appropriate therapy with calcium and exchange resins should be initiated. Patients with persistently low calcium should be considered for calcitriol (Calcijex, Rocaltrol) therapy.[28] Finally, these patients may also need empiric antibiotic therapy for opportunistic infections.

Hemodialysis may be required in situations wherein conservative management fails. Overt renal failure may develop with associated volume overload and life-threatening hyperkalemia. Hemodialysis is preferred over peritoneal dialysis because it is more effective in removing uric acid and phosphorus. Daily dialysis is usually required because cellular products accumulate rapidly. Renal insufficiency is usually reversible if treated early; late intervention may result in permanent renal insufficiency and dependence on dialysis.

SIADH

The syndrome of inappropriate secretion of antidiuretic hormone (SIADH) is characterized by hyponatremia with inappropriately concentrated urine; it is observed in 1% to 2% of patients with cancer. Small-cell lung cancer is by far the most common cause; it is responsible for 60% of all cases of SIADH.[29] The differential diagnosis of SIADH includes adverse effects of cytotoxic chemotherapy agents, notably cyclophosphamide and vincristine, and ectopic production of atrial natriuretic factor.[29]

Clinical symptoms depend on the level of hyponatremia and the rapidity with which it has occurred. Patients with a slow onset or mild hyponatremia demonstrate subtle mental status and cognitive changes such as memory loss, apathy, impaired abstract thinking, fatigue, anorexia, myalgias, and headache. Severe hyponatremia (serum sodium less than 115 mEq/L) or rapid onset of hyponatremia is characterized by asterixis, altered mental status, confusion, lethargy, seizures, and ultimately, coma. The physical examination may demonstrate papilledema, pathologic reflexes, and focal findings.

The differential diagnosis of hyponatremia includes liver disease, congestive heart failure, renal failure, hypothyroidism, and adrenal insufficiency. Normal thyroid and adrenal function and establishment of euvolemia must be demonstrated prior to a diagnosis of SIADH.[30] The volume status should be assessed by measurement of serum and urine electrolytes and osmolality. In SIADH, the urine sodium level is usually greater than 20 mmol/L and the urine osmolality commonly exceeds that of plasma.

Therapy involves treating the tumor producing the antidiuretic hormone or atrial natriuretic factor along with fluid management, usually fluid restriction or induced diuresis. Appropriate combination chemotherapy should be initiated, and brain metastases, if present, should be treated with radiotherapy.

Fluid intake should be limited to less than 1,000 mL/d and less than 500 mL/d if the patient responds poorly. Refractory cases of hyponatremia or patients who

TABLE 4

*Clinical Manifestations of
Cancer-Related Hypercalcemia*

General
  Dehydration
  Weight loss
  Anorexia
  Pruritus
  Polydipsia

Neuromuscular
  Fatigue
  Lethargy
  Muscle weakness
  Hyporeflexia
  Confusion
  Psychosis
  Seizure
  Obtundation
  Coma

Gastrointestinal
  Nausea
  Vomiting
  Constipation
  Obstipation
  Ileus

Genitorenal
  Polyuria
  Renal insufficiency

Cardiac
  Bradycardia
  Prolonged PR interval
  Shortened QT interval
  Wide T wave
  Atrial or ventricular arrhythmias

Adapted, with permission, from Thomas CR, Dodhia N.[33]

can be treated as outpatients can be managed with 600 to 1,200 mg/d of demeclocycline (Declomycin) in divided doses. Patients who are symptomatic with coma or seizures can be treated with 3% hypertonic saline by *slow* infusion at a rate sufficient to increase the serum sodium level by 0.5 to 1.0 mEq/L/h. Rapid correction (greater than 2 mEq/L/h) may be associated with central pontine myelinolysis. Normal saline with IV furosemide may also be effective.[27,30]

Hypercalcemia of Malignancy

Hypercalcemia is the most common metabolic emergency seen in cancer patients. Between 10% to 20% of patients with known malignancies experience this complication during the course of their disease. The most common tumor types associated with hypercalcemia include those of the breast, lung, kidney, and esophagus, hematologic malignancies (notably multiple myeloma), and cancer of the head and neck.[27] Hypercalcemia confers a grave prognosis; survival rate at 3 months is only 44%,[27] with mean survival times of 1 to 6 months.[31]

The serum calcium concentration is normally controlled by parathyroid hormone (PTH) and calcitonin. Vitamin D in the dihydroxylated form regulates intestinal absorption of calcium. PTH promotes calcium reabsorption in the distal nephron and enhances conversion of 25-hydroxycholecalciferol to calcitriol. PTH also activates both osteoblasts and osteoclasts, enhancing the rate of bony calcium turnover. Calcitonin counters these effects by suppressing osteoclast activity and stimulating deposition of calcium in the skeleton.[31]

In contrast, hypercalcemia in malignancy is caused by the tumor's elaboration of systemically acting humoral factors, which alter calcium metabolism in the bones, kidney, or intestine (humoral hypercalcemia of malignancy) and by stimulation of bone resorption at sites of tumor metastases to bone. Both mechanisms may operate simultaneously in some patients.

Humoral hypercalcemia of malignancy mimics primary hyperparathyroidism in many aspects. It is characterized by increased bony reabsorption, hypercalciuria, increased renal absorption of calcium despite increased filtered calcium, increased nephrogenous cAMP, hypophosphatemia, and hyperphosphaturia. The similarity of this syndrome to primary hyperparathyroidism led to the discovery of parathyroid hormone-related protein, which plays a central role in mediating the syndrome. This protein can be detected in the circulation by radioimmunoassays. Other substances known to be involved in calcium homeostasis include calcitriol; interleukins 1, 4, and 6; tumor necrosis factor-alpha; transforming growth factors-alpha and -beta; leukemia inhibitory factor; and prostaglandins (PG), notably PGE_2.[32]

Clinically, patients present with nonspecific symptoms, and the differential diagnosis is often difficult. Symptoms involve many bodily systems and are delineated in Table 4.[33]

Laboratory test findings include high serum calcium level (can be greater than 14 mg/dL), low serum chloride level, elevated or normal serum phosphate and bicarbonate levels, and elevated alkaline phosphatase levels. In contrast, only 25% of patients with primary hyperparathyroidism have a serum calcium level greater than 14 mg/dL, and the serum phosphate and bicarbonate levels are usually decreased while the serum chloride level is elevated to greater than 112 mmol/L.[27]

Acute therapy begins with aggressive saline rehy-

TABLE 5

Agents Frequently Used to Treat Hypercalcemia

Drug	Dosage	Onset of effect	Adverse effects	Comments
Saline	100–250 mL/h IV	Rapid	Volume overload, hypokalemia	More rapid initial infusuion (250–500 mL/h) required to correct volume depletion
Furosemide	80–120 mg IV every 2–6 h	4 h	Volume depletion, hypokalemia, hypomagnesemia	Use only after correction of volume depletion
Calcitonin	4–8 U/kg IM or SC every 6–12 h	2–4 h	Nausea and vomiting, hypersensitivity	Test dose of 1 unit recommended before therapy; duration of effect only 2–3 days in many patients
Etidronate disodium	7.5 mg/kg IV qd for 3–7 d	24–72 h	Nephrotoxicity	Infuse over at least 2 hours to reduce toxicity; use with caution in patients with renal dysfunction
Pamidronate disodium	30–90 mg IV over 24 h; 4-h infusions can be used also	24–48 h	Fever	Doses up to 90 mg are recommended by manufacturer; use with caution in patients with renal dysfunction
Gallium nitrate	100–200 mg/m²/d by continuous infusion for 5 d	24–48 h	Nephrotoxicity	Avoid in patients whose serum creatinine is > 2.5 mg/dL or who are receiving other nephrotoxic agents
Plicamycin	15–25 µg/kg IV over 4 h, every 48–72 h; 12.5 µg/kg in patients with renal or hepatic diseases	12–24 h	Hemorrhage, hepatotoxicity, nephrotoxicity, nausea, and vomiting	Avoid in patients with bleeding disorders; use with caution and reduce dosage in patients with renal or hepatic diseases; observe extravasation precautions

Adapted, with permission, from Hall TG, Burns-Schaiff R.A.[35]

dration. Patients have large volume deficits, and replacement of 5 to 8 L of saline in the first 24 hours is recommended. Patients should then maintain a urine output of 3 to 4 L/d until chronic therapy becomes effective, usually over several days.

Serum electrolytes should be monitored closely and replaced as needed. Hypokalemia is common. Patients with severe hypercalcemia should undergo cardiac monitoring. Patients unable to tolerate large volume replacement can be treated with loop diuretics in doses of 20 to 100 mg every 1 to 2 hours, with the goal of generating a urine output of 300 to 500 mL/h. Thiazide diuretics are to be avoided as they can increase serum calcium levels. Also, vitamin preparations or parenteral nutrition formulas with vitamin D are to be avoided, and close monitoring is required with the use of hormonal agents such as tamoxifen.

Some of the numerous pharmacologic agents available for the chronic treatment of hypercalcemia are outlined in Table 5. Agents may be classified into those that strongly inhibit bone reabsorption (plicamycin [Mithracin], bisphosphonates, and gallium nitrate [Ganite]) and those that act by other mechanisms.

Gallium Nitrate: Gallium acts to lower serum calcium levels by binding to bone and reducing the solubility of hydroxyapatite crystals. It does not alter the function of osteoclasts. The mean half-life of gallium is approximately 24 hours. The drug is not available for oral administration because it is poorly absorbed.

After the first dose, the serum calcium concentration in the patient's blood falls slowly, reaching a nadir at 7 to 10 days. Adverse effects include nephrotoxicity manifested as elevation in BUN and creatinine. The reported incidence is 8% to 15%. Other side effects of gallium include pulmonary effusions and infiltrates, optic neuritis, and reduced visual and auditory acuity.[34,35] Gallium has a direct antineoplastic effect on lymphoma and thus may be particularly effective against hypercalcemia resulting from this disease.

Plicamycin: Plicamycin is an antineoplastic antibiotic that induces hypocalcemia by directly inhibiting bone reabsorption and osteoclast function. It may also inhibit the function of vitamin D and PTH. Toxic effects occur with repeated doses and include hemorrhage, thrombocytopenia, qualitative platelet defects, renal insufficiency, hepatic injury, nausea, and vomiting. Plicamycin is contraindicated in patients with compromised renal function.[36]

Calcitonin: Calcitonin is the drug of choice for rapid reduction of a patient's serum calcium level. It acts within minutes to decrease renal tubular calcium reabsorption. Calcitonin also inhibits osteoclast activity and decreases skeletal release of calcium.

Unlike other pharmacologic agents, calcitonin is used safely in patients with organ failure. Coadministration of glucocorticoids may prolong the action of calcitonin. Administration of calcitonin as a single agent rarely returns serum calcium levels completely to normal; tachyphylaxis develops within 72 hours of administration. Calcitonin is thus best given as temporizing therapy in cases of life-threatening hypercalcemia until longer-acting agents can take effect.[36]

Bisphosphonates: Bisphosphonates are synthetic analogs of pyrophosphate; they inhibit osteoclast activity. Multiple agents have been developed, which differ in potency, activity, and side effects. Etidronate (Didronel) and pamidronate (Aredia) are the agents most commonly used in clinical practice.

Etidronate can be administered orally or parenterally, but its oral absorption is low. Adverse effects of etidronate include enhanced phosphate absorption by the kidney with hyperphosphatemia, metallic taste, bone demineralization after continued high doses, and nephrotoxicity. Use of etidronate is contraindicated in patients with a serum creatinine level of greater than 5 mg/dL.[37]

Pamidronate is more potent than etidronate and lacks the unwanted side effect of bone demineralization. Adverse effects include fever in up to 25% of patients, hypocalcemia and hypophosphatemia in 10% to 20% of patients, lymphopenia, phlebitis at the infusion site, nausea, and renal dysfunction.

HEMATOLOGIC EMERGENCIES

Hyperviscosity Syndrome

Hyperviscosity syndrome is characterized by sludging and decreased perfusion of the microvasculature and by vascular stasis brought on by markedly increased paraproteins or poorly deformable cells in the blood. Sludging is observed most frequently in retinal, cerebral, cardiac, and peripheral vessels. The syndrome is observed in conjunction with polycythemia vera, Waldenström's macroglobulinemia, multiple myeloma, chronic or acute leukemia with high cell counts, dysproteinemias, and very rarely with solid tumors. Waldenström's macro-

globulinemia accounts for 85% to 90% of cases, and myeloma for 5% to 10% of cases.[31] Hyperviscosity syndrome may also be observed in light chain disease where the light chain is highly polymerized.[38]

Clinically, the syndrome is characterized by three symptoms: bleeding, visual signs and symptoms, and neurologic defects. Patients may also present with congestive heart failure. Bleeding diatheses are usually manifested by epistaxis, ecchymoses, and mucosal bleeding. Tortuous, distended, "sausage-like" retinal veins are pathognomonic findings of the syndrome. Hemorrhages, exudates, and papilledema can occur as hyperviscosity syndrome progresses.[39]

Bleeding is multifactorial and is observed most commonly with IgM and IgA paraproteins.[39] Laboratory test results may reveal thrombocytopenia and defects in platelet function manifested as prolonged bleeding time, abnormal clot retraction, and abnormal platelet aggregation studies. Coating of platelets by the paraprotein inhibits aggregation and the release of platelet factor 3.[40]

Paraproteins have also been reported to act as inhibitors of coagulation factors V, VII, and VIII and prothrombin complex. Reduced levels of coagulation factors are also observed. Amyloid can directly bind to factor X, causing neutralization of the protein. Finally, the paraprotein can inhibit fibrin monomer polymerization resulting in prolonged thrombin time.

Thrombosis may also occur with hyperviscosity syndrome; it primarily involves the limbs or central nervous system. Polycythemia vera is commonly associated with thrombosis. Large-vessel thrombosis is related to significantly elevated hematocrits, whereas small-vessel thrombosis is likely to result from platelet abnormalities.

Diagnosis is clinical and is confirmed by determination of the serum viscosity. The normal range for serum viscosity (compared with water) is 1.4 to 1.8. Most patients begin to develop symptoms at serum viscosities greater than 4.0.[39] Other laboratory test findings commonly observed include the presence of anemia and iron deficiency, an elevated red blood cell mass in relation to the blood volume, renal dysfunction with azotemia, rouleaux formation, high serum M protein measurements, and thrombocytopenia.

Plasmapheresis is the acute therapy of choice for symptomatic hyperviscosity. A plasma exchange of 3 to 4 L of plasma in 24 hours is recommended. Maintenance plasmapheresis of 1 to 2 L once or twice a week may be needed until definitive therapy is effective. Replacement is usually with fresh frozen plasma as it replaces immunoglobulins and clotting factors. Hypocalcemia related to citrate anticoagulants may be observed. Plasma exchange is more effective for IgM paraproteinemias as 80% of the protein is intravascular. Definitive cytoreductive chemotherapy should be initiated as soon as possible. The prognosis for a symptomatic patient depends on that for the underlying disease.[39]

Hyperleukocytosis Syndrome

Patients with leukemia who have markedly elevated white blood cell (WBC) counts are at risk for end-organ damage related to leukemic infiltration and to the effects of leukemic cells on the vasculature. Intravascular sludging and leukostasis can develop along with white thrombus formation. Tissue damage occurs as a result of local hypoxia, hyperpermeability, and the release of lysosomes and procoagulants.

Diseases that predispose patients to leukostasis include acute myelogenous leukemia and chronic myelogenous leukemia in blast crisis with peripheral WBC counts greater than 100,000/mL or with rapidly increasing counts.[41] It is less likely that symptomatic hyperleukocytosis will develop in patients with lymphoblastic malignancies. There is no absolute threshold WBC count above which this syndrome develops.

Pathogenetic mechanisms involve poor deformability of leukemic blasts with sludging in the microvasculature, local hypoxia caused by blast cell consumption of oxygen, affinity of neoplastic cells for the pulmonary epithelium, and blast cell invasiveness.[42] Hyperviscosity usually does not occur as the hematocrit is reduced.[43]

The pulmonary and neurologic systems are most frequently clinically involved. Neurologic symptoms include dizziness, blurred vision, tinnitus, ataxia, confusion, delirium, somnolence, papilledema, retinal vein distension, retinal hemorrhages, coma, and intracranial hemorrhage.[41] Pulmonary symptoms include fever, tachypnea, dyspnea, hypoxia, pulmonary infiltrates, and respiratory failure. Hyperleukocytosis syndrome should be part of the differential diagnosis in all patients whose respiratory failure is associated with minimal findings on physical examination and chest x-ray.[44] Other manifestations of the syndrome include congestive heart failure, priapism, and peripheral vascular occlusion.[45]

Interpretation of laboratory test results is complicated by the fact that values may be spuriously altered by metabolically active WBCs. Platelet counts may be falsely elevated as automated counters may interpret WBC fragments as platelets. Manual platelet counts should be performed. The Po_2 and serum glucose may be artificially lowered by oxygen consumption and glycolysis by the white cells in the blood sample.[46] Pseudohyperkalemia may also be observed. Blood samples should be placed on ice immediately and kept cold until processed. Correlation should be obtained with pulse oximetry to assess the adequacy of oxygen replacement.[41,44,46]

Management of the syndrome includes supplemental oxygen, allopurinol, urinary alkalinization, hydration, and immediate cytoreductive therapy.[47,48] Initial management should include leukapheresis because cytotoxic chemotherapy induces cell lysis and can temporarily worsen symptoms. If leukapheresis is not available, hydroxyurea in doses of 50 to 100 mg/kg/d (3 to 5 g/m²)[49] may be used to effect rapid cytoreduction. The goal is to reduce total WBC counts by 20% to 60% in the first few hours of treatment.[41,43] Whole brain irradiation in doses of 4 to 6 Gy is recommended for CNS involvement. Correction of hemoglobin concentration to greater than 10 g/dL is contraindicated as it may worsen symptoms.[41] Definitive antileukemic chemotherapy can be given after initial therapy has reduced the risk to the patient.

HEMOSTATIC EMERGENCIES

Bleeding

The hemostatic system can be significantly altered by malignant disease and its treatment. A list of some of the causes of bleeding in patients with cancer is provided in Table 6. Abnormal hemostatic laboratory test values can be detected in 50% of patients with metastatic disease. Significant hemorrhage can occur in up to 10% of patients with cancer.[50]

Overall, the most common cause of hemorrhage is thrombocytopenia (50%). Usually, thrombocytopenia is the result of chemotherapy or marrow involvement by a tumor, but it may also be caused by consumptive coagulopathy, immune-mediated mechanisms, infection, or sequestration.[51]

Severe hemorrhage is uncommon with platelet counts higher than 10,000 to 20,000/mm³ or with slowly decreasing platelet counts. Use of prophylactic platelet infusions in such cases is controversial as there are no prospective randomized studies that establish a threshold above which platelets should be maintained to avoid bleeding.[52] However, because hemorrhage can be life threatening, platelet infusions of 6 to 8 units every 1 to 2 days are recommended until platelet counts consistently remain above 10,000 mm³.[51]

Patients who receive multiple transfusions often develop alloantibodies to human leukocyte antigen (HLA) class I determinants on platelets, which contribute to rapid clearance of transfused platelets. The incidence of alloimmunization in leukemic patients is 40% to 60% and approaches 80% to 90% in aplastic anemia patients.[53]

TABLE 6

Some Hemorrhagic Syndromes Occurring with Metastastic Malignancy [a]

Thrombocytopenia
   Immune thrombocytopenia

Disseminated intravascular coagulation
   Leukemia cell procoagulant activity
   Bacteremia
   Massive transfusions
   Shock

Decreased clotting factors/coagulation factor abnormalities
   Liver infiltration
   Cholestasis
   Drug-induced
   Acquired von Willebrand's disease

Primary fibrinolysis/fibrinogenolysis
   Leukemia cell proteolytic activity
   Drug-induced

Platelet dysfunction
   Myeloproliferative syndromes
   Acute leukemia
   Preleukemia
   Hairy-cell leukemia

Vascular defects
   Infiltration
   Hyperviscosity/leukostasis
   Extramedullary hematopoiesis

Circulating anticoagulants
   Factor inhibitors
   Heparin-like anticoagulants

---

[a] In descending order of probability
Adapted, with permission, from Bick RL: Coagulation abnormalities in malignancy: A review. Semin Thromb Hemost 18(4):359,365, 1992, and Ey FS, Goodnight SH: Bleeding disorders in cancer. Semin Oncol 17(2):188, 1990.

Patients in whom this condition develops should receive HLA-matched platelets from a family member or a single donor. Use of leukocyte-depleted platelets, leukocyte filters, single donor platelets, and UV-irradiated platelets can reduce the incidence of alloimmunization. These measures also reduce febrile transfusion reactions and the incidence of transfusion transmitted diseases such as cytomegalovirus (CMV).[54] The use of IV immune globulin is controversial because the data on platelet response is inconclusive.[53]

Abnormal platelet function also predisposes patients to bleeding. Platelet dysfunction is most commonly observed in myeloproliferative disorders such as chronic myelogenous leukemia (CML), essential thrombocythemia, myelofibrosis, and polycythemia vera as well as in diseases associated with paraproteins such as multiple myeloma, Waldenström's macroglobulinemia, and amyloidosis. Bleeding in these disorders is usually mucosal in nature and can be life threatening, as in gastrointestinal hemorrhage.

Platelet dysfunction associated with elevated platelet counts (greater than 700,000/mm^3) can be corrected by platelet pheresis. The most common platelet functional defects noted include impaired aggregation to adenosine diphosphate (ADP) and epinephrine, deficiency of alpha granules, and defective platelet factor 3 release.[51]

Paraproteins may be directed to platelet antigens and cause immune-mediated platelet destruction. Paraproteins may also interfere with platelet aggregation, fibrinogen binding, conversion of fibrinogen to fibrin (causing increased thrombin time), and inhibit clotting factor activity.[55] The patients at greatest risk are those with kappa light chains and markedly increased serum protein and viscosity.[55]

Malignancy involving the liver can cause defective or decreased synthesis of coagulation factors II, VII, IX, X, XI, XII, XIII, prekallikrein, high-molecular-weight kininogen, plasminogen, antithrombin III, protein S, and protein C. Bleeding can be corrected by replacement of vitamin K or the appropriate coagulation factors.

Acquired von Willebrand's disease is also seen in association with many hematologic malignancies. The disease usually improves with treatment of the underlying malignancy; other therapeutic measures include infusion of cryoprecipitate or desmopressin.[51,55]

Primary fibrinolysis can be seen in solid tumors and in hematologic malignancies and is characterized by local or systemic activation of the fibrinolytic system resulting in plasmin degradation of fibrin, fibrinogen, factor V, and factor VIII. It is much less common than secondary fibrinolysis seen with disseminated intravascular coagulation, which should be excluded first. Solid tumors with tissues capable of inducing fibrinolytic activity include sarcomas and tumors of the breast, thyroid, colon, and stomach. Therapy involves giving tranexamic acid or epsilon-aminocaproic acid to inhibit fibrinolysis. The recommended dose of tranexamic acid is 500 mg orally or IV, every 8 to 12 hours; epsilon-aminocaproic acid can be given as a 5- to 10-g slow IV loading dose followed by 1 to 2 g/h for 24 hours. Patients may then receive oral therapy.[51]

Many drugs can contribute to bleeding in cancer patients. Mechanisms of bleeding include defects in fibrin formation, platelet dysfunction, loss of vitamin K dependent factors, and development of coagulation factor inhibitors. Certain cephalosporins (for example, cefamandole [Mandol]) have an *N*-methylthiotetrazole side chain that induces a warfarin like gamma-decarboxylation of clotting factors. Many beta-lactam antibiotics impair aggregation of platelets by blocking ADP receptor activity. Amphotericin B (Fungizone), plicamycin, vincristine, and nitrofurantoin (Furadantin) also affect platelet function. Patients who are given antibiotic therapy should have regular monitoring of prothrombin time (PT), activated partial thromboplastin time (aPTT), and bleeding time, and vitamin K replacement should be considered. Bleeding can be treated with factor replacement or platelet infusions.

Asparaginase (Elspar) therapy for acute leukemia has been associated with bleeding and thrombotic events similar to those seen in disseminated intravascular coagulation (DIC). Bleeding is mediated by inhibition of hepatic protein synthesis with decreases in fibrinogen and factors V and VIII and increased fibrin degradation products. Thrombosis can result from acquired protein S and protein C deficiencies.[56] Bleeding can be corrected by halting asparaginase therapy and administering cryoprecipitate and fresh frozen plasma.[55] Other antineoplastic agents associated with bleeding include plicamycin, suramin, cyclosporine (Sandimmune), mitomycin, cisplatin, carboplatin (Paraplatin), and bleomycin.[56]

Acute leukemias may be complicated by the development of DIC in up to 50% of patients. Myeloblasts, promyelocytes, monocytes, and lymphoblasts contain procoagulant materials capable of initiating DIC and fibrinolysis. This is well characterized in acute promyelocytic leukemia, the M3 variant of acute nonlymphocytic leukemia. Solid tumors and sepsis cause injury to tissues and vascular endothelium, which may initiate DIC by exposure of tissue factor. Some malignancies commonly associated with DIC are gastric, prostate, breast, and lung cancers.[51]

Clinical manifestations of DIC may be varied and may include both bleeding and thrombosis. Mild bleeding can involve mucosal surfaces or skin with spontaneous bruising, petechiae, purpura, gingival bleeding, and bleeding from the sites of indwelling catheters. Fulminant DIC can be complicated by bleeding in multiple sites simultaneously and bleeding in pulmonary, CNS, gastrointestinal, or genitourinary sites. Thrombotic manifestations include deep venous thrombosis, pulmonary embolism, migratory thrombophlebitis (Trousseau's syndrome), or microangiopathic hemolytic anemia.[57] Chemotherapy may trigger or worsen DIC; initiation of low-dose heparin therapy may ameliorate these effects.[51]

Confirmation of DIC can be difficult; many laboratory tests show abnormal results only when applied to samples from cases of fulminant DIC. Low-grade or subacute DIC may be characterized by only subtly abnormal parameters or normal laboratory test results. Decreased quantities of platelets and fibrinogen and prolonged PT are together highly suggestive of the diagnosis.[57] It must be recognized that sepsis and neoplasia both act to elevate fibrinogen levels, thus, a normal fibrinogen level may actually represent a relative decrease of fibrinogen by a consumptive process. An increase in the PT is due to decreased quantities of factors II, V, X, and fibrinogen. Other abnormal test results include prolonged aPTT and thrombin time, decreased antithrombin III levels, increased fibrin degradation products, elevated D-dimer assay, and the presence of fragmented cells or schistocytes in the peripheral blood.

Therapy must address initiating mechanisms and should also include treatment of the underlying malignancy or sepsis. Treatment of the clinical syndrome is governed by its manifestations and severity. Patients whose laboratory test results are abnormal but who have no clinical manifestations (such cases are common in cancers where antineoplastic therapy induces cell lysis, as in acute promyelocytic leukemia) should be treated with antineoplastic chemotherapy and antibiotics only. Close observation is necessary as these patients can clinically deteriorate. Heparin, in therapeutic doses of 1,000 U/h during induction chemotherapy, may decrease morbidity and mortality.[57] Heparin should also be used in documented cases of thrombosis. Patients with thrombosis may also be given antiplatelet agents. Patients with Trousseau's syndrome often require chronic subcutaneous heparin.

Use of heparin in patients with bleeding in DIC is much more controversial. Heparin can interrupt the consumption of coagulation proteins and platelets by inhibiting thrombin formation but can cause bleeding by its own anticoagulant activity. No controlled trials have focused on heparin use in these patients, and heparin therapy must be individualized.[57]

Patients with significant bleeding benefit from replacement of clotting factors and platelets. Cryoprecipitate and fresh frozen plasma are the replacement products of choice. Patients with fibrinogen levels of less than 125 mg/dL should receive cryoprecipitate.

Thrombosis

Thromboembolic events occur in 5% to 10% of patients with cancer and are manifested as deep venous thrombosis, arterial thrombosis, migratory thrombophlebitis, pulmonary embolism, and nonbacterial thrombotic endocarditis.[58] Thromboembolic events rank second to infections as a cause of death in patients with solid tumors. Some malignancies that are often associated with thrombotic events are colon, gallbladder, gastric, lung (any cell type), myeloproliferative syndromes, ovary, pancreas, and paraprotein disorders.

Nonbacterial thrombotic endocarditis can occur in patients with lung, pancreatic, and colon cancers. The aortic valve is most frequently involved, and the spleen is the most commonly infarcted organ.

Hypercoagulability is mediated by several mechanisms. Increased levels of clotting factors are described, including fibrinogen and factors I, V, VIII:C, IX, and XI, and are manifested as shortened aPTT and PT. Low-grade DIC is manifested by increased titers of fibrin degradation products and D-dimer. Decreases in coagulation inhibitors are also revealed by acquired protein C, protein S, and antithrombin III defects. Of the two expressions of DIC, thrombosis is more common than bleeding in patients who have solid tumors, with an incidence as high as 40% to 50%.[51]

Solid tumors may cause tissue injury and elaboration of the tissue factor that initiates local thrombosis. Mucinous adenocarcinomas contain a sialic acid moiety that can nonenzymatically activate factor X.

Platelet abnormalities can also contribute to hypercoagulability with thrombocytosis and increased platelet adhesion. Thrombocytosis is most commonly associated with carcinoma of the pancreas, lung, gastrointestinal tract, ovary, and breast and with myeloproliferative syndromes.

Clinicians must carefully monitor patients for thrombotic complications. Appropriate testing includes impedance plethysmography, venography, arteriography, and ventilation/perfusion scanning. Full coagulation profiles should include PT, aPTT, platelet counts, D-dimer, fibrin split products, fibrinogen, antithrombin III, protein S, and protein C.

Therapy is directed at treating the acute event and reducing risk for subsequent events. All patients should receive antineoplastic therapy for the underlying malignancy. Asymptomatic patients may receive antiplatelet agents such as enteric-coated aspirin or dipyridamole.

Life-threatening thrombotic events can be treated with surgery (embolectomy or vena cava interruption) or thrombolytic therapy with streptokinase, urokinase, or plasminogen activators. Therapy for the acute condition should then be followed by anticoagulation with heparin.

Heparin and warfarin can be used to treat severe thrombosis and to minimize recurrent events. High doses of heparin are no more effective than low doses and are associated with increased risk of bleeding. Warfarin and heparin are generally contraindicated in patients with CNS disease. Heparin may be given for 7 to 10 days to maintain an aPTT of 1.5 to 2.0 times control. Oral warfarin can be started on day 5 and should overlap the heparin therapy for several days.[59] Less intensive regimens of warfarin with an international normalized ratio (INR) of 2.0 remain effective against thromboembolism and confer less risk of bleeding. The recommended target range is an INR of 2.0 to 3.0 (equivalent to a PT of 1.3 to 1.5 times control).[59] The duration of oral anticoagulant therapy is controversial; patients should be treated for 3 months or for the duration of the time they are at risk.[60]

CHEMOTHERAPY-INDUCED EMERGENCIES

Extravasation

Chemotherapeutic agents are classified as nonvesicants, irritants, or vesicants. By definition, vesicants can cause necrosis if extravasation occurs. If extravasation takes place, the drug should be immediately discontinued. The treatment for extravasation caused by daunorubicin (Cerubidine), doxorubicin, epirubicin (Farmorubicin), intravenous or intramuscular actinomycin, and mitomycin involves cooling the site with ice packs for approximately 24 hours and elevation of the limb. For the vinca alkaloids vincristine and vinblastine, the therapy consists of the application of warm compresses and local injection of hyaluronidase (Wydase). Immediate consultation with a plastic surgeon should be obtained because rapid debridement may minimize the overall injury.

REFERENCES

1. Byrne TN: Spinal cord compression from epidural metastases. N Engl J Med 327:614–619, 1992.
2. Perrin RG: Metastatic tumors of the axial spine. Curr Opin Oncol 4:525–532, 1992.
3. Markman M: Common complications and emergencies associated with cancer and its therapy. Cleve Clin J Med 61:105–114, 1994.
4. Willson JKV, Masaryl TJ: Neurologic emergencies in the cancer patient. Semin Oncol 16:490–503, 1989.
5. Choucair AK: Myelopathies in the cancer patient: Incidence, presentation, diagnosis, and management. Oncology 5(6):71–80, 1991.
6. Boogerd W, van der Sande JJ: Diagnosis and treatment of spinal cord compression in malignant disease. Cancer Treat Rev 19:129–150, 1993.
7. Bates T: A review of local radiotherapy and cord compression. Int J Radiat Oncol Biol Phys 23:217–221, 1992.
8. Thomas CR, Edmondson EA: Common emergencies in cancer medicine: Cardiovascular and neurologic syndromes. J Natl Med Assoc 83:1001–1017, 1991.
9. Lyons MK, Meyer FB: Cerebrospinal fluid physiology and the management of increased intracranial pressure. Mayo Clin Proc 65:684–707, 1990.
10. Schiller JH, Jones JC: Paraneoplastic syndromes associated with lung cancer. Curr Opin Oncol 5:335–342, 1993.
11. Chamberlain MC:. Current concepts in leptomeningeal metastasis. Curr Opin Oncol 4:533–539, 1992.
12. Choucair AK: Myelopathies in the cancer patient: Incidence, presentation, diagnosis, and management. Oncology 5(7):25–37, 1991.
13. Vaitkus PT, Herrmann HC, LeWinter MM: Treatment of malignant pericardial effusion. JAMA 272:59–64, 1994.
14. Helms SR, Carlson MD: Cardiovascular emergencies. Semin Oncol 16:463–470, 1989.

15. Escalante CP: Causes and management of superior vena cava syndrome. Oncology 7(6):61–77, 1993.

16. Kreisman H, Wolkove N: Pulmonary toxicity of antineoplastic therapy, in Perry MC (ed): The Chemotherapy Source Book, pp 598–619. Baltimore, Williams & Wilkins, 1992.

17. DeVries CR, Freiha FS: Hemorrhagic cystitis: A review. J Urol 143:1–9, 1990.

18. Shepherd JD, Pringle LE, Barnett MJ, et al: Mesna versus hyperhydration for the prevention of cyclophosphamide-induced hemorrhagic cystitis in bone marrow transplantation. J Clin Oncol 9:2016–2020, 1991.

19. Donahue LA, Frank IN: Intravesical formalin for hemorrhagic cystitis: Analysis of therapy. J Urol 141:809–812, 1989.

20. Levine LA, Jarrard DF: Treatment of cyclophosphamide-induced hemorrhagic cystitis with intravesical carboprost tromethamine. J Urol 149:719–723, 1993.

21. Liu YK, Harty JI, Steinbock GS, et al: Treatment of radiation or cyclophosphamide induced hemorrhagic cystitis using conjugated estrogen. J Urol 144:41–43, 1990.

22. Dosik GM, Luna M, Valdivieso M, et al: Necrotizing colitis in patients with cancer. Am J Med 67:646–656, 1979.

23. Pestalozzi BC, Sotos GA, Choyke PL, et al: Typhlitis resulting from treatment with taxol and doxorubicin in patients with metastatic breast cancer. Cancer 71:1797–1800, 1992.

24. Wade DS, Nava HR, Douglass HO: Neutropenic enterocolitis. Clinical diagnosis and treatment. Cancer 69:17–23, 1992.

25. Stellato TA, Shenk RR: Gastrointestinal emergencies in the oncology patient. Semin Oncol 16:521–531, 1989.

26. Arrambide K, Toto RD: Tumor lysis syndrome. Semin Nephrol 13:273–280, 1993.

27. Silverman P, Distelhorst CW: Metabolic emergencies in clinical oncology. Semin Oncol 16:504–515, 1989.

28. Dunlau RW, Camp MA, Allon M, et al: Calcitriol in prolonged hypocalcemia due to the tumor lysis syndrome. Ann Intern Med 110: 162–164, 1989.

29. Pierce ST. Paraendocrine syndromes. Curr Opin Oncol 5:639–645, 1993.

30. Moses AM, Scheinman SJ: Ectopic secretion of neurohypophyseal peptides in patients with malignancy. Endocrinol Metab Clin North Am 20:489–506, 1991.

31. Pimentel L: Medical complications of oncologic disease. Emerg Med Clin North Am 11:407–419, 1993.

32. Rosol TJ, Capen CC: Mechanisms of cancer-induced hypercalcemia. Lab Invest 67:680–702, 1992.

33. Thomas CR, Dodhia N: Common emergencies in cancer medicine: Metabolic syndromes. J Natl Med Assoc 83:809–818, 1991.

34. Kinirons MT: Newer agents for the treatment of malignant hypercalcemia. Am J Med Sci 305:403–406, 1993.

35. Hall TG, Burns Schaiff RA: Update on the medical treatment of hypercalcemia of malignancy. Clin Pharm 12:117–125, 1993.

36. Nussbaum SR: Pathophysiology and management of severe hypercalcemia. Endocrinol Metab Clin North Am 22:343–362, 1993.

37. Averbuch SD: New bisphosphonates in the treatment of bone metastases. Cancer 72:3443–3452, 1993.

38. Carter PW, Cohen HJ, Crawford J: Hyperviscosity syndrome in association with kappa light chain myeloma. Am J Med 86:591–595, 1989.

39. Geraci JM, Hansen RM, Kueck BD: Plasma cell leukemia and hyperviscosity syndrome. South Med J 83:800–805, 1990.

40. Patterson WP, Caldwell CW, Doll DC: Hyperviscosity syndromes and coagulopathies. Semin Oncol 17:210–216, 1990.

41. Baer MR: Management of unusual presentations of acute leukemia. Hematol Oncol Clin North Am 7:275–292, 1993.

42. Ringenberg QS, Doll DC: Acute nonlymphocytic leukemia: The first 48 hours. South Med J 83:931–940, 1990.

43. Soares FA, Landell GAM, Carduso MC: Pulmonary leukostasis without hyperleukocytosis: A clinicopathologic study of 16 cases. Am J Hematol 40:28–32, 1992.

44. Goenka P, Chait M, Hitti IF, et al: Acute leukostasis pulmonary distress syndrome. J Fam Pract 35:445–449, 1992.

45. Campbell J, Mitchell CA: Acute leg ischemia as a manifestation of the hyperleukocytosis syndrome in acute myeloid leukaemia. Am J Hematol 46:167, 1994.

46. Gartrell K, Rosenstrauch W: Hypoxaemia in patients with hyperleukocytosis: True or spurious, and clinical implications. Leuk Res 17:915–919, 1993.

47. Lascari AD: Improvement of leukemic hyperleukocytosis with only fluid and allopurinol therapy. Am J Dis Child 145:969–970, 1991.

48. Nelson SC, Bruggers CS, Kurtzberg J, et al: Management of leukemic hyperleukocytosis with hydration, urinary alkalinization, and allopurinol. Are cranial irradiation and invasive cytoreduction necessary? Am J Pediat Hematol Oncol 15: 351–355, 1993.

49. Dabrow MB and Wilkins JC: Management of hyperleukocytic syndrome, DIC, and thrombotic thrombocytopenic purpura. Postgrad Med 93:193–202, 1993.

50. Nand S, Messmore H: Hemostasis in malignancy. Am J Hematol 35: 45–55, 1990.

51. Bick RL: Coagulation abnormalities in malignancy: A review. Sem in Thromb and Hemost 18:353–372, 1992.

52. Heyman MR, Schiffer CA: Platelet transfusion therapy for the cancer patient. Semin Oncol 17:198–209, 1990.

53. Nugent DJ: Alloimmunization to platelet antigens. Semin Hematol 29:83–88, 1992.

54. Bensan K, Fields K, Hiemenz J, et al: The platelet-refractory bone marrow transplant patient: Prophylaxis and treatment of bleeding. Semin Oncol 20:102–109, 1993.

55. Ey FS, Goodnight SH: Bleeding disorders in cancer. Semin Oncol 17:187–197, 1990.

56. Rosen PJ: Bleeding problems in the cancer patient. Hematol Oncol Clin North Am 6:1315–1328, 1992.

57. Colman RW and Rubin RN: Disseminated intravascular coagulation due to malignancy. Semin Oncol 17:172–186, 1990.

58. Steingart RH: Coagulation disorders associated with neoplastic disease. Recent Resul Can Research 108:37–43, 1988.

59. Levine M, Hirsh J: The diagnosis and treatment of thrombosis in the cancer patient. Semin Oncol 17:160–171, 1990.

60. Scates SM: Diagnosis and treatment of cancer-related thrombosis. Semin Thromb Hemost 18:373–379, 1992.

CHAPTER 43

Epidemiology of Cancer and Prevention Strategies

L. Arlene Nazario, MD, Janet E. Macheledt, MD, MS, MPH, *and* Victor G. Vogel, MD, MHS

Department of Clinical Cancer Prevention, The University of Texas M. D. Anderson Cancer Center, Houston, Texas

Cancer epidemiology is the study of the distribution, determinants, and frequency of malignant disease in specific populations.[1] The objective is to define causative factors to formulate preventive strategies for control of the disease. Epidemiologic assessment provides the clinician with a quantification of cancer risk, outlines the basis for screening modalities for high-risk populations, and determines the efficacy of any preventive intervention.

Three types of epidemiologic research apply to the field of cancer. Descriptive epidemiology focuses on the trends and frequency of disease in a given population. Analytic epidemiology deals with identifying causes and the predisposing risk associated with the development of disease. Clinical epidemiology outlines screening programs and evaluates the impact of prevention strategies on overall outcome.

DESCRIPTIVE EPIDEMIOLOGY

The American Cancer Society estimates that, during 1995, there will be 1,252,000 new cancer cases and 547,000 deaths from cancer in the United States. In addition, about 120,000 new cases of carcinoma in situ (uterine, cervix, breast, and melanoma) plus more than 800,000 basal- and squamous-cell skin cancers will be diagnosed.[2]

Cancer incidence and mortality rates are higher among males than females.[2] In addition, Americans over 65 years old have a tenfold greater risk of developing cancer than younger individuals. Despite an increase in the overall cancer mortality rate between 1950 and 1990, the mortality rates for all cancers combined have declined substantially for individuals under 45 years old but increased for individuals over 55 years old. Most of the increase is attributable to deaths from lung cancer. African-Americans have a higher cancer mortality rate than whites.[3]

Currently, the leading cancers—those of the lung, breast, prostate, colon and rectum, and ovary—account for nearly 61% of the cancer burden in the United States (Table 1). If lung cancer is excluded, overall cancer deaths have declined over 14% since 1950.[3]

ANALYTIC EPIDEMIOLOGY

The goal of analytic epidemiology is to identify the factors that predispose individuals to the development of disease and to quantitate risk. Cancer risk factors include environmental exposures, genetic susceptibility, and immunosuppressive state but may be secondary to prior history of malignancy, viral infection, or therapy. These risk factors can act at different steps during carcinogenesis. Some risk factors linked to the development of cancer are listed in Tables 2 and 3. Established risk factors for site-specific malignancies will be discussed below.

Cancer of the Head and Neck

Between 1973 and 1989, the incidence rates of oral and pharyngeal cancer declined in white males of all ages while they increased in African-American males. African-American males younger than 65 have almost twice the incidence of oral and pharyngeal cancer seen in white males, but the trend changes for white men older than 65, who have higher rates than African-American men older

TABLE I

Estimated New Cancer Cases and Deaths for Leading Cancer Sites, United States, 1995

Site	Estimated new cases	Estimated deaths
Lung	169,900	157,400
Breast	183,400	46,240
Prostate	244,000	40,400
Colon and rectum	138,200	55,300
Ovary	26,600	14,500
All sites	1,252,000	547,000

Adapted from Macheledt JE, Vogel VG: The epidemiology of cancer, in Medical Oncology: A Comprehensive Review, pp 501–510. Huntington, PRR Inc, 1993, with data from Wingo PA, Tong T, Bolden S: Cancer statistics, 1995. CA Cancer J Clin 45:8–30, 1995.

TABLE 2

Known Cancer Risk Factors for Human Malignancy

Tobacco
  Smokeless tobacco, environmental tobacco smoke

Alcohol

Diet
  High animal-fat intake; aflatoxins; deficiencies in
  vitamins A and C and beta-carotene

Occupational exposures
  Aromatic amines, arsenic, asbestos, nickel, pesticides,
  polycyclic hydrocarbons, vinyl chloride, wood dusts, others

Radiation
  Ionizing and ultraviolet radiation, radon and its byproducts

Medications
  See Table 3

Infection
  Bacterial (*Helicobacter pylori*)
  Parasites (*Schistosoma haematobium, Clonorchis sinensis*)
  Viral (Epstein-Barr virus, hepatitis B and C viruses,
    human immunodeficiency virus, human papillomavirus,
    human T-lymphotropic virus type I)

Genetic susceptibility

Adapted from Macheledt JE, Vogel VG: The epidemiology of cancer, in Medical Oncology: A Comprehensive Review, pp 501–510. Huntington, PRR Inc, 1993; and from Fraumeni JF Jr, Devesa SS, Hoover RN, et al: Epidemiology of cancer, in DeVita VT Jr, Hellman S, Rosenberg SA (eds): Cancer: Principles & Practice of Oncology, pp 150–181. Philadelphia, JB Lippincott Co, 1993.

than 65. The incidence rates of laryngeal cancer are significantly higher for African-American males of all ages than for white males[4] and are continuing to rise for females.[3]

The most common head and neck malignancies are squamous-cell carcinomas of the upper aerodigestive tract. Tobacco exposure is a major etiologic factor. A 5- to 25-fold increased cancer risk has been documented for heavy smokers, compared with nonsmokers.[4] A clear dose-response relationship exists, and when smoking is combined with alcohol consumption, their effects on cancer risk appear to be synergistic. On the other hand, smoking cessation is associated with a declining risk.[5]

Cigar and pipe smokers, as well as users of smokeless tobacco, are at increased risk for developing head and neck malignancies. Cigar and pipe smoking is associated with oral, pharyngeal, and laryngeal cancers.[4] Pipe smokers are predisposed to developing cancer of the lip.[6] Smokeless tobacco, primarily chewing tobacco and snuff, is known to cause cancer of the oral cavity, perhaps because of the high concentrations of tobacco–specific *N*-nitrosamines in smokeless tobaccos.[6]

Marijuana smoking may be a carcinogen to the upper aerodigestive tract, possibly because the smoking increases exposure of the respiratory tract to tar and because of the rapid, deep inhalation used in marijuana smoking, which leads to particulate deposition.[7]

Alcohol use has been associated with cancers of the oral cavity, pharynx, and larynx as well. The effect of alcohol use is multiplicative to that of tobacco smoking, particularly for laryngeal cancers.[4]

Several epidemiologic studies have suggested an inverse relationship between micronutrient intake and cancer incidence. A protective effect has been reported for vitamin C against oral and pharyngeal cancer,[8] vitamin A against oral cancer,[9] and beta-carotene against laryngeal cancer.[10]

Additional risk factors for head and neck malignancies include occupational exposure to wood dust, organic compounds, and coal products.[4] An increased risk of developing laryngeal cancer has been related to asbestos exposure, exposure to nickel in smelting operations, occupational exposure to sulfuric acid, and the manufacture of mustard gas.[4]

The occurrence of a head and neck malignancy itself places the affected individual at higher risk for a secondary primary cancer.

Cancer of the Lung

Cancer of the lung is the second most common malignancy affecting both sexes. In the early 1950s, it became the leading cause of cancer deaths in men. In the mid-1980s, women's lung cancer mortality rates surpassed those from breast cancer. For 1995, it is estimated that 169,900 new cases of lung cancer will be diagnosed and that 157,400 patients with lung cancer will die of the disease.[2] Lung cancer is considered the most rapidly increasing cause of death from cancer.[11]

Cigarette smoking is a well-established pulmonary carcinogen. It is responsible for 90% of male and 78% of female lung cancer deaths.[12] A dose–response effect has been demonstrated between number of cigarettes per day smoked, duration of smoking, and subsequent cancer risk. This risk is 20-fold higher for one-pack-a-day smokers with over 30 years of tobacco use than it is for nonsmokers.[6] Younger age at initiation of smoking increases risk because it increases the overall duration of smoking, not because young people have an increased susceptibility.[13] Lifetime tar exposure is another good index of cancer risk.[12] There is an increased risk of developing airway obstruction[11,13] related to smoking unfiltered cigarettes.[13] Smoking cessation reduces the risk of lung cancer in former smokers, although the risk remains higher than the risk for those who have never smoked.[13]

Environmental tobacco smoke or passive exposure to smoking has been linked to lung cancer. The risk of developing lung cancer in a nonsmoker married to a smoker has been estimated to be increased by about 30%.[11,13]

Other environmental carcinogens include polycyclic hydrocarbons generated from the combustion of fossil fuels, radionuclides, and diesel exhaust.[13] Exposure to radon and its byproducts has been established as a cause of lung cancer. Radon interacts synergistically with cigarette smoke.[11,13] Annually, approximately 14,000 lung cancer deaths in the United States are attributable to radon exposure among smokers, making radon the second most important etiologic agent for lung cancer.[13]

Among the occupational carcinogens, past exposure to asbestos predisposes to the development of mesothelioma in the absence of tobacco use.[11] Among cigarette smokers, the risk for lung cancer is 50-fold higher in workers exposed to asbestos without protection, than in the nonsmoking, unexposed population.[11] Workers exposed to asbestos include those in the shipbuilding, fireproofing, acoustic-control, and pipe-insulation industries.[12] Other workplace exposures are listed in Table 4.

As discussed for head and neck malignancies, an inverse association between beta-carotene intake and lung cancer risk has been established.[11]

Cancer of the Esophagus

During the past two decades, the incidence rates of squamous-cell carcinoma of the esophagus have remained stable, whereas a steady increase for esophageal adenocarcinomas has been documented.[14-16] In the United States, esophageal cancer occurs most often in black men.[15] Mortality rates among blacks are three times higher than among whites.[3]

The risk of squamous-cell carcinoma of the esophagus is increased by agents that cause chronic irritation of the epithelial lining. Alcohol and tobacco use are the main etiologic factors; their interaction is multiplicative.[14] Thermal injuries from hot drinks, fungal toxins in pickled vegetables, achalasia, radiation, and strictures from swallowing lye may predispose to the development of cancer of the esophagus. This cancer has also been associated with poor nutritional status (particularly deficiencies of vitamins A and C and riboflavin), tylosis, and Plummer-Vinson syndrome.[14,15] In the Asian esophageal cancer belt, smoked opiates have a strong etiologic role.[14]

However, adenocarcinoma of the esophagus is more

TABLE 3

Drugs That May Induce Cancer in Humans

Drug	Cancer site
Antineoplastic agents	
Alkylating agents	Leukemia
Cyclophosphamide	Urinary bladder
Androgen-anabolic steroids	Liver
Immunosuppressants	
Azathioprine, cyclosporine	Non-Hodgkin's lymphoma
Phenacetin-containing analgesics	Renal pelvis
Estrogens	
Synthetic (diethylstilbestrol)	Vagina, cervix (adenocarcinoma)
Conjugated	Endometrium
Steroid contraceptives	Liver

Adapted from Macheledt JE, Vogel VG: The epidemiology of cancer, in Medical Oncology: A Comprehensive Review, pp 501–510. Huntington, PRR Inc, 1993; and from Fraumeni JF Jr, Devesa SS, Hoover RN, et al: Epidemiology of cancer, in DeVita VT Jr, Hellman S, Rosenberg SA (eds): Cancer: Principles & Practice of Oncology, pp 150–181. Philadelphia, JB Lippincott Co, 1993.

common in white individuals. The risk for its development is 30 to 125 times higher in individuals with Barrett's esophagus.[15]

Cancer of the Stomach

The incidence of gastric carcinoma in the United States has been declining for the past 50 years.[17] Mortality rates have also been declining and may be leveling off.[3] *Helicobacter pylori* infection and conditions that result in achlorhydria with intragastric bacterial overgrowth and formation of *N*-nitroso compounds have been implicated in the development of gastric carcinoma.[18]

Cancer of the Liver

Infection with hepatitis B virus has been causally related to the development of hepatocellular carcinoma. The relationship is limited to chronically active forms of the hepatitis B virus, that is, those that have hepatitis B surface antigen.[19] In populations with a high incidence of hepatocellular carcinoma, the risk for its development is more than 200 times greater in hepatitis B surface antigen carriers than among noncarriers.[20]

TABLE 4

Some Occupational Exposures Categorized as Bronchogenic Carcinogens

Arsenic

Chloromethyl compounds

Chromium

Ionizing radiation, gamma radiation

Certain man-made mineral fibers

Mustard gas

Nickel

Polycyclic aromatic hydrocarbons

Vinyl chloride

Adapted from Macheledt JE, Vogel VG: The epidemiology of cancer, in Medical Oncology: A Comprehensive Review, pp 501–510. Huntington, PRR Inc, 1993; and from Beckett WS: Epidemiology and etiology of lung cancer. Clin Chest Med 14(1):1–15, 1993.

Another etiologic factor is infection with hepatitis C virus, which progresses to chronic hepatitis and cirrhosis, ultimately leading to the development of hepatocellular carcinoma.[21]

Environmental exposures linked to hepatic malignancies include exposure to aflatoxins in contaminated food and to vinyl chloride, consumption of alcoholic beverages, medications such as androgen-anabolic steroids and steroid contraceptives, and parasitic infection with *Clonorchis sinensis*.[22]

Cancer of the Colon and Rectum

In the United States, the colon and rectum are among the leading sites of cancer. An individual's lifetime risk for developing colorectal cancer is 1 in 20. The risk increases with age, with only 3% of cases occurring before age 40.[23] Between 1973 and 1990, the mortality rates decreased significantly among whites and increased significantly among African-Americans.[3]

The sigmoid colon is the most common site of colon cancer in both sexes in industrialized countries. The disease moves proximally to the right side of the colon with increasing age.[23]

Diet is a well-established risk factor. Diets high in fat, particularly from animal sources, are associated with increased risk, whereas high fiber intake is associated with reduced risk. Diets rich in calcium, vitamin D, fruits, and vegetables also have a protective effect.[23] Alcohol consumption is related to rectal cancer and, less consistently, to colon cancer.[24]

Adenomatous polyps are thought to be premalignant lesions for colorectal cancer. Risk of developing colorectal cancer is associated with the number and size of adenomas, their degree of dysplasia, and their histology, with villous polyps indicating a higher risk.[23] Patients with chronic ulcerative colitis are at higher risk of developing colorectal cancer. The degree of predisposition is proportional to the extent of disease involvement and the duration of active disease. First-degree relatives of colorectal cancer patients are more susceptible to developing the disease themselves.[23]

About 1% of these cases have specific genetic disorders. Familial adenomatous polyposis is an autosomal dominant condition characterized by the tendency to develop hundreds of polyps. If left untreated, the polyps may become invasive cancer. The genetic defect has been traced to chromosome 5q21–q22, where a tumor-suppressor gene is presumed to reside. The same defect is found in patients with Gardner's syndrome (familial adenomatous polyposis with extracolonic manifestations). Patients with hereditary nonpolyposis colorectal cancer have family histories of colorectal cancer and are affected at an early age, often with right-sided mucinous tumors. These patients are predisposed to developing second malignancies of the breast, ovary, and endometrium.[23,25]

A history of colorectal cancer increases the risk for a second colorectal primary tumor by about 5%.[23]

Cancer of the Kidney and Renal Pelvis

The incidence and mortality rates for cancer of the kidney and renal pelvis are two times higher for males than for females. Most kidney malignancies arise in the renal parenchyma.[3] Individuals with hypertension or obesity, those who have been exposed to tobacco smoke or asbestos or have used phenacetin, and perhaps those with previous renal injury are at higher risk of developing renal-cell carcinoma. The risk for developing carcinoma of the renal pelvis increases by two- to threefold with exposure to tobacco smoke and by tenfold with abuse of phenacetin-containing analgesics. Upper urinary tract infections and stones may predispose to cancer of the renal pelvis as well.[26]

Patients with von Hippel-Lindau syndrome are also predisposed to developing renal-cell carcinoma.[22]

Cancer of the Bladder

Bladder cancer predominantly affects elderly people and tends to have a different natural history in younger patients.[27] Males are affected four times more often than females.[3]

Cigarette smoking is the most important cause of

bladder cancer, accounting for 25% to 60% of cases in industrialized countries. This activity has a clear dose-response effect on the development of transitional-cell, squamous-cell, and adenocarcinoma histologic subtypes.[27]

Occupational exposures in the dye, leather, textile, rubber, paint, petroleum, and chemical industries increase the risk of developing bladder cancer.[27]

Infection with *Schistosoma haematobium* with secondary chronic inflammatory response is causally related to the development of bladder cancer, particularly squamous-cell carcinomas.[27]

Exposure to the antineoplastic drug cyclophosphamide (Cytoxan, Neosar) predisposes an individual to bladder cancer. The association between bladder cancer and the artificial sweeteners cyclamate and saccharin, however, is derived from animal studies and has not been supported by human data.[27]

Cancer of the Prostate

In the United States, prostate cancer is the most common malignancy and the second leading cause of cancer death affecting the male population.[3] It is a disease of elderly men; less than 1% of cases are men younger than age 50. The incidence increases 50-fold in whites and 30-fold in African-Americans between the ages of 50 and 85.[28]

African-Americans have the highest incidence of prostate cancer in the world,[28,29] whereas Japan has one of the lowest rates.[28] Japanese migrants to Hawaii develop a risk for prostate cancer higher than that of native Japanese but only half that of American whites.[28]

African-American men tend to have metastatic disease at diagnosis, indeed, 40% more often than whites do. The overall survival rate for African-American men is 10% lower than that for white men, even when they are diagnosed at the same stage of disease.[29]

Neither smoking nor alcohol consumption affect the risk of developing prostate cancer.[29,30] Cadmium exposure, at work or in the diet, has been etiologically related to prostate cancer.[29] A familial tendency for prostate cancer exists, and members of such families are affected at an earlier age.[31]

Cancer of the Ovary

One in 70 American women will develop ovarian cancer in her lifetime. Epithelial ovarian cancer is infrequent before the age of 35, after which incidence rates progressively increase up to the age of 75.[32] Ovarian cancer is the most often fatal gynecologic malignancy.[2] Factors associated with increased risk include infertility, nulliparity, and use of fertility drugs. Tubal ligation and

hysterectomy with ovarian conservation and oral contraceptive use have been shown to have a protective effect. A risk reduction of about 50% has been documented after 5 years of oral contraceptive use.[32] The effect increases with duration of use and persists for 10 to 15 years after discontinuation.[33]

Familial clustering of ovarian cancer poses an increased risk on the basis of genetic susceptibility. Three different entities—site-specific ovarian cancer, breast-ovarian cancer, and Lynch syndrome II (hereditary non-polyposis colon cancer with proximal colonic predominance, endometrial cancer, and ovarian cancer)—are jointly referred to as hereditary ovarian cancer syndrome.[25] An autosomal dominant mode of inheritance with variable penetrance has been suggested for these diseases. Therefore, the probability of a woman in an affected family developing ovarian cancer is about 50%. Two to four generations of a family are usually affected. In such families, the disease develops at an earlier age than sporadic cases do, but there is no difference in prognosis given similar stage at diagnosis.[34] The tumors are usually serous cystadenocarcinomas.[33]

Hereditary ovarian cancer cases account for less than 1% of all cases.[32] Recent genetic studies located a gene on chromosome 17q21 (*BRCA1*) that predisposes to familial breast-ovarian cancer.[35] However, the lifetime risk of a 35-year-old woman developing ovarian cancer ranges from 1.6% if she has no affected relative members to 5% if she has one affected first-degree relative to 7% if she has two affected relatives.[33,36]

Genetic susceptibility for developing ovarian neoplasms has been documented. Women with Peutz-Jeghers syndrome have a 5% risk of developing ovarian tumors, patients with gonadal dysgenesis (46XY) may develop gonadoblastomas, and benign ovarian fibromas develop in patients who have inherited basal-cell nevus syndrome.[22]

Cancer of the Endometrium

Endometrial carcinoma is the most common gynecologic malignancy.[2] Its incidence is highest among white women, whereas its mortality rates are higher among African-American women. For the past two decades, the incidence rates have been declining, except among African-American women over 50 years old. Mortality rates have decreased for all ages.[3] Endometrial cancer, like ovarian cancer, is uncommon in before age 40; subsequently, incidence increases until age 70.

Established risk factors include use of unopposed estrogen replacement therapy, use of sequential oral contraceptives, obesity, nulliparity, and late menopause.[35]

Breast cancer patients are at increased risk of developing endometrial carcinoma, among other cancers, probably because of a shared hormonal effect.[37] Furthermore, there is very clear evidence that tamoxifen given as adjuvant treatment for breast cancer increases the risk of endometrial cancer by three- to sevenfold.[38] Polycystic ovarian disease and estrogen-secreting ovarian tumors are also associated with an increased risk.[35]

Use of combination oral contraceptives, which increase exposure to progesterone, and cigarette smoking, which may lower circulating estrogen levels, probably play a protective role.[35]

Cancer of the Cervix

In the United States, the incidence and mortality rates for cancer of the cervix have decreased by more than 70% in the last 40 years.[39] The highest rates of invasive cervical cancer are found in Latin America, where women have a sixfold greater risk than do American white women. In the United States, the incidence rates for African-Americans and Hispanics are twice those of whites and Asians.[40]

Cervical cancer tends to occur in women of lower socioeconomic classes. The risk is higher for women with multiple sexual partners; it has been reported to be three times higher for women who have had 10 or more partners than for women who have had one or no partners. Early age at first sexual intercourse increases the risk, perhaps because of increased susceptibility of the cervical epithelium to carcinogen exposure. Several studies have demonstrated that women who begin having sexual intercourse before age 16 have about twice the risk as those who begin after age 20. Multiparity has been related to cervical cancer risk, possibly because of cervical trauma during delivery and hormonal and nutritional changes during pregnancy. The risk is four times greater for Latin-American women who have borne 12 or more children than for those who have had only one child or no children.[40]

Human papillomavirus types 16 and 18 have been causally related to cervical intraepithelial neoplasia. A history of genital warts (condyloma acuminatum), which are linked to human papillomavirus types 6 and 11, may explain the increased risk associated with multiple sexual partners.[40] Warts may also be a marker of infection with other types of human papillomavirus that are carcinogenic.[41] Other sexually transmitted viruses, like herpes simplex virus 2, may interact as etiologic factors.[40]

Cancer of the Breast

Breast cancer is the most commonly diagnosed malignancy among women in the United States. For 1995, it is estimated that 182,000 women will be diagnosed with breast cancer and that 46,000 will die of the disease. Women's mortality rates for cancer of the breast are second only to those of cancer of the lung. Breast cancer incidence is low for women under age 40; only 6.5% of all such patients are less than 40 years old. However, the incidence rates triple by age 49 and double once again by age 69. Almost half of all cases of breast cancer are diagnosed in women age 65 and older.[42] The lifetime probability of a woman's developing breast cancer is one in eight, as determined by the revised methodology designed by the National Cancer Institute in collaboration with the American Cancer Society.[42]

Between 1940 and 1982, breast cancer incidence rates in the United States increased by approximately 1% per year, largely in women over 40 years old. From 1982 through 1987, the rate of increase accelerated to around 4% per year and then leveled off. The rising rate is mainly attributable to early detection, due to the increase in breast cancer screening. The increase in breast cancer cases (with no change in incidence rates) among women 20 to 39 years old during 1970 to 1990 was due to a shift in the age distribution of the population. However, breast cancer mortality rates have remained fairly stable, with almost no change from 1950 to 1990,[42] increasing only about 0.2% per year.[3]

Established hormone-related risk factors for breast cancer include early age at menarche, late age at menopause, nulliparity in women over age 40, and advanced age at first full-term pregnancy. The number of full-term pregnancies may increase the risk of breast cancer at younger ages but may be protective for women after the age of 50. Breast feeding and oophorectomy before menopause appear to be protective. Obesity in postmenopausal women elevates breast cancer risk, possibly due to peripheral conversion of androstenedione to estrogen in adipose tissue.[35]

In premenopausal women, biopsy-proven proliferative benign breast disease with atypical hyperplasia is a marker for increased risk and has the potential for evolving into breast cancer.[43] A history of breast cancer predisposes to the development of a contralateral second primary,[35] particularly if the initial tumor was lobular.[37,44]

Breast cancer patients are at increased risk of developing malignant melanoma and cancers of the ovary, endometrium, colon, thyroid, and salivary glands because of similar hormonal and genetic factors. Elevated risks of leukemia, non-Hodgkin's lymphoma (NHL), and cancers of the lung and kidneys are believed to be a result of the treatment modalities used in breast cancer patients. Whereas hormonal treatment for an initial breast tumor reduces the risk in the contralateral breast by 50%,[37,45] ionizing radiation at moderate to high doses increases the risk for breast cancer.[35] The risk depends on the woman's age at the time of exposure, and there is no increase in risk among women who were exposed after age 40.[22]

A family history of breast cancer predisposes members of affected families. Individuals with a history of premenopausal bilateral disease in first-degree relatives have the highest risk. The susceptibility is inherited in an autosomal dominant fashion with high penetrance and is manifested in both females and males.[31] A gene mapped to chromosome 17q21 (BRCA1) has been associated with early-onset familial breast cancer with a penetrance of 85% through age 70.[36,46]

Cancer of the Thyroid

Thyroid carcinoma is a rare malignancy with a high cure rate. It accounts for about 1% of all new cancers.[3] Women are affected two to three times more frequently than men.[47] Deaths from thyroid cancer account for only 0.2% of all cancer deaths per year.[3]

Exposure to ionizing radiation (up to 2,000 cGy) for the treatment of head and neck ailments predisposes to the development of cancer of the thyroid. There is a linear dose-response relationship, and risk is inversely related to age at exposure. A number of excess cases are seen 5 to 9 years after the insult, and increased risk persists even 35 years after exposure.[47]

Benign thyroid disease, specifically adenomas and goiters, are also risk factors for cancer of the thyroid. Follicular carcinomas are more common in iodine-deficient areas, while papillary histology predominates in areas with high iodine intake. Medullary thyroid carcinoma is familial and occurs as part of multiple endocrine neoplasia II. The gene for this disease has been mapped to chromosome 10.[47]

Cancer of the Skin

Nonmelanoma skin cancer, the most common malignancy in the United States,[48] refers collectively to basal-cell carcinoma and squamous-cell carcinoma of the skin. The incidence rates for nonmelanoma skin cancer, particularly squamous-cell carcinoma, increase with age. Men are affected twice as often as women.[49]

Nonmelanoma lesions tend to develop at sites of prior inflammation or scars. Environmental exposure to arsenic or radiation, prior therapy with psoralen plus ultraviolet A light, infection with human papillomavirus, and immune suppression may predispose to these malignancies.[48] Cigarette smoking increases the risk for squamous-cell carcinoma.[49]

Ultraviolet radiation is the most important risk factor.

It accounts for most cases and interacts with other factors as an etiologic agent.[48] Squamous-cell carcinoma is thought to be related to cumulative sun exposure, whereas basal-cell carcinoma is related to intermittent exposure, particularly before age 40.[49] The risk of nonmelanoma and melanoma skin cancers is higher for whites and for people with poor tanning ability or a tendency to sunburn, fair skin, red or blond hair, and blue eyes.[49,50]

Individuals with nonmelanoma skin cancer are at increased risk for developing new primary lesions.[48] The risk remains stable over time and increases with the number of skin cancers diagnosed. New lesions tend to be of the same histology as the original tumor. These patients may be at increased risk for cutaneous melanoma.[49]

The incidence of cutaneous malignant melanoma has been increasing. Australia has the highest incidence rate worldwide. The incidence is highest among persons in high socioeconomic classes. Having pale skin or a large number of melanocytic nevi and freckles, sunburn from intermittent intense solar ultraviolet irradiation (particularly early in life), and living near the equator are risk factors for cutaneous melanoma.[50,51] Ultraviolet irradiation from sunlamps or sunbeds increases the risk for melanoma as well.[51]

Patients treated with cytotoxic therapy and those with transplant-associated immunosuppression or xeroderma pigmentosum are at increased risk for melanoma.[50,51] Patients with albinism and those previously exposed to psoralen and ultraviolet A radiation are at high risk for nonmelanoma skin cancer, but the risk for melanoma is not significantly increased.[51]

There is a familial tendency toward dysplastic nevi. It is inherited in an autosomal dominant fashion with high penetrance, located in chromosome 1p36.[50]

Leukemias

Leukemias are a diverse group of hematologic malignancies. In general, the incidence rates of leukemias decreased slightly between 1973 and 1986. Leukemias tend to afflict more men than women and more whites than nonwhites. Acute myelogenous leukemia (AML) usually occurs after age 40, whereas acute lymphocytic leukemia is common during childhood, and its rates increase again after about age 60. After 1970, mortality rates for leukemias leveled off.[52]

Exposure to benzene has been etiologically linked to leukemias; such exposure is estimated to increase leukemia risk 2 to 4.5 times. Workers in the rubber and shoe leather industries are exposed to benzene, which was a greater hazard before 1970, when occupational safety standards were implemented.[52]

Radiation exposure at moderate to high doses increases the risk for leukemia. The effect of ionizing radiation was determined by studies of atomic bomb survivors and patients irradiated for medical purposes.[52] The increased risk for leukemia begins 2 to 4 years after exposure, peaks at 6 to 8 years, and declines to normal within 25 years.[22] Development of chronic lymphocytic leukemia (CLL) is not influenced by exposure to ionizing radiation.[52]

A small increase in leukemia risk has been noted for residents living near power plants. Childhood leukemia, but not adult leukemia, has been linked to exposure to electromagnetic fields. However, it seems that the actual wiring configuration is a better indirect measure of exposure than is residency near power plants. Cigarette smoking increases the risk for AML by 1.5- to twofold.[52]

Cytotoxic therapy increases the risk for developing a secondary leukemia, usually AML or a dysplastic syndrome. Older patients may be at increased risk, and risk decreases 10 years after treatment. Prolonged therapy with epipodophyllotoxins increases the risk, which is dependent on dose and schedule of administration. The latency period for acute leukemias related to epipodophyllotoxin therapy is shorter than for those associated with alkylating therapy. While abnormalities at chromosome 11q23 have been noted in patients treated with epipodophyllotoxins, exposure to alkylating agents has been related to abnormalities on chromosomes 5 and 7. Overall, 70% to 90% of patients with secondary leukemias related to prior cytotoxic chemotherapy display clonal aberrations and chromosomal deletions, including del 5, del 7, del 5q, and del 7q. Another cytogenetic abnormality related to prior therapy is acquired monosomy 7.[53]

Infection with human T-lymphotropic virus type I accounts for the high incidence of adult T-cell leukemia and lymphoma in areas of Japan and the Caribbean.[22]

Patients with aplastic anemia are at increased risk for leukemia. A family history of NHL, Hodgkin's disease, or CLL increases the risk as much as five times.[53] Genetic susceptibility for leukemia is seen in patients with Down's syndrome, autosomal recessive syndromes with chromosomal instability such as Bloom's and Fanconi's anemia, and ataxia telangiectasia.[22]

Lymphomas

Hodgkin's disease is the most common malignancy in young adulthood (ages 15 to 24 years). The incidence rates of lymphomas have declined for Americans age 65 and older.[3] The disease is more common in males than in females; reproductive and hormonal factors may have a protective effect against Hodgkin's disease among females.[54] High socioeconomic status, white race, and a family history of Hodgkin's disease increase the predisposing risk. The risk is also higher in families with few children and for individuals born earliest within the family. Epstein-Barr virus is found in approximately half of affected patients.

In the United States, the incidence of NHL has increased approximately 60% in the past two decades. Although acquired immunodeficiency syndrome (AIDS) has contributed to this increase, it is not solely responsible. The patients with AIDS who develop NHL are usually young men, whereas an overall increased incidence of NHL has been noted in elderly people of both genders. Among patients with NHL, the survival rates are better for whites and females.[55]

Patients treated with cytotoxic drugs, particularly alkylating agents and ionizing radiation for a prior neoplasia, have a three- to ninefold increased risk for NHL. The latency period is about 5 to 6 years.[55]

Environmental exposures that may cause NHL include exposure to pesticides, which particularly increase the risk for intermediate-grade NHL. Workers exposed to organic solvents may have a three times greater risk for NHL, and prolonged exposure increases that risk. Exposure to wood and cotton dust also predispose to the development of NHL. Use of hair dyes, especially long duration of use and young age at first use, increases risk as well. Smoking may also be a predisposing factor.[55] Agricultural laborers are exposed to oncogenic animal viruses that may be linked to NHL.[56]

Infection with *H pylori* is associated with a sixfold increased risk for gastric NHL.[55] Epstein-Barr virus infection is strongly associated with Burkitt's lymphoma in areas where the latter is endemic. Concurrent malarial infection in patients with the African form of Burkitt's lymphoma induces an immunodeficiency state that potentiates the oncogenic effect of Epstein-Barr virus.[22]

Immunodeficiency syndromes, autoimmune diseases with persistent antigenic stimulation, organ transplantation, and immunosuppressive therapy with azathioprine or cyclosporine are associated with increased risk for developing NHL.[22,56]

CLINICAL EPIDEMIOLOGY

Epidemiologic research plays an important role in the development of cancer screening modalities and prevention strategies. Cancer prevention focuses on decreasing incidence by lowering risk through changes in lifestyle patterns and behavior. Primary prevention attempts to stop the development of cancer. Secondary prevention aims to improve cure rates by cancer screening and early diagnosis and treatment.

Cancer Screening

Cancer screening involves testing to detect early-stage cancer in asymptomatic individuals. Ideally, screening tests should be easily administered, noninvasive, and inexpensive. To be beneficial, early detection should alter prognosis and improve survival.

Cervical Cancer: Cytologic screening for cervical cancer by Pap smears has had a major impact on the mortality rates for this malignancy. Successful screening relies on the detection of preinvasive lesions. When cervical cancer is diagnosed in situ, the cure rate is about 99%.[39] The current recommendation is that screening for cervical cancer (annual Pap smears) should start at age 18, or earlier in sexually active women. Examinations can be performed less frequently after three consecutive exams are deemed normal by a physician and can be discontinued at age 65 if findings were previously normal.[39] Screening at intervals of 2 years offers the same protection as annual exams, but intervals of longer than 2 years between screenings are associated with an increased risk for invasive cervical cancer.[57]

Breast Cancer: The combination of mammographic screening and clinical breast examination may reduce mortality rates from breast cancer by 30% to 40% in women over 50 years old. Nevertheless, guidelines for breast cancer screening vary. The American Cancer Society and the National Cancer Institute recommend annual clinical breast exams starting at age 40 and mammography every 1 to 2 years until age 50. Women older than 50 should have mammograms every year. The American College of Physicians, the American College of Surgeons, and the US Preventive Services Task Force recommend that mammography screening begin at age 50 and be performed at 1- to 2-year intervals until age 75 and more frequently if any abnormalities are diagnosed. Earlier breast cancer screening is advisable for those with increased risk for the disease.[39]

Colorectal Cancer: The goal of screening tests for colorectal cancer is to detect adenomatous polyps that might become invasive so that these can be removed, thus improving overall survival through the detection of early-stage disease. Fecal occult blood testing has reduced mortality from colorectal cancer by 38%,[58] and having a screening flexible sigmoidoscopic examination at least once every 10 years may decrease an individual's risk of death from rectal or distal colon cancer by 60% to 70%.[59,60]

Prostate Cancer: Digital rectal examination has been the traditional method of detecting abnormal areas in the prostate gland, but when used as a screening modality for prostate cancer, its effectiveness in diagnosing tumors confined to the prostate is uncertain.[61] Digital rectal examination plus measurement of serum prostate-specific antigen concentrations has been shown to enhance the detection rate for prostate cancer, but an optimal screening strategy for this disease has not yet been developed.[62] Transrectal ultrasonography and guided biopsy may be used in cases with abnormal findings.[63]

Other Malignancies: The efficacy of screening programs for other malignancies has not been determined. Screening strategies for other cancer sites are under investigation. Special attention must be paid to patients who have had a malignancy and who may, therefore, need screening for second malignancies at other sites.[64]

Chemoprevention

A relatively new approach to cancer prevention is under investigation through chemoprevention trials. Cancer chemoprevention is defined as the reversal of carcinogenesis in the premalignant phase.[65] The observation that retinoids, acting as modulators of cell differentiation, are effective in suppressing oral carcinogenesis and, therefore, in preventing second primary tumors in squamous-cell carcinoma of the head and neck has led to the evaluation of these agents as chemopreventive therapy for tumors of the upper aerodigestive tract in high-risk populations.[65,66] Studies of adjuvant hormonal therapy with tamoxifen for breast cancer have shown a 50% reduction of contralateral disease.[37] A national tamoxifen chemoprevention trial is being conducted to evaluate risk reduction for primary breast cancer in women at high risk.[67] With the development of new molecular techniques, chemoprevention trials will be aided by the identification of markers for premalignant lesions.

REFERENCES

1. Hennekens CH, Buring JE: Epidemiology in Medicine, pp 3–15. Boston, Little Brown & Co, 1987.

2. Wingo PA, Tong T, Bolden S: Cancer statistics, 1995. CA Cancer J Clin 45:8–30, 1995.

3. Miller BA, Ries LAG, Hankey BF, et al (eds): SEER Cancer Statistics Review: 1973–1990. Bethesda, Maryland, National Cancer Institute. NIH Publication No. 93–2789, 1993.

4. Spitz MR: Epidemiology and risk factors for head and neck cancer. Semin Oncol 21(3):281–288, 1994.

5. Blot WJ, McLaughlin JK, Winn DM, et al: Smoking and drinking in relation to oral and pharyngeal cancer. Cancer Res 48: 3282–3287, 1988.

6. Tobacco, in Tomatis L, Aitio A, Day NE, et al (eds): Cancer: Causes, Occurrence and Control, pp 169–180. Lyon, International Agency for Research on Cancer, IARC Publication No. 100, 1990.

7. Caplan GA, Brigham BA: Marijuana smoking and carcinoma of the tongue: Is there an association? Cancer 66:1005–1006, 1990.

8. Block G: Vitamin C status and cancer: Epidemiologic evidence

of reduced risk. Ann NY Acad Sci 669:280–290, 1992.

9. Marshall J, Graham S, Mettlin C, et al: Diet in the epidemiology of oral cancer. Nutr Cancer 3:145–149, 1982.

10. Mackerras D, Buffler PA, Randall DE, et al: Carotene intake and the risk of laryngeal cancer in coastal Texas. Am J Epidemiol 128:980–988, 1988.

11. Beckett WS: Epidemiology and etiology of lung cancer. Clin Chest Med 14(1):1–15, 1993.

12. Szabo E, Mulshine J: Epidemiology, prognostic factors, and prevention of lung cancer. Curr Opin Oncol 5(2):302–309, 1993.

13. Samet JM: The epidemiology of lung cancer. Chest 103(suppl 1):20–29S, 1993.

14. Muñoz N: Epidemiological aspects of oesophageal cancer. Endoscopy 25(9):609–612, 1993.

15. Mayer RJ: Overview: the changing nature of esophageal cancer. Chest 103(suppl 4):404–405S, 1993.

16. Cameron AJ: Epidemiologic studies and the development of Barrett's esophagus. Endoscopy 25(9):635–636, 1993.

17. Parsonnet J, Friedman GD, Vandersteen DP, et al: *Helicobacter pylori* infection and the risk of gastric carcinoma. N Engl J Med 325:1127–1131, 1991.

18. Stockbrugger RW: Epidemiology and pathology of precancerous lesions of the stomach. Eur J Cancer Prev 2(suppl 2):59–63, 1993.

19. Viruses and other biological agents, in Tomatis L, Aitio A, Day NE, et al (eds): Cancer: Causes, Occurrence and Control, pp 184–200. Lyon, International Agency for Research on Cancer, IARC Publication No. 100, 1990.

20. Beasley RP, Hwang LY, Lin CC, et al: Hepatocellular carcinoma and hepatitis B virus. Lancet 2:1129–1133, 1981.

21. Kiyosawa K, Furuta S: Clinical aspects and epidemiology of hepatitis B and C viruses in hepatocellular carcinoma in Japan. Cancer Chemother Pharmacol 31(suppl 1):S150–156, 1992.

22. Fraumeni JF Jr, Devesa SS, Hoover RN, et al: Epidemiology of cancer, in DeVita VT Jr, Hellman S, Rosenberg SA (eds): Cancer: Principles and Practice of Oncology, pp 150–181. Philadelphia, JB Lippincott, 1993.

23. DeCosse JJ, Tsioulias GJ, Jacobson JS: Colorectal cancer: Detection, treatment, and rehabilitation. CA Cancer J Clin 44: 27–42, 1994.

24. Willett WC: Micronutrients and cancer risk. Am J Clin Nutr 59 (suppl):1162–1165S, 1994.

25. Rustgi AK: Hereditary gastrointestinal polyposis and nonpolyposis syndromes. N Engl J Med 331:1694–1702, 1994.

26. McCredie M: Epidemiology of kidney cancer in Australia. Med J Aust 157(8):508–510, 1992.

27. Cohen SM, Johansson SL: Epidemiology and etiology of bladder cancer. Urol Clin North Am 19(3):421–428, 1992.

28. Karr JP: Prostate cancer in the United States and Japan. Adv Exp Med Biol 324:17–28, 1992.

29. Burks DA, Littleton RH: The epidemiology of prostate cancer in black men. Henry Ford Hosp Med J 40(1–2):89–92, 1992.

30. Talamini R, Franceschi S, LaVecchia C, et al: Smoking habits and prostate cancer: A case-control study in northern Italy. Prev Med 22(3):400–408, 1993.

31. Li FP: Molecular epidemiology studies of cancer in families. Br J Cancer 68:217–219, 1993.

32. Herbst AL: The epidemiology of ovarian carcinoma and the current status of tumor markers to detect disease. Am J Obstet Gynecol 170(4):1099–1105, 1994.

33. Kerlikowske K, Brown JS, Grady DG: Should women with familial ovarian cancer undergo prophylactic oophorectomy? Obstet Gynecol 80:700–707, 1992.

34. Bewtra C, Watson P, Conway T, et al: Hereditary ovarian cancer: A clinicopathological study. Int J Gynecol Pathol 11(3):180–187, 1992.

35. Kelsey JL, Whittemore AS: Epidemiology and primary prevention of cancers of the breast, endometrium, and ovary. A brief overview. Ann Epidemiol 4(2):89–95, 1994.

36. Miki Y, Swensen J, Shattuck-Eidens D, et al: A strong candidate for the breast and ovarian cancer susceptibility gene BRCA1. Science 266:66–71, 1994.

37. Horn-Ross PL: Multiple primary cancers involving the breast. Epidemiol Rev 15(1):169–176, 1993.

38. Fisher B, Costantino JP, Redmond CK, et al: Endometrial cancer in tamoxifen–treated breast cancer patients: Findings from the National Surgical Adjuvant Breast and Bowel Project (NSABP) B-14. J Natl Cancer Inst 86:527–537, 1994.

39. The National Strategic Plan for the early detection and control of breast and cervical cancers, pp 5–9. Washington, DC, US Department of Health and Human Services, 1993.

40. Brinton LA: Epidemiology of cervical cancer—overview, in Muñoz N, Bosch FX, Shah KV, et al (eds): The Epidemiology of Human Papillomavirus and Cervical Cancer, pp 3–23. Lyon, International Agency for Research on Cancer, IARC Scientific Publication No. 119, 1992.

41. Muñoz N, Bosch FX: HPV and cervical neoplasia: Review of case-control and cohort studies, in Muñoz N, Bosch FX, Shah KV, et al (eds): The Epidemiology of Human Papillomavirus and Cervical Cancer, pp 251–261. Lyon, International Agency for Research on Cancer, IARC Scientific Publication No. 119, 1992.

42. Miller BA, Feuer EJ, Hankey BF: The significance of the rising incidence of breast cancer in the United States, in DeVita VT Jr, Hellman S, Rosenberg SA (eds): Important Advances in Oncology 1994, pp 193–207. Philadelphia, JB Lippincott, 1994.

43. Bodian CA: Benign breast diseases, carcinoma in situ, and breast cancer risk. Epidemiol Rev 15(1):177–187, 1993.

44. Vandenbroucke A, Bourdon C: Epidemiological survey of preinvasive breast cancer. Eur J Cancer Prev 2(suppl 3):3–10, 1993.

45. Early Breast Cancer Trialists' Collaborative Group: Systemic treatment of early breast cancer by hormonal, cytotoxic, or immune therapy. Lancet 339:1–15, 1992.

46. Easton DF, Bishop DT, Ford D, et al: Genetic linkage analysis in familial breast and ovarian cancer: Results from 214 families. Am J Hum Genet 52:678–701, 1993.

47. Franceschi S, Boyle P, Maisonneuve P, et al: The epidemiology of thyroid carcinoma. Crit Rev Oncog 4(1):25–52, 1993.

48. Weinstock MA: Epidemiology of nonmelanoma skin cancer: Clinical issues, definitions, and classification. J Invest Dermatol 102(6):4–5S, 1994.

49. Karagas MR: Occurrence of cutaneous basal cell and squamous cell malignancies among those with a prior history of skin cancer. J Invest Dermatol 102(6):10S–13S, 1994.

50. Franceschi S, Cristofolini M: Cutaneous malignant melanoma: Epidemiological considerations. Semin Surg Oncol 8(6):345–352, 1992.

51. Elwood JM: Recent developments in melanoma epidemiology, 1993. Melanoma Res 3(3):149–156, 1993.

52. Sandler DP: Epidemiology and etiology of acute leukemia: An update. Leukemia 6 (suppl 4):3–5, 1992.

53. Vogel VG, Fisher RE: Epidemiology and etiology of leukemia. Curr Opin Oncol 5(1):26– 34, 1993.

54. Glaser SL: Reproductive factors in Hodgkin's disease in women: A review. Am J Epidemiol 139(3):237–246, 1994.

55. Weisenburger DD: Epidemiology of non-Hodgkin's lymphoma: Recent findings regarding an emerging epidemic. Ann Oncol 5 (suppl 1):19–24, 1994.

56. Pearce N, Bethwaite P: Increasing incidence of non-Hodgkin's lymphoma: Occupational and environmental factors. Cancer Res 52 (suppl 19):5496–5500S, 1992.

57. Shy K, Chu J, Mandelson M, et al: Papanicolaou smear screening interval and risk of cervical cancer. Obstet Gynecol 74:838–843, 1989.

58. Mandel JS, Bond JH, Church TR, et al: Reducing mortality from colorectal cancer by screening for fecal occult blood. N Engl J Med 328:1365–1371, 1993.

59. Selby JV, Friedman GD, Quesenberry CP, et al: A case-control study of screening sigmoidoscopy and mortality from colorectal cancer. N Engl J Med 326:653–657, 1992.

60. Levin B: Screening sigmoidoscopy for colorectal cancer. N Engl J Med 326:700–702, 1992.

61. Friedman GD, Hiatt RA, Quesenberry CP, et al: Case-control study of screening for prostatic cancer by digital rectal examinations. Lancet 337:1526–1529, 1991.

62. Krahn MD, Mahoney JE, Eckman MH, et al: Screening for prostate cancer. A decision analytic view. JAMA 272:773–780, 1994.

63. Catalona WJ, Smith DS, Ratliff TL, et al: Measurement of prostate-specific antigen in serum as a screening test for prostate cancer. N Engl J Med 324:1156–1161, 1991.

64. Offit K, Brown K: Quantitating familial cancer risk: A resource for clinical oncologists. J Clin Oncol 12:1724–1736, 1994.

65. Lippman SM, Hong WK: Retinoid chemoprevention of upper aerodigestive tract carcinogenesis, in DeVita VT Jr, Hellman S, Rosenberg SA (eds): Important Advances in Oncology 1992, pp 93–109. Philadelphia, JB Lippincott, 1992.

66. Hong WK, Lippman SM, Itri LM, et al: Prevention of second primary tumors with isotretinoin in squamous–cell carcinoma of the head and neck. N Engl J Med 323:795–801, 1990.

67. Nayfield SG, Karp JE, Ford LG, et al: Potential role of tamoxifen in prevention of breast cancer. J Natl Cancer Inst 83: 1450–1459, 1991.

Index

A

Acute lymphocytic leukemia, 3
  classification, 6
    French-American-British Working
      Group, 7
    immunophenotypic, 6
    morphologic, 6
  clinical features, 4
  epidemiology, 3
  etiology, 3
  investigations, biologic and
    prognostic, 16
    expression of *bcl-2*, 17
    minimal residual disease, 16
    multidrug resistance detection, 17
  laboratory features and workup, 4
    diagnostic workup, 6
    histochemical techniques, 5
  prognosis, 8
  survival, 16
  treatment, 11
    allogeneic bone marrow
      transplantation, 15
    autologous bone marrow
      transplantation, 16
    CNS prophylaxis and treatment, 14
    consolidation therapy, 13
    induction therapy, 12
    maintenance therapy, 13
Acute myelogenous leukemia, 27
  diagnosis and classification, 27
    cytogenetics, 28
    French-American-British Working
      Group, 27
    immunophenotyping, 29
  presentation, 27
  prognostic factors, 29
  treatment, 30
    acute promyelocytic leukemia, 33
    bone marrow transplantation, 32
    consolidation and intensification, 31
    postremission therapy, 30
    relapsed or refractory disease, 33
    remission induciton, 30
Adoptive cellular immunotherapy, 572
  chronic myelogenous leukemia, 573
  hairy-cell leukemia, 572
    interferon, 572
    purine analogs, 573
    splenectomy, 572
  Hodgkin's disease, 577
  Kaposi's sarcoma, 577
  lymphomas, cutaneous T-cell, 578
  lymphomas, non-Hodgkin's, 577
  melanoma, 578
  multiple myeloma, 574

combined with chemotherapy, 575
  maintenance therapy, 576
  previously untreated patients, 575
  relapsed patients, 575
  renal-cell carcinoma, 578
  thrombocytosis, severe, 574
Adrenal gland neoplasms, 488
  adrenocortical carcinoma, 488
    clinical presentation, 489
    epidemiology, 488
    treatment, 489
  pheochromocytoma, adrenal
    medulla, 489
    clinical features, 490
    diagnosis, 490
    epidemiology and incidence, 489
    preoperative medical
      management, 491
  pheochromocytoma, malignant, 491
AIDS-associated malignancies (*see* Retrovirus-associated malignancies)
Allogeneic marrow transplantation, 139
  age limitations, 147
  alternative donor, 146
  complications, 140
    graft failure, 141
    infection, 141
    late complications, 142
    myelosuppression, 140
    regimen-related, 140
  graft-vs-host disease, 142
    acute GVHD, 143
    chronic GVHD, 145
    HLA typing, 142
    immunobiology, 142
  marrow harvest and processing, 140
    alternative sources of hematopoietic
      stem cells, 140
    marrow transplantation, 140
  outcome, 145
    long-term survival, 146
    relapse, 145
  preparative regimens, 139
Antiemetic therapy, 629
  anticipatory emesis, 637
  antiemetic agents, 632
    antihistamines, 636
    benzodiazepines, 635
    butyrophenones, 636
    cannabinoids, 636
    corticosteroids, 635
    phenothiazines, 632
    serotonin-receptor antagonists, 633
    substituted benzamides, 632
  combination regimens, 636
  delayed emesis, 636
  factors influencing emesis, 630

methodology of trials, 632
  other management considerations, 637
  physiology, 629
  types of emesis, 629
Autologous transplantation, 151
  controversies, 152
    autologous vs allogeneic, 152
    integration with posttransplantation
      therapy, 153
    optimal dose-intensive
      preparation, 153
    progenitor cells derived from bone
      marrow vs peripheral blood, 152
    role of purging, 153
  future directions, 160
  general procedure, 151
    colony-stimulating factors, 152
    induction chemotherapy, 151
    patient assessment, 151
    preparative regimens, 151
    reinfusion of stem cells, 151
    stem-cell collection, 151
  health-care implications, 160
  potential complications of high-dose
    chemotherapy, 153
    hematologic toxicity, 154
    organ toxicity, 154
  results, 155
    acute myelogenous leukemia, 155
    acute lymphoblastic leukemia, 156
    breast cancer, 159
    chronic lymphocytic leukemia, 156
    chronic myelogenous leukemia, 156
    Hodgkin's disease, 157
    lymphoma, 157
    multiple myeloma, 158
    other solid tumors, 159
    pediatric solid tumors, 158

B

Biologic therapy (*see* Adoptive cellular
  immunotherapy, Colony-stimulating
  factors, Interferons, Interleukin-2,
  Monoclonal antibodies, Retinoids)
Bladder cancer, 449
  clinical presentation, 451
  diagnosis, 451
  epidemiology and etiology, 449
  molecular biology, 449
    chromosomal aberrations, 449
    oncogenes, 450
    suppressor genes, 450
  pathology, 450
  staging, 451
    Jewett-Marshall classification, 451
    TNM classification, 451, 452

treatment, 451
  carcinoma in situ, 452
  invasive disease, 453
  metastatic bladder cancer, 454
  superficial disease, 452
Bone marrow transplantation (*see* Allogeneic marrow transplantation, Autologous transplantation)
Brain tumors, 469
  acoustic schwannomas, 477
  cerebral metastases, 477
  clinical features, 471
  ependymomas, 475
  epidemiology and pathogenesis, 469
  gliomas/astrocytomas, 473
  medulloblastomas, 475
  meningeal carcinomatosis, 478
  meningiomas, 477
  neuroimaging, 471
  oligodendrogliomas, 475
  pineal region tumors, 476
  primary CNS lymphomas, 476
  spinal tumors, 471
  syndromes, by location, 470
  treatment, general concepts, 472
    radiation injury, 473
    radiation therapy, 472
Breast cancer, dose-intensive therapy for, 329
  background, 329
  calculating dose intensity, 330
    cumulative dose, 330
    dose rate, 331
    peak drug dose, 331
  high-dose chemotherapy with or
  without hematopoietic support, 332
    adjuvant therapy, 335
    cytokines, 337
    inflammatory breast cancer, 335
    metastatic disease, 333
    micrometastases, 336
    other issues, 336
    peripheral stem cells, 337
  early studies of, 331
Breast cancer, early stage, 301
  adjuvant therapy, 303
    node-negative disease, 303
    node-positive disease, 303
    other endocrine agents, 305
    ovarian ablation, 304
    tamoxifen therapy, 303
  chemotherapy, 305
    biological therapies, 307
    chemohormonal combinations, 307
    combination chemotherapy, 305
    dose-intensive chemotherapy, 307
    duration of therapy, 305
    non-cross-resistant therapies, 306
    regimens with and without
    anthracycline, 305
  prognostic factors, 301
    angiogenesis markers, 303
    application of, 303
    cathepsin D, 302
    HER-2/neu expression, 302

histologic subtypes, 303
hormone-receptor status, 302
lymphatic invasion, 303
nuclear/histologic grade, 302
S-phase fraction and DNA
  ploidy, 302
tumor size, 302
Breast cancer, estrogen replacement
therapy in, 337
  effects of estrogens, 338
  future studies, 341
  mammographic changes, 339
  relapse, 340
  tamoxifen, 339
Breast cancer, male, 307, 341
  clinical features, 342
  diagnosis, 342
  epidemiology and etiology, 341
  pathology, 342
  prognosis, 343
  staging, 343
  treatment, 344
    local-regional disease, 344
    metastatic disease, 344
Breast cancer, metastatic, 311
  diagnosis, 311
    history, 311
    imaging, 312
    laboratory tests, 312
    pathology, 312
    physical examination, 312
  molecular biology, 311
  treatment, 312
    bone metastases, 321
    brain metastases, 322
    chemotherapy, 313
    epidural metastases, 323
    evaluation of treatment
    response, 323
    hepatic metastases, 321
    hormonal therapy, 319
    leptomeningeal disease, 322
    stage IV, 322
Breast cancer, pregnancy and, 345
  diagnosis, 345
  pathology, 346
  prognosis, 346
  staging, 346
  subsequent pregnancy, 347
  treatment, 346
    chemotherapy, 347
    hormonal therapy, 347
    radiation therapy, 347

C

Cancer pain, 615
  definition and anatomic correlates, 615
    pain syndromes, 616
    pathophysiology, 616
  management, 618
    nonpharmacologic treatment, 624
    ongoing care, 625
    patient evaluation, 618

patient subgroups, 620
pharmacologic treatment, 620
psychosocial assessment, 619
Cervical carcinoma (*see* Uterine cervix,
carcinoma of the)
Chronic lymphocytic leukemia, 37
  associated disorders, 46
    autoimmune disorders, 46
    hairy-cell leukemia, 48
    large granular lymphocyte
    proliferation, 47
    prolymphocytic leukemia, 47
    secondary malignancies, 46
    T-cell chronic lymphocytic
    leukemia, 47
    transformation, 46
  clinical and laboratory features, 38
  diagnosis, 39
  epidemiology, 37
  etiology, 37
    cell of origin, 38
    chromosomal anomalies, 37
  staging and prognosis, 39
  transformation in,
  treatment, 40
    chlorambucil, 41
    combination chemotherapy, 42
    cyclophosphamide, 41
    nucleoside analogs, 42
    other treatment modalities, 44
Chronic myelogenous leukemia, 57
  blastic phase, 67
  clinical characteristics, 57
  cytogenetic and molecular changes, 59
  epidemiology, 57
  etiology, 57
  laboratory features, 58
    bone marrow, 58
    other laboratory findings, 58
    peripheral blood, 58
  minimal residual disease, 66
  molecular and physiopathologic
  phases, 58
  Ph-negative, 67
  staging, 59
  treatment, 61
    allogeneic bone marrow
    transplantation, 64
    autologous bone marrow
    transplantation, 66
    conventional, 61
    interferon, 61
Colony-stimulating factors, 587
  biology, 587
  clinical applications, 588
    anemia, 590
    autologous bone marrow
    transplantation, 589
    acute myeloid leukemia, 590
    chemotherapy-induced
    myelosuppression, 588
    myelodysplastic syndromes, 589
    other hematologic disorders, 590
    postchemotherapy, 588

toxicity, 591
Colorectal cancer, 263
  clinical presentation, 267
  etiology and risk factors, 265
    cancer history, 267
    diet, 266
    familial factors, 266
    inflammatory bowel disease, 267
    NSAIDs, 266
    other predisposing factors, 267
    polyps, 267
  molecular genetics and biology, 263
    adenoma caracinoma sequence, 265
  pathology, 267
  prognostic factors, 270
  screening and diagnosis, 268
    average-risk individuals, 268
    high-risk patients, 269
    initial diagnostic workup, 269
  staging, 270
    Dukes', 270
    Modified Astler Coller, 270
    TNM, 270
  treatment, 271
    advanced colorectal cancer, 275
    adjuvant therapy for colon
      cancer, 273
    adjuvant therapy for rectal
      cancer, 274
    surgery, 271

E

Endocrine malignancies (see Adrenal gland
  neoplasms, Parathyroid carcinoma,
  Thyroid carcinoma)
Endometrial carcinoma (see Uterine corpus, tumors of the)
Epidemiology of cancer, 661
  analytic epidemiology, 661
    bladder, 664
    breast, 666
    cervical, 666
    colorectal, 664
    endometrial, 665
    esophageal, 663
    head and neck, 661
    hepatic, 663
    kidney, 664
    leukemia, 667
    lung, 662
    lymphoma, 668
    ovarian, 665
    prostatic, 665
    renal pelvis, 664
    skin, 667
    stomach, 663
    thyroid, 667
  clinical epidemiology, 668
    chemoprevention, 669
    screening, 669
  descriptive epidemiology, 661
  risk factors, 662
    occupational exposure, 664

pharmaceuticals, 663
trends in incidence and mortality, 661
Esophageal carcinoma, 225
  pathogenesis, 225
  prognostic factors, 226
  staging, 226
    TNM classification, 227
  treatment, 226
    cost, 231
    multimodality therapy, 227
    palliative therapy, 230
    single-modality therapy, 226

G

Gallbladder carcinoma, 256
  clinical features, 257
  diagnosis, 257
  epidemiology and etiology, 256
  natural history, 257
  pathology, 256
  staging, 258
    TNM classification, 257
  treatment, 258
    chemotherapy, 258
    radiotherapy, 258
    surgery, 258
Gastric carcinoma, 235
  adjuvant therapy for resectable
    disease, 239
    chemoimmunotherapy, 240
    chemotherapy, 239
    radiotherapy, 239
  chemotherapy for advanced
    disease, 241
  diagnosis, 237
  epidemiology, 235
    predisposing factors and pre-
      malignant disease, 235
  future directions, 243
  molecular biology of, 236
  pathology and prognosis, 236
  radiotherapy for advanced disease, 240
  staging, 237
    TNM classification, 238
  surgery, 237
  treatment, 237
    localized unresectable disease, 240
    metastatic disease, 242
    resectable disease, 237
Gastrointestinal cancers (see Colorectal
  cancer, Esophageal cancer, Gastric carcinoma, Neuroendocrine tumors of the
  gastrointestinal tract, and Pancreatic
  carcinoma)
Gestational trophoblastic tumors, 377
  clinical presentation, 380
    complete mole, 380
    metastatic trophoblastic disease, 381
    partial mole, 381
  diagnostic studies, 381
    laboratory studies, 382
    radiologic studies, 382
  epidemiology and etiology, 377

pathogenesis and cell biology, 378
  cytogenetics, 379
  growth factors and oncogenes, 380
  pathology, 378
staging, 382
treatment, 383
  chemotherapy regimens, 385, 387
  CNS choriocarcinoma, 388
  metastatic disease, 386
  molar pregnancy, 383
  pulmonary metastases, 387
  salvage therapy, 387

H

Head and neck cancer, 207
  anatomy, 209
  biology, 208
  diagnosis, 209
  epidemiology, 207
  staging, 209
    TNM classification, 212
  treatment, 210
    adjuvant chemotherapy, 216
    cervical nodes, 213
    chemoprevention, 217
    chemoradiotherapy, 216
    combined modality for local or
      regional advanced disease, 214
    hypopharynx, 213
    larynx, 213
    metastatic or recurrent disease, 214
    nasopharynx, 211
    neoadjuvant chemotherapy, 215
    oral cavity, 212
    oropharynx, 212
    salivary glands, 213
Hematopoietic growth factors (see Colony-
  stimulating factors)
Hepatocellular carcinoma, 253
  clinical features, 253
  diagnosis, 253
  pathology, 253
  risk factors, 253
  staging, 253
    TNM system, 255
  treatment, 254
    chemotherapy, 255
    cryosurgery, 255
    liver transplantation, 256
    radiotherapy, 256
    surgery, 254
Hodgkin's disease, 111
  AIDS-associated,
    epidemiology, 111
    evaluation, 112
    histology, 111
  staging, 112
    Ann Arbor classification, 112
    recommended procedures, 113
  treatment, 113
    clinically staged disease, 115
    infradiaphragmatic presentation, 116
    laparotomy-staged disease, 113

salvage therapy, 117
stage III disease, 116
stage IV disease, 117
treatment complications, 118
cardiovascular, 121
endocrine, 121
miscellaneous, 123
pulmonary, 123
secondary malignancies, 118

I

Infections in cancer patients, 599, 607
fungal infections, 607
aspergillosis, 609
candidiasis, 607
treatment, 610
neutropenic patients, 599
bacterial pathogens, 599
duration of therapy, 602
initial management, 600
prevention of infection, 603
viral infections, 611
adenovirus, 612
cytomegalovirus, 611
herpes simplex virus, 612
respiratory RNA virus, 613
varicella zoster virus, 612
Interferons, 569
alpha interferon, 569
cervical cancer, 402
chronic lymphocytic leukemia, 49
chronic myelogenous leukemia, 61
endometrial cancer, 413
Kaposi's sarcoma, AIDS-
associated, 538
melanoma, 502
metastatic breast cancer, 313
multiple myeloma, 131
renal-cell carcinoma, 462
beta interferon, 569
biologic activity, 570
cell-surface receptors, 570
interferon antibodies, 570
gamma interferon, 570
renal-cell carcinoma, 463
toxicity, 570
acute effects, 570
chronic effects, 570
Interleukin-2, 571
biologic activity, 571
melanoma, 503
renal-cell carcinoma, 463
toxicity, 571

K

Kaposi's sarcoma (see Retrovirus-
associated malignancies)

L

Leukemia (see Acute lymphocytic leukemia, Acute myelogenous leukemia,

Chronic lymphocytic leukemia,
Chronic myelogenous leukemia)
Lung cancer, non-small-cell, 181
clinical presentation, 187
paraneoplastic syndromes, 188
diagnosis, 188
solitary pulmonary nodule, 18
epidemiology, 181
histology, 185
adenocarcinoma, 185
large-cell carcinoma, 186
squamous-cell carcinoma, 186
molecular biology, 186
risk factors/etiology, 181
asbestos exposure, 183
chemistry of carcinogenesis, 182
cigarette smoking, 181
diet, 184
genetic predisposition, 185
passive smoking, 183
radon exposure, 184
staging, 189
TNM classification, 193
treatment, 189
stage I/II disease, 189
stage III disease, 192
stage IV disease, 197
Lung cancer, small-cell, 169
biology, 169
autocrine factors, 170
drug resistance, 170
proto-oncogenes, 170
tumor-suppressor genes, 169
clinical evaluation, 173
clinical presentation, 172
etiology and epidemiology, 169
natural history, 172
pathology, 171
prognostic factors, 173
staging, 173
treatment, 174
brain irradiation, 177
chemoprevention, 177
combination chemotherapy, 175
induction therapy, 175
salvage regimens, 176
single-agent chemotherapy, 174
surgery, 177
thoracic irradiation, 176
Lymphomas (see Non-Hodgkin's lymphoma, indolent; Non-Hodgkin's lymphoma, intermediate- and high-grade;
Retrovirus-associated malignancies)

M

Melanoma, malignant, 493
biology, 494
diagnosis and staging, 496
AJCC system, 496
WHO system, 496
epidemiology, 493
future prospects, 505
genetics, 493

immunology, 494
metastatic disease,
prognosis, 497
treatment, 497
adjuvant therapy, 498
biochemotherapy, 503
biologic therapy, 502
combination chemotherapy, 500
high-dose chemotherapy with
autologous bone marrow
transplantation, 502
hormonal therapy, 501
metastatic disease, 498
primary melanoma, 497
single-agent therapy, 499
vaccines and monoclonal
antibodies, 505
types of, 495
Monoclonal antibodies, 593
clinical trials, 593
pancreatic carcinoma, 252
Myeloma, multiple, 127
biology, 127
clinical features, 128
anemia, 129
bone disease, 128
hypercalcemia, 128
infection, 129
renal failure, 128
diagnosis, 129
etiology, 127
response criteria, 130
staging and prognosis, 129
Durie-Salmon system, 130
M. D. Anderson system, 130
treatment, 131
bone marrow and stem-cell
transplantation, 132
previously untreated patients, 131
relapsing and refractory
disease, 132
remission maintenance, 131

N

Neuroendocrine tumors of the gastrointestinal tract, 285
epidemiology, 285
etiology, 285
gastrinomas, 290
localization techniques, 290
glucagonoma, 291
insulinomas, 290
natural history and diagnosis, 287
carcinoid syndrome, 288
carcinoid tumors, 288
imaging studies, 289
survival rates, 289
pancreatic polypeptideoma, 292
pathology, 285
cytoplasmic constituents, 287
diagnostic features, 286
electron microscopy, 286
granule contents, 287

gross histology, 286
growth factors and nuclear antigens, 287
histochemical analysis, 286
immunohistochemical markers, 286
neuroendocrine concept, 285
plasma membrane constituents, 287
secretory vesicle membrane constituents, 287
somatostatinoma, 291
treatment, 292
  biologic therapy, 294
  carcinoid tumors, 294
  chemotherapy and biochemo-therapy, 294
  future directions, 295
  islet-cell carcinomas, 294
  local-regional therapy with hepatic arterial embolization, 295
  management of hormonal excess, 292
  octreotide, 292
  omeprazole, 293
vipomas, 291
Non-Hodgkin's lymphoma, indolent, 73
basic concepts, 73
classification, 75
follicular lymphomas, 73
  biology, cytogenetics, and immuno-phenotypic characteristics, 76
  clinical features, diagnostic workup, and staging, 78
  cytology and pathology, 74
  prognostic factors, 79
future directions, 91
histologic progression and clinical transformation, 91
mantle-cell lymphoma, 82
small lymphocytic lymphomas, 80
  from mucosa-associated lymphoid tissue, 80
therapy, 83
  advanced-stage follicular, 84
  high-dose chemotherapy with autologous bone marrow transplantation, 89
  interferon, 88
  limited-stage follicular, 83
  mantle-cell lymphoma, 88
  PCR to assess response, 90
Non-Hodgkin's lymphoma, intermediate- and high-grade, 99
classification, 101
clinical features, 102
  sites of presentation, 102
  systemic features, 103
diagnosis, 103
epidemiology and etiology, 99
high-grade, 107
  HIV-related, 107
  T-cell-related, 107
intermediate-grade, 104
  advanced disease, 105
  localized and good prognosis, 104

relapse and primary refractory disease, 106
staging, 104
staging and treatment, 103

O

Oncologic emergencies, 643
cardiovascular, 646
  cardiac tamponade, 646
  superior vena cava syndrome, 646
chemotherapy-induced, 658
  extravasation, 658
gastrointestinal, 650
  gastrointestinal bleeding, 650
  neutropenic enterocolitis, 650
genitourinary, 648
  hemorrhagic cystitis, 648
  urinary tract obstruction, 649
hematologic, 654
  hyperleukocytosis syndrome, 655
  hyperviscosity syndrome, 654
hemostatic, 655
  bleeding, 655
  thrombosis, 657
metabolic, 650
  hypercalcemia of malignancy, 652
  SIADH, 651
  tumor lysis syndrome, 650
neurologic, 643
  altered mental status, 645
  increased intracranial pressure, 644
  leptomeningeal disease, 645
  seizures, 644
  spinal cord compression, 643
respiratory emergencies, 647
  airway obstruction, 647
  hemoptysis, massive, 647
  toxic lung injury, 648
Ovarian cancer, 359
etiology, 359
future directions,
pathology and staging, 363
  FIGO classification, 365
  histologic grading, 364
  secondary cytoreduction, 365
  surgery, 365
risk factors, 359
screening, 360
  abdominal/transvaginal ultrasound, 360
  CA125, 360
  DNA ploidy analysis, 362
  growth factors and cytokines, 361
  oncogenes, 361
  other prognostic factors, 362
  physical examination, 360
  steroid hormones, 361
  ultrasound plus CA125, 360
treatment, 366
  autologous bone marrow transplantation, 371
  biologic therapy, 371
  chemotherapy, 366

drug resistance, 370
gene therapy, 371
immunotherapy, 371
peripheral blood stem-cell support, 371
radiotherapy, 370

P

Pain (see Cancer pain)
Pancreatic cancer, 247
clinical features, 248
epidemiology and etiology, 247
diagnosis, 248
  serologic markers, 249
pathology, 248
staging, 249
  AJCC system, 250
treatment, 249
  adjuvant chemotherapy, 250
  adjuvant radiotherapy, 249
  biologic therapy, 252
  chemotherapy, 252
  future targets, 252
  hormonal therapy, 251
  pain control, 252
  radiotherapy, 252
  resectable disease, 249
  unresectable disease, 250
Parathyroid carcinoma, 487
clinical presentation, 487
incidence and etiology, 487
pathology, 487
treatment, 487
Pheochromocytoma (see Adrenal gland neoplasms)
Plasma-cell dyscrasias, 133
amyloidosis, 134
asymptomatic myeloma, 133
common laboratory features, 133
immunoglobulin heavy-chain disease, 134
monoclonal gammopathy of unknown significance, 133
solitary plasmacytoma of bone, 133
Waldenström's macroglobulinemia, 134
Prevention strategies (see Epidemiology of cancer)
Prostate cancer, 419
epidemiology, 419
diagnosis, 422
  prostate-specific antigen, 422
  screening, 423
  transrectal ultrasonography, 422
natural history, 421
pathogenesis, 420
pathology, 421
staging, 423
  TNM classification, 424
treatment, 425
  antiandrogen therapy, 426
  chemotherapy, 428
  early-stage disease, 425

flutamide withdrawal, 427
hormone-refractory disease, 427
ketoconazole, 428
metastatic disease, 426
radiation therapy, 426
radical prostatectomy, 425
stage C, 426
strontium-89, 428
surgery vs radiation for localized
disease, 425
watchful waiting, 425

R

Rectal cancer (*see* Colorectal cancer)
Renal-cell carcinoma, 459
angio-infarction, 462
clinical presentation, 460
epidemiology, 459
etiology, 459
immunotherapy, 462
alpha interferon, 462
combination biochemotherapy, 462
gamma interferon, 463
interleukin-2, 463
pathology, 459
prognosis, 461
radiographic evaluation, 460
radiotherapy, 462
staging, 461
Robson's staging system, 460
TNM staging, 461
surgical treatment, 461
local disease, 461
metastatic disease, 461
systemic therapy, 462
cytotoxic chemotherapy, 462
hormonal therapy, 462
Retinoids, 591
clinical applications, 591
acute promyelocytic leukemia, 592
chemoprevention, 591
other malignancies, 592
retinoic acid syndrome, 593
toxicity, 593
Retrovirus-associated malignancies, 531
adult T-cell leukemia/lymphoma, 552
clinical features and diagnosis, 553
diagnosis, 554
epidemiology, 552
etiologic agent, 552
pathogenesis, 553
prognostic factors, treatment,
and survival, 554
anorectal carcinoma, 551
disease features, 552
epidemiology, 551
pathogenesis, 551
screening, 552
therapy, 552
cervical neoplasia, 549
cervical cytology, 550
epidemiology, 549

gynecologic manifestations
of HIV disease, 550
invasive cervical carcinoma, 551
therapy, 551
HIV-associated, 531
Hodgkin's disease, 549
Kaposi's sarcoma, 532
clinical features, 535
combination chemotherapy, 538
cryotherapy, 536
epidemiology, 532
future therapies, 539
intralesional therapy, 537
laser and surgical therapies, 536
local therapy, 536
pathogenesis, 534
pathology, 533
radiation therapy, 537
single-agent therapy, 537
staging and prognostic factors, 535
systemic therapy, 537
non-Hodgkin's lymphoma, 539
clinical presentation, 542
epidemiology, 539
pathogenesis, 541
pathologic subtypes of
lymphoma, 541
staging and prognostic features, 542
therapy, 543
other malignancies, 552
primary CNS lymphoma, 547
clinical presentation and
diagnosis, 547
epidemiology, 547
pathogenesis, 548
prognostic factors and survival, 549
staging, 548
therapy, 549

S

Sarcomas, bone, 517
chondrosarcoma, 521
evaluation, 517
biopsy, 517
imaging techniques, 517
Ewing's sarcoma, 521
clinical presentation, prognostic
factors, and staging, 522
treatment, 522
histiocytoma, malignant fibrous, 521
osteosarcoma, 518
treatment of localized disease, 518
treatment of metastatic disease, 520
variants of, 520
staging of bone tumors, 517
Sarcomas, soft-tissue, 511
clinical presentation, 512
disease grade and staging, 513
AJCC system, 514
epidemiology and pathogenesis, 511
evaluation, 512
pathology, 512

alveolar soft-part sarcoma, 513
angiosarcoma, 513
botryoid sarcoma, 513
embryonal sarcoma, 512
epithelioid sarcoma, 513
histiocytoma, malignant fibrous, 513
leiomyosarcoma, 513
liposarcoma, 513
neurofibrosarcoma, 513
rhabdomyosarcoma, 512
synovial sarcoma, 513
treatment, 513
adjuvant chemotherapy, 515
local disease, 513
recurrent disease, 516
Stomach cancer (*see* Gastric carcinoma)

T

Testicular cancer, 433
diagnosis, 436
cytogenetic abnormalities, 436,
tumor markers, 436
epidemiology and etiology, 433
pathology and natural history, 433
carcinoma in situ, 434
extragonadal germ-cell tumors, 436
lymphomas and leukemias, 435
metastatic neoplasms, 435
nonseminomatous germ-cell
tumors, 434
rhabdomyosarcomas, 435
seminoma, 434
sex cord-stromal tumors, 435
staging and treatment, 437
carcinoma in situ, 437
nonseminomatous germ-cell
tumors, 440
salvage chemotherapy, 444
seminoma, 438
TNM classification, 441
Thyroid carcinoma, 483
classification of unusual tumors, 485
clinical presentation and course, 485
epidemiology, incidence, and
distribution, 483
etiology, 483
pathology, 484
therapy, 486

U

Unknown primary carcinomas, 559
biology, 559
chemotherapy, 564
clinical evaluation, 560
diagnosis, 560
epidemiology, 559
histopathologic evaluation, 561
treatment recommendations, 561
clinicopathologic subgroups, 562
axillary adenopathies, 562
bony metastases, 564

brain metastases, 564
cervical and supraclavicular
adenopathies, 562
disease limited to lymph nodes, 562
extragonadal germ-cell
syndrome, 562
hepatic metastases, 564
inguinal adenopathies, 563
malignant ascites, 563
multiple-site visceral disease, 564
neuroendocrine tumors, 563
pulmonary metastases and pleural
effusions, 563
single sites discovered on
resection, 564
Uterine cervix, carcinoma of the, 393
etiology, 393
natural history, 394
cervical intraepithelial neoplasia, 394
invasive cervical carcinoma, 395
pathology, 393

prognosis, 398
screening and diagnosis, 395
cervical cytologic screening, 395
management of abnormal smears/
preinvasive lesions, 396
staging, 397
FIGO staging system, 397
treatment, 398
carcinoma in situ, 399
chemotherapy, 400
during pregnancy, 400
invasive carcinoma found at simple
hysterectomy, 400
posttherapy surveillance, 402
radiotherapy, 399
recurrent disease, 400
stage IA, 399
stages IB and IIA, 399
stages IIB, III, and IV, 399
surgery, 398
ureteral obstruction, 400

Uterine corpus, tumors of the, 407
adenocarcinoma variants, 409
clinical findings, 410
staging and prognosis, 410
clinical features, 409
diagnosis, 408
epidemiology, 407
pathology, 409
recurrent disease, 412
chemotherapy, 413
hormonal therapy, 412
treatment, 411
stage I and stage II occult, 411
stage III, 411
stage IV, 412
diagnosed after hysterectomy, 412
uterine sarcomas, 413
natural history and clinical
presentation, 414
treatment, 415

Notes

Notes